Biomedical Ethics

Second Edition

Thomas A. Mappes
Professor of Philosophy
Frostburg State College

Jane S. Zembaty
Associate Professor of Philosophy
University of Dayton

McGraw-Hill Book Company

New York   St. Louis   San Francisco   Auckland   Bogotá   Hamburg
Johannesburg   London   Madrid   Mexico   Montreal   New Delhi
Panama   Paris   São Paulo   Singapore   Sydney   Tokyo   Toronto

This book was set in Times Roman by Publication Services.
The editor was Emily G. Barrosse;
the production supervisor was Diane Renda;
the cover was designed by Infield, D'Astolfo Associates.
Project supervision was done by Publication Services.
R. R. Donnelley & Sons Company was printer and binder.

BIOMEDICAL ETHICS

1 2 3 4 5 6 7 8 9 0   DOCDOC   8 9 8 7 6 5

ISBN 0-07-040124-1

Library of Congress Cataloging in Publication Data
Main entry under title:

Biomedical ethics.

    Reprinted from various sources.
    Includes bibliographies.
    1. Medical ethics—Addresses, essays, lectures.
    2. Bioethics—Addresses, essays, lectures.
I. Mappes, Thomas A.   II. Zembaty, Jane S.   [DNLM:
1. Bioethics—collected works.   2. Ethics, Medical—
collected works.   W 50 B6153]
R724.B49   1986   174'.2   85-9846
ISBN 0-07-040124-1

Contents

Preface

The second edition of *Biomedical Ethics*, like the first, is designed to provide an effective teaching instrument for courses in biomedical ethics. With this end in mind, and responsive to suggestions made by instructors using the book, we have made two major changes in the second edition. First, in an effort to enhance coherence and clarity in our introductory chapter, we have revamped it in such a way that our own exposition of some of the ethical theories central in biomedical ethics has replaced readings on ethical theory. This presentation of ethical theories is followed by a discussion of the major concepts and principles relevant to developing an understanding of the issues in biomedical ethics. Second, we have added an appendix of case studies for analysis and discussion. We have, of course, retained those features of the first edition that made it an effective teaching instrument. Thus we have maintained the comprehensive character of the text, organized the subject matter so that it unfolds in an efficient and natural fashion, and retained a number of helpful editorial features, such as the argument sketches that precede each selection and the annotated bibliographies at the end of each chapter. Finally, inasmuch as the value of any textbook anthology is largely dependent upon the quality of its readings, we have assembled a set of readings characterized by high-quality analysis and, to the greatest extent possible, clarity of writing style. We have also taken care to choose readings that reflect diverse viewpoints with regard to the leading issues in biomedical ethics. Although many of the selections are written by philosophers, the collection also includes writings by lawyers, physicians, scientists, and theologians, as well as relevant judicial opinions and official codes. Such a distribution reflects the interdisciplinary nature of biomedical ethics.

As the table of contents makes clear, this book is extremely comprehensive. We have placed a premium on comprehensiveness in order to allow individual instructors wide latitude regarding the choice of subject matter. In aiming at comprehensiveness, we have been especially concerned to widen the discussion of the professional-patient relationship (Chapters 2 and 3) so that it does not focus exclusively on the physician-patient relationship but also reflects the significant role of nurses in medical care. We have also thought it important in this second edition to incorporate chapter subsections on such topics as geriatric patients (Chapter 3), the mentally retarded (Chapter 6), and surrogate motherhood (Chapter 10). As for the overall organization and development of subject matter, subsection by subsection, chapter by chapter, we are confident that it unfolds in an efficient and natural fashion. We believe that our organization forestalls some of the perplexities and confusions that students often experience in biomedical ethics. For example, it seems important to us that students consider the concept of mental illness (Chapter 5) before discussing involuntary civil commitment (Chapter 6). Similarly, it seems important that students discuss the morality of suicide and the right to refuse lifesaving treatment (Chapter 7) before discussing the morality of euthanasia (Chapter 8), and so on. Still, we wish to emphasize the relative detachability of our various subsections and chapters. The issues of biomedical ethics are in many ways intertwined and overlapping. Thus there may be many reasons why an individual instructor would prefer to rearrange the order of presentation of our subsections and chapters.

The introductions to each chapter of this book provide one of its most important editorial features. In the introductions we explicitly identify the central issues in each chapter and scan the various positions on these issues together with their supporting argumentation. Whenever possible, we draw out the relationship between the arguments that appear in a certain chapter and the ethical theories, concepts, and principles discussed in our introductory chapter. Whenever necessary, we also provide conceptual and factual information. In this vein, as a matter of course, we explicate the meaning of technical biomedical terms and introduce relevant biomedical information. The purpose of the chapter introductions is to enhance the effectiveness of the book as a teaching instrument. This same central purpose is shared by the book's other editorial features, which include biographical as well as argument sketches preceding each selection and annotated bibliographies at the end of each chapter. The annotated bibliographies provide substantial guidance for further reading and research. The various entries in the bibliographies, like the various readings in each chapter, reflect diverse viewpoints.

We wish to thank the University of Dayton Department of Philosophy and Frostburg State College for their support of this project. We are indebted to the Kennedy Institute, Georgetown University, whose bioethics library has been a significant ally in our research efforts. We are also indebted to the reference librarians at both the University of Dayton and Frostburg State College. We are especially grateful to Lawrence P. Ulrich, University of Dayton, Joy Kroeger Mappes, Frostburg State College, and Mark Wicclair, West Virginia University, for their valuable criticisms and advice. Lawrence P. Ulrich also provided much of the material in the case studies and served as a critical reviewer of the cases. Finally, we must express our thanks to Linda McKinley, Betty Hume, and Shelley Drees for their help with manuscript preparation.

Thomas A. Mappes
Jane S. Zembaty

Chapter 1

Biomedical Ethics and Ethical Theory

A number of ethical issues (or problem areas) may be identified as associated with the practice of medicine and/or the pursuit of biomedical research. This set of ethical issues constitutes the subject matter of biomedical ethics. The proper task of biomedical ethics is to advance reasoned analysis in an effort to clarify and resolve such issues. What we term "biomedical ethics" is also commonly termed "bioethics." Although both terms have some measure of currency, we prefer "biomedical ethics" in order to make explicit the concern with issues associated with the practice of medicine.

THE NATURE OF BIOMEDICAL ETHICS

In order to properly situate biomedical ethics as a subdiscipline within the more general discipline of ethics, it is necessary to briefly discuss the nature of ethics as a philosophical discipline. Ethics, understood as a philosophical discipline, can be conveniently defined as the *philosophical* study of morality. As such, it must be immediately distinguished from the *scientific* study of morality, often called "descriptive ethics." The goal of descriptive ethics is to attain empirical knowledge about morality. The practitioner of descriptive ethics is dedicated to describing actually existing moral views and, subsequently, explaining such views by advancing an account of their causal origin. Moral views, no less than other aspects of human experience, provide behavioral and social scientists a range of phenomena that stand in need of explanation. For example, why does a certain individual have such a Victorian view of sexual morality? A Freudian psychologist may attempt an explanation in terms of basic Freudian categories and early childhood experience. Why does a particular group of people manifest such a high incidence of moral opposition to abortion? A sociologist may attempt an explanation in terms of relevant socialization factors. If most of the members of the group were raised as Roman Catholics, this fact is probably relevant to the desired explanation.

Ethics as a philosophical discipline stands in contrast to descriptive ethics. (Hereafter, the expression "ethics" will be used to designate the philosophical discipline, as distinct from descriptive ethics.) Philosophers commonly subdivide ethics into (1) normative ethics and (2) metaethics (analytic ethics), although the precise relationship of these two branches is a matter of some dispute. In normative ethics, philosophers attempt to establish what is morally right and what is morally wrong with regard to human action. In metaethics, philosophers are said to be concerned with an analysis of both moral concepts (e.g., the concept of duty or the concept of a right) and moral reasoning. It seems plausible to maintain that deliberations in normative ethics are to some extent dependent upon and cannot be completely detached from metaethical considerations. But whatever the precise relationship between normative ethics and metaethics, it is important to see that *normative ethics* is logically distinct from *descriptive ethics*. Whereas descriptive ethics attempts to describe (and explain) those moral views which in fact *are accepted*, normative ethics attempts to establish which moral views are *justifiable* and thus *ought to be accepted*. In *general* normative ethics, the task is to advance and provide a reasoned justification of an overall theory of moral obligation, thereby establishing an ethical theory that provides a general answer to the question: What is morally right and what is morally wrong? In *applied* normative ethics, as opposed to general normative ethics, the task is to resolve particular moral problems—for example: Is abortion morally justifiable?

In light of the distinctions just made, it is now possible to identify biomedical ethics as one branch of applied (normative) ethics. The task of biomedical ethics is to resolve ethical problems associated with the practice of medicine and/or the pursuit of biomedical research. Clearly, since there are ethical problems associated with other aspects of life, there are other branches of applied ethics. Business ethics, for example, is concerned with the ethical problems associated with the transaction of business. Importantly, in all branches of applied ethics, the particular issues under discussion are *normative* in character. Is this particular practice right or wrong? Is it morally justifiable? In applied ethics, the concern is not to establish which moral views people do in fact have. That is a descriptive matter. The concern in applied ethics, as in general normative ethics, is to establish which moral views people *ought* to have.

The following questions are typically raised in biomedical ethics. Is a physician morally obligated to tell a terminally ill patient that he or she is dying? Are breaches of medical confidentiality ever morally justifiable? Is abortion morally justifiable? Is euthanasia morally justifiable? Normative ethical questions such as these are concerned with the morality of certain practices. Other questions in biomedical ethics focus on the ethical justifiability of laws. It is one thing to discuss the morality of suicide but quite another thing (although related) to discuss the justifiability of laws that would sanction suicide intervention. Is society justified in enacting laws that would compel an individual, against his or her will, to submit to lifesaving medical treatment? Is society justified in enacting laws that would allow others to commit an individual, against his or her will, to a mental institution? The appearance of questions of this latter type signifies that biomedical ethics must rely not only on the theories of general normative ethics but also on the theories of social-political philosophy and philosophy of law. In these latter disciplines, a central theoretical question concerns the justifiable limits of law. Strictly speaking, if biomedical ethics is a type of applied ethics, ethics must be broadly understood as encompassing social-political philosophy and the philosophy of law.

Although many of the ethical issues falling within the scope of biomedical ethics have historical roots, especially insofar as they are related to various codes of medical ethics, biomedical ethics did not crystallize into a full-fledged discipline until very recently. Only since about 1970 have the various trappings of a relatively autonomous discipline become manifest. Centers for research in biomedical ethics have emerged, most notably the Institute of Society, Ethics, and the Life Sciences (located in Hastings-on-Hudson, New York and usually called "The Hastings Center") and the Kennedy Institute, Center for Bioethics, Georgetown University (Washington, D.C.). Journals such as the *Hastings Center Report* and the *Journal of Medicine and Philosophy* have sprung into existence. Bibliographies have been produced, conferences abound, and the field has its own encyclopedia, *The Encyclopedia of Bioethics* (1978). An increasing number of philosophers, as well as theologians, now identify biomedical ethics as an area of specialization.

If, as is clear, many of the ethical issues falling within the scope of biomedical ethics are not historically unprecedented, why is it that biomedical ethics has emerged as a vigorous and highly visible discipline only recently? Two cultural developments are at the root of the contemporary prominence of biomedical ethics: (1) the awesome advance of biomedical research as attended by the resultant development of biomedical technology; and (2) the practice of medicine in an increasingly complicated institutional setting.

Consider first the impact of recent biomedical research. It has been responsible not only for the creation of historically unprecedented ethical problems but also for adding new dimensions to old problems and making the solving of those old problems a matter of greater urgency. Some developments—for example, those associated with reproductive technologies such as *in vitro* fertilization and cloning—seem to present us with ethical problems that are genuinely unprecedented. More commonly, however, the advance of biomedical research has simply added complexity to old problems and created a sense of urgency with regard to their solution. Euthanasia is not a new problem; but our ability to save the lives of severely defective newborns who would have died in the past and our ability to sustain the biological processes of irreversibly comatose individuals have added new dimensions and, surely, a new urgency. Abortion is not a new problem, but the development of various techniques of prenatal diagnosis has created the new possibility of genetic abortion. Indeed, the many successes of biomedical research in our own time, as manifested in the associated technological developments, call attention to the value of systematic biomedical research on human subjects and thus occasion reexamination of ethical limitations with regard to human experimentation.

The practice of medicine in an increasingly complicated institutional setting is, along with the advance of biomedical research, largely responsible for the contemporary prominence of biomedical ethics. In the past, the practice of medicine was largely confined within the bounds of the physician-patient relationship. Now, however, hospitals and other medical institutions are intimately intertwined with physicians and other medical personnel in the delivery of medical care. Moreover, we have become increasingly conscious of issues of social justice. We hear talk of a right to health care and are confronted with numerous problems of allocation.

It is frequently said that biomedical ethics is an interdisciplinary field, and some explication of its interdisciplinary character might prove helpful. There is a sense in which biomedical ethics is interdisciplinary within philosophy itself, that is, inasmuch as it applies the theories of social-political philosophy and philosophy of law as well as those of ethics narrowly defined. There is also a sense in which biomedical ethics is interdisciplinary precisely because the issues under discussion are frequently approached not only from the vantage point of moral philosophy (the dominant vantage point in the collection of readings in this text), but also from the vantage point of moral theology. Whereas philosophical analysis proceeds on the basis of *reason alone,* theological analysis proceeds on the basis of *faith,* within a framework of "revealed truth." There is yet a third sense in which biomedical ethics is said to be interdisciplinary. In this sense, the most prominent one, biomedical ethics is interdisciplinary in that it necessarily requires the input of medicine and biology. (It also utilizes, where relevant, the empirical findings of the social sciences.) Medical and biological facts are an essential part of the grist for the mill of ethical evaluation. But it is also important to recognize that the *experience* of medical personnel and researchers is often essential to ensure that ethical discussions retain firm contact with the concrete realities that permeate the practice of medicine and the pursuit of biomedical research.

Although the issues of biomedical ethics are essentially normative, they are often intertwined with both conceptual issues and factual (i.e., empirical) issues. For example, suppose we are concerned with the ethical acceptability of intervention for the sake of preventing a person from committing suicide. Our basic concern is with a normative question; however, we must face the problem of clarifying the nature of suicide, a conceptual issue. For example, if a Jehovah's Witness, on the basis of religious principle, refuses a lifesaving blood transfusion, is the resultant death to be classified as a suicide? In addition to facing conceptual perplexities, we are also faced with an important factual question. Do those who typically attempt suicide really want to die? Presumably psychologists and sociologists have important things to tell us on this score. In the end, of course, we want to apply relevant ethical principles to the issue of the ethical acceptability of intervention for the sake of preventing a person from committing suicide. But ethical principles are applied in the light of conceptual structures and factual beliefs. In the case of some issues in biomedical ethics, underlying factual issues are especially prominent. For example, in addressing the normative question of whether it is ever morally permissible to use children as research subjects, it is important to consider a factual question. To what extent can therapeutic techniques be developed for children in the absence of research employing children as research subjects? In the case of other issues in biomedical ethics, associated conceptual issues command special attention. For example, one could hardly discuss the normative issue of whether the involuntary civil commitment of the mentally ill is a justifiable social practice without closely examining the concept of mental illness. To give a second example, in considering the morality of euthanasia, the distinction between active and passive euthanasia invites conceptual clarification.

It is helpful to approach the literature of biomedical ethics with an eye toward distinguishing conceptual, factual, and normative issues. Furthermore, with regard to normative issues, the central issues of biomedical ethics, one cannot hope to properly situate argumentation in biomedical ethics without some awareness of the various types of ethical theory developed in general normative ethics. Such theories provide the frameworks within which many of the arguments in biomedical ethics are formulated.

ETHICAL THEORIES

An ethical theory provides an ordered set of moral standards (in some cases, simply one *ultimate* moral principle) that is to be used in assessing what is morally right and what is morally wrong regarding human action in general. An ethical theory, in this sense, is a theory of moral obligation. A proponent of any such theory puts it forth as a framework within which a person can correctly determine, on any given occasion, what he or she (morally) ought to do.

The Critical Assessment of Competing Ethical Theories

Since a number of competing ethical theories may be identified, the question immediately arises, what criteria are relevant to an assessment of these competing theories? There is no easy way to answer this very fundamental and very controversial question, but let us start with those considerations whose relevance is unlikely to be disputed. Any theory in any field is rightly expected to be internally consistent. Thus a theory can be faulted on the basis of lack of coherence. In a similar vein, any theory is surely flawed to the extent that it is either unclear and/or incomplete. It might also be claimed that lack of simplicity should count against a theory, but the relevance of this consideration is somewhat more problematic. Perhaps simplicity should be understood as a subsidiary criterion, one whose relevance is limited to the case of deciding between two theories otherwise judged to be equally defensible. Surely a theory that exhibits simplicity is more elegant, more aesthetically pleasing, than one that does not. But if the latter theory is otherwise more adequate, it would seem to retain a superiority over the former.

If the above considerations are relevant to a critical assessment of theories in any field, we must yet identify considerations relevant to our particular concern, the critical assessment of (normative) ethical theories. Responsive to this task, it is suggested that the following criteria should be identified as embodying the two most important considerations. (1) The implications of an ethical theory must be reconcilable with our experience of the moral life. (2) An ethical theory must provide effective guidance where it is most needed, that is, in those situations where substantive moral considerations can be advanced on both sides of an issue. Although many philosophers would endorse the relevance of these two criteria, perhaps not so many would be willing to assign them the exclusive prominence suggested here. Nevertheless, in support of identifying (1) and (2) as the principal criteria relevant to a critical assessment of competing ethical theories, it can be pointed out that analogous considerations are clearly relevant (and prominent) in the critical assessment of empirical (i.e., scientific) theories. When competing empirical theories are under critical examination, it is surely relevant to ask which of the competitors gives a better account of the facts. It is also relevant to ask which of the competitors is superior in terms of heuristic value, that is, which can function to guide future research most effectively. In embracing the priority of (1) and (2), we are saying that an adequate ethical theory must achieve two major goals, analogous to the goals that must be achieved by an adequate empirical theory. An adequate ethical theory must accord with the "facts" of the moral life as we experience it, and it must function heuristically by guiding us when we are confronted with moral perplexity. An ethical theory should, on one hand, make sense out of the moral life by exhibiting the structure underlying our ordinary moral thinking. On the other hand, it should illuminate our moral judgment precisely where it is experienced to falter—in the face of moral dilemmas.

There is certainly no suggestion here that the standards embodied in (1) and (2) can be applied in some mechanical-like fashion to assess the relative adequacy of a proposed ethical theory. Intellectual judgments on these matters are necessarily complex and subtle. In saying, for example, that an adequate ethical theory must accord with our experience of the moral life, we certainly do not want to insist that each and every divergence from the verdict of "commonsense morality" must be interpreted as counting against an ethical theory. Perhaps we would be better advised to revise our moral judgment in light of the theory. (In empirical science, fact-theory mismatches are sometimes resolved not by modifying the theory but by reinterpreting the facts in the light of the theory.) In embracing (1), we undoubtedly commit ourselves to a point of view incompatible with the acceptance of an ethical theory that is revisionary in some wholesale sense, but we do not commit ourselves to the view that "commonsense morality" is sacrosanct. If an ethical theory successfully captures the underlying structure of our ordinary moral thinking, it will of course be true that its implications in large measure accord with our ordinary moral thinking. If the theory, however, cannot be reconciled with a relatively smaller range of our ordinary moral judgments, we may decide to interpret this disharmony as the product of inconsistency in "commonsense morality" rather than as an inadequacy in the proposed theory.

Teleological versus Deontological Theories

With the introduction of criteria (1) and (2), we are now prepared to undertake a survey of alternative ethical theories. Our immediate concern is the identification, articulation, and critical consideration of those ethical theories that are at once both prominent in general normative ethics and frequently reflected in argumentation advanced in biomedical ethics.

In contemporary discussions, ethical theories are frequently grouped into two basic, and mutually exclusive, classes—*teleological* and *deontological.* Any ethical theory that claims the rightness and wrongness of human action is *exclusively* a function of the goodness and badness of the consequences resulting directly or indirectly from that action is a teleological theory. Consequences are all-important here. A deontological theory maintains, in contrast, that the rightness and wrongness of human action is *not exclusively* (in the extreme case, not at all) a function of the goodness and badness of consequences. In accordance with this specification, a theory is deontological (rather than teleological) if it places limits on the relevance of teleological considerations. Thus an ethical theory in which the moral rightness and wrongness of human action is construed as totally independent of the goodness and badness of consequences would be only one kind, albeit the strongest or most extreme kind of deontological theory.

The most prominent teleological ethical theory is the theory known as "utilitarianism." The adequacy of utilitarianism and the issue of its proper explication continue to be dominant concerns in contemporary discussions of ethical theory. For this reason, and especially because much argumentation in biomedical ethics is based on utilitarian reasoning, utilitarianism warrants our detailed attention. However, it should first be noted that utilitarianism is not the only ethical theory that is rightly categorized as teleological. One other notable teleological theory is the theory known as "ethical egoism." The basic principle of ethical egoism can be phrased as follows: *A person ought to act so as to promote his or her own self-interest.* An action is morally right if, when compared to possible alternatives, its consequences are such as to generate the greatest balance of good over evil *for the agent.* (The impact of action on other people is irrelevant except as it may indirectly affect the agent.) Ethical egoism is a teleological theory precisely because, by the terms of the theory, the rightness and wrongness of human action is exclusively a function of the goodness and badness of consequences.

Ethical egoism is an enormously problematic theory, a theory whose implications seem to be intensely at odds with our ordinary moral thinking. Under certain conditions, ethical egoism leads us to the conclusion that it is a person's moral obligation to perform an action that is flagrantly antisocial in nature. Consider this example. Mr. *A* loves to set buildings on fire; nothing makes him happier than watching a building burn down. He recognizes that arson destroys property and subjects human life to serious risk, but he happens to be a thoroughly unsympathetic person, one whose well-being is not negatively affected by the misfortune of others. Of course, it would not be in *A*'s best self-interest (and thus would not be *A*'s moral obligation) to burn down a building if there is a good chance that he will be caught. (The punishment for arson is severe.) But if *A* is very clever, and it is virtually certain that he will not be caught, ethical egoism seems to imply that arson is the morally right thing for him to do.

Another problematic feature of ethical egoism is that it cannot be publicly advocated without inconsistency. Suppose that Ms. *B* embraces ethical egoism. Accordingly, she considers it her moral obligation always to act in such a way as to promote her individual self-interest. Can she now publicly advocate ethical egoism, that is, encourage others to adopt the view that each person's moral obligation is to act in such a way as to promote his or her individual self-interest? No. Since it is to *her* advantage that others *not* act egoistically, it follows that it would be immoral for her to publicly advocate ethical egoism.

In reducing morality to considerations of personal prudence, it can be argued, ethical egoism destroys the very sense behind morality. Morality, it would seem, functions (at least in part) to restrict the pursuit of personal self-interest. It is not that morality prohibits the pursuit of personal self-interest; rather it functions to place limits on this pursuit. In "collapsing" morality into prudence, ethical egoism does not accord with a commonly experienced phenomenon of the moral life, the tension between self-interest and morality, between "what would be best for me" and "what is the morally right thing."

In fairness to ethical egoism, it must be noted that its proponents have sometimes devised ingenious arguments in an attempt to minimize the sort of difficulties just discussed. However, ethical egoism is not widely defended in contemporary discussions of ethical theory, and it surely plays an insignificant role in discussions of biomedical ethics. It has been introduced primarily as a notable instance of a teleological yet nonutilitarian theory. Attention will now be focused on utilitarianism.

In its classical formulation, utilitarianism is found most prominently in the works of two English philosophers, Jeremy Bentham (1748–1832) and John Stuart Mill (1806–1873). In contemporary discussions, a distinction is made between two kinds of utilitarianism—*act-utilitarianism* and *rule-utilitarianism*. Although it is somewhat controversial whether a significant distinction can be maintained between these two versions of utilitarianism, it will be presumed for the sake of exposition that two distinct utilitarian ethical theories can indeed be articulated.

Act-Utilitarianism

Human action typically takes place within the fabric of our social existence. Thus an action performed by one person often impacts not only on the agent but on the lives of many others. Consider a man who refuses to stop smoking even though he suffers from emphysema. He will not be the only one to suffer the consequences; certainly those who care about him will also. His refusal to give up smoking, since it has the effect of further damaging his health, also produces a higher level of anxiety among the members of his family. Among the other detrimental consequences of his continuing to smoke is the negative impact, although small, on the productivity of those around him when he smokes. But the various consequences of a single action are seldom uniformly good or uniformly bad. In addition to the bad consequences already indicated, there are also a number of good consequences that result from the refusal to stop smoking. Most notably, the emphysema patient continues to derive the satisfaction associated with cigarette smoking. In addition, it is likely that his continuing to smoke will make him less irritable around others. When the various consequences of a single action are fully analyzed, more often than not we find ourselves confronted with a mixture of good and bad. If a person throws a late-night party, it is true that those in attendance may derive a great deal of pleasure, but it is also true that the neighbors may lose out on some much-needed sleep.

The basic principle of act-utilitarianism can be stated as follows: *A person ought to act so as to produce the greatest balance of good over evil, everyone considered.* Act-utilitarianism stands in vivid contrast to ethical egoism, which directs a person always to act so as to produce the greatest balance of good over evil *for oneself* (i.e., the agent). The act-utilitarian is committed to the proposition that the interests of everyone affected by an action are to be weighed in the balance along with the interests of the agent. Everyone's interests are entitled to an impartial consideration. According to the act-utilitarian, an action is morally right if, when compared to possible alternatives, its likely consequences are such as to generate the greatest balance of good over evil, everyone considered. If we refer to the net balance of good over evil (everyone considered) that is likely to be produced by a certain action as its (overall) *utility,* then we can say that act-utilitarianism directs a person always to choose that alternative which has the greatest utility. Thus we can express the basic principle of act-utilitarianism as follows: A person ought to act so as to maximize utility.

For the act-utilitarian, calculation is a paramount element in the moral assessment of action. The question is always, what is the utility of each of my alternatives in this particular set of circumstances? But any system of utilitarian calculation must ultimately be anchored in some conception of "intrinsic value" (i.e., that which is good or desirable in and of itself). The act that will maximize utility (by our definition) is the act that is likely to produce the greatest balance of good over evil, everyone considered. But what is to count as "good" and what as "evil" in our calculations? The answers provided within the framework of classical utilitarianism reflect a so-called "hedonistic" theory of intrinsic value. According to Bentham, only pleasure (understood broadly to include any type of satisfaction or enjoyment) has intrinsic value; only pain (understood broadly to include any dissatisfaction, frustration, or displeasure) has intrinsic disvalue. According to Mill, only happiness has intrinsic value; only unhappiness has intrinsic disvalue. To what extent there is substantive disagreement between Bentham and Mill on this matter is a complex question that cannot be dealt with here. It should be mentioned, however, that many contemporary utilitarian thinkers have embraced more elaborate and nonhedonistic theories of intrinsic value. Nevertheless, for the sake of exposition, we shall presume that a hedonistic theory of intrinsic value, in the spirit of Bentham and Mill, underlies utilitarian calculation.

In the spirit of act-utilitarianism, in order to determine what I should do in a certain situation, I must first attempt to delineate alternative paths of action. Next I attempt to foresee the consequences (sometimes numerous and far-reaching) of each alternative action. Then I attempt, in each case, to evaluate the consequences and to weigh the good against the bad, considering the impact of my action on everyone whom it is likely to affect. Such a reckoning will reveal the act that is likely to produce the greatest balance of good over evil, and this act is the morally right act for me in my particular circumstances. (If it appears likely that two competing actions would produce the same balance of good over evil, then either action will qualify as the morally correct action.) In some situations, it is true, no matter what I do, more evil (pain or unhappiness) will come into the world than good (pleasure or happiness). In such unfortunate situations, according to the act-utilitarian, the morally right act is that one which will bring the least amount of evil into the world.

Act-utilitarianism can rightly be understood as a form of "situation ethics." The act-utilitarian has no sympathy for the notion that certain kinds of actions are intrinsically wrong, that is, wrong by their very nature. Rather, a certain kind of action (e.g., lying) may be wrong in one set of circumstances, yet right in a different set of circumstances. The circumstances in which an action is to be performed are relevant to its morality (i.e., its rightness or wrongness) because the consequences of the action will vary depending on the circumstances. Thus the morality of action is a function of the situation confronting the agent—"situation ethics."

The situational character of act-utilitarianism is reflected in the act-utilitarian attitude toward moral rules. Among the "commonsense rules of morality" are the following: "do not kill," "do not injure," "do not steal," "do not lie," "do not break promises," and so forth. According to the act-utilitarian, these rules are to be understood merely as rules of thumb. They are, for the most part, reliable guides for human action, especially relevant when time constraints undermine the possibility of careful calculation. In most circumstances, acting in accordance with a moral rule is the way to maximize utility, but in some cases this is not so. In these latter cases, whenever there is good reason to believe that breaking a moral rule will produce a greater balance of good over evil (everyone considered), the right thing to do is to break it. In such a case, it would be wrong to follow the rule. Lying is usually wrong, breaking promises is usually wrong, killing is usually wrong, but whenever circumstances are such that there is good reason to believe that breaking a certain moral rule will maximize utility, the rule should be broken. Of course, the act-utilitarian insists, one must be cautious in concluding that any given exception to a moral rule is indeed justified. One must be wary of rationalization and not allow one's own interests to weigh more heavily than the interests of others in the utilitarian calculation. And most importantly, one must not be simple-minded in a consideration of the likely consequences of breaking a moral rule. Indirect and long-term consequences must be considered as well as direct and short-term consequences. Lying on a certain occasion may seem to promote most effectively the interests of those immediately involved, but perhaps the lie will provide a bad example for less reflective people, or perhaps it will contribute to a general breakdown of trust among human beings. In this same vein, one prominent contemporary act-utilitarian emphasizes the significance of the long-term, indirect consequences of promise breaking, while at the same time exhibiting the underlying act-utilitarian attitude toward moral rules:

> The rightness or wrongness of keeping a promise on a particular occasion depends only on the goodness or badness of the consequences of keeping or of breaking the promise on that particular occasion. Of course part of the consequences of breaking the promise, and a part to which we will normally ascribe decisive importance, will be the weakening of faith in the institution of promising. However, if the goodness of the consequences of breaking the rule is *in toto* greater than the goodness of the consequences of keeping it, then we must break the rule.... [1]

Act-utilitarianism has often been criticized on the grounds that, due to the extensive sort of calculations it seems to demand, it cannot function as a useful guide for human action. In the spirit of this criticism, the following questions are asked: How can I possibly predict all the consequences of my actions? How am I to assign weights to the various kinds of human satisfactions—for example, the pleasure of eating a cheeseburger versus the aesthetic enjoyment of the ballet? How am I to weigh the anxiety of one person against the inconvenience of another? And besides, how am I supposed to have time to do these extensive calculations? Act-utilitarians, in response to such questions, usually appeal rather directly to "common sense." They say, typically: There is no escape from a consideration of probabilities in rational decision making; predict as best you can, weigh as best you can, considering the time you have available for deliberation. All that can be expected is that you come to grips with the likely consequences of your alternatives in a serious-minded, sensible way, and then act accordingly.

Examples of Act-Utilitarian Reasoning in a Biomedical Context   The following examples are provided in an effort to exhibit act-utilitarian reasoning as it might arise in a biomedical context. It is not claimed that an act-utilitarian must necessarily reach the conclusion suggested in each case. It is only claimed that an act-utilitarian might plausibly reach the stated conclusion. In fact, an act-utilitarian can always assert that some likely consequence, either overlooked or insufficiently emphasized in a particular case, is the decisive one.

(1) A severely defective newborn, believed to have no realistic chance of surviving more than a few weeks, has contracted pneumonia. (The treatment of defective newborns is discussed in Chapter 8.) A physician, in conjunction with the parents of the infant, must decide whether to fight off the pneumonia with antibiotics, thereby prolonging the life of the infant. The alternative is simply to allow the infant to die. It seems clear that the interests of all those immediately involved are best served by deciding not to treat the pneumonia. Surely the infant has nothing to gain, and something to lose, by a slight extension of a pain-filled life. The parents, whose suffering cannot be eradicated whatever action is taken, nevertheless will find some relief knowing that their child's suffering has ended. In addition, hospital resources can be better utilized than to prolong the dying process of an infant who cannot benefit from further treatment. But there may be decisive consequences of an indirect, long-term nature. Perhaps allowing this infant to die will contribute to a breakdown of protective attitudes toward infants in general. No, the risk of this untoward consequence seems minimal. Withholding antibiotics, thereby allowing the infant to die, is the right thing to do in this particular case.

(2) A biomedical researcher, on the basis of animal studies she has conducted, believes that a certain drug therapy has great promise for the treatment of a particular kind of cancer in human beings. At present, however, her primary concern is to establish an appropriate dosage level for human beings; there have been several troublesome side effects exhibited by the animals who received large doses of the drug. Over the years, the researcher has found that students at her university are very willing to volunteer themselves as research subjects in experiments that can be identified as presenting only minimal risks to themselves. They are, however, understandably reluctant to volunteer for experiments that seem to present more substantial risks. The researcher in this particular case cannot honestly say that there are no substantial risks for research subjects. She expects, in particular, that perhaps 30 to 40 percent of the research subjects will have to contend with very prolonged nausea. But, if she is honest in conveying this information to potential research subjects, it is unlikely that they will volunteer in sufficient numbers. (The ethics of experimentation on human subjects is discussed in Chapter 4.) Perhaps, she reasons, it is justifiable in this particular case to withhold information about the risk of very prolonged nausea. After all, it is very likely that numerous people will eventually derive great benefit from the therapeutic technique under study. Surely this likely benefit far outweighs the short-term discomfort of a much smaller number. But suppose the deception comes to light. If those who routinely volunteer as research subjects are given a reason to distrust those conducting the experiments, the overall research effort will be impaired, and human welfare will be damaged greatly. This seems to be a decisive consideration. In this particular case, then, deception would be wrong. (If there were no realistic chance of the deception being discovered, it seems that the conclusion would be different.)

(3) In the 1960s when kidney dialysis machines were scarce, it was not possible for all who needed them to be accorded access. A hospital administrator or perhaps a committee has been charged with the responsibility of deciding, in essence, whose lives will be saved. (Such "microallocation decisions" are discussed in Chapter 11.) On a particular occasion, when there is room for one more patient, there are two candidates in great need. One of the candidates, a civic-minded woman of 40, is married and the mother of four children. The other candidate, an unmarried man of the same age, is known to be a drifter and an alcoholic. It seems clear, at first glance, that the consequences of saving the woman's life

are far superior to those of saving the man's life. Her husband, her children, and the community in general would be negatively affected in very substantial ways by her death. But is it not problematic to accord a person access to a scarce medical resource on the basis of his or her social role? If a precedent of this sort is set, will not those whose lives are less "socially useful" become somewhat anxious and fearful? On the other hand, perhaps this negative consequence will be balanced by a positive consequence, that is, people will be more inclined to become "socially useful." It still seems clear that the woman in this case should have priority over the man.

Critical Assessment of Act-Utilitarianism Act-utilitarianism seems to fare poorly when measured against a previously identified standard: The implications of an ethical theory must be reconcilable with our experience of the moral life. In a number of ways, it can be argued, act-utilitarianism clashes with our experience of the moral life. This failure to accord with our ordinary moral thinking is reflected in the following well-known objections to act-utilitarianism.

(1) *Act-utilitarianism confronts individuals with an overly demanding moral standard.* We are accustomed to thinking that at least some of our decisions are matters of "mere prudence," rightly decided on the basis of "what is best for me." Which major a college student should choose is a good example of a choice that we are inclined to consider essentially a nonmoral matter, a matter of "mere prudence." According to the act-utilitarian, however, a person is continually under a moral obligation to produce the greatest balance of good over evil, everyone considered. Whereas ethical egoism seems to wrongly "collapse" morality into prudence, it would seem that act-utilitarianism "expands" morality so as to destroy the realm of prudence. No aspect of a person's life can be considered merely a matter of prudence. Every decision is a moral decision, to be made on the basis of utilitarian calculation. But, however noble it might be for a college student to decide his or her major on the basis of a utilitarian calculation, it would seem that one is certainly not under an obligation to proceed in this manner. Doing so, we would ordinarily say, is not one's duty but, rather, is something "above and beyond the call of duty." Act-utilitarianism, in directing a person always to act so as to maximize utility, seems problematically to imply that it is one's duty to act in a way that we ordinarily consider "above and beyond the call of duty."

(2) *Act-utilitarianism does not accord with our experience of particular, morally significant relationships.* In our experience of the moral life, we are continually aware of highly particular, morally significant relationships that exist between ourselves and others. We are related to particular individuals in a host of morally significant ways, such as spouse to spouse, parent to child, creditor to debtor, promiser to promisee, employer to employee, teacher to student, physician or nurse to patient. In view of such relationships, it is ordinarily thought, we have special obligations—obligations that function to restrict the effort to maximize utility. Parents, we are strongly inclined to say, are obligated to care for their children even if there is good reason to think that the time and energy necessary for this task would maximize utility if redirected to some other task. In the same way, by virtue of the special relationship that exists between a physician and a patient, would it not be wrong for a physician to make decisions regarding patient treatment in the manner of an act-utilitarian? For a physician to damage the interests of an individual patient in an effort to maximize utility surely seems wrong. W. D. Ross, who has vigorously pressed this overall line of criticism against act-utilitarianism, asserts that the "essential defect of the...theory is that it ignores, or at least does not do full justice to, the highly personal character of duty."[2]

(3) *Act-utilitarianism does not accord with our conviction that individuals have rights.*
The notion of rights plays an important part in our ordinary moral thinking, but act-
utilitarianism seems incapable of accommodating this notion. Moreover, in certain circumstances, the action that would maximize utility (and thus the right action according to
the act-utilitarian) is one that we are inclined to consider seriously immoral precisely
because it entails the violation of some person's right. For example, it seems that act-
utilitarianism would allow an innocent person to be unjustly punished, as long as circumstances were such as to make this line of action the one that would generate the greatest
balance of good over evil. Suppose extreme social unrest has been created by a wave of
unsolved crimes. The enraged crowd will violently erupt, bringing massive evil into the
world, unless the authorities punish someone (anyone) in an effort to appease the appetite
for vengeance. So act-utilitarianism seems to allow the unjust treatment of a person as a
scapegoat, as a mere means to a social end. But surely an innocent person has a right not to
be punished, and it is by reference to this right that the wrongness of "scapegoating" is most
naturally understood. Similarly, "the common moral opinion that painless undetected
murders of old unhappy people are wicked, no matter what benefits result"[3] can be thought
to rest on the contention that people, however old and unhappy, nevertheless have a *right*
to life. It is often asserted against act-utilitarianism that it is a defective theory because it
allows "the end to justify the means." At least part of the sense behind this charge can be
made out in reference to the notion of rights. Certain means of achieving a desirable social
end are simply wrongful because they entail the violation of a person's right. Contra
act-utilitarianism, such means cannot be justified by the end.

Act-utilitarians have responded in two different ways to the overall claim that the theory
cannot be reconciled with our ordinary moral thinking. Some say, in essence, "so much the
worse for our ordinary moral thinking." In their view, we must simply overhaul our
collective moral consciousness and embrace the mind-set of the act-utilitarian. Most
act-utilitarians, however, do not adopt this revisionary stance. Rather, they seek to
demonstrate that the clash between act-utilitarianism and our ordinary moral thinking is
not nearly so severe as the above criticisms suggest. They argue that, when act-utilitarianism
is properly applied, when all the significant long-term, indirect consequences are taken into
account, the theory does not give rise to conclusions that seem so patently objectionable. It
is very doubtful, however, that this strategy of argument can completely rescue act-
utilitarianism from its difficulties.

Perhaps act-utilitarianism fares better when measured against the second of our previously
identified standards: An ethical theory must provide effective guidance where it is most
needed. At the very least, it must be said in favor of act-utilitarianism that it provides a
reasonably clear decision procedure, a sense of direction, for the resolution of moral
dilemmas. In the face of moral considerations that incline our judgment in conflicting
ways, act-utilitarianism counsels us to analyze the likely consequences of alternative
actions, in order to determine the alternative that will maximize utility. Still, however well
act-utilitarianism might be thought to fare with regard to our second standard, it seems to
be a seriously defective theory as measured against our first standard. Indeed, in contemporary times, most utilitarian thinkers have rejected act-utilitarianism in favor of a theory
known as rule-utilitarianism.[4]

Rule-Utilitarianism

The basic principle of act-utilitarianism has previously been formulated as follows: A
person ought to act so as to produce the greatest balance of good over evil, everyone
considered. In contrast, the basic principle of rule-utilitarianism can be formulated as

follows: *A person ought to act in accordance with the rule that, if generally followed, would produce the greatest balance of good over evil, everyone considered.* If the demand to produce the greatest balance of good over evil, everyone considered, is referred to as the principle (standard) of utility, then the principle of utility is the basic ethical principle in both the act-utilitarian and the rule-utilitarian systems. However, in the act-utilitarian system, determining the morally correct action is a matter of assessing alternative actions directly against the standard of utility; whereas in the rule-utilitarian system, determining the morally correct action involves an *indirect* appeal to the principle of utility. In the spirit of rule-utilitarianism, a moral code is first established by reference to the principle of utility. That is, a set of valid moral rules is established by determining which rules (as opposed to conceivable alternatives), if generally followed, would produce the greatest balance of good over evil. In rule-utilitarianism, individual actions are morally right if they are in accord with those rules.

The difference between act-utilitarian reasoning and rule-utilitarian reasoning can be represented schematically as follows:

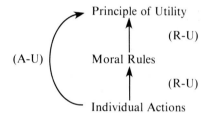

Act-utilitarian reasoning embodies a single-stage procedure, rule-utilitarian reasoning a two-stage procedure. Because the act-utilitarian is committed to assessing individual actions strictly on the basis of utilitarian considerations, act-utilitarianism is often referred to as "extreme" or "unrestricted" utilitarianism. Because the rule-utilitarian is committed to developing a moral code (a set of moral rules) on the basis of utilitarian considerations and then assessing individual actions not on the basis of utilitarian considerations but on the basis of accordance with the moral rules that have been established, rule-utilitarianism is often referred to as "restricted" utilitarianism.

For the act-utilitarian, moral rules have a very subordinate status. They are merely "rules of thumb," providing some measure of practical guidance. For the rule-utilitarian, moral rules assume a much more fundamental status, indeed a theoretical primacy. Only in reference to established moral rules can the moral assessment of individual actions be carried out. Thus the first and most crucial step for the rule-utilitarian is the articulation of a set of moral rules, themselves justified on the basis of utilitarian considerations. Underlying this task is the question of which rules (as opposed to conceivable alternatives), if generally followed, would produce the greatest balance of good over evil, everyone considered. That is, which rules, if adopted or recognized in our moral code, would maximize utility?

As a first approximation of a set of moral rules that could be justified on the basis of utilitarian considerations, consider the "commonsense rules of morality," rules such as "do not kill," "do not steal," "do not lie," "do not break promises." It is not difficult to visualize such rules as resting upon a utilitarian foundation. Surely the consequences of the adoption of the rule "do not kill" are dramatically better than the consequences of the adoption of the rule "kill whenever you want." If the latter rule were generally followed, society would be reduced to a profoundly uncivilized level. Similarly, the consequences of the adoption of the rule "do not steal" are dramatically better than the consequences of the adoption of the rule "steal whenever you want." If the former rule is generally followed, individuals will enjoy an important measure of personal security. If the latter rule were adopted by a society, anxiety and tension would dominate social existence. As for lying and promise breaking, if people felt free to engage in such behavior, the numerous advantages that derive from human trust and cooperation would evaporate. But the rules thus far exhibited as having a utilitarian foundation are essentially prohibitions. Are there not also rules of a more positive sort that could also be justified on the basis of utilitarian considerations? It would seem so. Consider rules such as "come to the aid of people in distress," and "prevent innocent people from being harmed." It surely seems that human welfare would be enhanced by the adoption of such rules as part of the overall fabric of our moral code.

According to the rule-utilitarian, an individual action is morally right when it accords with the rules or moral code established on a utilitarian basis. But the account of moral rules thus far presented is too simplistic. In order to be plausible, the rules that constitute the moral code must be understood as incorporating certain exceptions. The need to recognize justified exceptions is perhaps most apparent when we remember that moral rules, if stated unconditionally, can easily come into conflict with each other. When an obviously agitated person waves a gun and inquires as to the whereabouts of a third party, it may not be possible to act in accordance with both the rule "do not lie" and the rule "prevent innocent people from being harmed." Indeed, it is precisely this sort of situation that inclines us to consider incorporating an exception into our rule against lying. Suppose we say, "Do not lie *except* when necessary to prevent an innocent person from being harmed." When the possibility of a justified exception is raised, the rule-utilitarian employs the following decision procedure. The question is posed, Would the adoption of the rule with the exception have better consequences than the adoption of the rule without the exception? If so, the exception is a justified one; the rule incorporating the exception has greater utility than the rule without the exception. In the face of our proposed exception to the rule against lying, the rule-utilitarian would probably conclude that it does constitute a justified exception. The adoption of the rule "do not lie *except* when necessary to protect an innocent person from being harmed" would seem to preserve essentially all the social benefits provided by the adoption of the rule "do not lie," while at the same time bringing about an additional social benefit, an increased measure of personal security for potential victims of assault.

Examples of Rule-Utilitarian Reasoning in a Biomedical Context   (1) A substantive problem in biomedical ethics (discussed in Chapter 2) has to do with the morality of a physician lying to a patient, in particular, whether it is right for a physician to lie to a patient, saying that the patient's illness is not terminal when it is believed to be so. The rule-utilitarian would conceptualize this issue as raising the possibility of a justified exception to the rule against lying. (Notice that an act-utilitarian, in contrast, would insist on assessing every individual case on its own utilitarian merits.) Suppose we consider incorporating into the rule against lying an exception to this effect: "*except* when in the judgment of a physician it would be better for a patient that he or she not know that his or her illness is believed to be terminal." Would the adoption of the rule incorporating this exception have better consequences than the adoption of the rule without the exception? The correct answer to this question is perhaps arguable, but it would seem that the rule-utilitarian would conclude that the proposed exception is an unjustified one. It is perhaps true that adoption of a rule incorporating the proposed exception would result in many patients being spared (at least temporarily) the distress that accompanies knowledge of one's impending death. On the other hand, it seems that this gain would be dwarfed by

act → break a moral rule (usually one that is stated unconditionally)
rule → justifiable exceptions to a rule in the moral code

the distress and anxiety that would emerge from the erosion of trust within the confines of the physician-patient relationship. Whether a more limited exception could be formulated to a rule-utilitarian's satisfaction remains an open question.

(2) Another substantive problem in biomedical ethics (discussed in Chapter 8) has to do with the morality of mercy killing. Suppose a terminally ill patient, in great pain, requests that a physician terminate his or her life by administering a lethal dose of a drug. Such a case can be said to raise the issue of voluntary (active) euthanasia. The rule-utilitarian would conceptualize this issue (and other issues such as suicide and abortion) as raising the possibility of a justified exception to our rule against killing. Notice that at least one exception to our rule against killing is relatively uncontroversial. Killing in self-defense is justifiable, according to the rule-utilitarian, because although the adoption of the rule "do not kill" has dramatically better consequences than the adoption of the rule "kill whenever you want," adoption of the rule "do not kill *except* in self-defense" has still better consequences. As for voluntary (active) euthanasia, perhaps we should say that strong rule-utilitarian arguments can be advanced on both sides of the issue. Rule-utilitarian proponents of voluntary (active) euthanasia emphasize that social acceptance of this practice would result in great benefits—the primary one being that many dying people would be able to escape an extension of an anguished dying process. On the other side of the issue, however, we find, among a number of important concerns, insistence that availability of the lethal dose would create a climate of fear and anxiety among the elderly. Will dying people not come to feel that their families, to whom they have become a burden, expect them to ask for the lethal dose?

(3) A final illustration of rule-utilitarian reasoning in a biomedical context can be presented in reference to the principle of medical confidentiality (discussed in Chapter 3). This principle, which has an obvious basis in a rule-utilitarian structure, demands that information revealed within the context of a therapeutic relationship be held confidential. If patients could not rely on this expectation, they would be reluctant to communicate information that is essential to their proper treatment. Still, are there not justifiable exceptions to the principle of medical confidentiality? Suppose, for example, a patient reveals to his or her psychiatrist an intention to kill or injure a third party. Is it not incumbent upon the psychiatrist to break medical confidentiality in an effort to ensure protection for the third party? The situation just described is the basis of the *Tarasoff* case considered in Chapter 3, and rule-utilitarian arguments on both sides of the issue can be found in the judicial opinions presented. There is an obvious benefit associated with the recognition of an exception to medical confidentiality based on the interests of innocent third parties. Namely, threatened people will sometimes be saved from injury and death. On the other hand, it is argued, emotionally disturbed patients are likely to become more inhibited in communicating with psychiatrists; thus their cures will be inhibited, and a greater incidence of violence against innocent people will result.

Critical Assessment of Rule-Utilitarianism Rule-utilitarianism, it would seem, goes a long way toward alleviating the perceived difficulties of act-utilitarianism. Although act-utilitarians have charged rule-utilitarians with "superstitious rule-worship,"[5] it is act-utilitarianism rather than rule-utilitarianism that seems to clash with our ordinary moral thinking on this score. Indeed, rule-utilitarianism, in somewhat vivid contrast to act-utilitarianism, seems to fare reasonably well when measured against the standard that the implications of an ethical theory must be reconcilable with our experience of the moral life.

Whereas act-utilitarianism seems to confront individuals with an overly demanding moral standard, placing each of us under a continuing obligation to maximize utility with each of our actions, rule-utilitarianism is far less demanding of individuals. It requires only that individuals conform their actions to the rules that constitute a utilitarian-based moral code, and this requirement accords well with our ordinary moral thinking. Rule-utilitarianism also seems to accord reasonably well with our experience of particular, morally significant relationships. We commonly perceive ourselves as having special obligations arising out of our various morally significant relationships, and we think of these obligations as incompatible with functioning in the manner of an act-utilitarian. Parents have a special obligation to care for their children, physicians have a special obligation to act in the interests of their patients, and so forth. But such special obligations can be understood as having a rule-utilitarian foundation, as deriving from rules that, if generally followed, would maximize utility. Thus rule-utilitarianism seems to remedy another perceived difficulty of act-utilitarianism.

It is less clear that rule-utilitarianism is capable of providing a complete remedy for another perceived difficulty of act-utilitarianism, that is, its inability to provide an adequate theoretical foundation for individual rights. Surely rule-utilitarianism does not lead us so easily as does act-utilitarianism to conclusions that are incompatible with our ordinary moral thinking about the rights of individuals. For example, in suggesting that the painless murder of an old, unhappy person is the right thing as long as it can be done in complete secrecy, act-utilitarianism seems to clash violently with our conviction that such an action is patently objectionable, inasmuch as it constitutes a violation of a person's right to life. Rule-utilitarianism, in contrast, would never lead us to the conclusion that this sort of killing is morally legitimate. Surely the consequences of adopting the rule "do not kill *except* in the case of old, unhappy people who can be killed in complete secrecy" are dramatically worse than the consequences of adopting the rule without such an exception. If the rule with the exception were adopted, the lives of elderly people would be filled with anxiety and fear. In addition to rescuing utilitarian thinking from such obvious clashes with our ordinary moral thinking, rule-utilitarianism does suggest a way of accommodating the notion of individual rights. Just as our special obligations can be understood as deriving from rules in a utilitarian-based moral code, so too can an individual's rights be understood in this fashion. A person's right to life, for example, can be understood as a correlate of our utilitarian-based rule against killing. Of course, whatever exceptions are properly incorporated into our rule against killing will factor out as limitations on a person's right to life. Whether rule-utilitarianism in this manner can provide an adequate theoretical foundation for individual rights is a very controversial matter. Its critics charge that it cannot.

Closely related to the claim that rule-utilitarianism does not provide an adequate theoretical foundation for individual rights is the somewhat broader claim that rule-utilitarianism fails to provide an adequate theoretical grounding for what we take to be the obligations of justice. This broader criticism, which is also vigorously advanced against act-utilitarianism, is surely the principal residual difficulty confronting rule-utilitarianism. Critics of rule-utilitarianism allege, for example, that the theory is compatible with the blatant injustice of enslaving one segment of a society's population or at least discriminating against this segment. The idea is that social rules discriminating against an explicitly identified minority group might function to maximize utility by bringing about more happiness in the advantaged majority than unhappiness in the disadvantaged minority. Rule-utilitarians are inclined to argue in response to this line of criticism that when the consequences of adopting "unjust rules" are completely analyzed, it is never true that their adoption can be justified on utilitarian grounds. Rather, the rule-utilitarian contends, "the rules of justice" rest on a secure utilitarian foundation. Whether rule-utilitarianism, in this manner, can adequately be reconciled with the perceived obligations of justice is a matter of contemporary debate.

Rule-utilitarianism also seems to fare reasonably well when measured against the second of our suggested standards: An ethical theory must provide effective guidance where it is most needed. In the dilemma situation, where one moral rule, or principle, inclines us one way, another moral rule, or principle, inclines us another way, the rule-utilitarian instructs us to establish relative priority by considering the consequences of incorporating appropriate exceptions into the rules that are in conflict. The dilemma is to be resolved by adoption of a rule that will maximize utility. Although this decision procedure sometimes entails very complex factual analysis and deliberation, it does seem to provide us a substantial measure of explicit guidance. Since rule-utilitarianism also seems to be reasonably harmonious with our ordinary moral thinking, it is an ethical theory that cannot easily be dismissed.

Kantian Deontology

The most prominent of the classical deontological theories is that developed by the German philosopher, Immanuel Kant (1724–1804). Kantian deontology continues to command substantial attention in contemporary discussions of ethical theory and, importantly, is the underlying framework of much argumentation in biomedical ethics. In both of these respects, Kantian deontology is similar to utilitarianism and, like utilitarianism, warrants our detailed attention.

Kant sees utilitarianism as embodying a radically wrong approach in ethical theory. He emphasizes the need to avoid the "serpent-windings" of utilitarian thinking and refers to the Principle of Utility as "a wavering and uncertain standard." There is indeed a single, fundamental principle that is the basis of all moral obligation, but this fundamental principle is *not* the Principle of Utility. The "supreme principle of morality," the principle from which all of our various duties derive, is called by Kant the "Categorical Imperative."

Our present objective is an exposition of Kantian deontology. But the enormous complexity of Kant's moral philosophy is a formidable obstacle to any concise exposition of the structure of Kant's ethical system. In particular, we are faced with the problem that Kant formulated the basic principle of his system, the Categorical Imperative, in a number of different ways. Although Kant insists that his various formulations are all equivalent, this contention is explicitly denied by many of his expositors and critics. Thus, if we are to provide a coherent account of Kantian deontology, mindful of the need to provide an account that is especially useful in dealing with issues in biomedical ethics, it seems advisable to settle on a favored formulation of the Categorical Imperative. Since two of Kant's formulations of the Categorical Imperative are especially prominent, it will suffice for our purposes to choose a favored formulation from these two.

According to what we will call the "first formulation," the Categorical Imperative tells us: "Act only on that maxim through which you can at the same time will that it should become a universal law."[6] According to what we will call the "second formulation," the Categorical Imperative tells us: "Act in such a way that you always treat humanity, whether in your own person or in the person of any other, never simply as a means, but always at the same time as an end."[7] The first formulation of the Categorical Imperative has often been compared with the Golden Rule ("do unto others as you would have them do unto you"), and it may be true that both of these principles, when suitably interpreted, have roughly the same implications. At any rate, it is apparently the case that Kant considered the first formulation to be the most basic of all his formulations. Yet, despite this fact, and despite the fact that ethical theorists have tended to pay more attention to the first formulation than the second, it is the second formulation that we take to have greater promise for the task at hand. Two major reasons can be advanced for choosing to exhibit the structure of

Kant's ethical system in reference to the second formulation of the Categorical Imperative. First, the second formulation embodies a central notion—respect for persons—that is somewhat easier to grasp and apply than the more formalistic notion of universalizability, which is the core element of the first formulation. Second, when argumentation in biomedical ethics reflects a Kantian viewpoint, it is almost always couched in terms of the second formulation rather than the first.

Kantian deontology is an ethics of respect for persons. In Kant's view, every person, by virtue of his or her humanity (i.e., rational nature) has an inherent dignity. All persons, as rational creatures, are entitled to respect, not only from others but from themselves as well. Thus the Categorical Imperative directs each of us to "act in such a way that you always treat humanity, whether in your own person or in the person of any other, never simply as a means, but always at the same time as an end." From this fundamental principle, according to Kant, a host of particular duties can be derived. The resultant system of duties includes duties to self as well as duties to others. And in each of these cases, "perfect duties" must be distinguished from "imperfect duties," thus generating a fourfold classification of duties: (1) perfect duties to self, (2) imperfect duties to self, (3) perfect duties to others, (4) imperfect duties to others. Although the distinction between perfect and imperfect duties is not a transparent one, its structural importance in the Kantian system is hard to overemphasize. Perfect duties require of us that we do or abstain from certain acts. *There are no legitimate exceptions to a perfect duty.* Such duties are binding in all circumstances, because certain kinds of action are simply incompatible with respect for persons, hence strictly impermissible. Imperfect duties, by contrast, require of us, in some overall sense, that we pursue or promote certain goals (e.g., the welfare of others). However, action in the name of these goals must never be at the expense of a perfect duty. One of Kant's most prominent commentators relates the distinction between perfect and imperfect duties to the Categorical Imperative in the following way: "We transgress perfect duties by treating any person *merely* as a means. We transgress imperfect duties by failing to treat a person as an end, even though we do not actively treat him as a means."[8]

Our discussion of Kant's fourfold classification of duties will begin with a consideration of perfect duties to others. A transgression in this category of duty occurs whenever one person treats another person merely as a means. It is strictly impermissible for person A to treat person B merely as a means because such treatment is incompatible with respect for B as a person. Notice that Kant does not claim that it is morally wrong for one person to use another as a means. His claim is that it is morally wrong for one person to use another *merely* as a means. In the ordinary course of life, it is surely unavoidable (and morally unproblematic) that each of us in numerous ways uses others as means to achieve our various ends. A college teacher uses students as a means to achieve his or her livelihood. A college student uses instructors as a means of gaining knowledge and skills. Such human interactions, presumably based on the voluntary participation of the respective parties, are quite compatible with a principle of respect for persons. But respect for persons entails that each of us recognize the rightful authority of other persons (as rational beings) to conduct their individual lives as they see fit. We may legitimately recruit others to participate in the satisfaction of our personal ends, but they are used merely as a means whenever we undermine the voluntary or informed character of their consent to interact with us in some desired way. Person A coerces person B at knifepoint to hand over \$200. A uses B merely as a means. If A had requested of B a gift of \$200, leaving B free to determine whether or not to make the gift, A would have proceeded in a manner compatible with respect for B as a person. Person C deceptively rolls back the odometer of a car and thereby manipulates person D's decision to buy the car. C uses D merely as a means. C has acted in a way that is strictly incompatible with respect for D as a person.

In the Kantian system, among the most notable of our perfect duties to others are: (1) the duty not to kill an innocent person, (2) the duty not to lie, and (3) the duty to keep promises. Murder (the killing of an innocent person), lying, and promise breaking are actions that are intrinsically wrong. However beneficial the consequences of such an action might be in a given circumstance, the action is strictly impermissible. (Notice the anti-utilitarian character of Kant's thinking.) The murderer exhibits obvious disrespect for the person of the victim. The liar, in misinforming another person, violates the respect due to that person as a rational creature, with a fundamental interest in the truth. A person who makes a promise issues a guarantee upon which the recipient of the promise is entitled to rely in his or her future planning. The promise breaker shows disrespect for a person in undermining the effort to conduct the affairs of one's life. By murdering, lying, or promise breaking, an agent uses another person merely as a means to the agent's own ends.

According to Kant, each person has not only perfect duties to others but also perfect duties to self. The Categorical Imperative demands that no person (including oneself) be treated merely as a means. It is no more permissible to manifest disrespect for one's own person than to do so for the person of another. Kant insists, for example, that each person has a perfect duty to self to avoid drunkenness. Since drunkenness undermines a person's rational capacities, it is incompatible with respect for oneself as a rational creature. Kant believes that individuals debase themselves in the effort to achieve pleasure via inebriation. Inebriates treat themselves merely as a means (to the end of pleasure). But surely the foremost example of a perfect duty to self in the Kantian system is the duty not to commit suicide. To terminate one's own life, Kant insists, is strictly incompatible with respect for oneself as a person. In eradicating one's very existence as a rational creature, a person treats oneself merely as a means (ordinarily to the end of avoiding discomfort or distress). Suicide is an action that is intrinsically wrong, and there are no circumstances in which it is morally permissible.

In addition to the notion of perfect duties (both to self and others), the Kantian system also incorporates the notion of imperfect duties. Whereas perfect duties require, in essence, strict abstention from those actions that involve using a person merely as a means, imperfect duties have a very different underlying sense. Imperfect duties require the promotion of certain goals. In broad terms, there are two such goals—an agent's personal perfection (i.e., development) and the happiness or welfare of others. Respect for oneself as a person requires commitment to the development of one's capacities as a rational being. Thus Kant spoke of an imperfect duty to self to develop one's talents. The sense of this duty is that, by and large, it is up to each individual to decide which talents to cultivate and which to deemphasize. But a person is not free to abandon the goal of personal development. Although the duty to develop one's talents requires no *specific* actions, it does require each individual to formulate a plan of life that embodies a commitment to the goal of personal development.

Before discussing Kant's final category of duty, imperfect duty to others, it will prove helpful to introduce the notion of *beneficence*.[9] If one acts in such a way as to further the happiness or welfare of another, then one acts beneficently. (A benevolent person is one who is inclined to act beneficently.) Beneficence may be contrasted with *nonmaleficence*, which is ordinarily understood as the noninfliction of harm on others. One who harms ("does evil" to) another acts in a maleficent fashion. One who *refrains* from harming others acts in a nonmaleficent fashion. One who acts, in a more positive way, to contribute to the welfare of others acts in a beneficent fashion. Beneficence is a generic notion that can best be understood as including the following types of activity: (1) preventing evil or harm from befalling someone; (2) removing an evil that is presently afflicting someone; (3) providing benefits ("doing good") for someone. Although it is sometimes difficult to decide which of these categories is the most appropriate classification for a particular beneficent action, the following examples seem relatively straightfoward. Pushing someone out of the path of an oncoming car is an example of (1). Curing a patient's disease is an example of (2). Giving someone a $100 gift is an example of (3).

According to Kant, respect for other persons requires not only that we avoid using them merely as a means (by the observance of our perfect duties to others) but also that we commit ourselves in some general way to furthering their happiness or welfare. Thus Kant considers what we will call the "duty of beneficence" to be an imperfect duty to others. As with the duty to develop our talents, an imperfect duty to self, the duty of beneficence requires no *specific* actions. One does not violate the duty of beneficence by refusing to act beneficently in any individual case where the opportunity arises. What is required instead of specific actions is that each person incorporate in his or her life plan a commitment to promoting the well-being of others. Individuals are free to choose the sorts of actions they will embrace in an effort to further the well-being of others (e.g., contributing to the relief of famine victims); they are not free to abandon the general goal of furthering the well-being of others.

Since the duty of beneficence is an imperfect duty in the Kantian system, action in the name of beneficence must never be taken at the expense of a perfect duty. For example, it is impermissible to lie or break a promise in an effort to save a third party from harm. The same is true with regard to the imperfect duty to develop one's talents. For example, if one has resolved (quite properly) to develop one's creative powers, it is nevertheless impermissible to do so by "creatively" defrauding others.

The Kantian Framework in a Biomedical Context   With our exposition of Kantian deontology now complete, we are in a position to exhibit some of the more important applications of this ethical theory in the realm of biomedical ethics. To begin with, the theory has an obvious relevance to the much-discussed problem of whether or not a physician may justifiably lie to a patient (an issue discussed in Chapter 2). Since every person has a perfect duty to others not to lie, a straightforward implication of Kantian deontology is that a physician may *never* lie to a patient. If a patient, diagnosed as terminally ill by a physician, inquires about his or her prognosis, the physician may be much inclined to lie, motivated by a desire to protect the patient from the psychological turmoil that would accompany knowledge of his or her true condition; but action in the name of beneficence (an imperfect duty) may never be at the expense of a perfect duty. This same analysis is applicable to the use of placebos by physicians. Sometimes a patient becomes psychologically dependent on a certain medication. When the medication is discontinued, because the physician is convinced it is no longer needed and because its continued use represents a threat to health, the patient complains of the reemergence of symptoms. If such a patient is given a placebo, that is, a therapeutically inert but harmless substance, misrepresented as a medication, the patient may feel fine. Nevertheless, despite the fact that placebos may be capable of enhancing patient welfare, their employment entails lying and thus is morally impermissible.

Kantian deontology has some very important and very direct implications for the ethics of experimentation with human subjects (the topic of Chapter 4). Since it is morally wrong for any person to use any other person merely as a means, it follows that it is morally wrong for a biomedical researcher to use a human research subject merely as a means. And from this consideration it is but a short step to the requirement of voluntary informed consent as a basic principle of research ethics. If a researcher is engaged in a study that involves human subjects, we may presume that the immediate "end" being sought by the researcher is the successful completion of the study. But notice that the researcher may desire this particular end for any number of reasons: the speculative understanding it will provide; the technology it will make possible; the eventual benefit of humankind; personal recognition in the eyes of the scientific community; a raise in pay; and so forth. This mixture of self-centered and benevolent motivations may be considered the researcher's less immediate ends. Now, if researchers are to avoid using their research subjects merely as means (to the ends of the researchers), surely they must refrain from coercing the participation of their subjects and, in addition, provide information about the research project (most notably, risks to the subjects) sufficient for the subjects to make a rational decision with regard to their personal participation. Thus respect for persons demands that researchers honor the requirement of voluntary informed consent.

Suppose a researcher explains to a potential research subject how important it is that he or she consent to participate. There is no question but that the research project at issue, if brought to a successful conclusion, will provide substantial benefit to humankind. Does the potential subject have a moral obligation to participate? Surely not. Within the framework of Kantian deontology, the duty of beneficence is an imperfect duty. A person must on occasion act beneficently, but there is no obligation to perform any *specific* beneficent action. Interestingly enough, the same line of thought would seem to apply to the question, does a physician have a moral obligation to come to the aid of a seriously injured person (not by prior agreement the physician's patient) in an emergency situation?

Critical Assessment of Kantian Deontology   Are the implications of Kantian deontology reconcilable with our experience of the moral life? Can this theory function to provide effective guidance in the face of perceived moral dilemmas? These two questions reflect the criteria suggested earlier as most central to the assessment of the relative adequacy of an ethical theory.

Before indicating some of the ways in which Kantian deontology can be thought to be at odds with our ordinary moral thinking, it is important to emphasize that the theory does successfully account for crucial aspects of our experience of the moral life. To begin with, Kantian deontology provides an obvious foundation for the "commonsense rules of morality." The wrongfulness of actions that fly in the face of these rules—actions such as killing, injuring, stealing, lying, breaking promises—can very plausibly be understood as flowing from the Categorical Imperative. The Kantian deontologist maintains that these actions are wrong because they involve treating another person merely as a means, and there is something very compelling about the notion of respect for persons as the core notion of morality.

Kantian deontology also seems to provide a secure foundation for the notion of individual rights, a notion that is very prominent in our ordinary moral thinking. Individual rights, in the Kantian system, are to be understood as the correlates of our perfect duties to others. (Imperfect duties, in contrast, do not generate rights.) For example, each of us has a perfect *duty* not to kill an innocent person; thus every innocent person has a *right* not to be killed. More generally, every person has a right not to be used by another merely as a means. An innocent person has a right not to be punished, no matter how socially desirable the consequences might be in a certain set of circumstances. A potential research subject has a right not to be coerced or deceived into participation, even if the satisfactory completion of the study promises great benefit for humankind. In its insistence that individual rights cannot be overridden by "utilitarian" considerations, Kantian deontology achieves accord with our firmly entrenched (if somewhat vague) conviction that the "end does not justify the means."

Yet, there are aspects of Kantian deontology that cannot be easily reconciled with our experience of the moral life. One very prominent difficulty has to do with the Kantian contention that keeping promises and not lying are both duties of perfect obligation. We are quite at home, in our ordinary moral thinking, with both a duty to keep promises and a duty not to lie, but it is the exceptionless character of these duties in the Kantian system that we find troublesome. Surely in extreme cases, we are inclined to say, these duties must yield to more weighty moral considerations. For example, if a person breaks a rather trivial promise (say, to return a book at a certain time) in order to respond to the needs of a person in serious distress, surely he or she has not acted immorally. Or again, if a person lies to a would-be murderer about the whereabouts of the intended victim, surely the liar has not (all things considered) acted immorally. The Kantian deontologist sees in such examples a clash between a perfect duty and the imperfect duty of beneficence, and the Kantian teaching is that the former may never yield to the latter. But it would seem that a theory with such implausible implications stands in need of revision. Perhaps the problem is not only that Kantian deontology overstates the significance of certain "perfect" duties but that it understates the significance of the duty of beneficence, at least that aspect of beneficence that has to do with preventing serious harm from befalling another or alleviating the serious distress of another.

In our everyday existence as moral agents, we are accustomed to the idea that we have a number of important duties to others. It is less clear that the Kantian notion of duties to self can be reconciled with our experience of the moral life. This is difficult territory. For one thing, the issue of suicide (discussed in Chapter 7) seems to confound our moral "common sense" in a way that blatant wrongs such as murder, rape, and slavery do not. Still, despite significant disagreement, suicide is widely held to be morally wrong. But the issue is this: Do those who consider suicide morally wrong experience the duty not to commit suicide as a duty to self? It seems more likely that this duty is experienced as a duty to others (who may be negatively affected by one's suicide) or, in the case of religious believers, as a duty to God. A similar argument could be made with regard to the imperfect duty to develop one's talents.

It cannot be denied that Kantian deontology, to a substantial degree, is reconcilable with our experience of the moral life. On the other hand, it appears that the theory is attended with some significant and unresolved difficulties. How does Kantian deontology fare when measured against the second of our standards, the requirement that an ethical theory provide effective guidance in the face of moral dilemmas? Once again, it seems, the verdict is somewhat mixed.

It might be argued that Kantian deontology, by sorting our various duties into the categories of perfect and imperfect and assigning priority to perfect duties, provides us with a structure in terms of which moral dilemmas can be resolved. And this is perhaps true to the extent that our perplexity can be analyzed in terms of perfect duties marshalled against imperfect duties, but even here it is difficult to overlook the fact that the priority of perfect over imperfect duties is itself a somewhat problematic feature of Kantian deontology. One is tempted to say that even if the theory provides reasonably *clear* guidance, it fails to provide *correct* guidance. And what is one to do when confronted with a perfect duty in conflict with another perfect duty? Kantian deontology does not even seem to recognize the possibility of such conflicts, but consider the following example. Suppose a patient discusses a certain sensitive matter (e.g., euthanasia) with a nurse, who promises not to tell the patient's family that the matter was discussed. The next day a family member directly asks the nurse if this matter was discussed. Thus the perfect duty to tell the truth seems to come into direct conflict with the perfect duty to keep a promise. Is it possible that the guiding idea of respect for persons could somehow resolve the question of which of these duties must be preferred? Or must one resort, perhaps in utilitarian fashion, to a consideration of consequences?

W. D. Ross's Theory of Prima Facie Duties

In a book entitled *The Right and the Good* (1930), the English philosopher W. D. Ross proposed a deontological theory that has received considerable attention among ethical theorists. The point of departure for the development of Ross's theory is his concern to provide a defensible account of "cases of conscience," that is, situations that confront us with a conflict of duties. One perceived line of obligation pulls us in one direction, another perceived line of obligation pulls us in a contrary direction. We find ourselves unsettled and uncertain, but cannot avoid a choice. Which duty takes precedence over the other? The parent of a young child has promised to attend a community meeting, but the child seems to need special attention. Since our social existence is complex, conflict-of-duty situations are a recurrent feature of our daily life. In the biomedical context, such situations are pervasive.

For understandable reasons, Ross maintains that neither the Kantian nor the utilitarian can provide an account of conflict-of-duty situations that harmonizes with what he calls "ordinary moral consciousness." We have recently considered the relevant deficiency in the Kantian approach. It is implausible to maintain that the duty of beneficence can never take precedence over the duty to keep promises or the duty not to lie. As for the utilitarian approach, and here it is clear that Ross has act-utilitarianism in mind, this theory's insistence that in reality we have only the one duty of maximizing utility clashes with our conviction that we have distinct lines of obligation to distinct people. In order to provide an adequate account of conflict-of-duty situations, Ross maintains, it is essential to introduce the notion of "prima facie duty." The Latin phrase "prima facie," now commonplace in moral philosophy, literally means "at first glance." But the word "conditional" best expresses the sense of the phrase as Ross intends it. A prima facie duty is a conditional duty. A prima facie duty (as opposed to an absolute duty) can be overridden by a more stringent duty.

According to Ross, there are no absolute, or unconditional, duties, only prima facie duties. But what is the basis of our prima facie duties? Both the utilitarian and the Kantian assert that our various duties have a unitary basis in a fundamental principle of morality. The utilitarian believes that our various duties can be derived from the Principle of Utility. The Kantian believes that our various duties can be derived from the Categorical Imperative. Ross, in vivid contrast, maintains that our various prima facie duties have no unitary basis. Rather, they emerge out of our numerous "morally significant relations," relations such as promisee to promiser, creditor to debtor, spouse to spouse, child to parent, friend to friend, citizen to the state, fellow human being to fellow human being. "Each of these relations is the foundation of a *prima facie* duty, which is more or less incumbent on me according to the circumstances of the case."[10]

In unproblematic circumstances, where we are bound by only one prima facie duty, this particular prima facie duty is our *actual* duty. In conflict-of-duty situations, where two (or more) prima facie duties compete for priority, only one of these duties, the more stringent one in the circumstances, can be our actual duty. We have, for example, both a prima facie duty to keep promises and a prima facie duty to assist those who are in need. According to Ross, when these two duties come into conflict, it is clear (in terms of our "ordinary moral consciousness") that the duty to keep promises is usually more incumbent upon us than the duty to assist those who are in need. But if the promise is relatively trivial and the need of another is compelling—a matter of serious distress—then it is equally clear that the priority is reversed. In the difficult cases, Ross maintains, there is in principle no hard and fast rule to apply. In his view, the best anyone can do is to make a reflective, "considered decision" as to which of the competing prima facie duties has the priority in any given situation.

According to Ross, "there is nothing arbitrary about [our] *prima facie* duties. Each rests on a definite circumstance which cannot seriously be held to be without moral significance."[11] Accordingly, he proposes the following division of our prima facie duties.

(1) *Duties of fidelity* include keeping promises, honoring contracts and agreements, and telling the truth. Duties in this class rest on a person's previous acts. In giving one's word to do something, a person creates the duty to do so. (Ross thinks that by entering a conversation, a person implicitly agrees to tell the truth.) Notice that a person's so-called role responsibilities can be identified as an important subclass of duties of fidelity. A teacher has certain responsibilities as a teacher, a physician certain responsibilities as a physician, a nurse certain responsibilities as a nurse. In taking on a certain social role, a person brings into existence various duties of fidelity. In addition, further duties of fidelity arise out of agreements (both explicit and implicit) that a person enters into while functioning in a professional capacity.

(2) *Duties of reparation* also rest on a person's previous acts. Any person, by wrongfully treating someone else, creates the duty to rectify the wrong that has been perpetrated. For example, if *A* steals a certain amount of money from *B, A* thereby brings into existence the duty to repay this amount. (3) *Duties of gratitude* rest on previous acts of other persons, that is, beneficial services provided by them. If *A* has provided a good service for *B* when *B* was in need, *B* thereby stands under a duty to provide a good service for *A* when *A* is in need.

(4) *Duties of beneficence* "rest on the mere fact that there are other beings in the world whose condition we can make better."[12] (5) *Duties of nonmaleficence* rest on the complementary fact that we can also make the condition of our fellow human beings worse. The duties in this category, which Ross recognizes as especially stringent, can be summed up under the heading of "not injuring others." The duty not to kill and the duty not to steal are obvious examples.

(6) *Duties of justice* "rest on the fact or possibility of a distribution of pleasure or happiness (or of the means thereto) which is not in accordance with the merit of the persons concerned."[13] Benefits are to be distributed in accordance with personal merit, and existing unjust patterns of distribution are to be rectified. (7) *Duties of self-improvement* "rest on the fact that we can improve our own condition."[14]

Prima Facie Duties in a Biomedical Context Ross's framework of prima facie duties is helpful for conceptualizing many of the moral dilemmas that arise in a biomedical context. In analyzing such dilemmas as they arise from the point of view of health-care professionals, the category of duties of fidelity is especially important. Consider, for example, the physician-patient relationship (a topic under discussion in Chapter 2). The social understanding or implicit agreement that underlies this relationship undoubtedly includes a number of important provisions. Among these are the provision that the physician is to act in the best medical interest of the patient and the provision that the physician is to keep confidential any personal information that comes to light within the context of the physician-patient relationship. In the very act of accepting a patient for treatment, a physician thereby incurs a number of important prima facie duties of fidelity.

Suppose a physician is convinced that lying to a patient is in the best medical interest of the patient. In Ross's scheme, the prima facie duty not to lie, itself a duty of fidelity, comes into conflict with another duty of fidelity, the prima facie duty to act in the best medical interest of the patient. Since neither duty is unconditional, in one case the duty not to lie might be more incumbent upon the physician, whereas in another case the duty to act in the best interest of the patient might be the more stringent duty. Suppose, in a different case, a physician is treating a patient suffering from a condition that renders the patient in his or her occupation a danger to others. The patient, for example, is a bus driver subject to blackouts. The patient is desperate to keep his or her job and refuses to divulge the problem to his or her employer. Should the physician break medical confidentiality and notify the patient's employer, in an effort to ensure the public safety? In this case, the prima facie duty of beneficence comes into conflict with a duty of fidelity, the prima facie duty to keep medical confidentiality. (Justifiable exceptions to the duty to keep medical confidentiality are discussed in Chapter 3.)

Among the explicit role responsibilities of a typical hospital nurse is the obligation to follow physician's orders in the treatment of patients. By the simple act of accepting employment in the hospital setting, a nurse thereby incurs, among other numerous duties of fidelity, the prima facie duty to obey physicians' orders. But an important moral dilemma for the hospital nurse arises when, in the judgment of the nurse, following a physician's order would be detrimental to the patient. (This dilemma is discussed in Chapter 3.) Thinking in terms of Ross's theory, we can structure the dilemma as follows. The prima facie duty to follow physician's orders comes into conflict with two other prima facie duties. First there is a relevant duty of nonmaleficence. A nurse should not act in a way that would, in effect, injure another person. Second, there is another relevant duty of fidelity, deriving from the fact that a nurse has an implicit contract or agreement with the patient to act in his or her best medical interest. Is the collective force of these two prima facie duties more incumbent upon the nurse than the prima facie duty to follow a physician's orders? Since the duty of nonmaleficence is recognized by Ross (and "ordinary moral consciousness") as especially stringent, it seems that in most cases, at least where the potential harm to patients is significant, the nurse must conclude that it would be wrong to follow the physician's order.

Abstracting from any relevant role responsibilities on the part of health-care professionals, the issue of the moral justifiability of mercy killing (discussed in Chapter 8) might be conceptualized, in accordance with Ross's scheme, as a moral dilemma involving the conflict between a duty of beneficence and a duty of nonmaleficence. A terminally ill person suffering unbearable pain, it would seem, would benefit from an immediate and painless death. Thus we have on one hand a duty of beneficence—the prima facie duty to come to the assistance of a person in serious distress—and on the other hand we have a duty of nonmaleficence—the prima facie duty not to kill.

Critical Assessment of Ross's Theory   Since Ross developed his theory of prima facie duties explicitly in reference to the promptings of "ordinary moral consciousness," it would be surprising if his theory could not be reconciled with our experience of the moral life. Indeed, let us put aside whatever worries might be expressed on this score, for there is a much more obvious deficiency in Ross's theory. Recall that we have asked not only that an ethical theory be reconcilable with our experience of the moral life but also that it provide us with effective guidance where it is most needed, in the face of moral dilemmas. And despite the fact that Ross's theory provides us with a helpful framework for conceptualizing our moral dilemmas, it provides us with virtually no substantive guidance for resolving them.

In the difficult cases, where two prima facie duties come into strong conflict, Ross holds that there are no principles we can appeal to in an effort to make an appropriate decision. The most we can do, in his view, is render a "considered decision" as to which duty is more incumbent upon us in a certain situation. Although it is fine to be told to make a considered decision, what exactly is worthy of consideration in reaching a decision? Can we resist, however vaguely, falling back on some sort of utilitarian standard?

Ross would probably say, in response to the complaint just registered, that it is too to ask of an ethical theory that it provide the resources for the resolutio dilemmas. Morality, in his view, is somewhat indeterminate when the prima facie duties (themselves clearly determinate) come into conflict. But most moral philosophers would be unwilling to embrace this aspect of Ross's thinking. A rule-utilitarian, in particular, might argue that Ross's entire system of prima facie duties could be exhibited on the basis of a rule-utilitarian foundation. And in this way, the advantages of thinking in terms of prima facie duties could be combined with a utilitarian methodology for mediating among conflicting duties.

RELEVANT CONCEPTS AND PRINCIPLES

The foregoing examination of some major normative ethical theories provides the groundwork for a brief exploration of several important concepts in biomedical ethics. The most central of these concepts are autonomy, paternalism, and rights. Closely associated with these concepts is a set of principles, called "liberty-limiting principles," which are often invoked in order to justify limitations on individual liberty. This section provides a brief examination of these relevant concepts and principles.

Autonomy

Many discussions in biomedical ethics presume the importance of individual autonomy, stressing the right of autonomous decision makers to determine for themselves what will be done to their bodies. This "right of self-determination" is said to limit what physicians, nurses, and other professionals can justifiably do to patients. In fact, this right is often taken so seriously that professionals who act against their patients' wishes, even to save their patients' lives, are condemned as morally blameworthy and leave themselves open to charges of battery. In view of all this, it is useful to discuss the following questions, the first a conceptual question, the second an ethical one. (1) What sense of autonomy is operative in the widespread presumption that individual autonomy is an important value? and (2) What is the ethical basis for the value accorded to individual autonomy?

The Concept of Autonomy   In discussions of ethics, autonomy is typically defined as self-governance or self-determination. Individuals are said to act autonomously when they, and not others, make the decisions that affect their lives and act on the basis of their decisions. This general characterization needs to be explicated, however, since autonomy is a complex notion. Writers in biomedical ethics often conceptually distinguish several senses of autonomy in order to clarify some of the issues raised when questions are asked about justified infringements or limitations of individual autonomy: (1) autonomy as liberty of action; (2) autonomy as freedom of choice; and (3) autonomy as effective deliberation.[15] A brief consideration of these three senses of autonomy will also serve to emphasize the various ways in which an individual's action, thought, or choice may be less than fully autonomous.

1 Autonomy as Liberty of Action   Think of a would-be-physician, Mark, who sits under a tree waiting for medical knowledge to permeate his being. No one is forcing Mark to sit under the tree. He is free to leave anytime he chooses. His action results from his conscious intention to sit under the tree. (He does not mistakenly believe, for example, that he is sitting in medical school.) His action is also voluntary in the sense that it is not the result of coercion or duress. If autonomy is treated simply as a synonym for "liberty of action," then Mark is acting autonomously insofar as his action is intentional and voluntary. Mark's autonomy would be violated, however, if he were physically forced to sit under the tree or if someone were to coerce him into sitting there by threatening him with

When autonomy is identified with liberty of action, the primary contrast drawn is between autonomy and coercion. Coercion always involves the deliberate use of force or the threat of harm. The coercer's purpose is to get the person being coerced to do something he or she would not otherwise be willing to do. "Occurrent" coercion involves the use of physical force. "Dispositional" coercion involves the threat of harm.[16] An unscrupulous medical researcher, for example, might literally force individuals to participate as research subjects, as was done in Nazi Germany. This is occurrent coercion. But the researcher might also bring about the desired participation by threatening reluctant patients with some harm, such as the withdrawal of care essential for the patient's recovery. This is dispositional coercion. Moreover, with regard to the threat of harm, human beings can coerce other human beings either directly or by enacting laws that threaten them with harm. So laws as well as individuals can be coercive. For example, a physician is constrained from performing some late abortions by laws that threaten harm (in the form of punishment) to those who perform such operations.

2 Autonomy as Freedom of Choice   Suppose that a pregnant woman decides, after carefully weighing all the alternatives, that abortion is the best alternative in her situation. If she is very poor and public funds to pay for the abortion are not forthcoming, she is not free to act on her decision. Note that her lack of freedom is not due to coercion. Nevertheless, her autonomy is limited because her range of choices is narrowed. The same might be true of a weak, terminally ill patient who wants to speed the dying process but may be unable to do so because physical weakness makes any act, such as jumping out of a window, impossible. If others are unwilling to help hasten the patient's death, the patient's freedom of choice is limited. Or consider the patient who does not want to go through the process of choosing between alternative forms of treatment (surgery versus chemotherapy, for example) and asks the physician to make the choice without giving the patient any details about the risks and benefits of each. If the physician does not accede to the request and insists upon giving the patient the requisite information, the patient's liberty of action is not being constrained by coercion. Nonetheless, the patient's freedom of choice is narrowed insofar as the way he or she is treated is not in accordance with the preferred choice.

3 Autonomy as Effective Deliberation   The accounts of limitations on autonomy provided in the discussions of autonomy as liberty of action and autonomy as freedom of choice focus on factors external to the agent which limit his or her autonomy. The first focuses on the coercion exerted on the agent by others, either directly or indirectly. The second focuses on the unavailability of options which the agent might have chosen. By contrast, autonomy as effective deliberation focuses on the agent's internal states and on related internal constraints.

In most discussions in biomedical ethics, autonomy is closely allied with rationality. An autonomous individual is characterized as one who is capable of making *rational* and *unconstrained* decisions and acting accordingly. An individual *exercises* autonomy in this sense when he or she acts without constraint on the basis of rational and unconstrained decisions. The criteria of rationality and constraint are central here. Under what conditions are individuals and their decisions and actions unconstrained? We have already discussed some of the constraints on an individual's actions. Our present discussion focuses on autonomy and constraints in relation to the agent's decision-making process. This requires distinguishing between two senses of rationality.

According to the first sense of rationality, individuals are properly described as rational when they are capable of choosing the best means to some chosen end. In this sense of rationality, someone in our society who wants to be a physician and attends medical school in order to attain this end is acting rationally. Someone with the same desire who, like

Mark in our earlier example, sits under a tree and meditates for twelve hours a day, waiting for medical knowledge to "permeate his being," is acting irrationally. To be rational in this sense entails being capable of reasoning well on the basis of good evidence about the best means to achieve some end. Someone in our society, for example, who does not use contraceptives during intercourse because she believes that an amulet she wears will keep her from getting pregnant is acting irrationally. To be rational in this sense also entails being able to postpone immediate gratification when such postponement is necessary to achieve chosen goals. Would-be physicians in medical school who party every night because they desire the pleasures of partying, even though this seriously jeopardizes their chances of succeeding in school, are acting irrationally.

A second sense of rationality involves choosing ends rather than means to those ends. All thinking beings have goals or ends they believe are in their interest to pursue. Being able to select and identify appropriate goals or interests is an important aspect of rationality. In this sense of rationality, an individual is properly described as rational if he or she is capable of choosing appropriate ends, although what counts as an appropriate end is a notorious matter of dispute. One who chooses unprofitable or self-destructive ends, for example, may be characterized as irrational. Would-be suicides are often described as irrational in this sense, as are masochists. Would-be suicides might sometimes be rational in the first sense, that is, capable of choosing the most efficient and painless way to end their lives. However, those who hold that the choice of death as an end is always inappropriate would consider all would-be suicides irrational in the second sense.

If rational acts must be based on decisions concerning the best means to maximize appropriately chosen ends, a fully rational person will have to have a number of abilities:

1 The ability to formulate appropriate goals, especially long-term goals.
2 The ability to establish priorities among these goals.
3 The ability to determine the best means to achieve chosen goals.
4 The ability to act effectively to realize these goals.
5 The ability to either abandon the chosen goals or modify them if the consequences of using the available means are undesirable or if the means are inadequate.

To sum up the discussion of autonomy as effective deliberation thus far, an individual is autonomous in this sense only if he or she possesses the abilities requisite for effective reasoning and the disposition to exercise those abilities. But these abilities can be limited in many ways. When they are, decisions and actions may be less than fully rational. First, some individuals may not have sufficiently developed the necessary abilities or may even be incapable of sufficiently developing them. Second, even individuals who have the requisite abilities may be unable to *exercise* them on a particular occasion due to various internal factors. Emotions such as fear may make the impartial weighing of information impossible. Laziness may keep an individual from learning all the pertinent information. The presence of pain or the use of drugs may also affect the exercise of reasoning abilities. It may be best, therefore, to speak of *degrees* of rationality and irrationality since many factors can make decisions and actions less than fully rational without pushing them to the irrational end of the spectrum.

Furthermore, autonomy as effective deliberation may be constrained in ways that do not affect the "rationality" of the decision. A lack of appropriate information, lies, and deception can all limit the effective exercise of the abilities required for rational deliberation. Physicians, for example, can constrain their patients' decision-making processes by deliberately withholding information. A patient who is told about only one possible kind of therapy and lacks information about alternatives cannot weigh the relative risks and benefits of all possible therapies in relation to long-term ends. In that situation a patient's "choice" of the therapy recommended by the physician is less than fully autonomous. Yet the choice might be rational both because the patient's deliberative process has been logical and because it may actually be in the latter's best interests in light of long-term goals. But to the extent that the patient's decision-making processes are constrained by the lack of information, the patient is not free to effectively exercise his or her autonomy.

In summary, to be completely autonomous or self-determining, an individual must possess the characteristics necessary for effective deliberation, be free of internal constraints in the exercise of those abilities, and be neither coerced by others nor have his or her range of options narrowed by them. A person's autonomy can be infringed upon, limited, or usurped by others in many ways including coercion, deception, lying, failing to supply necessary information, and narrowing the individual's range of options, for example, by refusing to act in accordance with his or her expressed desires. It can also be diminished by internal factors, such as strong emotions, the lack of appropriate capacities, fever, compulsion, and severe pain. To respect others' autonomy or right of self-determination is to treat them as individuals having the abilities required to be rational decision makers, capable of identifying their own interests and making their own reflective choices about the best means to advance these. An individual (*A*) fails to respect a person's (*B*'s) autonomy if *A* imposes constraints on *B*'s deliberative process or liberty of action or if *A* narrows *B*'s range of choices. In each of these cases, *A* interferes in some way with the effective exercise of *B*'s autonomy, and this is prohibited by the principle of respect for autonomy.

Autonomous Decisions and Appropriate Ends   Concern is often expressed in biomedical ethics about the ends or values appropriate for human beings to pursue. This concern was mentioned in the discussion of autonomy as effective deliberation. The principle of respect for persons requires noninterference with others' autonomy and exercise of autonomy. But when an individual chooses ends that seem inappropriate or irrational or makes a decision whose implementation is likely to bring about such ends, others question the competency of the decision maker and thus his or her autonomy (in the third sense). What does the principle of respect for autonomy require of medical personnel when a patient's expressed choices are inconsistent with the professionals' conceptions of appropriate human goals?

One way of approaching the issue is to distinguish between actions and choices that are in keeping with an individual's usual choices and those that are not. Individuals have a history of choices and decision making. The values that shape some lives may be considered irrational and inappropriate by others and yet be firmly held and carefully thought out. For example, a Jehovah's Witness on religious grounds risks his life by refusing blood transfusions deemed essential by his physician. This refusal is consistent with the values and beliefs that govern his life. There are no good grounds for questioning the rationality of the refusal when it is understood in the context of his ultimate values. And there are no good grounds for rejecting those ultimate values as inconsistent with the choices of an autonomous agent. In another case a 22-year-old patient who has no history of strong religious belief is in severe pain and has a temperature of 103°. When told she needs surgery and possibly blood transfusions, she refuses both, saying she wants to die so she can go to heaven where there is no pain. This case is clearly different from the Jehovah's Witness case. First, her physical condition provides good grounds for questioning the rationality and, therefore, autonomy of her decision. Second, her statement is not in accordance with her past history of decisions and values. If prior to the illness, she had expressed strong religious beliefs that made her present "decision" intelligible, her present physical condition might not provide sufficient grounds for questioning her autonomy. If there is good reason to believe that her new goal was "chosen" when her abilities for effective deliberation were severely constrained by her physical condition, however, then we have grounds for questioning the rationality of that goal in her case. Here, the principle of respect for autonomy does not seem to require treating her expressed wishes as those of an autonomous agent. But suppose she remained in pain for a prolonged period and her temperature fluctuated and was often normal. Suppose that knowing the prognosis and the future pain she would be experiencing, she has gone through a long reflective process culminating in the adoption of religious beliefs that give her great hope of an afterlife. In light of this hope and an evaluation of a very negative prognosis provided by medical professionals, she decides not to have the surgery. Here, her decision may not be in keeping with her history of decisions since she has chosen new ultimate values. Nonetheless, there may be good reason to hold that her decisions are autonomous ones, which should be respected in keeping with the principle of respect for persons.

One way of rephrasing the issue is as follows. Under what conditions are the ultimate ends or values that guide a patient's decisions to be accepted as those of an autonomous decision maker by medical professionals and accorded the respect that is required by the principle of autonomy? A possible answer is that either (1) the values must be firmly and consistently held over a long period of time; or (2) if there is a change in ultimate ends or values, there must be good grounds for thinking that the change is the result of a reflective reassessment of ends and values.

The Value of Autonomy   What is the basis for the moral value accorded to individual autonomy? The strongest claims regarding its moral primacy come from Kant and from certain other deontologists. In Kant's view, persons, unlike things, must always be accorded respect as self-determining subjects. They must be treated as ends in themselves and never merely as objects. For Kant, the fundamental principle of morality, respect for persons as moral agents, entails respect for personal autonomy. Such respect is due them as a right—autonomous agents are entitled to respect. If persons were not taken to be autonomous agents, there would be no basis for the moral responsibility we have toward other human beings, which precludes our using them, as we do cattle, chickens, rocks, land, and trees, simply to serve our own ends. But how does Kant understand autonomy?

Kant's primary focus is on the autonomy of the will. For Kant, "Autonomy of the will is the property the will has of being a law to itself."[17] What Kant calls the "dignity of man as a rational creature" is due to human beings possessing just that property that enables them to govern their own actions in accordance with rules of their own choosing. Putting aside many complexities in Kant's own thinking, a Kantian position central in biomedical ethics describes autonomy in terms of self-control, self-direction, or self-governance. The individual capable of acting on the basis of effective deliberation, guided by reason, and neither driven by emotions or compulsions nor manipulated or coerced by others, is, on a Kantian position, the model of autonomy.

For utilitarians, autonomy is an important value. John Stuart Mill, who speaks of individuality rather than autonomy, argues, for example, that liberty of action and thought is essential in developing both the intellectual and character traits necessary for truly human happiness:

> The human faculties of perception, judgment, discriminative feeling, mental activity, and even moral preference, are exercised only in making a choice. He who does anything because it is the custom makes no choice. He gains no practice either in discerning or in desiring what is best. The mental and moral, like the muscular powers, are improved by being used....
> He who lets the world, or his own portion of it, choose his plan of life for him, has no need of any other faculty than the ape-like one of imitation. He who chooses his plan for

himself employs all his faculties. He must use observation to see, reasoning and judgment to foresee, activity to gather materials for decision, discrimination to decide, and when he has decided, firmness and self-control to hold to his deliberate decision....

Where, not the person's own character, but the traditions or customs of other people are the rule of conduct, there is wanting one of the principal ingredients of human happiness.[18]

For Mill, persons possessing "individuality" are autonomous in a very strong sense, reflectively choosing their own plans of life, making their own decisions without manipulation by others, and exercising firmness and self-control in acting on their decisions.

Despite the high value placed on autonomy by utilitarians, their interest in autonomy differs from the Kantian one. On a Kantian view, respect for the personal autonomy of rational agents is entailed by the fundamental principle of morality, which serves as a limiting criterion for all moral conduct. That is, it places limits on what one individual can do to another human being without acting immorally. As noted earlier, one person can never use another as a subject in a medical experiment without his or her consent, no matter what potential good consequences for society as a whole might result. For a utilitarian such as Mill, respect for individual autonomy has utility value. A society that fosters respect for persons as autonomous agents will be a more progressive and, on balance, a happier society because its citizens will have the opportunities to develop their capacities to act as rational, responsible moral agents. If it could be shown that respect for individual autonomy does not have sufficient utility value, the utilitarian might have no good grounds for objecting to practices that infringe upon that autonomy.

Liberty-Limiting Principles

Since autonomy is accorded such great moral significance, a moral justification must be given for any infringement on or limitation or usurpation of autonomy. Many of the discussions in biomedical ethics explore such *proposed* justifications. The following exposition will center on the most general kinds of reasons advanced in these discussions.

Six suggested general reasons, most frequently considered when limitations of liberty (one aspect of autonomy) are at issue, are embodied in six principles, often called "liberty-limiting principles," stated below.[19] It is important to note at the outset that while some writers advance these principles as legitimate liberty-limiting principles, others argue against the legitimacy of many, or even most, of them.

1 A person's liberty is justifiably restricted to prevent that person from harming others (the harm principle).

2 A person's liberty is justifiably restricted to prevent that person from offending others (the offense principle).

3 A person's liberty is justifiably restricted to prevent that person from harming himself or herself (the principle of paternalism).

4 A person's liberty is justifiably restricted to benefit that person (the principle of extreme paternalism).

5 A person's liberty is justifiably restricted to prevent that person from acting immorally (the principle of legal moralism).

6 A person's liberty is justifiably restricted to benefit others (the social welfare principle).

These liberty-limiting principles are most frequently discussed when questions are raised about the justification of coercive laws, such as laws limiting access to hallucinogenic drugs. But the considerations they embody are also pertinent when applied to individual acts and practices that infringe upon or limit others' *autonomy*. It should also be noted that more than one of these principles might be advanced to justify a proposed limitation or infringement.

The harm principle is the most widely accepted liberty-limiting principle. Few will dispute that the law is within its proper bounds when it constrains individuals from performing acts that will seriously harm other persons or will seriously impair important institutional practices. Laws that threaten thieves, murderers, and the like, with punishment, for example, are usually perceived as a necessary part of any social system. Individual acts of coercion whose intent is to prevent individuals from harming others are also usually considered morally permissible. A bystander, for example, who prevents a terrorist from killing or wounding someone, is praised and not blamed for interfering with the terrorist's action. Aside from the harm principle, however, the moral legitimacy of the liberty-limiting principles under discussion here is a matter of dispute.

According to the offense principle, the law may justifiably be invoked to prevent offensive behavior in public. "Offensive" behavior is understood as behavior that causes shame, embarrassment, or discomfort to onlookers. In the leading example of the relevance of the offense principle to biomedical ethics, individuals who behave offensively in public are sometimes involuntarily committed to mental institutions, even though their behavior poses no serious threat of harm to themselves or others. If individuals are committed to mental institutions simply because their behavior is considered offensively eccentric, then the offense principle is being invoked, at least implicitly. Attacks on the use of such grounds to deprive individuals of much of their autonomy are attacks on the legitimacy of the offense principle.

According to the principle of legal moralism, liberty may justifiably be limited to prevent immoral behavior or, as it is often expressed, to "enforce morals." Acts such as kidnapping, murder, and fraud are undoubtedly immoral, but the principle of legal moralism does not have to be invoked to justify laws against them. An appeal to the harm principle already provides a widely accepted independent justification. The principle of legal moralism usually comes to the fore only when so-called victimless crimes are at issue. Is it justifiable to legislate against homosexual acts, gambling, or prostitution simply on the grounds that such activities are thought to be morally unacceptable? In biomedical ethics, the principle of legal moralism is sometimes invoked, at least implicitly, when it is argued that suicide is an immoral act and that, therefore, it is justifiable to act to prevent suicide, even if the decision to commit it is the result of careful deliberation. Many do not accept the principle of legal moralism as a legitimate liberty-limiting principle, however. Mill holds, for example, that to accept the principle is tantamount to permitting a "tyranny of the majority."

The social welfare principle also has some relevance in biomedical ethics. According to this principle, individual autonomy can justifiably be restricted to benefit others. Such justifications are sometimes attempted in discussions of biomedical and behavioral research. It is argued, for example, that using human beings as research subjects without informing them (thus bypassing their consent) is morally justified if the research project promises some potentially great benefit to others in society. Those who find such justifications questionable may be wary about accepting the social welfare principle as a legitimate liberty-limiting principle.

The liberty-limiting principles that are most prominent in the literature of biomedical ethics are the paternalistic principles. Disagreements about the legitimacy of paternalistic justifications affect the resolution of a number of important issues in biomedical ethics. Physicians or nurses, for example, who lie to patients in order to spare them pain are often accused of acting on questionable (i.e., paternalistic) grounds. The paternalistic justifications offered for certain laws that are of special concern in biomedical ethics are also frequently attacked. Among such laws are those that allow courts to commit individuals to mental institutions either in order to keep them from harming themselves or in order to force them to receive treatment. Because of the centrality of paternalism in biomedical ethics, it is essential to examine the concept of paternalism as well as some of the arguments offered both for and against paternalistic actions and practices.

Paternalism

The definition of paternalism most widely cited is Gerald Dworkin's:

> [Paternalism is] the interference with a person's liberty of action justified by reasons referring exclusively to the welfare, good, happiness, needs, interests, or values of the person being coerced.[20]

When paternalism in the legal system is at issue, this definition is acceptable since laws, backed by force or the threat of harm, are by nature coercive. However, many of the actions considered paternalistic in biomedical ethics do not fit this definition. Consider the following examples, which are similar to some discussed in our earlier presentation of autonomy.

 1 A physician decides not to tell a patient that he has Alzheimer's disease. The patient had frequently asserted that if he were ever to receive such a diagnosis, he would immediately proceed to commit suicide as efficiently and painlessly as possible because the life of an Alzheimer's disease victim was antithetical to everything he valued. The physician, who believes that the patient will commit suicide if informed of his condition, considers deliberate premature death a morally unacceptable harm to the patient and, therefore, withholds the information.

 2 A physician refuses to perform an abortion on a woman who lives in a small, isolated town with no other physicians. They both know that the woman cannot afford to travel elsewhere to have the abortion. The physician refuses to perform the abortion because she believes that the woman will eventually regret the decision and become seriously depressed about it.

 3 A patient asks a physician not to give him information about relevant alternative treatments, but to make the choice for him. The physician insists upon giving the patient the information because the physician believes the patient will be better off if he makes his own decision.

Note that none of these cases involve coercion; yet they can all be correctly described as paternalistic interferences, limitations, or infringements on autonomy. In each of the cases, a physican has in one way or another infringed upon or limited a patient's autonomy. In both the second and third cases, a physician has narrowed a patient's range of choices to exclude the preferred choices, ostensibly for the patient's own good. In the first case, a physician has denied a patient information vital to effective deliberation about the balance of his life, again for his own good (i.e., to keep him from harming himself). In the first and second cases physicians have treated patients as individuals incapable of making the correct judgments about their own best interests. In all three cases, a physician has effectively usurped a patient's decision-making power, substituting his or her judgment for the patient's. While it is difficult to capture this sense of paternalism in a precise definition, a rough definition can be given as follows:

Paternalism is the interference with, limitation of, or usurpation of individual autonomy justified by reasons referring exclusively to the welfare or needs of the person whose autonomy is being interfered with, limited, or usurped.

Is such paternalistic behavior ever morally justified? If yes, under what conditions do paternalistic grounds constitute good reasons, either for coercion or for effectively taking decisions out of the individuals' hands for their own good? In considering the justifiability of paternalistic actions, keep in mind the difference between the principle of paternalism and the principle of extreme paternalism. The latter would apply to paternalistic actions whose intent is to benefit individuals; whereas the former would apply to paternalistic actions whose intent is to keep individuals from harm.

In the framework of Kantian ethical theory, the moral fundamentality of individual autonomy seems to prohibit any paternalistic actions when the individuals affected are capable of self-governance or self-determination. It would always be morally wrong, for example, for physicians to withhold information about surgical procedures from patients simply because the physicians believed that their patients would refuse to undergo potentially beneficial procedures if informed of all the risks. Charles Fried, a contemporary ethicist who adopts a Kantian approach to paternalism in the medical context, maintains that patients must never be denied relevant information. By withholding it, physicians fail to treat patients as ends in themselves. In Fried's view, patients can never be treated simply as means to ends, even when the ends in question are their own ends (e.g., their restored health).[21]

John Stuart Mill provides the classical utilitarian statement on the illegitimacy of paternalistic actions. This statement is frequently cited in court opinions concerning the right of self-determination in medical matters. Mill argues:

> [O]ne very simple principle [is] entitled to govern absolutely the dealings of society with the individual in the way of compulsion and control, whether the means used be physical force in the form of legal penalties, or the moral coercion of public opinion. That principle is, that the sole end for which mankind are warranted, individually or collectively, in interfering with the liberty of action of any of their number, is self-protection. That the only purpose for which power can be rightfully exercised over any member of a civilized community, against his will, is to prevent harm to others. His own good, either physical or moral, is not sufficient warrant. He cannot rightfully be compelled to do or forbear because it will be better for him to do so, because it will make him happier, because, in the opinions of others, to do so would be wise, or even right.[22]

In this statement, Mill asserts that while prevention of harm to others is sometimes sufficient justification for interfering with another's autonomy, the individual's own good never is. Mill rejects paternalistic interventions because of the high utility value that he assigns to individual autonomy. In assigning it this value, Mill assumes that individuals are, on the whole, better judges of their own interests than anyone else, so that minimizing paternalistic interventions will maximize human happiness. Mill himself qualified his strong rejection of paternalism, stating:

> [T]his doctrine is meant to apply only to human beings in the maturity of their faculties. We are not speaking of children, or of young persons below the age which the law may fix as that of manhood or womanhood. Those who are still in a state to require being taken care of by others, must be protected against their own actions as well as external injury.[23]

In the kinds of cases he cites, Mill assumes that people are justified in acting paternalistically because they are better judges of an individual's interests than is the individual himself or herself. Arguing in this way, Mill seems to open the door for the justification of paternalism in the case of individuals who may not be able to correctly identify and advance their own interests because they lack the required level of ability for effective deliberation. Such individuals, often described as having "diminished autonomy" insofar as they lack the necessary abilities or capacities for self-determination, include infants, young children, and the severely mentally retarded. It is important to see that the paternalistic restrictions Mill allows may limit autonomy as liberty of action since they may involve coercion. They may also limit autonomy in the second sense discussed earlier since they narrow the range of available choices. But they do not limit autonomy in the sense central to Mill's, as well as Kant's, moral position since those with diminished autonomy lack what is essential for an appropriate level of effective rational deliberation.

Many contemporary attempts to justify *some* paternalistic actions adopt an approach similar to Mill's, stressing the apparently diminished autonomy of those who are treated paternalistically. If they were fully autonomous, the argument runs, they would want the benefits involved and would want to avoid the harms. Those who argue in this way must deal with an underlying conceptual issue. They must identify the criteria that should be used in determining whether a person's autonomy is sufficiently diminished to justify paternalism. In light of our earlier discussion of rationality, constraint, and autonomy, it seems plausible to hold the following view regarding diminished autonomy. When a person's autonomy (in the third sense) is *severely* constrained by intellectual lacks (e.g., lack of reasoning ability or ignorance of relevant facts), and when acting on decisions made under such constraints will probably result in some serious, irrevocable harm, the individual's autonomy would seem to be sufficiently impaired to justify paternalistic acts. Two examples may be helpful here. People under the influence of hallucinogenic drugs who decide to leap from twentieth-floor windows in order to get home more quickly, believing that they (like Superman) can fly, are hardly acting in an autonomous manner. Their decisions are grossly inconsistent with the best inductive evidence we possess regarding what happens to human beings who leap out of windows. Severely retarded individuals who decide to go out alone in a busy city but are incapable of understanding traffic signals would also seem to be acting in a much less than fully autonomous way. They are unaware of the kind of risk they would be running by going out alone. In both cases, there is good reason to assume that the individuals are incapable, whether temporarily or permanently, of the level of reasoning required for sufficiently autonomous decision making. Paternalistic interventions seem to be justified here in light of the high value placed on life and the permanent or temporary inability of the individuals involved to understand that acting on their decisions could be fatal.

Does the fact that a decision will result in death or some other serious, irrevocable harm *always* provide sufficient grounds for the claim that autonomy is so severely diminished that paternalism is justified? Some especially problematic cases involve decisions to commit suicide. Many suicide attempts are the result of temporary disorientation associated with drugs, alcohol, or extreme, but temporary, depression. In accordance with our earlier discussion of rationality and autonomy, decisions to commit suicide in these cases are far from fully rational and autonomous. Cases involving individuals who are so severely constrained in their reasoning that they are temporarily or permanently incapable of correctly assessing the probable severely harmful results of their acts would seem to provide clear instances of sufficiently diminished autonomy. As already noted, however, some decisions to end or risk life may be based on carefully thought-out reasons and may be either consistent with the person's own long-term conception of a satisfying or meaningful life or the result of a new but reflective reassessment of ultimate values and goals. It would beg the question to call these latter decisions irrational and, therefore, nonautonomous, in order to justify paternalistic interventions, simply on the grounds that the person's intended act will probably result in serious self-harm. It may be that in the case of those ends that are usually considered highly undesirable (e.g., death or the possibility of severe injury), it should be presumed that the individual's choice is not rational and, therefore, not an autonomous one. This presumption would justify, at best, temporarily constraining someone from certain acts in order to establish the rationality of the choice. In summary, paternalistic actions are justified when they are necessary either (1) to keep persons with severely diminished autonomy from doing themselves serious, irrevocable harm or (2) to temporarily constrain persons from acting to bring about *presumably* irrational self-harming ends until it can be determined whether the individuals are acting autonomously. This kind of paternalism, often called "weak paternalism," is consistent with the position of those who agree with Mill's criticism of paternalism. The interventions do not show a lack of respect for individual autonomy. Rather, they are attempts either to prevent individuals from seriously harming themselves when they are acting non-autonomously or to prevent them from harming themselves until it can be determined whether their acts are indeed autonomous ones. Such weak paternalism stands in contrast to strong paternalism, which maintains that paternalistic treatment is sometimes justified even when (1) and (2) do not apply.

The severely or even mildly mentally retarded may pose special problems when questions of justified paternalism are raised, precisely because they *may* lack the abilities necessary for autonomy as effective deliberation. Whether the mildly retarded lack such abilities is a matter of dispute, however. Some of the readings in Chapter 6 argue, for example, that many people classified as mildly mentally retarded are capable of effective deliberation if they are given appropriate training and information. In the case of mentally retarded individuals who are capable of effective deliberation, paternalistic treatment would seem to be justified only if strong paternalism is justified. But if strong paternalism is not justified in the case of the nonmentally retarded, then it would also not be justified in the case of mildly mentally retarded individuals capable of effective deliberation. On the other hand, in the case of mentally retarded individuals whose autonomy is diminished to the point that paternalistic interferences in their lives would be instances of weak paternalism, paternalistic actions whose intent is to benefit these individuals could be as justifiable as those whose intent is to keep them from harm.

Is strong paternalism ever justified? One defense of strong paternalism rests on a prudential argument that itself appeals to the importance of autonomy. We are aware that we often act in ignorance and that we are often tempted to act in ways incompatible with what we see as our long-term interests. Acting in ignorance, or too weak-willed to resist temptation, we may do ourselves serious irreversible harm of a sort that would severely diminish our autonomy. We are also aware that accidents, illnesses, diseases, and emotional pressures may diminish our rational capacities and thus our autonomy. We should be willing, therefore, to accept those paternalistic acts, laws, and practices whose intent is either to protect individual autonomy from being severely diminished or, if it has already been diminished, to restore it. This argument is advanced in order to justify the following kinds of laws: (1) laws, such as those against the sale of laetrile, that protect us against our own ignorance; (2) laws, such as those against the sale of hallucinogenic drugs (without prescription), that protect us against our own weaknesses of the will and/or ignorance; and (3) laws that allow courts and psychiatrists to commit the "mentally ill" to institutions against their will in order to cure them (restore their autonomy) or to keep them from the kind of self-harm that might further reduce their autonomy. The same sort of prudential argument is sometimes invoked to justify paternalistic acts by physicians when these acts are performed to prevent some serious deterioration of the patient's autonomy. However, some of the constraining interventions that would seem to be justified by this line of argument are very problematic. Some individuals, for example, might prefer to give in to temptations, weighing the pleasures of using hallucinogenic drugs more highly than its dangers or risks. Others might want to have access to laetrile, hoping that it will help and willing to risk the possibility that it might not. The involuntary civil commitment of the mentally ill for their own good is perhaps even more questionable, as some of the readings in Chapter 6 bring out.

A radically different defense of paternalism on the part of the state is offered by critics of the liberal individualist tradition, which is associated with both natural right theorists such as John Locke and utilitarians such as Mill. These critics question the need to justify laws and government practices whose intent is to benefit or keep from self-harm the members of society being constrained. In this view, a need to justify the state's interference with individual autonomy arises from a social-political theory that misunderstands the relation between the state and the individual and mistakenly stresses the primacy of individual interests rather than the interests of the social whole. The ideal of the liberal-individualist tradition in social-political theory is a society with a minimal amount of state interference with individual autonomy. Critics of this social-political ideal reject the justifications that are offered in defense of the primacy accorded individual autonomy as simply expressions of an ideological commitment to "Western liberal thought." The ideology of the critics stresses the primacy of the interests of society as a whole. A social-political system committed to the latter ideal perceives all individual acts as significant for society at large and government regulation of any of those acts as part of the state's legitimate role. Any final assessment of such a defense of state paternalism, of course, is intimately intertwined with the resolution of fundamental questions about the relation between the individual and the state.

In a totally different vein, indirect support for opposition to paternalism comes from certain sociologists, psychologists, and other social theorists who offer analyses to explain the recent emphasis on antipaternalism in American society. They attribute much of the recent stress on antipaternalism to a growing awareness of both the class differences in our society and the fact that those who perform paternalistic acts (e.g., psychiatrists, judges, physicians, and the administrators and staffs of mental institutions) are usually members of the upper middle-class, while those who are treated paternalistically are usually members of the poorer, less-privileged classes. An awareness of this class difference, and of the related differences in interests and values, gives rise to serious doubts about both the ability and the willingness of those wielding paternalistic authority to act in the interests of those whom they typically constrain. On this analysis, it is not the moral legitimacy of the principle of paternalism that is really at issue when paternalistic acts and practices are increasingly rejected. Rather, what is at issue are the abuses resulting from so-called paternalistic acts that do not in fact serve to benefit (or keep from harm) the individuals constrained, but do serve the ends of the members of the professions wielding paternalistic authority. This line of argument is intended to point out that the current antipaternalistic stress is probably not the result of conscious deliberation about the legitimacy of central ethical principles but a rejection of what passes as justified paternalism in a class society in which the "constrainers" are neither knowledgeable nor altruistic enough to perceive correctly the interests of those they constrain. However, the factual claims, if correct, tend to support a Mill-like claim that unless the interests and values of constrainers and constrainees coincide, individual self-interest is better served in the long run if paternalism is rejected rather than accepted.

The Language of Rights

Many discussions in biomedical ethics, including discussions of autonomy and paternalism, are couched in the language of rights. People are said, for example, to have rights to health, privacy, or life. It is also said that our most fundamental right is the right to self-determination. Paternalistic medical practices are described as "infringements" on this fundamental right. Those who defend the legalization of euthanasia appeal to a "right to death with dignity," antiabortionists to a "fetus's right to life," and advocates of national health insurance to a "right to health care." Such appeals may sometimes invoke constitutional or legal rights, but more often they appeal to purported *moral* rights which, it is said, *must* be acknowledged by all moral agents and by society, and which ought, sometimes, to be guaranteed by being enacted as legal rights. One example of a document that invokes the language of rights is the "UN Declaration of Human Rights." This document announces that all persons have a right to medical treatment as well as to many other things, such as a decent standard of living. "Human Rights" here may be understood as one species of moral rights. The rights asserted by the UN Declaration are certainly not legal ones since there is no international system of laws that recognizes and guarantees them for all human beings. A citizen of the United States, for example, cannot walk into a hospital, demand and receive treatment simply on the basis of the claim that the UN Declaration proclaims his or her right to such care. Those who argue that the United States should have a national health insurance system do, however, often claim that there is a "moral" right to adequate health care that our society must recognize and guarantee through its legal system.

Although talk of moral rights is commonplace in biomedical ethics, some ethicists argue that using the language of rights may hinder rather than help us in our attempts to develop an understanding of the moral issues that arise in the biomedical context. Rights talk, it is said, often engenders confusions that result, at least in part, from a lack of agreement regarding answers to the following types of questions about moral rights: (1) How do we determine what kinds of entities have rights and what kinds do not? Do fetuses have rights? Animals? Children? The mentally retarded? (2) When there is a conflict of rights, how should we resolve the conflict? Do the rights of the fetus take precedence over the rights of the woman bearing it? (3) When there is a disagreement about the existence of a specific right, how do we determine whether such a right exists? Is there a right to health care?

Conflicting claims using the language of rights cannot be resolved in a rational way unless these types of questions are answered. If legal or constitutional rights are at issue, we can answer such questions by examining the laws and constitutional decisions bearing on the rights in question. If moral rights are at issue, however, answering them requires agreement about the system of moral rules and principles that should be used as a basis for determining what moral rights must be recognized by all moral individuals and societies. In the absence of such agreement, disagreements over conflicting claims using the language of rights would seem to be disguised and confused disagreements about the more fundamental issues discussed earlier in this introduction—issues centering on the correctness of competing ethical theories, principles, and values. Suppose two individuals disagree about the existence of a moral right to death with dignity, for example. That dispute, it seems, can be resolved only if both individuals lay out the reasons supporting their claims. These reasons must include statements of the ethical principles and rules that support the conflicting views about rights. In attempting to determine which of the claimants is correct, we will have to examine the merits of any competing principles and rules and choose among them. If a choice cannot be made, it seems that the debate about rights cannot be settled.

Rights talk is also often criticized for very different reasons than those just discussed. An overemphasis on establishing legal rights, such as the right to adequate medical care, for example, is said to obscure the "emptiness" of many such rights in practice. Critics of some of the mainstream articles in biomedical ethics sometimes argue that the emphasis on rights ignores the social-cultural reality that makes the exercise of many rights problematic for the poor, the uneducated, and the otherwise disadvantaged members of our society. What is needed, they argue, is not a proliferation of government-backed rights but a radical reorganization of the existing institutions and social structures that are responsible for many of the moral dilemmas discussed in biomedical ethics.

Given the problems mentioned above, it might seem more useful to avoid the language of rights in our disputes and phrase our problems in terms of conflicting ethical theories, principles, rules, and values. However, since so many disputes in biomedical ethics invoke the language of rights, a brief examination of the concept of a right is a necessary prerequisite to understanding and evaluating many of the arguments in this text.

What is involved in the claim that someone has a right to X? Several theses, which are not all mutually compatible, are prominent in contemporary philosophical discussions.

(1) *The Correlativity Thesis: Any right entails a correlative obligation on others either not to interfere with one's liberty or to provide something.* On this thesis, A has a right to X only if others have a correlative obligation to provide A with X or to not interfere with A's pursuit of X. A has a right to health care, for example, only if others (individuals or groups) have a correlative obligation to provide A with health care. A has a right to privacy only if others have a correlative obligation not to interfere with A's privacy. The rights in question may be legal ones (those recognized and guaranteed by some system of laws) or moral ones (those required by a system of moral principles and rules).

(*a*) *The Correlativity Thesis and Positive Rights.* When the rights at issue carry correlative obligations to provide the rights holder with some benefit, good, opportunity, or service, they are often called "positive rights," or sometimes, "welfare rights." If A has a positive right to a minimum income, for example, then someone has a correlative obligation to provide it. Note that on the correlativity view, if A has a right to be provided with X, the bearer of the correlative obligation must be specifiable. If A has a right to health care, it would be useless to claim simply that someone somewhere has an obligation to provide that care. On the correlativity thesis, there must be some definite person or group who must acknowledge A's right and provide the necessary care on demand. If the state recognizes such a right through appropriate legislation, then a legal right is established, and the state through its legitimate agencies and representatives takes on the legal obligations involved. If the rights in question are only moral rights, however, then on the correlativity thesis, a full-fledged account of rights (given perhaps from a Kantian or utilitarian perspective) would involve specifying the individuals or groups who are morally obligated to fulfill the requisite obligations.

(*b*) *The Correlativity Thesis and Negative Rights.* When the rights at issue carry correlative obligations of noninterference, they are often called "negative rights," or sometimes, "liberty rights." If A has a negative right to X, no one should prevent A from pursuing X. Here again there is a correlation between rights and obligations. For example, if A has negative rights to privacy, then others have an obligation to refrain from interfering with A's privacy. Here there is no correlative obligation to provide some benefit but only an obligation, incumbent on all, not to interfere with the exercise of some rights. As in the case of positive rights, rights of noninterference may be either legal or moral or both. Negative rights are the kinds of rights that were proclaimed and defended in the seventeenth and eighteenth centuries by upholders of natural rights, such as John Locke. They asserted natural rights to life, liberty, and property, for example. Holders of this view perceived the natural negative rights they asserted as moral rights belonging to all rational agents independently of any legal system. In contrast, twentieth-century defenders of moral rights have often been concerned primarily with positive rights, such as the right to health care. In biomedical ethics, both negative and positive rights are invoked. When considering claims about rights, it is sometimes important to ask whether the writer is treating a right as a negative or positive right. A right to life, for example, may be read as a negative right if it is understood as asserting that others have an obligation not to interfere with an individual by taking his life. A right to life is sometimes asserted as a positive right, however. Here the claim is that others have an obligation to provide the rights holder with the necessities needed to maintain life.

(2) *The Only Rights that Exist Are Legal Rights. A* has a right to *X* if and only if it is specifically granted by law. In this view, all other rights talk is simply rhetorical. As Jeremy Bentham, a noted utilitarian, argued in the nineteenth century, "Right . . . is the child of law: from *real* laws come *real* rights; but from *imaginary* laws, from laws of nature, . . . come *imaginary* rights."[24] Upholders of this view often argue that appeals to any rights other than legal or constitutional rights are simply disguised appeals to *values.* Rights exist only where there are correlative obligations assigned to specific individuals or groups and where there is a system of codified rules—a system that includes rules regarding both the enforcement of obligations and the provision of redress for persons whose rights are infringed. Asssertions of rights, such as natural rights or the human rights asserted in the UN Declaration, that are not recognized and guaranteed by some legal system are simply assertions of values and are binding on no one. Sometimes a value held by a particular society is used as the basis for establishing a legal right in that society. If it is, the value and the right (a legal right) coincide; but if it is not, the value in question is mistakenly described if it is characterized as a right. (If, for example, enough value is placed on the health of all our citizens, we may eventually enact the legislation that will guarantee all Americans a legal right to equal access to medical care. It would simply be rhetorical, however, to claim that such a legal right *must* be established because all human beings have a "moral right" to health care.) If this position on rights is correct, all appeals to moral rights to bolster claims in biomedical ethics would be pointless except as rhetorical devices used to underscore the moral importance of the values being asserted.

(3) *Legal rights are not the only kinds of rights, but not all rights entail correlative duties.* Declarations of human rights, such as the one proclaimed by the United Nations, are statements of moral ideals that all societies should strive to realize. These moral ideals do not entail correlative duties. Recently, for example, a resolution introduced in Congress asserted a "right to food" for all human beings. A protester, understanding rights in sense 1(*a*), argued that guaranteeing food for everyone in the world would severely lower American living standards. The sponsoring congressman, understanding rights in sense 3, responded that the resolution would impose *no* correlative obligations on the United States to guarantee food to everyone either at home or abroad. It would merely provide a guideline for future policy—a goal toward which to strive. This concept of a right is one possible interpretation of the language of human rights. To the extent that such ideals are acknowledged and guaranteed by a legal system, of course, they become legal rights entailing correlative duties and, therefore, fall under either 1(*a*) or 1(*b*).

The charge is sometimes made that only a deontological ethical theory is capable of providing a theory of moral rights that will include a theory of correlative obligations binding on all moral agents. A utilitarian theory, it is said, can at best provide only a theory of values and goals. This is debatable, and many rule-utilitarians would not agree. It is not surprising, however, that utilitarians often advocate the second and third positions on moral rights, whereas deontologists usually support the correlativity view, at least in the case of those rights considered most fundamental, such as the right of self-determination.

THE RESOLUTION OF MORAL DISAGREEMENTS

Moral issues in biomedical ethics have generated a great deal of controversy. Disagreements are common; moral consensus relatively rare. Sometimes, in regard to the morally correct approach to frozen embryos, for example, the relevant questions are just beginning to be asked, and the relevant issues are just beginning to be explored. However, in other cases (e.g., abortion) the issues have been explored in depth. Various writers have presented positions, others have responded, and more carefully thought-out views have emerged through dialectical exchange. Anyone approaching biomedical ethics for the first time by using this text, presented with opposing positions strongly defended by their upholders, cannot help but wonder whether any moral agreement on the issues is possible. When there is so much disagreement, can we hope to resolve moral controversies? If yes, what procedures should we use? On what principles can we rely? Several ways of approaching moral disagreements, presented below, may facilitate the resolution of controversies or, at the very least, clarify the nature of the disagreements.

(1) *Getting clear about the relevant facts.* Many times, moral disagreements can be traced to disagreements about relevant facts. People may disagree, for example, about whether cancer patients should be told the truth about their condition. Sometimes, discussion may show that the disputants agree on the principle that the truth should always be given to patients who want it and can handle it appropriately. In such cases, the disagreement may be due to a radical difference in the disputants' beliefs about the effect of such information on patients' psychological states or about patients' desires to be told the truth. Sissela Bok's article in Chapter 2 gets to the heart of this *factual* disagreement. She presents the results of relevant factual studies in order to challenge physicians who claim that many cancer patients do not want the truth and that truthful information often harms patients. A lack of appropriate factual information or a disagreement about the facts is often present in other controversies as well. Utilitarians may disagree about the possible good and bad effects that establishing a right to health care or legalizing euthanasia may have on society. Critics of medical paternalism may overestimate the ability of the seriously ill to effectively deliberate about their care. It is useful, therefore, in thinking about issues in biomedical ethics, to examine the possibility that factual considerations may have to be explored and relevant information acquired. This is not an easy task since in many instances it will require a knowledge of psychology, sociology, and, even, economics. But a recognition of the nature of the problem—that the problem is a factual one and not a disagreement on moral principles—is a first step toward a resolution.

(2) *Conceptual clarification.* Controversies can sometimes be settled or clarified if the disputants can agree about the meaning of a relevant concept (e.g., paternalism or autonomy). In our earlier discussion of rights, for example, the dispute between the congressman advocating a right to food and his opponent was due in part to a very different understanding of rights. Disagreements in regard to abortion are sometimes disagreements about just what is involved in the concept of person. The disputants might agree that there are some things it is never acceptable to do to persons but, given their

different conceptions of personhood, disagree about whether the fetus is a person. In the case of euthanasia, conceptual clarification is essential since many of the pro and con arguments are unclear to the disputing parties when expressions such as "euthanasia," "passive euthanasia," and "active euthanasia" are understood differently. Conceptual clarification will not resolve a disagreement when the conceptual differences are effectively the result of differences in moral beliefs, but, even then, such clarification can help to bring out the nature of the disagreement more clearly.

(3) *Agreement on ethical theory, moral principles, or values.* If the disputants can agree on a moral theory or a set of moral principles or the centrality of certain values, many disputes can be resolved. For example, if individuals can agree that the offense principle is *not* an acceptable liberty-limiting principle, then they would agree that committing those diagnosed as mentally ill to institutions *solely* on the grounds that their behavior is offensive to others is not morally permissible. Or if they can agree that rule utilitarianism is the strongest ethical theory, then they can approach all moral issues from that standpoint. It is important to see, however, that even without agreement on the best ethical theory, it is possible to agree on the correctness of crucial moral principles, such as the principle of respect for persons, or the centrality of certain values. The President's Commission for the Study of Ethical Problems in Medicine and Biomedical and Behavioral Research, for example, recently completed the task of determining just what values ought to guide decision making in the provider-patient relationship. Commission members agreed that two values were central: promotion of a patient's well-being and respect for a person's self-determination. Having reached this agreement, they were able to proceed to explore the relevant concepts and develop more specific recommendations about moral decision making in the health-care context. (Chapter 2 contains a selection from their report.)

It is important to see, however, that even when there is agreement on some principles, rules, or values, disagreements can still arise in a particular context. Different values, rules, or principles may conflict, for example. Our earlier discussion of W. D. Ross illustrates the kinds of conflicts that can arise among prima facie duties. Thus individuals might agree on the correctness of rules asserting that both beneficence and nonmaleficence are prima facie duties, and yet they may disagree about which takes precedence in a particular context, when acting in accordance with one duty means violating the other. When this occurs, further discussion is necessary to determine whether agreement can be secured on which value, rule, or principle should have priority in a given context. Disagreement can also arise about whether a principle or rule applies in a particular case. As noted earlier, for example, there is a general agreement that the harm principle is a legitimate liberty-limiting principle. Invoking the harm principle, then, two individuals might agree that persons who pose a serious threat of harm should be committed to institutions. Yet they might hold opposing views on the question of whether the majority of those diagnosed as mentally ill should be committed to hospitals without their consent. The reason for this difference of opinion might be due to very different beliefs regarding the extent of potential harm to others posed by the majority of those diagnosed as mentally ill. If they pose no serious threat of harm to others, then the harm principle does not apply, and their commitment cannot be justified on such grounds. Thus resolution of the controversy here hinges on the evaluation of relevant factual material in order to determine whether the harm principle can be legitimately applied to justify commitment.

As the articles in this text demonstrate, attempts at factual and conceptual clarification play an important role in the ongoing exploration of issues in biomedical ethics. They also demonstrate the importance of agreeing on ethical principles, rules, and fundamental values. Also worth noting are some typical philosophical methods writers use both to show the inadequacies of an opposing position and to explore possible problems in a position they themselves are developing. One such method involves using examples and opposing counterexamples to show that a proposed conceptual account is inadequate because it is either too narrow or too broad. For example, suppose paternalism is defined in such a way that coercion is a necessary component of any paternalistic action. The inadequacies of this definition can be shown by providing examples of actions appropriately characterized as paternalistic that do not involve coercion. In contrast, suppose a paternalistic act is defined as any act that benefits someone. That definition can be shown to be too broad by providing examples of actions satisfying the definition that would not be considered paternalistic. In a simple business transaction, for example, Jones buys a chair from Smith rather than Caldwell, simply because Smith has a better product at a fair price. Smith benefits from the transaction by making a profit. But there is no reason to consider Jones's action paternalistic. Other methods used by philosophers include pointing out either the inconsistencies in a position or the, perhaps unexpected, consequences following from a line of argument. It was pointed out to Mary Anne Warren, whose article on abortion is reprinted in Chapter 9, for example, that the arguments she offers in defense of abortion would also justify infanticide. Warren was faced with the need to either (1) rethink her original line of argument; (2) accept the morality of infanticide; or (3) develop a new argument that would enable her to maintain that abortion is moral but infanticide is not. Her postscript, also reprinted in Chapter 9, is Warren's response to this line of criticism. In conclusion, when reading the articles in this text, it is useful both to recognize the stratagems the authors employ in their arguments and to use the stratagems just discussed to evaluate and criticize the arguments they advance.

T.A.M. and J.S.Z.

NOTES

1 J. J. C. Smart, "Extreme and Restricted Utilitarianism," in Michael D. Bayles, ed., *Contemporary Utilitarianism* (New York: Doubleday, 1968), p. 100.
2 W. D. Ross, *The Right and the Good* (Oxford: The Clarendon Press, 1930), p. 22.
3 Alan Donagan, "Is There a Credible Form of Utilitarianism?" in *Contemporary Utilitarianism,* p. 189. Donagan's point is that act-utilitarianism is "monstrous" and "incredible" because it seems to recommend such murders.
4 The distinction between act-utilitarianism and rule-utilitarianism is a distinction that has become prominent only in contemporary times. Accordingly, the writings of Bentham and Mill are somewhat ambiguous with regard to these categories. Although Bentham is probably rightly understood as an act-utilitarian, a very strong case can be made for interpreting Mill as a rule-utilitarian. See, for example, J. O. Urmson, "The Interpretation of the Moral Philosophy of J. S. Mill," in *Contemporary Utilitarianism,* pp. 13–24.
5 Smart, "Extreme and Restricted Utilitarianism," p. 107.
6 Immanuel Kant, *Groundwork of the Metaphysic of Morals,* trans. H. J. Paton (New York: Harper & Row, 1964), p. 88.
7 *Ibid.,* p. 96.
8 H. J. Paton, *The Categorical Imperative: A Study in Kant's Moral Philosophy* (Chicago: University of Chicago Press, 1948), p. 172.

9 The account of beneficence suggested here follows an analysis presented by Tom L. Beauchamp and James F. Childress in chapters 4 and 5 of *Principles of Biomedical Ethics,* 2d ed. (New York: Oxford University Press, 1983).

10 Ross, *The Right and the Good,* p. 19.

11 *Ibid.,* p. 20.

12 *Ibid.,* p. 21.

13 *Ibid.*

14 *Ibid.*

15 Writers in biomedical ethics and social philosophy characterize autonomy differently. Bruce L. Miller, for example, distinguishes four senses of autonomy, including: autonomy as liberty of action, autonomy as authenticity, autonomy as effective deliberation, and autonomy as moral reflection. (The discussion in this chapter follows Miller to some extent, but diverges in important ways.) Gerald Dworkin prefers to distinguish between liberty and freedom on the one hand and autonomy on the other, using "autonomy" much more narrowly than Miller. See Bruce L. Miller, "Autonomy and the Refusal of Lifesaving Treatment," *Hastings Center Report* 11 (August 1981), pp. 25–28; and Gerald Dworkin, "Autonomy and Informed Consent," in President's Commission: *Making Health Care Decisions,* Appendix G (1982), pp. 63–81.

16 The distinction between occurrent and dispositional coercion is made by Michael D. Bayles in "A Concept of Coercion," in J. Roland Pennock and John D. Chapman, eds., *Coercion: Nomos XIV* (Chicago: Aldine-Atherton, 1972), pp. 16–29.

17 Kant, *Groundwork,* p. 108.

18 John Stuart Mill, *Utilitarianism, On Liberty, Essay on Bentham,* ed. Mary Warnock (New York: New American Library, 1962), pp. 187, 185. All quotations in this chapter are from *On Liberty* in this edition.

19 Joel Feinberg's discussion of such principles served as a guide for the formulations adopted here. See Joel Feinberg, *Social Philosophy* (Englewood Cliffs, N.J.: Prentice-Hall, 1973), Chapter 2.

20 Gerald Dworkin, "Paternalism," *The Monist* 56 (January 1972), p. 65.

21 Charles Fried, *Medical Experimentation: Personal Integrity and Social Policy* (New York: American Elsevier, 1974), p. 101.

22 Mill, *On Liberty,* p. 135.

23 *Ibid.*

24 Jeremy Bentham, *Anarchical Fallacies,* ed. John Bowring, Vol. 2 (New York: Russell and Russell, 1962; as reproduced from the 1843 edition), p. 220.

ANNOTATED BIBLIOGRAPHY: CHAPTER 1

Bayles, Michael D., ed.: *Contemporary Utilitarianism* (New York: Doubleday, 1968). This volume includes ten articles by contemporary philosophers. Various points of view on the nature and justifiability of utilitarian theory are represented.

Callahan, Daniel: "Bioethics as a Discipline," *Hastings Center Studies* 1 (no. 1, 1973), pp. 66–73. Callahan specifies three tasks for the bioethicist: (1) identifying ethical issues, (2) providing a systematic means of thinking through these issues, and (3) helping physicians and scientists make correct decisions. He calls for the development of a unique methodology for bioethics and emphasizes that the discipline must serve the needs of physicians and scientists, "at whatever cost to disciplinary elegance."

Caplan, Arthur L.: "Ethical Engineers Need Not Apply: The State of Applied Ethics Today," *Science, Technology, & Human Values* 6 (Fall 1980), pp. 24–32. Caplan presents criticisms of what he calls the "engineering model" of applied ethics. According to this model, applied ethics is only a technical process whereby existing theory is used to solve particular moral problems.

Childress, James F.: *Who Should Decide?: Paternalism in Health Care* (New York: Oxford, 1982). In this extended discussion of paternalism, Childress examines the metaphors and principles underlying the disputes about professional paternalism in health care.

Clouser, K. Danner: "Bioethics," *Encyclopedia of Bioethics* (1978), vol. 1, pp. 115–127. In this article, written for those who are "seeking a conceptual grasp of the field itself," Clouser situates medical ethics within the broader field of bioethics. Against those who contend that bioethics will have to develop new ethical principles, he argues that it simply involves "ordinary morality applied to new areas of concern."

Donagan, Alan: *The Theory of Morality* (Chicago: University of Chicago, 1977). In this book, Donagan provides a theory of morality whose philosophical basis is Kant's "second formulation" of the Categorical Imperative.

Feinberg, Joel: *Social Philosophy* (Englewood Cliffs, N.J.: Prentice-Hall, 1973). Feinberg gives a detailed account of legal and moral rights and of liberty-limiting principles.

Gorovitz, Samuel: "Bioethics and Social Responsibility," *The Monist* 60 (January 1977), pp. 3–15. Calling attention to a number of philosophical topics that cut across a variety of bioethical issues, Gorovitz contends that philosophers have a unique and essential role to play in bioethics. He also attempts to identify some of the genuinely new ethical problems that have arisen out of recent developments in biomedical research.

Jonsen, Albert R., and Lewis H. Butler: "Public Ethics and Policy Making," *Hastings Center Report* 5 (August 1975), pp. 19–31. After a suggested analysis of communication difficulties between ethicists and policy makers, three tasks are identified for "public ethics" (ethics applied to public policy): (1) the articulation of relevant moral principles in a given policy problem, (2) the elucidation of proposed policy options in light of these principles, and (3) the display of a ranked order of moral options for policy choice. These three tasks are then illustrated by reference to the case of fetal research and the case of national health insurance.

Kant, Immanuel: *Groundwork of the Metaphysic of Morals,* translated and analyzed by H. J. Paton (New York: Harper & Row, 1964). In this work, a basic reference point, Kant offers an overall statement and defense of his ethical theory.

Macklin, Ruth: "Moral Concerns and Appeals to Rights and Duties: Grounding Claims in a Theory of Justice," *Hastings Center Report* 6 (October 1976), pp. 31–38. Macklin criticizes contemporary appeals to rights in debates in biomedical ethics, arguing that we cannot settle disputes about rights until we work out a theory of rights.

Mill, John Stuart: *Utilitarianism, On Liberty, Essay on Bentham,* edited by Mary Warnock (New York: New American Library, 1962). In his famous essay *Utilitarianism,* Mill offers a classic statement of the utilitarian position. In his equally well-known essay *On Liberty,* he defends the classic libertarian position rejecting strong paternalism and all liberty-limiting principles other than the harm principle.

Sartorius, Rolf, ed.: *Paternalism* (Minneapolis: University of Minnesota Press, 1983). The papers in this two-part collection of articles were all written by participants in a conference on paternalism held in 1980. The papers in the first part were all published previously and include, for example, Gerald Dworkin's frequently reprinted article "Paternalism." The second part contains papers prepared for the conference.

Taylor, Paul W.: *Principles of Ethics: An Introduction* (Encino, Calif.: Dickenson, 1975). Chapter 4 of this book provides a very valuable discussion of utilitarianism. Also helpful is the exposition of ethical egoism in Chapter 3 and the exposition of Kant's ethical system in Chapter 5.

APPENDIX: Selected Reference Sources in Biomedical Ethics

The Hastings Center's Bibliography of Ethics, Biomedicine, and Professional Responsibility (Frederick, Md.: University Publications of America, 1984). This selective and partially annotated bibliography is organized by topic. The compiler of this bibliography is also responsible for the *Hastings Center Report,* the leading journal in biomedical ethics.

Reich, Warren T., ed. in chief: *Encyclopedia of Bioethics* (New York: Macmillan, 1978). This four-volume set, an invaluable basic reference source in biomedical ethics, contains 314 articles. Each article is followed by a selected bibliography.

Walters, LeRoy, ed.: *Bibliography of Bioethics* (volumes 1–6 published by Gale Research Co.; subsequent volumes published by Macmillan, Free Press.) This bibliography, whose volumes are issued annually, features an extensive cross-referencing system.

Chapter 2

Physicians' Obligations and Patients' Rights

INTRODUCTION

What moral rules should govern the physician in dealing with patients? Are physicians ever morally justified in acting paternalistically to their patients? Are they ever morally justified in withholding information from patients, lying to them, or treating them without their consent? This chapter deals with such questions as it examines some of the fundamental moral issues associated with the physician-patient relationship and, consequently, with many of the other issues in this book.

Codes of Medical Ethics

The "Hippocratic Oath," reprinted in this chapter, reflects the traditional paternalism of the medical profession. The oath requires physicians to act so as to "benefit" the sick and "keep them from harm," but says nothing about patients' rights. Most of the medical codes of ethics designed by the American Medical Association exemplify a similar approach. They state the standards that should guide physicians in their professional relationships with patients and others but remain silent on patients' rights. According to the 1957 AMA code, for example, the objective of the medical profession is to use its scientifically based expertise to "render service to humanity."[1] Physicians are expected to promote the well-being of their patients, but nothing is said about any patient right to participate knowledgeably in making the decisions that define that "well-being." In contrast, the discussions that have taken place over the last twenty years in biomedical ethics have frequently emphasized patients' rights, especially their right of self-determination. This emphasis reflects a growing change in lay attitudes toward health-care professionals, especially physicians.

For a long time physicians were viewed as dedicated, hardworking, selfless individuals who could be expected to do everything in their power to benefit their patients. Patients, on the other hand, were viewed as dependent individuals having an obligation to trust their physicians who were assumed to be personally concerned with their patients' well-being. It was often taken for granted that doctors, because of their purported wisdom, objectivity, benevolence, and skill were in the best position to decide what was in their patients' best interests. Professional codes of medical ethics reflected this view of the physician-patient relationship, affirming that physicians would act to benefit their patients and would not exploit the often vulnerable patients over whom they frequently held great influence and power.

Current attitudes toward physicians are very different, due to many factors including the following. First, the physician-patient relationship has become increasingly impersonal as the growth of medical knowledge and technology has made modern medicine more complex. Growing complexity has led to an increase in specialization and the growth of large, depersonalized medical institutions. Second, the rise of "iatrogenic illnesses," illnesses resulting from medical interventions, has sometimes raised doubts about the skills of physicians. Publicity about medical mistakes and questionable medical practices has further eroded some of the lay trust in both the judgments of physicians and in their selfless dedication to their patients' well-being. Third, a growing awareness of the economic and educational differences between physicians and many of their patients has resulted in doubts about the capacity of physicians to perceive the best interests of their clients and to act accordingly.

In keeping with such changes in lay attitudes toward physicians, many recent discussions of medical ethics, including Robert M. Veatch's in this chapter, have attempted first to make explicit and then to criticize the paternalism implicit in traditional codes of medical ethics. Veatch and others reject as morally unacceptable professional codes that seem to sanction using paternalistic reasons to justify medical practices (e.g., lying or withholding relevant information for a "patient's own good") that violate a patient's right of self-determination. The most recent statement of the American Medical Association's "Principles of Medical Ethics," reprinted in this chapter, takes account of some of these criticisms, and for the first time, explicitly affirms the physician's commitment to "dealing honestly with patients" and respecting their rights. In view of the centrality of paternalism in the traditional medical model, however, two related questions continue to be addressed: "Is medical paternalism always morally unacceptable?" and "Is medical paternalism always incompatible with respect for patients' rights?"

Paternalism and Respect for Patient Autonomy

As presented in Chapter 1, paternalism is the interference with, limitation of, or usurpation of individual autonomy justified by reasons referring exclusively to the welfare or needs of the person whose autonomy is being interfered with, limited, or usurped. In acting paternalistically, physicians in effect act as if they, and not their patients, are best able to identify what is in their patients' best interests as well as the best means to advance those interests. Veatch, who in this chapter discusses four possible models of the physician-patient relationship, sees the paternalistic (or "priestly") model as incompatible with the values of individual freedom and individual dignity, or, to use the language of Chapter 1, as incompatible with the principle of respect for another's autonomy or right of self-determination. However, as Jane S. Zembaty points out in a reading in this chapter, paternalistic actions whose intent is to preserve individual autonomy would sometimes seem to be justified. Terrence F. Ackerman, in this chapter, goes even further, arguing that real respect for patient autonomy may require physicians to engage in paternalistic practices in order to assist patients in regaining some of the autonomy lost because of the constraining effects of illness. While affirming the importance of honesty and respect for patients' rights, Ackerman criticizes the above mentioned "Principles of Medical Ethics," questioning their adequacy as a moral framework designed to guide physician-patient interaction. To understand his concern, it is helpful to discuss two kinds of cases in which the values perceived as fundamental in physician-patient interactions—promotion of a patient's medical well-being and respect for patient autonomy—only appear to conflict.

First, a patient's abilities for any effective deliberation may be so severely constrained by illness (e.g., high fever, delirium) that autonomous decisions are virtually impossible and "apparent" decisions may not even be in accordance with the patient's history of decisions and values. In such cases, the promotion of a patient's well-being may require acting against his or her expressed wishes. This would appear to violate the principle of respect for autonomy. But the conflict between the two values may not be real. If the patient's autonomy as effective deliberation is so severely diminished and the desires expressed are also inconsistent with the patient's history and values, the principle of respect for autonomy would not even seem to apply. When there are compelling reasons for believing that a patient's decisions are not autonomous and that as a result the patient cannot exercise the right of self-determination, no paternalistic usurpation of that right is involved when decisions are made for the patient.

Second, the patient and physician may disagree about just what constitutes a patient's well-being. A physician, for example, might insist on continuing aggressive treatment in the case of a cancer patient, even though past treatment has brought no positive results. The patient might have a strong desire to discontinue the therapy advocated by the physician and to let life end without the additional discomforts caused by the therapy. To foster the patients' well-being then, the physician might think it necessary to resort to paternalistic practices intended to circumvent the patient's decision. Here the physician may see a conflict between two obligations—an obligation to promote the patient's well-being and an obligation to respect the patient's right of self-determination. But this may not be the locus of the conflict; rather, the conflict may be between the physician's values and the patient's. The physician may believe that any chance of prolonging a life, no matter how slight, justifies continuing treatment. The patient may believe that a few extra days or weeks of uncomfortable in-hospital life, with an infinitely small chance of prolonging life further, are not worth the price. If the patient's decision is the result of reflection and in keeping with the patient's history of decisions and values, respect for autonomy would seem to require the physician to act in accordance with the *patient's* perception of his or her well-being. If the patient's decision is not in accordance with the patient's history of decisions and values but *is* the result of a careful reflective reevaluation of those values, respect for autonomy would again seem to require the physician to act in accordance with the patient's choices. The conflict here is not between an obligation to respect autonomy and an obligation to promote a patient's well-being but between two different conceptions of "well-being." The physician is not faced with having to choose to violate either the principle of respect for a patient's autonomy or the obligation to promote the patient's well-being; rather, he or she is faced with having to accept the patient's conception of what constitutes the patient's well-being and acting accordingly. The problem arises because whether something promotes an individual's well-being is to some extent a subjective judgment. This is true in health care as well as in other areas of human life. There is no good reason to believe that physicians' medical knowledge gives them the expertise to decide just what patients should value in making their health-care decisions, although physicians' medical knowledge can give patients the information they need to make decisions in keeping with their own goals and values.

The problematic cases that concern Ackerman arise because of the constraining effects illness has on autonomy. In relation to the first kind of case, for example, it is sometimes difficult to judge whether a patient's capacity for effective deliberation is sufficiently undermined by illness so that the question of an infringement of the right of self-determination does not arise. In the face of such uncertainty, does the physician's obligation to promote the patient's well-being entail an obligation to act so as to "restore the patient's autonomy" to the greatest extent possible, given the nature of the patient's illness, even if this involves some measure of paternalism? Ackerman holds that it does; but physicians who act as Ackerman recommends run the danger exemplified by the second kind of case. As Mark Perl and Earl E. Shelp point out in this chapter, physicians sometimes fail to see that a disagreement with a patient about some course of treatment may not be due to the constraining effects that illness has on a patient's competency to make decisions but to a disagreement about values.

Truth-Telling

As noted above, traditional codes of medical ethics have little to say about deception, lying, or truth-telling. Yet some of the most widely disputed issues in biomedical ethics center on the physician's obligation to be truthful with the patient and on the patient's right to know the truth. Until recently, it was not unusual for physicians to lie to seriously ill patients about their illnesses for paternalistic reasons. Nor was it unusual for physicians to prescribe alternating injections of sterilized water with injections of pain-killing drugs for patients who were told that all the injections contained some opiate. In the first kind of case, physicians often argued that patients did not want to know the truth or that the truth would harm the patient. In the second kind of case, they often argued that the deceptive practices were justified because water does have a psychotherapeutic effect and yet is much less dangerous to the patient than too-frequent injections of opiates. This latter view is succinctly expressed in a letter written to *The Lancet:*

> Whenever pain can be relieved with a ml of saline, why should we inject an opiate? Do anxieties or discomforts that are allayed with starch capsules require administration of a barbiturate, diazepam, or propoxyphene?[2]

Are physicians ever morally justified in such lies and deceptive practices? If yes, under what conditions are their lies and deceptions justified?

One way to approach these questions is to begin with the more general questions: Is it always morally wrong to lie? Is it always morally correct to tell the truth? In answering these questions, of course, we must give reasons to justify the position taken. If it is *always* wrong to lie or to intentionally deceive others, then it is wrong for anyone, including physicians, to do so. If lies and intentional deception are *sometimes* morally acceptable, then it is necessary to specify the conditions that make them acceptable. Once these conditions are determined, we can then explore the particular physician-patient situation to see if it satisfies them.

Rule-utilitarians, for example, faced with deciding under what conditions, if any, lies and intentionally deceptive practices are justified, would have to consider the possible consequences of adopting and following a particular rule. In the medical context, for example, they would ask, "What would be the effect on the physician-patient relationship if physicians followed the rule, 'Lie to your patients whenever you believe that doing so is in the patient's best interests'?" In weighing the potential consequences of following such a rule, they would have to take account of the erosive effect that following it would have on patients' trust in the veracity of physicians.

How would the rule-utilitarian respond to a physician who argued as follows: Physicians ought to lie to patients because (1) most patients do not want to know the truth, and (2) the truth can be harmful to patients. Thus moral rules that forbid lying to patients are not in keeping with the Principle of Utility. First the utilitarian would have to examine the two factual claims underpinning this view, a task carried out by Sissela Bok in this chapter. Bok argues that (1) many patients do want to know the truth, and (2) physicians tend to overestimate the possible harmful consequences of telling patients the truth and to underestimate the possible good ones. The rule-utilitarian who agreed with Bok's analysis would still be faced with determining whether exceptions should be built into a rule prohibiting lying to patients. These exceptions would be designed to cover cases where there is very strong evidence to show that a patient does not want to know or would be seriously harmed by knowing. The rule-utilitarian would then have to determine whether the harm done to these patients would be outweighed by the balance of good consequences generated by adopting and following a rule that prohibits all lying in the physician-patient relationship.

Deontologists, of course, take a different approach. Immanuel Kant, whose deontological position is discussed in Chapter 1, is usually read as defending an "absolutist" position: All lies, including those done out of altruistic motives, are wrong. Not all deontologists agree with this absolutist position. As noted in Chapter 1, W. D. Ross maintains, for example, that there is a prima facie obligation not to lie or intentionally deceive but that this obligation can sometimes be overridden by some other prima facie obligation. In the physician-patient relationship, the overriding obligation might sometimes be the physician's obligation to promote the patient's medical well-being. Contrary to Ross, Joseph S. Ellin, in this chapter, takes an absolutist position in his prohibition against all lying in the physician-patient relationship. Ellin argues that it is always wrong for the physician to lie to patients but that the physician does not have even a prima facie obligation not to deceive. He bases his argument on his conception of the physician-patient relationship, seeing it as a fiduciary relationship. A "fiduciary relationship" is one of trust, often between unequals, where one party (e.g., the physician), is committed to promoting the well-being of the dependent party (e.g., the patient). Since trust is an essential element in a fiduciary relationship and lying seriously undermines trust, all lying is morally unacceptable. But, Ellin argues, this is not true of deceptive practices such as the use of placebos. In the medical context, deceptive practices may be simply one tool used by physicians to achieve the aims of the fiduciary relationship.

Informed Consent

Discussions about truth-telling and lying in medical ethics frequently arise in conjunction with discussions of the requirement of informed consent. It is now widely accepted that both law and morality require that no medical interventions be performed on competent adults without their informed and voluntary consent. But lying to patients or even withholding information from them can seriously undermine their ability to make informed decisions and, therefore, to give informed consent. In order to be able to give such consent, and thereby to exercise their right of self-determination, patients must have access to the necessary relevant information, and physicians are usually the only ones in a position to supply it. Judge Spotswood W. Robinson III affirms this point in a judicial opinion reprinted in this chapter, when he argues that physicians have a duty to "satisfy the vital informational needs of the patient."

The informed consent requirement is a relatively recent addition to the ethical constraints governing the physician-patient relationship. Traditional codes of medical ethics have nothing to say about any physician obligation to inform patients about the risks and benefits of alternative diagnostic and treatment techniques. As Jay Katz emphasizes in a reading in this chapter, the doctrine of informed consent was first introduced into case law in 1956. Since then, however, it has received a great deal of attention in biomedical ethics as both a legal and an ethical requirement. In 1982, for example, Congress assigned the task of determining the ethical and legal implications of the informed consent requirement to the President's Commission for the Study of Ethical Problems in Medicine and Biomedical and Behavioral Research. In its report, the Commission described ethically valid consent "as an ethical obligation that involves a process of shared decisionmaking based upon the mutual respect and participation [of patients and health professionals]."[3]

What is the moral basis of the informed consent requirement? The Commission, some of whose recommendations are reprinted in this chapter, identified two values as providing the ethical foundation of the requirement: respect for the patient's autonomy, or the right of self determination, and the promotion of the patient's well-being. Katz, who begins his article with a discussion of the legal development of the informed consent requirement, notes that its "avowed purpose" was to protect patients' rights to self-determination. Katz then details some of the ambivalences in court decisions dealing with the requirement of informed consent due to the possible tensions between the obligations entailed by the right of self-determination and the obligations entailed by physicians' commitments to promote their patients' medical well-being.

Much of the literature on informed consent focuses on several difficulties that affect the application of the requirement: (1) Who is *competent* to give consent? (2) When is consent *informed* consent? That is, how much information must a patient receive and understand before his or her consent is informed rather than partially informed or uninformed? (3) When is consent *voluntary* consent? Each of these questions will be briefly examined in order to show some of the difficulties that affect the application of the requirement. It is important to note that the problems here are both conceptual and empirical. The meaning of the concepts "informed," "competent," and "voluntary" must be explicated so that it can be determined just what counts as voluntary and informed consent. Then in a particular case, it must be determined whether the individual in question is capable of giving voluntary and informed consent.

(1) Who is competent to give consent? The patient who is sick enough to be in a hospital or institution may not be functioning normally enough to be a rational decision maker. Patients who are under great emotional stress, who are frightened or in severe pain, are often considered to be less than competent decision makers. In a burn center in California, for example, the following procedure is used when a patient with burns over sixty percent of his or her body is admitted. During the first two hours after the patient is severely burned there is no pain since the nerve endings are anesthetized. Patients during this time are given a choice. They can opt either to start a course of treatment, which will be prolonged and excruciatingly painful but may save their lives, or to simply receive pain-killing medication and care until they die. Can a patient in such circumstances, even if free from pain, be considered rational enough to weigh these alternatives? Recent work on the topic of competency stresses that it is not "all or nothing." The Commission's report, for example, maintains that individuals should be judged to be incapable of decision making only when

they lack the ability to make decisions that promote their well-being in keeping with their own previously expressed values and preferences.

(2) How much information must patients be given before their consent is informed? Suppose a patient suffering from breast cancer agrees to have a radical mastectomy. She is not told that studies indicate that this radical surgery is no more effective than much less radical surgery. Has the patient been given sufficient information to guarantee that her decision is a fully informed one? What criteria must the physician use in determining when sufficient information has been given? Is more information better than less? Studies have shown that patients receiving long, detailed explanations of the risks and purposes of a procedure may comprehend and retain very little of the significant information. In contrast, those who are given less detailed information may be able to comprehend and retain more of the important facts.[4] It is sometimes argued that lay persons, unlike medical professionals, cannot understand enough about the procedures, the risks, and other factors to ever give fully informed consent. In many cases, it is asserted, the most that can be hoped for is that the patient will *assent* to the procedure. (A parallel point is developed in the context of experimentation in Chapter 4 by Franz J. Ingelfinger.) An additional complication here is that physicians often make their own decisions in conditions of uncertainty. They cannot give patients information that they themselves do not possess.

(3) When is consent really voluntary? It is often argued that it is very easy to manipulate even highly competent patients into giving consent when the request is made by someone in a position of authority. For example, it has been shown that physicians, whose patients sometimes see them as "god" figures, and psychiatrists, whose judgments patients trust, find it very easy to get the consent they request. When patients are influenced in this way, is their consent sufficiently voluntary?

Recent work on informed consent, such as that of the President's Commission, stresses the importance of the process of communication and of the patient's cognitive-information processing. Studies have been undertaken to both understand and improve the procedures used to get "informed consent."[5] If the goal is informed consent, it seems insufficient to simply hand over information to patients via a form or a short conversation listing possible risks and alternatives; rather, it is necessary to determine how much the patient has understood and, perhaps, even some of the other factors that may be affecting the patient's decision, such as concern about a physician's reaction to a refusal. Take the example of a terminally ill, diabetic, cancer-ridden patient who, after repeatedly rejecting amputation of his gangrenous left foot, suddenly assented. His consent appeared to be both voluntary and informed. However, given his past history and the staff's knowledge of his values, a decision was made to call in an ethical counselor to determine the reasons for the patient's change of mind. After a long conversation with the patient, the counselor learned that the patient had consented to the amputation only because he erroneously believed that without this consent the physician and the hospital would refuse to continue their care. Once he understood that his belief was incorrect, he withdrew his assent to the amputation. The staff members' knowledge of this patient's character and values as well as their concern that the consent be truly informed and voluntary may not be the norm, but this case illustrates that informed consent requires something more than forms and cursory rituals. It also shows the need for medical professionals to better understand the communication processes they use to achieve informed consent.

The readings in this chapter provide only a few samples of the extensive literature on medical paternalism, truth-telling, and informed consent. The issues they raise about the physician-patient relationship continue to be widely discussed in biomedical ethics.

J.S.Z.

NOTES

1 American Medical Association, "Principles of Medical Ethics," *Journal of the American Medical Association,* vol. 164, no. 10 (July 6, 1957), p. 1119.
2 J. Sice: "Letter to the Editor," *The Lancet* 2 (1972), p. 651.
3 President's Commission for the Study of Ethical Problems in Medicine and Biomedical and Behavioral Research, *Making Health Care Decisions,* vol. 1, p. 2.
4 On this point, see Ralph J. Alfidi, "Controversy, Alternatives, and Decisions in Complying with the Legal Doctrine of Informed Consent," *Radiology* 114 (January 1975), pp. 231–234.
5 Barrie R. Cassileth, et al.: "Informed Consent—Why Are Its Goals Imperfectly Realized?" *New England Journal of Medicine* 302 (1980), pp. 896–900; and T. M. Grundner, "On the Readability of Surgical Consent Forms," *ibid.,* pp. 900–902.

Medical Codes of Ethics

The Hippocratic Oath

Little is known about the life of Hippocrates, a Greek physician born about 460 B.C.. We know that he was a widely sought, well-known, and influential healer who is said to have lived 85, 90, 104, or 109 years. A collection of documents known as the *Hippocratic Writings* (largely written from the fifth to the fourth century, B.C.) is believed to represent the remains of the Hippocratic school of medicine. Some of the works in this collection are credited to Hippocrates. The oath reprinted here, however, is believed to have been written by a philosophical sect known as the Pythagoreans in the latter part of the fourth century, B.C.

For the Middle Ages and later centuries, the Hippocratic Oath embodied the highest aspirations of the physician. It sets forth two sets of duties: (1) duties to the patient and (2) duties to the other members of the guild (profession) of medicine. In regard to the patient, it includes a set of absolute prohibitions (e.g., against abortion and euthanasia) as well as a statement of the physician's obligation to help and not to harm the patient.

I swear by Apollo Physician and Asclepius and Hygieia and Panaceia and all the gods and goddesses, making them my witnesses, that I will fulfil according to my ability and judgment this oath and this covenant:

To hold him who has taught me this art as equal to my parents and to live my life in partnership with him, and if he is in need of money to give him a share of mine, and to regard his offspring as equal to my brothers in male lineage and to teach them this art—if they desire to learn it—without fee and covenant; to give a share of precepts and oral instruction and all the other learning to my sons and to the sons of him who has instructed me and to pupils who have signed the covenant and have taken an oath according to the medical law, but to no one else.

I will apply dietetic measures for the benefit of the sick according to my ability and judgment; I will keep them from harm and injustice.

I will neither give a deadly drug to anybody if asked for it, nor will I make a suggestion to this effect.

Reprinted with permission of the publisher from *Ancient Medicine: Selected Papers of Ludwig Edelstein*, edited by Owsei Temkin and C. Lilian Temkin, p. 6. Copyright © 1967 by the Johns Hopkins Press: Baltimore.

Similarly I will not give to a woman an abortive remedy. In purity and holiness I will guard my life and my art.

I will not use the knife, not even on sufferers from stone, but will withdraw in favor of such men as are engaged in this work.

Whatever houses I may visit, I will come for the benefit of the sick, remaining free of all intentional injustice, of all mischief and in particular of sexual relations with both female and male persons, be they free or slaves.

What I may see or hear in the course of the treatment or even outside of the treatment in regard to the life of men, which on no account one must spread abroad, I will keep to myself holding such things shameful to be spoken about.

If I fulfil this oath and do not violate it, may it be granted to me to enjoy life and art, being honored with fame among all men for all time to come; if I transgress it and swear falsely, may the opposite of all this be my lot.

Principles of Medical Ethics (1980)

American Medical Association

This 1980 version of the ethical code of the American Medical Association states the standards that should guide physicians in their relationships with (1) patients, (2) colleagues, (3) members of allied health professions, and (4) society. Unlike the Hippocratic Oath, it does not expressly assert the physician's obligation to help patients and keep them from harm. Rather, it asserts that a physician "shall be dedicated to providing competent medical service with compassion and respect for human dignity." Unlike earlier codes it explicitly calls for both honesty in dealing with patients and colleagues and respect for patients' rights.

PREAMBLE

The medical profession has long subscribed to a body of ethical statements developed primarily for the benefit of the patient. As a member of this profession, a physician must recognize responsibility not only to patients, but also to society, to other health professionals, and to self. The following Principles adopted by the American Medical Association are not laws, but standards of conduct which define the essentials of honorable behavior for the physician.

PRINCIPLES

I A physician shall be dedicated to providing competent medical service with compassion and respect for human dignity.

II A physician shall deal honestly with patients and colleagues, and strive to expose those physicians deficient in character or competence, or who engage in fraud or deception.

III A physician shall respect the law and also recognize a responsibility to seek changes in those requirements which are contrary to the best interests of the patient.

IV A physician shall respect the rights of patients, of colleagues, and of other health professionals, and shall safeguard patient confidences within the constraints of the law.

V A physician shall continue to study, apply and advance scientific knowledge, make relevant information available to patients, colleagues, and the public, obtain consultation, and use the talents of other health professionals when indicated.

VI A physician shall, in the provision of appropriate patient care, except in emergencies, be free to choose whom to serve, with whom to associate, and the environment in which to provide medical services.

VII A physician shall recognize a responsibility to participate in activities contributing to an improved community.

Reprinted with permission of the publisher from *American Medical News*, August 1/8, 1980, p. 9.

Physician-Patient Models, Paternalism, and Patient Autonomy

Models for Ethical Medicine in a Revolutionary Age

Robert M. Veatch

Robert M. Veatch is professor of medical ethics at the Kennedy Institute of Ethics, Georgetown University. He has a Ph.D. in medical ethics as well as an M.S. in pharmacology. Veatch's edited books include *The Teaching of Medical Ethics* (1973) and *Ethics and Health Policy* (1976). He is the author of *Value-Freedom in Science and Technology* (1976), *Death, Dying and the Biological Revolution: Our Last Quest for Responsibility* (1976), *Case Studies in Medical Ethics* (1977), and *A Theory of Medical Ethics* (1981).

Veatch presents four possible models for the moral relationship between the physician and the patient: (1) *The Engineering Model:* The physician is an applied scientist who presents the facts to the lay person but leaves all the decisions to the latter; (2) *The Priestly Model:* The physician, guided by the principle "Benefit and do no harm," plays a paternalistic role in relation to the patient; (3) *The Collegial Model:* The physician and lay person are seen as equal colleagues sharing common interests and striving for a common goal; and (4) *The Contractual Model:* The physician and lay person are not perceived as equals but as having some mutual interests and sharing ethical authority and responsibility. Veatch draws out the ethical implications of these different models.

Most of the ethical problems in the practice of medicine come up in cases where the medical condition or desired procedure itself presents no moral problem. Most day-to-day patient contacts are just not cases which are ethically exotic. For the woman who spends five hours in the clinic waiting room with two screaming children waiting to be seen for the flu, the flu is not a special moral problem; her wait is. When medical students practice drawing blood from clinic patients in the cardiac care unit—when teaching material is treated as material—the moral problem is not really related to the patient's heart in the way it might be in a more exotic heart transplant. Many more blood samples are drawn, however, than hearts transplanted. It is only by moving beyond the specific issues to more basic underlying ethical themes that the real ethical problems in medicine can be dealt with.

Most fundamental of the underlying themes of the new medical ethics is that health care must be a human right, no longer a privilege limited to those who can afford it. It has not always been that way, and, of course, is not anything near that in practice today. But the norm, the moral claim, is becoming increasingly recognized. Both of the twin revolutions have made their contribution to this change. Until this century health care could be treated as a luxury, no matter how offensive this might be now. The amount of real healing that went on was minimal anyway. But now, with the biological revolution, health care really is essential to "life, liberty, and the pursuit of happiness." And health care is a right for everyone because of the social revolution which is really a revolution in our conception of justice. If the obscure phrase "all men are created equal" means anything in the medical context where biologically it is clear that they are not equal, it means that they are equal in the legitimacy of their moral claim. They must be treated equally in what is essential to their humanity: dignity, freedom, individuality. The sign in front of the prestigious, modern hospital, "Methadone patients use side door" is morally offensive even if it means nothing more than that the Methadone Unit is located near that door. It is strikingly similar to "Coloreds to the back of the bus." With this affirmation of the right to health care, what are the models of

Reprinted with permission of the author and the publisher from *Hastings Center Report*, vol. 2 (June 1972), pp. 5–7.

professional-lay relationships which permit this and other basic ethical themes to be conveyed?

1 The Engineering Model One of the impacts of the biological revolution is to make the physician scientific. All too often he behaves like an applied scientist. The rhetoric of the scientific tradition in the modern world is that the scientist must be "pure." He must be factual, divorcing himself from all considerations of value. It has taken atomic bombs and Nazi medical research to let us see the foolishness and danger of such a stance. In the first place the scientist, and certainly the applied scientist, just cannot logically be value-free. Choices must be made daily—in research design, in significance levels of statistical tests, and in perception of the "significant" observations from an infinite perceptual field, and each of these choices requires a frame of values on which it is based. Even more so in an applied science like medicine choices based upon what is "significant," what is "valuable," must be made constantly. The physician who thinks he can just present all the facts and let the patient make the choices is fooling himself even if it is morally sound and responsible to do this at all the critical points where decisive choices are to be made. Furthermore, even if the physician logically could eliminate all ethical and other value considerations from his decision-making and even if he could in practice conform to the impossible value-free ideal, it would be morally outrageous for him to do so. It would make him an engineer, a plumber making repairs, connecting tubes and flushing out clogged systems, with no questions asked. Even though I strongly favor abortion reform, I am deeply troubled by a physician who really believes abortion is murder *in the full sense* if he agrees to either perform one or refer to another physician. Hopefully no physician would do so when confronted with a request for technical advice about murdering a post-natal human.

2 The Priestly Model In proper moral revulsion to the model which makes the physician into a plumber for whom his own ethical judgments are completely excluded, some move to the opposite extreme, making the physician a new priest. Establishment sociologist of medicine Robert N. Wilson describes the physician-patient relationship as religious. "The doctor's office or the hospital room, for example," he says, "have somewhat the aura of a sanctuary, ...the patient must view his doctor in a manner far removed from the prosaic and the mundane."

The priestly model leads to what I call the "As-a syndrome." The symptoms are verbal, but the disease is moral. The chief diagnostic sign is the phrase "speaking-as-a...." In counseling a pregnant woman who has taken Thalidomide, a physician says, "The odds are against a normal baby and 'speaking-as-a-physician' that is a risk you shouldn't take." One must ask what it is about medical training that lets this be said "as-a-physician" rather than as a friend or as a moral man or as a priest. The problem is one of generalization of expertise: transferring of expertise in the technical aspects of a subject to expertise in moral advice.

The main ethical principle which summarizes this priestly tradition is "Benefit and do no harm to the patient." Now attacking the principle of doing no harm to the patient is a bit like attacking fatherhood. (Motherhood has not dominated the profession in the Western tradition.) But Fatherhood has long been an alternative symbol for the priestly model; "Father" has traditionally been a personalistic metaphor for God and for the priest. Likewise, the classical medical sociology literature (the same literature using the religious images) always uses the parent-child image as an analogy for the physician-patient relationship. It is this paternalism in the realm of values which is represented in the moral slogan "Benefit and do no harm to the patient." It takes the locus of decision-making away from the patient and places it in the hands of the professional. In doing so it destroys or at least minimizes the other moral themes essential to a more balanced ethical system. While a professional group may affirm this principle as adequate for a professional ethic, it is clear that society, more generally, has a much broader set of ethical norms. If the professional group is affirming one norm while society affirms another for the same circumstances, then the physician is placed in the uncomfortable position of having to decide whether his loyalty is to the norms of his professional group or to those of the broader society. What would this larger set of norms include?

a Producing Good and Not Harm Outside of the narrowest Kantian tradition, no one excludes the moral duty of producing good and avoiding harm entirely. Let this be said from the start. Some separate producing good and avoiding evil into two different principles placing greater moral weight on the latter, but this is also true within the tradition of professional medical ethics. The real difference is that in a set of ethical norms used more universally in the broader society producing good and avoiding harm is set in a much broader context and becomes just one of a much larger set of moral obligations.

b   Protecting Individual Freedom   Personal freedom is a fundamental value in society. It is essential to being truly human. Individual freedom for both physician and patient must be protected even if it looks like some harm is going to be done in the process. This is why legally competent patients are permitted by society to refuse blood transfusions or other types of medical care even when to the vast majority of us the price seems to be one of great harm. Authority about what constitutes harm and what constitutes good (as opposed to procedures required to obtain a particular predetermined good or harm) cannot be vested in any one particular group of individuals. To do so would be to make the error of generalizing expertise.

c   Preserving Individual Dignity   Equality of moral significance of all persons means that each is given fundamental dignity. Individual freedom of choice and control over one's own life and body contribute to that dignity. We might say that this more universal, societal ethic of freedom and dignity is one which moves beyond B. F. Skinner.

Many of the steps in the hospitalization, care, and maintenance of the patient, particularly seriously ill patients, are currently an assault on that dignity. The emaciated, senile man connected to life by IV tubes, tracheotomy, and colostomy has difficulty retaining his sense of dignity. Small wonder that many prefer to return to their own homes to die. It is there on their own turf that they have a sense of power and dignity.

d   Truth-Telling and Promise-Keeping   As traditional as they sound, the ethical obligations of truth-telling and promise-keeping have retained their place in ethics because they are seen as essential to the quality of human relationships. It is disturbing to see these fundamental elements of human interaction compromised, minimized, and even eliminated supposedly in order to keep from harming the patient. This is a much broader problem than the issue of what to tell the terminal carcinoma patient or the patient for whom there has been an unanticipated discovery of an XYY chromosome pattern when doing an amniocentesis for mongolism. It arises when the young boy getting his measles shot is told "Now this won't hurt a bit" and when a medical student is introduced on the hospital floor as "Doctor." And these all may be defended as ways of keeping from harming the patient. It is clear that in each case, also, especially if one takes into account the long-range threat to trust and confidence, that in the long run these violations of truth-telling and promise-keeping may do more harm than good. Both the young boy getting the shot and the medical student are being taught what to expect from the medical profession in the future. But even if that were not the case, each is an assault on patient dignity and freedom and humanity. Such actions may be justifiable sometimes, but the case must be awfully strong.

e   Maintaining and Restoring Justice   Another way in which the ethical norms of the broader society move beyond concern for helping and not harming the patient is by insisting on a fair distribution of health services. What we have been calling the social revolution, as prefigurative as it may be, has heightened our concern for equality in the distribution of basic health services. If health care is a right then it is a right for all. It is not enough to produce individual cases of good health or even the best aggregate health statistics. Even if the United States had the best health statistics in the world (which it does not have), if this were attained at the expense of inferior health care for certain groups within the society it would be ethically unacceptable.

At this point in history with our current record of discriminatory delivery of health services there is a special concern for restoring justice. Justice must also be compensatory. The health of those who have been discriminated against must be maintained and restored as a special priority.

3   The Collegial Model   With the engineering model the physician becomes a plumber without any moral integrity. With the priestly model his moral authority so dominates the patient that the patient's freedom and dignity are extinguished. In the effort to develop a more proper balance which would permit the other fundamental values and obligations to be preserved, some have suggested that the physician and the patient should see themselves as colleagues pursuing the common goal of eliminating the illness and preserving the health of the patient. The physican is the patient's "pal." It is in the collegial model that the themes of trust and confidence play the most crucial role. When two individuals or groups are truly committed to common goals then trust and confidence are justified and the collegial model is appropriate. It is a very pleasant, harmonious way to interact with one's fellow human beings. There is an equality of dignity and respect, an equality of value contributions, lacking in the earlier models.

But social realism makes us ask the embarrassing question. Is there, in fact, any real basis for the assumption of mutual loyalty and goals, of common interest which would permit the unregulated community of colleagues model to apply to the physician-patient relationship?

There is some proleptic sign of a community of real common interests in some elements of the radical health movement and free clinics, but for the most part we have to admit that ethnic, class, economic, and value differences make the assumption of common interest which is necessary for the collegial model to function a mere pipedream. What is needed is a more provisional model which permits equality in the realm of moral significance between patient and physician without making the utopian assumption of collegiality.

4   The Contractual Model   The model of social relationship which fits these conditions is that of the contract or covenant. The notion of contract should not be loaded with legalistic implications, but taken in its more symbolic form as in the traditional religious or marriage "contract" or "covenant." Here two individuals or groups are interacting in a way where there are obligations and expected benefits for both parties. The obligations and benefits are limited in scope, though, even if they are expressed in somewhat vague terms. The basic norms of freedom, dignity, truth-telling, promise-keeping, and justice are essential to a contractual relationship. The premise is trust and confidence even though it is recognized that there is not a full mutuality of interests. Social sanctions institutionalize and stand behind the relationship, in case there is a violation of the contract, but for the most part the assumption is that there will be a faithful fulfillment of the obligations.

Only in the contractual model can there be a true sharing of ethical authority and responsibility. This avoids the moral abdication on the part of the physician in the engineering model and the moral abdication on the part of the patient in the priestly model. It also avoids the uncontrolled and false sense of equality in the collegial model. With the contractual relationship there is a sharing in which the physician recognizes that the patient must maintain freedom of control over his own life and destiny when significant choices are to be made. Should the physician not be able to live with his conscience under those terms the contract is not made or is broken. This means that there will have to be relatively greater open discussion of the moral premises hiding in medical decisions before and as they are made.

With the contractual model there is a sharing in which the patient has legitimate grounds for trusting that once the basic value framework for medical decision-making is established on the basis of the patient's own values, the myriads of minute medical decisions which must be made day in and day out in the care of the patient will be made by the physician within that frame of reference.

In the contractual model, then, there is a real sharing of decision-making in a way that there is realistic assurance that both patient and physician will retain their moral integrity. In this contractual context patient control of decision-making on the individual level is assured without the necessity of insisting that the patient participate in every trivial decision. On the social level community control of health care is made possible in the same way. The lay community is given and should be given the status of contractor. The locus of decision-making is thus in the lay community, but the day-to-day medical decisions can, with trust and confidence, rest with the medical community. If trust and confidence are broken the contract is broken.

Medical ethics in the midst of the biological and social revolutions is dealing with a great number of new and difficult ethical cases: in vitro fertilization, psychosurgery, happiness pills, brain death, and the military use of medical technology. But the real day-to-day ethical crises may not be nearly so exotic. Whether the issue is in an exotic context or one which is nothing more complicated medically than a routine physical exam, the ethos of ethical responsibility established by the appropriate selection of a model for the moral relationship between the professional and the lay communities will be decisive. This is the real framework for medical ethics in a revolutionary age.

A Limited Defense of Paternalism in Medicine

Jane S. Zembaty

Jane S. Zembaty is associate professor of philosophy at the University of Dayton. She is the coeditor of *Social Ethics: Morality and Social Policy* (2nd ed. 1982) and the author of "Plato's *Timaeus*: Mass and Sortal Terms and Identity Through Time in the Phenomenal World."

Zembaty argues that physicians may sometimes be justified in acting paternalistically in regard to their patients. She maintains that it is important to distinguish between two kinds of cases: (1) those cases where physicians deny the patient's autonomy and act paternalistically in order to prevent patients from choosing to act in ways that are incompatible with the physicians' values; (2) those cases where physicians act paternalistically in order to protect the autonomy of the individual when that autonomy might be destroyed if the physician were to act nonpaternalistically. In Zembaty's view, even if it is morally unacceptable for physicians to act paternalistically in the first kind of case, they may be justified in acting paternalistically in the second kind of case.

Criticisms of medical paternalism are commonplace today. Paternalistic medical practices are perceived as violations of patients' rights, especially their right of self-determination. Robert M. Veatch, for example, criticizes such practices because they take "the locus of decision-making away from the patient and [place] it in the hands of the professional."[1] In this paper, I argue that medical professionals may *sometimes* be justified in acting paternalistically *even if* most cases of medical paternalism are morally unacceptable. I first isolate the kind of case in which the physician may be morally justified in acting paternalistically. I then make explicit the ethical grounds which could be used to justify the physician's actions in this kind of case.

I

The following cases illustrate the kinds of actions performed by physicians which are often labeled "paternalistic." I have deliberately constructed these cases to bring out some important differences between them. In order to highlight these differences, some of the cases present the extreme rather than the everyday situations faced by most physicians and other medical professionals. For the same reason, the physicians in the cases are credited with a more thorough knowledge of their patients than today's medical professionals usually have.

1 A physician has determined that John W. has amyotrophic lateral sclerosis. This is a progressive degenerative disease of the motor tracts of the lateral columns and anterior horns of the spinal cord. The disease causes progressive muscular atrophy and usually fatality within two to three years. The physician knows John W. well and has a good understanding of his personality, character, ideas, and beliefs. She withholds information about John's condition from him believing that if John knew the correct diagnosis and prognosis, he would choose suicide over the indignities and pain that would be a part of the last few months of his life. The physician does not believe that learning the truth about his physical condition would make it impossible for John to continue to function rationally. She is convinced, however, that John's deliberations about his future would culminate in a decision to commit suicide before his physical condition deteriorated to

such an extent that he would need the assistance of others to end his life.

2 Mary H., a woman in her mid-forties, is in a hospital for some tests related to what for her are abnormalities in her menstrual cycle. The gynecologist, without telling Mary, orders a certain test in addition to the tests indicated by her present problem. (He routinely orders this test for women patients having other tests associated with menopausal irregularities.) On the basis of the results of this particular test, the physician informs Mary at seven in the morning that she must be prepared for surgery as soon as possible. She is to undergo a complete hysterectomy later in the day just as soon as the necessary preparations can be made. Mary questions the need for the surgical procedure and asks for more information as well as another medical opinion. The gynecologist reacts angrily, but he eventually explains that the test in question is used as a means of determining whether ovarian cancer will develop *before* there are any *overt* symptoms of such a malignant growth. He informs her that hysterectomies are routinely performed simply on the basis of the results of this test. Mary refuses to have the hysterectomy without further information.

Mary H. then consults other physicians, including a close friend whose specialization is urology but who has access to medical experts knowledgeable about the test in question. The urologist tells her about a recently published report which questions the "accuracy" of the test as a predictor of cancer. Although the test shows that there is some sort of abnormality in some of the cells, it has never been proven that these abnormalities are indicators of a precancerous condition. With one exception, all the women whose tests had shown the presence of such abnormalities had had the recommended surgery. In none of these cases did the examinations of the tissue removed show the presence of any cancer. In the case of the one exception, the woman who did not have the surgery did develop cancer fifteen years later. The long span of time between the test and the appearance of the actual symptoms of cancer precluded reaching any conclusion about the efficacy of the test in determining the future development of cancer. Having gathered all this information, Mary H. decides against the operation. She reasons that there is no evidence to show that such a procedure is necessary and decides that she is willing to run the risk that fifteen years hence cancer *might develop.* Her original

gynecologist believes that his decision is still the correct one and that a patient should not run the risk that Mary is willing to run. He grants that, as a rule, he effectively takes the decision out of the patient's hands by not informing her about the controversial state of the evidence used in making the decision to perform the recommended surgery.

3 George Z. has amyotrophic lateral sclerosis. His physician knows him well and has a good understanding of his personality, character, ideas, and beliefs. He knows that George has seen three cancer-stricken members of his family die long painful deaths. He knows that George is a very religious person whose religious beliefs preclude his committing suicide. He also believes, on the basis of his knowledge of George's character, that if George is given the information about his physical condition and understands what he will have to face before he dies, George will deteriorate mentally to such an extent that he will be unable to function at all. He will be reduced to the same dependent status as a severely mentally-retarded individual who is incapable of taking care of even his simplest physical needs. The physician lies to George about his condition so that George can have at least one relatively good year before the disease reaches its final debilitating stages.

4 Dorothy N., diagnosed as a schizophrenic, has been able to function outside of an institution for ten years although she is on medication, routinely visits a psychiatrist, and avoids stressful situations as much as possible. She is self-supporting and has no immediate family. Dorothy is experiencing severe back pain as well as other symptoms which lead her physician to decide that she has a ruptured disc and that a laminectomy is in order. A laminectomy is the surgical removal of the posterior arch of a vertebra. In about one percent of the cases, such surgery results in partial paralysis. In his conversations with Dorothy about the proposed surgery, the physician does not tell her that there is a one percent chance that partial paraplegia will result from the surgical procedure. In fact, he talks to Dorothy about the laminectomy as if the procedure were no more risky than an appendectomy. He reaches his decision about what information to withhold from Dorothy after consulting with her psychiatrist. The physician is convinced that the additional emotional stress caused by the fear of paraplegia and of other possible complications will result in Dorothy's retreat into a world of her own creation, rendering her incapable, at least temporarily, of making any rational decisions about the measures to be taken to alleviate her physical condition.

In each of the four cases just outlined, the physician either lies or withholds information in order to keep the patient from what the physician perceives as a possible harm that would be produced by the patient to himself or herself. John W.'s physician wants to keep him from committing suicide. Mary H.'s physician does not want to give Mary the chance to make a decision which he believes will probably result in her eventual death from ovarian cancer. George Z.'s physician wants to keep George from deteriorating mentally to such an extent that George becomes completely dependent on others for both his physical care and any future decisions about his well-being. Dorothy N.'s physician wants to keep her from regressing into the kind of schizophrenic state which might, at least temporarily, take all decision-making power about her future out of her hands and require her involuntary commitment to a mental institution, to be followed by subsequent legal procedures to permit the required surgery. All of these cases could be said to provide instances of paternalism, as paternalism is described in contemporary ethical theory.

In contemporary ethical discussions, the most widely cited definition of paternalism is Gerald Dworkin's:

> [Paternalism is] the interference with a person's liberty of action justified by reasons referring exclusively to the welfare, good, happiness, needs, interests, or values of the person being coerced.[2]

When paternalism in the legal system is at issue, this definition is acceptable since laws, backed by force or the threat of harm, are by nature coercive. However, as other writers on paternalism have pointed out, many paternalistic actions involve neither force nor the threat of harm.[3] A more useful definition, therefore, is the following:

> Paternalism is the interference with a person's autonomy justified by reasons referring exclusively to the welfare, good, happiness, needs, interests, or values of the person being constrained.[4]

An individual's autonomy can be constrained in various ways. To be an autonomous individual is to be capable of weighing choices rationally and of acting on the basis of those rationally-made choices. Limits can be placed on an individual's autonomy either by interfering with the individual's freedom to exercise choice or by interfering with the choice-making process. The freedom to exercise choice is restricted whenever individuals are constrained from performing actions which they intentionally want to perform. Individuals, for example, who are locked in a room with barred windows are unable to leave that room even if they should decide to do so. The choice-making process can be restricted in many ways. Some drugs, for example, directly affect an individual's capacity for rational thinking. But the choice-making process is also restricted when the decision maker is given information (relevant to a particular decision) which is inadequate, distorted, or false.[5] All of the cases presented above provide instances of this last sort of restriction. Critics of medical paternalism maintain that intentional restrictions of this sort are incompatible with a respect for the patient's autonomy and the patient's right of self-determination.

In contrast, an individual's autonomy is respected when the individual is recognized as someone having the right of self-determination. A patient's autonomy is respected when the medical professional acts in recognition of this right. According to a recent court ruling, the recognition of the right of self-determination entails that the patient have "an opportunity to evaluate knowledgeably the options available and the risks dependent upon each."[6] By acting paternalistically and withholding information which is relevant to a patient's decision about what shall be done to him or her, the medical professional *seems* to show a lack of respect for a patient's autonomy. In the cases presented above, for example, John W.'s and Mary H.'s physicians, in effect, usurp their patient's decision-making power. They limit their patients' choices by deliberately withholding information which could affect those choices. George Z.'s and Dorothy N.'s physicians also withhold information which *might* affect their choices *if* the physicians are wrong about their patients' emotional and mental states. (George Z. might commit suicide despite his religious beliefs. Dorothy N. might not regress mentally and might decide against the laminectomy.)

The difference between the two sets of cases lies in the physicians' reasons for limiting individual autonomy by withholding information. In examples 1 and 2, the physicians are determined to prevent John W. and Mary H. from making choices the physicians consider unacceptable. In examples 3 and 4, the professionals are concerned *to prevent an even greater loss of individual autonomy* which they believe will result if the pertinent information is disclosed—a loss which could shut out the possibility of any rational decision-making permanently for George Z. and at least temporarily for Dorothy N. This difference in reasons is relevant in isolating the kind of case in which the physician might be justified in acting paternalistically. In what follows, I will attempt to show why the paternalistic actions exemplified by cases 3 and 4 may be justified even if most instances of medical paternalism are morally unacceptable.

II

Critics of medical paternalism advance two main types of arguments. The first type rests on the relation between some theory of morality and the principle of respect for individual autonomy. Here the argument is primarily theoretical. The second type attempts to show that medical professionals do not have the knowledge required to accurately predict the harmful consequences for the patient if the physician fails to act paternalistically. Here the argument is primarily empirical. In this section, I focus on some of the theoretical justifications offered for the rejection of medical paternalism in order to show that these justifications themselves open the door for the justification of *some* paternalistic actions. In the last section of this paper, I briefly discuss the empirically-based type of argument.

Many of those who reject paternalism and stress the physician's duty to recognize and respect the patient's autonomy argue from either a deontological or a utilitarian perspective. I will address each of these positions in turn, beginning with the utilitarian one. Utilitarians stress the social value of autonomy; but for them, autonomy is one value among others—albeit a very important one. John Stuart Mill, one of the foremost utilitarians, argues that the exercise of individual autonomy is essential in developing both the intellectual and character traits which give human beings their worth and which contribute to society's progress:

> ...The human faculties of perception, judgment, discriminative feeling, mental activity, and even moral preference, are exercised only in making a choice. He who does anything because it is the custom makes no choice. He gains no practice either

in discerning or in desiring what is best. The mental and moral, like the muscular powers, are improved by being used.... He who lets the world, or his own portion of it choose his plan of life for him, has no need of any other faculty than the ape-like one of imitation.... Where not the person's own character, but the traditions or custom of other people are the rule of conduct, there is wanting one of the principal ingredients of human happiness and quite the chief ingredient of individual and social progress....[7]

On a view such as Mill's, respect for individual autonomy has *utility value*. A society which fosters respect for persons as autonomous agents will be a more progressive and, on balance, a happier society because its citizens will have the opportunities to develop their capacities to act as rational, responsible moral agents. Paternalism is morally unacceptable because it functions to stifle the individual's development as a rational decision maker. For Mill, an individual's good, "either physical or moral, is not a sufficient warrant" for interfering with his or her freedom of action precisely because such interference keeps individuals from becoming experienced, rational choosers.[8]

Contemporary rule-utilitarian critics of medical paternalism argue in accordance with Mill's position. They maintain that freedom of choice is such an important social value that patients should be allowed to choose for themselves whether they will be treated, what kind of treatment they will receive, whether they will continue to live with a debilitating disease or die. If harm results to patients as a result of these choices, that is a price that must be paid in the interest of protecting the individual's freedom of choice. If individual autonomy is given that much value by the rule-utilitarian, any paternalistic attempt to limit choice by lying or deception in a single case would seem to be morally unacceptable. On this line of reasoning, both John W.'s and Mary H.'s physicians would be guilty of immoral behavior. But the actions of physicians in regard to George Z. and Dorothy N. would not be ruled morally unacceptable simply on this line of reasoning. In order to demonstrate the moral unacceptability of paternalistic actions whose intent is to prevent a much more severe loss of autonomy, the utilitarian would have to advance arguments to show that in these cases some equally or more significant moral rule comes into conflict with, and takes precedence over, those rules which protect autonomy. In the absence of such arguments, the utilitarian could consistently maintain that some paternalistic actions are morally unjustified while others are justified. As long as the high value placed on individual autonomy serves as the ground for the utilitarian rejection of medical paternalism, it would seem incoherent to claim that paternalistic actions *intended to preserve that autonomy* are ethically unacceptable.[9] On a utilitarian view, then, a distinction between justified and unjustified paternalism could be made in medical ethics in accordance with the difference noted between the two sets of cases. Paternalistic actions whose intent is to limit individual autonomy by limiting choice would continue to stand condemned as long as respect for individual autonomy continued to be accorded high utility value. But paternalistic actions whose intent is to preserve an individual's capacity for autonomous decisions would seem to be not only compatible with a rule asserting the medical professional's obligation to respect the patient's autonomy, but might even be required by it.

A Kantian deontologist maintains, in contrast to the utilitarian, that respect for persons as free moral agents is not simply one value among others, but the very foundation of morality. On this view, acting paternalistically with regard to patients could never be justified simply by appeal to the possible good consequences for the patients. It would always be morally wrong, for example, for physicians to withhold information about surgical procedures from patients because the physicians believed that the patients would refuse to undergo potentially beneficial surgery if informed of all the risks. Charles Fried, a contemporary ethicist, adopts such a Kantian approach to paternalism in the medical context. He maintains that patients must never be denied relevant information. By withholding it, physicians fail to treat their patients as ends-in-themselves and treat them merely as objects. On Fried's view, patients can never be treated simply as means to ends, even when the ends in question are those of the patients themselves (e.g., the patients' restored health):

> The patient has a right to know all the relevant details about the situation he finds himself in.... Thus lucidity is not just an instrumental benefit, contingently useful to a patient.... To deny a patient an opportunity for lucidity is to treat him not as a person but as a means to an end. And even if the ends are the patient's own ends, to treat him as a means to them is to undermine his humanity insofar

as humanity consists in choosing and being able to judge one's own ends, rather than being a machine which is used to serve ends, even one's own ends.[10]

This is a puzzling statement. If the patient's humanity or personhood consists in "choosing and being able to judge his own ends," then paternalistic actions whose intent is to preserve the individual's ability to choose or judge his own ends would again seem to be justified. In fact, if a nonpaternalistic action (e.g., telling the truth to George Z. or Dorothy N.) would serve to destroy that personhood which is supposed to be the ground for morality, it is difficult to see how in such cases the *failure to act paternalistically* could be justified.

I realize that I am now advancing a consequentialist argument against the deontologist. I maintain, however, that a deontologist does not necessarily have to reject consequences of this kind as irrelevant to morality. Rather, the deontologist needs to distinguish between the *kinds* of bad consequences the physicians are trying to avoid in the two sets of cases. In the first set, physicians are trying to limit their patients' choices in order to keep them from making choices incompatible with the physicians' values. This would be ethically unacceptable to a deontologist such as Fried. Fried stresses the importance of individual autonomy because he sees the individual as the center of values, as someone who has the right both to choose those values and to act in accordance with them. The actions of the physicians in the first set of cases are inconsistent with this kind of reasoning. In the second set of cases, however, the physicians are trying to protect that very characteristic of the persons involved—their capacity for making rational choices—which on the deontological view makes each person the center of values. Physicians who act in this way may be acting *mistakenly* since they may be too pessimistic in their assessments of their patients' emotional stability, but it is difficult to see why the deontologist would want to accuse them of acting immorally if they are acting to preserve that which is supposed to serve as the very ground of the respect owed to patients by physicians. *perhaps mistakenly but not immorally!*

III

As noted earlier, the physicians in the above examples are credited with a knowledge of their patients that few physicians actually possess. In actual practice, the knowledge that medical professionals have of their patients is much more skimpy. Furthermore, physicians often make their decisions about what to tell patients on the basis of very general and questionable empirical generalizations about the effects of distressing information on patients.[1] Those who offer empirical arguments against medical paternalism emphasize both the inadequacy of the usual medical professional's knowledge of a patient's psychological makeup and the questionable validity of many psychiatric generalizations about patients' reactions. Such empirical arguments serve a useful purpose. First, they focus attention on the need for medical professionals to become better informed about their patients' psychic makeup before acting paternalistically. Second, they bring out into the open the tendency of medical professionals to impose their values on patients whose own values may be very different. However, if these empirical arguments are to provide good reasons for rejecting *all* medical paternalism, they will have to show that physicians are *always* wrong about the effect of distressing information on patients. Since such certainty seems to be an impossible goal, these critics of medical paternalism should explore the difference between (1) the paternalistic actions of physicians who want to impose their values on their patients or simply assume that their patients share their values and (2) the paternalistic actions of physicians who respect their patients' autonomy and right of self-determination but who act paternalistically on the basis of all the knowledge they can gather about their patients' values and emotional makeup out of a respect for that very autonomy.

To summarize, I have argued that some cases of medical paternalism may be morally justified even if most cases are morally unjustifiable. My central claim is that paternalism is justified (at least) when autonomy is protected to a much greater degree than it would be if a nonpaternalistic position were accepted. My argument for this claim rests on a brief exploration of the reasons advanced by utilitarians and deontologists against paternalism. If it is the case that for both utilitarians and deontologists, respect for individual autonomy provides the basis for the rejection of paternalism, then at least one set of paternalistic actions should be exempt from this rejection. Paternalistic actions which do in fact infringe on individual autonomy to some extent but whose intent is to prevent a much more severe loss of autonomy would seem to be in keeping with that respect for autonomy which provides a basis for rejecting other instances of medical paternalism.

NOTES

1 Robert M. Veatch, "Models for Ethical Medicine in a Revolutionary Age," *Hastings Center Report* 2 (June 1972), p. 2. Veatch does admit that medical paternalism is justified sometimes; but, he maintains, "the case must be awfully strong." In this paper, I try to bring out the kind of situation which Veatch might see as involving justified medical paternalism.

2 Gerald Dworkin, "Paternalism," *The Monist* 56 (January 1972), p. 65.

3 Bernard Gert and Charles M. Culver, "Paternalistic Behavior," *Philosophy and Public Affairs* 6 (Fall 1976), pp. 45–47; Allen Buchanan, "Medical Paternalism," *Philosophy and Public Affairs* 7 (Summer 1978), pp. 370–390.

4 On some interpretations of paternalism, paternalistic actions do not always interfere with a person's autonomy. Those which do not are instances of weak paternalism as weak paternalism is explicated in Joel Feinberg, *Social Philosophy* (Englewood Cliffs, N.J.: Prentice-Hall, 1973), p. 52. Weak paternalism is explained as follows: "The state has the right to prevent self-regarding harmful conduct only when it is substantially nonvoluntary, or when intervention is necessary to establish whether it is voluntary or not." Strong paternalism, in contrast, is simply paternalism "unmediated by the voluntariness standard." When individuals are prevented from performing actions which will result in harm to themselves but which are substantially nonvoluntary, then their autonomy is not being infringed upon since the individuals are not really choosing to perform those particular actions. I am not concerned with *this* "weak" form of paternalism in this paper.

5 Allen Buchanan (see earlier citation) would disagree with the claim that withholding information interferes with the decision-making process. He argues that an individual can be deprived of information and still be free to decide and to act although his decision will not be an informed one. Since on my view, as on Joel Feinberg's, "lacks" can serve as

constraints on freedom of action and choice, with-holding or distorting information does constrain the decision-making process.

6 *Canterbury v. Spence,* No. 22099, U.S. Court of Appeals, District of Columbia Circuit, May 19, 1972. 464 *Federal Reporter,* 2nd series, 772.

7 John Stuart Mill, *Utilitarianism, On Liberty, Essay on Bentham,* ed. Mary Warnock (New York: New American Library, 1962), pp. 187, 185.

8 *Ibid.,* p. 135.

9 Some rule-utilitarians argue, of course, that they do not reject paternalism *in principle.* Rather, their

rejection of what Joel Feinberg calls "strong pater-nalism" is based on the empirical claim that on balance the total bad consequences of accepting and following rules which allow paternalistic behav-ior far outweigh the good ones. See Tom L. Beau-champ, "Paternalism and Bio-behavioral Control," *The Monist* 60 (January 1977).

10 Charles Fried, *Medical Experimentation: Personal Integrity and Social Policy* (New York: American Elsevier Publishing Co., 1974), p. 101.

11 Allen Buchanan, in the article cited earlier, presents empirical arguments against medical paternalism.

Why Doctors Should Intervene

Terrence F. Ackerman

Terrence F. Ackerman is director of the Program for Human Values and Ethics at the University of Tennessee Center for the Health Sciences and an adjunct member in medical ethics at St. Jude Children's Hospital. He is the author of "Medical Ethics and the Two Dogmas of Liberalism" and "Experimentation in Bioethics Research."

Ackerman criticizes the notion of respect for autonomy that identifies it with noninterference. He argues that noninterference fails to respect patient autonomy because it does not take account of the transforming effects of illness. Ackerman's major contention is that the autonomy of those who are ill is limited by all kinds of constraints—physical, cognitive, emotional, and social. Ackerman argues in favor of medical paternalism, where appropriate, maintaining that real respect for the autonomy of patients requires physicians to actively attempt to neutralize the impediments that interfere with patients' choices, helping them to restore control over their lives.

Patient autonomy has become a watchword of the medical profession. According to the revised 1980 AMA Principles of Medical Ethics,[1] no longer is it permissible for a doctor to withhold information from a patient, even on grounds that it may be harmful. Instead the physician is expected to "deal honestly with patients" at all times. Physicians also have a duty to respect the confidentiality of the doctor-patient relationship. Even when disclosure to a third party may be in the patient's interests, the doctor is instructed to release information only when required by law. Respect for the autonomy of patients has given rise to many specific patient

rights—among them the right to refuse treatment, the right to give informed consent, the right to privacy, and the right to competent medical care provided with "respect for human dignity."

While requirements of honesty, confidentiality, and patients' rights are all important, the underlying moral vision that places exclusive emphasis upon these factors is more troublesome. The profession's notion of respect for autonomy makes noninterference its essential fea-ture. As the Belmont Report has described it, there is an obligation to "give weight to autonomous persons' considered opinions and choices while refraining from

Reprinted with permission of the author and the publisher from *Hastings Center Report,* vol. 12 (August 1982), pp. 14–17.

obstructing their actions unless they are clearly detrimental to others."[2] Or, as Tom Beauchamp and James Childress have suggested, "To respect autonomous agents is to recognize with due appreciation their own considered value judgments and outlooks even when it is believed that their judgments are mistaken." They argue that people "are entitled to autonomous determination without limitation on their liberty being imposed by others."[3]

When respect for personal autonomy is understood as noninterference, the physician's role is dramatically simplified. The doctor need be only an honest and good technician, providing relevant information and dispensing professionally competent care. Does noninterference really respect patient autonomy? I maintain that it does not, because it fails to take account of the transforming effects of illness.

"Autonomy," typically defined as self-governance, has two key features. First, autonomous behavior is governed by plans of action that have been formulated through deliberation or reflection. This deliberative activity involves processes of both information gathering and priority setting. Second, autonomous behavior issues, intentionally and voluntarily, from choices people make based upon their own life plans.

But various kinds of constraints can impede autonomous behavior. There are physical constraints—confinement in prison is an example—where internal or external circumstances bodily prevent a person from deliberating adequately or acting on life plans. Cognitive constraints derive from either a lack of information or an inability to understand that information. A consumer's ignorance regarding the merits or defects of a particular product fits the description. Psychological constraints, such as anxiety or depression, also inhibit adequate deliberation. Finally, there are social constraints—such as institutionalized roles and expectations ("a woman's place is in the home," "the doctor knows best") that block considered choices.

Edmund Pellegrino suggests several ways in which autonomy is specifically compromised by illness:

In illness, the body is interposed between us and reality—it impedes our choices and actions and is no longer fully responsive.... Illness forces a reappraisal and that poses a threat to the old image; it opens up all the old anxieties and imposes new ones—often including the real threat of death or drastic alterations in life-style. This ontological as-

sault is aggravated by the loss of...freedoms we identify as peculiarly human. The patient...lacks the knowledge and skills necessary to cure himself or gain relief of pain and suffering....The state of being ill is therefore a state of "wounded humanity," of a person compromised in his fundamental capacity to deal with his vulnerability.[4]

The most obvious impediment is that illness "interposes" the body or mind between the patient and reality, obstructing attempts to act upon cherished plans. An illness may not only temporarily obstruct long-range goals; it may necessitate permanent and drastic revision in the patient's major activities, such as working habits. Patients may also need to set limited goals regarding control of pain, alteration in diet and physical activity, and rehabilitation of functional impairments. They may face considerable difficulties in identifying realistic and productive aims.

The crisis is aggravated by a cognitive constraint—the lack of "knowledge and skills" to overcome their physical or mental impediment. Without adequate medical understanding, the patient cannot assess his or her condition accurately. Thus the choice of goals is seriously hampered and subsequent decisions by the patient are not well founded.

Pellegrino mentions the anxieties created by illness, but psychological constraints may also include denial, depression, guilt, and fear. I recently visited an eighteen-year-old boy who was dying of a cancer that had metastasized extensively throughout his abdomen. The doctor wanted to administer further chemotherapy that might extend the patient's life a few months. But the patient's nutritional status was poor, and he would need intravenous feedings prior to chemotherapy. Since the nutritional therapy might also encourage tumor growth, leading to a blockage of the gastrointestinal tract, the physician carefully explained the options and the risks and benefits several times, each time at greater length. But after each explanation, the young man would say only that he wished to do whatever was necessary to get better. Denial prevented him from exploring the alternatives.

Similarly, depression can lead patients to make choices that are not in harmony with their life plans. Recently, a middle-aged woman with a history of ovarian cancer in remission returned to the hospital for the biopsy of a possible pulmonary metastasis. Complications ensued and she required the use of an artificial respirator for several days. She became severely depressed and soon refused further treatment. The behavior was entirely out of character with her previous full commitment to treatment. Fully supporting her overt wishes might have robbed her of many months of relatively comfortable life in the midst of a very supportive family around which her activities centered. The medical staff stalled for time. Fortunately, her condition improved.

Fear may also cripple the ability of patients to choose. Another patient, diagnosed as having a cerebral tumor that was probably malignant, refused life-saving surgery because he feared the cosmetic effects of neurosurgery and the possibility of neurological damage. After he became comatose and new evidence suggested that the tumor might be benign, his family agreed to surgery and a benign tumor was removed. But he later died of complications related to the unfortunate delay in surgery. Although while competent he had agreed to chemotherapy, his fears (not uncommon among candidates for neurosurgery) prevented him from accepting the medical intervention that might have secured him the health he desired.

Social constraints may also prevent patients from acting upon their considered choices. A recent case involved a twelve-year-old boy whose rhabdomyosarcoma had metastasized extensively. Since all therapeutic interventions had failed, the only remaining option was to involve him in a phase I clinical trial. (A phase I clinical trial is the initial testing of a drug in human subjects. Its primary purpose is to identify toxicities rather than to evaluate therapeutic effectiveness.) The patient's course had been very stormy, and he privately expressed to the staff his desire to quit further therapy and return home. However, his parents denied the hopelessness of his condition, remaining steadfast in their belief that God would save their child. With deep regard for his parents' wishes, he refused to openly object to their desires and the therapy was administered. No antitumor effect occurred and the patient soon died.

Various social and cultural expectations also take their toll. According to Talcott Parsons, one feature of the sick role is that the ill person is obligated "...to seek *technically competent* help, namely, in the most usual case, that of a physician and to *cooperate* with him in the process of trying to get well."[5] Parsons does not describe in detail the elements of this cooperation. But clinical observation suggests that many patients

relinquish their opportunity to deliberate and make choices regarding treatment in deference to the physician's superior educational achievement and social status ("Whatever you think, doctor!"). The physical and emotional demands of illness reinforce this behavior.

Moreover, this perception of the sick role has been socially taught from childhood—and it is not easily altered even by the physician who ardently tries to engage the patient in decision making. Indeed, when patients are initially asked to participate in the decision-making process, some exhibit considerable confusion and anxiety. Thus, for many persons, the institutional role of patient requires the physician to assume the responsibilities of making decisions.

Ethicists typically condemn paternalistic practices in the therapeutic relationship, but fail to investigate the features that incline physicians to be paternalistic. Such behavior may be one way to assist persons whose autonomous behavior has been impaired by illness. Of course, it is an open moral question whether the constraints imposed by illness ought to be addressed in such a way. But only by coming to grips with the psychological and social dimensions of illness can we discuss how physicians can best respect persons who are patients.

RETURNING CONTROL TO PATIENTS

In the usual interpretation of respect for personal autonomy, noninterference is fundamental. In the medical setting, this means providing adequate information and competent care that accords with the patient's wishes. But if serious constraints upon autonomous behavior are intrinsic to the state of being ill, then noninterference is not the best course, since the patient's choices will be seriously limited. Under these conditions, real respect for autonomy entails a more inclusive understanding of the relationship between patients and physicians. Rather than restraining themselves so that patients can exercise whatever autonomy they retain in illness, physicians should actively seek to neutralize the impediments that interfere with patients' choices.

In *The Healer's Art,* Eric Cassell underscored the essential feature of illness that demands a revision in our understanding of respect for autonomy:

If I had to pick the aspect of illness that is most destructive to the sick, I would choose the loss of control. Maintaining control over oneself is so vital to all of us that one might see all the other phenomena of illness as doing harm not only in their own right but doubly so as they reinforce the sick person's perception that he is no longer in control.[6]

Cassell maintains, "The doctor's job is to return control to his patient." But what is involved in "returning control" to patients? Pellegrino identifies two elements that are preeminent duties of the physician: to provide technically competent care and to fully inform the patient. The noninterference approach emphasizes these factors, and their importance is clear. Loss of control in illness is precipitated by a physical or mental defect. If technically competent therapy can fully restore previous health, then the patient will again be in control. Consider a patient who is treated with antibiotics for a routine throat infection of streptococcal origin. Similarly, loss of control is fueled by lack of knowledge—not knowing what is the matter, what it portends for life and limb, and how it might be dealt with. Providing information that will enable the patient to make decisions and adjust goals enhances personal control.

If physical and cognitive constraints were the only impediments to autonomous behavior, then Pellegrino's suggestions might be adequate. But providing information and technically competent care will not do much to alter psychological or social impediments. Pellegrino does not adequately portray the physician's role in ameliorating these.

How can the doctor offset the acute denial that prevented the adolescent patient from assessing the benefits and risks of intravenous feedings prior to his additional chemotherapy? How can he deal with the candidate for neurosurgery who clearly desired that attempts be made to restore his health, but feared cosmetic and functional impairments? Here strategies must go beyond the mere provision of information. Crucial information may have to be repeatedly shared with patients. Features of the situation that the patient has brushed over (as in denial) or falsely emphasized (as with acute anxiety) must be discussed in more detail or set in their proper perspective. And the physician may have to alter the tone of discussions with the patient, emphasizing a positive attitude with the overly depressed or anxious patient, or a more realistic, cautious attitude with the denying patient, in order to neutralize psychological constraints.

The physician may also need to influence the beliefs or attitudes of other people, such as family members,

that limit their awareness of the patient's perspective. Such a strategy might have helped the parents of the dying child to conform with the patient's wishes. On the other hand, physicians may need to modify the patient's own understanding of the sick role. For example, they may need to convey that the choice of treatment depends not merely upon the physician's technical assessment, but on the quality of life and personal goals that the patient desires.

Once we admit that psychological and social constraints impair patient autonomy, it follows that physicians must carefully assess the psychological and social profiles and needs of patients. Thus, Pedro Lain-Entralgo insists that adequate therapeutic interaction consists in a combination of "objectivity" and "cooperation." Cooperation "is shown by psychologically reproducing in the mind of the doctor, insofar as that is possible, the meaning the patient's illness has for him."[7] Without such knowledge, the physician cannot assist patients in restoring control over their lives. Ironically, some critics have insisted that physicians are not justified in acting for the well-being of patients because they possess no "expertise" in securing the requisite knowledge about the patient.[8] But knowledge of the patient's psychological and social situation is also necessary to help the patient to act as a fully autonomous person.

BEYOND LEGALISM

Current notions of respect for autonomy are undergirded by a legal model of doctor-patient interaction. The relationship is viewed as a typical commodity exchange—the provision of technically competent medical care in return for financial compensation. Moreover, physicians and patients are presumed to have an equal ability to work out the details of therapy, *provided that* certain moral rights of patients are recognized. But the compromising effects of illness, the superior knowledge of physicians, and various institutional arrangements are also viewed as giving the physician an unfair power advantage. Since the values and interests of patients may conflict with those of the physician, the emphasis is placed upon noninterference.[9]

This legal framework is insufficient for medical ethics because it fails to recognize the impact of illness upon autonomous behavior. Even if the rights to receive adequate information and to provide consent are secured, affective and social constraints impair the

not a contractual relationship!
contractual equal

ability of patients to engage in contractual therapeutic relationships. When people are sick, the focus upon equality is temporally misplaced. The goal of the therapeutic relationship is the "development" of the patient—helping to resolve the underlying physical (or mental) defect, and to deal with cognitive, psychological, and social constraints in order to restore autonomous functioning. In this sense, the doctor-patient interaction is not unlike the parent-child or teacher-student relationship.

The legal model also falls short because the therapeutic relationship is not a typical commodity exchange in which the parties use each other to accomplish mutually compatible goals, without taking a direct interest in each other. Rather, the status of patients as persons whose autonomy is compromised constitutes the very stuff of therapeutic art. The physician is attempting to alter the fundamental ability of patients to carry through their life plans. To accomplish this delicate task requires a personal knowledge about and interest in the patient. If we accept these points, then we must reject the narrow focus of medical ethics upon noninterference and emphasize patterns of interaction that free patients from constraints upon autonomy.

I hasten to add that I am criticizing the legal model only as a *complete* moral framework for therapeutic interaction. As case studies in medical ethics suggest, physicians and patients *are* potential adversaries. Moreover, the disability of the patient and various institutional controls provide physicians with a distinct "power advantage" that can be abused. Thus, a legitimate function of medical ethics is to formulate conditions that assure noninterference in patient decision making. But various positive interventions must also be emphasized, since the central task in the therapeutic process is assisting patients to reestablish control over their own lives.

In the last analysis, the crucial matter is how we view the patient who enters into the therapeutic relationship. Cassell points out that in the typical view "...the sick person is seen simply as a well person with a disease, rather than as qualitatively different, not only physically but also socially, emotionally, and even cognitively." In this view, "...the physician's role in the care of the sick is primarily the application of technology...and health can be seen as a commodity."[10] But if, as I believe, illness renders sick persons "qualitatively different," then respect for personal autonomy requires a therapeutic interaction considerably more complex than the noninterference strategy.

Thus the current "Principles of Medical Ethics" simply exhort physicians to be honest. But the crucial requirement is that physicians tell the truth in a way, at a time, and in whatever increments are necessary to allow patients to effectively use the information in adjusting their life plans.[11] Similarly, respecting a patient's refusal of treatment maximizes autonomy only if a balanced and thorough deliberation precedes the decision. Again, the "Principles" suggest that physicians observe strict confidentiality. But the more complex moral challenge is to use confidential information in a way that will help to give the patient more freedom. Thus, the doctor can keep a patient's report on family dynamics private, and still use it to modify attitudes or actions of family members that inhibit the patient's control.

truth

confidential

At its root, illness is an evil primarily because it compromises our efforts to control our lives. Thus, we must preserve an understanding of the physician's art that transcends noninterference and addresses this fundamental reality.

REFERENCES

1 American Medical Association, *Current Opinions of the Judicial Council of the American Medical Association* (Chicago, Illinois: American Medical Association, 1981), p. ix. Also see Robert Veatch, "Professional Ethics: New Principles for Physicians?," *Hastings Center Report* 10 (June 1980), 16–19.

2 The National Commission for the Protection of Human Subjects of Biomedical and Behavioral Research, *The Belmont Report: Ethical Principles and Guidelines for the Protection of Human Subjects of Research* (Washington, D.C.: U.S. Government Printing Office, 1978), p. 58.

3 Tom Beauchamp and James Childress, *Principles of Biomedical Ethics* (New York: Oxford University Press, 1980), p. 59.

4 Edmund Pellegrino, "Toward a Reconstruction of Medical Morality: The Primacy of the Act of Profession and the Fact of Illness," *The Journal of Medicine and Philosophy* 4 (1979), 44–45.

5 Talcott Parsons, *The Social System* (Glencoe, Illinois: The Free Press, 1951), p. 437.

6 Eric Cassell, *The Healer's Art* (New York: Lippincott, 1976), p. 44. Although Cassell aptly describes the goal of the healer's art, it is unclear whether he considers it to be based upon the obligation to

respect the patient's autonomy or the duty to enhance the well-being of the patient. Some parts of his discussion clearly suggest the latter.

7 Pedro Lain-Entralgo, *Doctor and Patient* (New York: McGraw-Hill, 1969), p. 155.

8 See Allen Buchanan, "Medical Paternalism," *Philosophy and Public Affairs* 7 (1978), 370–90.

9 My formulation of the components of the legal model differs from, but is highly indebted to, John Ladd's stimulating analysis in "Legalism and Medical Ethics," in John Davis et al., editors, *Contemporary Issues in Biomedical Ethics* (Clifton, N.J.: The Humana Press, 1979), pp. 1–35. However, I would not endorse Ladd's position that the moral principles that define our duties in the therapeutic setting are of a different logical type from those that define our duties to strangers.

10 Eric Cassell, "Therapeutic Relationship: Contemporary Medical Perspective," in Warren Reich, editor, *Encyclopedia of Bioethics* (New York: Macmillan, 1978), p. 1675.

11 Cf. Norman Cousins, "A Layman Looks at Truthtelling," *Journal of the American Medical Association* 244 (1980), 1929–30. Also see Howard Brody, "Hope," *Journal of the American Medical Association* 246 (1981), pp. 1411–12.

Psychiatric Consultation Masking Moral Dilemmas in Medicine

Mark Perl and Earl E. Shelp

Mark Perl, a psychiatrist, is assistant professor of psychiatry and director, Consultation-Liaison Service Department of Psychiatry at the University of Texas at Houston. Earl E. Shelp is assistant professor of bioethics, Institute of Religion and Baylor College of Medicine at the Texas Medical Center, Houston, Texas. Shelp is editor of *Justice and Health Care* (1981), *Beneficence and Health Care* (1982), and *The Clinical Encounter: The Moral Fabric of the Patient-Physician Relationship* (1983). His articles include "Justice: A Moral Test for Health Care and Health Policy."

Perl and Shelp point out that physicians who are faced with some moral dilemma in their dealings with patients or their families may sometimes call in a psychiatrist as a consultant. In doing so they may expect the psychiatrist to resolve the issue in accordance with the physician's wishes. Both the physicians and the patients in such cases tend not to see the psychiatrists consulted as moral arbiters but, rather, as experts in resolving intrapsychic and interpersonal conflict. But Perl and Shelp maintain that when psychiatrist-consultants act as the physicians expect, they may be acting in the former capacity rather than the latter. Perl and Shelp argue that the correct role for psychiatrists in such cases is to help patients arrive at decisions autonomously, even when those decisions are not in accordance with physicians' wishes.

Psychiatric consultations are a legitimate and necessary clinical activity in any general medical hospital or clinic. At times, however, psychiatrists are consulted when their fellow physicians face moral dilemmas related to patient care. In this article, we attempt to show that such moral issues may be masked as requests for help for a "depressed patient" or a "management problem."

Reprinted by permission of the *New England Journal of Medicine*. Vol. 307, pp. 618–21; 1982.

The practice of medicine abounds with value-laden decisions. Although this has generally been recognized, it has recently received increased attention in the press and the medical literature. Discussion has focused on the care of the dying, transplantation, abortion, genetic manipulation, behavior control, and other such visible morally debatable and troublesome problems. In addition, as Cassell[1] and Goldworth[2] have pointed out, even the day-to-day practice of medicine can be viewed as a predominantly moral activity supported by technical procedures. Most authors agree with Kass's opinion that medicine is more than merely "a technical service that is delivered, like auto repair or plumbing."[3] It is an enterprise encompassing human agents and wills; at times it touches the most dramatic and difficult situations and choices that people ever face. Medical schools, residency training programs, and continuing-education programs have increasingly recognized the importance of the teaching and discussion of ethics,[4-8] although there is controversy about how to approach the topic.[4,9-11]

Ethical dilemmas in medical care arise when a particular course of action involves a conflict between competing moral values. The patient and the physician may disagree about what is right, proper, or good, or the physician alone may face a choice between two or more difficult options. The opinions or demands of other interests—the patient's family, the law, and society at large—may further complicate the situation.

Sometimes nonpsychiatric physicians turn to their psychiatric colleagues for help and guidance with morally troublesome cases. In these contexts, psychiatrists are not necessarily seen as moral arbiters; rather, we believe they are regarded as experts in mediating and resolving conflict, both intrapsychic and interpersonal. The primary physician is often acutely aware of the patient's psychic distress and of the interpersonal tensions that accompany the medical-moral problems. The psychiatrist is expected to fill a mediating role, often with a mandate to resolve the situation in a particular direction, to persuade the patient or family to act in a certain way. In the process, unfortunately, a moral consideration of the proposed or expected actions and a consideration of the ethical dimensions of the case are often overlooked or ignored by both the primary physician and the psychiatrist.

We have examined three instances of such a series of events as they occurred in a large general hospital. We have no incidence or prevalence figures to quote, but we believe that the problem is regrettably common. In the following discussion, we will highlight the ethical aspects of each case, without undertaking a complete analysis. We will focus on the limitations of the psychiatrist's role and on the constructive part that he or she might properly play in the management of difficult cases that present moral dilemmas.

CASE 1: METASTATIC OSTEOSARCOMA

A 70-year-old man with no previous psychiatric history was treated surgically for metastatic osteosarcoma of the right hand. After several amputations had failed to arrest the disease, a further procedure was recommended in which the right arm would be disarticulated at the shoulder joint. The patient declined all further treatment and asked to be discharged. A psychiatric consultation was called for "depression." It was apparent that the primary physician had sought the psychiatrist's help in persuading the patient to have additional surgery.

At issue were conflicting notions of what action was morally required, given the circumstances of the case. Whereas the patient had exercised his moral and legal autonomy by his refusal of additional surgery, the surgeon viewed the situation in terms of professional duty rather than as an occasion to respect individual liberty or rights. He tended to give greater emphasis to the patient's putative duty to live and to his own understanding of the physician's duty to prolong life to the extent possible.

The psychiatrist was asked to address the patient's decision to refuse surgery; implicitly, the consultant was expected either to persuade the patient to consent or to find some basis for mental incompetence. The surgeon's unstated assumption seemed to be that this patient would not rationally choose to discontinue treatment and that his choice was largely the product of depression or some other emotional condition. We at the psychiatry service could not assume a priori that such was the case without examining the situation; furthermore, we were uncomfortable in the role that had (apparently) been assigned to us.

One could argue, however, that a range of activities might have been considered within the psychiatrist's realm in this case. For instance, it would have seemed appropriate to assess how the patient was coping with his situation and to offer him the opportunity to share with an interested and understanding professional the web of complex feelings leading up to his decision. The patient's family might have welcomed the opportunity to receive counseling during this distressing period of crisis. There may also have been good reason to work with the primary physician (and other staff members) to help them sort out their feelings about this dying patient and his decision to stop treatment. Perhaps the psychiatrist could best have been of service by helping to sort out the sources of discomfort of all the various parties and pointed out that there were difficult ethical questions to be considered, which did not necessarily fall within the expertise of the psychiatrist. Ethical issues do not necessarily submit to psychiatric resolution.

We interviewed the patient, and found that although he was distressed by his circumstances, his decision-making ability was not impaired. He and his family were offered counseling by our staff but declined further psychiatric contact. Other support services—pastoral care and social services—were made available. Eventually, the patient's wishes were respected, and he was discharged to his home.

CASE 2: REQUEST FOR STERILIZATION

A 21-year-old single woman, who had had two unwanted pregnancies, requested tubal ligation to prevent further pregnancies. She had tried using contraceptive pills and a diaphragm but seemed to have difficulty employing them correctly. She was unwilling to use an intrauterine device. Her gynecologist referred her to a psychiatrist on the grounds that "no competent person would seek sterilization so early in life."

The gynecologist's dilemma turned on questions about the proper use of medical technology. Is the purpose of medicine to cure disease only, or does it encompass procedures to facilitate better living as defined by the patient? What are the indications for medical intervention in this sort of circumstance, and what are the indications for nonintervention, even when intervention is requested? The age of the patient, her marital status, the irreversible nature of the procedure, and the belief that in general elective sterilizations were immoral contributed to the gynecologist's discomfort at the request. His personal biases regarding reproduction tended to prejudice his view regarding the mental competency of the patient.

It seemed appropriate for our service to offer this patient psychotherapy in order to discuss her difficulties in the past. It also seemed likely that she might appreciate the presence of a sympathetic, nonjudgmental counselor in grappling with the pros and cons of undergoing this almost irreversible procedure. Furthermore, it is routine in many settings to ensure that such a decision is an informed one—that the patient understands the procedure and its consequences, as well as alternative means of contraception. (We wonder, though, whether a psychiatrist should necessarily be consulted for this, or whether another physician or layperson could make that determination.)

It is important to note that the issues of therapy and evaluation of the capacity to give informed consent are clearly separable and distinct from the above-mentioned moral questions and not related to them. In the current case, the patient was judged able to give fully informed consent and did not wish to be counseled. The gynecologist accepted our assessment but referred her elsewhere for sterilization, since he was unwilling to operate.

CASE 3: BRAIN DEATH

A 35-year-old man involved in a motor-vehicle accident sustained severe head injuries and was declared brain-dead by the neurosurgeon. The family was so advised, and permission was sought to turn off the patient's respirator and other life supports. At this time the organ-transplantation team requested permission to obtain the patient's kidneys. His wife refused both requests, wanting instead to take the patient home and maintain him on a respirator for as long as possible. She was referred for psychiatric consultation.

The neurosurgeon seemed to be facing a dilemma related to the decision to cease life support. In such cases, decisions of the next of kin are usually respected. In this case, however, the decisions of the spouse were at odds with the wishes of the primary physician. The neurosurgeon was uncomfortable with the idea of allowing the patient to suffer biologic death at home at a later time. It is impossible to isolate a single reason for the neurosurgeon's discomfort. Perhaps he acted out of a benevolent desire to relieve the stress on the family in dealing with the final hours. Perhaps he perceived the patient's wife as extraordinarily distressed and trying to deny the medical facts of her husband's case and wishing for a miracle cure. Perhaps, too, he was under pressure from his colleagues to obtain the kidneys.

There was, of course, an appropriate place for professional counseling of the patient's relatives. Families weighing the unpleasant alternatives before them may welcome the chance to explore their feelings before making their decision. There is much latitude in deciding whether to refer such families to a psychiatrist or to another professional, for example, a member of the clergy or a social worker. In some centers the psychiatry service routinely sees the relatives of every patient in the intensive-care unit. In this case, however, calling in a psychiatrist was unusual. As in all the cases discussed above, there was a danger that the primary physician would implicitly invalidate a decision that conflicted with the physician's own wishes or value system, by suggesting that it did not have a rational basis.

We advised the neurosurgeon that the decision to discontinue life support was a moral and legal issue, not necessarily a psychiatric issue. We counseled the patient's wife and other family members to help them cope with their distress. Eventually, the patient's wife and other relatives decided against taking the patient home and in favor of ceasing mechanical life support; we hope that this was not because of any subtle coercion on our part. Kidney donation was refused.

DISCUSSION

One might wonder whether psychiatrists should acquire a mantle of expertise in moral and ethical matters. Certainly Freud[12] was delighted by the prospect that psychiatrists might become "secular pastoral workers" using science to guide human choices and values. More recently, Breggin[13] reiterated this theme, going so far as to refer to psychotherapy as "applied ethics." Confusion has arisen in some professional circles and in the public mind about the proper role of the psychiatrist in medicine and society. Being an expert in the science of human behavior tends to be equated with knowing which behavior is morally right. Psychiatrists are customarily called in to render opinions on what are, in fact, ethical and legal questions—in schools, courts, prisons and the military.[14–16]

Not surprisingly, then, internists, surgeons, and other nonpsychiatric physicians may call on psychiatrists when facing an ethical quandary. Psychiatrists are seen by their colleagues as having added training in dealing with conflict, including moral conflict, as being more reflective, and as having more time to assess the situation. Many authors suggest that the presence of a psychiatric consultant on the medical team has a humanizing, moral influence. This ascription is applied even more strongly to the liaison psychiatrist. Thus, Krakowski sees the psychiatrist as a guardian of the psychosocial and holistic approach to the patient, and

by implication, as being more approachable than other physicians on moral questions as well.[17]

There is a danger in artificially demarcating physicians' roles in this way. If the psychiatrist is seen as more humanistic, is the surgeon less so? Such an approach militates against, rather than in favor of, the biopsychosocial unity of medicine. Can any physician learn to understand and constructively deal with moral conflict by routinely calling in a stranger to make the decision for him or her? To some degree at least, moral choices are personal, with effects on others. It appears to serve no legitimate purpose for medicine to mask moral choices as psychiatric problems—that is, as merely belonging to another field of medicine. In some cases the act of calling in a psychiatrist communicates a threat to the patient of being labeled mentally incompetent or insane. The consultation thus acts as a subtle lever to coerce patients to comply with the primary physician's moral judgments or treatment preference.

Much has been written about the value of psychiatric consultation in the general medical setting. Little has been said, however, about what is outside the proper role and expertise of the psychiatrist. The temptation is great for the psychiatrist to assume the role of moral guide or moral decision maker. But the psychiatrist's mission has traditionally been one of helping patients arrive at decisions autonomously, of providing the opportunity to discuss and explore complex issues and feelings in a nonjudgmental setting. It would seem imprudent for the psychiatrist in cases like those discussed above to lend authority to another physician in influencing a patient's decisions (so as to conform to that physician's desires) when the patient is competent to choose among morally defensible options.

REFERENCES

1 Cassell, E. J., Moral thought in clinical practice: applying the abstract to the usual. In: Engelhardt, H. T., Callahan, D., eds., *Science, ethics, and medicine*. Vol. 1. The foundation of ethics and its relationship to science. Hastings-on-Hudson, N.Y.: The Hastings Center, Institute of Society, Ethics and the Life Sciences. 1976:147–60.

2 Goldworth, A., Moral questions in a clinical setting. In: Engelhardt, H. T., Callahan, D., eds. *Science, ethics and medicine*. Vol. 1. The foundation of ethics and its relationship to science. Hastings-on-

Hudson, N.Y.: The Hastings Center, Institute of Society, Ethics and the Life Sciences, 1976:161–6.

3 Kass, L. R., Ethical dilemmas in the care of the ill. I. What is the physician's service. *JAMA*. 1980; 244:1811–6.

4 Shelp, E. E., Russell, M. L., Grose, N. P., Students' attitudes to ethics in the medical school curriculum. *J Med Ethics*. 1981; 7:70–3.

5 Levine, M. D., Scott, L., Curran, W. J., Ethics rounds in a children's medical center: evaluation of a hospital-based program for continuing education in medical ethics. *Pediatrics*. 1977; 60:202–8.

6 Keller, A. H., Ethics/human values education in the family practice residency. *J Med Educ*. 1977; 52:107–16.

7 Jellinek, M., Parmelee, D., Is there a role for medical ethics in postgraduate psychiatry courses? *Am J Psychiatry*. 1977; 134:1438–9.

8 Appelbaum, P. S., Reiser, S. J., Ethics rounds: a model for teaching ethics in the psychiatric setting. *Hosp Community Psychiatry*. 1981; 32:555–60.

9 White, R. J., Is formal ethics training really needed? *Am Med News*. 1981; August 14:16.

10 Boisaubin, E. V., Ethical training of M.D.s is imperative. *Am Med News*. 1981; October 23:22.

11 Barthel, J. S., Ethical physicians are made from ethical medical students. *Am Med News*. 1981; October 16:5.

12 Freud, S., The question of lay analysis (1926); Postscript (1927). In: Strachey, J., ed. *Standard edition of the complete psychological works of Sigmund Freud*. London: Hogarth, 1959: vol. 20, 179–258.

13 Breggin, P. R., Psychotherapy as applied ethics. *Psychiatry*. 1971; 34:59–74.

14 Shelp, E. E., Reflections on the morality of psychiatry. In: Hall, R. C. W., ed. *Psychiatry in crisis*. New York: Spectrum, 1982:11–24.

15 The Hastings Center. In the service of the state: the psychiatrist as double agent: a conference on conflicting loyalties by the American Psychiatric Association and the Hastings Center/ March 24–26, 1977. *Hastings Center Rep*. 1978; 8: Suppl 1–24.

16 Menninger, K., *Whatever became of sin?* New York: Hawthorne, 1973.

17 Krakowski, A. J., Liaison psychiatry: a service for averting dehumanization of medicine. *Psychother Psychosom*. 1979; 32:164–9.

Truth-Telling

Lies to the Sick and Dying

Sissela Bok

Sissela Bok teaches ethics at the Harvard Medical School. She has written numerous articles on medical ethics including "The Ethics of Giving Placebos." Bok has served on human-experimentation committees in hospitals and on the Ethics Advisory Board to the Secretary of Health, Education, and Welfare (1979–1980). She is the author of *Lying: Moral Choice in Public and Private Life* (1978), from which this article is excerpted, and *Secrets: On the Ethics of Concealment and Revelation* (1983).

Bok challenges the following claims that physicians often make: (1) patients do not want bad news; and (2) truthful information harms patients. Against (1) Bok argues: (a) studies have shown that physicians and patients differ widely on the factual question of whether patients want to know the truth in the case of serious illness; and (b) physicians are only partly correct in their claim that patients who *say* they want to know the truth deny the truth even when given it repeatedly. Against (2) Bok argues: (a) the harm resulting from the disclosure of bad news or risks to patients is much less than physicians think; and (b) the benefits resulting from such disclosures are much more substantial than physicians believe. In responding to the two claims, Bok also brings out some of the other possible bad consequences of lying to patients with serious illnesses.

A forty-six-year-old man, coming to a clinic for a routine physical check-up needed for insurance purposes, is diagnosed as having a form of cancer likely to cause him to die within six months. No known cure exists for it. Chemotherapy may prolong life by a few extra months, but will have side effects the physician does not think warranted in this case. In addition, he believes that such therapy should be reserved for patients with a chance for recovery or remission. The patient has no symptoms giving him any reason to believe that he is not perfectly healthy. He expects to take a short vacation in a week.

For the physician, there are now several choices involving truthfulness. Ought he to tell the patient what he has learned, or conceal it? If asked, should he deny it? If he decides to reveal the diagnosis, should he delay doing so until after the patient returns from his vacation? Finally, even if he does reveal the serious nature of the diagnosis, should he mention the possibility of chemotherapy and his reasons for not recommending it in this case? Or should he encourage every last effort to postpone death?

In this particular case, the physician chose to inform the patient of his diagnosis right away. He did not, however, mention the possibility of chemotherapy. A medical student working under him disagreed; several nurses also thought that the patient should have been informed of this possibility. They tried, unsuccessfully, to persuade the physician that this was the patient's right. When persuasion had failed, the student elected to disobey the doctor by informing the patient of the alternative of chemotherapy. After consultation with family members, the patient chose to ask for the treatment.

Doctors confront such choices often and urgently. What they reveal, hold back, or distort will matter profoundly to their patients. Doctors stress with corresponding vehemence their reasons for the distortion or concealment: not to confuse a sick person needlessly, or cause what may well be unnecessary pain or discomfort, as in the case of the cancer patient; not to leave a patient without hope, as in those many cases where the dying are not told the truth about their condition; or to improve the chances of cure, as where unwarranted optimism is expressed about some form of therapy. Doctors use information as part of the therapeutic regimen; it is given out in amounts, in admixtures, and according to timing believed best for patients. Accuracy, by comparison, matters far less.

Lying to patients has, therefore, seemed an especially excusable act. Some would argue that doctors, and *only* doctors, should be granted the right to manipulate the truth in ways so undesirable for politicians, lawyers, and others.[1] Doctors are trained to help patients; their relationship to patients carries special obligations, and they know much more than laymen about what helps and hinders recovery and survival.

Even the most conscientious doctors, then, who hold themselves at a distance from the quacks and the purveyors of false remedies, hesitate to forswear all lying. Lying is usually wrong, they argue, but less so than allowing the truth to harm patients. B.C. Meyer echoes this very common view:

> [O]urs is a profession which traditionally has been guided by a precept that transcends the virtue of uttering truth for truth's sake, and that is, "so far as possible, do no harm."[2]

Truth, for Meyer, may be important, but not when it endangers the health and well-being of patients. This has seemed self-evident to many physicians in the past—so much so that we find very few mentions of veracity in the codes and oaths and writings by physicians through the centuries. This absence is all the more striking as other principles of ethics have been consistently and movingly expressed in the same documents.

The two fundamental principles of doing good and not doing harm—of beneficence and nonmaleficence—are the most immediately relevant to medical practitioners, and the most frequently stressed. To preserve life and good health, to ward off illness, pain, and death—these are the perennial tasks of medicine and nursing. These principles have found powerful expression at all times in the history of medicine. In the Hippocratic Oath physicians promise to:

> use treatment to help the sick...but never with a view to injury and wrong-doing.[3]

And a Hindu oath of initiation says:

> Day and night, however thou mayest be engaged, thou shalt endeavor for the relief of patients with all thy heart and soul. Thou shalt not desert or injure the patient even for the sake of thy living.[4]

But there is no similar stress on veracity. It is absent from virtually all oaths, codes, and prayers. The Hippocratic Oath makes no mention of truthfulness to patients about their condition, prognosis, or treatment. Other early codes and prayers are equally silent on the subject. To be sure, they often refer to the confidentiality with which doctors should treat all that patients tell them; but there is no corresponding reference to honesty toward the patient. One of the few who appealed to such a principle was Amatus Lusitanus, a Jewish physician widely known for his skill, who, persecuted, died of the plague in 1568. He published an oath which reads in part:

> If I lie, may I incur the eternal wrath of God and of His angel Raphael, and may nothing in the medical art succeed for me according to my desires.[5]

Later codes continue to avoid the subject. Not even the Declaration of Geneva, adopted in 1948 by the World Medical Association, makes any reference to it. And the Principles of Medical Ethics of the American Medical Association[6] still leave the matter of informing patients up to the physician.

Given such freedom, a physician can decide to tell as much or as little as he wants the patient to know, so long as he breaks no law. In the case of the man mentioned at the beginning of this chapter, some physicians might feel justified in lying for the good of the patient, others might be truthful. Some may conceal alternatives to the treatment they recommend; others not. In each case, they could appeal to the A.M.A. Principles of Ethics. A great many would choose to be able to lie. They would claim that not only can a lie avoid harm for the patient, but that it is also hard to know whether they have been right in the first place in making their pessimistic diagnosis; a "truthful" statement could therefore turn out to hurt patients unnecessarily. The concern for curing and for supporting those who cannot be cured then runs counter to the desire to be completely open. This concern is especially strong where the prognosis is bleak; even more so when patients are so affected by their illness or their medication that they are more dependent than usual, perhaps more easily depressed or irrational.

Physicians know only too well how uncertain a diagnosis or prognosis can be. They know how hard it is to give meaningful and correct answers regarding health and illness. They also know that disclosing their own uncertainty or fears can reduce those benefits that depend upon faith in recovery. They fear, too, that revealing grave risks, no matter how unlikely it is that these will come about, may exercise the pull of the "self-fulfilling prophecy." They dislike being the bearers of uncertain or bad news as much as anyone else. And last, but not least, sitting down to discuss an illness truthfully and sensitively may take much-needed time away from other patients.

These reasons help explain why nurses and physicians and relatives of the sick and dying prefer not to be bound by rules that might limit their ability to suppress, delay, or distort information. This is not to say that they necessarily plan to lie much of the time. They merely want to have the freedom to do so when they believe it wise. And the reluctance to see lying prohibited explains, in turn, the failure of the codes and oaths to come to grips with the problems of truth-telling and lying.

But sharp conflicts are now arising. Doctors no longer work alone with patients. They have to consult with others much more than before; if they choose to lie, the choice may not be met with approval by all who take part in the care of the patient. A nurse expresses the difficulty which results as follows:

> From personal experience I would say that the patients who aren't told about their terminal illness have so many verbal and mental questions unanswered that many will begin to realize that their illness is more serious than they're being told.[...]
>
> Nurses care for these patients twenty-four hours a day compared to a doctor's daily brief visit, and it is the nurse many times that the patient will relate to, once his underlying fears become overwhelming. [...]This is difficult for us nurses because being in

constant contact with patients we can see the events leading up to this. The patient continually asks you, "Why isn't my pain decreasing?" or "Why isn't the radiation treatment easing the pain?"[...]We cannot legally give these patients an honest answer as a nurse (and I'm sure I wouldn't want to) yet the problem is still not resolved and the circle grows larger and larger with the patient alone in the middle.[7]

The doctor's choice to lie increasingly involves co-workers in acting a part they find neither humane nor wise. The fact that these problems have not been carefully thought through within the medical profession, nor seriously addressed in medical education, merely serves to intensify the conflicts.[8] Different doctors then respond very differently to patients in exactly similar predicaments. The friction is increased by the fact that relatives often disagree even where those giving medical care to a patient are in accord on how to approach the patient. Here again, because physicians have not worked out to common satisfaction the question of whether relatives have the right to make such requests, the problems are allowed to be haphazardly resolved by each physician as he sees fit.

THE PATIENT'S PERSPECTIVE

The turmoil in the medical profession regarding truth-telling is further augmented by the pressures that patients themselves now bring to bear and by empirical data coming to light. Challenges are growing to [two] major arguments for lying to patients:... Patients do not want bad news; and truthful information harms them....

The [first] argument for deceiving patients refers specifically to giving them news of a frightening or depressing kind. It holds that patients do not, in fact, generally want such information, that they prefer not to have to face up to serious illness and death. On the basis of such a belief, most doctors in a number of surveys stated that they do not, as a rule, inform patients that they have an illness such as cancer.

When studies are made of what patients desire to know, on the other hand, a large majority say that they *would* like to be told of such a diagnosis.[9] All these studies need updating and should be done with larger numbers of patients and non-patients. But they do show that there is generally a dramatic divergence between physicians and patients on the factual question of whether patients want to know what ails them in cases of serious illness such as cancer. In most of the studies, over 80 percent of the persons asked indicated that they would want to be told.

Sometimes this discrepancy is set aside by doctors who want to retain the view that patients do not want unhappy news. In reality, they claim, the fact that patients say they want it has to be discounted. The more someone asks to know, the more he suffers from fear which will lead to the denial of the information even if it is given. Informing patients is, therefore, useless; they resist and deny having been told what they cannot assimilate. According to this view, empirical studies of what patients say they want are worthless since they do not probe deeply enough to uncover this universal resistance to the contemplation of one's own death.

This view is only partially correct. For some patients, denial is indeed well established in medical experience. A number of patients (estimated at between 15 percent and 25 percent) will give evidence of denial of having been told about their illness, even when they repeatedly ask and are repeatedly informed. And nearly everyone experiences a period of denial at some point in the course of approaching death.[10] Elisabeth Kübler-Ross sees denial as resulting often from premature and abrupt information by a stranger who goes through the process quickly to "get it over with." She holds that denial functions as a buffer after unexpected shocking news, permitting individuals to collect themselves and to mobilize other defenses. She describes prolonged denial in one patient as follows:

> She was convinced that the X-rays were "mixed up"; she asked for reassurance that her pathology report could not possibly be back so soon and that another patient's report must have been marked with her name. When none of this could be confirmed, she quickly asked to leave the hospital, looking for another physician in the vain hope "to get a better explanation for my troubles." This patient went "shopping around" for many doctors, some of whom gave her reassuring answers, others of whom confirmed the previous suspicion. Whether confirmed or not, she reacted in the same manner; she asked for examination and reexamination....[11]

But to say that denial is universal flies in the face of all evidence. And to take any claim to the contrary as "symptomatic" of deeper denial leaves no room for reasoned discourse. There is no way that such universal denial can be proved true or false. To believe in it is a metaphysical belief about man's condition, not a statement about what patients do and do not want. It is true that we can never completely understand the possibility of our own death, any more than being alive in the first place. But people certainly differ in the degree to which they can approach such knowledge, take it into account in their plans, and make their peace with it.

Montaigne claimed that in order to learn both to live and to die, men have to think about death and be prepared to accept it.[12] To stick one's head in the sand, or to be prevented by lies from trying to discern what is to come, hampers freedom—freedom to consider one's life as a whole, with a beginning, a duration, an end. Some may request to be deceived rather than to see their lives as thus finite; others reject the information which would require them to do so; but most say that they want to know. Their concern for knowing about their condition goes far beyond mere curiosity or the wish to make isolated personal choices in the short time left to them; their stance toward the entire life they have lived, and their ability to give it meaning and completion, are at stake.[13] In lying or withholding the facts which permit such discernment, doctors may reflect their own fears (which, according to one study,[14] are much stronger than those of laymen) of facing questions about the meaning of one's life and the inevitability of death.

Beyond the fundamental deprivation that can result from deception, we are also becoming increasingly aware of all that can befall patients in the course of their illness when information is denied or distorted. Lies place them in a position where they no longer participate in choices concerning their own health, including the choice of whether to be "patient" in the first place. A terminally ill person who is not informed that his illness is incurable and that he is near death cannot make decisions about the end of his life; about whether or not to enter a hospital, or to have surgery; where and with whom to spend his last days; how to put his affairs in order—these most personal choices cannot be made if he is kept in the dark, or given contradictory hints and clues.

It has always been especially easy to keep knowledge from terminally ill patients. They are most vulnerable, least able to take action to learn what they need to know, or to protect their autonomy. The very fact of being so ill greatly increases the likelihood of control by others. And the fear of being helpless in the face of such control is growing. At the same time, the period of dependency and slow deterioration of health and strength that people undergo has lengthened. There has been a dramatic shift toward institutionalization of the aged and those near death. (Over 80 percent of Americans now die in a hospital or other institution.)

Patients who are severely ill often suffer a further distancing and loss of control over their most basic functions. Electrical wiring, machines, intravenous administration of liquids, all create new dependency and at the same time new distance between the patient and all who come near. Curable patients are often willing to undergo such procedures; but when no cure is possible, these procedures merely intensify the sense of distance and uncertainty and can even become a substitute for comforting human acts. Yet those who suffer in this way often fear to seem troublesome by complaining. Lying to them, perhaps for the most charitable of purposes, can then cause them to slip unwittingly into subjection to new procedures, perhaps new surgery, where death is held at bay through transfusions, respirators, even resuscitation far beyond what most would wish.

Seeing relatives in such predicaments has caused a great upsurge of worrying about death and dying. At the root of this fear is not a growing terror of the *moment* of death, or even the instants before it. Nor is there greater fear of *being* dead. In contrast to the centuries of lives lived in dread of the punishments to be inflicted after death, many would now accept the view expressed by Epicurus, who died in 270 B.C.:[15]

Death, therefore, the most awful of evils, is nothing to us, seeing that, when we are, death is not come, and, when death is come, we are not.

The growing fear, if it is not of the moment of dying nor of being dead, is of all that which now precedes dying for so many: the possibility of prolonged pain, the increasing weakness, the uncertainty, the loss of powers and chance of senility, the sense of being a burden. This fear is further nourished by the loss of trust in health professionals. In part, the loss of trust results from the abuses which have been exposed—the Medicaid scandals, the old-age home profiteering, the commercial exploitation of those who seek remedies for their ailments;[16] in part also because of the deceptive practices patients suspect, having seen how friends and relatives were kept in the dark; in part, finally, because of the sheer numbers of persons, often strangers, participating in the care of any one patient. Trust which might have gone to a doctor long known to the patient goes less easily to a team of strangers, no matter how expert or well-meaning.

It is with the working out of all that *informed consent*[17] implies and the information it presupposes that truth-telling is coming to be discussed in a serious way for the first time in the health professions. Informed consent is a farce if the information provided is distorted or withheld. And even complete information regarding surgical procedures or medication is obviously useless unless the patient also knows what the condition is that these are supposed to correct.

Bills of rights for patients, similarly stressing the right to be informed, are now gaining acceptance.[18] This right is not new, but the effort to implement it is. Nevertheless, even where patients are handed the most elegantly phrased Bill of Rights, their right to a truthful diagnosis and prognosis is by no means always respected.

The reason why even doctors who recognize a patient's right to have information might still not provide it brings us the [second] argument against telling all patients the truth. It holds that the information given might hurt the patient and that the concern for the right to such information is therefore a threat to proper health care. A patient, these doctors argue, may wish to commit suicide after being given discouraging news, or suffer a cardiac arrest, or simply cease to struggle, and thus not grasp the small remaining chance for recovery. And even where the outlook for a patient is very good, the disclosure of a minute risk can shock some patients or cause them to reject needed protection such as a vaccination or antibiotics.

The factual basis for this argument has been challenged from two points of view. The damages associated with the disclosure of sad news or risks are rarer than physicians believe; and the *benefits* which result from being informed are more substantial, even measurably so. Pain is tolerated more easily, recovery from surgery is quicker, and cooperation with therapy is greatly improved. The attitude that "what you don't know won't hurt you" is proving unrealistic; it is what patients do not know but vaguely suspect that causes them corrosive worry.

It is certain that no answers to this question of harm from information are the same for all patients. If we look, first, at the fear expressed by physicians that informing patients of even remote or unlikely risks connected with a drug prescription or operation might shock some and make others refuse the treatment that would have been best for them, it appears to be unfounded for the great majority of patients. Studies show that very few patients respond to being told of such risks by withdrawing their consent to the procedure and that those who do withdraw are the very ones who might well have been upset enough to sue the physician had they not been asked to consent beforehand.[19] It is possible that on even rarer occasions especially susceptible persons might manifest physical deteriorations from shock; some physicians have even asked whether patients who die after giving informed consent to an operation, but before it actually takes place, somehow expire because of the information given to them.[20] While such questions are unanswerable in any one case, they certainly argue in favor of caution, a real concern for the person to whom one is recounting the risks he or she will face, and sensitivity to all signs of distress.

The situation is quite different when persons who are already ill, perhaps already quite weak and discouraged, are told of a very serious prognosis. Physicians fear that such knowledge may cause the patients to commit suicide, or to be frightened or depressed to the point that their illness takes a downward turn. The fear that great numbers of patients will commit suicide appears to be unfounded.[21] And if some do, is that a response so unreasonable, so much against the patient's best interest that physicians ought to make it a reason for concealment or lies? Many societies have allowed suicide in the past; our own has decriminalized it; and some are coming to make distinctions among the many suicides which ought to be prevented if at all possible, and those which ought to be respected.[22]

Another possible response to very bleak news is the triggering of physiological mechanisms which allow death to come more quickly—a form of giving up or of preparing for the inevitable, depending on one's outlook. Lewis Thomas, studying responses in humans and animals, holds it not unlikely that:

> [...]there is a pivotal movement at some stage in the body's reaction to injury or disease, maybe in aging as well, when the organism concedes that it is finished and the time for dying is at hand, and at this moment the events that lead to death are launched, as a

coordinated mechanism. Functions are then shut off, in sequence, irreversibly, and, while this is going on, a neural mechanism, held ready for this occasion, is switched on....[23]

Such a response may be appropriate, in which case it makes the moments of dying as peaceful as those who have died and been resuscitated so often testify. But it may also be brought on inappropriately, when the organism could have lived on, perhaps even induced malevolently, by external acts intended to kill. Thomas speculates that some of the deaths resulting from "hexing" are due to such responses. Lévi-Strauss describes deaths from exorcism and the casting of spells in ways which suggest that the same process may then be brought on by the community.[24]

It is not inconceivable that unhappy news abruptly conveyed, or a great shock given to someone unable to tolerate it, could also bring on such a "dying response," quite unintended by the speaker. There is every reason to be cautious and to try to know ahead of time how susceptible a patient might be to the accidental triggering—however rare—of such a response. One has to assume, however, that most of those who have survived long enough to be in a situation where their informed consent is asked have a very robust resistance to such accidental triggering of processes leading to death.

When, on the other hand, one considers those who are already near death, the "dying response" may be much less inappropriate, much less accidental, much less unreasonable. In most societies, long before the advent of modern medicine, human beings have made themselves ready for death once they felt its approach. Philippe Ariès describes how many in the Middle Ages prepared themselves for death when they "felt the end approach." They awaited death lying down, surrounded by friends and relatives. They recollected all they had lived through and done, pardoning all who stood near their deathbed, calling on God to bless them, and finally praying. "After the final prayer all that remained was to wait for death, and there was no reason for death to tarry."[25]

Modern medicine, in its valiant efforts to defer disease and to save lives, may be dislocating the conscious as well as the purely organic responses allowing death to come when it is inevitable, thus denying those who are dying the benefits of the traditional approach to death. In lying to them, and in pressing medical efforts to cure them long past the point of possible recovery, physicians may thus rob individuals of an autonomy few would choose to give up.

Sometimes, then, the "dying response" is a natural organic reaction at the time when the body has no further defense. Sometimes it is inappropriately brought on by news too shocking or given in too abrupt a manner. We need to learn a great deal more about this last category, no matter how small. But there is no evidence that patients in general will be debilitated by truthful information about their condition.

Apart from the possible harm from information, we are coming to learn much more about the benefits it can bring patients. People follow instructions more carefully if they know what their disease is and why they are asked to take medication; any benefits from those procedures are therefore much more likely to come about.[26] Similarly, people recover faster from surgery and tolerate pain with less medication if they understand what ails them and what can be done for them....[27]

NOTES

1 Plato, *The Republic*, 389 b.

2 B. C. Meyer, "Truth and the Physician," *Bulletin of the New York Academy of Medicine* 45 (1969): 59–71. See, too, the quotation from Dr. Henderson in Chapter I of this book [original source of this selection], p. 12.

3 W. H. S. Jones, trans., *Hippocrates*, Loeb Classical Library (Cambridge, Mass.: Harvard University Press, 1923), p. 164.

4 Reprinted in M. B. Etziony, *The Physician's Creed: An Anthology of Medical Prayers, Oaths and Codes of Ethics* (Springfield, Ill.: Charles C. Thomas, 1973), pp. 15–18.

5 See Harry Friedenwald, "The Ethics of the Practice of Medicine from the Jewish Point of View," *Johns Hopkins Hospital Bulletin*, no. 318 (August 1917), pp. 256–261.

6 "Ten Principles of Medical Ethics," *Journal of the American Medical Association* 164 (1957): 1119–20.

7 Mary Barrett, letter, *Boston Globe*, 16 November 1976, p. 1.

8 Though a minority of physicians have struggled to

bring them to our attention. See Thomas Percival, *Medical Ethics*, 3d ed. (Oxford: John Henry Parker, 1849), pp. 132–41; Worthington Hooker, *Physician and Patient* (New York: Baker and Scribner, 1849), pp. 357–82; Richard C. Cabot, "Teamwork of Doctor and Patient Through the Annihilation of Lying," in *Social Service and the Art of Healing* (New York: Moffat, Yard & Co., 1909), pp. 116–70; Charles C. Lund, "The Doctor, the Patient, and the Truth," *Annals of Internal Medicine* 24 (1946): 955; Edmund Davies, "The Patient's Right to Know the Truth," *Proceedings of the Royal Society of Medicine* 66 (1973): 533–36.

9 For the views of physicians, see Donald Oken, "What to Tell Cancer Patients," *Journal of the American Medical Association* 175 (1961): 1120–28; and tabulations in Robert Veatch, *Death, Dying, and the Biological Revolution* (New Haven and London: Yale University Press, 1976), pp. 229–38. For the view of patients, see Veatch, *ibid.*; Jean Aitken-Swan and E.C. Easson, "Reactions of Cancer Patients on Being Told Their Diagnosis," *British Medical Journal*, 1959, pp. 779–83; Jim McIntosh, "Patients' Awareness and Desire for Information About Diagnosed but Undisclosed Malignant Disease," *The Lancet* 7 (1976): 300–303; William D. Kelly and Stanley R. Friesen, "Do Cancer Patients Want to Be Told?," *Surgery* 27 (1950): 822–26.

10 See Avery Weisman, *On Dying and Denying* (New York: Behavioral Publications, 1972); Elisabeth Kübler-Ross, *On Death and Dying* (New York: The Macmillan Co., 1969); Ernest Becker, *The Denial of Death* (New York: Free Press, 1973); Philippe Ariès, *Western Attitudes Toward Death*, trans. Patricia M. Ranum (Baltimore and London: Johns Hopkins University Press, 1974); and Sigmund Freud, "Negation," *Collected Papers*, ed. James Strachey (London: Hogarth Press, 1950), 5: 181–85.

11 Kübler-Ross, *On Death and Dying*, p. 34.

12 Michel de Montaigne, *Essays*, bk. 1, chap. 20.

13 It is in literature that these questions are most directly raised. Two recent works where they are taken up with striking beauty and simplicity are May Sarton, *As We Are Now* (New York: W.W. Norton & Co., 1973); and Freya Stark, *A Peak in Darien* (London: John Murray, 1976).

14 Herman Feifel et al., "Physicians Consider Death," *Proceedings of the American Psychoanalytical Association*, 1967, pp. 201–2.

15 See Diogenes Laertius, *Lives of Eminent Philosophers*, p. 651. Epicurus willed his garden to his friends and descendants, and wrote on the eve of dying:
"On this blissful day, which is also the last of my life, I write to you. My continual sufferings from strangury and dysentery are so great that nothing could augment them; but over against them all I set gladness of mind at the remembrance of our past conversations." (Letter to Idomeneus, *Ibid.*, p. 549).

16 See Ivan Illich, *Medical Nemesis* (New York: Pantheon, 1976), for a critique of the iatrogenic tendencies of contemporary medical care in industrialized societies.

17 The law requires that inroads made upon a person's body take place only with the informed voluntary consent of that person. The term "informed consent" came into common use only after 1960, when it was used by the Kansas Supreme Court in *Nathanson vs. Kline,* 186 Kan. 393,350, p.2d,1093 (1960). The patient is now entitled to full disclosure of risks, benefits, and alternative treatments to any proposed procedure, both in therapy and in medical experimentation, except in emergencies or when the patient is incompetent, in which case proxy consent is required.

18 See, for example, "Statement on a Patient's Bill of Rights," reprinted in Stanley Joel Reiser, Arthur J. Dyck, and William J. Curran, *Ethics in Medicine* (Cambridge, Mass. and London: MIT Press, 1977), p. 148.

19 See Ralph Alfidi, "Informed Consent: A Study of Patient Reaction," *Journal of the American Medical Association* 216 (1971): 1325–29.

20 See Steven R. Kaplan, Richard A. Greenwald, and Arvey I. Rogers, Letter to the Editor, *New England Journal of Medicine* 296 (1977): 1127.

21 Oken, "What to Tell Cancer Patients"; Veatch, *Death, Dying, and the Biological Revolution*; Weisman, *On Dying and Denying*.

22 Norman L. Cantor, "A Patient's Decision to Decline Life-Saving Treatment: Bodily Integrity Versus the Preservation of Life," *Rutgers Law Review*, 26: 228–64; Danielle Gourevitch, "Suicide Among the Sick in Classical Antiquity," *Bulletin of the History of Medicine* 18 (1969): 501–18; for bibliography, see Bok, "Voluntary Euthanasia."

23 Lewis Thomas, "A Meliorist View of Disease and Dying," *The Journal of Medicine and Philosophy*, I (1976): 212–21.

24 Claude Lévi-Strauss, *Structural Anthropology* (New York: Basic Books, 1963), p. 167; See also Eric Cassell, "Permission to Die," in John Behnke and Sissela Bok, eds., *The Dilemmas of Euthanasia* (New York: Doubleday, Anchor Press, 1975), pp. 121–31.

25 Ariès, *Western Attitudes Toward Death*, p. 11.

26 Barbara S. Hulka, J. C. Cassel, et al. "Communication, Compliance, and Concordance between Physicians and Patients with Prescribed Medications," *American Journal of Public Health*, Sept. 1976, pp. 847–53. The study shows that of the nearly half of all patients who do not follow the prescriptions of the doctors (thus foregoing the intended effect of these prescriptions), many will follow them if adequately informed about the nature of their illness and what the proposed medication will do.

27 See Lawrence D. Egbert, George E. Batitt, et al., "Reduction of Postoperative Pain by Encouragement and Instruction of Patients," *New England Journal of Medicine* 270 (1964), pp. 825–827. See also: Howard Waitzskin and John D. Stoeckle, "The Communication of Information about Illness," *Advances in Psychosomatic Medicine*, vol. 8, 1972, pp. 185–215.

Lying and Deception: The Solution to a Dilemma in Medical Ethics

Joseph S. Ellin

Joseph S. Ellin is professor of philosophy at Western Michigan University. His specializations are philosophy of law and ethics. Ellin is the coeditor of *Profits and Professions* (1983) and author of "Special Professional Morality and the Duty of Veracity."

Ellin poses the following apparent dilemma: "Either we say that veracity is an absolute duty, which is too strict; or we admit that it is prima facie only, which seems ad hoc, useless, and mushy." Ellin suggests that the resolution of the dilemma lies in the distinction drawn in morality between lying and deception. Conceiving the relationship between the patient and the physician as a "fiduciary" relationship, on the model of the lawyer-client relationship, Ellin proceeds to argue that physicians have an absolute duty not to lie to patients; however, they do not have even a prima facie duty not to deceive.

Should doctors deceive their patients? Should they ever lie to them? Situations arise in the practice of medicine in which it appears that a medically desirable course of treatment cannot be undertaken, or cannot succeed, unless the patient is deceived; or that a patient's health or state of mind would be damaged unless some information is concealed from him, at least temporarily. Sometimes medical personnel feel justified in practicing deceit for reasons which do not directly benefit patients; for example, Veatch's case of the medical students who are instructed to introduce themselves to hospital patients as "Doctor Smith" (instead of "Medical Student Smith") so as to overcome more quickly the anxiety they feel as they begin the transformation from layperson to physician.[1] Since in such cases most writers concede that patients ought not to be deceived unless something more important than truth is at stake, the problem is typically analyzed as determining the relative

Reprinted with permission of the publisher from *Westminster Institute Review*, vol. 1 (May 1981), pp. 3–6.

weight of the rights and interests involved: the patient's interest in the truth versus his or her interest in health and peace of mind, or perhaps the patient's right to the truth versus someone else's right to or interest in something else. When, however, the problem is posed in this way, the patient's right to the truth seems relatively unimportant, especially compared to an interest as obviously important as health, so that it seems evident that deception is justified, or even obligatory. The principle of not deceiving patients seems to have little weight when deception is thought necessary to achieve some desirable end.

The alternative, however, would seem to be to adopt the rigorist position that the duty of veracity is absolute, and this seems even less attractive. Most writers concede that the duty of veracity is prima facie only, at least as a principle of medical ethics where life and suffering are at stake; it does not appear plausible to adopt an ethic in which it is made obligatory to inflict avoidable anguish on someone already sick, especially where hope and good spirits, in addition to being desirable in themselves, may promote healing and help prolong life. One could hope to avoid this dilemma by holding that the duty of veracity, though not absolute, is to be given very great weight, and may be overridden only in the gravest cases; but this line conflicts with many of our intuitions about actual cases and will probably prove useless because ad hoc. There is a temptation to deceive, or at the very least to conceal information and blur the truth, not only to prevent anxiety and stimulate hope and good spirits, but to make possible the use of placebos, to persuade patients to abandon harmful habits, to generate confidence in the medical team and the like. The whole problem is to determine what counts as a sufficiently important end to justify an exception to the veracity principle. Hence the dilemma: either we say that veracity is an absolute duty, which is too strict; or we admit that it is prima facie only, which seems ad hoc, useless, and mushy.

I would like to suggest that the solution to this dilemma is to be found in the simple distinction between lying and deception. Writers on medical ethics do not seem to acknowledge this distinction, though it is commonly made in ordinary morality. But if we allow it, assuming also that we adopt a certain conception of the doctor-patient relationship, we can say that the duty not to lie is indeed absolute, but that there is no duty at all not to practice deception. Deception, on this view, is not even wrong prima facie, but is simply one tool the doctor may employ to achieve the ends of medicine. The conception of the doctor-patient relationship which allows us to reach this result is that of a fiduciary relationship, and the argument I wish to make is that two principles, the one prohibiting lying and the other allowing deception, may be defended through this conception.

A little reflection will make clear that in ordinary morality we do distinguish between lying and deception. Most of us would not lie, but we are much less scrupulous about deceiving. We might even make it a point of honor not to actually lie when we feel justified in planting false ideas in other people's minds. You ask me how my book is coming. I have done nothing on it in a month. I reply, "The work is very difficult." This is not a lie (the work *is* very difficult); but I have managed to convey a false impression. I prefer such evasion even to a white lie or harmless fiction ("Very well." "Slowly."). Countless examples suggest themselves. An amusing story is told of a certain St. Athanasius. His enemies coming to kill him, but mistaking him for another, asked, "Where is the traitor Athanasius?" The Saint replied, "Not far away."[2]

One reason we do not distinguish between lying and deception in the medical context is that deception is sometimes used for unacceptable ends. An example of such malignant deception is given by Marsha Millman. A doctor performs a liver biopsy (a procedure not without risk) under circumstances in which the procedure is probably not justified. He avoids telling the patient the results for some days. Finally he says, "Don't worry, the biopsy didn't show anything wrong with your liver." When the patient after much agitation is allowed to read her chart, she discovers that the report on the biopsy reads, "No analysis, specimen insufficient for diagnosis."[3]

When doctors deceive for self-interested motives, to cover up their bad judgment or their failures, we are apt to think the distinction between lying and deception is mere hair-splitting. Millman asserts that the doctor "had evasively lied." Though strictly speaking inaccurate, this characterization is correct from the moral point of view, since because of the doctor's bad motive, the evasion may be considered morally no different from a lie. But the situation is different when the motives are benevolent. James Childress gives the interesting case of a patient who, due to constant pain caused by chronic intestinal problems, injects himself six times daily with a strong (but allegedly non-addictive) pain-killer. When the patient is admitted to the hospital with another complaint, the staff decides to wean him from the drug by gradually diluting the dosage with saline solution. After a time, when the pain does not recur, the patient is told that he is no longer receiving the medication.[4]

Here we have a treatment plan that can work only through deception; if the patient knows he is not receiving the usual dosage, his pain will recur. Hence the staff does not have the option of simply telling him what they intend to do and then doing it over his objections. The staff's alternatives therefore are: comply with the patient's wishes and administer medication they believe to be unnecessary and harmful; promise to do what he wants and then follow their withdrawal plan anyway, i.e., lie; avoid telling him what they are doing without actually lying about it. If it were not possible to carry out the plan without lying, if for example the patient asked direct questions about his medication, the choice thus posed between abandoning the plan and lying to him would seem far more difficult than the choice between abandoning the plan and simply deceiving him. It seems preferable to carry out the plan without actually lying; so much so that we are tempted to say that if the staff could not avoid lying, it would be better to abandon the plan, whereas employing the plan using deception is quite justifiable, given the alternative.

The distinction between lying and deception may, however, seem unjustified from what Sissela Bok has called "the perspective of the deceived." As far as the deceived is concerned, deception can be just as bad as a lie. Both give rise to resentment, disappointment and suspicion. Those deceived, as Bok says, "feel wronged; ... They see that they were manipulated, that the deceit made them unable to make choices for themselves ... unable to act as they would have wanted to act."[5] The deceived has been led to have false beliefs, has been deprived of control of a situation, has been subjected to manipulation, and so suffers a sense of betrayal and wounded dignity. Like lying, deception harms many interests. We have an interest in acquiring true beliefs, in having the information needed to make wise decisions about our lives, in being treated as trustworthy and intelligent persons, in being able to trust those in whom we put our trust. The deceiver, either intention-

ally or inadvertently, harms these interests. To the person whose interests are harmed by deceit, it is small comfort that the deceit did not involve an actual lie.

Those who find the lying/deception distinction objectionable are probably thinking of the harm each does to the deceived. Their argument is that if it is equally harmful to deceive and to lie, then no distinction between the two should be allowed. However, such a view oversimplifies the moral situation, as analysis of deception will reveal.

Intentional deception, short of lying, involves two elements: a statement or action from which it is expected that the person who is the target of the deception will draw a false conclusion, and failure to provide information which would prevent the conclusion from being drawn. The important thing is that the false information itself is not actually presented to the person deceived: everything said and done is in a sense innocent and within the rights of the deceiver. Because of this, it is possible to take the view that intentional deception is no moral wrong at all. No less a moralist than Kant writes: "I can make believe, make a demonstration from which others will draw the conclusion I want, though they have no right to expect that my action will express my real mind. In that case, I have not lied to them ... I may, for instance, wish people to think that I am off on a journey, and so I pack my luggage."[6] Kant evidently sees nothing wrong with this; his view seems to be that he has every right to pack his luggage if he chooses and if others draw certain conclusions (however reasonable) which turn out to be false, they have only themselves to blame. This, however, is too lenient on deceivers. If a person says or does something, knowing or believing that others are likely to draw false conclusions from it, and if the person refrains from providing them information he knows would prevent the false conclusions from being drawn, then he is at least in part responsible for the deception. But though he is partly responsible, he is not as responsible as he would be were he to present the false conclusion himself. Even when there is a lie, of course, the victim must bear some of the blame for being deceived, since he has imprudently trusted the liar and failed to confirm the statements made. But when a victim is deceived without a lie, he is more to blame, since he has not only failed to investigate a situation, but has also drawn or jumped to a conclusion which goes beyond the statements made to him. Even where the conclusion is a very natural inference from the statements or actions, the fact that it is an inference shows that the deceived participates in his own deception.

However, this is not the only reason why deception is considered less bad than lying. When I lie, I tell you something which, since it is false, ought not to be believed; this harms your interest in having true beliefs. When I deceive, however, I merely give you grounds for an inference which does not actually follow; this harms your interest in having good grounds for inferences, but does not directly harm your interest in having true beliefs.

The third reason why deception is not as bad as lying is that lying violates the social contract in a way that deception does not. In a sense, the social contract is renewed by every act of speech (more properly by every assertion), since to speak is implicitly to give an assurance that what one says is true. Every statement implies a promise or certification of its truth. A lie, which with a single act both implies a promise and violates it, thus involves a self-contradiction. It could be said that the social contract prohibits deception generally, on the rule-utilitarian ground that social life would be unduly burdened if, as in a spy novel, every apparently innocent action were a potential source of misinformation. But though deception may be a violation of the rules (lying, too, is a violation of the rules in this sense), it is not at the same time a reaffirmation of the rules, and hence is not an implicit self-contradiction. We can understand this when we see that although the social contract may prohibit deception, it cannot prohibit deceptive statements, since deceptive statements which are not lies are true, and the social contract cannot prohibit true statements. The contract does prohibit making true statements with the intent to deceive, or in circumstances such that the speaker does or should realize that the statement is likely to deceive. But an intention is not a promise, not even an implicit promise, hence there is nothing self-contradictory about deception. To the extent that the deceiver affirms the contract by his statement, he also obeys the contract, since his statement is true.

This analysis has an important consequence for the theory of professional morality I am defending here, since it enables us to see the difference between lying and deception with regard to trust. In everyday life we have the feeling that the liar is less trustworthy than the deceiver. Why is this, since they both intend to mislead?

The conceptual basis of this perception is that the liar reaffirms the promise of the social contract in the very act (the lie) by which he violates that promise. The deceiver may violate the social contract but does not promise to obey it in the very act of violation. Doubtless a deceiver should not be trusted, but it seems reasonable that we would be even more wary, more on guard against a person who not only deceives, but breaks a promise in the very act of reaffirming it. The significance of this distinction for professional morality I shall explain shortly.

So far I have argued that morality draws a distinction between lying and intentional deception. Now I must address the more controversial question of what the doctor's obligations are with respect to the duty of veracity. I will argue that if we conceive the doctor-patient relationship as a fiduciary relationship, then the doctor has an absolute duty not to lie, but not even a prima facie duty not to deceive. This is different from the view of ordinary morality which condemns both lying and deception, holds both wrong prima facie only, but holds lying morally worse. My defense of the above propositions as principles of medical ethics rests partly on conceptual points, and partly on contingent psychological facts having to do with the conditions of trust. It is because trust is more important in the doctor-patient relationship, conceived as fiduciary, than in ordinary life, that there is a difference between ordinary and professional morality.

As is well-known, there are many conceptions of the doctor-patient relationship. One can think of doctors as priests, friends, engineers, business partners, or partners in health. One can think of the relationship with patients as contractual, philanthropic, collegial, even exploitive. Doubtless there is merit in each of these points of view; each represents some significant truth about some doctor-patient relationships. Such conceptions or models are useful because they illuminate ethical principles; there are connections between the model of the relationship and the ethical principles which should govern it. A doctor who thinks of himself as a body mechanic will have different views about providing information to patients than one who thinks of himself as engaged with the patient in a partnership in healing. (It is unlikely that the doctors in the previous examples thought of themselves as engaged in a partnership with their patients.) Similarly, a doctor who imagines himself to be a patient's friend takes a different view of how much time he should spend with a patient than one who believes he is merely fulfilling a contract for services.

Undoubtedly many medical personnel think of themselves as having a fiduciary relationship, or something like it, with their patients or clients. The fiduciary conception is based on the legal notion of someone, the fiduciary, who has certain responsibilities for the welfare of another, the beneficiary. It is important to recognize that a fiduciary's responsibilities are limited to the specific goals of the relationship. A lawyer, for example, has responsibility for the client's legal affairs (or some of them), an accountant for his financial affairs, etc. Every beneficiary will have many interests which are external to the responsibilities of the fiduciary. This is not to say that these other interests might not impinge on the content of that relationship, but only that since the relationship was established for certain purposes relative to the specific competencies of the professional, the professional's responsibilities stop at the edges of these purposes.

If I seek legal assistance, it is because I want my legal interests to be protected; I do not expect my lawyer to take responsibility for my emotional stability, the strength of my marriage, how I use my leisure time, etc., though of course these other interests of mine might be affected by my legal condition. Where my legal interests conflict with some of my other interests, it is up to me, not my lawyer, to make the necessary choices. Those who expect their lawyer or doctor to look after a broad range of their interests, perhaps even their total welfare, obviously do not have a fiduciary conception of the professional relationship; they think of the professional as priest, friend, or some similarly broad model.

Since a fiduciary relationship is limited by specific defining goals, it is not a contractual relationship, although a legal contract may be the instrument that binds the relationship. A contractual relationship is more open, in that the parties may write anything they please into the contract. The responsibilities of the professional are exactly those stated in the contract, neither more nor less. In a contractual relationship, the professional's decisions will be guided by his interpretation of what the contract requires. Thus if a doctor believes he has agreed with the patient to do everything possible to restore the patient's health and preserve the patient's life, he will take one course of action. If,

however, he believes he has also agreed to protect the patient's family from prolonged worry and exhaustion of resources, though these are not strictly speaking medical goals, he may well do or recommend something else.

Now in addition to one's interests in health, financial condition, etc., a person has moral interests. I have an interest not to be lied to, not to be manipulated, not to be treated with contempt. There is no theoretical reason why these moral interests could not conflict with other interests such as health. But since under the fiduciary conception a professional's responsibility is to foster only those interests which define the relationship, the professional is not obligated to foster the client's moral interests. Normally, of course, there will not be a conflict, and no doubt in certain professions, such as law, opportunity for conflict is small. But such conflicts do arise in the practice of medicine (the Childress example is a clear case). The fiduciary conception imposes no professional obligation on the doctor to be concerned with these interests. This is not to say that a doctor ought not to be concerned with such interests. But if he should be, this is either because the doctor-patient relationship ought not to be construed as fiduciary, or because under certain circumstances, the commands of ordinary morality ought to override the commands of medical ethics.

Since a patient's interest in not being deceived is a moral interest and not a health interest, the doctor-patient relationship, construed as fiduciary, does not even prima facie exclude deception. To argue that it does, is to construe the relationship as priestly, friendly, contractual or something else. One could hold that if general moral obligations take precedence over professional obligations, the doctor has a general moral obligation not to deceive, even if he has no such professional obligation. That general moral obligations take precedence over profesional obligations is a proposition many professionals would dispute, however; lawyers for example will argue that their general moral obligation not to harm or pain innocent people is overridden by their professional obligation to do everything possible to protect their client's legal interests.[7]

It may seem to follow from this that doctors also have no obligation to avoid actual lying when, in their best judgment, a patient's health might be injured were he to learn some truth. To see why this is not the case we have to distinguish between the obligations *of* the doctor-patient relationship, and the obligations which make the relationship possible. In a fiduciary relationship, the only obligation *of* the relationship is to do whatever is necessary to further the goals by which the relationship is defined. But it might be the case that the relationship could not be established unless other obligations were respected. If this is the case, it follows that obligations which make the relationship possible override, in cases of conflict, obligations *of* the relationship, since the latter could not exist without the former (if the relationship is not established, then neither are any of its obligations). Hence, if the obligation not to lie is an obligation which makes the relationship possible, it follows that this obligation overrides even the obligation to protect health, and is thus an absolute.

The argument that lying destroys the doctor-patient relationship, conceived as fiduciary, is partly a conceptual argument, partly an argument based on judgment and experience. It is often said that the doctor-patient relationship depends heavily on trust. The patient puts himself (often literally) in the hands of his doctor. Although this could be true to an extent of any interpretation of the relationship, it is less true of some interpretations than others. Contracts, for example, do not depend on trust so much as on an understanding of mutual self-interest; a contractual relationship succeeds when each party understands that it is not in either party's best interest to violate the contract. Even the priest or friend roles do not require trust as their foundation, though they do generate trust. A priest is someone who has a special calling or vocation; his entire life is dedicated to an ideal of service. We trust him because his life witnesses his trustworthiness.[8] A friendship relation is based on personal satisfactions and mutual compatibility; these generate trust but do not rest on it. It is the fiduciary relationship which depends heavily on trust. A fiduciary must be trusted to act with the true interests of the beneficiary in view; the law recognizes this by defining trust as "a fiduciary relationship."[9] If, however, we were to allow the fiduciary to lie, the trust basis of the relationship would be undermined and the relationship itself jeopardized. A lie, it will be recalled, violates a kind of implicit assurance we give when we speak, namely, that our words will be used to state the truth. Deception through evasive or misleading statements which are nonetheless true, does not violate such an assurance but accords with it. The deceiver can thus be trusted at least to

speak the truth, while the liar violates the very assurance he is giving with his speech.

Although the argument that the liar undermines the basis of the fiduciary relationship by showing himself to be untrustworthy is empirical, it is not open to one kind of objection commonly brought against empirical arguments in ethics. The objection is that if the only reason to avoid a certain practice is that the practice leads to undesirable consequences, then the solution is to employ the practice anyway, but do so in such a way that the consequences are avoided. Thus Alan Goldman criticizes arguments which oppose lying or deceiving by "appeal to certain systematic disutilities that might be projected, e.g., effects upon the agent's trustworthiness and upon the trust that other people are willing to accord him if his lies are discovered." According to Goldman, "The only conclusion that I would draw from the empirical points...is that doctors should perhaps be better trained in psychology in order to be able to judge the effects..." of the decision to lie or not.[10]

Goldman's argument is good not against those who oppose lying on the ground that it destroys trust, but only against those who hold this and *also* hold (as Goldman himself holds) that lying would be wrong even if it didn't affect trust. If lying is wrong whether it affects trust or not, then the fact that it affects trust obviously cannot be the reason why it is wrong. But as I do not claim that lying is wrong (in the professional-client relationship) if it does not affect trust, I need not deny that the tendency of lying to destroy trust might from time to time be countered by certain clever psychological tactics on the part of liars. This does not in the least show that lying does not tend to destroy trust. However, I maintain that the tendency of lying to destroy trust is considerably greater than the tendency of deception to destroy trust, and this I argue partly on the basis of the conceptual difference between lying and deception, partly on the basis of experience. Lying is more destructive to trust than deception because lying is a greater violation of the social contract. The liar by his false speech violates the very promise that he makes in speaking, the promise to speak the truth. And it is for this reason, as I think experience reveals, that we find ourselves less trusting of someone who has lied to us, than of someone who has misled us or created a false impression.

Given this threat to trust, it seems plausible to hold

that lying is too dangerous ever to be allowed in a relationship founded on trust. Suppose we adopted a rule which made lying only prima facie wrong, and thus permitted lying in certain very serious cases. The patient would know that the doctor could not be trusted to tell the truth, even in response to a direct question, when the doctor deemed it unwise to do so; and therefore the patient would know that the doctor could never be believed, since even an apparently trivial matter might in fact be serious enough for the doctor to feel justified in lying about. Of course the fact that the patient would know this does not necessarily mean that the patient would not trust the doctor anyway. But a patient who has been lied to has been given very strong grounds to conclude that the doctor is not to be trusted, so that even a single justified lie is likely to undermine the patient's trust.

Let us test the prohibition of lying against a case where our intuitions seem to lead us to the opposite conclusion. Gert and Culver give the following case: "Mrs. E is in extremely critical condition after an automobile accident which has taken the life of one of her four children and severely injured another. Dr. P believes that her very tenuous hold on life might be weakened by the shock of hearing of her children's conditions, so he decides to deceive her for a short period of time."[11] According to these authors, a rational person would choose to be deceived in such circumstances, so there is nothing wrong with the doctor's decision to deceive her. As is typical of the medical ethics literature, the authors do not distinguish between lying and deception. On our principles, there is nothing even prima facie wrong with the doctor's use of evasive or misleading statements to conceal the truth. But suppose Mrs. E demands a straight answer from which evasion offers no escape. Gert and Culver seem to propose that the question to be answered is whether a rational person would want to be lied to in these circumstances, but as there does not seem to be any way to arrive at an answer to this question, their proposal does not really advance beyond our intuitions. In this case, our intuitions strongly suggest that lying would be justified in order to protect the woman's health, but on the principles advanced in this essay, lying is not permitted, since if Dr. P lies in response to Mrs. E's direct question, she will eventually discover that he cannot be trusted, and that therefore they cannot enjoy a relationship based on trust. Of course

this is not to say that the doctor must tell her the truth in the bluntest or most painful way, but only that he must not lie. Where a harmful truth cannot be concealed, it is up to the doctor to reveal it in a way least damaging to the patient. To take a different view is to hold that the doctor-patient relationship is not a fiduciary relationship based on trust, but something else, friendship perhaps, or maybe some form of paternalism, in which the doctor has the responsibility of balancing all of the patient's interests and making decisions in light of his conception of the patient's total welfare. If, however, these conceptions of the relationship seem unattractive to us (and I have not argued that they should seem unattractive) we will have to take the view, intuitions to the contrary notwithstanding, that even in the situation just described, the doctor's duty is to tell the truth.

NOTES

1 Robert Veatch, *Case Studies in Medical Ethics* (Cambridge: Harvard University Press, 1977), pp. 147f.

2 I found this example in an unpublished paper by James Rachels, "Honesty." Rachels evidently borrowed it from P.T. Geach, *The Virtues* (Cambridge: Cambridge University Press; 1977), p. 115.

3 Marcia Millman, *The Unkindest Cut* (New York: William Morrow and Co., 1977), pp. 138f.

4 James Childress, "Paternalism and Health Care," in *Medical Responsibility*, ed. Wade L. Robison and Michael S. Pritchard (New York: Humana Press, 1979), pp. 15–27.

5 Sissela Bok, *Lying* (New York: Pantheon Books, 1978), ch. 2.

6 Immanuel Kant, *Lectures on Ethics*, trans. Louis Infeld (New York: Harper and Row, 1963), pp. 147–154.

7 The contention that, as a general rule, professional obligations override ordinary moral obligations, is critically examined and disputed by Alan H. Goldman, *The Moral Foundations of Professional Ethics* (Totowa, N.J.: Littlefield, Adams and Co., 1980).

8 On the idea of medicine as a calling founded on "covenant" which transforms the doctor, see William F. May, "Code, Covenant, Contract or Phi-

lanthropy," *Hastings Center Report* 5, 6 (December, 1975): 29–38.

9 "Trust. Noun: a fiduciary relationship; a matter of confidence." *Ballantine's Law Dictionary*, 3rd ed.

10 Goldman, *Professional Ethics*, p. 176.

11 Bernard Gert and Charles Culver, "The Justification of Paternalism" in Robison and Pritchard, *Medical Responsibility*, p. 7.

Informed Consent

Opinion in *Canterbury v. Spence*

Judge Spotswood W. Robinson III

Spotswood W. Robinson III is a circuit court judge serving on the U.S. Court of Appeals, District of Columbia. Prior to his appointment to the bench, Judge Robinson served as an associate professor of law at Howard University (1939–1949) and as the dean of the Law School (1960–1963).

A 19-year-old man, John W. Canterbury, developed paraplegia after a laminectomy (a surgical procedure). Prior to the surgery, his physician, William Thornton Spence, did not inform Canterbury that the operation involved the risk of paralysis. Canterbury brought an action against the physician and the hospital. In defending his decision to withhold the information from the patient, Dr. Spence testified that communicating the 1 percent risk "is not good medical practice because it might deter patients from undergoing needed surgery and might produce adverse psychological reactions which could preclude the success of the operation." In this selection, Judge Robinson argues that an adult patient of sound mind has the right to determine what should be done to his or her body. Because of this right, a physician has the duty to inform the patient about those dangers that "are material" to the patient's decision. The Court allows two exceptions to this rule of disclosure. It holds, however, that a physician cannot remain silent simply because divulgence might prompt the patient to forego therapy that the physician perceives as necessary.

Suits charging failure by a physician adequately to disclose the risks and alternatives of proposed treatment are not innovations in American law. They date back a good half-century, and in the last decade they have multiplied rapidly. There is, nonetheless, disagreement among the courts and the commentators on many major questions, and there is no precedent of our own directly in point. For the tools enabling resolution of the issues on this appeal, we are forced to begin at first principles.

The root premise is the concept, fundamental in American jurisprudence, that "[e]very human being of adult years and sound mind has a right to determine what shall be done with his own body...." True consent to what happens to one's self is the informed exercise of a choice, and that entails an opportunity to evaluate knowledgeably the options available and the risks attendant upon each. The average patient has little or no understanding of the medical arts, and ordinarily has only his physician to whom he can look for

U.S. Court of Appeals, District of Columbia Circuit; May 19, 1972. 464 Federal Reporter, 2nd Series, 772. Reprinted with permission of West Publishing Company.

enlightenment with which to reach an intelligent decision.[1] From these almost axiomatic considerations springs the need, and in turn the requirement, of a reasonable divulgence by physician to patient to make such a decision possible.[2]

A physician is under a duty to treat his patient skillfully, but proficiency in diagnosis and therapy is not the full measure of his responsibility. The cases demonstrate that the physician is under an obligation to communicate specific information to the patient when the exigencies of reasonable care call for it. Due care may require a physician perceiving symptoms of bodily abnormality to alert the patient to the condition. It may call upon the physician confronting an ailment which does not respond to his ministrations to inform the patient thereof. It may command the physician to instruct the patient as to any limitations to be presently observed for his own welfare, and as to any precautionary therapy he should seek in the future. It may oblige the physician to advise the patient of the need for or desirability of any alternative treatment promising greater benefit than that being pursued. Just as plainly, due care normally demands that the physician warn the patient of any risks to his well-being which contemplated therapy may involve.

The context in which the duty of risk-disclosure arises is invariably the occasion for decision as to whether a particular treatment procedure is to be undertaken. To the physician, whose training enables a self-satisfying evaluation, the answer may seem clear, but it is the prerogative of the patient, not the physician, to determine for himself the direction in which his interests seem to lie. To enable the patient to chart his course understandably, some familiarity with the therapeutic alternatives and their hazards becomes essential.

A reasonable revelation in these respects is not only a necessity but, as we see it, is as much a matter of the physician's duty. It is a duty to warn of the dangers lurking in the proposed treatment, and that is surely a facet of due care. It is, too, a duty to impart information which the patient has every right to expect.[3] The patient's reliance upon the physician is a trust of the kind which traditionally has exacted obligations beyond those associated with arms-length transactions. His dependence upon the physician for information affecting his well-being, in terms of contemplated treatment, is well-nigh abject. As earlier noted, long before the instant litigation arose, courts had recognized that the physician had the responsibility of satisfying the vital informational needs of the patient. More recently, we ourselves have found "in the fiducial qualities of [the physician-patient] relationship the physician's duty to reveal to the patient that which in his best interests it is important that he should know." We now find, as a part of the physician's overall obligation to the patient, a similar duty of reasonable disclosure of the choices with respect to proposed therapy and the dangers inherently and potentially involved. . . .

Once the circumstances give rise to a duty on the physician's part to inform his patient, the next inquiry is the scope of the disclosure the physician is legally obliged to make. The courts have frequently confronted this problem but no uniform standard defining the adequacy of the divulgence emerges from the decisions. Some have said "full" disclosure, a norm we are unwilling to adopt literally. It seems obviously prohibitive and unrealistic to expect physicians to discuss with their patients every risk of proposed treatment—no matter how small or remote—and generally unnecessary from the patient's viewpoint as well. Indeed, the cases speaking in terms of "full" disclosure appear to envision something less than total disclosure, leaving unanswered the question of just how much.

The larger number of courts, as might be expected, have applied tests framed with reference to prevailing fashion within the medical profession. Some have measured the disclosure by "good medical practice," others by what a reasonable practitioner would have bared under the circumstances, and still others by what medical custom in the community would demand. We have explored this rather considerable body of law but are unprepared to follow it. The duty to disclose, we have reasoned, arises from phenomena apart from medical custom and practice. The latter, we think, should no more establish the scope of the duty than its existence. Any definition of scope in terms purely of a professional standard is at odds with the patient's prerogative to decide on projected therapy himself. That prerogative, we have said, is at the very foundation of the duty to disclose, and both the patient's right to know and the physician's correlative obligation to tell him are diluted to the extent that its compass is dictated by the medical profession.[4]

In our view, the patient's right of self-decision shapes the boundaries of the duty to reveal. That right can be effectively exercised only if the patient possesses enough information to enable an intelligent choice. The scope of the physician's communications to the patient, then, must be measured by the patient's need, and that need is the information material to the decision. Thus the test for determining whether a particular peril must be divulged is its materiality to the patient's decision: all risks potentially affecting the decision must be unmasked. And to safeguard the patient's interest in achieving his own determination on treatment, the law must itself set the standard for adequate disclosure.

Optimally for the patient, exposure of a risk would be mandatory whenever the patient would deem it significant to his decision, either singly or in combination with other risks. Such a requirement, however, would summon the physician to second-guess the patient, whose ideas on materiality could hardly be known to the physician. That would make an undue demand upon medical practitioners, whose conduct, like that of others, is to be measured in terms of reasonableness. Consonantly with orthodox negligence doctrine, the physician's liability for nondisclosure is to be determined on the basis of foresight, not hindsight; no less than any other aspect of negligence, the issue on nondisclosure must be approached from the viewpoint of the reasonableness of the physician's divulgence in terms of what he knows or should know to be the patient's informational needs. If, but only if, the fact-finder can say that the physician's communication was unreasonably inadequate is an imposition of liability legally or morally justified.

Of necessity, the content of the disclosure rests in the first instance with the physician. Ordinarily it is only he who is in position to identify particular dangers; always he must make a judgment, in terms of materiality, as to whether and to what extent revelation to the patient is called for. He cannot know with complete exactitude what the patient would consider important to his decision, but on the basis of his medical training and experience he can sense how the average, reasonable patient expectably would react. Indeed, with knowledge of, or ability to learn, his patient's background and current condition, he is in a position superior to that of most others—attorneys, for example—who are called upon to make judgments on pain of liability in damages for unreasonable miscalculation.

From these considerations we derive the breadth of the disclosure of risks legally to be required. The scope of the standard is not subjective as to either the physician or the patient; it remains objective with due regard for the patient's informational needs and with suitable leeway for the physician's situation. In broad outline, we agree that "[a] risk is thus material when a reasonable person, in what the physician knows or should know to be the patient's position, would be likely to attach significance to the risk or cluster of risks in deciding whether or not to forego the proposed therapy."

The topics importantly demanding a communication of information are the inherent and potential hazards of the proposed treatment, the alternatives to that treatment, if any, and the results likely if the patient remains untreated. The factors contributing significance to the dangerousness of a medical technique are, of course, the incidence of injury and the degree of the harm threatened. A very small chance of death or serious disablement may well be significant; a potential disability which dramatically outweighs the potential benefit of the therapy or the detriments of the existing malady may summon discussion with the patient.

There is no bright line separating the significant from the insignificant; the answer in any case must abide a rule of reason. Some dangers—infection, for example—are inherent in any operation; there is no obligation to communicate those of which persons of average sophistication are aware. Even more clearly, the physician bears no responsibility for discussion of hazards the patient has already discovered, or those having no apparent materiality to patients' decision on therapy. The disclosure doctrine, like others marking lines between permissible and impermissible behavior in medical practice, is in essence a requirement of conduct prudent under the circumstances. Whenever nondisclosure of particular risk information is open to debate by reasonable-minded men, the issue is for the finder of the facts.

Two exceptions to the general rule of disclosure have been noted by the courts. Each is in the nature of a physician's privilege not to disclose, and the reasoning underlying them is appealing. Each, indeed, is but a recognition that, as important as is the patient's right to know, it is greatly outweighed by the magnitudinous circumstances giving rise to the privilege. The first comes into play when the patient is unconscious or otherwise incapable of consenting, and harm from a failure to treat is imminent and outweighs any harm threatened by the proposed treatment. When a genuine emergency of that sort arises, it is settled that the impracticality of conferring with the patient dispenses with need for it. Even in situations of that character the physician should, as current law requires, attempt to secure a relative's consent if possible. But if time is too short to accommodate discussion, obviously the physician should proceed with the treatment.

The second exception obtains when risk-disclosure poses such a threat of detriment to the patient as to become unfeasible or contraindicated from a medical point of view. It is recognized that patients occasionally become so ill or emotionally distraught on disclosure as to foreclose a rational decision, or complicate or hinder the treatment, or perhaps even pose psychological damage to the patient. Where that is so, the cases have generally held that the physician is armed with a privilege to keep the information from the patient, and we think it clear that portents of that type may justify the physician in action he deems medically warranted. The critical inquiry is whether the physician responded to a sound medical judgment that communication of the risk information would present a threat to the patient's well-being.

The physician's privilege to withhold information for therapeutic reasons must be carefully circumscribed, however, for otherwise it might devour the disclosure rule itself. The privilege does not accept the paternalistic notion that the physician may remain silent simply because divulgence might prompt the patient to forego therapy the physician feels the patient really needs. That attitude presumes instability or perversity for even the normal patient, and runs counter to the foundation principle that the patient should and ordinarily can make the choice for himself. Nor does the privilege contemplate operation save where the patient's reaction to risk information, as reasonably foreseen by the physician, is menacing. And even in a situation of that kind, disclosure to a close relative with a view to securing consent to the proposed treatment may be the only alternative open to the physician....

NOTES

1 Patients ordinarily are persons unlearned in the medical sciences. Some few, of course, are schooled in branches of the medical profession or in related fields. But even within the latter group variations in degree of medical knowledge specifically referable to particular therapy may be broad, as for example, between a specialist and a general practitioner, or between a physician and a nurse. It may well be, then, that it is only in the unusual case that a court could safely assume that the patient's insights were on a parity with those of the treating physician.

2 The doctrine that a consent effective as authority to form therapy can arise only from the patient's understanding of alternatives to and risks of the therapy is commonly denominated "informed consent." The same appellation is frequently assigned to the doctrine requiring physicians, as a matter of duty to patients, to communicate information as to such alternatives and risks. See, *e.g.*, Comment, Informed Consent in Medical Malpractice, 55 Calif.L.Rev. 1396 (1967). While we recognize the general utility of shorthand phrases in literary expositions, we caution that uncritical use of the "informed consent" label can be misleading. See, *e.g.*, Plante, An Analysis of "Informed Consent," 36 Ford.L.Rev. 639, 671–72 (1968).

In duty-to-disclose cases, the focus of attention is more properly upon the nature and content of the physician's divulgence than the patient's understanding or consent. Adequate disclosure and informed consent are, of course, two sides of the same coin—the former a *sine qua non* of the latter. But the vital inquiry on duty to disclose relates to the physician's performance of an obligation, while one of the difficulties with analysis in terms of "informed consent" is its tendency to imply that what is decisive is the degree of the patient's comprehension. As we later emphasize, the physician discharges the duty when he makes a reasonable effort to convey sufficient information although the patient, without fault of the physician, may not fully grasp it. Even though the factfinder may have occasion to draw an inference on the state of the patient's enlightenment, the factfinding process on performance of the duty ultimately reaches back to what the physician actually said or failed to say. And while the factual conclusion on adequacy of the revelation will vary as between patients—as, for example, between a lay patient and a physician-patient—the fluctuations are attributable to the kind of divulgence which may be reasonable under the circumstances.

3 Some doubt has been expressed as to ability of physicians to suitably communicate their evaluations of risks and the advantages of optional treatment, and as to the lay patient's ability to understand what the physician tells him. Karchmer, Informed Consent: A Plaintiff's Medical Malpractice "Wonder Drug," 31 Mo.L.Rev. 29, 41 (1966). We do not share these apprehensions. The discussion need not be a disquisition, and surely the physician is not compelled

to give his patient a short medical education; the disclosure rule summons the physician only to a reasonable explanation. That means generally informing the patient in non-technical terms as to what is at stake: the therapy alternatives open to him, the goals expectably to be achieved, and the risks that may ensue from particular treatment and

no treatment. So informing the patient hardly taxes the physician, and it must be the exceptional patient who cannot comprehend such an explanation at least in a rough way.

4 For similar reasons, we reject the suggestion that disclosure should be discretionary with the physician.

Informed Consent in the Therapeutic Relationship: Law and Ethics

Jay Katz

Jay Katz, a psychiatrist, teaches law and psychiatry at Yale University Law School. He is coauthor of *Psychoanalysis, Psychiatry and Law* (1967), *Experimentation with Human Beings* (1972), and *Catastrophic Diseases: Who Decides What?* (1982). He is also the author of *The Silent World of Doctor and Patient* (1984) and numerous articles on informed consent.

Katz traces the legal history of the informed consent requirement, which initially developed in order to protect patients' right to "thoroughgoing self-determination." He discusses the ambivalence of the courts toward the informed consent doctrine and traces this ambivalence to two conflicting commitments: (1) a commitment to autonomy and the right of self-determination and (2) a commitment to protect some of the most important interests of otherwise responsible adults, when the exercise of the right of self-determination might hurt those interests. Katz discusses some of the tensions that result when the requirements of traditional medical paternalism seem to come into conflict with the requirement of informed consent.

The doctrine of informed consent, introduced into U.S. case law in 1957, represents judges' groping efforts to delineate physicians' duties to inform patients of the benefits and risks of diagnostic and treatment alternatives, including the consequences of no treatment, as well as to obtain patients' consent (*Salgo* v. *Stanford University*). The doctrine's avowed purpose was to protect patients' right to "thoroughgoing self-determination" (*Natanson* v. *Kline*). The legal implications of informed consent, however, remain unclear. The doctrine is in fact more of a slogan, which judges have been too timid or too wise to translate into law, at least as yet. It has been employed with little care but great

passion to voice a dream of personal freedom and individual dignity. Though its legal impact in protecting patients' right to self-decision making has been scant, the threat of informed consent has opened profound issues for the traditional practice of medicine.

THE MEDICAL FRAMEWORK

It has been insufficiently recognized, particularly by judges, that disclosure and consent, except in the most rudimentary fashion, are obligations alien to medical practice. Hippocrates' admonitions to physicians are still followed today: "Perform [these duties] calmly and adroitly, concealing most things from the patient while you are attending to him. Give necessary orders with cheerfulness and serenity, turning his attention away from what is being done to him; sometimes reprove sharply and emphatically, and sometimes comfort with solicitude and attention, revealing nothing of the patient's future or present condition" (Hippocrates). Thus it is not surprising that the Hippocratic Oath is silent on the duty of physicians to inform, or even converse with, patients. Similarly Dr. Thomas Percival, whose 1803 book *Medical Ethics* influenced profoundly the subsequent codifications of medical ethics in England and the United States, commented only once on the discourse between physicians and patients, restricting his remarks to "gloomy prognostications." Even in that context he advised that "friends of the patient" be primarily informed, though he added that the patient may be told "if absolutely necessary" (Percival, p. 91). The Code of Ethics of the American Medical Association, adopted in 1847, and the Principles of Medical Ethics of the American Medical Association, adopted in 1903 and 1912, repeat, in almost the same words, Percival's statement. The AMA Principles of Medical Ethics, endorsed in 1957, delete Percival's wording entirely and substitute the vague admonition that "physicians...should make available to their patients ...the benefits of their professional attainments." The pertinent sections of the *Opinions of the Judicial Council of the AMA*, interpreting the Principles, note only the surgeon's obligation to disclose "all facts relevant to the need and performance of the operation" and the experimenter's obligation, when using new drugs and procedures, to obtain "the voluntary consent of the person" (American Medical Association, Judicial Council, "Principles"). Nine years later, the AMA House of Delegates in endorsing, with modifications, the Declaration of Helsinki, asked that investigators, when engaged "in clinical [research] primarily for treatment," make relevant disclosures to and obtain the voluntary consent of patients or their legally authorized representative.

Thus in the context of therapy no authoritative statement encouraging disclosure and consent has ever been promulgated by the medical profession. The AMA's tersely worded surgical exception was compelled by the law of malpractice. Its experimental exception represented primarily an acquiescence to United States Public Health Service and the U.S. Department of Health, Education, and Welfare require-

ments, which in turn were formulated in response to congressional concerns about research practices. When disclosure and consent prior to the conduct of therapeutic research were endorsed by the AMA, it did not extend those requirements to *all* patient care but limited the exception to "clinical [research] primarily for treatment."

Two significant conclusions can be drawn: (1) "Informed consent" is a creature of law and not a medical prescription. A duty to inform patients has never been promulgated by the medical profession, though individual physicians have made interesting, but as a rule unsystematic, comments on this topic. Judges have been insufficiently aware of the deeply ingrained Hippocratic tradition against disclosure and, instead, seem to have assumed that individual physicians' lack of disclosure was aberrant with respect to standard medical practice, and hence "negligent," in the sense of "forgetful" or "inadvertent," conduct. (2) When judges were confronted with claims of lack of informed consent, no medical precedent, no medical position papers, and no analytic medical thinking existed on this subject. Thus physicians were ill prepared to shape judges' notions on informed consent with thoughtful and systematic positions of their own.

THE LEGAL FRAMEWORK

With the historical movement from feudalism to individualism, consent, respect for the dignity of human beings, and the right of individuals to shape their own lives became important principles of English common law and, in turn, of American common law. Yet, as these principles gained greater acceptance, questions arose in many areas of law about the capacity of human beings to make their own decisions and about the need to protect them from their "own folly." The tug of war between advocates of thoroughgoing self-determination and those of paternalism has continued unabated. The informed consent doctrine manifests this struggle. While in physician-patient interactions the legal trend during the past two decades has been to increase somewhat the right of patients to greater freedom of choice, the informed consent doctrine has not had as far-reaching an impact on patients' self-determination as many commentators have assumed. This fact has been insufficiently appreciated and has led to confusion, further compounded by the courts' rhetoric that seemed to promise more than it delivered.

Consent to medical and surgical interventions is an ancient legal requirement. Historically an intentional touching without consent was adjudicated in battery. The law has not changed at all in this regard, and a surgeon who operates on a patient without permission is legally liable, even if the operation is successful. In such instances any inquiry into medical need or negligent conduct becomes irrelevant, for what is at issue is the disregard of the person's right to exercise control over his body. The jurisprudential basis of these claims is personal freedom:

> ...under a free government at least, the free citizen's first and greatest right, which underlies all others— the right to himself—is the subject of universal acquiescence, and this right necessarily forbids a physician or surgeon, however skillful or eminent ...to violate without permission the bodily integrity of his patient by...operating on him without his consent...[Pratt v. Davis].

But what does consent mean? In battery cases it means only that the physician must inform the patient what he proposes to do and that the patient must agree. Medical emergencies and patients' incompetence are the only exceptions to this requirement.

In mid-twentieth century, judges gradually confronted the question whether patients are entitled not only to know what a doctor proposes to do but also to decide whether the intervention is advisable in the light of its risks and benefits and the available alternatives, including no treatment. Such awareness of patients' informational needs is a modern phenomenon, influenced by the simultaneous growth of product liability and consumer law.

The law of fraud and deceit has always protected patients from doctors' flagrant misrepresentations, and in theory patients have always been entitled to ask whatever questions they pleased. What the doctrine of informed consent sought to add is the proposition that physicians are now under an affirmative duty to offer to acquaint patients with the important risks and plausible alternatives to the proposed procedure. The underlying rationale for that duty was stated in Natanson v. Kline:

> Anglo-American law starts with the premise of thorough-going self-determination. It follows that each man is considered to be master of his own body, and he may, if he be of sound mind, expressly prohibit the performance of life-saving surgery, or other medical treatment. A doctor might well believe that an operation or form of treatment is desirable or necessary but the law does not permit him to substitute his own judgment for that of the patient by any form of artifice or deception [Natanson v. Kline].

The language employed by the Natanson court in support of an affirmative duty to disclose derives from the language of the law of battery, which clearly makes the patient the ultimate decision maker with respect to his body. Thus the courts reasoned, with battery principles very much in mind, that significant protection of patients' right to decide their medical fate required not merely perfunctory assent but a truly "informed consent," based on an adequate understanding of the medical and surgical options available to them.

Yet in the same breath judges also attempted to intrude as little as possible on traditional medical practices. In doing so their impulse to protect the right of individual self-determination collided with their equally strong desire to maintain the authority and practices of the professions. Law has always respected the arcane expertise of physicians and has never held them liable if they practiced "good medicine." The law of consent in battery represented no aberration from this principle since most physicians agree that patients at least deserve to know the nature of the proposed procedure. However, the new duty of disclosure that the law, in the name of self-determination, threatened to impose upon physicians was something quite different. For the vast majority of physicians significant disclosure is not at all part of standard medical practice. Most doctors believe that patients are neither emotionally nor intellectually equipped to be medical decision makers, that they must be guided past childish fears into "rational" therapy, and that disclosures of uncertainty, gloomy prognosis, and dire risks often seriously undermine cure. Physicians began to wonder whether law was now asking them to practice "bad" medicine.

In the early informed consent cases, judges simply did not resolve the conflict between self-determination and professional practices and authority. The result was distressing confusion. In obeisance to the venerable ideal of self-determination, courts purported to establish, as a matter of law, the physician's

> ...obligation...to disclose and explain to the patient in language as simple as necessary the nature of the

ailment, the nature of the proposed treatment, the probability of success or of alternatives, and perhaps the risks of unfortunate results and unforeseen conditions within the body [*Natanson* v. *Kline*].

The threat of such an obligation greatly disturbed the medical profession. It recognized that serious implementation of such a standard would significantly alter medical practice. Physicians argued that in order fully to serve patients' best interests, they must have the authority to exercise medical judgment in managing patients. Courts likewise bowed to this judgment. In the very sentence that introduced the ambiguous but exuberant new phrase, "informed consent," the court showed its deference to medical judgment and its hesitancy to disturb traditional practice:

> ...in discussing the element of risk a certain amount of discretion must be employed consistent with the full disclosure of facts necessary to an informed consent [*Salgo* v. *Stanford University*].

Thus the extent to which evolving case law, under the banner of individualism, was challenging traditional medical practice—which for millennia has treated patients paternally as children—remained confusing. In those earlier cases (*Salgo* v. *Stanford University*, *Natanson* v. *Kline*) judges were profoundly allegiant to both points of view, but the balance was soon tipped decisively in favor of protecting medical practices.

Battery or Negligence

The striking ambivalence of judges toward the doctrine of informed consent manifested itself in the competition between battery and negligence doctrines as a means of analyzing and deciding the claims of lack of informed consent. Battery offered a more rigorous protection of patients' right to self-determination. The inquiry into disclosure and consent would not be governed by professional practices but instead would rest on the question: Has the physician met his expanded informational responsibility so that the patient is able to exercise a choice among treatment options? A negative answer to this question would show that the physician's actions constitute trespass, rendering him liable for an unauthorized and "offensive" contact (*Dow* v. *Kaiser Foundation*).

However, in virtually every jurisdiction judges resolved the competition in favor of negligence law. In doing so, judges were able to defer to medical judgment

by evaluating the adequacy of disclosure against the medical professional standard of care, asserting that this standard will govern those duties as it does other medical obligations. As a consequence, physicians remain free to exercise the wisdom of their profession and are liable only for failure to disclose what a reasonable doctor would have revealed. Furthermore, negligence theory does not redress mere dignitary injuries, irrespective of physical injuries, and requires proof that the patient, fully informed, would have refused the proposed treatment. Interferences with self-determination, standing alone, are not compensated.

In rejecting battery, judges made much of the fact that such an action required "intent," while negligence involved "inadvertence"; it was the latter, they believed, that accounted for the lack of disclosure. They overlooked that the withholding of information on the part of physicians is generally quite intentional, dictated by the very exercise of medical judgment that the law of negligence seeks to respect. In stating that the nondisclosures were "collateral" to the central information about the nature of the proposed procedure and hence not required for a valid consent, judges discarded the very idea of informed consent—namely, that absence of expanded disclosure vitiates consent. They refused to extend the inquiry to the total informational needs of patients, without which patients' capacity for self-decision making remains incomplete. At bottom, the rejection of an expanded battery theory and of its proposed requirement of informed consent followed from the threat they posed to the authority of doctors and traditional medical practice.

Thus informed consent, based on patients' thoroughgoing self-determination, was a misnomer from the time the phrase was born. To be sure, a new cause of action has emerged for failure to inform of the risks of, and in most jurisdictions alternatives to, treatment. Some duty to disclose risks and alternatives, the courts were willing to say, exists; the extent of that duty is defined by the disclosure practice of a reasonable physician in the circumstances of the case. The new claim is firmly rooted in the law of negligent malpractice, in that plaintiffs are still required to prove the professional standard of care by means of medical expert witnesses. In these, the majority of jurisdictions, traditional medical practice—which generally opposes disclosure—has scarcely been threatened at all in legal reality. The legal life of informed consent, except for dicta about self-determination and the hybrid negligence law promulgated in a handful of jurisdictions, was almost over as soon as it began. Judges had briefly toyed with the idea of patients' self-determination and then largely cast it aside. Good medicine, as defined by doctors, remains good law almost everywhere.

Modifications in Professional Standard of Care

In a few jurisdictions, beginning in 1972 in the District of Columbia with the decision in *Canterbury* v. *Spence*, the new cause of action for failure to inform combined elements of battery with negligence, creating a legal hybrid. The court purported to abandon the professional standard of care with respect to disclosure, asserting that

> ...respect for the patient's right of self-determination on particular therapy demands a standard set by law for physicians rather than one which physicians may or may not impose upon themselves [*Canterbury* v. *Spence*].

Thus the court laid down a judge-made rule of disclosure of risks and alternatives, which for all practical purposes resembled an expanded battery standard of disclosure.

The preoccupation with risk disclosure, however, continued unabated. From the very beginning, despite all the talk about "informed consent," judges did not lay down any rules for a careful inquiry into the nature and quality of consent, which on its face any meaningful implementation of the doctrine required. Instead major emphasis was placed on risk disclosures. Since in the cases before courts plaintiff-patients only complained of the injurious results of treatment, this emphasis is understandable. Yet to focus solely on risks is to bypass the principal issue of self-determination—namely, whether the physician kept the patient from arriving at his own decision. The *Canterbury* court, too, restricted its concerns largely to risk disclosures; and added the requirement that

> an unrevealed risk that should have been made known must materialize for otherwise the omission, however, unpardonable, is legally without consequence [ibid.].

Thus the court foreclosed legal redress for the patient who, fully informed of the potential effects of, for example, a maiming operation, would have chosen an alternative medical course, even though some of the risks did not materialize.

But to the extent these jurisdictions have abandoned the professional standard of disclosure, traditional medical practice has been challenged; "good medicine," in the eyes of the profession, may no longer be a sufficient defense. Seemingly, in these jurisdictions self-determination has begun to encroach upon the province of medical paternalism. That encroachment, however, may be substantially an illusion, for the touted abandonment of the professional standard of disclosure in *Canterbury* was far from complete. Medical judgment to truncate full disclosure must be "given its due," the court said, when "it enters the picture." The court left ambiguous when the plaintiff must establish the appropriate standard of disclosure by an expert witness, or when he must produce such a witness in order to rebut a defendant-physician's claim that good medical judgment was exercised.

What is clear is that the physician has a "therapeutic privilege" not to disclose information where such disclosure would pose a threat to the "well-being" of the patient. But the ambit of this privilege as well as the relationship of its invocation to a directed verdict is not clear, and this for "good" reasons: Even in these most liberal jurisdictions with respect to patients' rights, courts still cannot face squarely the question of how much they are willing to challenge the traditional medical wisdom of nondisclosure. The law remains ambiguous with respect to this, the core issue of informed consent.

Tensions Between Self-Determination and Paternalism

Beyond its allegiance to medical paternalism, noted above, the *Canterbury* court showed its preference for paternalism in another way. Under negligence law, the courts have stated that lack of disclosure cannot be said to have caused the patient's injury unless the patient, if adequately informed, would have declined the procedure; this is the crucial problem of causation in informed consent cases. Such an approach to causation is quite appropriate where law seeks not to compensate interference with self-determination, but only physical injuries resulting from inadequate disclosure. Yet the *Canterbury* court, and every court that has considered the matter subsequently, held that the decision whether or not to undertake therapy must be examined not from the point of view of the patient-plaintiff but from that of a "prudent person in the patient's position," limiting the inquiry to whether a "reasonable patient" would have agreed to the procedure. This substitution of a community standard of a "reasonable" person cuts the heart out of the courts' purported respect for individual self-determination. Questions of the influence of hindsight and bitterness are familiar to juries, as is the problem of self-serving testimony generally. While those are delicate problems, they do not justify abrogating the very right at issue in cases of informed consent: the right of individual choice, which may be precisely the right to be an "unreasonable" person.

Epilogue on Law

Thus law has proceeded feebly toward the objective of patients' self-determination. While a new cause of action, occasionally hybridized with battery, has emerged for the negligent failure to disclose risks and alternative treatments, it remains a far cry from the avowed purpose of the informed consent doctrine, namely, to secure patients' autonomy and right to self-determination. In not tampering significantly with the medical wisdom of nondisclosure, yet creating a new cause of action based on traditional disclosure requirements, courts may have accomplished a different result, very much in line with other purposes of tort law—namely, to provide physically injured patients with greater opportunities for seeking compensation whenever it can be argued that disclosure might have avoided such injuries. In doing so judges may have hoped, through the anticipatory tremors of dicta, to urge doctors to consider modifying their traditional disclosure practices. But judges have been unwilling, at least as yet, to implement earnestly patients' right to self-determination.

WHITHER INFORMED CONSENT?

The disquiet that the doctrine of informed consent has created among physicians cannot be fully explained by the small incremental step courts have taken to assure greater patient participation in medical decision making. More likely it was aroused by the uncertainty over the scope of the doctrine and by an appreciation that medical practice, indeed all professional practice, would be radically changed if fidelity to thoroughgoing self-determination were to prevail. In what follows, some

of the issues raised by the idea of an informed consent doctrine, based on a premise of self-determination, will be discussed.

Patients

Traditionally patients have been viewed as ignorant about medical matters, fearful about being sick, childlike by virtue of their illness, ill-equipped to sort out what is in their best medical interest, and prone to make decisions detrimental to their welfare (Parsons). Thus physicians have asserted that it makes little sense to consult patients on treatment options; far better to interact with them as beloved children and decide for them. In the light of such deeply held convictions, many physicians are genuinely puzzled by any informed consent requirement. Moreover, its possible detrimental impact on compassion, reassurance, and hope—ancient prescriptions for patient care—has raised grave ethical questions for the medical profession.

Those concerns should not be dismissed lightly. What may be at issue, however, is not an intrinsic incapacity of patients to participate in medical decision making. For not all patients, and probably not even most, are too uneducated, too frightened, or too regressed to understand the benefits and risks of treatment options available to them. Moreover, their capacities for decision making are affected to varying degrees, for example, by the nature of the disease process, its prognosis, acuteness, painfulness, etc., as well as by the personality of patients. The medical literature is largely silent on the question of who—under what circumstances and with what conditions—should or should not be allowed to participate fully in medical decision making.

But why has not the sorting-out process, distinguishing between those patients who do and those who do not have the capacity for decision making, been undertaken long ago? One answer suggests itself: Once those patients have been identified who, in principle, can make decisions on their own behalf, physicians would be compelled to confront the questions of whether to interact with them on a level of greater equality; whether to share with them the uncertainties and unknowns of medical diagnosis, treatment, and prognosis; and whether to communicate to them their professional limitations as well as the lack of expert consensus about treatment alternatives. Such an open dialogue would expose the uncertainties inherent in most medical interventions; and to the extent medicine's helpful and curative power depends on the faith and confidence which the physician projects, patients may be harmed by disclosure and consent.

Physicians' objections to informed consent, therefore, may have less to do with the incompetence of patients as such than with an unrecognized concern of the doctrine's impact on the dynamics of cure. Put another way, the all too sweeping traditional view of patients has misled doctors into believing that medicine's opposition to informed consent is largely based on patients' incompetence, rather than on an apprehension, however dimly perceived, that disclosure would bring into view much about the practice of medicine that physicians seek to hide from themselves and their patients; for example, the uncertainties and disagreements about the treatments employed; the curative impact of physicians' and patients' beliefs in the unquestioned effectiveness of their prescriptions rather than the prescriptions themselves; the difficulty in sorting out the contributions that *vis medicatrix naturae* ("the healing power of nature") makes to the healing process; the impact of patients' suggestibility to cure, etc. Thus the question: When does informed consent interfere with physicians' effectiveness and with the dynamics of cure?

Little attention has been paid to the fact that the practice of Hippocratic medicine makes patients more incompetent than they need be. Indeed patients' incompetence can become a self-fulfilling prophecy as a consequence of medical practices. That the stress of illness leads to psychological regression, to chronologically earlier modes of functioning, has been recognized for a long time. Precious little, however, is known about the contributions that physicians' attitudes toward and interactions with their patients make to the regressive pull. Also, little is known about the extent to which regression can be avoided by not keeping patients in the dark, by inviting them to participate in decision making, and by addressing and nurturing the intact, mature parts of their functioning. This uncharted territory requires exploration in order to determine what strains will be imposed on physicians and patients alike, if Anna Freud's admonition to students of the Western Reserve Medical School is heeded:

...you must not be tempted to treat [the patient] as a child. You must be tolerant toward him as you would be toward a child and as respectful as you would be towards a fellow adult because he has only gone back to childhood as far as he's ill. He also has another part of his personality which has remained intact and that part of him will resent it deeply, if you make too much use of your authority [quoted in Katz, p. 637].

Physicians

Traditionally physicians have asserted that their integrity, training, professional dedication to patients' best medical interests, and commitment to "doing no harm" are sufficient safeguards for patients. The complexities inherent in medical decision making, physicians maintain, require that trust be patients' guiding principle. The idea of informed consent does not question the integrity, training, or dedication of doctors. Without them, informed consent would be of little value. What the idea of informed consent does question is the necessity and appropriateness of physicians' making all decisions for their patients; it calls for a careful scrutiny of which decisions belong to the doctor and which to the patient.

Physicians have preferences about treatment options that may not necessarily be shared by patients. For example, no professional consensus exists about the treatment of breast cancer. The advantages and disadvantages of lumpectomy, simple mastectomy, radical mastectomy, radiation therapy, chemotherapy, and various combinations among these are subject to much controversy. Dr. Bernard Fisher, chairman of the National Surgical Adjuvant Breast Cancer Project, has said that we simply do not know which method is best (Fisher). Thus the question must be answered: How extensive an opportunity must patients be given to select which alternative? Informed consent challenges the stereotypical notion that physicians should assume the entire burden of deciding what treatment *all* patients, *whatever* their condition, should undergo. Indeed, can the assumption of this burden be defended purely on medical grounds in the first place? Is not the decision in favor of one treatment for breast cancer over another, like many other treatment decisions, a combination of medical, emotional, aesthetic, religious, philosophical, social, interpersonal, and personal judgments? Which of these component judgments belong to the physician and which to the patient?

Much needs to be investigated in order to learn the practical human limits of any new obligations to disclose and to obtain consent:

1. Informing patients for purposes of decision making requires learning new ways of interacting and communicating with patients. Such questions as the following will have to be answered: What background information must patients receive in order to help them formulate their questions? How should physicians respond to "precipitous" consents or refusals? How deeply should doctors probe for understanding? What constitutes irrelevant information that only tends to confuse? What words and explanations facilitate comprehension? Physicians have not been in the habit of posing such questions.

2. Underlying informed consent is the assumption that physicians have considerable knowledge about their particular specialties, keep abreast of new developments, and are aware of what is happening in other fields of medicine that impinge on their area of professional interest. This is not so; indeed, it may be asking too much. Moreover, since physicians have their preferences for particular modes of treatment, can they be expected to present an unbiased picture of alternative treatments?

3. Physicians have consistently asserted that informed consent interferes with compassion (Silk). Doctors believe that, in order to maintain hope or to avoid the imposition of unnecessary suffering, patients in the throes of a terminal illness, and other patients as well, should not be dealt with honestly. But the evidence for such allegations is lacking. When physicians are asked to support them with clinical data, they are largely unable to do so (Oken). Indeed, the few studies that have been conducted suggest that most patients do not seem to yearn for hope based on deception, but for hope based on a reassurance that they will not be abandoned, that everything possible will be done for them, and that physicians will deal truthfully with them. Moreover, evidence is accumulating that informed patients become more cooperative, more capable of dealing with discomfort and pain, and more responsible. Whether the often alleged conflict between "compassionate" silence and "cruel" disclosure is myth or reality remains to be seen. Disclosure may turn out to be a greater burden to those who have to interact with patients than to the patients themselves.

4. Informed consent confronts the role of faith in the cure of disease and the complex problems created by the uncertainties inherent in medical practice. To some extent the two issues are intertwined. The effectiveness of a therapeutic program, it has often been said, depends on three variables: the "feeling of trust or faith the patient has in his doctor and therefore in his therapy..., the faith or confidence the physician has in himself and in the line of therapy he proposes to use..., and the therapy [itself]" (Hoffer, p. 124). Informed consent could interfere with the first two variables and thus undermine the effectiveness of treatment. Precisely because of the uncertainties in medical decision making, the physician, to begin with, defends himself against those uncertainties by being more certain about what he is doing than he realistically can be. There is perhaps some unconscious wisdom in what he has been doing since Hippocrates' days, for the unquestioned faith the doctor has in his own therapy is also therapeutic in its own right. Thus, to be a more effective healer, a physician may need to defend himself against his uncertainties by believing himself to be more powerful than he is. That defense will be threatened by informed consent, for it would now require him to be more aware of what he does not know, and therapeutic effectiveness in turn might suffer. Finally, patients' response to treatment also depends on faith in the physician and his medicines. Knowing of the "ifs" and "buts" may shake patients' faith and undermine the therapeutic impact of suggestibility, which contributes so much to recovery from illness.

Physicians' traditional counterphobic reaction to uncertainty, adopting a sense of conviction that what seems right to them is the only correct thing to do, has other consequences as well. Defensive reactions against uncertainty have led to overenthusiasm for particular treatments that have been applied much more widely than an unbiased evaluation would dictate. The ubiquitous tonsillectomies performed to the psychological detriment of untold children is a classical example. Moreover, by not acknowledging uncertainty to themselves, doctors cannot acknowledge it to their patients. Thus consciously and unconsciously physicians avoid the terrifying confrontation of uncertainty, particularly when associated with poor prognosis. As a result, communications with patients take the form of an evasive monologue. The dialogue that might reveal these uncertainties is discouraged (Davis).

While disclosure of information would reduce patients' ignorance, it would also diminish doctors' power within the physician-patient relationship. As Waitzkin and Stoeckle have observed, the "physician enhances his power to the extent that he can maintain the patient's uncertainty about the course of illness, efficacy of therapy, or specific future actions of the physician himself" (p. 187). Thus new questions arise: What consequences would a diminution of authority have on physicians' effectiveness as healers? How would patients react to less powerful doctors? Would they accept them or turn to new faith healers?

Limits of Self-Determination

Patients' capacity for self-determination has been challenged on the grounds that neither total understanding nor total freedom of choice is possible (Ingelfinger). This of course is true. Any informed consent doctrine, to be realistic, must take into account the biological, psychological, intellectual, and social constraints imposed upon thought and action. But those inherent constraints, which affect all human beings, do not necessarily justify treating patients as incompetents. Competence does not imply total understanding or total freedom of choice.

What needs to be explored is the extent to which medicine, like law, should presume competence rather than incompetence, in interactions with patients. Neither presumption comports fully with the psychobiology of human beings; both of them express value judgments on how best to interact with human beings. Once the value judgment is made, one can decide on the additional safeguards needed to avoid the harm that any fiction about human behavior introduces.

The idea of informed consent asks for a presumption in favor of competence. If that is accepted, it may also follow that human beings should be allowed to strike their own bargains, however improvident. The then Circuit Judge Warren E. Burger, in commenting on a judicial decision to order a blood transfusion for a Jehovah's Witness had this to say: "Nothing in [Justice Brandeis' 'right to be let alone' philosophy suggests that he] thought an individual possessed these rights only as to *sensible* beliefs, *valid* thought, *reasonable* emotions or *well-founded* sensations. I suggest he intended to include a great many foolish, unreasonable and even absurd ideas which do not conform such as refusing medical treatment even at great risk" (*Application of President of Georgetown College*). A physician may wish, and even should try, to persuade his patients to agree to what he believes would serve their medical interests best; but ultimately he may have to bow to his patients' decision, however "senseless" or "unreasonable," or withdraw from further participation.

The alternatives, deception or coercion, may be worse, for either would victimize not only patients but physicians as well.

CONCLUSION

The narrow scope that courts have given to the informed consent doctrine may reflect a deeply held belief that the exercise of self-determination by patients is often against the best interests of otherwise responsible adults and that those interests deserve greater protection than personal freedom. It may also reflect a judicial recognition of law's limited capacity to regulate effectively the physician-patient relationship. Therefore, once having suggested that patients deserve at least a little openness in communication, courts may have concluded that they had gone as far as they could. Judges, at least for the time being, have largely left it up to the medical profession to confront the question of patients' greater participation in medical decision making.

Despite their snail's pace, the courts' approach may have merit. Implementing a right of self-determination has tremendous consequences for medical practice. Many difficult problems, each with vast ethical implications, need to be considered by the medical profession. Thus introspection and education, responsive to the legal and professional problems that new patterns of physician-patient interaction will create, may ultimately provide firmer foundations for new patterns of physician-patient interactions than forced change through outside regulation. The latter, however, may increase if the profession does not rise to the challenge of addressing these long-neglected problems.

BIBLIOGRAPHY

American Medical Association, Judicial Council: *Opinions and Reports of the Judicial Council.* Chicago: 1969.

———, Judicial Council: "Principles of Medical Ethics:" *Opinions and Reports of the Judicial Council*, pp. vi–vii.

Burger, Warren E.: "Reflections on Law and Experimental Medicine." *UCLA Law Review* 15 (1968): 436–442.

Davis, Fred: "Uncertainty in Medical Prognosis: Clinical and Functional." *American Journal of Sociology* 66 (1960): 41–47.

Fisher, Bernard: "The Surgical Dilemma in the Primary Therapy of Invasive Breast Cancer: A Critical Appraisal." *Current Problems in Surgery*, October 1970, pp. 1–53.

Glass, Eleanor S.: "Restructuring Informed Consent: Legal Therapy for the Doctor-Patient Relationship." *Yale Law Journal* 79 (1970): 1533–1576.

Henderson, L. J.: "Physician and Patient as a Social System." *New England Journal of Medicine* 212 (1935): 819–823.

Hippocrates: "Decorum." *Hippocrates*. 4 vols. Translated by W. H. S. Jones. The Loeb Classical Library. London: William Heinemann; New York: G. P. Putnam's Sons, 1923, vol. 2, pp. 278–301, especially par. 16, pp. 296–299.

Hoffer, A.: "A Theoretical Examination of Double-Blind Design." *Canadian Medical Association Journal* 97 (1967): 123–127.

Ingelfinger, F. J.: "Informed (But Uneducated) Consent." *New England Journal of Medicine* 287 (1972): 465–466.

Katz, Jay, ed.: *Experimentation with Human Beings: The Authority of the Investigator, Subject, Professions, and State in the Human Experimentation Process*. New York: Russell Sage Foundation, 1972.

Katz, Jay, and Capron, Alexander Morgan: *Catastrophic Diseases: Who Decides What? A Psychosocial and Legal Analysis of the Problems Posed by Hemodialysis and Organ Transplantation*. New York: Russell Sage Foundation, 1975.

McCoid, Allan H.: "A Reappraisal of Liability for Unauthorized Medical Treatment." *Minnesota Law Review* 41 (1957): 381–434.

Oken, Donald: "What to Tell Cancer Patients: A Study of Medical Attitudes." *Journal of the American Medical Association* 175 (1961): 1120–1128.

Parsons, Talcott: *The Social System*. Glencoe, Ill.: Free Press, 1951.

Percival, Thomas: *Medical Ethics*. Edited by Chauncey D. Leake. Baltimore: Williams & Wilkins Co., 1927.

Plante, Marcus L.: "An Analysis of 'Informed Consent'." *Fordham Law Review* 36 (1968): 639–672.

Silk, Arthur D.: "A Physician's Plea: Recognize Limitations of Informed Consent." *American Medical News*, 12 April 1976, p. 19.

Waitzkin, H., and Stoeckle, J. D.: "The Communication of Information about Illness: Clinical, Sociological, and Methodological Considerations." *Advances in Psychosomatic Medicine* 8 (1972): 180–215.

COURT DECISIONS

Application of President of Georgetown College. 331 F. 2d 1010 (D.C. Cir. 1964). Certiorari denied. 377 U.S. 978. 12 L. Ed. 2d 746. 84 S. Ct. 1883 (1964).

Canterbury v. Spence. 464 F.2d 772 (D.C.C.A. 1972).

Cobbs v. Grant. 104 Cal. Rptr. 505. 502 P.2d 1 (1972).

Dow v. Kaiser Foundation. 12 Cal. App.3d 488. 90 Cal. Rptr. 747 (Ct. App. 1970).

In re Estate of Brooks. 32 Ill. 2d 361. 205 N.E.2d 435 (1965).

Mohr v. Williams. 104 N.W. 12 (Minn. 1905).

Natanson v. Kline. 186 Kan. 393. 350 P.2d 1093 (1960). 187 Kan. 186. 354 P.2d 670 (1960).

Pratt v. Davis. 118 Ill. App. 161 (1905). Aff. 224 Ill. 300. 79 N.E. 562 (1906).

Salgo v. Stanford University. 317 P.2d 170 (Cal. 1st Dist. Ct. App. 1957).

Schloendorff v. New York Hospital. 105 N.E. 92 (N.Y. 1914).

Wilkinson v. Vesey. 295 A.2d 676 (R.I. 1972).

Conclusions and Recommendations Regarding Informed Consent

President's Commission for the Study of Ethical Problems in Medicine and Biomedical and Behavioral Research

The President's Commission, created in 1978, began its deliberations early in 1980 and ended them in 1983. Its task was to deal with several specific issues raised by

Reprinted from President's Commission for the Study of Ethical Problems in Medicine and Biomedical and Behavioral Research, *Making Health Care Decisions*, Volume One: Report (1982), pp. 2–6.

the practice of medicine and the distribution of health care. The Commission issued reports on the informed consent requirement, the definition of death, genetic screening and counseling, the compensation of research subjects, and the distribution of health care. During its life, the Commission included twenty-one commissioners. It was chaired by Morris B. Abram; its executive director was Alexander Morgan Capron, who is professor of law, ethics, and public policy at Georgetown University Law Center.

In making its recommendations, the Commission rejects the idea that obtaining informed consent is simply a matter of reciting the contents of a form and getting a signature. It sees ethically valid consent as a *process* of shared decision making based on mutual respect and participation. Although stressing the importance of self-determination, the Commission recognizes that some people may be permanently incapable of making their own decisions and that others may be temporarily unable to exercise their right of self-determination. It, therefore, provides some recommendations about making decisions for those unable to do so.

Before the Commission could consider means of improvement, it had to address the underlying theoretical issues. The ethical foundation of informed consent can be traced to the promotion of two values: personal well-being and self-determination. To ensure that these values are respected and enhanced, the Commission finds that patients who have the capacity to make decisions about their care must be permitted to do so voluntarily and must have all relevant information regarding their condition and alternative treatments, including possible benefits, risks, costs, other consequences, and significant uncertainties surrounding any of this information. This conclusion has several specific implications:

(1) Although the informed consent doctrine has substantial foundations in law, it is essentially an ethical imperative.

(2) Ethically valid consent is a process of shared decision-making based upon mutual respect and participation, not a ritual to be equated with reciting the contents of a form that details the risks of particular treatments.

(3) Much of the scholarly literature and legal commentary about informed consent portrays it as a highly rational means of decisionmaking about health care matters, thereby suggesting that it may only be suitable for and applicable to well-educated, articulate, self-aware individuals. Whether this is what the legal doctrine was intended to be or what it has inadvertently become, it is a view the Commission unequivocally rejects. Although subcultures within American society differ in their views about autonomy and individual choice and about the etiology of illness and the roles of healers and patients,[1] a survey conducted for the Commission found a universal desire for information, choice, and respectful communication about decisions.[2] Informed consent must remain flexible, yet the process, as the Commission envisions it throughout this Report, is ethically required of health care practitioners in their relationships with all patients, not a luxury for a few.

(4) Informed consent is rooted in the fundamental recognition—reflected in the legal presumption of competency—that adults are entitled to accept or reject health care interventions on the basis of their own personal values and in furtherance of their own personal goals. Nonetheless, patient choice is not absolute.

• Patients are not entitled to insist that health care practitioners furnish them services when to do so would violate either the bounds of acceptable practice or a professional's own deeply held moral beliefs or would draw on a limited resource on which the patient has no binding claim.

• The fundamental values that informed consent is intended to promote—self-determination and patient well-being—both demand that alternative arrangements for health care decisionmaking be made for individuals who lack substantial capacity to make their own decisions. Respect for self-determination requires, however, that in the first instance individuals be deemed to have decisional capacity, which should not be treated as a hurdle to be surmounted in the vast majority of cases, and that incapacity be treated as a disqualifying factor in the small minority of cases.

• Decisionmaking capacity is specific to each particular decision. Although some people lack this capacity for all decisions, many are incapacitated in more limited ways and are capable of making some decisions but not others. The concept of capacity is best understood and applied in a functional manner. That is, the presence or absence of capacity does not depend on a person's status or on the decision reached, but on that individual's actual functioning in situations in which a decision about health care is to be made.

• Decisionmaking incapacity should be found to exist only when people lack the ability to make decisions that promote their well-being in conformity with their own previously expressed values and preferences.

• To the extent feasible people with no decisionmaking capacity should still be consulted about their own preferences out of respect for them as individuals.

(5) Health care providers should not ordinarily withhold unpleasant information simply because it is unpleasant. The ethical foundations of informed consent allow the withholding of information from patients only when they request that it be withheld or when its disclosure per se would cause substantial detriment to their well-being....

(6) Achieving the Commission's vision of shared decisionmaking based on mutual respect is ultimately the responsibility of individual health care professionals. However, health care institutions such as hospitals and professional schools have important roles to play in assisting health care professionals in this obligation. The manner in which health care is provided in institutional settings often results in a fragmentation of responsibility that may neglect the human side of health care. To assist in guarding against this, institutional health care providers should ensure that ultimately there is one readily identifiable practitioner responsible for providing information to a particular patient. Although pieces of information may be provided by various people, there should be one individual officially charged with responsibility for ensuring that all the necessary information is communicated and that the patient's wishes are known to the treatment team.

(7) Patients should have access to the information they need to help them understand their conditions and make treatment decisions....

(8) As cases arise and new legislation is contemplated, courts and legislatures should reflect this view of ethically valid consent. Nevertheless, the Commission does not look to legal reforms as the primary means of bringing about changes in the relationship between health care professionals and patients.

(9) The Commission finds that a number of relatively simple changes in practice could facilitate patient participation in health care decisionmaking. Several specific techniques—such as having patients express, orally or in writing, their understanding of the treatment consented to—deserve further study. Furthermore, additional societal resources need to be committed to improving the human side of health care, which has apparently deteriorated at the same time there have been substantial gains in health care technology....

(10) Because health care professionals are responsible for ensuring that patients can participate effectively in decisionmaking regarding their care, educators have a responsibility to prepare physicians and nurses to carry out this obligation....

(11) Family members are often of great assistance to patients in helping to understand information about their condition and in making decisions about treatment. The Commission recommends that health care institutions and professionals recognize this and judiciously attempt to involve family members in decisionmaking for patients, with due regard for the privacy of patients and for the possibilities for coercion that such a practice may entail.

(12) The Commission recognizes that its vision of health care decisionmaking may involve greater commitments of time on the part of health professionals. Because of the importance of shared decisionmaking based on mutual trust, not only for the promotion of patient well-being and self-determination but also for the therapeutic gains that can be realized, the Commission recommends that all medical and surgical interventions be thought of as including appropriate discussion with patients. Reimbursement to the professional should therefore take account of time spent in discussion rather than regarding it as a separate item for which additional payment is made.

(13) To protect the interests of patients who lack decisionmaking capacity and to ensure their well-being and self-determination, the Commission concludes that:

• Decisions made by others on patients' behalf should, when possible, attempt to replicate the ones patients would make if they were capable of doing so. When this is not feasible, decisions by surrogates on behalf of patients must protect the patients' best interests. Because such decisions are not instances of personal self-choice, limits may be placed on the range of acceptable decisions that surrogates make beyond those that apply when a person makes his or her own decisions.

• Health care institutions should adopt clear and explicit policies regarding how and by whom decisions are to be made for patients who cannot decide.

• Families, health care institutions, and professionals should work together to make health care decisions for patients who lack decisionmaking capacity. Recourse to courts should be reserved for the occasions when concerned parties are unable to resolve their disagreements over matters of substantial import, or when adjudication is clearly required by state law. Courts and legislatures should be cautious about requiring judicial review of routine health care decisions for patients who lack capacity.

• Health care institutions should explore and evaluate various informal administrative arrangements, such as "ethics committees," for review and consultation in nonroutine matters involving health care decisionmaking for those who cannot decide.

• As a means of preserving some self-determination for patients who no longer possess decisionmaking capacity, state courts and legislatures should consider making provision for advance directives through which people designate others to make health care decisions on their behalf and/or give instructions about their care.

The Commission acknowledges that the conclusions contained in this Report will not be simple to achieve. Even when patients and practitioners alike are sensitive to the goal of shared decisionmaking based on mutual respect, substantial barriers will still exist.[3] Some of these obstacles, such as long-standing professional attitudes or difficulties in conveying medical information in ordinary language, are formidable but can be overcome if there is a will to do so. Others, such as the dependent condition of very sick patients or the ever-growing complexity and subspecialization of medicine, will have to be accommodated because they probably cannot be eliminated. Nonetheless, the Commission's vision of informed consent still has value as a measuring stick against which actual performance may be judged and as a goal toward which all participants in health care decisionmaking can strive.

NOTES

1 Robert A. Hahn, *Culture and Informed Consent: An Anthropological Perspective* (1982), Appendix F in Vol. 3 of this Report.
2 The Commission's survey of the public broke down these responses on the basis of variables such as age, gender, race, education, and income.
3 Jay Katz, *Informed Consent—A Fairy Tale?: Law's Vision*, 39 U. Pitt. L. Rev. 137 (1977).

ANNOTATED BIBLIOGRAPHY: CHAPTER 2

Ad Hoc Committee on Medical Ethics, American College of Physicians: "American College of Physicians Ethics Manual," *Annals of Internal Medicine* 101 (1984), pp. 129–137 (Part I), pp. 263–274 (Part II). This is a position paper published by the American College of Physicians. It is an extended presentation of the college's thinking on the physician-patient relationship, the physician-society relationship and on other ethical issues including the ethics of research. The document can be seen as the fruition of much of the reflection that has taken place during the last 10 to 15 years in the field of biomedical ethics.

Alfidi, Ralph J.: "Informed Consent: A Study of Patient Reaction," *Journal of the American Medical Association* 216 (May 24, 1971), pp. 1325–1329. Alfidi reports on a statistical study of informed consent. This study showed, contrary to the expectations of those conducting it, that patients did not refuse angiography after being informed of its possible complications. Alfidi was surprised to learn that patients seem to prefer a straightforward and perhaps even harsh statement of the possible complications of medical procedures.

Edelstein, Ludwig: *Ancient Medicine* (Baltimore: Johns Hopkins, 1967). In this book, Edelstein discusses "The Hippocratic Oath" and shows that it contains two distinct sets of obligations—those pertaining to the patient and those owed to the physician's teacher and the teacher's progeny.

Etziony, M. B., ed.: *The Physician's Creed* (Springfield, Ill.: Charles C Thomas, 1973). This is subtitled "An Anthology of Medical Prayers, Oaths and Codes of Ethics Written and Recited by Medical Practitioners through the Ages." The collection reveals the aims and ethical orientation of medicine during its history.

Ladd, John: "Legalism in Medical Ethics," *Journal of Medicine and Philosophy* 4 (March 1979), pp. 70–80. Ladd criticizes the recent trend in biomedical ethics that tends to reduce all moral relationships to rule-following and rights claims. He proposes an alternative "ethic of responsibility."

Masters, Roger D.: "Is Contract an Adequate Basis for Medical Ethics?" *Hastings Center Report* 5 (December 1975), pp. 24–28. Masters argues that contract theory is not an adequate basis for medical ethics. He examines the differences between the physician-patient relationship and the contractual relationship that usually holds between buyers and sellers of other types of services. Masters argues that we should not base medical ethics on some "presumed rights" of isolated individuals. We must focus instead on the entire social context and formulate theories about patients' rights and professional obligations within a broader ethical theory that will balance the interests and obligations of human beings as they relate to the whole community.

Oken, Donald: "What to Tell Cancer Patients," *Journal of the American Medical Association* 175 (1961), pp. 1120–1128. Oken presents research data about physicians' attitudes and policies in regard to "telling" cancer patients the truth.

President's Commission for the Study of Ethical Problems in Medicine and Biomedical and Behavioral Research: *Making Health Care Decisions: The Ethical and Legal Implications of Informed Consent in the Patient-Practitioner Relationship Vol. 1: Report* (Washington, D.C.: U.S. Government Printing Office, 1982). This report presents the Commission's conclusions and recommendations regarding both the role of informed consent in the patient-practitioner relationship and the means which might be used to promote a fuller understanding by patients and professionals of their common enterprise.

——: *Making Health Care Decisions Vol. 2 Appendices: Empirical Studies of Informed Consent.* This volume contains the empirical studies used by the President's Commission in formulating its conclusions.

——: *Making Health Care Decisions Vol. 3: Studies in the Foundations of Informed Consent.* Viewpoints represented in this volume are those of a psychologist, a historian, an anthropologist, a sociologist, a pediatrician-oncologist, a philosopher, and a medical student.

Ramsey, Paul: *The Patient as Person* (New Haven: Yale University Press, 1970). Ramsey's book has been one of the most influential works in contemporary discussions of medical ethics. It covers a wide variety of topics, such as the ethics of experimentation and the ethics of transplantation. In this book, Ramsey puts forth his often-quoted view on the physician-patient relationship. He describes this relationship in terms of a covenant and sees the principle of informed consent as the "cardinal canon of loyalty," which joins people together in medical practice and investigations.

Reiser, Stanley Joel, Arthur J. Dyck, and William J. Curran: *Ethics in Medicine: Historical Perspectives and Contemporary Concerns* (Cambridge, Mass.: M.I.T., 1977), Chapter

4. This chapter, entitled "Truth-Telling in the Physician-Patient Relationship," includes articles scanning the period from 1803 to 1974.

Rosoff, Arnold J.: *Informed Consent: A Guide for Health Care Providers* (Rockville, Md.: Aspen, 1981). This is a reference book that contains a great deal of practical information. It (1) sets forth the law in the informed consent area; (2) provides a philosophical framework for understanding legal developments; and (3) lays a foundation for researching questions of patient-consent law in particular states.

Chapter 3

Professionals' Obligations, Institutions, and Patients' Rights

INTRODUCTION

Many who receive medical care today do so in hospitals, nursing homes, clinics, and other large institutions. Providers of health care include nurses, interns, staff physicians, operating room technicians, and other health-care professionals and paraprofessionals. Many medical care providers are not private practitioners but employees of the kinds of institutions mentioned above. Under these circumstances, a discussion of patients' rights and health professionals' responsibilities must encompass much more than the moral considerations raised in Chapter 2, which center primarily on the physician-patient relationship. This chapter explores some of the rights of hospital patients, the correlative responsibilities of professionals, and some ethical issues raised regarding geriatric patients in both hospitals and nursing homes. It also examines some of the moral dilemmas faced by nurses and other health-care professionals because of possible conflicts of obligation.

Patients' Rights

What rights do hospital patients have? Recent statements of patients' rights, such as the American Hospital Association's "A Patient's Bill of Rights," included in this chapter, attempt to answer this question. These documents, however, usually say nothing about the nature of the rights in question. They do not specify whether the statements of "rights" function: (1) as analogues of professional codes of ethics intended to provide moral guidelines for professional behavior, (2) as explicit formulations of moral rights, carrying correlative obligations, which the framers of these statements believe to be among the moral rights of all autonomous individuals, or (3) simply as statements of legal rights granted by a particular legal system. Despite this ambiguity, statements of patients' rights do serve as reminders to both hospital patients and health professionals that patients are persons; they are neither "mere objects" to be manipulated by professionals nor subservient beings who have waived their right of self-determination and other rights simply by becoming hospital patients.

Statements of hospital patients' rights have been explicitly formulated only recently. Most of us would take the rights asserted for granted. They include, for example, patients' rights to confidentiality and to adequate information regarding their condition. The apparent need to make these rights explicit, however, may be due to an increased awareness of their importance and of their almost routine institutional abuses. Any recent hospital patient suspects that hospital routines are often organized around staff convenience rather than patient comfort and that patients are often treated as "cases" rather than as "persons." One critic of hospital practices, Willard Gaylin, describes the situation as follows:

> A stay in a hospital exposes an individual to a condition of passivity and impotence unparallelled in adult life, this side of prison. You are dressed in an uncomfortable garment, leaving you exposed and ludicrous; told when you must sleep and when you must rise; informed of what you may eat and when you have to eat it; notified as to when you can have visitors, who they shall be, and how long they can stay. You are discussed in the third person in your presence as though you were some idiot child or inanimate object. If you are unfortunate enough to have an interesting case, you will be presented to a group of strangers who may take the invasion of your privacy as their privilege. Your chart, at the foot of the bed, will contain all the vital information that you would seem to be entitled to have; yet, should you attempt to examine it, you will be treated like a pre-pubescent caught with a copy of *Portnoy's Complaint*.
>
> Some of this may be necessary for health and some for convenience, but most of it is simply the inevitable result of an authoritative person dealing with people who unquestionably accept his authority.[1]

Gaylin is not impressed by the American Hospital Association's statement of rights. He considers it a weak document that simply reminds patients of their rights but does not take hospitals to task for their failure to respect patients' rights. As George Annas points out in a reading in this chapter, however, although the document can be criticized on grounds of incompleteness, lack of specificity, and unenforceability, it does have tremendous symbolic value, especially since the rights it espouses are currently under attack. Critics question both the advisability of asserting these rights and patients' interest in exercising them. For Annas, the grounds for the attack lie in the tension, discussed in Chapter 2, between health professionals' desires to promote patients' medical well-being, *as it is perceived by those professionals,* and patients' right of self-determination. Annas, arguing that patients do have rights and do want to exercise them, proposes and discusses five rights intended to humanize hospitals and to promote hospital patients' self-determination.

The Nurse: Professional Obligations and Patients' Rights

Nurses face both a special set of moral problems with regard to patients' rights and a set of moral problems similar to those faced by physicians. Nurses, like physicians, for example, are sometimes forced to choose between doing what they believe will promote patients' well-being and respecting patients' right of self-determination. In this chapter, Sheri Smith discusses three possible models of the nurse-patient relationship, analogous to three of the models of the physician-patient relationship presented by Robert Veatch in Chapter 2. Rejecting paternalism, she argues for a contracted-clinician model, which respects both a patient's right of self-determination and a nurse's right of conscientious refusal. She notes, however, that nurses often face moral dilemmas that are not faced by physicians. These dilemmas result from the nurse's position in the hospital health-care hierarchy. Nurses in hospitals care for patients and supervise others giving that care. Usually, they are directly responsible both for patient care and for the implementation of therapy. At the same time, nurses have very little influence in decision making regarding patients. Furthermore, they are subordinate to doctors who make diagnoses and issue orders that nurses are obligated to carry out. Under these circumstances, nurses are sometimes confronted with situations in which their obligations to patients seem to conflict with their obligations to physicians. The following questions exemplify the kinds of problems nurses face: (1) Should nurses follow physicians' orders when (*a*) they have good reason to believe that the orders are mistaken, (*b*) the physicians refuse to admit that they might be mistaken, and (*c*) following orders will jeopardize a patient's safety or well-being? (2) What should nurses do if they have good reason to believe that physicians are violating their patients' right of self-determination? For example, what should a nurse do when a physician lies or withholds information from a patient? E. Joy Kroeger Mappes focuses on these sorts of questions in this chapter. She stresses the difficulties faced by nurses in our society when protecting patients' interests requires them to "buck" the hierarchical system. Mappes attributes a major part of this difficulty to the classist and sexist forces in society.

Nurses frequently agree with Mappes, expressing concern about the impact of sexism and the nurse's powerlessness on hospital patient care. They note, for example, that nurses usually lack the power to enforce staffing standards even when understaffing endangers patients' lives. Those who argue that nurses should have more power sometimes ask whether nurses themselves have an obligation to support collective professional efforts to change a hierarchical system that often works to the patient's detriment. James L. Muyskens deals with such questions in this chapter as he discusses the collective responsibility of the nursing profession.

Privacy, Confidentiality, and Conflicting Loyalties

Whatever the full complement of patients' rights may be, the right of privacy and the related principle of confidentiality deserve special discussion. The importance of the principle of confidentiality in the medical context has long been recognized. It is affirmed in the "Hippocratic Oath" as well as in more recent medical ethical codes such as those of the American Medical Association and the American Nurses' Association. It is also recognized by the ethical codes of medical record librarians and medical social workers. Even the law recognizes the importance of the patient's right to retain control of the information held by health professionals. It does so in two ways: (1) Physicians and psychotherapists are subject to legal sanctions if they reveal confidential information about patients; (2) Physicians and psychotherapists are exempt from giving testimony about their patients before a court of law. Most discussions of the moral significance of the principle of confidentiality in the health-care context stress either the importance of protecting the trust essential to the professional-patient relationship or the patient's right of privacy.

The right of privacy is broader than the right of patients to have confidential information kept confidential by health-care personnel. Observation of hospitalized patients without their consent, for example, is seen as one very important violation of privacy. Why is so much moral significance attached to this broader right of privacy? Discussions of privacy, like discussions of informed consent, stress the relation between the right of privacy and individual autonomy. Richard Wasserstrom's analysis of the right of privacy in this chapter, for example, includes the claim that the diminution of privacy suffered by hospitalized patients affects their sense of being autonomous individuals deserving the respect accorded to such individuals. Others argue that the right of privacy is one of our most basic rights, since to acknowledge another's right of privacy is to acknowledge that the other is an autonomous individual with exclusive control over access to certain core aspects of himself or herself.

The selection by LeRoy Walters in this chapter and the opinions in *Tarasoff v. Regents of the University of California* raise a different issue regarding the patient's right to retain control over certain kinds of information. They focus on the moral dilemmas posed for physicians and psychotherapists by conflicting obligations. In *Tarasoff,* for example, the psychologist had to choose between respecting the confidence of a patient, Prosenjit Poddar, and warning a young woman, Tatiana Tarasoff, that Poddar might try to kill her. He did not warn the woman or her family, and Poddar did kill her. Should the psychologist have violated the principle of confidentiality in respect to his patient? Did he have an obligation to protect the life of a woman who was not his patient? If he did, should this obligation have taken precedence over his duty to respect Poddar's confidences? The contrast between the majority and the dissenting opinions in the case serves to heighten awareness of the moral dilemmas raised for the professional who must choose between violating a patient's rights and failing to perform an act that might save the life of another human being.

Other problems are raised for the traditional right to confidentiality by current developments in medical care. Hospital medicine, the need to share information among the members of health-care teams, the existence of third-party insurance programs, and the expanding limits of medicine all result in a fairly wide dissemination of "confidential" information about patients. Mark Siegler, in this chapter, discusses some of these problems.

Geriatric Patients

Literature in biomedical ethics dealing with patients' rights has been relatively silent on the rights of patients in nursing homes and other extended-care facilities.[2] Ethical issues centering on geriatric patients, who make up the bulk of the population in such institutions, have not received much attention in the literature thus far. Is there a need to deal more extensively with ethical issues revolving around the rights of geriatric patients, specifically with issues raised by care in extended-care facilities? Ruth Macklin explores such questions in an article in this chapter. Much of her discussion centers on questions of patient autonomy and competence and on some often unexamined assumptions that underlie the paternalistic treatment of geriatric patients. Both Macklin and George A. Kanoti discuss some of the moral questions raised regarding the treatment of geriatric patients in nursing homes.

                                                                                     J.S.Z.

NOTES

1 Willard Gaylin, "The Patient's Bill of Rights," *Saturday Review of the Sciences* 1 (February 24, 1973), p. 22.

2 The major exception to this generalization about extended-care facilities is the mental institution or hospital. The rights of those institutionalized as mentally ill have been extensively discussed.

Hospitals and Patients' Rights

A Patient's Bill of Rights

American Hospital Association

This statement, issued by the American Hospital Association, was affirmed by the AHA House of Delegates on February 6, 1973. It makes explicit some "moral rights" that many would take for granted (such as the right to considerate and respectful care) and some legal rights that hospitals, as well as other institutions, must respect.

The American Hospital Association presents a Patient's Bill of Rights with the expectation that observance of these rights will contribute to more effective patient care and greater satisfaction for the patient, his physician, and the hospital organization. Further, the Association presents these rights in the expectation that they will be supported by the hospital on behalf of its patients, as an integral part of the healing process. It is recognized that a personal relationship between the physician and the patient is essential for the provision of proper medical care. The traditional physician-patient relationship takes on a new dimension when care is rendered within an organizational structure. Legal precedent has established that the institution itself also has a responsibility to the patient. It is in recognition of these factors that these rights are affirmed.

(1) The patient has the right to considerate and respectful care.

(2) The patient has the right to obtain from his physician complete current information concerning his diagnosis, treatment, and prognosis in terms the patient can be reasonably expected to understand. When it is not medically advisable to give such information to the patient, the information should be made available to an appropriate person in his behalf. He has the right to know, by name, the physician responsible for coordinating his care.

(3) The patient has the right to receive from his physician information necessary to give informed consent prior to the start of any procedure and/or treatment. Except in emergencies, such information for informed consent should include but not necessarily be limited to the specific procedure and/or treatment, the medically significant risks involved, and the probable duration of incapacitation. Where medically significant alternatives for care or treatment exist, or when the patient requests information concerning medical alternatives, the patient has the right to such information. The patient also has the right to know the name of the person responsible for the procedures and/or treatment.

(4) The patient has the right to refuse treatment to the extent permitted by law and to be informed of the medical consequences of his action.

(5) The patient has the right to every consideration of his privacy concerning his own medical care program. Case discussion, consultation, examination, and treatment are confidential and should be conducted discreetly. Those not directly involved in his care must have the permission of the patient to be present.

(6) The patient has the right to expect that all communications and records pertaining to his care should be treated as confidential.

(7) The patient has the right to expect that within its capacity a hospital must make reasonable response to the request of a patient for services. The hospital must provide evaluation, service, and/or referral as indicated by the urgency of the case. When medically permissible, a patient may be transferred to another facility only after he has received complete information and explanation concerning the needs for and alternatives to such a transfer. The institution to which the patient is to be transferred must first have accepted the patient for transfer.

(8) The patient has the right to obtain information as to any relationship of his hospital to other health care and educational institutions insofar as his care is concerned. The patient has the right to obtain information as to the existence of any professional relationships among individuals, by name, who are treating him.

(9) The patient has the right to be advised if the hospital proposes to engage in or perform human experimentation affecting his care or treatment. The patient has the right to refuse to participate in such research projects.

(10) The patient has the right to expect reasonable continuity of care. He has the right to know in advance what appointment times and physicians are available and where. The patient has the right to expect that the hospital will provide a mechanism whereby he is informed by his physician or a delegate of the physician of the patient's continuing health care requirements following discharge.

(11) The patient has the right to examine and receive an explanation of his bill regardless of source of payment.

(12) The patient has the right to know what hospital rules and regulations apply to his conduct as a patient.

No catalog of rights can guarantee for the patient the kind of treatment he has a right to expect. A hospital has many functions to perform, including the prevention and treatment of disease, the education of both health professionals and patients, and the conduct of clinical research. All these activities must be conducted with an overriding concern for the patient, and, above all, the recognition of his dignity as a human being. Success in achieving this recognition assures success in the defense of the rights of the patient.

The Emerging Stowaway, Patients' Rights in the 1980s

George J. Annas

George J. Annas teaches law and medicine in the Department of Socio-Medical Sciences and Community Medicine at the Boston University School of Medicine. Annas is the author of *The Rights of Hospital Patients* (1975), coauthor of *Informed Consent to Human Experimentation* (1977) and *The Rights of Doctors, Nurses and Allied Health Professionals* (1981), and coeditor of *Genetics and the Law* (1976). He also writes a regular column on "Law and the Life Sciences" for the *Hastings Center Report*.

Annas maintains that the majority of physicians favor medical paternalism because they value their patients' health and continued life more than patients' right to self-determination. This general view, he argues, affects their attitudes to "patients' rights" and tends to make them accept the conclusions of sloppy studies that downgrade the importance of some of the rights asserted and throw doubt on patients' interest in exercising them. Annas discusses some of these studies to bring out their inadequacies and then asserts five rights intended to humanize the hospital environment and give patients more of a voice regarding their treatment.

At one point in Edgar Allan Poe's *Narrative of Arthur Gordon Pym of Nantucket*, Pym, who has stowed away in the hold of a whaling vessel, believes he has been abandoned and that the hold will be his tomb. He expressed sensations of "extreme horror and dismay," and "the most gloomy imaginings, in which the dreadful deaths of thirst, famine, suffocation, and premature interment, crowded in as the prominent disasters to be encountered."

It is probably uncommon for hospitalized patients to feel as gloomy as Pym. Nevertheless, installed in a strange institution, separated from friends and family, forced to wear a degrading costume, confined to bed, and attended to by a variety of strangers who may or may not keep the patient informed of what they are doing, the average patient is intimidated and disoriented. Such an atmosphere encourages dependence and discourages the assertion of individual rights.

As the physician-director of Boston's Beth Israel Hospital has warned: "today's hospital stands increasingly to become a jungle, whose pathways to the uninitiated are poorly marked and fraught with danger...."[1] In this jungle the notion that patients have rights that demand respect is often foreign.

The movement for enhanced patients' rights is based on two premises: (1) citizens possess certain rights that are not automatically forfeited by entering into a relationship with a physician or health care facility; and (2) most physicians and health care facilities fail to recognize these rights, fail to provide for their protection or assertion, and limit their exercise without recourse.[2]

The primary argument against patients' rights is that patients have "needs" and defining these needs in terms of rights leads to the creation of an unhealthy adversary relationship.[3] It is not, however, the creation of rights, but the disregard of them, that produces adversaries. When provider and patient work together in an atmosphere of mutual trust and understanding, the articulation of rights can only enhance their relationship....

THE AHA BILL OF RIGHTS

It must strike most people as ironic that the first major health care organization to put forward a patients' bill of rights was the American Hospital Association (AHA), an organization composed primarily of hospital administrators. One would not expect landlords to pen a bill of rights for tenants, police for suspects, or wardens for prisoners. Nor would one reasonably expect that the hospital administrator's view on rights for patients would be the same as either the patient's or society's. Nevertheless, physicians and nurses should be ashamed that the administrators were well out in front of them on this issue. Even though it leaves much to be desired in terms of completeness, specificity, and enforceability, the AHA Bill has tremendous symbolic value in legitimizing the notion of rights in the health care institution.[4] On the other hand, fewer than half of all AHA member hospitals have formally adopted even this bill, and the symbolic victory of the 1970s is currently under attack.

THE ATTACK ON PATIENTS' RIGHTS

Physicians, who perhaps value their own professional autonomy more than any other group, nevertheless devalue it for their own patients. Instead, paternalism is the norm with the majority of physicians believing that the health and continued life of their patients is much more important than their patients' right to self-determination. This belief system not only leads to conflicts with individual patients about their own care, but also to a general view that sees patients' rights as being a luxury item in medicine rather than a necessity.

A few examples illustrate the point. Two particular rights of patients have recently come under attack in the medical literature: access to medical records and informed consent. In an attack on "record reading," four psychiatrists at Boston's Peter Bent Brigham Hospital interviewed the 11 out of 2,500 patients at that hospital in a one year period who asked to see their medical records.[5] It is doubtful that anything of general importance about a patient's reactions to reading their charts can be learned from an uncontrolled, nonblind, clinically impressionistic study of those few individuals who, for whatever reason, buck a system that routinely fails to inform them of their right of access to their records. Nonetheless, the authors' conclusion that such patients have a variety of personality defects, usually manifesting themselves in mistrust of and hostility toward the hospital staff, should not be permitted to go uncontested. In a setting where trusting patients are not routinely told of their right to access, it seems reasonable to assume that only the least trusting or most angry will ask to see their records. To locate the source of mistrust in the patient's personality style or in the stress of illness and hospitalization is to forget, as Dr. Lipsett perceptively suggests, that "the doctor-patient relationship cannot be understood simply in terms of the patient's side of the equation."[6] Altman et al. thus fall into what Professor Robert Burt of the Yale Law School has referred to as "the conceptual trap of attempting to transform two-party relationships, in which mutual self-delineations are inherently confused and intertwined, by conceptually obliterating one party...."[7] Thus, it would seem that the ten women who asked to read their charts "to confirm the belief that the staff harbored negative personal attitudes toward them..." were correct in the belief; the psychiatrists labelled them "of the hysterical type with demanding, histrionic behavior and emotional over-involvement with the staff."

Altman et al. also seem unaware of the wide variety of settings in which patients have *benefited* from routine record access, and incorrectly assert that there were no strikingly beneficial effects in the two studies they do cite. In the first study, for example, two patients expressed their completely unfounded fear that they had cancer only after their record was reviewed with them, and one pregnant patient noted an incorrect Rh typing that permitted RhoGam to be administered at the time of delivery.[8] In the other study they cite, 50 percent of the patients made some factual correction in the record.[9]

In short, the study seems to have been done and published for the primary purpose of proving that the right to record access is unimportant since it is only exercised by "mentally disturbed" people who are not improved by reading their charts. It fails to prove this, and even if it succeeded, I would still be unwilling to deprive the other 2,489 patients of their right to access in the future. If we believe in individual freedom and the concept of self-determination, we must give all citizens the right to make their *own* decisions and to have access to information that is widely available to those making decisions about them. It is as irrelevant in this connection that 2,489 patients at the Peter Bent Brigham Hospital did not ask to see their records as it is that more than 200 million Americans never have had to exercise their right to remain silent when arrested. Rights serve us all, whether we exercise them or not.

The attack on informed consent, which many physicians have long considered a "legal fiction,"[10] most recently surfaced in a study often used to "prove" that informed consent was not an important patients' right in practice, because patients could not remember what they were informed of.[11] The methodology involved interviewing 200 consecutive cancer patients who had consented to chemotherapy, surgery, or radiation therapy for their cancers within 24 hours after they had signed consent forms. Upon questioning, most could not recall the procedure consented to, its major risks, or the alternatives to it. From this the authors conclude that the process is not working and that informed consent itself is suspect. Although this may seem to be a reasonable conclusion (an alternative one is simply that patients have poor recall), it turns out that the authors presumed their major premise. Approximately two-thirds of their sample group (66 percent) opted for radiation therapy. That group signed a consent form that said "the procedure, its risks and benefits and alternatives have been explained to me." Maybe they were, but maybe they were not. The authors did not know, so their entire study was based on a premise that was unsubstantiated. Such a poorly designed study, it

seems to me, could only be published if the editors agreed so strongly with the conclusion that they did not even review the methodology.

A perhaps more interesting part of the study asked the patients some general questions about informed consent. The first was, "What are consent forms for?" Approximately 80 percent responded: "To protect the physicians' rights." The authors were upset at this response, but the patients of course were correct. That *is* the primary function of *forms*. If one wants these forms also to protect the patient, three simple steps are necessary: (1) the forms must be complete; (2) they must be in lay language; and (3) the patients must be given a copy of the form and time to think over the information it contains.[12] The reason none of these is usually done is clear: Informed consent is not taken seriously in the hospital setting. It is, like record access, a luxury that is secondary to caring for the medical "needs" of the patient, and besides, it really doesn't matter anyway because patients can't remember anything they've been told....

Other significant findings that indicate the extent to which patients understand and appreciate the consent process are: 80 percent thought the forms were necessary; 76 percent thought they contained just the right amount of information; 84 percent understood all or most of the information; 75 percent thought the explanations given were important; and 90 percent said they would try to remember the information contained on the forms. To me, this suggests that the patients surveyed, understood, and appreciated the informed consent process much better than the researchers did. Their data are certainly not flawless, but one can conclude from the data just the opposite of what the researchers did: For almost all patients, informed consent is seen as very important.

Related to this general attack on rights is an attack on the patient population itself. The notion is that the major problems with the health care delivery system are not problems with providers, but with patients. We eat too much, smoke too much, do not exercise enough, take too many risks, and it serves us right if we get sick. The American health care enterprise must deal with a bad class of patients that (on top of everything) now not only wants access to care, but also wants some say in what kind of care is provided! As Lewis Thomas has put it in a related vein, this is "becoming folk doctrine about disease. You become ill because of not living right. If you get cancer it is, somehow or other, your own fault. If you didn't cause it by smoking or drinking, or eating the wrong things, it came from allowing yourself to persist with the wrong kind of personality in the wrong environment."[13]

This attitude would be humorous if it was not so pervasive and did not affect patient care so profoundly. Martha Lear has given us some excellent and telling examples in her deeply moving book, *Heartsounds*, that chronicles the final four years of life of her physician-husband who goes through eight operations and eleven hospitalizations during that period. Together they identify the "it's your fault ploy," which means that no matter what goes wrong in the hospital setting, it is the fault of the patient, not the health care system.

Why did the operation take so long?
Because you lost so much blood.
Not: Because the surgeon blew it.
Why do you keep making these tests?
Because you have a very stubborn infection.
Not: Because I can't diagnose your case.
Why did I get sick again?
Because you were very weak.
Not: Because I did not treat you competently the first time.[14]

Dr. Lear is constantly asking himself if he treated patients that way, and usually admits that he did. He suggests that every physician be required to spend at least a week a year in a hospital bed: "That would change some things in a hurry."[15]

AN AGENDA FOR THE 80s

Since patients *do* have rights and *do* want to exercise them, and since the major attacks on the notion of patients' rights have been based on sloppy studies and false premises, the patients' rights movement is likely to gain momentum. Indeed, the 1970s can be most properly viewed as a decade in which the notion of rights has become legitimized through basic education of health care providers to the existence of patients' rights. I suggest that the 1980s will be a decade in which the primary thrust will be working on ways to directly enhance the status of patients in the hospital as a means of humanizing the hospital environment so that patients can have a greater voice in how they are treated.

I suggest the following five point Patients' Rights Agenda for the 1980s:

1 No Routine Procedures
2 Open Access to Medical Records
3 Twenty-Four-Hour-a-Day Visitor Rights
4 Full Experience Disclosure
5 Effective Patient Advocate

1. *No Routine Procedures.*   It is all too common for nurses and others to respond to the question, "Why is this being done?" with, "Don't worry, it's routine." This should not be an acceptable response. No procedure should *ever* be performed on a patient because it is routine; it should only be performed if it is *specifically* indicated for that patient. Thus, routine admission tests, routine use of johnnies, routine use of wheelchairs for in-hospital transportation, and routine use of sleeping pills, to name a few notable examples, would be abolished. Use of these procedures means patients are treated as fungible robots rather than individual human beings. These procedures are often demeaning and unnecessary.

2. *Open Access to Medical Records.*   Although currently provided for by federal law and many state statutes and regulations, open access to medical records by patients remains difficult, and patients often assert their right to see their records at the peril of being labeled "distrustful" or "trouble-maker." The information in the hospital chart is about the patient and properly belongs to the patient. The patient must have access to it, both to enhance his or her own decision-making ability and to make it clear that the hospital is an "open" institution that is not trying to hide things from the patient. Surely if hospital personnel are making decisions about the patient on the basis of information in the chart, the patient also deserves access to the information.

3. *Twenty-Four-Hour-a-Day Visitor Rights.*   One of the most important ways to both humanize the hospital and enhance patient autonomy is to ensure that at least one person of the patient's choice has unlimited access to the patient at any time of the day or night. This person should also be permitted to stay with the patient during any procedure (e.g., childbirth, induction of anesthesia), as long as the person does not interfere with the care of other patients.

4. *Full Experience Disclosure.*   The most important gain of the past decade has been the almost universal acknowledgment of the need for the patient's informed

consent. Nevertheless, some information that is material to the patient's decision is still withheld: the experience of the person doing the procedure.[16] Patients have a right to know if the person asking permission to draw blood, take blood gases, do a bone marrow aspiration, or do a spinal tap has ever performed the procedure before, and if so, what the person's complication rate is. This applies not only to student nurses, but also to board certified surgeons—we all do things for the first time, and not every patient wants to take such an active role in our education.

5. *An Effective Patient Advocate.* Although a patients' bill of rights is necessary, it is not sufficient. Rights are not self-actualizing. Patients are sick and desire relief from pain and discomfort more than they demonstrate a desire to exercise their rights; they are also anxious, and may hold back complaints for fear of retaliation. It is critical that patients have access to a person whose job it is to work *for the patient* to help the patient exercise the rights outlined in the institution's bill of rights. This person should sit in on all major hospital committees that deal with patient care, have authority to obtain medical records for patients, call consultants, launch complaints directly with all members of the hospital, medical, nursing, and administrative staff, and be able to delay discharges. Although there appear to be some successful "patient representatives" that are hired by the hospitals, it is not fair to give them this title since they must represent the hospital, and it is likely that ultimately effective representation can only be obtained by someone who is hired by a consumer group or governmental agency outside of the hospital in which the representative works.

CONCLUSION

We have made a beginning in the long journey toward humanizing the hospital and promoting patient self-determination in it. But more specific measures are needed before patients will be assured that they can effectively exercise their rights in institutional settings.

Like Poe's Arthur Gordon Pym, the notion that patients have rights has survived the days of darkness, isolation, and starvation. It is now generally accepted (although sporadically attacked), and it is up to patients and providers alike to see to it that these rights become a reality for every citizen.

NOTES

1 M. Rabkin, quoted in G. J. Annas, "The Hospital: A Patient Rights Wasteland," *Civil Liberties Review* (Fall 1974): 11.

2 See generally, G. J. Annas, *The Rights of Hospital Patients* (New York: Avon, 1975).

3 E. G. Margolis, "Conceptual Aspects of a Patient's Bill of Rights," *Connecticut Medicine Supplement* 43, no. 9 (October 1979): 9–11. Also see Ladd, "Legalism and Medical Ethics," in Davis, Hoffmaster, and Shorten, eds., *Contemporary Issues in Biomedical Ethics* (New Jersey, Humana Press, 1978), pp. 1–35.

4 Reprinted in Annas, pp. 25–27.

5 J. H. Altman, P. Reich, M. J. Kelly and M. P. Rogers, "Patients Who See Their Medical Record," *New England Journal of Medicine* 302, no. 3 (1980): 169.

6 D. Lipsett, "The Patient and the Record," *New England Journal of Medicine* 302, no. 3 (1980): 167.

7 R. Burt, *Taking Care of Strangers: The Rule of Law in Doctor-Patient Relations* (New York: The Free Press, 1979), p. 43.

8 D. P. Stevens, R. Staff, and I. MacKay, "What Happens When Hospitalized Patients See Their Own Records," *Annals of Internal Medicine* 86 (1977): 474, 476.

9 A. Golodetz, J. Ruess, and R. Milhous, "The Right to Know: Giving the Patient His Medical Record," *Archives of Physical Medicine and Rehabilitation* 57 (1976): 78, 81. And experience under the new record access regulation enacted by the Board of Registration in Medicine indicates that patients want access to their records for a variety of reasons. In the period from October 13, 1978 (when the regulation went into effect) to January 31, 1980, the Medicine Board received more phone calls from consumers asking about the medical records regulation (approximately ten a month) than about any other single issue dealt with by the Board. There were also 33 formal complaints filed concerning record access during this period. Of this number, almost half (16) needed help from the Board to get their physician to forward a copy of their record directly to another physician. Of the remaining 17, 6 needed information for insurance purposes, 6 wanted to review the record for various reasons,

one alleged negligence, one wanted the record sent to a school nurse, one was moving to another state, one wanted a second opinion, and one wanted her contact lens prescription. (Statistics compiled by Judy Miller, a student at Boston College Law School.)

10 See, for example, E. G. Laforet, "The Fiction of Informed Consent," *Journal of the American Medical Association* 235 (April 12, 1976): 1579.

11 B. R. Cassileth et al., "Informed Consent—Why Are Its Goals Imperfectly Realized?" *New England Journal of Medicine* 302, no. 16 (1980): 896.

12 See, generally, chapter on informed consent in G. J. Annas, L. H. Glantz, and B. F. Katz, *The Rights of Doctors, Nurses and Allied Health Professionals* (New York: Avon, 1981); and G. J. Annas, L. H. Glantz, and B. F. Katz, *Informed Consent to Human Experimentation: The Subject's Dilemma* (Cambridge, Mass.: Ballinger, 1977). And see D.

Rennie, "Informed Consent by 'Well-Nigh Abject' Adults," *New England Journal of Medicine* 302, no. 16 (1980): 916. I suggest that the physician accept far more than simply the duty to improve consent forms. Physicians should accept education of the patient through the process of consent as a worthwhile therapeutic goal. To deny the possibility of informed consent is to ensure that it will never be achieved—an attitude that is immoral and illegal.

13 L. Thomas, "On Magic in Medicine," *New England Journal of Medicine* 299 (August 31, 1978): 461, 462.

14 M.L. Lear, *Heartsounds* (New York: Simon and Schuster, 1980), p. 47.

15 *Ibid.*, p. 44.

16 G. J. Annas, "The Care of Private Patients in Teaching Hospitals: Legal Implications," *Bulletin of the New York Academy of Medicine* 56, no. 4 (May 1980): 403–11.

Nurses' Obligations and Patients' Rights

American Nurses' Association Code for Nurses

This code of ethics, adopted by the American Nurses' Association in 1976, states some of the obligations nurses have to (1) their patients, (2) the nursing profession, and (3) the public. The word "patient," however, is never used. Throughout the document, the recipient of nurses' professional services is referred to as the "client." Unlike other codes of nursing ethics, this code does not explicitly assert any obligation "to carry out physicians' orders." Rather, it emphasizes nurses' obligations to clients and views both nurses and clients as the bearers of both basic rights and responsibilities.

PREAMBLE

The *Code for Nurses* is based on belief about the nature of individuals, nursing, health, and society. Recipients and providers of nursing services are viewed as individuals and groups who possess basic rights and responsibilities and whose values and circumstances command respect at all times. Nursing encompasses the promotion and restoration of health, the prevention of illness, and the alleviation of suffering. The statements of the *Code* and their interpretation provide guidance for conduct and relationships in carrying out

nursing responsibilities consistent with the ethical obligations of the profession and quality in nursing care.

CODE FOR NURSES

1 The nurse provides services with respect for human dignity and the uniqueness of the client unrestricted by considerations of social or economic status, personal attributes, or the nature of health problems.

Reprinted with the permission of the American Nurses' Association.

2 The nurse safeguards the client's right to privacy by judiciously protecting information of a confidential nature.

3 The nurse acts to safeguard the client and the public when health care and safety are affected by the incompetent, unethical, or illegal practice of any person.

4 The nurse assumes responsibility and accountability for individual nursing judgments and actions.

5 The nurse maintains competence in nursing.

6 The nurse exercises informed judgment and uses individual competence and qualifications as criteria in seeking consultation, accepting responsibilities, and delegating nursing activities to others.

7 The nurse participates in activities that contribute to the ongoing development of the profession's body of knowledge.

8 The nurse participates in the profession's efforts to implement and improve standards of nursing.

9 The nurse participates in the profession's efforts to establish and maintain conditions of employment conducive to high quality nursing care.

10 The nurse participates in the profession's effort to protect the public from misinformation and misrepresentation and to maintain the integrity of nursing.

11 The nurse collaborates with members of the health professions and other citizens in promoting community and national efforts to meet the health needs of the public.

Three Models of the Nurse-Patient Relationship

Sheri Smith

Sheri Smith is associate professor of philosophy at Rhode Island College. Her areas of specialization are ethics and professional ethics. Smith runs medical ethics conferences monthly as a member of the scientific staff at the Roger Williams General Hospital in Providence, Rhode Island. She is also a member of the hospital's Ethics and Clinical Investigations Committee. Smith is a founding member of the Society for the Study of Professional Ethics and served as its first president (1978–1982).

Smith presents three possible models of the nurse-patient relationship. (1) *The Surrogate Mother Model*: On this model—analogous to Robert Veatch's priestly model of the physician—the nurse, like a mother, stands in a "paternalistic" relation to the patient. (2) *The Nurse-Technician Model*: On this model—analogous to Veatch's engineering model—the nurse is an ethically neutral provider of technical assistance paid for by patients, with patients retaining ultimate responsibility for identifying their needs and determining their best interests. (3) *The Contracted-Clinician Model*: On this model—analogous to Veatch's contractual model—both the patient's right of self-determination and the nurse's right of conscientious objection are emphasized. Smith concludes by arguing in favor of the contracted-clinician model. She notes, however, that although both the physician-patient and nurse-patient relationships may be conceptualized in contractual terms, there may be a significant difference between the two sets of relationships because of nurses' obligations to obey physicians.

A critical philosophical issue about nursing is raised in several of the essays in this volume [*Nursing: Images and Ideals*], but it has been left unresolved. That issue is the question of the nature of the nurse-patient relationship. The failure to resolve the issue is critical, for the solution of ethical dilemmas in nursing practice often depends upon the definition of nursing and the responsibilities and rights thought to be inherent in the nurse-patient relationship.[1] My purpose in this [article] is to characterize three views of the nature of the nurse-patient relationship—the surrogate mother, nurse technician, and contracted clinician models—and to show the strengths and weaknesses of those models and their consequences for nursing practice. I will contend that assumptions about the nature of the nurse-patient relationship pervade the discussion of ethical dilemmas in nursing practice. In order to support that contention I will use examples from the essays by Dan Brock, who argues for the contracted clinician model; Mila Aroskar, who discusses the surrogate mother model in commenting on historical images of nurses; and Sally Gadow, whose conceptualizations of nursing can be shown to provide a philosophical basis for the models presented herein. My discussion of nursing models owes much to Robert Veatch's description of analogous models for the patient-physician relationship.[2] The question of how far the analogy between nurse-patient and physician-patient relationships can be drawn, and how the nature of the nurse-patient relationship might be altered by the relationship the patient has with his physician, is one on which I will comment briefly at the end of this discussion.

THE NURSE AS SURROGATE MOTHER

We can distinguish the three major models of the nurse-patient relationship by their conceptualizations of the extent and nature of the nurse's ethical responsibility and the assumptions made concerning patients and illness. In the surrogate mother model the nurse's primary responsibility and commitment is to the patient. (It should be noted here that, for the purposes of this discussion, "patient" will be understood to mean a competent adult.) The ethical responsibility of the nurse is defined by this commitment to the patient, as it is spelled out in nursing codes of ethics such as the American Nurses' Association Code. The nurse is even urged by the ANA code to serve as protector of the patient when his care and safety are in jeopardy through the actions of others. Other ethical responsibilities which nurses have, for example, in relation to physicians, are derived from this primary commitment to the patient.

It is the model of the nurse as a surrogate mother which has exerted greatest influence in the history of nursing and nursing education.[3] On this model, the nurse's ethical responsibility is understood as an unlimited commitment to the patient. It is the nurse's obligation to provide nursing care, to take care of the patient, and to act in his or her best interests at all times. The nurse has ultimate responsibility for the care which the patient receives. This means that the nurse also has an obligation to determine what constitutes the best care for the patient, and to act in his or her behalf if that care is not being provided. The nurse, then, has a kind of total commitment to patient care and ultimate responsibility for determining that the patient's best interests are served.

However, this commitment to the patient alone would not give rise to the surrogate mother model. It is only when joined with observations about the nature of sickness and patients that the model is derived. Patients, generally, are sick, suffering, fearful, dependent individuals. Because of illness and hospitalization, patients may be unable to exercise emotional control or to make important decisions, and, in at least some respects, may be irrational.[4] Consequently, the patient cannot be trusted to make the best decisions about his or her care, if able to make decisions at all. The patient needs someone to provide care and to make the decisions, i.e., decisions for his or her own good. The nurse's commitment to care for the patient, then, is a commitment to an individual who is sick, dependent, and perhaps unable to understand what his or her best interests are. The nurse's relationship to the patient should be that of a surrogate mother to her child.

It should be noted here that, on this model, the values of the nurse carry great weight, since nurses will make critical decisions in terms of their own values, i.e., their ideas about what constitutes the best interests of the patient. For example, a nurse might attempt to persuade a patient to accept a treatment for the patient's own good. She might withhold information if she believed that a patient would make the "wrong" choice if the information were provided. She might even make decisions concerning the appropriate goals for a patient's treatment. In short, acting on her responsibility for the care of the patient, the nurse may impose her own judgments and decisions about care.

On this model, then, the nurse's concern for the patient's welfare and intervention in his life are similar to a parent's concern for a child's welfare and intervention in the child's life. It is this conceptualization of nursing that is revealed by the stereotype of the nurse as mother described by Mila Aroskar in her essay "The Fractured Image: The Public Stereotype of Nursing and the Nurse." She suggests that traditionally nursing has implied a mother's relationship to her children, caring for her family and managing her home.[5] Moreover, Aroskar points out, in the first American nursing schools, the family was the model for the hospital, a model in which the nurse is seen as mother, the physician as father and patients as children.[6]

In her comments on the image of the nurse Aroskar supports the conclusions of JoAnn Ashley in *Hospitals, Paternalism, and the Role of the Nurse.* Ashley observes, "The role of women (nurses) was very early conceived as that of caring for the 'hospital family.' Their purpose was to provide efficient economical production in the form of patient care; they were to be loyal to the institution and devoted to preserving its reputation. Through service and self-sacrifice, they were to work continuously to keep the 'family' happy ... Like mothers in a household, nurses were responsible for meeting the needs of all members of the hospital 'family'—from patients to physicians."[7]

Thus, traditionally, the "mother" image has been the prevailing image of the nurse. The corresponding philosophical assumption is that the nature of the nurse-patient relationship is fundamentally like that of a mother to a child. This assumption has had profound impact on our beliefs about the character of nursing dilemmas, and our expectations concerning appropriate solutions of ethical issues in nursing practice, for it includes the belief that the nurse should always act in what is perceived to be the patient's interest.

This belief, that the nurse should always act in the patient's interest, as Sally Gadow points out, implies a conceptualization of nursing as paternalism. She notes that paternalism is often defended as the belief that, for an individual's own good, decisions should be made by those most capable of knowing what is in his best interest.[8] In actuality, however, paternalistic acts and attitudes limit the rights or freedom of individuals in their own interests.[9] Paternalism thus involves the intent

to obtain what is believed to be a good for the other person, with the effect of violating his known wishes.[10] To accept the surrogate mother model of the nurse-patient relationship, therefore, with its assumptions about the extent of the nurse's ethical responsibility to the patient, and the helplessness and need of the patient, is to conceive of nursing as paternalism.

THE NURSE AS TECHNICIAN

If the two primary assumptions of the surrogate mother model concerning the extent of the nurse's ethical responsibility and the nature of patients are rejected, the resulting model of the nurse-patient relationship is a view which could be called the technical model. This model is derived from the contemporary view of nursing as a clinical science.[11] The nurse, it is suggested, should provide scientific care; that is, the nurse should apply scientific methods and scientific treatment to the care of patients. The nurse's commitment to the patient is a commitment to provide the best nursing care possible, meeting the patient's needs to the best of her ability. Further, the nurse is committed to the objective, nonjudgmental, noninterfering application of nursing knowledge and skills in treating patients. The nurse must respect the values and beliefs of patients, and be fair and unbiased in the treatment of patients. A nurse should not impose her own values or make value judgments in administering nursing care; on the contrary, she must remain ethically neutral. Thus the extent of the nurse's ethical responsibility is limited to the correct application of knowledge and skills to meet the needs of the patient.

The needs of the patient are biological phenomena with which a nurse must deal factually and objectively by providing care as requested by the patient. It is assumed that the patient's ability to make decisions and to judge his own best interests is not impaired by illness or hospitalization. Consequently, the patient retains ultimate responsibility for identifying his needs and determining his best interests. The nurse has no role in determining those interests and needs, either by attempting to influence the patient, or by refusing to help him attain his goals.

If the patient is regarded as completely capable of making his own decisions about what is good for him, and the nurse's obligation to the patient is to provide the scientific care he requests (or the physician requests for him), then the model of the nurse-patient relationship is as follows. It is a relationship between a technician, the nurse, and an individual who receives technical assistance, the patient. The nurse should merely apply knowledge and technical skills as requested by the patient. Her only concern as a professional should be to apply those skills correctly and objectively. That is to say, she should not be concerned with the decisions which the patient might make about his treatment or health, even if her involvement in his decisions would be for the patient's own good.[12] She should just provide the patient with any information and technical advice which he needs in order to make decisions concerning his health. It is a consequence of this model that the nurse would simply supply nursing care as requested, regardless of the foolishness or moral repugnance of the patient's requests and decisions. The nurse's moral values and judgments would be irrelevant to her function as a provider of nursing care.[13]

Belief in the nurse's ethical neutrality, her concern and obligation to provide the best, correct care, and the unimpaired rational abilities of the patient produce this model of the nurse-patient relationship. If the nurse's responsibility on this model is construed to include protecting the patient's interests as he has determined them, then the nurse's role is to serve as an advocate for the patient. This image of nursing as technical assistance to patients is the conceptualization which Gadow calls consumerism.[14]

THE NURSE AS CONTRACTED CLINICIAN

The third model of the nurse-patient relationship follows from the assumption that the patient is capable of determining his own best interests, a premise about patients which is also assumed by the technical model, and the belief that the ethical responsibility of the nurse is defined by the rights of the patient. The patient's right to self-determination is essential to the rights-based moral view of the nurse-patient relationship which Dan Brock develops in his essay "The Nurse-Patient Relation: Some Rights and Duties." Brock argues that a nurse's unique relation to the patient can be explained only by viewing the nurse-patient relationship as arising from an agreement between nurse and patient, an agreement in which the patient contracts to have specified care provided by the nurse and the nurse incurs an obligation to the patient to provide that care.[15] On this model of the nurse-patient relationship, the patient has the right to control both what happens to his body and

the role which the nurse takes with him in providing nursing care;[16] "...the right to determine what is done to and for the patient, and to control, within broad limits, the course of the patient's treatment and care, originates and generally remains with the patient."[17] Thus the nurse's commitment to the patient is a commitment to provide the nursing care which he chooses. Nurses are not justified in doing something because it is in the best interests of the patient, moreover, since the right to act in the patient's interest is "...*created* and *limited* by the permission or consent (from the patient-nurse/physician agreement) the patient has given."[18] Therefore, it is the patient's right to control the course of his treatment, his right to self-determination, which defines the ethical responsibility of the nurse.

An important consequence of the contracted clinician model is that the nurse is not required to be ethically neutral. Since the nurse-patient relationship arises from an agreement, the nurse can refuse to participate in the relationship, if her own ethical values would be compromised. For example, the nurse can refuse to care for abortion patients if she believes abortion is unethical. Therefore, the nurse's commitment to the patient is limited by her own permission or consent as well as by the rights of the patient.

The patient's right to self-determination, which is essential in this model, is also essential for Sally Gadow's conceptualization of nursing as existential advocacy. This conceptualization is based on the belief that "freedom of self-determination is the most fundamental and valuable human right, and therefore is a greater good than any which health care can provide."[19] Nurses must assist patients in authentically exercising that freedom of self-determination, that is, in making decisions which express the full complexity of their values.[20] The nurse is obligated to act in the patient's interest, but she cannot define what the patient's "best interest" is. She must assist patients to determine their best interests and to become clear about what they want to do.[21] "Existential advocacy, as the essence of nursing, is the nurse's participation with the patient in determining the unique meaning which the experience of health, illness, suffering, or dying is to have for that individual."[22]

Gadow argues for existential advocacy as the philosophical foundation of nursing. This conceptualization of nursing supports Brock's model of the nurse-patient relationship in its central features. Both Brock and

Gadow agree that the fundamental value to be preserved in the nurse-patient relationship is the patient's right to self-determination. They are agreed that the patient determines what his best interests are and that the patient has the right to decide which role the nurse takes with him.[23] The conceptualization of nursing as advocacy, in Gadow's sense, could therefore serve as a basis for the contracted clinician model of the nurse-patient relationship. It is important to note here that it is not patients' rights advocacy which supports the contracted clinician model. For, as Gadow suggests, patients' rights advocacy is really what she calls consumerism, that is, the belief that the nurse should just obey the patient's wishes. Consumerism thus forces the patient to make a decision autonomously. It involves the paternalistic assumption that patients should make important decisions with only technical assistance and information.[24] However, Brock and Gadow both argue that the patient's right to self-determination is inviolate. That is, it is the patient's right to determine what he needs from the nurse; whether he makes a decision autonomously is his choice. The patient can, if he wishes, receive advice from the nurse; he can even choose a paternalistic relationship with the nurse. The patient's freedom to determine his relationship with the nurse is the key to the contracted clinician model.

AN ETHICAL DILEMMA

I have attempted to show that different beliefs about the ethical responsibilities of nurses and assumptions about patients yield three models of the nurse-patient relationship. These models have implications for nursing practice which are of critical importance. I will argue that, on the basis of these ethical implications, the contracted clinician model should be accepted. In order to establish that, it will be necessary to consider an example. The implications for nursing practice will be most clearly revealed if we consider a case which will show the essential differences concerning the responsibility of the nurse with regard to the patient's best interests, and the role of the nurse's personal values and beliefs.

Mr. A. is a 56-year-old man who has had leukemia for one year. He has again voluntarily admitted himself for control of hemorrhaging and intractable pain. He also suffers from very high fevers and an oral infection with open sores. He is depressed and anxious about the future. During the past six months he has been hospitalized frequently to receive chemotherapy and blood transfusions. On recent hospitalizations, however, the chemotherapy has been discontinued because of Mr. A.'s lowered white blood count. Though he is aware of his deteriorating condition, he is optimistic about the possibility of another remission.

When he is examined by the physician, the physician informs him that he is in the terminal phase of leukemia. The physician explains that he will receive painkillers and will be treated with intravenous fluids to combat the dehydration. Blood transfusions and a bone marrow aspiration will also be used to stabilize the progress of the disease. The physician, however, does not hold out any hope of prolonging Mr. A.'s life for a significant period of time. He indicates that there is only a remote hope of remission.

Mr. A., extremely upset at this prognosis, exclaims that he cannot bear the pain any longer, and expresses a wish to die. Mr. A. explains his situation to his family and again expresses his wish to die without any prolonged suffering. Mrs. A. disagrees vehemently with him, and argues that any means available should be used to prolong Mr. A.'s life.

Consequently, Mr. A. is admitted to the hospital, the intravenous treatment is begun, and he is left to rest. Several minutes later Nurse B., who has been present throughout Mr. A.'s examination and treatment, enters his room to discover that Mr. A. is unconscious; the flow of intravenous fluids has been mistakenly adjusted so that all of the intravenous fluids have been absorbed. As a result it is very unlikely that Mr. A. will regain consciousness. Moreover, the rapid infusion of the fluids will have immediate fatal consequences if action is not taken. What should Nurse B. do?[25]

As with all case descriptions, there is some ambiguity in this situation. It is unclear why Mr. A. voluntarily admitted himself under the circumstances or why he consented to the treatment. Since there are many aspects of this case that deserve more careful description and analysis, it cannot be adequately discussed within the scope of this [article]. It will serve, however, to illustrate the ethical implications of the three nurse-patient models.

It is necessary for the purposes of clarifying the implications of these models to make an assumption about the judgments and personal moral values of Nurse B. Let us assume that she disagrees with Mr. A.; she is convinced Mr. A. has valuable life remaining, and she believes that preserving life is a duty. In this situation there are essentially two options open to Nurse B. Nurse B. can respect Mr. A.'s wish to die and refrain from initiating any treatment, or Nurse B. can do everything possible to keep Mr. A. alive—for example, she can page the physician and immediately begin extraordinary emergency procedures. The critical element in Nurse B.'s decision in this case will be her own philosophical view of the nature of the nurse-patient relationship, that is, the role which she believes her values should play in that relationship, as well as her beliefs about her ethical responsibility for the patient.

If Nurse B. assumes the surrogate mother model of the nurse-patient relationship, there are important consequences for her practice of nursing. The strength of this model is that it clearly recognizes the vulnerability, suffering, and need of the patient. It recognizes that patients may not make the best decisions in situations such as Mr. A.'s situation. Nurse B., consequently, will be aware of Mr. A.'s vulnerability; she will be sympathetic, understanding, and willing to provide the mothering care and concern which Mr. A. may need.

Moreover, Nurse B. will regard her ethical commitment to the patient, Mr. A., as an all-encompassing responsibility to do what she believes is in Mr. A.'s best interests. Consequently, in this situation, she will act according to her perception of what is best for Mr. A. Even though Mr. A. has expressed a wish to die, she will page the physician and initiate emergency procedures in an attempt to save Mr. A.'s life.

If Nurse B. accepts the technical model, on the other hand, her action in this situation will be quite different. On the technical model, Nurse B.'s own beliefs about the sanctity of life are irrelevant, since she is required to be ethically neutral in her practice of nursing. Her skills are to be utilized to satisfy the patient's wishes and requests. If a patient requests an abortion, for example, the nurse's obligation is to supply good nursing care, regardless of her own judgments about the desirability or morality of abortion. In this case, since Mr. A. has expressed a wish to die, Nurse B. would ignore her own judgment about the best interests of Mr. A. and the immorality of letting him die. Nurse B. has no obligation to undertake any actions aimed at saving his life, for Mr. A. clearly does not wish to have

his life saved. Therefore, Nurse B. will not initiate treatment.

Similarly, if Nurse B. accepts the contracted clinician model, she will not initiate treatment. On this model her ethical responsibility will be defined by Mr. A.'s right to control and determine what happens to him. Though Nurse B. disagrees with Mr. A.'s wish to die, she will not impose her own judgments and values in this situation. She will allow Mr. A. to die.

The differences between the technical model and the contracted clinician model are not obvious in this case, for though they involve quite different assumptions, they result in the same action. The key difference between these models is the role of the nurse's values in the nurse-patient relationship. On the technical model, the nurse's values are irrelevant, for she must remain ethically neutral. However, on the contracted clinician model, the nurse's values are important factors in the relationship with the patient. The nurse can refuse to participate in that relationship if her values are compromised. Thus this model allows the nurse's values to become an important aspect of the relationship with the patient.

Only the general features of the surrogate mother, technical, and contracted clinician models of the nurse-patient relationship have been outlined here. However, some significant conclusions can be drawn. First, the surrogate-mother model of the nurse-patient relationship is inadequate for the same reasons that a paternalistic model of the physician-patient relationship is unacceptable, i.e., it condones actions which violate a patient's right to self-determination. It is clearly ethically objectionable for the nurse to impose her beliefs about the patient's best interests and in effect to make an important decision for the patient. Secondly, it seems evident to me that the technical model is also inadequate. The nurse, in caring for patients and making decisions about nursing care, is not functioning solely as a technician. An acceptable model for the nurse-patient relationship must recognize the ethical aspects of nursing practice.

Because it recognizes the ethical aspects of nursing practice and the patient's right to self-determination, the contracted clinician model is the best of these three models. There is, however, one consequence of this which deserves comment. As Brock points out, the implication of his model is that the nurse-patient relationship is essentially the same as the physician-patient relationship. It seems to me, though, that there is a significant difference. Though both nurse and physician are viewed as having a contractual relationship with the patient, there is an additional factor which complicates the nurse-patient relationship. The nurse is obligated to provide nursing care because of her agreement with the patient; furthermore, she is also obligated to obey the physician because of her agreement with the patient. That is, this obligation is imposed by the agreement with the patient because the nurse agrees to provide the nursing care necessary to the patient's needs as he or she identifies them. She is therefore obligated to assist the physician in providing care necessary to the patient's needs. The physician, however, does not have a similar obligation to the nurse. This suggests to me that these relationships may be significantly different in some respects. The question of how the nature of the nurse-patient relationship is altered by the relationship the patient has with his physician is an issue which deserves careful analysis, for these relationships are central to some of the most difficult ethical dilemmas in nursing practice.

NOTES

1 Sally Gadow argues that nursing can be defined in terms of the nurse-patient relationship in "Existential Advocacy: Philosophical Foundation of Nursing," in Stuart F. Spicker and Sally Gadow, eds., *Nursing: Images and Ideals*, New York: Springer, 1980, chapter 4.

2 Robert Veatch discusses his models of the patient-physician relationship in "Models for Ethical Medicine in a Revolutionary Age," *Hastings Center Report*, June 1972, pp. 5–7.

3 The influence of this image of nurses as surrogate mothers has been reported by several nurses and sociologists. For example, Hans O. Mauksch, "Nursing: Churning for Change," in Freeman, Howard E., *et al.* (eds.), *Handbook of Medical Sociology*, 2nd ed., Englewood Cliffs, N.J.: Prentice-Hall, Inc., 1972, and most recently Myra E. Levine

in "Nursing Ethics and the Ethical Nurse," *American Journal of Nursing*, May 1977, p. 845.

4 Some interesting observations concerning patients are made by Henry J. Lederer, "How the Sick View Their World," in *The Journal of Social Issues*, 8(4), 1952, pp. 4–15.

5 Mila Aroskar, "The Fractured Image: The Public Stereotype of Nursing and the Nurse," in Spicker and Gadow, *Nursing*, chapter 2.

6 *Ibid.*

7 JoAnn Ashley, *Hospitals, Paternalism, and the Role of the Nurse* (New York: Teachers College Press, 1976), p. 17.

8 Gadow, "Existential Advocacy."

9 *Ibid.*

10 *Ibid.*

11 The view presented here about the nature of the nurse-patient relationship is that expressed by Gerene Major in her paper "The Abortion Patient and the Nurse." My thinking concerning the issues discussed herein was developed in response to her paper.

12 Gadow, "Existential Advocacy."

13 *Ibid.*

14 *Ibid.*

15 Dan Brock, "The Nurse-Patient Relation: Some Rights and Duties," in Spicker and Gadow, *Nursing*, chapter 5.

16 *Ibid.*

17 *Ibid.*

18 *Ibid.*

19 Gadow, "Existential Advocacy."

20 *Ibid.*

21 *Ibid.*

22 *Ibid.*

23 Gadow believes that the patient and nurse can freely decide what their relationship will be.

24 *Ibid.*

25 This case is based upon a case presented to me by Gertrude Mulvey, R.N.

Ethical Dilemmas for Nurses: Physicians' Orders versus Patients' Rights

E. Joy Kroeger Mappes

E. Joy Kroeger Mappes teaches in the department of philosophy at Frostburg State College (Maryland). Her areas of specialization are ethics and social philosophy. Mappes also serves as a member of a hospital ethics committee. In the past, she has worked as a registered nurse.

Mappes identifies two kinds of ethical dilemmas that arise for the hospital nurse. One kind of ethical dilemma arises in cases in which following physicians' orders (explicit or implicit) would violate the patient's right to adequate medical treatment. Although Mappes makes clear that the nurse can be faced with some difficult matters of judgment, she argues that the nurse is morally obligated to act on behalf of the patient in those cases in which there is good reason to think that the physician's orders are not in the best medical interest of the patient. A second kind of ethical dilemma arises in cases in which following physicians' orders would violate the patient's right of self-determination. In Mappes' view, this second class of cases is less problematic than the first, since the nurse is not faced with problematic judgments about the patient's best medical interest. She contends that the nurse is morally obliged to act to protect the patient's right of self-determination. However, emphasizing the classist and sexist forces that typically make it difficult for the nurse to act on behalf of the patient, she goes on to suggest that "changes must be made in the workplace."

The American Hospital Association in a widely promulgated statement entitled "A Patient's Bill of Rights," makes explicit a number of the generally recognized rights of hospitalized patients.[1] Among the rights expressly articulated in the AHA statement is a cluster of rights closely associated with a more general right, the right of self-determination. The "self-determination cluster" includes: (1) the right to information concerning diagnosis, treatment, and prognosis; (2) the right to information necessary to give informed consent; and (3) the right to refuse treatment. The AHA statement duly recognizes several other important patient rights but, importantly, fails to explicitly recognize the patient's right to adequate medical care.[2] Surely, if the purpose of a statement of patients' rights is to catalogue patients' rights, we ought not to overlook this one. After all, the patient has agreed to enter the hospital setting precisely for the purpose of obtaining medical treatment. To the extent that adequate medical care is not forthcoming, the patient has been done an injustice.

That is, the patient's right to adequate medical care has been violated.

This paper explores two types of ethical dilemmas related to patients' rights that arise for the hospital nurse.[3] (1) The first set of dilemmas is related to the patient's basic right to adequate medical care. (2) The second set of dilemmas is related to the cluster of rights closely associated with the patient's right of self-determination. Dilemmas arise for a nurse if adequate medical care for a patient would be jeopardized by following the expressed or understood orders of a physician. Dilemmas also arise for a nurse if the patient's right to self-determination would be violated by following the expressed or understood orders of a physician. In each case, the logic of the dilemma is similar. The dilemma arises because the nurse's apparent obligation to follow the physician's order conflicts with his or her obligation to act in the interest of the patient. To carry out the physician's order would be to act against the interest of the patient. To act in the interest of the patient would be to disobey the physician's order.[4] I will argue that when this conflict arises the nurse's obligation to the patient is overriding and that nurses must act and be allowed and encouraged to act to protect the rights of the patient.

I NURSING DILEMMAS AND THE PATIENT'S RIGHT TO ADEQUATE MEDICAL CARE

In a hospital the primary responsibility for a patient's care rests with a physician. Physicians determine the medical diagnosis, treatment, and prognosis of patients' illnesses and write orders to arrive at and effect these determinations. In general, physicians' orders govern what a patient is to do and what is to be done for a patient, i.e., the degree of activity, diet, medication, diagnostic and treatment procedures to be performed. Nurses carry out physicians' orders themselves, delegate tasks to others, or make the orders known to those responsible for carrying them out. They are not generally allowed by law to diagnose or prescribe.[5] Although this is a greatly oversimplified picture of what goes on, as anyone familiar at all with the functioning of a hospital will realize, at least some of the complexities involved in the interaction among physicians, nurses, and patients in a hospital setting will emerge as we proceed.

The complexity of the ethical dilemmas arising for nurses regarding the patient's right to adequate medical care can best be understood by examining various examples. The following are suggested as being not atypical of situations arising in hospitals:

(1) A patient who has had emphysema for a number of years is admitted to a cardiac unit for observation with a tentative diagnosis of myocardial infarction. Oxygen is ordered in a concentration commonly given for patients with this diagnosis. The nurse, knowing that oxygen is contraindicated for patients with emphysema, must decide whether to carry out or question the order through appropriate channels.

(2) A patient admitted to the hospital for a diagnostic work-up has been on a special and fairly extensive drug therapy regimen. This regimen is common to patients of a particular private physician, seemingly regardless of their diagnosis. The private physician orders the drug therapy program continued after admission. However, accepted medical practice would ordinarily call for ceasing as many drugs as is safely possible, thus avoiding unnecessary variables in arriving at an

accurate diagnosis. In general the private physician is viewed by other physicians as incompetent. The nurse is aware that the orders do not reflect good medical practice, but also realizes that she[6] will be dealing with this physician as long as she works at that hospital. The nurse must decide whether to follow the orders or refuse to carry out the orders, attempting through channels to have the orders changed.

(3) A frail patient recovering from recent surgery has been receiving intra-muscular antibiotic injections four times a day. The injection sites are very tender, and though the patient now is able to eat without problems, the intern refuses to change the order to an oral route of administration of the antibiotic because the absorption of the medication would be slightly diminished. The nurse must decide whether to follow the order as it stands or continue through channels to try to have the order changed.

(4) A nurse on the midnight shift of a large medical center is closely monitoring a patient's vital signs (blood pressure, pulse rate, respiratory rate). The physicians have been unable to diagnose the patient's illness. In reviewing the patient's record, the nurse thinks of a possible diagnosis. The patient's condition begins to worsen and the nurse phones the intern-on-call to notify him of the patient's condition. The nurse mentions that the record indicates that diagnosis X is possible. The intern dismisses the nurse's suggested diagnosis and instructs the nurse to follow existing orders. Concerned that the patient's condition will continue to deteriorate, the nurse contacts her supervisor who concurs with the intern. The patient's blood pressure gradually but steadily falls and the pulse increases. The nurse has contacted the intern twice since the initial call but the orders remain unchanged. The nurse must decide whether to pursue the matter further, e.g., calling the resident-on-call and/or the patient's private physician.[7]

What are the obligations of nurses in such cases? Under what circumstances are nurses obligated to rely on their judgment and to question the physician's order? To what extent must nurses pursue the questioning when, in their view, the patient's right to adequate medical care is being violated? It is often taken for granted that when the medical assessments of physician and nurse differ, "the physician knows best." In order to see both why this is thought, perhaps correctly so, to be generally true and yet why it is surely not always true, it is necessary to consider some of the factors that account for the difference in physician and nurse assessments.

A nurse's assessment of what constitutes adequate medical treatment may differ from a physician's assessment for at least three reasons. *(a)* There is a difference in the amount and the content of their formal training. Physicians generally have a number of years more formal training than nurses, though that difference is not as great as it once was. More nurses now continue formal training in various ways, i.e., by pursuing graduate work and/or by becoming nurse practitioners, nurse clinicians, or nurse anesthetists. In addition, proportionately more nurses than ever before are college graduates. However, a physician's formal training is more extensive and detailed. Moreover, and perhaps most importantly, physicians are explicitly trained in the diagnosis and treatment of illness, with the emphasis of the training placed on the hard sciences. Nurses are trained to be knowledgeable about illness in general, the symptoms and treatment of illness, and the complications and side effects of various forms of therapy. While this formal training includes both the hard sciences and the social (primarily behavioral) sciences, there is an emphasis on the behavioral sciences. Nurses are trained to concentrate on the overall well-being of the patient. *(b)* There may be a difference in the length or concentration of their experience. For example, nurses who have worked in special care units (in medical and surgical cardiac units, burn units, renal units, intensive care units) for a number of years acquire a great deal of knowledge which may not be possessed by interns, and perhaps even residents and nonspecialty private physicians. Nurses who have worked for years in small community hospitals may well be more knowledgeable in some areas than some physicians. *(c)* There may be a difference in their knowledge of the patient. Nurses often have more detailed knowledge about patients than do physicians, who often see a patient only once a day. Nurses who are "at the bedside" are thus in a position to recognize small changes as they happen. Because of the possibility of more detailed knowledge, nurse assessments may be more accurate than physician assessments. Where physician and nurse assessments differ then, it is not necessarily the case that the physician's assessment is the correct one simply because of the amount and content of the physician's formal training. Physicians do make mistakes and, when they do, nurses must be in a position to protect the patient.[8]

Ethical dilemmas of the kind typified in the above four examples arise when to follow physician's orders would be to act against the medical interest of the patient. Given the fact that the *basic* obligation of both the physician and the nurse is to act in the medical interest of the patient, it is rather striking that anyone should suppose that the nurse's obligation to follow the physician's orders should ever take precedence. What, after all, is the foundation of the nurse's obligation to follow the physician's orders? Presumably, the nurse's obligation to follow the physician's orders is grounded on the nurse's obligation to act in the medical interest of the patient. The point is that the nurse has an obligation to follow physicians' orders because, ordinarily, patient welfare (interest) thereby is ensured. Thus when a nurse's obligation to follow a physician's order comes into *direct* conflict with the nurse's obligation to act in the medical interest of the patient, it would seem to follow that the patient's interests should always take precedence.

For instance, Example 1 provides a clear case of a medically unsound order. In fact, it is such a clear case that a nurse not questioning the order would be judged incompetent. The medically unsound order may be the result of a medical mistake or of medical incompetence. If the order is the result of an oversight, the physician is likely to be grateful when (if) a nurse questions the order. If the order is a result of incompetence, the physician is not likely to be grateful. Whatever the reason for the medically unsound order, the nurse is obligated to question an order if it is clearly medically unsound. The nurse must refuse to carry out the order if it is not changed, and to press the matter through channels in order to protect the medical interest of the patient. Example 2 is similar to Example 1 in that it involves a medical practice that is clearly unsound. If the orders are questioned, the physician here again is not likely to be grateful. Indeed, since the physician's practice may ultimately be at stake, the pressures brought to bear on a nurse may be overwhelming, particularly if the physician's colleagues choose to defend him or her. It is undeniable, however, that medical incompetence is not in the best medical interest of patients, and thus that the nurse's obligation is to question the order. It is of course true that a nurse acting on behalf of the patient in this situation may pay a heavy price, perhaps his or her job, for protecting the medical interests of patients. However, the nurse's moral obligation is no less real on this account.

With Example 3 the murkiness begins, since it does not provide a clear case of unsound medical practice, though perhaps it presents us with a case in which the physician is operating with a too-narrow view of good medical practice. As I mentioned earlier, nurses often are more concerned with the overall well-being of the patient. Physicians often are concerned only with identifying the illness, treating it, and determining how responsive the illness is to the treatment. To the extent that Example 3 resembles Example 1, i.e., the lumps are very bad and the difference in the absorption of the medication in the two routes of administration is small, the nurse has an obligation to question the order. Example 4 is like Example 3 in that it does not provide a clear case of a medically unsound order. However, in Example 4, much more is at stake. Since life itself is involved, any decision must be considered very carefully. The problem here is not a problem of weighing or balancing but a problem of being either right or wrong. Both Examples 3 and 4 force a nurse to assess this question: "How strong are my grounds for thinking that the orders are not in tune with the patient's best medical interest?" The murkiness comes in knowing exactly when the physician's order is in direct conflict with the patient's medical interest. As the last two examples illustrate, it can be very difficult to know exactly what is in the best medical interest of the patient. To the extent that the nurse has carefully considered the situation and is sure that his or her view is in accord with good medical care, the order should be questioned. The less sure one is, the less clear it becomes whether the order should be questioned and the matter pressed through channels.

In arguing the above, I am not advocating uncritical questioning. Clearly, questioning at some point must cease. Otherwise, hospitals could not function efficiently and as a result the medical interest of all patients would suffer. But if there is little or no opportunity for nurses and other health professionals to contribute their knowledge to the care of the patient, or if they are directly or indirectly discouraged from contributing, it would seem that they will find it difficult, if not impossible, to fulfill their obligations with respect to the patient's right to adequate medical care.

II NURSING DILEMMAS AND THE PATIENT'S RIGHT OF SELF-DETERMINATION

The complexity of the ethical dilemmas arising for nurses regarding the patient's right of self-determination can best be understood by examining various cases. Again, the following are suggested as being not atypical of situations arising in hospitals:

(1) A patient is scheduled for prostate surgery (prostatectomy) early in the morning. Because he is generally unaware of what is happening to him due to senility, he is judged incompetent to give informed consent for surgery. The patient's sister visits him in the evenings, but the physicians have not been available during those times for her to give consent. The physicians have asked the nurses to obtain consent from the patient's sister. When she arrives the evening before surgery is scheduled, the nurses explain to her that her brother is to have surgery and what it would entail. The sister had not been told that surgery was being considered and questions its necessity for her brother who has not experienced any real problems due to an enlarged prostate. She does not feel she can sign the consent form without talking with one of his physicians. Should the nurses encourage her to sign the consent form, as the physicians have requested, or call one of the physicians to speak with the patient's sister?

(2) A patient in the cardiac unit who was admitted with a massive myocardial infarction begins to show signs of increased cardiac failure. The patient and the family have clearly expressed their desire to the medical and nursing staff to refrain from "heroics" should complications arise. The patient stops breathing and the intern begins to intubate the patient, requests the nurse's assistance, and orders a respirator. Should the nurse follow orders or attempt to convince the intern to reconsider, calling the resident-on-call should the intern refuse?

(3) A patient is hospitalized for a series of diagnostic tests. The tests, history, and physical pretty clearly indicate a certain diagnosis. The physicians only tell the patient that they are not yet sure of the diagnosis, reassuring the patient that he is in good hands. Each day after the physicians leave, the patient asks the nurse, coming in to give medications, what the tests have shown and what his diagnosis is. When the nurse encourages the patient to ask the physicians these questions, he says he feels intimidated by them and that when he does ask questions they simply say that everything will be fine. Should the nurse reinforce what the physicians have said or attempt to convince the physicians that the patient has a right to information about his illness, pressing the matter through channels if they do not agree?

(4) A patient suffering from cancer is scheduled for

surgery in the morning. While instructing the patient not to eat or drink after a certain hour, the nurse realizes that the patient is unaware of the risks involved in having the surgery and of those involved in not having the surgery. In talking further, the nurse sees clearly that the option of not having surgery was never presented and that the patient has only a vague idea of what the surgery will entail. She also appears to be unaware of her diagnosis. The patient has signed the consent form for surgery. Should the nurse proceed in preparing the patient for surgery, or, proceeding through channels, attempt to provide for a genuinely informed consent for the surgery?

What are the obligations of nurses in examples such as these? To what extent must nurses pursue questioning when, in their view, the patient's right of self-determination is being violated? Unless we are willing to say that a patient upon entering a hospital surrenders the right of self-determination, it seems clear that physicians' orders, explicit and implied, should be questioned in all of the above examples. After all, in each of the above examples, one of the rights expressly outlined by the American Hospital Association is in danger of being abridged. The rights involved are (or should be) known by all to be possessed by all. Here a difference in the formal training and knowledge based on experience is not relevant in any difference between a physician's and a nurse's assessment. No formal training in medicine is necessary to arrive at the conclusion that the patient's right of self-determination is endangered.

The tension that exists for nurses in situations typified in the above four examples is not really that of a moral dilemma, but rather, a tension between doing what is morally right and what is least difficult practically, a tension common in everyday life. The problem is not that the nurse's obligation is unclear, but that in actual situations fulfilling this moral obligation is extremely difficult. What we must consider now in some detail are the social forces that make it so difficult for a nurse to act on behalf of the patient.

III NURSING DILEMMAS AND THE IMPORTANCE OF A CLASSIST AND SEXIST CONTEXT

I have argued that when following a physician's order would violate the patient's right to adequate medical care or the patient's right of self-determination, the nurse's moral obligation is to question the order. If necessary, the matter should be pressed through chan-

nels. It is well and good to say what nurses should do. It is quite another thing, given the forces at work in the everyday world in which nurses must work, to expect nurses to do what they ought to do.

To begin with, we must recognize that there is an important class difference between physicians and nurses, the difference between the upper middle class or upper class of physicians and the lower middle class of nurses.[9] A large proportion of physicians both start out and end their lives in the upper class. Though the economic status of a physician is not as high as that of a high-level corporation executive, the social status of a physician is very high because of the prestige of the profession of medicine in the United States today.[10] Physicians have a high social status in American society and they understand and identify with people who have a similarly high status.[11] "Physicians talked with physicians; nurses talked with nurses," is an observation of one sociological study.[12] Generally physicians do not understand or identify with nurses (or with most patients), in part because of a difference in social status. Correspondingly there is an educational difference between physicians and nurses. As mentioned earlier, the formal educational training necessary for a physician is generally much longer than that necessary for a nurse, and their training differs in content.

The differences in the composition of each profession on the basis of sex is clear. Most physicians are male (93.1 percent) and most nurses are female (97.3 percent).[13] In accordance with traditional sex roles, physicians are encouraged to be decisive and to act with authority. Studies indicate that physicians view themselves as omnipotent.[14] Nurses are encouraged to be tactful, sensitive, and diplomatic. Tact and diplomacy are necessary to make a physician feel in control. Put another way, nurses' recommendations for patient treatment must take a particular form. These recommendations must appear to be initiated by the physician. Nurses are expected to take the initiative and are responsible for making recommendations, but at the same time must appear passive.[15] Nurses who see their roles, partially at least, as one of consultant must follow certain rules of the "game."[16] If they refuse to follow the rules, they will be made to suffer consequences such as snide remarks, ostracism, harassment, or job termination.

Again, in accordance with traditional sex roles, nurses in hospitals are viewed much the same as are wives and mothers in the family. This is the view of nursing held both by society and by physicians. Nurses as women are expected to be subservient to physicians as men, to provide "tender loving care" to whoever may be in need, and to be responsible and competent in the absence of physicians but to relinquish that responsibility upon request, i.e., when physicians are present.[17]

As in society, women in hospitals (here women nurses) are typically viewed as sex objects, a situation which encourages physicians to discount the input of nurses with regard to patient care. The observation that women are viewed by male physicians as sexual objects was prevalent in a project which studied the discriminatory practices and attitudes against women in forty-one United States medical schools as seen from questionnaires completed by 146 women medical students. As the author notes, "The open expression of the notion that any woman—even if she is a patient—is fair game for lecherous interests of all men (including physicians) is in some ways the most distressing fact of these student observations."[18] Responses showing the prevalent attitude of physicians toward women in general or toward women as patients included: "[I] often hear demeaning remarks, usually toward nurses offered by clinicians.... " "[There is] superficial discussion of topics related to women...Basic assumption: women are not worth serious consideration." "[The] most frequent remarks concern female patients—women's illnesses are assumed psychosomatic until proven otherwise."[19] Perhaps the most frequent response of women medical students depicting the attitudes of male medical students, professors, and clinicians centered around the use of slides in class of parts of women's anatomy and slides of nude women from magazine centerfolds. Those slides were introduced by medical-student colleagues or instructors often to bait women medical students or belittle them. One student relates, "My own experience with [a professor who had included a "nudie" slide in his lecture] was an interesting and emotional comment ending on, 'Men need to look down on women, and that's why I show the slide.'"[20] The response of the male members of the class to the slides was generally one of unmitigated laughter and approval. With such a negative and restricted view of women as persons, nurses, not to mention all women, are at a disadvantage in dealing with most male physicians.

Another aspect of the sexism that permeates the physician-nurse relationship is reflected in divergent standards of mental health for men and women. A study of thirty-three female and forty-six male psychi-atrists, psychologists, and social workers showed that they held a different standard of mental health for women and men. The standard agreed upon for mentally healthy men was basically the same as the standard for mentally healthy adults. The standard for mentally healthy women included being more easily influenced, less objective, etc., in general characteristics which are less socially desirable.[21] Women then who are mentally healthy women are mentally unhealthy adults and women who are mentally healthy adults are mentally unhealthy women. This is clearly a "no win" situation for all women. Women nurses are no exception.

It is the just described classist and sexist economic and social context of the physician-nurse relationship that often inhibits the nurse from effectively functioning on behalf of the patient. Nurses have a moral responsibility to act on behalf of the patient, but in order to expect them to carry out that responsibility, changes must be made in the workplace. Nurses must be in a position to act to protect the rights of patients. They must be allowed and encouraged to do so. Therefore, those operating and managing hospitals and those responsible for hospital policies must establish policies which make it possible for nurses to protect patients' rights without risking their present and future employment. Those operating and managing hospitals cannot eradicate classism and sexism, but they must be aware of the impact it has on patient care, for again the ultimate goal of everyone connected with hospitals is adequate medical care within the framework of patients' rights. As potential patients it is important to all of us.[22]

NOTES

1 The statement can be found, for example, in *Hospitals*, vol. 4 (Feb. 16, 1973).

2 I am aware of the difficulties in determining what constitutes adequate medical care. For example, is adequate medical care determined solely by reference to past and present medical practices, by the established wisdom of knowledgeable health professionals, or by knowledgeable recipients of medical care? And how is the standard for knowledgeability determined? I am presuming that problems such as these, though difficult, are not insoluble. I am also aware of the related difficulty in distinguishing medical care from health care. And what distinguishes medical care and health care from

nursing care? In this paper, "medical care" will refer to the diagnosis and treatment of illness. Health professionals then, who aid physicians in the process of diagnosing and treating illness, aid in providing medical care.

3 A large majority of all working nurses work in hospitals.

4 The International Code of Nursing Ethics is ambiguous in addressing such a dilemma. The relevant section (#7) of the code merely states: "The nurse is under an obligation to carry out the physician's orders intelligently and loyally and to refuse to participate in unethical procedures." What exactly is the nurse supposed to do when to carry out the physician's orders is in effect to participate in unethical procedures? The most recent (1976) version of the *Code for Nurses* (available from the American Nurses' Association) adopted by the American Nurses' Association directly addresses this problem. Section 3 states, "The nurse acts to safeguard the client and the public when health care and safety are affected by the incompetent, unethical, or illegal practice of any person." The interpretive statement of section 3 begins, "The nurse's primary commitment is to the client's care and safety. Hence, in the role of client advocate, the nurse must be alert to and take appropriate action regarding any instances of incompetent, unethical, or illegal practice(s) by any member of the health-care team or the health-care system itself, or any action on the part of others that is prejudicial to the client's best interests."

5 The area of practice which is solely that of the nurse and the area of practice which is solely that of the physician is presently in a state of flux. The submissive role that nursing has held in relation to the physician's practice of medicine is being rejected by the nursing profession. Nurse practice acts, which regulate the practice of nursing, in many states reflect the change toward an expanded and more independent role for nurses. For example, a definition of a nursing diagnosis, as distinct from a medical diagnosis, is a part of some nurse practice acts. Daniel A. Rothman and Nancy Lloyd Rothman, *The Professional Nurse and the Law* (Boston: Little, Brown, 1977), pp. 65–81.

6 The overwhelming majority of nurses are women and the overwhelming majority of physicians are men. Because the examples are intended to reflect the hospital situation as it exists, I will use the feminine pronoun to refer to nurses and the masculine pronoun to refer to physicians.

7 In an actual case of this description, the intern dismissed the nurse's diagnosis by asking if her woman's intuition told her that diagnosis X was the correct one. The nurse's decision was to not pursue the matter, and early in the morning the patient sustained a cardiac arrest and was unresponsive to resuscitation efforts by the resuscitation team.

8 Obviously, nurses also make mistakes, but physicians are clearly in a position to protect the patient when they become aware of nurses' mistakes.

9 Vicente Navarro, "Women in Health Care," *New England Journal of Medicine*, vol. 292 (Feb. 20, 1975), p. 400.

10 Barbara Ehrenreich and John Ehrenreich, "Health Care and Social Control," *Social Policy*, vol. 5 (May/June 1974), p. 33.

11 Raymond S. Duff and August Hollingshead, *Sickness and Society* (New York: Harper & Row, 1968), p. 371.

12 *Ibid.*, p. 376.

13 Navarro, p. 400.

14 Robert L. Kane and Rosalie A. Kane, "Physicians' Attitudes of Omnipotence in a University Hospital," *Journal of Medical Education*, vol. 44 (August 1969), pp. 684–690; and Trucia Kushner, "Nursing Profession: Condition Critical," *Ms*, vol. 2 (August 1973), p. 99.

15 Kushner, p. 99.

16 Leonard I. Stein, "The Doctor-Nurse Game," in Edith R. Lewis, ed., *Changing Patterns of Nursing Practice: New Needs, New Roles* (New York: American Journal of Nursing Company, 1971), p. 227.

17 JoAnn Ashley, *Hospitals, Paternalism, and the Role of the Nurse* (New York: Teachers College, 1976), p. 17.

18 Margaret A. Campbell, *Why Would A Girl Go into Medicine?* (Old Westbury, N.Y.: Feminist Press, 1973), p. 73.

19 *Ibid.*, p. 74.

20 *Ibid.*, p. 26.

21 Inge K. Broverman, Donald M. Broverman, Frank E. Clarkson, Paul S. Rosenkrantz, and Susan R. Vogel, "Sex-Role Stereotypes and Clinical Judgments of Mental Health," *Journal of Consulting*

and Clinical Psychology, vol. 34 (February 1970), pp. 1–7.

22 I wish to thank Jorn Bramann, Marilyn Edmunds, Jane Zembaty, and especially Tom Mappes for their helpful comments on earlier versions of this paper.

Collective Responsibility and the Nursing Profession

James L. Muyskens

James L. Muyskens is professor of philosophy at Hunter College. He is the author of *Moral Problems in Nursing: A Philosophical Investigation* (1982). His recent articles include "Religious-Belief as Hope," "Kant's Moral Argument," "Life after Death: An Idle Wish or a Reasonable Hope?," and "Nurses Collective Responsibility and the Strike Weapon."

Muyskens argues that there are cases of *collective responsibility* that are not reducible to statements that ascribe responsibility to *individuals*. Professions, such as nursing, that promulgate an ideal standard of professional behavior (a code of ethics) are the kinds of groups to which collective responsibility can be attributed. Muyskens discusses some of the issues within the nursing profession today to emphasize the following: (1) Even though performances, actions, or conditions within the nursing profession are undesirable, particular members of the profession *are not individually responsible*. They cannot be expected to be either heroes or saints. (2) Even though the behavior of individual nurses does not fall below the standards we can reasonably require individuals to meet, the *group's* conduct is below the professional standards we can reasonably expect the group to meet. For Muyskens, the notion of collective responsibility is a strong weapon for those who are working to upgrade the nursing profession and the health-care delivery system.

Members of the nursing profession, for a variety of reasons including the nature of the profession but also economic exploitation and sexism,[1] have been "caught in the middle." On the one hand, for example, the nurse is hired to carry out the directives of the physician and to support the policy of the hospital administration. The system cannot function as presently constituted without such cooperation and support in carrying out the decisions and policies of those higher up in the hierarchy. Yet, on the other hand, the nurse is legally and morally accountable for her or his judgments exercised and actions taken. "Neither physician's prescriptions nor the employing agency's policies relieve the nurse of ethical or legal accountability for actions taken and judgments made."[2]

A common predicament of nurses is expressed in the April issue of *Nursing 78* by a nurse at a West Coast university hospital. She says:

> Our biggest problem right now is that our nursing leadership at the administrative level is completely impotent. They have no voting rights on any committee that has direct control over the hospital and/or nursing. Worse, the acting director and her associate have no idea of taking any power into their own hands, where it rightfully belongs. They ask permission to improve staffing ratios, by increasing or closing beds, and when they're turned down, say to us "Sorry girls! Work doubles."...[3]

The overwork and understaffing not only make working conditions less than desirable for the nurse, they clearly endanger patients. When, for example, one registered nurse and an aide must try to care for thirty to thirty-six patients who have just undergone surgery, the situation is very dangerous and health care cannot be delivered in accordance with acceptable standards.

We can all sympathize with the nurse who wrote the following:

> I am supposed to be responsible for the control and safety of techniques used in the operating theatre. I have spent many hours teaching the technicians and the aides the routines necessary for maintaining aseptic conditions during surgery. They have learned to prepare materials and to maintain an adequate supply for all needs. They have learned to handle supplies with good technique.
>
> I find it is extremely difficult to have these appropriate routines carried out constantly by employees with little theoretical background or understanding. The surgeons are frequently breaking techniques and respond in a belligerent manner when breaks in technique are brought to their attention. I find a reminder of techniques often brings a determined response to ignore the reminder and proceed with surgery. For a male surgeon to be questioned by a female nurse is a serious breach of respect to them.
>
> One day a surgeon wore the same gown for two successive operations even though there were other gowns available. I quietly called this to his attention, but I had no authority which really allowed me to control his behavior for the good of the patient. In this situation even the hospital administrator was of no help to me.[4]

This nurse is responsible for the control and safety of techniques used in the operating rooms. The conditions over which she is responsible have fallen below acceptable standards. Although she has done her best, the assigned task has not been accomplished. The patients who have a right to expect, and have paid for, a safe and aseptic operating room have been let down.

Nursing is the largest group of health-care professionals within the vast health-care delivery system—a system that, despite some dramatic achievements, is increasingly under attack as dehumanizing, exploitative, and cost-ineffective. Despite the seeming powerlessness of any individual nurse, taken collectively nursing more than any other health-care profession is

a necessary component in the emergence of the present health-care delivery system. The present system could not have developed without nursing. If all nurses were to walk out tomorrow, the system would collapse. This cannot be said for any other group of health-care professionals, including physicians. Hence, if the health-care delivery system is substandard (as I believe it is), the nurse is not merely a victim of the system (along with the rest of us), but she or he is also an accomplice. As an accomplice she shares responsibility for the system's deficiencies. The nurse's plight is by no means unique. The paradoxical plight of the nurse of being both powerless and powerful, responsible yet not responsible, is a plight in which we almost all find ourselves in some aspects of our lives.

One way to try to make sense of these paradoxical situations—the way to be explored in this essay—is to introduce the notion of collective responsibility. Two dramatic and widely discussed illustrations of this are the prosecution's case against certain middle-level Nazis after World War II and the defense's case for First Lieutenant William Calley charged with murder at My-Lai.

In the prosecution case, blame for the actions of certain individual members of the collective is ascribed to all members. Karl Jaspers expressed this view when he said: "Every German is made to share the blame for the crimes committed in the name of the Reich… inasmuch as we let such a regime arise among us."[5] In condemning every German, Jaspers is not merely blaming each German for his or her active or passive tolerance of the Nazis. He is saying that "the world of German ideas," "German thought," and "national tradition" are to blame. Collective responsibility is used as a net from which no member of the collective can escape.

In the defense case, the individual whose behavior has fallen below the acceptable standard is shielded from the full weight of blame, because the weight is shifted to the collective. It is the collective, the system, that must bear the brunt of the burden rather than the individual. In the Calley case it was claimed that Americans as a group failed to perform as they could have been expected.

In a recent survey of nurses' attitudes[6] this defense strategy was tacitly used. It was reported that, although nurses saw themselves as performing well given the work conditions, they "felt they ought somehow to deliver even when the system won't let them." The writers of the report indicate that this blame is misplaced ("not deserved"). Although performing below the acceptable standard, they were not to be blamed because as individuals each was doing the best possible for her in the situation. The system itself was to be blamed.

If the blame appropriately ascribed in a situation is no greater than the sum of all the ascriptions of blame to the individuals, we do not have a case of collective responsibility except in a weak (distributive) sense. By collective responsibility in the strong (nondistributive) sense—as the term is to be used in this essay—we mean that the responsibility of the group is not equivalent to that of the individuals. That is, the whole is not equal to the sum of its parts.

It is incontrovertible that we do ascribe responsibility to collectives in this strong sense. To use an example of D.E. Cooper,[7] if we say that the local tennis club is responsible for its closure, we don't necessarily or usually mean that the officers of the club or any particular members are responsible for its closure. If you were to question the speaker, he or she may be unwilling to blame any particular individuals or the officers of the club. It is not that any person failed to do what was expected of him or her. Yet something was missing. "It was just a bad club as a whole."[8] From the claim that the local tennis club is responsible for its closure no statements about particular individuals follow. "This is so," as Cooper says, "because the existence of a collective is compatible with a varying membership. No determinate set of individuals is necessary for the existence of a collective."[9]

As R.S. Downie has argued, "...to provide an adequate description of the actions, purposes, and responsibilities of a certain range of collectives, such as governments, armies, colleges, incorporated business firms, etc., we must make use of concepts which logically cannot be analyzed in individualistic terms."[10] The reductionists who deny this have the principle of parsimony on their side, but little else. Although the reductionist says the ascriptions of collective responsibility could be reduced to statements about individuals, he or she does not do it. These reductionistic attempts suffer from the same problems and deserve the same fate as the discredited reductionist programs in theory of knowledge and philosophy of science.

The question to ask then is what set of conditions must obtain in order properly to ascribe nondistributive,

collective blame or responsibility. The conditions advanced by Cooper in his essay "Responsibility and the 'System'" are sufficiently accurate and refined for purposes of this essay. These conditions are:

1 Members of a group perform undesirable acts.

2 Their performing these acts is partly explained by their acting in accordance with the "way of life" of the group (i.e., the rules, mores, customs, etc., of the group).

3 These characteristics of the group's "way of life" are below standards we might reasonably expect the group to meet.

4 It is not necessarily the case that members of the group, in performing the acts, are falling below standards we can reasonably expect individuals to meet.[11]

A few comments about these conditions are in order. Clearly we do not *hold* an individual or a group responsible—that is, following its etymology: having liability to answer to a *charge*—if undesirable acts have not been performed. When no undesirable acts occur, the question of blame or responsibility in the sense of liability does not arise. Hence we see the need for Condition 1.

The second condition is not strictly necessary. It does seem, as Virginia Held has argued,[12] that when special conditions obtain, even a random collection of individuals can be held responsible (a claim denied by Condition 2). However, for present purposes—consideration of collective responsibility of members of a profession—this stronger claim need not be defended. The most plausible cases for ascribing collective responsibility are those cases in which the group has distinctive characteristics, has a sense of solidarity and cohesion (for example, feels "vicarious pride and shame"[13]), members identify themselves as members of the group (for example, "Who are you?" "I am a nurse."), and some of these group feelings or characteristics are appealed to in explaining the acts in question. For example, if the citizens of Syldavia can be characterized as being rather hostile and distrustful of foreigners and their customs, laws, and policies reflect this, then, when (say) some border guards—in over-zealously carrying out the Syldavian policy—kill some visiting dignitaries, we blame not only the border guards but the Syldavians. In contrast, if these border guards steal from the visiting dignitaries but in accounting for this behavior we would not be inclined to appeal to any larger group feelings or characteristics, we definitely would not wish to ascribe collective blame.

We have seen above in the variety of cases discussed that it is when a collective fails to live up to what can reasonably be expected of it—i.e., it falls below an acceptable standard—that it can incur collective blame. Hence we see the need for Condition 3.

Condition 4 is necessary because the standards applied to groups may be different from those applied to individuals. For example, we may feel that the nurse (in the case cited above) who was charged with responsibility for the control and safety of techniques used in the operating rooms adequately met her obligations. She did not fall below standards we can reasonably expect an individual to meet. After all, as Joel Feinberg has argued, "no individual person can be blamed for not being a hero or a saint." Yet, as Feinberg goes on to say, "a whole people can be blamed for not producing a hero when the times require it, especially when the failure can be charged to some discernible element in the group's 'way of life' that militates against heroism."[14] Although Feinberg was not talking about this case or collective responsibility of the nursing profession (he was talking about a Jesse James train robbery case), his remarks are especially apt for this case and many other situations within the nursing profession.

One can readily see that conditions outlined for properly ascribing nondistributive collective responsibility obtain in many situations within professions. Professions more than most other collectives are bound together by common aspirations, values, methodologies, and training. In too many cases, they also have similar socioeconomic backgrounds and are of the same sex and ethnic group. As we have seen, the more cohesive the group, the less problematic the ascription of collective responsibility. The fact that professions such as nursing promulgate codes of ethics or standards of behavior toward which they expect members to strive, provides a clear criterion for judging whether the actual practices of the profession fall below standards to which we can reasonably hold the group.

In addition to meeting these formal criteria for ascribing collective responsibility, there are several other reasons unique to professions for ascribing collective responsibility in certain situations.

A   There are several ways by which one becomes responsible. One can be *saddled* with it by circum-

stances, one can have responsibility *assigned* to one, or one can deliberately *assume* responsibility.[15] Typically a profession is chosen. In choosing the profession, one *assumes* the responsibility concomitant with being a professional. One chooses to adopt the values, methodology, and "way of life" of the profession. Such choice is much less prominent with most other basic group affiliations. One does not choose family membership, region of birth, usually not citizenship, and often not military service. Once in the profession, of course, as people go about their jobs, they will also sometimes be saddled with responsibility by circumstances and be assigned responsibility. But these assignments are all within the context of choice to assume professional responsibility. This choice to assume professional responsibility provides the backdrop for all one's professional activities. Hence, as a professional, more than most other group affiliations, one sees oneself as a member of the group and has—with eyes open—chosen the identification.

B   Nurses (as is, of course, also the case in several other professions) have been vested by the state with the power to regulate and control nursing practice. This collective power or right—given exclusively to the profession—has concomitant with it a collective responsibility or duty to see to it that acceptable standards are maintained. Since it is possible that each individual nurse, including officers of the American Nursing Association, is meeting acceptable standards in her or his own assignments and yet the group's "way of life" must be characterized as below an acceptable standard, appeal to collective responsibility is one of the tools the public has at its disposal to try to insure adequate nursing and general health care. Obviously in these cases (when no individual has failed to meet her or his legal obligation) the public does not have recourse to lawsuits against individuals.

C   Supposedly as a means to protect the public, the licensing statutes of the states allow only those who have passed certain requirements set down by the state to practice nursing. One result of this is that the profession which is by law also self-regulatory becomes a protected monopoly. If a person is going to receive nursing care, this care must be provided by a member of the profession. If nursing care is to be upgraded, it must be from within with at most prodding from without. Quite clearly one of the most effective tools for such prodding is that of demonstrating collective responsibility, a responsibility that goes beyond the sum of each individual's responsibility.

From the discussion thus far, it is evident that the appeal to collective responsibility when some substandard behavior or undesirable acts have occurred is a two-edged sword. It can be used to show that, despite undesirable performances or actions or conditions within a collective, a particular member of the collective is not individually responsible. However, it can also be used to show that, despite the fact that the behavior of individuals does not fall below standards we can reasonably require individuals to meet (given that we cannot *demand* that an individual be a hero), the group's conduct is below standards we can reasonably expect the group to meet. One of the reasons the weapon of collective responsibility looks suspect in the widely discussed World War II prosecution and Vietnam conflict defense cases is that only one edge of the sword is used while the other edge is conveniently ignored.

If conditions for properly ascribing collective responsibility are satisfied, to the extent that the individual is exonerated, the group is indicted. To the degree the individual *qua* individual is indicted, the group is exonerated. Either way the individual group member bears responsibility. For any member of a collective but especially (for reasons cited above) a professional, it is not enough just to know that one has done all that could be expected of him or her strictly as an individual. The arm of responsibility for a professional has a longer reach than that of the individual.

Specific situations within the nursing profession illustrate the two edges of the sword of collective responsibility. These situations should be seen within the context of the rapid evolution of the nursing profession in recent years. In recent years there has been considerable effort both within and outside the profession (e.g., the medical profession) to upgrade the requirements for licensure. These efforts have borne results. The scope of the professional nurse has expanded greatly as exemplified by medical-assistant programs and the use of nurses as paramedical practitioners to relieve the shortage of medical doctors in certain areas. The history of the struggle first to adopt a code of ethics for American nurses and then to revise it reflects this evolution. Tentative codes were presented in the twenties, thirties, and forties. These efforts were met by opposition from those who feared the professionalization of nursing. A striking instance of this is the advice given by a physician to one of the earliest advocates of a code of ethics for American nurses: "Be good women but do not have a code of ethics."[16] It was not until 1950 that a code of ethics was adopted.

The code has been changed several times since then, the most recent being in 1976. Two of the most interesting changes from our vantage point have been the following: Earlier versions stated that the nurse had an obligation to carry out physician's orders. The 1968 and 1976 versions of the code stress instead the nurse's obligation to the patient (called client in the 1976 version). The physician just mentioned who advised against having a code may have foreseen this development! Whereas earlier versions of the code point to an obligation to sustain confidence in associates, this has been replaced by the obligation to protect the patient from incompetent, unethical, or illegal practice from any quarter.[17]

With this background one can see why it is especially interesting to look at the nursing profession when speaking of collective responsibility in the professions. The fundamental issue in the ongoing struggle to upgrade the profession—reflected in the code changes—has been that of accountability, the willingness to make decisions and accept responsibility for these decisions. The crucial question in the attempt to upgrade the profession is that of the interface of individual and collective responsibility.

The author of an article in the *Quarterly Record of the Massachusetts General Hospital Nurses Alumnae Association* wrote about "blame avoidance" behavior in nurses. As explained, blame avoidance behavior is exhibited when the nurse says such things as "I did this because the supervisor told me to do it," or "the doctor ordered it," or "the hospital rules demanded it." The author maintains that accountability requires that the nurse can say, "I did this because in my best judgment it is what the patient needed."[18] Notwithstanding the many good qualities common to nurses, blame avoidance behavior does seem to be one of the more prevalent, endemic faults of the nursing profession. As we have seen, a concerted effort by many within the profession has made inroads on this "way of life" of the profession.

These efforts have been made without explicit appeal to the concept of collective responsibility. As a result, judgment in cases of blame avoidance and other unacceptable or undesirable behavior has tended either to be too harsh or too lenient. That is, either *(a)* one judges that the individual nurse caught in the middle and in difficult circumstances has done all one can reasonably expect her or him to do. After all, we can not expect or demand that such a person be a hero or a saint. Hence, the nurse is exonerated. Yet the unacceptable practice or condition continues unabated. Or *(b)* one focuses on professional responsibility and the fact that, if some individuals do not stand up against substandard practices—no matter what the odds of thereby improving the situation and no matter at what price to the individual—these practices likely will not be stopped. From this perspective the individual nurse who fails to do all within her or his power—including actions that will likely jeopardize the nurse's position—to insure the best care possible for patients in the nurse's care, is judged to be a moral coward.

For example, in the case of the nurse charged with responsibility for maintaining a safe and aseptic operating room, without appeal to the concept of collective responsibility we are likely to say either: (1) that she has done all we can require of her—(She has asked the surgeon to comply. She does not have the authority or status to demand compliance to proper procedures. The lack of compliance quite properly was followed by a report to the hospital administration) or (2) that she has not done all we can require of her—(She cannot allow dangerous violations of operating room aseptic standards to take place. In doing so, she is failing to carry out her assignment and is allowing the patient's life to be placed in jeopardy. She should not be cowed by the surgeon's arrogance and sexism. Even at the risk of losing her job, she cannot allow the operation to take place in these conditions).

The problem is that (1) is too lenient a judgment and (2) is too harsh. We cannot require the nurse *qua* individual to do more than she has done. But the nurse *qua* nurse shares blame with her colleagues in such cases despite the much greater blame which must be placed on the surgeon violating reasonable requirements. The lack of aggressive advocacy for the patient's welfare, the willingness to be dominated by the (usually male) physician or surgeon—unfortunate even if understandable "ways of life" of the nursing profession—which partially explain this nurse's behavior are below

the standard we can rightfully expect the group authorized to provide nursing services to meet. Appeal to collective responsibility yields a judgment neither too harsh nor too lenient.

This judgment conforms to the moral intuitions of the nurses surveyed who were mentioned earlier. Despite a feeling that as individuals they were doing all that could reasonably be required of them in their circumstances, they still felt dissatisfied with their performance. As nurses they felt blame for falling short of the mark set for the profession.

This dissatisfaction, when seen in the light of collective responsibility, can be turned to positive use. The nurse who has done all she is required to do as an individual need not suffer debilitating guilt. Guilt, in such cases, is misplaced. Her individual actions do not warrant guilt. And, in contrast to nondistributive collective responsibility, there is no nondistributive collective guilt. "Guilt," as Feinberg has said, "consists in the intentional transgression of a prohibition." "... there can be no such thing as vicarious guilt."[19] However, although rightfully free of guilt, she cannot be complacent. She is a member of a group that stands judged (i.e., is liable) and must, with her colleagues, take appropriate steps to alleviate the undesirable conditions. It is not enough for a professional to do all that is required of her or him as an individual. With the nurse having freely accepted the privileges and benefits of the profession, her or his responsibilities in the areas of professional competence are greater than would be those of an equally skilled and knowledgeable individual who was not a member of the profession.

In order to meet this larger responsibility, as the American Nursing Association has recognized, "there should be an established mechanism for the reporting and handling of incompetent, unethical, or illegal practice within the employment setting so that such reporting can go through official channels and be done without fear of reprisal. The nurse should be knowledgeable about the mechanism and be prepared to utilize it if necessary."[20]

Paradoxically if such machinery which collective responsibility requires were put in place, individual accountability would increase and the need to appeal to collective responsibility would decrease. If reporting incompetent, unethical, or illegal conduct could be done effectively through official channels and done without fear of reprisal, such reporting—which under more dangerous and less effective circumstances is not required—would be morally required of the individual. Hence, it may be that a profession should strive to organize itself and regulate itself to such a degree that the conditions for proper ascription of collective responsibility do not arise. But this is not the situation within the nursing profession at the present. Therefore, I conclude that the notion of collective responsibility is a timely weapon of considerable force for those who are working toward upgrading the nursing profession and the health-care delivery system.

NOTES

1 See JoAnn Ashley, *Hospitals, Paternalism, and the Role of the Nurse* (New York: Teachers, 1976), for a discussion of economic exploitation and sexism, which have plagued the nursing profession.

2 "Code for Nurses with Interpretive Statements" (Kansas City, Mo.: American Nurses' Association, 1976), p. 10.

3 Marjorie A. Godfrey, "Job Satisfaction—Or Should That Be Dissatisfaction? How Nurses Feel About Nursing," Part I, *Nursing 78* (April 1978), pp. 101–102.

4 Barbara L. Tate, ed., *The Nurse's Dilemma* (New York: American Journal of Nursing Company. 1977), pp. 47–48.

5 Quoted by D.E. Cooper, "Responsibility and the 'System,'" in Peter French, ed., *Individual and Collective Responsibility* (Cambridge, Mass.: Schenkman, 1972), p. 86.

6 Godfrey, ibid., Part II, *Nursing 78* (May 1978), p.110.

7 D.E. Cooper, "Collective Responsibility," *Philosophy*, vol. XLIII, no. 165 (July 1968), pp. 260–262.

8 Ibid., p. 262.

9 Ibid., p. 260.

10 R.S. Downie, "Responsibility and Social Roles," in French, op. cit., p. 69.

11 "Responsibility and the 'System,'" in French, op. cit., pp. 90–91.

12 Virginia Held, "Can a Random Collection of Individuals Be Morally Responsible?" *The Journal of Philosophy*, vol. LXVII, no. 14 (July 23, 1970), pp. 471–481.

13 Joel Feinberg, "Collective Responsibility," *The Journal of Philosophy*, vol. LXV, no. 21 (Nov. 7, 1968), p. 677.

14 Ibid., p. 687.

15 Kurt Baier, "Guilt and Responsibility," in French, op. cit., p. 52.

16 Lavinia L. Dock, *A History of Nursing*, vol. III (New York: Putnam, 1912), p. 129.

17 See Kathleen M. Sward, "An Historical Perspective," in *Perspectives on the Code for Nurses* (Kansas City, Mo.: American Nurses' Association, 1978), for a discussion of these and other changes in the versions of the code.

18 Quoted by Barbara Durand, "A Nursing Practice Perspective," in *Perspectives on the Code for Nurses* (Kansas City, Mo.: American Nurses' Association, 1978), p. 19.

19 Feinberg, ibid., p. 676.

20 Sward, ibid., p. 8.

Privacy and Confidentiality

The Legal and Philosophical Foundations of the Right to Privacy

Richard Wasserstrom

Richard Wasserstrom, who has an LL.B. as well as a Ph.D. in philosophy, is professor of philosophy at the University of California at Santa Cruz. Wasserstrom is the author of *The Judicial Decision: Toward a Theory of Legal Justification* (1961) and *Philosophy and Social Issues: Five Studies* (1980) and editor of *Morality and the Law* (1970), *War and Morality* (1970), and *Today's Moral Problems* (3rd ed., 1985). He has also published many articles on issues in ethics and the philosophy of law.

Wasserstrom argues that there are at least three distinct kinds of interests or claims that may be involved in our talk about the importance of privacy. He is especially interested in examining the sense of privacy implicit in the patient's bill of rights enacted by a Minnesota statute. The statute asserts a patient's right to "every consideration of his privacy and individuality as it relates to his social, religious, and psychological well-being." According to Wasserstrom, the root idea in this sense of privacy is that "of the control that an individual will be able to maintain over information about himself or herself." The patient's right to privacy protects the individual from the harm that could result from the exposure of the kind of information that makes an individual unusually vulnerable and exposed. Wasserstrom also examines the similar role played by the related principle of confidentiality in the physician-patient and psychiatrist-patient relationships.

I

If there is one thing that is undeniably true of privacy, it is that there are several different phenomena that have been and that can be discussed under the heading of "privacy." Almost all of the discussion has been of comparatively recent vintage. In legal scholarship, the classic reference to a right of privacy is the article by Brandeis and Warren entitled, "The Right of Privacy," which appeared in *The Harvard Law Review* in 1890. The first enunciation by the United States Supreme Court of an explicit constitutional right of privacy occurred in 1965 in the case of *Griswold v. Connecticut.* And almost all philosophical and public policy examinations of privacy have appeared within the past fifteen years.

The topic of privacy is very much in the air and in the news today; it is the subject of appreciable discussion and legislation. As witness, for example, the 1973 Minnesota statute which enacted a patient's "bill of rights" and which included within those rights two that explicitly mentioned privacy: "Every patient and resident shall have the right to every consideration of his privacy and individuality as it relates to his social, religious, and psychological well-being" and "Every patient and resident shall have the right to respectfulness and privacy as it relates to his medical care program.

Case discussion, consultation, examination, and treatment are confidential and should be conducted discreetly."

Part of the problem in thinking about privacy, and in deciding, for instance, what this statute means, is, as I have said, that the same thing is not always meant at all by the term "privacy." In fact, there are, I believe, at least three distinct kinds of interests or claims that may be involved when commentators, the courts, legislatures, and ordinary citizens talk about privacy and its importance.

The kind of thing that Brandeis and Warren were concerned with was the unconsented use by an individual of another's identity in order to secure some special advantage. The central focus here is upon the improper use of a person's name or likeness for commercial purposes, as, for example, when a person's name and picture are included in the advertising for a product in order to enhance the sale of the product. But I include within this category cases in which true facts of a certain sort about an individual are made public, as for instance when there is an unconsented public showing of the films of a particular Caesarian birth.

The United States Supreme Court was concerned with a rather different sense of "privacy" in the Griswold case. That case involved primarily the constitutionality of a Connecticut statute which made it a crime for any person to use any drug, medicinal article or instrument for the purpose of preventing conception. One reason some of the members of the Court gave for holding the statute unconstitutional was that the statute intruded improperly into a constitutionally protected zone of privacy. That zone of privacy existed, apparently, in virtue of the fact that the behavior covered by the statute included that of married persons in respect to their own sexual relationship. This idea—that certain relationships and certain behavior occuring within the home were immune from governmental regulation—was also utilized by the Court in the abortion decision and in a case involving an individual's right to possess and read pornographic literature in his home.

The third sense of "privacy" is reflected in the contemporary concern over the wrong, if any, that was done by the members of the plumber's squad who broke into the office of Daniel Ellsberg's psychiatrist to see what they could learn about Ellsberg from the notes of his psychiatrist. It is reflected, as well, in the worry many persons have over the development and use of sophisticated spying devices which make it possible surreptitiously to overhear another's conversations or observe another's behavior. And it is reflected, too, in the concern over the large scale accumulation of data which now exists about each one of us and which is capable of being stored in and retrieved from large scale data banks. Here, it seems to me, the root issue captured by this idea of privacy is that of the control that an individual will be able to maintain over information about himself or herself.

It is this third sense of "privacy" that I propose to concentrate upon. I think it is the one that is centrally involved in that section of the patient's bill of rights that gives to every patient and resident the right "...to every consideration of his privacy and individuality as it relates to his social, religious, and psychological well being." But my interest is not legislative interpretation. What I am convinced of is that this sense of "privacy" is an important one and that it does figure in problems of medicine, as well as those of social existence generally. So that the issue I want to concentrate upon is that of the kind and degree of control a person ought to be able to exercise in respect to knowledge of or the disclosure of information about himself or herself. I want to consider primarily what this kind of privacy is all about and why persons might think it is of importance.

II

Information about oneself is not all of the same type; as a result control over some kinds may be much more important than control over others. For this reason, I want to start by trying to identify some of the different types of information about oneself over which persons might desire to retain control, and I want to describe the situations in which this information comes into being. To do this, I shall consider three situations and look at the ways they resemble each other and differ from one another.

There is first of all the fact that you can, if you wish to, look "inward" and become aware of the ideas that are running through your mind, the various emotions you are experiencing, and the variety of bodily sensations you are having—an itch on your scalp or a pain in your side. One thing that is significant about one's mental states—about one's dreams, conscious thoughts, hopes, fears, an desires—is that the most direct, the best, and often the only evidence for another of what they are consists in my deliberately revealing them to you. To be sure, my nonverbal behavior may give an observer a clue as to what is going on in my mind. If, for example, I have a faraway look in my eyes you may infer that I am daydreaming about something and not paying very much attention to you. In addition, there is, no doubt, a more intimate and even conceptual connection between observable behavior and certain states of feeling. If I am blushing that may mean that I am embarrassed. If I am talking very fast that may lead you to infer correctly that I am excited or nervous. It is also sometimes the case that I will not know my own thoughts and feelings, etc., and that by saying what I think they are a skilled observer can, by listening to me and watching me as I talk, tell better than can I what is really going on inside my head.

But even taking all of these qualifications into account, it still remains the case, I believe, that the only way to obtain very detailed and accurate information about what I am thinking, fearing, imagining, desiring, or hating and how I am experiencing it is for me to tell you or show you. If I do not, the ideas and feeling remain within me and in some sense, at least, known only to me. Because people cannot read other people's minds, these things about me are known only to me in a way in which other things are not unless I decide to disclose them to you.

What about things that are going on in my body? In

some respects the situation is similar to that of my thoughts and in some respects different. There are things that are going on in my body that are like my thoughts, fears and fantasies. If I have a slight twinge of pain in my left big toe, there is no way for anyone else to know that unless I choose to disclose it. Of course, if the toe is swollen and red, and if I grimace whenever I put any weight on it, an observer could doubtless infer correctly that I was experiencing pain there. But in many other cases the only evidence would be my verbal report.

There are other things about my body concerning which this privileged position does not obtain. Even though they are *my* ribs, I cannot tell very well what they look like; even though it is *my* blood, I cannot tell with any precision how much alcohol is there. A person looking through a fluoroscope at my ribs or at an X-ray of my ribs can tell far better than can I (just from having them as *my* ribs or from looking down at *my* chest) what my ribs look like. A trained technician looking at a sample of my blood in combination with certain chemicals can determine far better than I can (just from it being *my* blood) what the alcoholic content is or whether I am anemic.

So there are some facts about my body that I know in a way others logically cannot know them, that can be known to others only if I disclose them by telling what they are. There are other facts about my body that cannot be known by others in the way I know them but that can be inferred from observation of my body and my behavior. And there are still other kinds of facts about my body that I don't know and that can be learned, if at all, only by someone or something outside of myself.

In the second place, there is some information that is private only in virtue of the setting in which the information is disclosed or communicated. For example, suppose that I have broken my arm and that I am in a room with the door closed, alone with the doctor while he or she sets the break. Or suppose instead that I am in an enclosed telephone booth, calling a hospital to make an appointment to donate some blood. In both of these cases it is the setting that makes the behavior distinctive and relevant for our purposes. In both of these cases I believe I have a substantial degree of present control over the information about myself—that my arm is broken and is being set, or that I want to donate blood to the hospital—because of the situation in which the information is being conveyed or disclosed.

If no one is in a position to see me and the doctor, then no one is in a position at that time to know about my arm. If no one is in a position to overhear (at my end) what I am saying to the person at the hospital, and if no one is tapping the telephone line, then no one is able at that time to hear what I am saying except for the person at the other phone. We can, I think, usefully describe cases of this kind as cases of things being done in private—meaning by that only that they are done in a setting in which there did not appear to be anyone other than the person to whom I was talking, etc., who was in a position to hear what was being said or to see what was being done. This is, of course, an extremely weak sense of privacy, and for at least two reasons. To begin with, the information is less within my control than is information about my mental states, not yet revealed to anyone, because the other person can if he or she chooses reveal what he or she has learned about me. And in addition, there is nothing about the character of the information which seems to make further revelation a source of concern.

It is this last point which leads to the third kind of case I want to discuss. Suppose that instead of having my broken arm set by a doctor, my wife and I are alone in a room engaged in sexual intercourse. Or suppose, that instead of calling the hospital to arrange to give blood, I have called my psychotherapist from a phone booth to tell her about some special problem I an having trouble dealing with right now. Both of these things are being done in private in the same sense in which the discussion with the hospital or the treatment of my broken arm were private, i.e., no one else could see or hear. But these also have an additional quality not possessed by the earlier two examples. When I call my therapist from a phone booth—or await her in her office—I certainly do expect that what I tell her is not being overheard by anyone else while I am telling her. In addition, though, I also reasonably expect that what I am telling her will be kept in confidence by her. Thus, it is private in the additional respect that the understanding between us is that it will not be subsequently disclosed to anyone—at least without my consent. It is what might be called a private kind of communication. And that is not the case with my phone call to the hospital. Absent special or unusual circumstances (like telling the hospital that I don't want anyone to know I am giving blood), I have no particular interest in retaining control over disclosure of this fact.

Similarly, engaging in sexual intercourse with my wife is private in the additional respect that it is the sort of intimate thing that is not appropriately observed by others or discussed with them—again, absent special or unusual circumstances, e.g., treatment at a Masters and Johnson clinic (and even here we would expect to be able to control quite specifically who would have access to this information, and under what circumstances). So, in addition to being done in private this act, too, is a private kind of thing. In this respect it seems unlike having my broken arm set by the doctor. For in that case there was no expectation on my part that what my arm looked like or how it was treated should not be made known to others. (This particular case is not a clear one, and I will return to it later to say more about why it is not. For the present, though, let us suppose that it is private only in the sense of having been made so by the setting.)

The most obvious and the important connection between the idea of doing something in private and doing a private kind of thing is that we typically do private things only in situations where we reasonably believe that we are doing them in private. That we believe we are doing something in private is, often, a condition that has to be satisfied before we are willing to disclose an intimate fact about ourselves or to engage in the doing of an intimate act. I would probably have called the hospital to arrange to donate blood even if I were phoning from a crowded room where there were lots of people who could overhear what I was saying. The telephone was a convenient way to make the arrangements. But the fact that I was making them in a setting that appeared to be private was not important to me. It did not affect what I disclosed to the person at the other end. Thus, even if I had suspected that the telephone line was tapped so that an unknown person overheard my conversation, I would probably have called the hospital. In the case of my conversation with my therapist, however, it was the belief that the conversation was in a private setting that made me willing to reveal a private kind of thing. If someone tapped that telephone line and overheard what I said to my therapist, they injured me in a way that is distinguishable on this basis alone from the injury, if any, done to me by tapping my conversation with the hospital. That is to say, at a minimum they would have gotten me to do or to reveal something that I would not have done or revealed if they had not hidden their presence from me.

It should be evident, too, that there are important similarities, as well as some differences, between the first and third cases—between my knowledge of my own mental states and my disclosure of intimate or otherwise confidential information to those to whom I choose to disclose it. What are they? Why might we believe that a special injury had been done to us if information of certain sorts became known, without our consent to others? Consider an extreme, somewhat fanciful case first.

III

Suppose existing technology made it possible for an outsider in some way to look into or monitor another's mind. What, if anything, would be especially disturbing or objectionable about that?

To begin with, there is a real sense in which we have far less control over when we shall have certain thoughts and what their content will be than we have over, for example, to whom we shall reveal them and to what degree. Because our inner thoughts, feelings, and bodily sensations are so largely beyond our control, we would, I think, feel appreciably more insecure in our social environment than we do at present were it possible for another to "look in" without our consent to see what was going on in our heads.

This is so at least in part because many, although by no means all, of our uncommunicated thoughts and feelings are about very intimate matters. Our fantasies and our fears often concern just those matters that in our culture we would least choose to reveal to anyone else. At a minimum we might suffer great anxiety and feelings of shame were the decisions as to where, when, and to whom to disclose, not to be wholly ours. Were access to our thoughts possible in this way we would see ourselves as creatures who are far more vulnerable than we are now.

In addition, there is always the more straightforward worry about accountability for our thoughts and feelings. As I mentioned, they are often not within our control. For all of the reasons that we ought not hold people accountable for behavior not within their control, we would not want the possibility of accountability to extend to uncommunicated thoughts and feelings.

Finally, one rather plausible conception of what it is to be a person carried with it, I believe, the idea of the existence of a core of thoughts and feelings that are the person's alone. If anyone else could know all that I am thinking or perceive all that I am feeling except in the form I choose to filter and reveal what I am and how I see myself—if anyone could, so to speak, be aware of all this at will I might cease to have as complete a sense of myself as a distinct and separate person as I have now. A significant, if not fundamental, part of what it is to be an individual person is to be an entity that is capable of being exclusively aware of its own thoughts and feelings.

Considerations such as these—and particularly the last one—help us to understand some of the puzzles concerning the privilege against self-incrimination, as well as some of the worries about coercive therapies. Because of the significance of exclusive control over our own thoughts and feelings, the privilege against self-incrimination can be seen to rest, ultimately, upon a concern that confessions never be coerced or required by the state. The point of the privilege is not primarily that the state must be induced not to torture individuals in order to extract information from them. Nor is the point even essentially that the topics of confession will necessarily (or even typically) be of the type that we are most unwilling to disclose because of the unfavorable nature of what this would reveal about us. Rather, the fundamental point is that required disclosure of one's thoughts by itself diminishes the concept of individual personhood within the society.

Similarly, non-consensual drug therapies which reduce if not destroy the patient's resistance to disclosing the things that he or she is thinking are subject to the same criticism. The objection to such therapies is not merely that the individuals involved will be led to say things which they would not have otherwise said, because they regarded such disclosures as shameful or otherwise reflecting badly on themselves (although this is certainly a substantial if not decisive consideration against ever doing this to individuals). The additional objection to such therapies is that they take away from the individual control over that one area which is for others exclusively within their control and by which they are helped to maintain a clear sense of their own selfhood and individuality.

The more prominent worry today does not, I think, concern intrusion into the domain of one's uncommunicated thoughts and feelings, but rather concerns the degree to which communications between persons about private things shall remain exclusively within

their control. What, for example, would be the wrong that was done to me were someone to have tapped my phone conversation with my therapist, or if my therapist had told other persons what I had told her? Or what would have been the injury that would have been done to us if, unknown to my wife and me, one of the walls in our room had really been one-way glass and we had been observed engaged in intercourse by a class of prospective sex therapists and counselors?

The most obvious point, I guess, is that because of our social attitudes toward the disclosure of intimate facts and behavior, most of us would be extremely pained were we to learn that these had become known to persons other than those to whom we chose to disclose them. It is important to see that the pain can come about in several different ways. If I do something private with somebody and I believe that we are doing it in private, I may very well be hurt or embarrassed if I learn subsequently that we were observed but didn't know it. Thus if I learn after the fact that my wife and I were observed while we were having intercourse, the knowledge that we were observed will cause us distress both because our expectations of privacy were incorrect and because we do not like the idea that we were observed during this kind of intimate act. People have the right, I think, simply to have the world be what it appears to be precisely in those cases in which they regard privacy as essential to the diminution of their own vulnerability.

Reasoning such as this lies behind, I think, a case that arose some years ago in California. A department store had complained to the police that homosexuals were using its men's room as a meeting place. The police responded by drilling a small hole in the ceiling over the enclosed stalls. A policeman then stationed himself on the floor above and peered down through the hole observing the persons using the stall for eliminatory purposes. Eventually the policeman discovered and apprehended two homosexuals who used the stall as a place to engage in forbidden sexual behavior. The California Supreme Court held the observations of the policeman to have been the result of an illegal search and ordered the conviction reversed. What made the search objectionably illegal, I believe, was that it occurred in the course of this practice which deceived all of the persons who used the stall and who believed that they were doing in private something that was socially regarded as a private kind of thing. They were entitled,

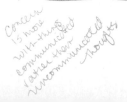

especially for this kind of activity, both to be free from observation and to have their expectations of privacy honored by the state.

There is an additional reason why the observation or disclosure of certain sorts of activity is objectionable. That is because the kind of spontaneity and openness that is essential to them disappears with the presence of an observer or the lack of a guarantee of confidentiality. To see that this is so, consider a different case. Suppose I know in advance that we will be observed during intercourse. Here there is no problem of defeated reasonable expectations. But there may be injury nonetheless. For one thing, I may be unwilling or unable to communicate an intimate fact or engage in intimate behavior in the presence of an observer. In this sense I will be quite directly prevented from going forward. For another thing, even if I do go ahead the character of the experience may very well be altered. Knowing that someone is watching or listening may render what would have been an enjoyable experience unenjoyable. Or, having someone watch or listen may so alter the character of the relationship that it is simply not the same kind of relationship it was before. The presence of the observer may make spontaneity impossible. Aware of the observer, I am engaged in part in viewing or imagining what is going on from his or her perspective. I thus cannot "lose" myself as completely in the activity.

Nor is this the only problem presented by a nondeceptive absence of privacy. Suppose that one is in a setting in which one can be certain that there will never be privacy, that virtually everything one does and virtually everything that happens to one will be recorded and known to others. Even if nothing particularly embarassing, incriminating or intimate goes on (or is apt to go on) there is, I think, something else that is troublesome and objectionable about such an environment. To begin with, it will be difficult for the individuals who are the objects of such scrutiny to continue to retain a sense of their own individuality and autonomy. Concomitantly, it will be difficult for the individuals who are conducting and maintaining the scrutiny to continue to retain a sense of the subjects as persons rather than objects.

This seems to me to be part of what is seriously wrong with the way medicine is often practiced, hospitals typically run, and patients almost always treated. Patients, and especially patients in hospitals, are observed, monitored, checked and the information

obtained thereby routinely and regularly recorded in accordance with notions of institutional regularity, thoroughness and convenience. Much if not all of the observation and the collection of information may be for the patient's welfare. And I am certainly not suggesting that any of this is done maliciously. But I do think it likely that the absence of these malevolent features tends to disarm and thereby to make the practices even more dangerous. In an environment of the sort I have described, it will, as I have suggested, be difficult for a patient to preserve his or her sense of autonomy and individuality. In this environment it will be easy for those of the institution who are not patients to see themselves as different in important respects from the patients. They are not continually under scrutiny; the patients as objects are. In such a setting, medical personnel all too often become both manipulative and paternalistic in their relationship with their patients. A lack of privacy, in this sense, is not the only reason for the dominance of these modes of interaction between the medical personnel and the patients. But it, coupled with a lack of sensitivity toward the harm that can be caused, is certainly one of the significant causes.

IV

I want to say a word, finally, about the law's special concern for the relationship between medicine and intimate kinds of things as that concern is manifested in the evidentiary privileges.

There are two distinct evidentiary privileges that relate to medicine. These two privileges—the physician-patient privilege and the psychotherapist-patient privilege—establish the right that a patient has to have kept confidential most information acquired by the doctor or psychotherapist in the course of treating the patient, even though the communication would constitute otherwise relevant evidence at a trial.

The case for the psychotherapist-patient privilege is the easier one to make out. Because of the nature of the things typically discussed in psychotherapy persons very often see themselves as rendering themselves extremely vulnerable through their revelation to another. This comes about in two ways. First, psychotherapy typically deals with many things that the patient has never disclosed to another; things of which previously he or she alone has been aware. So therapy often involves admission into what was previously the private self—the core of individuality. And second, the kinds of things revealed are often the sort that, individuals believe, would reflect badly upon them were these facts to become known to others. For psychotherapy almost always deals with the respects in which *our* person sees himself or herself as deficient. It is natural, therefore, that persons should want substantial guarantees of non-disclosure without which they would see themselves as having exposed themselves to unreasonable risk of injury from others. And it is appropriate that the law should provide those guarantees so that the processes of psychotherapy can go forward.

What is less clear and hence more instructive is why there should be a physician-patient privilege. Several alternative rationales present themselves. One is that the physician often plays the role of psychotherapist. Another is that diseases often *have* a "mental" or emotional component. Hence it is essential for the treatment of physical diseases that the physician be able to explore with the patient the related or underlying mental aspect. Both of these accounts fit comfortably into the kind of analysis already proposed, and if this were all there were to the physician-patient privilege it would not be much of a puzzle. But the privilege protects more than communications between the patient and physician about these sorts of intimate matters. It covers all of the things that the doctor discovers about the patient's body and all of the things the patient tells the doctor about his or her body. And this same concern is reflected in the sweeping language of that section of the patient's bill of rights which requires that "Case discussion, consultation, examination, and treatment are confidential and should be conducted discreetly." (The language is sweeping because it covers all case information and not just information about psychiatric or "intimate" details.)

What this reveals, I think, is that attitudes and beliefs concerning one's body, as well as one's diseases, are uncertain and varied in our culture. Much information about our bodies does not enjoy a privileged epistemic status. And much information about the physical condition of our bodies is not—it seems to me—the kind of information which is naturally seen as intimate and deserving of confidential status. Nevertheless, in our culture many persons do regard much, if

not all, information about the state of their bodies as the kind of information which ought to be kept largely under their control.

I suspect that the reasons for this are varied and deep. Some have to do with the connection between the fact that it is *our* body and our sense of ourselves as distinct individuals. For there is a long and respectable philosophical tradition which takes the body to be the individuating element in existence. Some of the reasons have to do, instead, with a rather different philosophical-religious tradition; namely, that which regards the body as the least human and most corrupt feature of human life. The body *per se* is a source of shame and evil. Clearly, then, the less said and known about it the better. And finally, there is the sense in which a diseased body is seen by many as a kind of imperfection and one which somehow reflects badly upon them. It is easy, I think, to see how natural it is to want to keep hidden imperfections and blemishes of any sort. It is not even very hard to see how the move is made from that concern to a stronger desire to keep hidden deficiencies that are in some way or other one's fault. Whether rational or not, our attitudes toward beliefs about both physical and mental disease still contain many of these features within them.

What all of this shows, in addition, is how socially contingent much, if not all, that is deemed to be intimate and private is. What the patient's bill of rights protects, what the evidentiary privileges protect, what the concern for privacy protects is information which is deemed by the culture to render the individual unusually vulnerable and exposed. It is information which if known to others, except in special contexts, is unusually capable of causing injury to the person involved. It is, I think, an important and fascinating question—but one that is beyond the scope of this paper: to ask whether there is any information that is, so to speak, intrinsically private, rather than contingently so, or to ask whether it is even socially necessary that in every culture there be some information that functions in this fashion. I think there is much that can be said on both sides of these questions. For the purposes of our inquiry, however, it is, I believe, sufficient to observe that for our culture at this time these concerns for and about privacy make very good moral sense.

The Principle of Medical Confidentiality

LeRoy Walters

LeRoy Walters is director of the Center for Bioethics, Kennedy Institute of Ethics, Georgetown University. He is also a member of Georgetown's department of philosophy. Walters is the editor of the annual *Bibliography of Bioethics* and coeditor of *Contemporary Issues in Bioethics* (2nd ed., 1982). In addition, he has published articles on topics such as fetal research, the just-war tradition, and technology assessment and genetics. Among these articles are "Technology Assessment and Genetics" and "Fetal Research and the Ethical Issues."

Walters presents (1) the philosophical arguments for the preservation of the principle of medical confidentiality and (2) the kinds of reasons that could justify violations of the principle. Walters, while insisting upon the importance of the principle, holds that the health-care professional has only a prima facie and not an absolute obligation to preserve the principle. In Walters' view, the following sorts of considerations are relevant in determining whether this prima facie obligation may be overriden in a particular case: (1) The principle may come into conflict with the rights of the patient; (2) it may conflict with the interests of an innocent third party; and (3) There may be a serious conflict between the principle and the rights of society in general.

I

...There are two primary philosophical arguments in favor of preserving medical confidentiality. The first argument is utilitarian and refers to possible long-term consequences. The second argument is non-utilitarian and speaks of respect for the rights of persons.

The utilitarian argument for the preservation of medical confidentiality is that without such confidentiality the physician-patient relationship would be seriously impaired. More specifically, the promise of confidentiality encourages the patient to make a full disclosure of his symptoms and their causes, without fearing that an embarrassing condition will become public knowledge.[1] Among medical professionals, psychotherapists have been particularly concerned to protect the confidentiality of their relationship with patients. In the words of one psychiatrist:

> The patient in analysis must learn to free associate and to break down resistances to deal with unconscious threatening thoughts and feelings. To revoke secrecy after encouraging such risk-taking is to threaten all future interactions.[2]

A second argument for the principle of medical confidentiality is that the right to a sphere of privacy is a basic human right. In what is perhaps the classic essay concerning the right of privacy, Samuel Warren and Louis Brandeis wrote in 1890 that the common law secured "to each individual the right of determining, ordinarily, to what extent his thoughts, sentiments, and emotions shall be communicated to others."[3] Present-day advocates of the right of privacy frequently employ the imagery of concentric circles or spheres. In the center is the "core self," which shelters the individual's "ultimate secrets"—"those hopes, fears, and prayers that are beyond sharing with anyone unless the individual comes under such stress that he must pour out these ultimate secrets to secure emotional release."[4] According to this image, the next largest circle contains intimate secrets which can be shared with close relatives or confessors of various kinds. Successively larger circles are open to intimate friends, to casual acquaintances, and finally to all observers.

The principle of medical confidentiality can be based squarely on this general right of privacy. The patient, in distress, shares with the physician detailed information concerning problems of body or mind. To employ the imagery of concentric circles, the patient admits the physician to an inner circle. If the physician, in turn, were to make public the information imparted by the patient— that is, if he were to invite scores or thousands of other persons into the same inner circle— we would be justified in charging that he had violated the patient's right of privacy and that he had shown disrespect to the patient as a human being.

These two arguments for the principle of medical confidentiality—the argument based on probable consequences of violation and the argument based on the right of privacy—seem to constitute a rather strong case for the principle. However, we have not yet faced the question whether the principle of confidentiality is a moral absolute, or whether it can be overridden by other considerations. . . .

II

There are, in my view, three general reasons which might conceivably justify violating the principle of confidentiality.[5] The first is that the principle may come into conflict with the rights of the patient himself. To illustrate, one can envision a situation in which a patient, in a temporary fit of depression, threatens to kill himself or herself or to perform an irrational act which will almost certainly destroy the patient's reputation. In the case of threatened suicide, one finds oneself weighing a secret vs. a life. Perhaps the physician should feel free, in such a case, to violate the principle of confidentiality and to involve a third party for the protection of the patient himself or herself.

A second possible ground for violating the principle of confidentiality is that it may conflict with the right of an innocent third party. In older textbooks of moral theology, one can discover hypothetical cases constructed to illustrate this dilemma. Often the case involves a physician and a young couple about to be married. Because of his professional relationship with the husband-to-be, the physician knows that the man is concealing a condition of infective syphilis or permanent impotence from his future wife. The question then arises whether the physician should violate the principle of confidentiality in order to warn the unsuspecting innocent party.[6]

In our own time the physician's dilemma is more likely to concern the case of a "battered child." If the abused child is brought to the physician by the battering parents, the physician faces an immediate conflict of loyalties. Does he or she owe it to his adult patients to keep confidential the fact that they have abused the child? Or, is the physician under the obligation to protect the child from further harm by disclosing the child's injuries to the proper public authorities? It should perhaps be noted in passing that most states in the United States require that the physician report child-abuse cases to the appropriate governmental agency.[7]

A third possible ground for violating the principle of confidentiality is a serious conflict between the principle and the rights or interests of society in general. The possibility of such a conflict was formally recognized in 1912, when the American Medical Association revised its code of ethics. A new clause was introduced into the confidentiality section of the code, specifically authorizing the physician to report communicable diseases, even if such reports were based on confidential information. The justification for this type of disclosure was, of course, the protection of society at large from the spread of infectious disease.[8]

At present, various states require reports of particular types of contagious disease. Almost universally, the physician is legally obligated to report cases of venereal disease to the proper government authorities. The reporting of tuberculosis is also frequently required. State provisions for protecting the confidentiality of such public health reports vary widely, with about half of the states taking measures to prevent public disclosure of the data.[9] Whenever states require physicians to report such data concerning communicable diseases, the general justification for the violation of physician-patient confidentiality is that society at large must be protected.

There is a second type of situation in which the principle of confidentiality and the public good seem to come into sharp conflict. In these cases the physician discovers a serious medical problem in a patient whose occupation makes him responsible for the lives of many other persons. Two standard examples are a railroad signalman who is discovered to be subject to attacks of epilepsy, or an airline pilot with failing eyesight. A case reported in a recent essay on medical secrecy reads as follows:

Last year, 30 people were killed when a bus driver had a heart attack and plunged his bus into the East River in New York City. The driver's physician had known about the bad heart, had cautioned him not to drive, but felt he could not report it to the company since the patient might lose his job.[10]

In cases involving such critical occupations, some would argue that the physician's duty to protect the lives of many persons overrides his obligation to observe the principle of medical confidentiality.

In the future we are likely to see vigorous battles waged over the question of medical confidentiality vs. the public good. Three examples can be briefly cited. Already one hears rhetoric which implies that genetic disorders are quasi-contagious diseases.[11] According to this viewpoint, members of future generations will be "infected" if decisive action is not taken now. Is it possible that such pressures will lead to the requirement that physicians routinely report genetic defects to public health authorities? To cite a second example, epidemiologists constantly pursue new correlations between chronic diseases and particular environmental factors or medical conditions. Their studies frequently require surveys of total populations or random samples of such populations.[12] Will the desire of patients to keep their medical records confidential and their refusal to take part in such epidemiological studies come to be seen as an anti-social act or as a failure to perform a civic duty? Third, it is at least conceivable that the concept of public health could be expanded to include "economic contamination." According to this view, any disease which prevents a person from being a fully-productive member of the labor force would be seen as a hazard to the society's overall economic health, particularly if public funds were being used to defray the expenses of the illness. Cost-benefit analysis would indicate that because of the illness, other persons in the society would need to work to subsidize the relatively-less-productive ill person. As one economist put it, well persons would become, at least partially, the "economic slaves" of the patient.[13] If the concept of public health is expanded in this economic direction, it seems likely that there will be tremendous pressure directed against maintaining the medical confidentiality of patients whose treatment is subsidized by public funds.

My own view is that the physician has a prima facie obligation to preserve the principle of medical confidentiality.[14] This obligation is based on the two considerations mentioned...above, a concern for protecting the physician-patient relationship and a desire to respect the patient's right of privacy. Thus, the burden of proof must be assumed by anyone who wishes to argue that the principle of medical confidentiality should be violated. However, there are some cases in which this prima facie obligation can be overridden because of other very weighty considerations, for example, the desire to protect the patient's own life or the lives of other persons. According to this view, then, the physician's duty to observe the principle of medical confidentiality is a very important moral obligation, but not an absolute obligation or one's only obligation....

NOTES

1 A similar line of argument was advanced in favor of testimonial privilege for physicians in *Randa v. Bear,* 50 Wash. 2d 415, 312 P. 2d 640 (1957); cited by William J. Curran and E. Donald Shapiro, *Law, Medicine, and Forensic Science* (2nd ed.; Boston: Little, Brown, 1970), p. 377.

2 Harvey L. Ruben and Diane D. Ruben, "Confidentiality and Privileged Communications: The Psychotherapeutic Relationship Revisited," *Medical Annals of the District of Columbia* 41 (6): 365, June 1972.

3 The Warren-Brandeis article appeared in the *Harvard Law Review,* vol. 4, 1890, at p. 193. This quotation is taken from Susan Beggs-Baker, *et al.,* "Individual Privacy Considerations for Computerized Health Information Systems," *Medical Care* 12 (1): 79, January 1974. For a perceptive recent treatment of the right to privacy see Charles Fried, *An Anatomy of Values: Problems of Personal and Social Choice* (Cambridge, Mass.: Harvard University Press, 1970), chap. 9. The constitutional right of privacy has recently been affirmed by the U.S. Supreme Court in the cases *Griswold v. Connecticut* [381 U.S. 479, 85 S. Ct. 1678 (1965)] and *Katz v. United States* [389 U.S. 347, 88 S. Ct. 507 (1967)].

4 Alan F. Westin, *Privacy and Freedom* (New York: Atheneum, 1967), p. 33.

5 The following analysis parallels, in part, Robert E. Regan's discussion of "various conflicts between the duty of medical secrecy and other rights and duties" in *Professional Secrecy in the Light of Moral Principles: with an Application to Several Important Professions* (Washington, D.C.: Augustinian Press, 1943), pp. 138–148.

6 This illustration is drawn from Regan, *Professional Secrecy,* pp. 143–147.

7 Dennis Helfman, *et al.,* "Access to Medical Records," in the *Appendix* to U.S. Department of Health, Education and Welfare, *Report of the Secretary's Commission on Medical Malpractice* (Washington, D.C.: U.S. Government Printing Office, 1973), pp. 180–181.

8 Regan, *Professional Secrecy,* p. 116. A similar, although more general, exception to the confidentiality obligation is included in the current AMA "Principles of Medical Ethics," (Judicial Council, *Opinions and Reports,* p. vii).

9 Helfman, *et al.,* "Access to Medical Records," p. 181. State laws requiring that cases of drug addiction be reported would be justified by means of analogous arguments *(ibid).*

10 Henry A. Davidson, "Professional Secrecy," in E. Fuller Torrey, ed., *Ethical Issues in Medicine: The Role of the Physician in Today's Society* (Boston: Little, Brown, 1968), p. 194.

11 See for example, Amitai Etzioni, *Genetic Fix* (New York: Macmillan, 1973), especially chap. 4.

12 Great Britain, Medical Research Council, "Responsibility in the Use of Medical Information for Research," *British Medical Journal* 1 (5847): 213–216, 27 January 1973.

13 See the comments of the economist Lester Thurow on a related issue in Betty Cochran, "Conference Report: Conception, Coercion, and Control," *Hospital and Community Psychiatry* 25 (5), 287, May 1974.

14 William Frankena, *Ethics* (2nd ed.; Englewood Cliffs, N.J.: Prentice-Hall, 1973), pp. 26–28.

Majority Opinion in *Tarasoff v. Regents of the University of California*

Justice Mathew O. Tobriner

Mathew O. Tobriner is an associate justice of the Supreme Court of California. Prior to his appointment to the Supreme Court of California, Justice Tobriner served as a judge in the District Court of Appeals, 1st District of California (1959–1962) and as a professor at the Hastings Law School (1958–59). Justice Tobriner contributes to legal journals.

Tatiana Tarasoff was murdered by Prosenjit Poddar, who was a patient of psychotherapists employed by the University of California Hospital. Her parents brought an action against the university regents, doctors, and campus police. The Tarasoffs complained that the doctors and police had failed to warn them that their daughter was in danger from Poddar. In finding for the Tarasoffs, Justice Tobriner argues that a doctor or psychotherapist treating a mentally ill patient has a duty to warn third parties of threatened dangers arising out of the patient's violent intentions. Responding to the defendants' appeal to the important role played by the principle of confidentiality in the psychotherapeutic situation, Tobriner argues that the public interest in safety from violent assault must be weighed against the patient's right to privacy.

On October 27, 1969, Prosenjit Poddar killed Tatiana Tarasoff. Plaintiffs, Tatiana's parents, allege that two months earlier Poddar confided his intention to kill Tatiana to Dr. Lawrence Moore, a psychologist employed by the Cowell Memorial Hospital at the University of California at Berkeley. They allege that on Moore's request, the campus police briefly detained Poddar, but released him when he appeared rational.

California Supreme Court; July 1, 1976. 131 California Reporter 14. Reprinted with permission of West Publishing Co.

They further claim that Dr. Harvey Powelson, Moore's superior, then directed that no further action be taken to detain Poddar. No one warned plaintiffs of Tatiana's peril....

We shall explain that defendant therapists cannot escape liability merely because Tatiana herself was not their patient. When a therapist determines, or pursuant to the standards of his profession should determine, that his patient presents a serious danger of violence to another, he incurs an obligation to use reasonable care to protect the intended victim against such danger. The discharge of this duty may require the therapist to take one or more of various steps, depending upon the nature of the case. Thus it may call for him to warn the intended victim or others likely to apprise the victim of the danger, to notify the police, or to take whatever other steps are reasonably necessary under the circumstances....

PLAINTIFFS' COMPLAINTS

...Plaintiffs' first cause of action, entitled "Failure to Detain a Dangerous Patient," alleges that on August 20, 1969, Poddar was a voluntary outpatient receiving therapy at Cowell Memorial Hospital. Poddar informed Moore, his therapist, that he was going to kill an unnamed girl, readily identifiable as Tatiana, when she returned home from spending the summer in Brazil. Moore, with the concurrence of Dr. Gold, who had initially examined Poddar, and Dr. Yandell, assistant to the director of the department of psychiatry, decided that Poddar should be committed for observation in a mental hospital. Moore orally notified Officers Atkinson and Teel of the campus police that he would request commitment. He then sent a letter to Police Chief William Beall requesting the assistance of the police department in securing Poddar's confinement.

Officers Atkinson, Brownrigg, and Halleran took Poddar into custody, but, satisfied that Poddar was rational, released him on his promise to stay away from Tatiana. Powelson, director of the department of psychiatry at Cowell Memorial Hospital, then asked the police to return Moore's letter, directed that all copies of the letter and notes that Moore had taken as therapist be destroyed, and "ordered no action to place Prosenjit Poddar in 72-hour treatment and evaluation facility."

Plaintiffs' second cause of action, entitled "Failure to Warn on a Dangerous Patient," incorporates the allegations of the first cause of action, but adds the assertion that defendants negligently permitted Poddar to be released from police custody without "notifying the parents of Tatiana Tarasoff that their daughter was in grave danger from Prosenjit Poddar." Poddar persuaded Tatiana's brother to share an apartment with him near Tatiana's residence; shortly after her return from Brazil, Poddar went to her residence and killed her.

Plaintiffs' third cause of action, entitled "Abandonment of a Dangerous Patient," seeks $10,000 punitive damages against defendant Powelson. Incorporating the crucial allegations of the first cause of action, plaintiffs charge that Powelson "did the things herein alleged with intent to abandon a dangerous patient, and said acts were done maliciously and oppressively."

Plaintiffs' fourth cause of action, for "Breach of Primary Duty to Patient and the Public," states essentially the same allegations as the first cause of action, but seeks to characterize defendants' conduct as a breach of duty to safeguard their patient and the public. Since such conclusory labels add nothing to the factual allegations of the complaint, the first and fourth causes of action are legally indistinguishable....

...We direct our attention...to the issue of whether plaintiffs' second cause of action can be amended to state a basis for recovery.

PLAINTIFFS CAN STATE A CAUSE OF ACTION AGAINST DEFENDANT THERAPISTS FOR NEGLIGENT FAILURE TO PROTECT TATIANA

The second cause of action can be amended to allege that Tatiana's death proximately resulted from defendants' negligent failure to warn Tatiana or others likely to apprise her of her danger. Plaintiffs contend that as amended, such allegations of negligence and proximate causation, with resulting damages, establish a cause of action. Defendants, however, contend that in the circumstances of the present case they owed no duty of care to Tatiana or her parents and that, in the absence of such duty, they were free to act in careless disregard of Tatiana's life and safety.

In analyzing this issue, we bear in mind that legal duties are not discoverable facts of nature, but merely conclusory expressions that, in cases of a particular type, liability should be imposed for damage done. "The assertion that liability must...be denied because defendant bears no 'duty' to plaintiff 'begs the essential question—whether the plaintiff's interests are entitled to legal protection against the defendant's conduct.-...[Duty] is not sacrosanct in itself, but only an expression of the sum total of those considerations of policy which lead the law to say that the particular plaintiff is entitled to protection.'"

In the landmark case of *Rowland v. Christian* (1968), Justice Peters recognized that liability should be imposed "for an injury occasioned to another by his want of ordinary care or skill" as expressed in section 1714 of the Civil Code. Thus, Justice Peters, quoting from *Heaven v. Pender* (1883) stated:"'Whenever one person is by circumstances placed in such a position with regard to another...that if he did not use ordinary care and skill in his own conduct...he would cause danger of injury to the person or property of the other, a duty arises to use ordinary care and skill to avoid such danger.'"

We depart from "this fundamental principle" only upon the "balancing of a number of considerations"; major ones "are the foreseeability of harm to the plaintiff, the degree of certainty that the plaintiff suffered injury, the closeness of the connection between the defendant's conduct and the injury suffered, the moral blame attached to the defendant's conduct, the policy of preventing future harm, the extent of the burden to the defendant and consequences to the community of imposing a duty to exercise care with resulting liability for breach, and the availability, cost and prevalence of insurance for the risk involved."

The most important of these considerations in establishing duty is foreseeability. As a general principle, a "defendant owes a duty of care to all persons who are foreseeably endangered by his conduct, with respect to all risks which make the conduct unreasonably dangerous." As we shall explain, however, when the avoidance of foreseeable harm requires a defendant to control the conduct of another person, or to warn of such conduct, the common law has traditionally imposed liability only if the defendant bears some special relationship to the dangerous person or to the potential victim. Since the relationship between a therapist and his patient satisfies this requirement, we need not here decide whether foreseeability alone is sufficient to create a duty to exercise reasonable care to protect a potential victim of another's conduct.

Although, as we have stated above, under the common law, as a general rule, one person owed no duty to control the conduct of another nor to warn those endangered by such conduct, the courts have carved out an exception to this rule in cases in which the defendant stands in some special relationship to either the person whose conduct needs to be controlled or in a relationship to the foreseeable victim of that conduct. Applying this exception to the present case, we note that a relationship of defendant therapists to either Tatiana or Poddar will suffice to establish a duty of care; as explained in section 315 of the Restatement Second of Torts, a duty of care may arise from either "(a) a special relation...between the actor and the third person which imposes a duty upon the actor to control the third person's conduct, or (b) a special relation...between the actor and the other which gives to the other a right of protection."

Although plaintiffs' pleadings assert no special relation between Tatiana and defendant therapists, they establish as between Poddar and defendant therapists the special relation that arises between a patient and his doctor or psychotherapist. Such a relationship may support affirmative duties for the benefit of third persons. Thus, for example, a hospital must exercise reasonable care to control the behavior of a patient which may endanger other persons. A doctor must also warn a patient if the patient's condition or medication renders certain conduct, such as driving a car, dangerous to others.

Although the California decisions that recognize this duty have involved cases in which the defendant stood in a special relationship *both* to the victim and to the person whose conduct created the danger, we do not think that the duty should logically be constricted to such situations. Decisions of other jurisdictions hold that the single relationship of a doctor to his patient is sufficient to support the duty to exercise reasonable care to protect others against dangers emanating from the patient's illness. The courts hold that a doctor is liable to persons infected by his patient if he negligently fails to diagnose a contagious disease, or having diagnosed the illness, fails to warn members of the patient's family.

Since it involved a dangerous mental patient, the decision in *Merchants Nat. Bank & Trust Co. of Fargo v. United States* (1967) comes closer to the issue. The Veterans Administration arranged for the patient to work on a local farm, but did not inform the farmer of the man's background. The farmer consequently permitted the patient to come and go freely during nonworking hours; the patient borrowed a car, drove to his wife's residence and killed her. Notwithstanding the lack of any "special relationship" between the Veterans Administration and the wife, the court found the Veterans Administration liable for the wrongful death of the wife.

In their summary of the relevant rulings Fleming and Maximov conclude that the "case law should dispel any notion that to impose on the therapists a duty to take precautions for the safety of persons threatened by a patient, where due care so requires, is *not* in any way opposed to contemporary ground rules on the duty relationship. On the contrary, there now seems to be sufficient authority to support the conclusion that by entering into a doctor-patient relationship the therapist becomes sufficiently involved to assume some responsibility for the safety, not only of the patient himself, but also of any third person whom the doctor knows to be threatened by the patient." [Fleming & Maximov, *The Patient or His Victim: The Therapist's Dilemma* (1974) 62 Cal. L. Rev. 1025, 1030.]

Defendants contend, however, that imposition of a duty to exercise reasonable care to protect third persons is unworkable because therapists cannot accurately predict whether or not a patient will resort to violence. In support of this argument amicus representing the American Psychiatric Association and other professional societies cites numerous articles which indicate that therapists, in the present state of the art, are unable reliably to predict violent acts; their forecasts, amicus claims, tend consistently to overpredict violence, and indeed are more often wrong than right. Since predictions of violence are often erroneous, amicus concludes, the courts should not render rulings that predicate the liability of therapists upon the validity of such predictions.

The role of the psychiatrist, who is indeed a practitioner of medicine, and that of the psychologist who performs an allied function, are like that of the physician who must conform to the standards of the profession and who must often make diagnoses and predictions based upon such evaluations. Thus the judgment of the therapist in diagnosing emotional disorders and in predicting whether a patient presents a serious danger of violence is comparable to the judgment which doctors and professionals must regularly render under accepted rules of responsibility.

We recognize the difficulty that a therapist encounters in attempting to forecast whether a patient presents a serious danger of violence. Obviously we do not require that the therapist, in making the determination,

render a perfect performance; the therapist need only exercise "that reasonable degree of skill, knowledge, and care ordinarily possessed and exercised by members of [that professional specialty] under similar circumstances." Within the broad range of reasonable practice and treatment in which professional opinion and judgment may differ, the therapist is free to exercise his or her own best judgment without liability; proof, aided by hindsight, that he or she judged wrongly is insufficient to establish negligence.

In the instant case, however, the pleadings do not raise any question as to failure of defendant therapists to predict that Poddar presented a serious danger of violence. On the contrary, the present complaints allege that defendant therapists did in fact predict that Poddar would kill, but were negligent in failing to warn. Amicus contends, however, that even when a therapist does in fact predict that a patient poses a serious danger of violence to others, the therapist should be absolved of any responsibility for failing to act to protect the potential victim. In our view, however, once a therapist does in fact determine, or under applicable professional standards reasonably should have determined, that a patient poses a serious danger of violence to others, he bears a duty to exercise reasonable care to protect the foreseeable victim of that danger. While the discharge of this duty of due care will necessarily vary with the facts of each case, in each instance the adequacy of the therapist's conduct must be measured against the traditional negligence standard of the rendition of reasonable care under the circumstances. As explained in Fleming and Maximov, *The Patient or His Victim: The Therapist's Dilemma* (1974), "...the ultimate question of resolving the tension between the conflicting interests of patient and potential victim is one of social policy, not professional expertise....In sum, the therapist owes a legal duty not only to his patient, but also to his patient's would-be victim and is subject in both respects to scrutiny by judge and jury,"...

The risk that unnecessary warnings may be given is a reasonable price to pay for the lives of possible victims that may be saved. We would hesitate to hold that the therapist who is aware that his patient expects to attempt to assassinate the President of the United States would not be obligated to warn the authorities because the therapist cannot predict with accuracy that his patient will commit the crime.

Defendants further argue that free and open communication is essential to psychotherapy; that "unless a patient...is assured that...information [revealed by him] can and will be held in utmost confidence, he will be reluctant to make the full disclosure upon which diagnosis and treatment...depends." The giving of a warning, defendants contend, constitutes a breach of trust which entails the revelation of confidential communications.

We recognize the public interest in supporting effective treatment of mental illness and in protecting the rights of patients to privacy and the consequent public importance of safeguarding the confidential character of psychotherapeutic communication. Against this interest, however, we must weigh the public interest in safety from violent assault. The Legislature has undertaken the difficult task of balancing the countervailing concerns. In Evidence Code section 1014, it established a broad rule of privilege to protect confidential communications between patient and psychotherapist. In Evidence Code section 1024, the Legislature created a specific and limited exception to the psychotherapist-patient privilege: "There is no privilege...if the psychotherapist has reasonable cause to believe that the patient is in such mental or emotional condition as to be dangerous to himself or to the person or property of another and that disclosure of the communication is necessary to prevent the threatened danger."

We realize that the open and confidential character of psychotherapeutic dialogue encourages patients to express threats of violence, few of which are ever executed. Certainly a therapist should not be encouraged routinely to reveal such threats; such disclosures could seriously disrupt the patient's relationship with his therapist and with the persons threatened. To the contrary, the therapist's obligations to his patient require that he not disclose a confidence unless such disclosure is necessary to avert danger to others, and

even then that he do so discreetly, and in a fashion that would preserve the privacy of his patient to the fullest extent compatible with the prevention of the threatened danger.

The revelation of a communication under the above circumstances is not a breach of trust or a violation of professional ethics; as stated in the Principles of Medical Ethics of the American Medical Association (1957), section 9: "A physician may not reveal the confidence entrusted to him in the course of medical attendance...*unless he is required to do so by law or unless it becomes necessary in order to protect the welfare of the individual or of the community.*" (Emphasis added.) We conclude that the public policy favoring protection of the confidential character of patient-psychotherapist communications must yield to the extent to which disclosure is essential to avert danger to others. The protective privilege ends where the public peril begins.

Our current crowded and computerized society compels the interdependence of its members. In this risk-infested society we can hardly tolerate the further exposure to danger that would result from a concealed knowledge of the therapist that his patient was lethal. If the exercise of reasonable care to protect the threatened victim requires the therapist to warn the endangered party or those who can reasonably be expected to notify him, we see no sufficient societal interest that would protect and justify concealment. The containment of such risks lies in the public interest. For the foregoing reasons, we find that plaintiffs' complaints can be amended to state a cause of action against defendants Moore, Powelson, Gold, and Yandell and against the Regents as their employer, for breach of a duty to exercise reasonable care to protect Tatiana....

Dissenting Opinion in *Tarasoff v. Regents of the University of California*

William P. Clark

William P. Clark, who began practicing law in 1958, served as associate justice of the Supreme Court of California from 1973 to 1981. Subsequently, he was assistant to the president of the United States for national security.

California Supreme Court; July 1, 1976. 131 California Reporter 14. Reprinted with permission of West Publishing Co.

Justice Clark, dissenting from Justice Tobriner's majority opinion, argues that confidentiality in the psychiatrist-patient relationship must be assured for three reasons. (1) Without the promise of such confidentiality, people needing treatment will be deterred from seeking it. (2) Effective therapy requires the patient's full disclosure of his or her innermost thoughts. Without the assurance that the thoughts disclosed will not be revealed by the therapist, the patient could not overcome the psychological barriers standing in the way of such revelations. (3) Successful treatment itself requires a relationship of trust between psychiatrist and patient. In light of these three reasons, Clark argues that if a duty to warn is imposed on psychiatrists, the result will be an increase in violent acts by persons who either don't seek help or whose therapy is unsuccessful. Furthermore, Clark holds, imposing such a duty on psychiatrists will result in an increase in the involuntary civil commitment of patients.

Until today's majority opinion, both legal and medical authorities have agreed that confidentiality is essential to effectively treat the mentally ill, and that imposing a duty on doctors to disclose patient threats to potential victims would greatly impair treatment. Further, recognizing that effective treatment and society's safety are necessarily intertwined, the Legislature has already decided effective and confidential treatment is preferred over imposition of a duty to warn.

The issue whether effective treatment for the mentally ill should be sacrificed to a system of warnings is, in my opinion, properly one for the Legislature, and we are bound by its judgment. Moreover, even in the absence of clear legislative direction, we must reach the same conclusion because imposing the majority's new duty is certain to result in a net increase in violence....

COMMON LAW ANALYSIS

Entirely apart from the statutory provisions, the same result must be reached upon considering both general tort principles and the public policies favoring effective treatment, reduction of violence, and justified commitment.

Generally, a person owes no duty to control the conduct of another. Exceptions are recognized only in limited situations where (1) a special relationship exists between the defendant and injured party, or (2) a special relationship exists between defendant and the active wrongdoer, imposing a duty on defendant to control the wrongdoer's conduct. The majority does not contend the first exception is appropriate to this case.

Policy generally determines duty. Principal policy considerations include foreseeability of harm, certainty of the plaintiff's injury, proximity of the defendant's conduct to the plaintiff's injury, moral blame attributable to defendant's conduct, prevention of future harm, burden on the defendant, and consequences to the community.

Overwhelming policy considerations weigh against imposing a duty on psychotherapists to warn a potential victim against harm. While offering virtually no benefit to society, such a duty will frustrate psychiatric treatment, invade fundamental patient rights and increase violence.

The importance of psychiatric treatment and its need for confidentiality have been recognized by this court. "It is clearly recognized that the very practice of psychiatry vitally depends upon the reputation in the community that the psychiatrist will not tell." [Slovenko, *Psychiatry and a Second Look at the Medical Privilege* (1960) 6 Wayne L. Rev. 175, 188.]

Assurance of confidentiality is important for three reasons.

Deterrence from Treatment

First, without substantial assurance of confidentiality, those requiring treatment will be deterred from seeking assistance. It remains an unfortunate fact in our society that people seeking psychiatric guidance tend to become stigmatized. Apprehension of such stigma—apparently increased by the propensity of people considering treatment to see themselves in the worst possible light—creates a well-recognized reluctance to seek aid. This reluctance is alleviated by the psychiatrist's assurance of confidentiality.

Full Disclosure

Second, the guarantee of confidentiality is essential in eliciting the full disclosure necessary for effective treatment. The psychiatric patient approaches treatment with conscious and unconscious inhibitions against revealing his innermost thoughts. "Every person, however well-motivated, has to overcome resistances to therapeutic exploration. These resistances seek support from every possible source and the possibility of disclosure would easily be employed in the service of resistance." (Goldstein & Katz, *Psychiatrist-Patient Privilege: The GAP Proposal and the Connecticut Statute,* 36 Conn. Bar J., 175, 179; see also, 118 Am. J. Psych. 734, 735.) Until a patient can trust his psychiatrist not to violate their confidential relationship, "the unconscious psychological control mechanism of repression will prevent the recall of past experiences." [Butler, *Psychotherapy and Griswold: Is Confidentiality a Privilege or a Right?* (1971) 3 Conn. L. Rev. 599, 604.]

Successful Treatment

Third, even if the patient fully discloses his thoughts, assurance that the confidential relationship will not be breached is necessary to maintain his trust in his psychiatrist—the very means by which treatment is effected. "[T]he essence of much psychotherapy is the contribution of trust in the external world and ultimately in the self, modelled upon the trusting relationship established during therapy" (Dawidoff, *The Malpractice of Psychiatrists,* 1966 Duke L. J. 696, 704.) Patients will be helped only if they can form a trusting relationship with the psychiatrist. All authorities appear to agree that if the trust relationship cannot be developed because of collusive communication between the psychiatrist and others, treatment will be frustrated.

Given the importance of confidentiality to the practice of psychiatry, it becomes clear the duty to warn imposed by the majority will cripple the use and effectiveness of psychiatry. Many people, potentially violent—yet susceptible to treatment—will be deterred from seeking it; those seeking it will be inhibited from making revelations necessary to effective treatment; and, forcing the psychiatrist to violate the patient's trust will destroy the interpersonal relationship by which treatment is effected.

VIOLENCE AND CIVIL COMMITMENT

By imposing a duty to warn, the majority contributes to the danger to society of violence by the mentally ill and greatly increases the risk of civil commitment—the total deprivation of liberty—of those who should not be confined. The impairment of treatment and risk of improper commitment resulting from the new duty to warn will not be limited to a few patients but will extend to a large number of the mentally ill. Although under existing psychiatric procedures only a relatively few receiving treatment will ever present a risk of violence, the number making threats is huge, and it is the latter group—not just the former—whose treatment will be impaired and whose risk of commitment will be increased.

Both the legal and psychiatric communities recognize that the process of determining potential violence in a patient is far from exact, being fraught with complexity and uncertainty.[1]

In fact precision has not even been attained in predicting who of those having already committed violent acts will again become violent, a task recognized to be of much simpler proportions.

This predictive uncertainty means that the number of disclosures will necessarily be large. As noted above, psychiatric patients are encouraged to discuss all thoughts of violence, and they often express such thoughts. However, unlike this court, the psychiatrist does not enjoy the benefit of overwhelming hindsight in seeing which few, if any, of his patients will ultimately become violent. Now, confronted by the majority's new duty, the psychiatrist must instantaneously calculate potential violence from each patient on each visit. The difficulties researchers have encountered in accurately predicting violence will be heightened for the practicing psychiatrist dealing for brief periods in his office with heretofore nonviolent patients. And, given the decision not to warn or commit must always be made at the psychiatrist's civil peril, one can expect most doubts will be resolved in favor of the psychiatrist protecting himself.

Neither alternative open to the psychiatrist seeking to protect himself is in the public interest. The warning itself is an impairment of the psychiatrist's ability to treat, depriving many patients of adequate treatment. It is to be expected that after disclosing their threats, a significant number of patients, who would not become violent if treated according to existing practices, will engage in violent conduct as a result of unsuccessful treatment. In short, the majority's duty to warn will not only impair treatment of many who would never become violent but worse, will result in a net increase in violence.[2]

The second alternative open to the psychiatrist is to commit his patient rather than to warn. Even in the absence of threat of civil liability, the doubts of psychiatrists as to the seriousness of patient threats have led psychiatrists to overcommit to mental institutions. This overcommitment has been authoritatively documented in both legal and psychiatric studies. This practice is so prevalent that it has been estimated that "as many as twenty harmless persons are incarcerated for every one who will commit a violent act." [Steadman & Cocozza, *Stimulus/Response: We Can't Predict Who Is Dangerous* (Jan. 1975) 8 Psych. Today 32, 35.]

Given the incentive to commit created by the majority's duty, this already serious situation will be worsened....

NOTES

1 A shocking illustration of psychotherapists' inability to predict dangerousness...is cited and discussed in Ennis, *Prisoners of Psychiatry: Mental Patients, Psychiatrists, and the Law* (1972): "In a well-known study, psychiatrists predicted that 989 persons were so dangerous that they could not be kept even in civil mental hospitals, but would have to be kept in maximum security hospitals run by the Department of Corrections. Then, because of a United States Supreme Court decision, those persons were transferred to civil hospitals. After a year, the Department of Mental Hygiene reported that one-fifth of them had been discharged to the community, and over half had agreed to remain as voluntary patients. During the year, only 7 of the 989 committed or threatened any act that was sufficiently dangerous to require retransfer to the maximum security hospital. Seven correct predictions out of almost a thousand is not a very impressive record.

"Other studies, and there are many, have reached the same conclusion: psychiatrists simply cannot predict dangerous behavior." (*Id.* at p. 227).

2 The majority concedes that psychotherapeutic dialogue often results in the patient expressing threats of violence that are rarely executed. The practical problem, of course, lies in ascertaining which threats from which patients will be carried out. As to this problem, the majority is silent. They do, however, caution that the therapist certainly "should not be

encouraged routinely to reveal such threats; such disclosures could seriously disrupt the patient's relationships with his therapist and with the persons threatened."

Thus, in effect, the majority informs the therapists that they must accurately predict dangerousness—a task recognized as extremely difficult—or face crushing civil liability. The majority's reliance on the traditional standard of care for professionals that "therapist need only exercise 'that reasonable degree of skill, knowledge, and care ordinarily possessed and exercised by members of [that professional specialty] under similar circumstances'" is seriously misplaced. This standard of care assumes that, to a large extent, the subject matter of the specialty is ascertainable. One clearly ascertainable element in the psychiatric field is that the therapist cannot accurately predict dangerousness, which, in turn, means that the standard is inappropriate for lack of a relevant criterion by which to judge the therapist's decision. The inappropriateness of the standard the majority would have us use is made patent when consideration is given to studies, by several eminent authorities, indicating that "[t]he chances of a second psychiatrist agreeing with the diagnosis of a first psychiatrist 'are barely better than 50–50; or stated differently, there is about as much chance that a different expert would come to some different conclusion as there is that the other would agree.'" (Ennis & Litwack, *Psychiatry and the Presumption of Expertise: Flipping Coins in the Courtroom,* 62 Cal. L. Rev. 693, 701, quoting Ziskin, Coping with Psychiatric and Psychological Testimony, 126.) The majority's attempt to apply a normative scheme to a profession which must be concerned with problems that balk at standardization is clearly erroneous.

In any event, an ascertainable standard would not serve to limit psychiatrist disclosure of threats with the resulting impairment of treatment. However compassionate, the psychiatrist hearing the threat remains faced with potential crushing civil liability for a mistaken evaluation of his patient and will be forced to resolve even the slightest doubt in favor of disclosure or commitment.

Confidentiality in Medicine—A Decrepit Concept

Mark Siegler

Mark Siegler is associate professor of medicine, Pritzker School of Medicine, University of Chicago and the director of the Center for Clinical Ethics at the university. His numerous published articles in biomedical ethics include "A Physician's Perspective on a Right to Health Care" and "Therapeutic Research Protocol: Should Patients Pay?"

Siegler argues that hospital medicine, the rise of health-care teams, the existence of third-party insurance programs, and the expanding limits of medicine will necessarily have to modify our traditional understanding of medical confidentiality. He identifies two functions of confidentiality in medicine: (1) respect for the patient's sense of individuality and privacy and (2) the improvement of the patient's health care, which requires a bond of trust between the health professional and the patient. Siegler then proposes possible solutions to the problems raised by the developments in medical care cited above. He concludes by criticizing those violations of a patient's right of privacy that are due to careless indiscretion on the part of professionals.

Medical confidentiality, as it has traditionally been understood by patients and doctors, no longer exists. This ancient medical principle, which has been included in every physician's oath and code of ethics since Hippocratic times, has become old, worn-out, and useless; it is a decrepit concept. Efforts to preserve it appear doomed to failure and often give rise to more problems than solutions. Psychiatrists have tacitly acknowledged the impossibility of ensuring the confidentiality of medical records by choosing to establish a separate, more secret record. The following case illustrates how the confidentiality principle is compromised systematically in the course of routine medical care.

A patient of mine with mild chronic obstructive pulmonary disease was transferred from the surgical intensive-care unit to a surgical nursing floor two days after an elective cholecystectomy. On the day of transfer, the patient saw a respiratory therapist writing in his medical chart (the therapist was recording the results of an arterial blood gas analysis) and became concerned about the confidentiality of his hospital records. The patient threatened to leave the hospital prematurely unless I could guarantee that the confidentiality of his hospital record would be respected.

This patient's complaint prompted me to enumerate the number of persons who had both access to his hospital record and a reason to examine it. I was amazed to learn that at least 25 and possibly as many as 100 health professionals and administrative personnel at our university hospital had access to the patient's record and that all of them had a legitimate need, indeed a professional responsibility, to open and use that chart. These persons included 6 attending physicians (the primary physician, the surgeon, the pulmonary consultant, and others); 12 house officers (medical, surgical, intensive-care unit, and "covering" house staff); 20 nursing personnel (on three shifts); 6 respiratory therapists; 3 nutritionists; 2 clinical pharmacists; 15 students (from medicine, nursing, respiratory therapy, and clinical pharmacy); 4 unit secretaries; 4 hospital financial officers; and 4 chart reviewers (utilization review, quality assurance review, tissue review, and insurance auditor). It is of interest that this patient's problem was straightforward, and he therefore did not

Reprinted by permission of the *New England Journal of Medicine.* Vol. 307, pp. 1518-1521; 1982.

require many other technical and support services that need multiple consultants and fellows, such specialized procedures as dialysis, or social workers, chaplains, the modern hospital provides. For example, he did not physical therapists, occupational therapists, and the like.

Upon completing my survey I reported to the patient that I estimated that at least 75 health professionals and hospital personnel had access to his medical record. I suggested to the patient that these people were all involved in providing or supporting his health-care services. They were, I assured him, working for him. Despite my reassurances the patient was obviously distressed and retorted, "I always believed that medical confidentiality was a part of a doctor's code of ethics. Perhaps you should tell me just what you people mean by 'confidentiality'!"

TWO ASPECTS OF MEDICAL CONFIDENTIALITY

Confidentiality and Third-Party Interests

Previous discussions of medical confidentiality usually have focused on the tension between a physician's responsibility to keep information divulged by patients secret and a physician's legal and moral duty, on occasion, to reveal such confidences to third parties, such as families, employers, public-health authorities, or police authorities. In all these instances, the central question relates to the stringency of the physician's obligation to maintain patient confidentiality when the health, well-being, and safety of identifiable others or of society in general would be threatened by a failure to reveal information about the patient. The tension in such cases is between the good of the patient and the good of others.

Confidentiality and the Patient's Interest

As the example above illustrates, further challenges to confidentiality arise because the patient's personal interest in maintaining confidentiality comes into conflict with his personal interest in receiving the best possible health care. Modern high-technology health care is available principally in hospitals (often, teaching hospitals), requires many trained and specialized workers (a "health-care team"), and is very costly. The existence of such teams means that information that previously had been held in confidence by an individual

physician will now necessarily be disseminated to many members of the team. Furthermore, since health-care teams are expensive and few patients can afford to pay such costs directly, it becomes essential to grant access to the patient's medical record to persons who are responsible for obtaining third-party payment. These persons include chart reviewers, financial officers, insurance auditors, and quality-of-care assessors. Finally, as medicine expands from a narrow, disease-based model to a model that encompasses psychological, social, and economic problems, not only will the size of the health-care team and medical costs increase, but more sensitive information (such as one's personal habits and financial condition) will now be included in the medical record and will no longer be confidential.

The point I wish to establish is that hospital medicine, the rise of health-care teams, the existence of third-party insurance programs, and the expanding limits of medicine all appear to be responses to the wishes of people for better and more comprehensive medical care. But each of these developments necessarily modifies our traditional understanding of medical confidentiality.

THE ROLE OF CONFIDENTIALITY IN MEDICINE

Confidentiality serves a dual purpose in medicine. In the first place, it acknowledges respect for the patient's sense of individuality and privacy. The patient's most personal physical and psychological secrets are kept confidential in order to decrease a sense of shame and vulnerability. Secondly, confidentiality is important in improving the patient's health care—a basic goal of medicine. The promise of confidentiality permits people to trust (i.e., have confidence) that information revealed to a physician in the course of a medical encounter will not be disseminated further. In this way patients are encouraged to communicate honestly and forthrightly with their doctors. This bond of trust between patient and doctor is vitally important both in the diagnostic process (which relies on an accurate history) and subsequently in the treatment phase, which often depends as much on the patient's trust in the physician as it does on medications and surgery. These two important functions of confidentiality are as important now as they were in the past. They will not be supplanted entirely either by improvements in medical technology or by recent changes in relations between some patients and doctors toward a rights-based, consumerist model.

POSSIBLE SOLUTIONS TO THE CONFIDENTIALITY PROBLEM

First of all, in all nonbureaucratic, noninstitutional medical encounters—that is, in the millions of doctor-patient encounters that take place in physicians' offices, where more privacy can be preserved—meticulous care should be taken to guarantee that patients' medical and personal information will be kept confidential.

Secondly, in such settings as hospitals or large-scale group practices, where many persons have opportunities to examine the medical record, we should aim to provide access only to those who have "a need to know." This could be accomplished through such administrative changes as dividing the entire record into several sections—for example, a medical and financial section—and permitting only health professionals access to the medical information.

The approach favored by many psychiatrists—that of keeping a psychiatric record separate from the general medical record—is an understandable strategy but one that is not entirely satisfactory and that should not be generalized. The keeping of separate psychiatric records implies that psychiatry and medicine are different undertakings and thus drives deeper the wedge between them and between physical and psychological illness. Furthermore, it is often vitally important for internists or surgeons to know that a patient is being seen by a psychiatrist or is taking a particular medication. When separate records are kept, this information may not be available. Finally, if generalized, the practice of keeping a separate psychiatric record could lead to the unacceptable consequence of having a separate record for each type of medical problem.

Patients should be informed about what is meant by "medical confidentiality." We should establish the distinction between information about the patient that generally will be kept confidential regardless of the interest of third parties and information that will be exchanged among members of the health-care team in order to provide care for the patient. Patients should be made aware of the large number of persons in the modern hospital who require access to the medical record in order to serve the patient's medical and financial interests.

Finally, at some point most patients should have an opportunity to review their medical record and to make informed choices about whether their entire record is to be available to everyone or whether certain portions of the record are privileged and should be accessible only to their principal physician or to others designated explicitly by the patient. This approach would rely on traditional informed-consent procedural standards and might permit the patient to balance the personal value of medical confidentiality against the personal value of high-technology, team health care. There is no reason that the same procedure should not be used with psychiatric records instead of the arbitrary system now employed, in which everything related to psychiatry is kept secret.

AFTERTHOUGHT: CONFIDENTIALITY AND INDISCRETION

There is one additional aspect of confidentiality that is rarely included in discussions of the subject. I am referring here to the wanton, often inadvertent, but avoidable exchanges of confidential information that occur frequently in hospital rooms, elevators, cafeterias, doctors' offices, and at cocktail parties. Of course, as more people have access to medical information about the patient the potential for this irresponsible abuse of confidentiality increases geometrically.

Such mundane breaches of confidentiality are probably of greater concern to most patients than the broader issue of whether their medical records may be entered into a computerized data bank or whether a respiratory therapist is reviewing the results of an arterial blood gas determination. Somehow, privacy is violated and a sense of shame is heightened when intimate secrets are revealed to people one knows or is close to—friends, neighbors, acquaintances, or hospital roommates—rather than when they are disclosed to an anonymous bureaucrat sitting at a computer terminal in a distant city or to a health professional who is acting in an official capacity.

I suspect that the principles of medical confidentiality, particularly those reflected in most medical codes of ethics, were designed principally to prevent just this sort of embarrassing personal indiscretion rather than to maintain (for social, political, or economic reasons) the absolute secrecy of doctor-patient communications. In this regard, it is worth noting that Percival's Code of Medical Ethics (1803) includes the following admonition: "Patients should be interrogated concerning their complaint in a tone of voice which cannot be overheard."[1] We in the medical profession frequently neglect these simple courtesies.

CONCLUSION

The principle of medical confidentiality described in medical codes of ethics and still believed in by patients no longer exists. In this respect, it is a decrepit concept. Rather than perpetuate the myth of confidentiality and invest energy vainly to preserve it, the public and the profession would be better served if they devoted their attention to determining which aspects of the original principle of confidentiality are worth retaining. Efforts could then be directed to salvaging those.[2]

NOTES

1 Leake, C. D., ed., *Percival's medical ethics.* Baltimore, Williams & Wilkins, 1927.

2 Supported by a grant (OSS-8018097) from the National Science Foundation and by the National Endowment for the Humanities. The views expressed are those of the author and do not necessarily reflect those of the National Science Foundation or the National Endowment for the Humanities.

Nursing Homes and the Rights of Geriatric Patients

The Geriatric Patient: Ethical Issues in Care and Treatment

Ruth Macklin

Ruth Macklin teaches bioethics at the Albert Einstein College of Medicine, Bronx, New York. She is the author of *Man, Mind and Morality: The Ethics of Behavior Control* (1981) and coeditor of *Mental Retardation and Sterilization* (1981), *Violence and the Politics of Research* (1981), and *Moral Problems in Medicine* (2nd ed., 1983). Macklin has also published numerous articles on biomedical ethics.

Macklin is concerned with two questions: Are there special ethical problems that arise in caring for elderly patients? Are there special ethical problems that arise in caring for them in an extended-care facility? In exploring these questions, she (1) discusses the complexity of making judgments about the competency of the elderly, (2) examines possible ways of testing competency, and (3) brings out some of the assumptions underlying judgments of diminished capacity in the elderly. Macklin concludes by raising questions about the paternalistic control exercised in extended-care facilities for the elderly and suggests the need for appropriate changes.

In any discussion about medical ethics, it is always fair to ask whether the ethical issues that arise in a particular setting or regarding a particular patient population are unique to that setting or population, or whether the same ethical concerns mark the care of patients in other facilities or from other special groups. It would be an easy, if not rather boring, exercise if we could simply transfer the moral problems and any proposed solutions to them from one setting, or one patient population, to another. Yet it would be surprising if there were no common ethical problems among different areas of medical practice. After all, medical treatment and research, nursing services, administration of health care facilities, and other activities in the sphere of medical and health care all focus on the patient: ill, ailing, or injured people. With regard to geriatric patients, these questions need reply: Are there special ethical problems that arise in caring for elderly patients, problems that never or rarely occur in general medicine or with other special populations? Are there special ethical problems that arise in caring for such patients in an extended care facility, problems that never or rarely exist in the context of ambulatory care or short-term medical facilities?

It should come as no surprise to learn that the answers to these questions are both "yes" and "no." Similarities and differences between the situations that give rise to ethical issues in the care and treatment of geriatric patients can be found elsewhere in medicine. It is only very recently, with the rise of the medical specialty of geriatrics, that medically related ethical problems of the elderly as a special patient population have begun to receive attention. Like the typical adult patient, many elderly persons are perfectly capable of granting (or refusing) consent for medical treatment, and of making life choices following their release from the hospital. Like other special populations, most notably mental patients, those elderly who suffer from senile dementia lack the capacity to grant informed consent or to participate in decisionmaking regarding their care and treatment.

Yet in spite of these evident similarities, the elderly differ in a number of relevant respects from other patient populations. Elderly patients, as they near the end of the life span, often have a different set of values in their assessments of the quality of life than do younger persons. Furthermore, elderly persons who have begun to decline in their mental capacity nevertheless have a lifetime of experiences and accomplishments that inform their wants and perceived needs relating to medical treatment and aftercare. Since there is no expectation that they will reenter the work force, or enjoy a return to productivity, their plight differs significantly from that of other hospitalized adults who are better able to exercise their autonomy as patients. Finally, like all residents of extended care facilities, the elderly in such settings are at risk for increased dependency and other typical consequences of institutionalization.

Key concepts in bioethics include paternalism, autonomy, and informed consent. These assume special importance in the care and treatment of geriatric patients because of the prevalence of dementing illness. When elderly persons suffer slight cognitive impairment, to what extent should they be permitted (or encouraged) to make decisions regarding their own medical care and treatment, as well as other life choices? Under what conditions is it justifiable to remove from people their decisionmaking autonomy about matters affecting primarily themselves, when they have enjoyed a lifetime of such autonomy? Should a finding of incompetence in one area automatically be transferred to or assumed to exist in, any other area? (Compare competency to manage one's financial affairs, competency to make a will, and competency to grant or refuse consent for a medical procedure.) Are the considerations that might support some form of paternalism (coercing people for their own good) the same for all special populations whose competency may be in doubt, or do special considerations obtain in the case of the elderly? When elderly persons of questionable capacity disagree with what others think is best for them regarding a medical or life choice decision, how should such differences be handled? What role should other family members play in the settlement of such disagreements? This last question is of crucial importance for geriatric patients, since if they have not been declared *legally* incompetent, family members are not automatically empowered to override their relative's medical decision (for example, a refusal of amputation).

According to one recent account, "estimates are that approximately 10% of persons older than 65 years have clinically important intellectual impairment. In a survey of nursing homes published in 1978, respondents to a questionnaire reported that 50% to 75% of the residents in their facilities were intellectually impaired."[1] Another set of figures reports that "one out of every six persons over the age of 65—about 1½ million people—is at least moderately demented. Sixty to eighty percent of nursing home patients are demented."[2] These figures are roughly the same, and they suggest that the problem of senile dementia is one of considerable magnitude.

The magnitude of the problem is only one dimension that gives rise to ethical concerns. Another is the uncertainty and variability of judgments about the mental status of elderly patients. Several factors contribute to the uncertainty and variability of such judgments, and at the risk of repeating what is well known, it is worth citing a number of those factors to illustrate the complexity of the problem of making judgments of competence.

The first factor is the reversibility or irreversibility of impaired intellectual function. Obviously, it is important to assess the causes of mental impairment whenever possible, whether or not there exist clear or uncontroversial criteria for determining what a person should be permitted to do or to decide at a particular level of competence. The fact that we lack such criteria points to still another problem, to be addressed shortly. It seems clear that if impaired mental functioning can be reversed, not only should efforts be made to reverse it, but also that an ethical requirement in such situations is that any decisions about life choices affecting the elderly should be postponed if possible until mental function is restored. Although these points may seem obvious, it remains true that demands on the time and resources of personnel in a hospital or extended care facility often prevent prompt or accurate diagnoses, especially in an area of emerging medical knowledge, such as the causes of dementia. Since these causes are numerous, and include everything from depression to deficiencies in nutrients, prompt and thorough diagnostic workups are vital for the prospects of reversing mental impairment.

A fact that bears directly on the broader ethical issues in treating geriatric patients in an extended care facility is that the most common causes of *reversible* impaired intellectual function are therapeutic drug intoxication, depression, and metabolic or infectious disorders.[3] This fact suggests that adequate knowledge on the part of physicians and other health care workers, and the devotion of sufficient time and effort to make timely and accurate diagnoses, can go a long way toward reversing this unfortunate condition in many elderly patients. Especially troubling are the facts about the adverse effects of medication. "An enormous number of drugs have been implicated, including diuretics, digitalis, oral antidiabetic drugs, analgesics, anti-inflammatory agents, sedatives, and psychopharmacologic agents."[4] Add to the sheer number of drugs having this effect the further consideration that the elderly metabolize drugs differently from younger persons and that they are often being treated with multiple drugs, leading to toxicity from drug interactions, and it is not hard to conclude that a significant cause of mental impairment in elderly patients is iatrogenic.

More problematic from another standpoint are the disorders that cause *irreversible* dementia. According to a report of the National Institute on Aging Task Force, two of them—Alzheimer's disease and multi-infarct dementia—account for approximately 80 percent of the dementias of old age.[5] Unlike the reversible causes of mental impairment, which must be diagnosed

and treated promptly, but in which actions or decisions on the part of the elderly can often await their improvement, cases of irreversible mental decline pose a different set of problems. A poignant moral dilemma in such cases is when, how much, and in what manner to disclose to a patient the prognosis of the disease and the facts about impending decline. We need to develop a sensitive and humane approach both to informing Alzheimer's patients of the details and prognosis of their disease, and to working with families in preparing for the patient's decline in mental capacity—a decline that has both short-term and long-term implications for decisions and actions concerning legal, financial, and other life circumstances. The ethical questions surrounding disclosure are linked with the more general issue of paternalism toward elderly persons who are in physical and mental decline, and whose growing dependence on others demands a morally sound approach.

Another factor lending complexity to the problem of making judgments of competency in the elderly is the existence of several different tests of competency—tests that may yield conflicting results when applied to elderly persons suffering from dementia. The above-noted report mentions several tests commonly used in the mental status examination: orientation for time, place, and persons; short-term memory, arithmetic calculation; ability to name objects; comprehension of spoken and written language; ability to write a spontaneous sentence; and ability to copy simple geometric figures. The report asserts that the impression of progressively deteriorating mental function can be confirmed and documented by such tests, but that assertion may be misleading. Even if these commonly used tests succeed in confirming a supposition that a patient is undergoing progressive mental decline, they yield no clear picture of the tasks or judgments that the patient is able or unable to perform beyond those specifically measured in the tests themselves. What does a test for a patient's ability to do arithmetic calculations have to do with that patient's understanding of a proposed medical procedure for which the patient's consent is sought? What does an inability to copy simple geometric figures tell us about a person's ability to make changes in his or her will? One problematic example is that of an elderly patient suffering from senile dementia who exhibits severe impairment of short-term memory, yet scores 110 on a standard psychometric instrument for measuring IQ. When two different tests of competency yield conflicting results, which one should be selected as a measure of the patient's competency? Or do they not conflict at all because they measure discrete capacities?

The existence of multiple measures for evaluating competency is one consideration contributing to the complexity of this issue. A related but quite different issue is the value question of how strong or how weak tests of competency should be—a factor that bears directly on the ethics of paternalistic treatment of elderly persons of questionable capacity. Since these conceptual and ethical issues surrounding judgments of competency are directly related to a patient's ability to grant or refuse consent for a wide variety of biomedical interventions, as well as to engage in a number of different life tasks, it is important to look carefully at current practices and knowledge in related fields. Recent research has concentrated largely on psychiatric patients in an attempt to gain a better understanding of competency as it relates to various tasks. The trend in both law and medicine in the last few years has been toward developing a notion of variable competence, and toward selecting situation-specific criteria for judging competence, rather than viewing it as a global attribute of people.

In a recent article discussing currently used tests of competency to consent to treatment, the authors describe five basic categories into which such tests fall.[6] These are: (1) evidencing a choice; (2) "reasonable" outcome of choice; (3) choice based on "rational" reasons; (4) ability to understand; and (5) actual understanding. Noting that these categories overlap, the authors point out that the tests range from the weakest test of competency to the strongest, with the tests at the lowest level being most respectful of the autonomy of patient decisionmaking. Just which of these tests ought to be used to determine the competence of elderly patients is a question not easy to answer, and one that probably would elicit some controversy among caregivers, family members, and elderly patients themselves. These same authors argue that

the test that is actually applied combines elements of all of the tests described above. However, the circumstances in which competency becomes an issue determine which elements of which tests are stressed and which are underplayed. Although in theory competency is an independent variable that determines whether or not the patient's decision to accept or refuse treatment is to be honored, in practice it

seems to be dependent on the interplay of two other variables, the risk/benefit ratio of treatment and the valence of the patient's decision, i.e., whether he or she consents to or refuses treatment.[7]

Since questions of individual preference and personal values are often bound up in treatment refusals, it is crucial to try to assess the reasons behind an elderly person's refusal to consent. The stricter the standard of competence, in the interest of protecting patients from their own unwise decisions, the more autonomy is traded for a gain in benevolent paternalism. It is generally assumed that when elderly patients suffer diminished capacity, and thus cannot speak on their own behalf, caregivers and family have their "best interests" at heart and will act in accordance with those interests; yet the validity of this and related assumptions has yet to be adequately explored. The question of where the presumption ought to lie regarding elderly persons of questionable competence is more a matter for decision than a matter of scientific discovery of the precise attributes that constitute competency. Should the presumption lie in their ability to judge and decide for themselves, suggesting the adoption of a weak test of competency? Or should the presumption lie on the side of impaired ability to judge, suggesting the adoption of a strong test of competency? We seek to avoid erring in either of two opposite directions: being too paternalistic with the elderly, taking their dependency and "childlike" attributes as grounds for coercing them for their own good; and on the other hand, being too permissive in respecting their autonomy, thereby opening the door to self-destructive or other irresponsible acts. The one evil consists of violating the cherished value of individual freedom; the other evil is to allow harm, destruction, or even death to befall a helpless, dependent person with declining mental and physical faculties.

These ethical dilemmas point to a research agenda for studying problems of competency and informed consent in the elderly. For elderly persons of doubtful or declining competence, the following problem areas deserve further study. Current practices surrounding disclosure by physicians, other health care workers, and family members to elderly patients with declining mental functioning need to be analyzed, focusing on the values to be attained by adhering to any particular policy or practice. What are the conditions under which full and frank disclosure about a patient's condition should take place? Are there special circumstances under which information should be withheld? How can such patients be helped to prepare themselves, psychologically and emotionally, for a deterioration in their cognitive capacities? What supports can be offered to the families of patients such as those suffering from Alzheimer's disease, especially in regard to assessing the appropriate time and method of disclosure?

Further work is also called for concerning the problem of paternalism toward the elderly who suffer from growing incompetence, and of the autonomy of aging individuals to make decisions and perform tasks both related and unrelated to biomedical procedures. Where ought the presumption lie: with the elderly themselves, to demonstrate their continued competence? Or with those who challenge their competence, to show that the principle of beneficence dictates treating those with senile dementia as incompetent, and therefore no longer autonomous, agents? There is a special poignancy to the problem of the growing incompetence of elderly persons, stemming from their own awareness of that decline, and the fact that having once been normally functioning adults, they are witness to their own mental and physical deterioration and to changes in the attitudes and behavior of others toward them. Even in cases where mental functioning is clearly impaired, a morally sound approach dictates enlisting the participation of elderly patients as much as possible in decisions regarding their own care and treatment.

At the outset I mentioned the prospect of special ethical problems that arise in caring for patients in an extended care facility. Although the characteristics of "total institutions"—to use Erving Goffman's term—are by now well-known, it is worth repeating here that especially in the case of elderly persons, residents of such facilities often respond to their environment in ways that exacerbate their already declining capacities. One writer describes the situation as follows:

> Many nursing homes, geriatric wards, and mental hospitals have the characteristics of total institutions: simply by their institutional structures and expectations, they determine the behavior of their residents.... According to one description (Citrin and Dixon, 1977), a radical alteration in life-style following institutionalization, joined with increasing demands by the institution's staff and decreasing physical functioning frequently brings about socially withdrawn, confused, or disoriented behavior among the elderly. Thus (Butler 1975), substantial numbers

of patients in mental hospitals develop a chronic state of psychological dependence and deterioration. Infantilization and loss of self-image are frequently the result of institutionalization and interaction with the institution's staff....[8]

The term "infantilization" is a key one here, and serves as a reminder that the elderly in decline are not, of course, literally "infants," in spite of many behavioral similarities. The ethical problem is to determine to what extent care and treatment of the elderly who exhibit "infantile behavior" in the metaphorical sense should be treated as we deem it proper to treat infants and small children—that is, in accordance with a justifiable pattern of paternalistic control. Insofar as the institutional structure of an extended care facility deepens those problems by reinforcing the dependency and childlike behavior of its residents, it seems possible—at least in principle—to make changes in that structure, and thereby lessen the ethical problems to some extent. Let me illustrate.

I recently learned of the existence of several nursing homes in Great Britain,[9] facilities that differ markedly from those in the United States and are not typical in Britain, either. One way of describing this difference is by reference to the overworked "medical model" as compared with a "social model" for setting policies and organizing practices and social life in the institution. Whereas the typical pattern of nursing home organization is largely similar to that of a hospital, or more generally, a medical facility, these British nursing homes are organized more as a social facility. As in the typical nursing home, the residents are ill, ailing, infirm, mentally impaired, or incontinent, yet are able to perform a variety of tasks for themselves, including, for some, meal preparation. The residents are not only allowed but encouraged to make virtually every decision that affects their daily life and activity, except, of course, those requiring medical expertise. Thus they have liberty to choose the furniture in their rooms, to decide for themselves when to wake up in the morning and when to retire at night (even if they wish to stay up as late as 2 A.M.), and to make various other choices and decisions in their everyday lives. These British nursing homes thus strive to maximize the privacy, the autonomy, and the decisionmaking of their residents in an effort to create an atmosphere as similar as possible to that which the elderly persons enjoyed prior to entering. One especially striking feature is that residents are allowed to fight and squabble with one another, which enables them to vent their frustrations and emotions in ways they have experienced all their lives.

This social model has its value trade-offs, of course: what is a gain for the residents in their freedom, autonomy, and privacy amounts to a loss for staff in being able to run things as smoothly and efficiently as possible. The more choices and decisions that are left to the residents, the harder it is for staff to plan and organize the daily routine, since individual residents' wants and needs may vary substantially. It is apparently also true that the bias against paternalism is frequently difficult for the staff to accept, accustomed as they are to the norm in extended care facilities and hospitals, where the staff gives orders and constructs a regimen, and patients are expected to comply. One very positive benefit for residents of these facilities is improvement in depression, one of the most troubling and intractable characteristics of elderly persons.

If careful, empirical observation reveals that changes of this sort in the social structure of a facility for the elderly do indeed yield such benefits, then it is ethically desirable to make an effort to bring about such changes. Benefits to the residents clearly would seem to outweigh inconvenience and reduced efficiency of the staff, and although practical difficulties must always be heeded in any recommendations for change, this particular experience suggests another area for further research that might improve care and treatment of the elderly in extended care facilities.

NOTES

1 National Institute on Aging Task Force, "Senility Reconsidered: Treatment Possibilities for Mental Impairment in the Elderly," *Journal of the American Medical Association* 244 (1980): 259.

2 G. B. Kolata, "Clues to the Cause of Senile Dementia," *Science* 211 (1981): 1032.

3 National Institute on Aging Task Force, "Senility Reconsidered," pp. 259–263.

4 *Ibid.,* p. 260.

5 *Ibid.*

6 L. H. Roth, et al. "Tests of Competency to Consent to Treatment," *American Journal of Psychiatry* 134 (1977): 279–284.

7 *Ibid.,* pp. 283–284.

8 W. T. Reich, "Ethical Issues Related to Research Involving Elderly Subjects," *Gerontologist* 18 (1978): 333.

9 Presentation by Dr. Marvin Rosenberg delivered at The Hastings Center, Institute of Society, Ethics and the Life Sciences, Project on Health Policy and Geriatrics, May 13, 1981.

Needed: A Geriatric Ethic

George A. Kanoti

George A. Kanoti is professor of religious ethics at John Carroll University. His published articles include "Ethical Implications in Psychotherapy," "Psychotherapy: The Priesthood?" and "Bioethics and Patient Care."

Kanoti's article is aimed at nursing home administrators. He asks them to examine some ethical issues faced by those who care for the elderly in extended-care institutions. Calling for a geriatric ethic founded on respect for the dignity of the elderly, Kanoti identifies three major means employed by the elderly to preserve their dignity: defiance, interdependence, and serenity. He then suggests a set of principles (developed by Drew Christiansen) as a guide in developing a geriatric ethic.

The status of social attitudes in North America concerning aging and the aged can be reflected via a tale Mark Twain reportedly told on himself. He said that as a young man of 17, "I was thoroughly embarrassed by my father. I thought he was the most stupid person I knew. I was amazed," he said, "when I became 18 at how much my father had learned in a year." Our society is probably at the age of 17 years and 9 months in its attitude toward aging and the aged. It is slowly emerging from a very negative, embarrassed, and fearful attitude toward the aged and aging. Media exposure, legislative activity, and "gray" power movements are contributing to this change. And yet society has a long way to go.

No one is more conscious of these changes and the import they will have on social institutions than nursing home administrators (NHAs). They stand in a unique and difficult position during this change because the institutions they administer grew out of society's inability to cope with aging and the aged person. For many years nursing homes were regarded as depositories for the healthy, senile, ill, and dying aged person. The NHA was (and by many persons, still is) regarded as a caretaker, that is, one who watches over and takes care of the basic survival needs of the home residents until they die—usually in a relatively short time.

The gathering of so many aged persons into these facilities, however, began both to create unique problems and to raise serious questions about the care of the aged. Furthermore, these gatherings began to provide a growing body of information about the reality of the aged person and the aging process itself that destroyed many of society's myths about the aged person—myths that society created to rationalize and assuage its feelings about removing the person of 65 years and older from the social and employment world. Nursing homes revealed that not all 65-year-old persons are senile, incompetent, and incontinent. The reality is that the aged are the most heterogeneous group in our society. The elderly are less and less alike, not at all like "peas in a pod." As persons mature they tend to separate themselves from the undifferentiated mass of their peers. The elderly are at the outer limits of maturation and reveal a great diversity. Some are intensely intelligent, capable persons; some are living at the edge of a vegetative state; some are almost comatose.

ROLE IDENTIFICATION HAMPERS NHAs

The NHAs have experienced and know this, but unfortunately they are hampered because their role identification still reflects society's assumptions and fears about the aged. Society would like to forget that nursing homes exist. The following quotations from articles in *Gerontologist* point to this. Joseph Eaton, in "The Art of Aging and Dying" (June 1964, p. 94), remarked:

> Each [society] provides its people with a system of values and expectations within which they can deal with life crises in an acceptable fashion. The denial of aging, when the facts are contrary, is one way of dealing with the problem.

Barney Glaser, in "Social Loss of Aged and Dying Patients" (June 1966, p. 77), commented:

> ...geriatric patients, along with lower class patients, tend to receive the full brunt of the consequences of being a low social loss...[they are regarded as] ...socially dead, while biologically alive...death [of the aged] is often regarded as a social gain to all involved...since vital funds, medical resources and human emotions are no longer drained away for such low social value.

These social attitudes and values influence both the NHAs and the elderly who come under their care. They handicap the professional-resident relationship and, at times, even prevent any true communication. Ideally, the professional-resident relationship should be one of openness, confidence, trust, and cooperation. Too often it is guarded, mistrustful, and uncooperative. It is my belief that at the root of this communication problem rests not a technical question such as, Did I choose the right words with this new resident? or Does my application form ask the right questions? but, rather, an ethical issue, the responsibility to preserve a sense of dignity for aging persons.

This ethical issue is especially important today because of society's expectations, fears, and embarrassments about aging. These societal attitudes have produced a serious problem for the elderly person: how to live and age in dignity in a society that is in love with youth, embarrassed by age, and frightened by death. Some of the tactics developed by the society's aged to preserve their sense of dignity will not only give insight into the way the elderly view nursing homes, but will also help establish ethical guidelines that will foster effective communications between NHAs, their staffs, and the elderly. Hence, those concerned with the aging must talk of a geriatric ethic.

The best way to explore this geriatric ethic is to ask, What is dignity? Dignity can be defined as a quality of a person that other persons respond to by recognizing the knowledge, skill, or position which that person has. When individuals possess certain knowledge, skills, or position, they can act with a sense of freedom or autonomy. A dignified person has power over others which must be deferred to and recognized. An example may be helpful. When individuals attend a national convention and are present at the keynote address delivered by a renowned participant of a White House Conference on Aging, they approach the speech with expectation and respect for the comments of the "distinguished speaker." Should the listeners find themselves yawning after the first five minutes of the speech, they would try to force themselves to stay awake and would be inclined to feel guilty about missing what the speaker is saying. Most would not ask whether the speech is really good. The dignity of the speaker based on knowledge and experience forces the listeners to look within themselves rather than find the speaker responsible. They would probably ask themselves, Why am I tired? Did I miss a key point?

On the other hand, when an elderly person bores a younger person, that is just boredom. No sense of the other's dignity forces self-questioning or worries about personal loss due to inattention. At most, studied politeness is given the old person.

The degree of dignity given to persons is in proportion to the range of their power. Because aged persons' ranges of autonomy are narrowing through enforced retirement, economic reduction, loneliness, etc., the respect they receive tends to be slight.

This loss of dignity and power is sensed by the elderly and frequently experienced in a dramatic way as sorrow, depression, feelings of worthlessness. Consequently, the elderly must struggle to retain their dignity and power. They employ various tactics to shore up their dignity in the face of society's increasing indifference to them. Drew Christiansen in "Dignity in Aging" (*Hastings Report*, February 1974, p.6) indicates three major means the elderly employ to preserve their dignity: defiance, interdependence, and serenity.

ELDERLY ATTEMPT TO PRESERVE DIGNITY

Defiance does not mean resisting law or authority; rather it refers to actions persons take to keep their sense of self-respect under pressure. Since most elderly are denied the usual sources of power (and of dignity)

that bring society's respect, such as money, beauty, and position, they employ defiance under this increasing pressure to deny them dignity. Thus, defiance helps them gain from others recognition of their value as persons. The elderly frequently employ this tactic by maneuvering to retain their own decision-making power instead of relinquishing these decisions to other persons. By surprise, boldness, and even studied aloofness elderly persons handle their own decisions. A sign of defiance at times may be elderly persons' own decisions to enter a hospital or a nursing home without any succumbing to familial pressure. By deciding to move into a total care facility, these elderly persons preserve their dignity.

Interdependence is another tactic by which dignity is preserved. Some elderly use defiance and extreme independence to preserve dignity. The recluse comes to mind—the elderly person with a houseful of cats. Many elderly, however, preserve their dignity by a sense of interdependence, i.e., they do so by sharing their lives with their families or others. As long as they can give and receive something, whether it be advice (what to look for in a career choice), skills (the procedures for home canning or how to stoke a coal furnace), or services (baby-sitting grandchildren), they are dignified by a sense of interdependence. When these tasks or services are denied them, their dignity slips, and frequently the elderly move to a tactic of avoidance or extreme independence because they do not wish to be undignified by being dependent.

Other elderly persons retain their dignity, not by power, defiance, or interdependence, but by serenity. They choose to take on some task with a sense of love and certain skill. The elderly person who invariably feeds the pigeons in the town square or waters the plants in the shopping mall is using this type of tactic. Giving care and concern to this chosen task involves no great power or wealth, but an inner strength, a spirit, which can be called dignity.

In summary, dignity is a complicated social reality. It is the respect given persons for the self-direction of their lives. Respect means to give value to such persons' actions and to allow these persons to direct their lives within the limits they have set for themselves. Dignity, then, results from a relationship between a person's deliberate actions and another person's witnessing and/or experiencing these actions. Dignity cannot exist in isolation. Dignity for the aged persons demands definite responses from all persons who witness and/or experience the aged person's actions. Therefore, the most important concept about dignity is that it is a social phenomenon that is empty without witnesses and acknowledgements.

When the elderly's tactics of dignity are recognized and responded to positively, communication can take place. Any conversation or action, however, that refuses to acknowledge or resists the tactics of the elderly to preserve dignity results in destructive action, the breakdown of communication.

Society has lost its sense of responsibility to the aged, its obligation to preserve and foster their dignity. A working set of principles can redirect its sight on the sense of dignity that is all-important to the elderly and thus help open communication between NHAs and the aging. Drew Christiansen's principles are very helpful toward developing a geriatric ethic ("Dignity in Aging," p. 8, paraphrased):

1. Losses are not to be compounded. Losses, which are inevitable in old age, such as physical, mental, social losses, do not necessarily mean indignity to the elderly. For example, only when dependency becomes humiliation, does dependency become indignity. Humiliation results when losses take more from the loser than is absolutely necessary. For example, physical loss of mobility, which requires the use of a wheelchair, should not demand refusal of opportunity for interdependence, serenity, or defiance. A plant lover confined to a wheelchair

should be provided with a chair-high potting table so that the elderly gardener can still care for plants, even though he or she is no longer able to kneel to turn the soil.

2. Opportunities for the elderly to determine their own lives should be extended and expanded. The opportunity for others to decide for them, e.g., "We know best, Dad," should be reduced. Undignifying submission to another's will must be reduced.

3. No one, because of age alone, should be deprived of the right to direct those areas of responsibility he or she chooses to take on, e.g., disposition of family heirlooms.

Growing sensitivity to the ethical responsibility of each person to meet the elderly's need to preserve dignity will help establish and keep open communication with the aging. Then the NHA can even more effectively assist aged persons in their waning days to exit life with a sense of dignity. Perhaps the greatest benefit of this insistence on an ethic of dignity will come not to today's aged, but to the current middle-aged generation, for they cannot escape the reality that they too will age and that when they are the elderly, the feelings they have shown toward aging will be reflected in their children's treatment of them.

ANNOTATED BIBLIOGRAPHY: CHAPTER 3

Annas, George N.: *The Rights of Hospital Patients* (New York: Avon, 1975). This American Civil Liberties Union handbook on the rights of hospital patients is intended to be used as a guide by those who are directly affected by the problems discussed. Using a question-and-answer approach, the book provides a statement of the rights patients had under the law at the time the guidebook was written.

Aroskar, Mila: "Ethics in the Nursing Curriculum," *Nursing Outlook* 25 (April 1977), pp. 260–264. This is a report on a survey of ethics teaching in nursing schools.

Aroskar, Mila, Josephine M. Flaherty, and James M. Smith: "The Nurse and Orders Not to Resuscitate," *Hastings Center Report* 7 (August 1977), pp. 27–28. Aroskar presents a factual case study to illustrate the kinds of ethical problems faced by nurses. Flaherty and Smith discuss the moral principles involved and make recommendations concerning the correct way for nurses to act in such cases.

Ashley, JoAnn: *Hospitals, Paternalism and the Role of the Nurse* (New York: Teachers College, 1976). This book is a study of the development of nursing in the United States. Ashley gives extensive historical documentation in showing that hospitals were established by male physicians and male hospital administrators to offer nursing care provided by women. Ashley amply documents the overt and covert efforts made to deny nurses any voice or control in establishing and changing hospital policies and nursing practices.

Benjamin, Martin, and Joy Curtis: *Ethics in Nursing* (New York: Oxford University Press, 1981). The intent of this book is to give nursing students and nurses an introduction to the identification and analysis of ethical issues in nursing. The book includes a large number of actual cases, many of which are discussed in detail.

Bok, Sissela: "The Limits of Confidentiality," *Hastings Center Report* 13 (February 1983), pp. 24–31. Bok admits that there are strong reasons for maintaining confidentiality in the professional context. However, she argues, these reasons do not support practices of secrecy, which undermine and contradict that respect for persons and for human bonds that confidentiality is supposed to protect.

Corea, Gena: *The Hidden Malpractice: How American Medicine Treats Women as Patients and Health Care Professionals* (New York: Morrow, 1977). Corea discusses the inferior position held by women in the health-care hierarchy. She attempts to explain how and why women were placed in this position and describes the effect of sexist medical practices on the health of women.

Daley, Dennis W.: "*Tarasoff v. Regents of the University of California* (Cal. 528 P2nd 553) and the Psychotherapist's Duty to Warn," *San Diego Law Review* 12 (July 1975), pp. 932–951. Daley provides an analysis of the practical problems and potential consequences for psychiatry stemming from the *Tarasoff* decision. He discusses in more detail the same types of issues set forth in Justice Clark's dissenting opinion in the case, such as the difficulty of predicting violence and the importance of confidentiality in the patient-therapist relationship.

De George, Richard T.: "The Moral Responsibility of the Hospital," *The Journal of Medicine and Philosophy* 7 (1982), pp. 87–100. De George addresses the question: Can a hospital be held morally responsible? He argues that hospitals do satisfy criteria for moral responsibility and, therefore, can have moral responsibilities. De George explores the ways that moral responsibility can be intelligibly attributed to a hospital as well as how the responsibilities of the hospital, which are assumed by those within it who act for it (e.g., physicians, administrators), can be separated from the professional moral responsibilities and the personal moral responsibilities of doctors, nurses, and others working in the hospital.

Gadow, Sally: "Medicine, Ethics, and the Elderly," *Gerontologist* 20 (December 1980), pp. 680–685. Gadow presents some of the ethical problems in the medical care of the elderly and discusses a spectrum of contemporary views on aging and some relevant ethical principles. She concludes by suggesting how the ethical problems might be addressed in view of the various social/medical views on aging and different ethical principles.

May, William F.: "Who Cares for the Elderly?" *Hastings Center Report* 12 (December 1982), pp. 31–37. May discusses the various strategies adopted by Americans in caring for the elderly as well as what these strategies show about American character and ideals. Having discussed the ethics of the care-givers, he proceeds to consider the ethics and the duties of the aged care-receivers.

Muyskens, James: *Moral Problems in Nursing: A Philosophical Investigation* (Totowa, N.J.: Rowman and Littlefield, 1982). This book is written primarily for nurses and nursing students. Muyskens presents and defends a specific moral stance and discusses the moral problems faced by nurses from that stance.

Parent, W. A.: "Privacy, Morality, and the Law," *Philosophy and Public Affairs* 12 (Fall 1983), pp. 269–288. Parent's five-part article focuses on the following: (1) the definition of privacy; (2) the value of privacy; (3) the moral right to privacy; (4) criteria of wrongful invasion; and (5) the legal right to privacy.

Veatch, Robert M.: *Case Studies in Medical Ethics* (Cambridge, Mass.: Harvard University Press, 1977). Veatch offers excellent studies of cases that pose ethical dilemmas for medical professionals. He also provides a general introduction on ethical theory as well as analyses of some of the cases presented.

Chapter 4

Ethical Issues in Human Experimentation

INTRODUCTION

This chapter explores some of the ethical issues raised by biomedical experimentation (or research) using human subjects. Analyses of these issues employ some of the same ethical concepts and principles discussed in the previous two chapters. Here, too, appeal is made to the value of individual autonomy, the requirement of informed consent, and antipaternalism. In addition, other questions are raised about social justice and about the obligations that individuals have to participate as experimental subjects.

Conceptual Issues

Before examining some of the ethical issues raised by human experimentation, we should clarify the meaning of "human experimentation" (or "research using human subjects") and the distinction often made between therapeutic and nontherapeutic experimentation (or research). In the biomedical context, "therapy" ordinarily refers to a set of activities the primary purpose of which is to relieve suffering and to restore or maintain health. Such therapy takes many forms. Medical treatment, diagnosis, and even some preventative measures (e.g., vaccine injections) are all considered forms of therapy. It is important to notice that the primary aim of therapy is to benefit the recipient. By contrast, "research" or "experimentation" refers to a set of scientific activities the primary purpose of which is to develop or contribute to generalizable knowledge about the chemical, physiological, or psychological processes involved in human functioning. But it is called "human experimentation" not simply because it attempts to expand our knowledge of human functioning but because it uses human beings as subjects.

In keeping with these explications of therapy and experimentation or research a distinction is often drawn between therapeutic and nontherapeutic research. *Therapeutic research*, like all research, is said to be concerned with the acquisition of generalizable knowledge. However, in therapeutic experimentation, the patient-subjects are themselves expected to benefit medically from the new drug, vaccine, treatment, or diagnostic procedure being tried. For example, the first patients on kidney dialysis machines and the first recipients of coronary bypass surgery were participants in medical experiments. The techniques involved had never been tried on human subjects, so the use of these techniques on these patient-subjects was experimental. Furthermore, the information gained by the medical professionals furthered their research and thus contributed to generalizable knowledge. At the same time, however, the new techniques provided a form of therapy designed to alleviate the patient-subjects' own medical problems. Thus the procedures were used on the patients for their benefit, because they promised to be more effective than any other therapy available, and not simply to provide information required by the research project. By contrast, *nontherapeutic research* is said to be research whose *sole* aim is to provide information required by the researchers. Nontherapeutic research is not concerned with providing therapy for the research subjects. An example will illustrate the difference between therapeutic and nontherapeutic research projects.

In 1963 three doctors injected live cancer cells into twenty-two seriously ill and debilitated patients in the Jewish Chronic Disease Hospital in Brooklyn, New York. The purpose of the experiment was to measure the subject's ability to reject foreign cells. These subjects were selected for the experiment because of their debilitated condition. During an earlier phase of the research project, two things had been established: (1) Healthy human subjects rejected the injected substance in four to six weeks; and (2) Human subjects already ill with advanced cancer took six weeks to several months to reject it. The researchers thought it necessary to use the patients in the Jewish Chronic Disease Hospital to test the following hypothesis: The slower rejection rate of the cancer patients used in the earlier phase of the study was due to the debilitated condition that usually accompanies chronic illness and not to their cancer. Since the test used in the research project was completely unrelated to the therapeutic program of the twenty-two patients in the Jewish Chronic Disease Hospital, this research project provides a clear example of nontherapeutic research.

Nontherapeutic research, of course, is not limited to projects that involve the use of new techniques, drugs, or vaccines. Some nontherapeutic research projects are designed simply to understand normal or abnormal physiological or psychological functions. In such projects, the research subjects may be required to do little more than contribute urine or blood samples, fill out forms, or take written or oral tests.

In practice, it is difficult to draw a clear-cut line between therapeutic and nontherapeutic research projects. Therapeutic research is not conducted *solely* to benefit the patient-subjects since the purpose of all research is to contribute to generalizable knowledge. In addition, the therapeutic project may require patient-subjects to undergo additional procedures unrelated to their own therapy. They may have to give blood samples or be catheterized, for example. Such additional procedures are nontherapeutic for the patients and may even carry some risks unrelated to their own therapy. Nontherapeutic research, in turn, may *indirectly* provide medical benefits for experimental subjects, such as better medical care. Because of these and other difficulties, some writers in biomedical ethics, including Gregory E. Pence in this chapter, reject the terminology that contrasts therapeutic and nontherapeutic research. They replace it with a three-fold classification: (1) research, (2) practice, and (3) nonvalidated practices (i.e., innovative therapy). Research, as noted previously, is designed to develop generalizable knowledge and is not intended to directly benefit the patient. *Practice* is directly intended to benefit patients and uses validated procedures to do so, that is, procedures known to carry a "reasonable expectation of success." Nonvalidated practices are also directly intended to benefit patient-subjects, but the therapies are innovative and may not have been tested sufficiently to have a reasonable expectation of success.[1] The therapeutic-nontherapeutic research distinction continues to be widely used, however, and is utilized in codes of research ethics in setting up guidelines for the conduct of research using human subjects.

The Research Imperative

Many biomedical research projects involve at least some risk to patient-subjects. Drugs being tested may turn out to be toxic, for example. In some experiments, subjects may have to be deliberately exposed to a disease such as malaria before they can be used to test the efficacy of a new treatment. What moral justification can be given for experimentation that puts human subjects at risk?

Little is said in response to this question in the literature of biomedical ethics. When it is discussed, the primary justification advanced for human experimentation is a utilitarian one. This justification features two central claims:

1 Human experimentation enhances the discovery of new diagnostic and therapeutic techniques. Past research, for example, has made possible cardio-vascular surgery, renal transplantation, and the control of poliomyelitis.

2 Controlled experimentation is necessary for sound medical practice. Possible iatrogenic illnesses will be prevented only if clinical research provides necessary knowledge about human reactions to specific therapies. In the past, physicians employed many techniques that were of no benefit and sometimes even harmed patients. For example, neither the blood-letting common in the eighteenth century nor the practice of freezing the stomachs of patients with ulcers in the twentieth century had any therapeutic value. Yet both practices were erroneously believed to be therapeutic. To take another example, X-rays in the twentieth century were much too widely used before it was learned that there was a connection between overexposure to X-rays and certain types of cancer. Well-designed, controlled research projects, it is argued, will help to minimize the employment of useless or harmful procedures.

The utilitarian conclusion is that human experimentation is not just morally permissible; rather, it is morally required because its harmful consequences for some will be far outweighed by its anticipated provision of future benefits and prevention of future harm to others. Maurice B. Visscher, in this chapter, argues in this vein in defense of a "Research Imperative."

Sometimes a different sort of argument, based on considerations of justice, is advanced to justify human experimentation and to defend the view that individuals have a duty to participate as research subjects in projects designed to advance medical knowledge. The argument is simple. We are the beneficiaries of the advances made by past biomedical research. Without the use of human subjects these advances would have been impossible. Since we have benefited from the sacrifices made by past research subjects, we have an obligation, in the interest of fairness, to see that such research continues. Since it cannot continue without research subjects, we ought to reciprocate for past sacrifices by serving as subjects ourselves. Hans Jonas attacks this argument in this chapter, claiming that we have no obligation to participate as research subjects, even if medical progress requires it. In his view, medical progress is only an optional goal and not an essential one.

Informed Consent

Most of the literature on the ethics of human experimentation is concerned with specifying the *conditions* under which human experimentation is ethically acceptable. Since World War II, at least thirty-three different guidelines and codes of ethics identifying these conditions have been formalized. Foremost among these are the two codes included in this chapter—"The Nuremberg Code" and the "Declaration of Helsinki." Common to all these codes is the principle that experimentation cannot be conducted on human subjects without their informed consent. Intensive discussions of this informed consent requirement are commonplace in the literature on human experimentation. Some writers offer justifications of the requirement. Others discuss the difficulties of applying it in practice. Still others focus on questions dealing with the use of research subjects who cannot meet the conditions for informed consent.

The *justifications* offered for the requirement that no human beings be used as experimental subjects without their informed consent are similar to those advanced to justify the requirement in the ordinary (nonresearch) biomedical context. (See Jay Katz's article in Chapter 2.) The primary argument, advanced from a deontological perspective, rests on the principle of respect for persons. Respect for human beings as persons requires that their autonomy be promoted and protected. Research that uses human subjects without their consent violates that autonomy and is, therefore, morally unacceptable. Paul Ramsey, one of the main proponents of this position, holds that informed consent is the "chief canon of loyalty" between two persons—the biomedical researcher and the patient-subject. It serves as a deontological check on any attempt to justify the use of human subjects solely on utilitarian grounds, insofar as it affirms that human beings are not objects to be used, without their consent, for others' benefit. In Ramsey's view only individuals who (1) are capable of knowingly involving themselves in a common cause with the researcher and (2) are willing to participate as research subjects may serve in that capacity.

The problems raised in *applying* the informed consent requirement in the research context are similar to those raised by the requirement in the ordinary (nonresearch) biomedical context and are discussed in Chapter 2. The problems stem from the requirement's three components: (1) The consentee must be informed; (2) The consentee must be competent to give consent; and (3) The consent must be voluntary. In this chapter, Franz J. Ingelfinger argues that most research subjects do not in fact meet these three requirements even when they are capable of signing the necessary forms or giving oral assent. Pence, on the other hand, challenges the claim that most medically uneducated adults cannot give real informed consent to sophisticated medical research. He cites a recent study said to demonstrate that adult subjects can be brought to a level of understanding superior to that of the average professor teaching in medical school. Such empirical claims about problems associated with the application of the informed consent requirement are parts of a larger discussion that has both conceptual and ethical dimensions. The meanings of concepts such as "voluntary" must be explicated, for example, before it can be determined what counts as "voluntary" consent. Then in a particular case, it must be empirically determined whether the individuals giving consent can meet the conditions required for "voluntary" consent. For example, in this chapter, Carl Cohen analyzes the concept of coercion prior to arguing that prison inmates can sometimes meet the conditions for voluntary consent. But ethical issues are also intertwined with the conceptual and empirical ones. Take the geriatric patient, mentioned by Ruth Macklin in Chapter 2, who suffers from Alzheimer's disease. Without research, the development of cures or preventive measures will not be possible. If it is necessary to use those suffering from Alzheimer's as research subjects, what rules should be adopted to gauge whether they are capable of giving consent? Someone in the earlier stages of the disease may fluctuate between periods of "competency" and "incompetency," complicated by the effects of the disease and the influence of medication. Should assent given during a "competent" period override dissent expressed during an "incompetent" one? Neither conceptual analysis alone nor empirical studies can answer this kind of question.

Who Should be a Research Subject?

If there is to be research, there must obviously be research subjects. Who should these subjects be? According to Hans Jonas, the first call for "volunteers" should go to the scientific community because its members identify with the purposes and the success of the research and can best understand the procedures and risks involved. Thus they are best able to give truly free and informed consent. This ideal is rarely practiced. Research subjects are often the economically and socially disadvantaged. Many of them are in public institutions such as prisons, homes for the mentally retarded, and public hospital wards. In addition, children, including infants (both in and out of institutions), are often used as research subjects, raising troubling questions about the use of those incapable of giving consent. It is not surprising, therefore, that there has been a great deal of debate about the ethical difficulties raised by research involving the above kinds of subject groups. These debates center on two concerns: (1) the requirement of informed consent and (2) the requirement of social justice. Several selections in this chapter, focusing on the use of children and prison inmates as research subjects, exemplify these concerns.

Children as Research Subjects Since children, especially young children, cannot give informed consent because they lack the competence to assess information about research procedures, any research using them as subjects apparently violates the informed consent requirement. When the research project is primarily therapeutic and is reasonably expected to benefit the child, it is less troublesome. Here, as in the case of validated therapies, it is usually agreed that proxies, such as parents and guardians, can legitimately consent on the child's behalf. However, when the procedure is not intended to directly benefit the child but to acquire knowledge that will benefit future patients, the child's participation in the research is morally problematic. Is it ever morally correct for parents and guardians to consent in their children's behalf to the latter's participation in nontherapeutic research?

Perhaps no one is more opposed to using children as subjects in nontherapeutic research than Paul Ramsey, whose argument is included in a reading in this chapter. In Ramsey's view, it is always wrong to subject children to procedures that are neither intended nor reasonably expected to be of direct benefit to them. Even if children as a group are the intended beneficiaries of the research, Ramsey will not allow it. His position is grounded in the claim (discussed earlier in this introduction) that all human experimentation must be a joint venture, freely undertaken by two autonomous persons. In keeping with this position, he refuses to recognize the validity of proxy consent to any nontherapeutic procedures.

Proponents of research using children cite its benefits to children as a group. Children are not just "little adults" in sickness or in health. Results of studies on adults cannot be simply extrapolated to children. To cite just one example, it would be disastrous to administer intravenous fluids to infants and children on the basis of adult requirements. Children would be given too much or too little. The requirements for specific age groups can only be identified by studying the normal constituents of body fluids and metabolism in normal infants and children. There are also a number of diseases, like infantile autism, that are unique to children. For these, as well as many other reasons, the use of children as research subjects is required for medical progress that will eventually benefit children as a group. In view of these potential gains, some proponents of research using children advance arguments to justify the validity of proxy consent.

One such proponent, Richard A. McCormick, in an article reprinted in this chapter, argues that all members of society, including children, have some minimal moral duties. These include the duty to participate in nontherapeutic research when the risks are minimal and the promise of future benefits great. Parents and guardians who give proxy consent to such participation are only making it possible for children to carry out their duties. McCormick's argument raises interesting questions regarding adult participation in research. If all members of society have an obligation to participate in research, can society legitimately draft them into service, thus bypassing the informed consent requirement altogether?

Gregory E. Pence approaches the issues differently, focusing on minors who are old enough to understand something about the research that requires their participation. Pence distinguishes between a subject's "consent" (short for informed consent), "assent," and "dissent." It is possible to either assent or dissent to something, without having either the information or the extent of competence required for informed consent. Pence argues that when minors are old enough to understand something about the project and their role in it, even if they cannot meet the conditions for informed consent, their assent should be sought and their dissent respected and safeguarded.

Prisoners as Research Subjects Most of the literature on the use of prisoners as subjects in primarily nontherapeutic research also centers on the informed consent requirement. The claim is often made that prisoners are so situated that their consent cannot be sufficiently free and informed. One approach taken is to argue that inmates in United States prisons today cannot give sufficiently free consent because of the conditions in these prisons. Critics of the prison system, such as Jessica Mitford, in this chapter, point to the following: crowded living conditions, inadequate medical care, very limited opportunities to make even small sums of money, and indeterminate sentences with unknown or nonobjective conditions for early release. All these factors, along with the coercive nature of the prisons, *in fact* make it impossible for the consent of prisoners to be sufficiently free. In addition, the precarious situation of prisoners makes it easy for researchers to abuse them and to withhold relevant information from them. It is impossible, therefore, to guarantee that the prisoners' consent will ever be sufficiently informed. These opponents of nontherapeutic research in prisons conclude that *in fact* prisoners can give neither sufficiently free nor sufficiently informed consent.

Another approach taken involves a stronger claim: prisoners cannot *in principle* give sufficiently free and informed consent. It is not simply that the conditions that in fact exist in our present system make the requisite consent impossible. Rather, the inherently coercive institutional environment of total institutions, such as prisons, makes voluntary consent impossible in principle. On this view, even if prisoners say that they "want" to be research subjects, their expressed desires can never be expressions of sufficiently voluntary consent.

Proponents of research in prisons respond that it is *not* in principle impossible for prisoners' consent to be sufficiently free and informed. Like Carl Cohen in this chapter, they grant that the precarious position of prisoners makes them especially vulnerable to manipulation and exploitation so that safeguards must be provided to prevent abuses. However, they maintain, a prisoner's desire to participate in research should be accorded the same respect as that given to any other volunteer. Furthermore, they point out, the requirement of informed consent is itself grounded in respect for an individual's autonomy and right of self-determination. To deny prisoners the right to decide for themselves whether they will participate in research is to treat them paternalistically and deny them this fundamental right. Prisoners themselves have argued in this vein, asserting a right to volunteer in the face of governmental attempts to end drug testing in prisons.[2]

Two other kinds of considerations are raised by proponents and opponents of nontherapeutic research in prisons. Proponents bring in utilitarian considerations. Opponents raise questions of social justice. Proponents cite both the benefits to society and the benefits to the prisoners. Society gains, for example, if drugs are first tested in a controlled situation. Prisoners also gain: (1) because they earn small sums of money and may receive better medical care and (2) because they have an opportunity to perform altruistic acts and to develop pride in their contribution. Opponents argue that prisoners are treated *unjustly* if as a group they carry a disproportionate share of the burdens and risks involved in nontherapeutic research in comparison with the population as a whole. Here it is pointed out, for example, that the population as a whole benefits by the drug testing, which according to United States law must be conducted before new drugs are made available to the public. The first phase of drug testing requires their use by "normal" subjects (subjects who do not have the disease, illness, or symptom related to the drug being tested). The purpose of this phase-one testing is to establish human tolerance and safety levels. Since World War II, most phase-one drug tests have been conducted in prisons. But prisoners are a minority of the population. Why should they as a group carry a disproportionate share of the risks of these tests? This objection to research in prisons raises wider questions of social justice about the fair distribution of burdens and benefits in a society.

Paying Research Subjects   In our society, as noted earlier, the economically deprived do carry a disproportionate share of the burdens and risks of research. One of the reasons they do so is that the monetary rewards offered to volunteers can provide a very strong incentive for participating, when opportunities to gain money in other ways are either limited or nonexistent. Is it morally wrong to offer money to potential research subjects? Federal regulations dealing with the protection of research subjects do not reject the use of money as an inducement to participate in research, but they forbid offering "undue inducements" to lure people into volunteering. Ruth Macklin, in this chapter, analyzes the concept of "undue inducement" and discusses some of the moral problems faced by attempts to determine the correct level of payment. Lisa Newton, in response, criticizes some of Macklin's arguments but agrees with Macklin that payments to research subjects should be low.

J. S. Z.

NOTES

1 On these distinctions, see Robert J. Levine, "Clarifying the Concepts of Research Ethics," *Hastings Center Report* 9 (June 1979), pp. 21–26.

2 Marjorie Sun, "Inmates Sue to Keep Research in Prisons," *Science* 212 (May 8, 1981), pp. 650–651.

Ethical Codes

The Nuremberg Code

"The Nuremberg Code of Ethics in Medical Research" was developed by the Allies after the Second World War. During the War Crimes Trials in Germany, this code provided the standards against which the practices of Nazis involved in human experimentation were judged. The Nuremberg Code emphasizes the essentiality of voluntary consent. Its first and longest article discusses consent in great detail. The code also sets forth other criteria that must be met before any experiment using human beings as subjects can be judged morally acceptable.

(1) The voluntary consent of the human subject is absolutely essential. This means that the person involved should have legal capacity to give consent; should be so situated as to be able to exercise free power of choice, without the intervention of any element of force, fraud, deceit, duress, overreaching, or other ulterior form of constraint or coercion; and should have sufficient knowledge and comprehension of the elements of the subject matter involved as to enable him to make an understanding and enlightened decision. This latter element requires that before the acceptance of an affirmative decision by the experimental subject there should be made known to him the nature, duration, and purpose of the experiment; the method and means by which it is to be conducted; all inconveniences and hazards reasonably to be expected; and the effects upon his health or person which may possibly come from his participation in the experiments.

The duty and responsibility for ascertaining the quality of the consent rests upon each individual who initiates, directs or engages in the experiment. It is a personal duty and responsibility which may not be delegated to another with impunity.

(2) The experiment should be such as to yield fruitful results for the good of society, unprocurable by other methods or means of study, and not random and unnecessary in nature.

(3) The experiment should be so designed and based on the results of animal experimentation and a knowledge of the natural history of the disease or other problem under study that the anticipated results [will] justify the performance of the experiment.

(4) The experiment should be so conducted as to avoid all unnecessary physical and mental suffering and injury.

(5) No experiment should be conducted where there is an a priori reason to believe that death or disabling injury will occur; except, perhaps, in those experiments where the experimental physicians also serve as subjects.

(6) The degree of risk to be taken should never exceed that determined by the humanitarian importance of the problem to be solved by the experiment.

(7) Proper preparations should be made and adequate facilities provided to protect the experimental subject against even remote possibilities of injury, disability, or death.

(8) The experiment should be conducted only by scientifically qualified persons. The highest degree of skill and care should be required through all stages of the experiment of those who conduct or engage in the experiment.

(9) During the course of the experiment the human subject should be at liberty to bring the experiment to an end if he has reached the physical or mental state where continuation of the experiment seems to him to be impossible.

(10) During the course of the experiment the scientist in charge must be prepared to terminate the experiment at any stage, if he has probable cause to believe, in the exercise of good faith, superior skill and careful judgment required of him that a continuation of the experiment is likely to result in injury, disability, or death to the experimental subject.

Reprinted from *Trials of War Criminals before the Nuremberg Military Tribunals* (Washington, D.C.: U.S. Government Printing Office, 1948).

Declaration of Helsinki

World Medical Association

In 1964 the Eighteenth World Medical Assembly meeting in Helsinki, Finland, adopted an ethical code to be used as a guide by medical doctors involved in biomedical research involving human subjects. This code was revised at the Twenty-Ninth World Medical Assembly held in Tokyo, Japan, in 1975. The code reprinted here is the revised version. It has much in common with the Nuremberg Code (e.g., the informed consent requirement and the requirement that animal experimentation must precede human experimentation). The Helsinki Code, however, goes beyond the Nuremberg Code in certain important respects. Two differences are especially noteworthy: (1) The Helsinki Code distinguishes between clinical (therapeutic) and nonclinical (nontherapeutic) biomedical research and sets forth specific criteria of ethical acceptability for each, as well as other basic principles common to both. (2) The Nuremberg Code is silent regarding the informed consent requirement in the case of the legally incompetent. The Helsinki Code addresses itself to such cases, asserting the ethical acceptability of what is sometimes called "proxy consent."

INTRODUCTION

It is the mission of the medical doctor to safeguard the health of the people. His or her knowledge and conscience are dedicated to the fulfillment of this mission.

The Declaration of Geneva of The World Medical Association binds the doctor with the words, "The health of my patient will be my first consideration," and the International Code of Medical Ethics declares that, "Any act or advice which could weaken physical or mental resistance of a human being may be used only in his interest."

The purpose of biomedical research involving human subjects must be to improve diagnostic, therapeutic and prophylactic procedures and the understanding of the aetiology and pathogenesis of disease.

In current medical practice most diagnostic, therapeutic or prophylactic procedures involve hazards. This applies *a fortiori* to biomedical research.

Medical progress is based on research which ultimately must rest in part on experimentation involving human subjects.

In the field of biomedical research a fundamental distinction must be recognized between medical research in which the aim is essentially diagnostic or therapeutic for a patient, and medical research, the essential object of which is purely scientific and without direct diagnostic or therapeutic value to the person subjected to the research.

Special caution must be exercised in the conduct of research which may affect the environment, and the welfare of animals used for research must be respected.

Because it is essential that the results of laboratory experiments be applied to human beings to further scientific knowledge and to help suffering humanity, The World Medical Association has prepared the following recommendations as a guide to every doctor in biomedical research involving human subjects. They should be kept under review in the future. It must be stressed that the standards as drafted are only a guide to physicians all over the world. Doctors are not relieved from criminal, civil and ethical responsibilities under the laws of their own countries.

I BASIC PRINCIPLES

(1) Biomedical research involving human subjects must conform to generally accepted scientific principles

and should be based on adequately performed laboratory and animal experimentation and on a thorough knowledge of the scientific literature.

(2) The design and performance of each experimental procedure involving human subjects should be clearly formulated in an experimental protocol which should be transmitted to a specially appointed independent committee for consideration, comment and guidance.

(3) Biomedical research involving human subjects should be conducted only by scientifically qualified persons and under the supervision of a clinically competent medical person. The responsibility for the human subject must always rest with a medically qualified person and never rest on the subject of research, even though the subject has given his or her consent.

(4) Biomedical research involving human subjects cannot legitimately be carried out unless the importance of the objective is in proportion to the inherent risk to the subject.

(5) Every biomedical research project involving human subjects should be preceded by careful assessment of predictable risks in comparison with foreseeable benefits to the subject or to others. Concern for the interests of the subject must always prevail over the interests of science and society.

(6) The right of the research subject to safeguard his or her integrity must always be respected. Every precaution should be taken to respect the privacy of the subject and to minimize the impact of the study on the subject's physical and mental integrity and on the personality of the subject.

(7) Doctors should abstain from engaging in research projects involving human subjects unless they are satisfied that the hazards involved are believed to be predictable. Doctors should cease any investigation if the hazards are found to outweigh the potential benefits.

(8) In publication of the results of his or her research, the doctor is obliged to preserve the accuracy of the results. Reports of experimentation not in accordance with the principles laid down in this Declaration should not be accepted for publication.

(9) In any research on human beings, each potential subject must be adequately informed of the aims, methods, anticipated benefits and potential hazards of the study and the discomfort it may entail. He or she should be informed that he or she is at liberty to abstain from participation in the study and that he or she is free to withdraw his or her consent to participation

at any time. The doctor should then obtain the subject's freely-given informed consent, preferably in writing.

(10) When obtaining informed consent for the research project the doctor should be particularly cautious if the subject is in a dependent relationship to him or her or may consent under duress. In that case the informed consent should be obtained by a doctor who is not engaged in the investigation and who is completely independent of this official relationship.

(11) In case of legal incompetence, informed consent should be obtained from the legal guardian in accordance with national legislation. Where physical or mental incapacity makes it impossible to obtain informed consent, or when the subject is a minor, permission from the responsible relative replaces that of the subject in accordance with national legislation.

(12) The research protocol should always contain a statement of the ethical considerations involved and should indicate that the principles enunciated in the present Declaration are complied with.

II MEDICAL RESEARCH COMBINED WITH PROFESSIONAL CARE (CLINICAL RESEARCH)

(1) In the treatment of the sick person, the doctor must be free to use a new diagnostic and therapeutic measure, if in his or her judgment it offers hope of saving life, reestablishing health or alleviating suffering.

(2) The potential benefits, hazards and discomfort of a new method should be weighed against the advantages of the best current diagnostic and therapeutic methods.

(3) In any medical study, every patient—including those of a control group, if any—should be assured of the best proven diagnostic and therapeutic method.

(4) The refusal of the patient to participate in a study must never interfere with the doctor-patient relationship.

(5) If the doctor considers it essential not to obtain informed consent, the specific reasons for this proposal should be stated in the experimental protocol for transmission to the independent committee (I, 2).

(6) The doctor can combine medical research with professional care, the objective being the acquisition of new medical knowledge, only to the extent that medical research is justified by its potential diagnostic or therapeutic value for the patient.

III NON-THERAPEUTIC BIOMEDICAL RESEARCH INVOLVING HUMAN SUBJECTS (NON-CLINICAL BIOMEDICAL RESEARCH)

(1) In the purely scientific application of medical research carried out on a human being, it is the duty of the doctor to remain the protector of the life and health of that person on whom biomedical research is being carried out.

(2) The subjects should be volunteers—either healthy persons or patients for whom the experimental design is not related to the patient's illness.

(3) The investigator or the investigating team should discontinue the research if in his/her or their judgment it may, if continued, be harmful to the individual.

(4) In research on man, the interest of science and society should never take precedence over considerations related to the well-being of the subject.

General Ethical Issues

Medical Research on Human Subjects as a Moral Imperative

Maurice B. Visscher

Maurice B. Visscher, M.D., is professor emeritus of physiology at the University of Minnesota Medical School. He is past president of the National Society for Medical Research. Visscher is the author of *Ethical Constraints and Imperatives in Medical Research* (1975), from which this selection is excerpted. He is also the editor of *Chemistry and Medicine* (1940) and *Humanistic Perspectives in Medical Ethics* (1972).

Visscher offers a justification for the use of human subjects in biomedical research. He maintains that such experimentation is necessary if physicians are to comply with the chief principle of traditional medical ethics, "First do no harm." If physicians are to avoid "unintentional" harm to their patients, Visscher argues, new therapies must be developed and tested. Since human beings differ physiologically from animals in other species, human subjects must ultimately be used as research subjects, even in those cases where animals can be used in the initial stages of research.

PRIMUM NON NOCERE

The use of human subjects in biomedical research is considered by scientists to be indispensible to progress in medical science and to consequent improvement in the art of medical practice, but the protection of the rights and welfare of every human being is equally a first priority of a civilized society. So long as these two basic precepts are not in conflict there are no major ethical problems in connection with scientific study on human subjects. However, there are situations in which the two objectives can clash, and then ethical problems arise.

In the practice of medicine the classic principle *primum non nocere* could be, if one knew what might be harmful, a simple rule to follow. Unfortunately even in

From Maurice B. Visscher, *Ethical Constraints and Imperatives in Medical Research,* 1975. Courtesy of Charles C. Thomas, Publisher, Springfield, Illinois.

ordinary medical practice such certainty is impossible. Intentional harm can be avoided, but unintentional harm cannot yet be avoided because of lack of adequate knowledge of human biology, broadly defined. Thus one comes, in attempting to fulfill the primary obligation of the medical profession, "first do no harm," to an ethical imperative to the profession as a whole and to the investigative physician specifically to make studies to learn how to avoid doing harm to patients. In other words, physicians frequently cannot properly perform their first function fully unless more research is done. This may be, to some, a different twist to the problem of ethics of medical practice, including the investigative use of human subjects, from the more simplistic views of the past. If it is, as seems obvious, obligatory upon physicians to learn how to do no harm, then scientific investigation, including that on human subjects, becomes a necessity for an ethical medical profession. Equally it becomes an activity [in] which society at large must, if it wishes to provide a milieu in which medicine can be practiced ethically, promote the conditions under which medical and related research can be carried out in harmony with humanistic ethics.

The learned pharmacologist, Nobel Laureate Professor B. N. Halpern,[1] who discovered and developed numerous widely used and important new therapeutic agents, has stated the case very convincingly. In a recent essay he wrote in connection with studies of drug toxicity and effectiveness:

> I should like to stress yet again most forcefully that, in the interests of science and even of the protection of society against the absolutely unpredictable collective damage that the introduction of a new drug may cause, it is indispensable that trials in man should be included in pharmacological research.

> The term "human experimentation" raises a sinister echo in each of us, for reasons known to us all. But fear solves no scientific problems. For my part, the recommendations...that safety tests of new drugs should be carried out on fully informed volunteers in conditions of almost absolute security—is more in conformity with the requirements of ethics than the thousands of such trials hypocritically carried out daily in hospitals in all countries on individuals who are totally ignorant of what is being done to them.

Writing on the topic, "Justification for the Human Trial," [Henry K.] Beecher[2] has said:

The importance of the project undertaken must be commensurate with the risk involved. The insurance of this is a cardinal responsibility of all who undertake experimentation in man. But having stated that important principle, there is still a vast area where judgment—one hopes sound judgment—must operate. Only the fanatic denies that animal experimentation must precede the human. As Sir Geoffrey Jefferson put it, "Man is too rare, too expensive, altogether too valuable an animal" to be first used in study of technical procedures or trial of even therapeutic agents. There are (nevertheless) species differences. Ultimately, the definitive test must be done in man. *but every human is an individual thus may react differently.*

This is obviously true because, although certain similarities are found in fundamental processes from the simplest organisms to man, as in the general mechanisms of information storage in the genetic apparatus, and in the basic building blocs of certain enzymes, there are also very important differences between species, becoming greater the farther they are apart in the phylogenetic tree. Even within a single genus the possibilities for variations in gene combinations are so great that aside from single ovum twins or the products of many generations of inbreeding important differences between individuals are evident in many characteristics. Histoincompatibility as a cause of the usual homograft rejection is evidence that even at the molecular level individuality is the rule. Fortunately for the applicability of blood transfusion in therapy is the existence, as first discovered by Landsteiner, of major blood types, within which differences in properties of agglutinins for red blood cells are ordinarily so small as to permit survival of the cells. An extension of Landsteiner's discovery, and others based upon it, into the field of tissue and organ transplantation is also yielding promising results.

It is, of course, not only in the area of immunology that individuality is important. Reactions to drugs of all sorts differ, not only in different species but among individuals of a single species or even a single genus. For example, the doses of digitalis glycosides required to produce a given effect in a rat are orders of magnitude higher than those needed per unit body weight in a cat or a man. Some drug effects seen in one species, or even in an entire family within a particular class, are not seen at all in another class. It is partly for these reasons that drug studies must be carried out in many species of lower animals before even planning to use them in man. And because of the intraspecies and intragenus variability of individuals, one must eventually study the effects of new agents on large numbers of humans in order to know what the limiting parameters for both efficacy and safety are. Furthermore the physician must know how to assess the idiosyncracies of individual patients in their responsiveness to pharmaceutical agents, and must understand as much as is known about the principles of action of such agents if he is to be a reliable physician.

There is also a need to study human subjects in connection with disease entities which are unique to man, or almost so. Likewise with respect to nervous and mental processes, although much can be learned by studies on lower animals, particularly with respect to basic neural mechanisms, there remain those features of function that are uniquely human which would forever remain shrouded in mystery if the scientific method were not to be employed to throw light upon them.

In other words, it is a fanciful dream concocted in the minds of scientific illiterates that medical science, or any other biological science, could progress without the study of actual living systems, and ultimately in the case of medicine, study of living human subjects.

There is a corollary to these lines of reasoning. It is that there is an ethical imperative for physicians as a group to promote medical research, including studies on human subjects. Obviously for various reasons not every physician can be an investigator, but at least every physician should give moral support to the enterprise of advancement of medical knowledge. The vast majority of physicians accept this view in principle, but in practice many fail to act to promote the medical research enterprise.

The conclusions of Claude Bernard[3] in his *Introduction to the Study of Experimental Medicine,* written a little more than a century ago, are undoubtedly pertinent today. He said, "For we must not deceive ourselves, morals do not forbid making experiments on one's neighbor or on one's self; in everyday life men do nothing but experiment on one another. Christian morals forbid only one thing, doing ill to one's neighbor. So, among the experiments that may be tried on man, those that can only harm are forbidden, those that are innocent are permissible, and those that may do good are obligatory."

REFERENCES

1 Halpern, B. N.: CIOMS round tables: 1. *Biomedical Science and the Dilemma of Human Experimentation.* Paris, UNESCO House, 1967, pp. 30, 31.
2 Beecher, Henry K.: *Experimentation in Man.* Springfield, Thomas, 1958, p. 32.
3 Bernard, Claude as translated by Henry Copley Greene: *An Introduction to the Study of Experimental Medicine.* U.S.A., Henry Schuman, 1927, p. 102.

Philosophical Reflections on Experimenting with Human Subjects

Hans Jonas

Hans Jonas is professor emeritus of philosophy at the New School for Social Research. His areas of specialization are ancient philosophy, metaphysics, and ethics. Jonas is the author of several works including *Gnostic Religion* (1963), *Phenomenon of Life* (1968), and *The Phenomenon of Life: Toward a Philosophical Biology* (1983). He has also published a collection of his essays, *Philosophical Essays: From Ancient Creed to Technological Man* (1974). This collection includes such articles as "Biological Engineering—A Preview" and "Against the Stream: Comments on the Definition and Redefinition of Death."

Jonas criticizes two arguments often given to justify using human beings as research subjects. (1) Medical experimentation is justified either because it will result in great benefits to society or because it will prevent great future harm. (2) Justice requires that we, who are the beneficiaries of past research, in turn accept the obligation to participate in such research. Jonas maintains against (1) that most of the biomedical research using human subjects is not essential to the well-being or survival of the species. Furthermore, he holds, we do not have a strict obligation to advance medical progress. Jonas maintains against (2) that past participants in medical research performed altruistic acts. If we owe *them* anything, we owe them a debt of gratitude. We do not owe any obligation to *society in general* to participate in medical research simply because we are the beneficiaries of past research. Jonas does not claim that all experimentation on human subjects is unjustified. He does hold, however, that the first volunteers for such experimentation should be the researchers themselves or other members of the scientific community. These are the individuals who are most capable of giving truly educated informed consent and who are best able to identify with the purposes of the research projects.

Experimenting with human subjects is going on in many fields of scientific and technological progress. It is designed to replace the over-all instruction by natural, occasional experience with the selective information from artificial, systematic experiment which physical science has found so effective in dealing with inanimate nature. Of the new experimentation with man, medical is surely the most legitimate; psychological, the most dubious; biological (still to come), the most dangerous. I have chosen here to deal with the first only, where the case *for* it is strongest and the task of adjudicating conflicting claims hardest....

THE PECULIARITY OF HUMAN EXPERIMENTATION

Experimentation was originally sanctioned by natural science. There it is performed on inanimate objects, and this raises no moral problems. But as soon as animate, feeling beings become the subjects of experiment, as they do in the life sciences and especially in medical research, this innocence of the search for knowledge is lost and questions of conscience arise. The depth to which moral and religious sensibilities can become aroused over these questions is shown by the vivisection issue. Human experimentation must sharpen the issue as it involves ultimate questions of personal dignity and sacrosanctity. One profound dif-

ference between the human experiment and the physical (besides that between animate and inanimate, feeling and unfeeling nature) is this: The physical experiment employs small-scale, artificially devised substitutes for that about which knowledge is to be obtained, and the experimenter extrapolates from these models and simulated conditions to nature at large. Something deputizes for the "real thing"—balls rolling down an inclined plane for sun and planets, electric discharges from a condenser for real lightning, and so on. For the most part, no such substitution is possible in the biological sphere. We must operate on the original itself, the real thing in the fullest sense, and perhaps affect it irreversibly. No simulacrum can take its place. Especially in the human sphere, experimentation loses entirely the advantage of the clear division between vicarious model and true object. Up to a point, animals may fulfill the proxy role of the classical physical experiment. But in the end man himself must furnish knowledge about himself, and the comfortable separation of non-committal experiment and definitive action vanishes. An experiment in education affects the lives of its subjects, perhaps a whole generation of school-children. Human experimentation for whatever purpose is always *also* a responsible, non-experimental, definitive dealing with the subject himself. And not even the noblest purpose abrogates the obligations this involves.

This is the root of the problem with which we are faced: Can both that purpose and this obligation be satisfied? If not, what would be a just compromise? Which side should give way to the other? The question is inherently philosophical as it concerns not merely pragmatic difficulties and their arbitration, but a genuine conflict of values involving principles of a high order. May I put the conflict in these terms? On principle, it is felt, human beings *ought* not to be dealt with in that way (the "guinea pig" protest); on the other hand, such dealings are increasingly urged on us by considerations, in turn appealing to principle, that claim to override those objections. Such a claim must be carefully assessed, especially when it is swept along by a mighty tide. Putting the matter thus, we have already made one important assumption rooted in our "Western" cultural tradition: The prohibitive rule is, to that way of thinking, the primary and axiomatic one; the permissive counter-rule, as qualifying the first, is secondary and stands in need of justification. We must justify the infringement of a primary inviolability, which needs no justification itself; and the justification of its infringement must be by values and needs of a dignity commensurate with those to be sacrificed....

HEALTH AS A PUBLIC GOOD

The cause invoked [for medical experimentation] is health and, in its more critical aspect, life itself—clearly superlative goods that the physician serves directly by curing and the researcher indirectly by the knowledge gained through his experiments. There is no question about the good served nor about the evil fought— disease and premature death. But a good to whom and an evil to whom? Here the issue tends to become somewhat clouded. In the attempt to give experimentation the proper dignity (on the problematic view that a value becomes greater by being "social" instead of merely individual), the health in question or the disease in question is somehow predicated on the social whole, as if it were society that, in the persons of its members, enjoyed the one and suffered the other. For the purposes of our problem, public interest can then be pitted against private interest, the common good against the individual good. Indeed, I have found health called a national resource, which of course it is, but surely not in the first place.

In trying to resolve some of the complexities and ambiguities lurking in these conceptualizations, I have pondered a particular statement, made in the form of a question, which I found in the *Proceedings* of the earlier *Daedalus* conference: "Can society afford to discard the tissues and organs of the hopelessly unconscious patient when they could be used to restore the otherwise hopelessly ill, but still salvageable individual?" And somewhat later: "A strong case can be made that society can ill afford to discard the tissues and organs of the hopelessly unconscious patient; they are greatly needed for study and experimental trial to help those who can be salvaged." [1] I hasten to add that any suspicion of callousness that the "commodity" language of these statements may suggest is immediately dispelled by the name of the speaker, Dr. Henry K. Beecher, for whose humanity and moral sensibility there can be nothing but admiration. But the use, in all innocence, of this language gives food for thought. Let me, for a moment, take the question literally. "Discarding" implies proprietary rights—nobody can discard what does not belong to him in the first place. Does society then own my body? "Salvaging" implies the same and, moreover, a use-value to the owner. Is the life-extension of certain individuals then a public interest? "Affording" implies a critically vital level of such an interest—that is, of the loss or gain involved. And "society" itself—what is it? When does a need, an aim, an obligation become social? Let us reflect on some of these terms.

WHAT SOCIETY CAN AFFORD

"Can society afford...?" Afford what? To let people die intact, thereby withholding something from other people who desperately need it, who in consequence will have to die too? These other, unfortunate people indeed cannot afford not to have a kidney, heart, or other organ of the dying patient, on which they depend for an extension of their lease on life; but does that give them a right to it? And does it oblige society to procure it for them? What is it that *society* can or cannot afford—leaving aside for the moment the question of what it has a *right* to? It surely can afford to lose members through death; more than that, it is built on the balance of death and birth decreed by the order of life. This is too general, of course, for our question, but perhaps it is well to remember. The specific question seems to be whether society can afford to let some people die whose death might be deferred by particular means if these were authorized by society. Again, if it is merely a question of what society can or cannot afford, rather than of what it ought or ought not to do, the answer must be: Of course, it can. If cancer, heart disease, and other organic, noncontagious ills, especially those tending to strike the old more than the young, continue to exact their toll at the normal rate of incidence (including the toll of private anguish and misery), society can go on flourishing in every way.

Here, by contrast, are some examples of what, in sober truth, society cannot afford. It cannot afford to let an epidemic rage unchecked; a persistent excess of deaths over births, but neither—we must add—too great an excess of births over deaths; too low an average life expectancy even if demographically balanced by fertility, but neither too great a longevity with the necessitated correlative dearth of youth in the social body; a debilitating state of general health; and things of this kind. These are plain cases where the whole condition of society is critically affected, and the public interest can make its imperative claims. The Black Death of the Middle Ages was a *public* calamity of the acute kind; the life-sapping ravages of endemic malaria or sleeping sickness in certain areas are a public calamity of the chronic kind. Such situations a society as a whole can truly not "afford," and they may call for extraordinary remedies, including, perhaps, the invasion of private sacrosanctities.

This is not entirely a matter of numbers and numerical ratios. Society, in a subtler sense, cannot "afford" a single miscarriage of justice, a single inequity in the dispensation of its laws, the violation of the rights of even the tiniest minority, because these undermine the moral basis on which society's existence rests. Nor can it, for a similar reason, afford the absence or atrophy in its midst of compassion and of the effort to alleviate suffering—be it widespread or rare—one form of which is the effort to conquer disease of any kind, whether "socially" significant (by reason of number) or not. And in short, society cannot afford the absence among its members of *virtue* with its readiness for sacrifice beyond defined duty. Since its presence—that is to say, that of personal idealism—is a matter of grace and not of decree, we have the paradox that society depends for its existence on intangibles of nothing less than a religious order, for which it can hope, but which it

cannot enforce. All the more must it protect this most precious capital from abuse.

For what objectives connected with the medico-biological sphere should this reserve be drawn upon—for example, in the form of accepting, soliciting, perhaps even imposing the submission of human subjects to experimentation? We postulate that this must be not just a worthy cause, as any promotion of the health of anybody doubtlessly is, but a cause qualifying for transcendent social sanction. Here one thinks first of those cases critically affecting the whole condition, present and future, of the community we have illustrated. Something equivalent to what in the political sphere is called "clear and present danger" may be invoked and a state of emergency proclaimed, thereby suspending certain otherwise inviolable prohibitions and taboos. We may observe that averting a disaster always carries greater weight than promoting a good. Extraordinary danger excuses extraordinary means. This covers human experimentation, which we would like to count, as far as possible, among the extraordinary rather than the ordinary means of serving the common good under public auspices. Naturally, since foresight and responsibility for the future are of the essence of institutional society, averting disaster extends into long-term prevention, although the lesser urgency will warrant less sweeping licenses.

SOCIETY AND THE CAUSE OF PROGRESS

Much weaker is the case where it is a matter not of saving but of improving society. Much of medical research falls into this category. As stated before, a permanent death rate from heart failure or cancer does not threaten society. So long as certain statistical ratios are maintained, the incidence of disease and of disease-induced mortality is not (in the strict sense) a "social" misfortune. I hasten to add that it is not therefore less of a human misfortune, and the call for relief issuing with silent eloquence from each victim and all potential victims is of no lesser dignity. But it is misleading to equate the fundamentally human response to it with what is owed to society: it is owed by man to man—and it is thereby owed by society to the individuals as soon as the adequate ministering to these concerns outgrows (as it progressively does) the scope of private spontaneity and is made a public mandate. It is thus that society assumes responsibility for medical care, research, old age, and innumerable other things not originally of the public realm (in the original "social contract"), and they become duties toward "society" (rather than directly toward one's fellow man) by the fact that they are socially operated.

Indeed, we expect from organized society no longer mere protection against harm and the securing of the conditions of our preservation, but active and constant improvement in all the domains of life: the waging of the battle against nature, the enhancement of the human estate—in short, the promotion of progress. This is an expansive goal, one far surpassing the disaster norm of our previous reflections. It lacks the urgency of the latter, but has the nobility of the free, forward thrust. It surely is worth sacrifices. It is not at all a question of what society can afford, but of what it is committed to, beyond all necessity, by our mandate. Its trusteeship has become an established, ongoing, institutionalized business of the body politic. As eager beneficiaries of its gains, we now owe to "society," as its chief agent, our individual contributions toward its *continued pursuit.* I emphasize "continued pursuit." Maintaining the existing level requires no more than the orthodox means of taxation and enforcement of professional standards that raise no problems. The more optional goal of pushing forward is also more exacting. We have this syndrome: Progress is by our choosing an acknowledged interest of society, in which we have a stake in various degrees; science is a necessary instrument of progress; research is a necessary instrument of science; and in medical science experimentation on human subjects is a necessary instrument of research. Therefore, human experimentation has come to be a societal interest.

The destination of research is essentially melioristic. It does not serve the preservation of the existing good from which I profit myself and to which I am obligated. Unless the present state is intolerable, the melioristic goal is in a sense gratuitous, and this not only from the vantage point of the present. Our descendants have a right to be left an unplundered planet; they do not have a right to new miracle cures. We have sinned against them, if by our doing we have destroyed their inheritance—which we are doing at full blast; we have not sinned against them, if by the time they come around arthritis has not yet been conquered (unless by sheer neglect). And generally, in the matter of progress, as humanity had no claim on a Newton, a Michelangelo, or a St. Francis to appear, and no right to the blessings

of their unscheduled deeds, so progress, with all our methodical labor for it, cannot be budgeted in advance and its fruits received as a due. Its coming-about at all and its turning out for good (of which we can never be sure) must rather be regarded as something akin to grace.

THE MELIORISTIC GOAL, MEDICAL RESEARCH, AND INDIVIDUAL DUTY

Nowhere is the melioristic goal more inherent than in medicine. To the physician, it is not gratuitous. He is committed to curing and thus to improving the power to cure. Gratuitous we called it (outside disaster conditions) as a *social* goal, but noble at the same time. Both the nobility and the gratuitousness must influence the manner in which self-sacrifice for it is elicited, and even its free offer accepted. Freedom is certainly the first condition to be observed here. The surrender of one's body to medical experimentation is entirely outside the enforceable "social contract."

Or can it be construed to fall within its terms—namely, as repayment for benefits from past experimentation that I have enjoyed myself? But I am indebted for these benefits not to society, but to the past "martyrs," to whom society is indebted itself, and society has no right to call in my personal debt by way of adding new to its own. Moreover, gratitude is not an enforceable social obligation; it anyway does not mean that I must emulate the deed. Most of all, if it was wrong to exact such sacrifice in the first place, it does not become right to exact it again with the plea of the profit it has brought me. If, however, it was not exacted, but entirely free, as it ought to have been, then it should remain so, and its precedence must not be used as a social pressure on others for doing the same under the sign of duty....

THE "CONSCRIPTION" OF CONSENT

...The mere issuing of the appeal, the calling for volunteers, with the moral and social pressures it inevitably generates, amounts even under the most meticulous rules of consent to a sort of *conscripting.* And some soliciting is necessarily involved....And this is why "consent," surely a non-negotiable minimum requirement, is not the full answer to the problem.

Granting then that soliciting and therefore some degree of conscripting are part of the situation, who may conscript and who may be conscripted? Or less harshly expressed: Who should issue appeals and to whom?

The naturally qualified issuer of the appeal is the research scientist himself, collectively the main carrier of the impulse and the only one with the technical competence to judge. But his being very much an interested party (with vested interests, indeed, not purely in the public good, but in the scientific enterprise as such, in "his" project, and even in his career) makes him also suspect. The ineradicable dialectic of this situation—a delicate incompatibility problem—calls for particular controls by the research community and by public authority that we need not discuss. They can mitigate, but not eliminate the problem. We have to live with the ambiguity, the treacherous impurity of everything human.

SELF-RECRUITMENT OF THE COMMUNITY

To whom should the appeal be addressed? The natural issuer of the call is also the first natural addressee: the physician-researcher himself and the scientific confraternity at large. With such a coincidence—indeed, the noble tradition with which the whole business of human experimentation started—almost all of the associated legal, ethical, and metaphysical problems vanish. If it is full, autonomous identification of the subject with the purpose that is required for the dignifying of his serving as a subject—here it is; if strongest motivation—here it is; if fullest understanding—here it is; if freest decision—here it is; if greatest integration with the person's total, chosen pursuit—here it is. With the fact of self-solicitation the issue of consent in all its insoluble equivocality is bypassed *per se*. Not even the condition that the particular purpose be truly important and the project reasonably promising, which must hold in any solicitation of others, need be satisfied here. By himself, the scientist is free to obey his obsession, to play his hunch, to wager on chance, to follow the lure of ambition. It is all part of the "divine madness" that somehow animates the ceaseless pressing against frontiers. For the rest of society, which has a deep-seated disposition to look with reverence and awe upon the guardians of the mysteries of life, the profession assumes with this proof of its devotion the role of a self-chosen, consecrated fraternity, not unlike the monastic orders of the past, and this would come nearest to the actual, religious origins of the art of healing. . . .

NOTE

1 *Proceedings of the Conference on the Ethical Aspects of Experimentation on Human Subjects,* November 3–4, 1967 (Boston, Massachusetts . . . pp. 50–51.

Informed (but Uneducated) Consent

Franz J. Ingelfinger

Franz J. Ingelfinger (1910–1980) was a physician who taught in the department of medicine, Boston University. He was also the editor of the *New England Journal of Medicine,* the journal of the Massachusetts Medical Society, from 1967 to 1977. In his capacity as editor, Ingelfinger frequently wrote editorials dealing with issues in biomedical ethics. He was the coeditor of *Controversy in Internal Medicine* (1974). His articles include "Medicine: Meritorious or Meretricious?" and "Arrogance."

Ingelfinger discusses some of the problems raised in *applying* the informed consent requirement. He questions the capacity of most patient-subjects to ade-

Reprinted by permission from the *New England Journal of Medicine,* vol. 287, no. 9 (August 31, 1972), pp. 465–466.

quately comprehend the information given by the physician-investigator. Ingel-finger also holds that any investigator-subject relation involves some coercion on the part of the investigator. If free choice requires the absence of all such coercion as well as adequate comprehension of the pertinent information, he contends, then in most cases the "process of obtaining informed consent is no more than elaborate ritual conferring no more than the semblance of propriety on human experimentation."

The trouble with informed consent is that it is not educated consent. Let us assume that the experimental subject, whether a patient, a volunteer, or otherwise enlisted, is exposed to a completely honest array of factual detail. He is told of the medical uncertainty that exists and that must be resolved by research endeavors, of the time and discomfort involved, and of the tiny percentage risk of some serious consequences of the test procedure. He is also reassured of his rights and given a formal, quasilegal statement to read. No exculpatory language is used. With his written signature, the subject then caps the transaction, and whether he sees himself as a heroic martyr for the sake of mankind, or as a reluctant guinea pig dragooned for the benefit of science, or whether, perhaps, he is merely bewildered, he obviously has given his "informed consent." Because established routines have been scrupulously observed, the doctor, the lawyer, and the ethicist are content.

But the chances are remote that the subject really understands what he has consented to—in the sense that the responsible medical investigator understands the goals, nature, and hazards of his study. How can the layman comprehend the importance of his perhaps not receiving, as determined by the luck of the draw, the highly touted new treatment that his roommate will get? How can he appreciate the sensation of living for days with a multi-lumen intestinal tube passing through his mouth and pharynx? How can he interpret the information that an intravascular catheter and radiopaque dye injection have an 0.01 per cent probability of leading to a dangerous thrombosis or cardiac arrhythmia? It is moreover quite unlikely that any patient-subject can see himself accurately within the broad context of the situation, to weigh the inconveniences and hazards that he will have to undergo against the improvements that the research project may bring to the management of his disease in general and to his own case in particular. The difficulty that the public has in understanding information that is both medical and stressful is exemplified by [a] report [in the *New England Journal of Medicine*, August 31, 1972, page 433]—only half the families given genetic counseling grasped its impact.

Nor can the information given to the experimental subject be in any sense totally complete. It would be impractical and probably unethical for the investigator to present the nearly endless list of all possible contingencies; in fact, he may not himself be aware of every untoward thing that might happen. Extensive detail, moreover, usually enhances the subject's confusion. Epstein and Lasagna showed that comprehension of medical information given to untutored subjects is inversely correlated with the elaborateness of the material presented.[1] The inconsiderate investigator, indeed, conceivably could exploit his authority and knowledge and extract "informed consent" by overwhelming the candidate-subject with information.

Ideally, the subject should give his consent freely, under no duress whatsoever. The facts are that some element of coercion is instrumental in any investigator-subject transaction. Volunteers for experiments will usually be influenced by hopes of obtaining better grades, earlier parole, more substantial egos, or just mundane cash. These pressures, however, are but fractional shadows of those enclosing the patient-subject. Incapacitated and hospitalized because of illness, frightened by strange and impersonal routines, and fearful for his health and perhaps life, he is far from exercising a free power of choice when the person to whom he anchors all his hopes asks, "Say, you wouldn't mind, would you, if you joined some of the other patients on this floor and helped us to carry out some very important research we are doing?" When "informed consent" is obtained, it is not the student, the destitute bum, or the prisoner to whom, by virtue of his condition, the thumb screws of coercion are most relentlessly applied; it is the most used and useful of all experimental subjects, the patient with disease.

When a man or woman agrees to act as an experimental subject, therefore, his or her consent is marked by neither adequate understanding nor total freedom of choice. The conditions of the agreement are a far cry from those visualized as ideal. Jonas would have the subject identify with the investigative endeavor so that he and the researcher would be seeking a common cause: "Ultimately, the appeal for volunteers should seek...free and generous endorsement, the appropriation of the research purpose into the person's [i.e., the subject's] own scheme of ends."[2] For Ramsey, "informed consent" should represent a "covenantal bond between consenting man and consenting man [that] makes them...joint adventurers in medical care and progress."[3] Clearly, to achieve motivations and attitudes of this lofty type, an educated and understanding, rather than merely informed, consent is necessary.

Although it is unlikely that the goals of Jonas and of Ramsey will ever be achieved, and that human research subjects will spontaneously volunteer rather than be "conscripted,"[2] efforts to promote educated consent are in order. In view of the current emphasis on involving "the community" in such activities as regional planning, operation of clinics, and assignment of priorities, the general public and its political leaders are showing an increased awareness and understanding of medical affairs. But the orientation of this public interest in medicine is chiefly socioeconomic. Little has been done to give the public a basic understanding of medical research and its requirements not only for the people's money but also for their participation. The public, to be sure, is being subjected to a bombardment of sensation-mongering news stories and books that feature "break-throughs," or that reveal real or alleged exploitations—horror stories of Nazi-type experimentation on abused human minds and bodies. Muckraking is essential to expose malpractices, but unless accompanied by efforts to promote a broader appreciation of medical research and its methods, it merely compounds the difficulties for both the investigator and the subject when "informed consent" is solicited.

The procedure currently approved in the United States for enlisting human experimental subjects has one great virtue: patient-subjects are put on notice that their management is in part at least an experiment. The deceptions of the past are no longer tolerated. Beyond this accomplishment, however, the process of obtaining "informed consent," with all its regulations and conditions, is no more than elaborate ritual, a device that, when the subject is uneducated and uncomprehending, confers no more than the semblance of propriety on human experimentation. The subject's only real protection, the public as well as the medical profession must recognize, depends on the conscience and compassion of the investigator and his peers.

REFERENCES

1 Epstein, L. C., Lasagna, L.: "Obtaining informed consent: form or substance." *Arch Intern Med* 123: 682–688, 1969.
2 Jonas, H.: "Philosophical reflections on experimenting with human subjects." *Daedalus* 98:219–247, Spring, 1969.
3 Ramsey, P.: "The ethics of a cottage industry in an age of community and research medicine." *N Engl J Med* 284:700–706, 1971.

Children as Research Subjects

Consent as a Canon of Loyalty with Special Reference to Children in Medical Investigations

Paul Ramsey

Paul Ramsey is Harrington Spear Paine Professor of Religion at Princeton University. His books include *The Patient as Person: Explorations in Medical Ethics* (1970), *Fabricated Man: The Ethics of Genetic Control* (1970), *Ethics at the Edges of Life* (1978), and *Deeds and Rules in Christian Ethics* (1980). Among his many published articles are "Protecting the Unborn" and "The Ethics of a Cottage Industry in an Age of Community and Research Medicine."

According to Ramsey, the principle of informed consent is the "cardinal canon of loyalty," which joins people together in medical practice and investigation. In his view, experimentation on a human subject, which is not for that subject's benefit, can never be justified if it is performed without the subject's free and informed consent. Since young children are incapable of giving such consent, research involving children should never be allowed unless participation in such research benefits the child. The use of an experimental procedure on children is morally justified only if the procedure is either (1) seen as the best means to effect the child's own recovery from an illness or disease or (2) intended to protect the child against some greater risk.

From consent as a canon of loyalty in medical practice it follows that children, who cannot give a mature and informed consent, or adult incompetents, should not be made the subjects of medical experimentation unless, other remedies having failed to relieve their grave illness, it is reasonable to believe that the administration of a drug as yet untested or insufficiently tested on human beings, or the performance of an untried operation, may further *the patient's own recovery*.

Now that is not a very elaborate moral rule governing medical practice in the matter of experiments involving children or incompetents as human subjects. It is a good example of the general claims of childhood specified for application in medical care and research. It is also a qualification immediately entailed by the meaning of consent in medical investigations as a joint undertaking between men. Again, one has to be prudent (which does not mean overcautious or scrupulous) in order to know how to care for child-patients in this way. One must know the possible relation of a proposed procedure to the child's own recovery, and also its

likely effectiveness compared with other methods that have been or could be tried. These considerations may provide the doctor with necessary and sufficient reason for investigations upon children, perhaps even very hazardous ones. One has to proportion the peril to the diagnostic or therapeutic needs of the child.

Practical medical judgment has undeniable and ominous room for its determinations, since a "benefit" is whatever is *believed* to be of help to the child. Still the limits this rule imposes on practice are essentially clear; where there is no possible relation to the child's recovery, a child is not to be made a mere object in medical experimentation for the sake of good to come. The likelihood of benefits that could flow from the experiment for many other children is an equally insufficient warrant for child experimentation. The individual child is to be tended in illness or in dying, since he himself is not able to donate his illness or his dying to be studied and worked upon solely for the advancement of medicine. Again, future experience may tell us more about the meaning of this particular rule expres-

Reprinted with permission of the publisher from Paul Ramsey, *The Patient as a Person* (New Haven, Conn.: Yale University Press, 1970).

sive of loyalty to a human child, and we may learn a great deal more about how to apply it in new situations with greater sensitivity and refinement—or we may learn more and more how to practice violations of it. But we are committed to refraining from morally significant exceptions to this rule defining impermissible medical experimentation upon children.

To experiment on children in ways that are not related to them as patients is already a sanitized form of barbarism; it already removes them from view and pays no attention to the faithfulness-claims which a child, simply by being a normal or a sick or dying child, places upon us and upon medical care. We should expect no morally significant exceptions to this canon of faithfulness to the child. To expect future justifiable exceptions is, in some sense, already to have forgotten the child....

To attempt to consent for a child to be made an experimental subject is to treat a child as not a child. It is to treat him as if he were an adult person who has consented to become a joint adventurer in the common cause of medical research. If the grounds for this are alleged to be the presumptive or implied consent of the child, that must simply be characterized as a violent and a false presumption. Nontherapeutic, nondiagnostic experimentation involving human subjects must be based on true consent if it is to proceed as a human enterprise. No child or adult incompetent can choose to become a participating member of medical undertakings, and no one else on earth should decide to subject these people to investigations having no relation to their own treatment. That is a canon of loyalty to them. This they claim of us simply by being a human child or incompetent. When he is grown, the child may put away childish things and become a true volunteer. This is the meaning of being a volunteer: that a man enter and establish a consensual relation in some joint venture for medical progress—where before he could not, nor could anyone else, "volunteer" him for submission to unknown possible hazards for the sake of good to come.

If the requirement of parents, investigators, and state authorities in regard to their wards is "Never subject children to the unknown possible hazards of medical investigations having no relation to their own treatment," we must understand that the maladies for which the individual needs treatment and protection need not already be resident within the compass of the child's own skin. He can properly be regarded as one of

a population, and we can add to the foregoing words: "except in epidemic conditions." Dr. Salk tried his polio vaccine on himself and his own children first. Then it was tested on selected children within a normal population. This involved some risk for the children vaccinated, and for other children as well, that the disease *might* be contracted from the vaccine itself, or that there might be unexpected injurious results. But the normal population of children was already subjected to waves of crippling epidemic summer after summer. A parent consenting for his child to be used in this trial was balancing the risks from the trial against the hazards from polio itself for that same child.

Physician-investigators are often in a quandary in which they are torn between the warrants for giving an experimental drug, and the warrants for withholding it from anyone in order to test it. Neither act seems justified, or both acts are equally warranted, when there is no available remedy and the indications are that a new drug may succeed. This situation also justifies a parent or guardian in consenting for a child, since we are supposing the hazard of the proposed treatment to be less or no greater than the hazard of the disease itself when treated by the established procedures. That would be a medical trial having clear relation to the treatment or protection of the child himself. He is not made, without his consent, the subject of medical investigations of possible benefit only to other children, other patients, or for the future advancement of medical science.

These may have been the circumstances surrounding the field trial of the vaccine for rubella (German measles) made in Taiwan, if this was in epidemic conditions, or in expectation of epidemic conditions, early in 1968 by a medical team from the University of Washington, headed by Dr. Thomas Grayston.[1] The vaccine was given to 3,269 young grade-school boys in the cities of Taipei and Taichung, while roughly an equal number were left unvaccinated for comparison purposes. The latter group were given Salk polio vaccine so that they would derive some benefit from the experience to which they were subjected. This generous "payment" does not alter the moral dilemma of withholding the rubella vaccine from a selected group. Yet there may have been an equipoise between the hazards of contracting rubella or other damage from the vaccine and the hazards of contracting it if not vaccinated. There could have been a likelihood favoring the vaccinated of the two comparison groups.

These considerations, we may suppose, produced the quandary in the conscience of the investigators that was partially relieved by giving the unrelated Salk vaccine to the control group. Such equipoise alone would warrant—and it would sufficiently warrant—a parent or guardian in consenting that his child or ward be used for these research purposes. In the face of actual or predictable epidemic conditions, this would be medical investigation having some measurable or immeasurable relation to a child's own treatment or protection, as surely as the catheterization of the heart of a child with congenital heart trouble may be needed in his own diagnosis and treatment; and to this type of treatment a parent may venture to consent in his child's behalf. If no gulf is to be fixed between maladies beneath the skin and diseases afflicting children as members of a population, then the consent-requirement means: "Never submit children to medical investigation not related to their own treatment, except in face of epidemic conditions, endangering also each individual child." This is simply the meaning of the consent-requirement in application, not a "quantity-of-benefit-to-come" exception clause or a violation of this canon of loyalty to child-patients.

Indeed, a stricter construction of the necessary connection between proxy consent and the foreseeable needs of the child would permit the use of only girl children in field trials of rubella vaccine. Rubella is not the most contagious type of measles. The benefit to the subjects used in these trials (which plus the consent of parents legitimated subjecting them to experiment) was mainly to prevent their giving birth to children with congenital malformations should they later contract rubella during pregnancy. Therefore, there was stronger argument for considering only girl children as part of a population in establishing the necessary connection between experiment and "treatment."

More questionable were the earlier trials of the rubella vaccine performed upon the inmates of a retarded children's home in Conway, Arkansas. These subjects were not specially endangered by an epidemic of rubella. Few of the girls among them will ever be able to become part of the population of child-bearing women, or be in danger of pregnancy while in institutions. Using them simply had the advantage that they were segregated from the rest of the population, and any degree of risk to them would not spread to other people, including women of child-bearing age.

If children are incapable of truly consenting to experiments having unknown hazards for the sake of good to come, and if no one else should consent for them in cases unrelated to their own treatment, then medical research and society in general must choose a perhaps more difficult course of action to gain the benefits we seek from medical investigations. Surely it was possible to secure normal adult volunteers to consent to segregate themselves from the rest of the population for the duration of a rubella trial.[2] That method was simply more costly and inconvenient. At the same time, this illustrates the general fact that if we as a society are to proceed to the conquest of diseases, indeed, if we are to teach medical skills with fairness and justice to the poor and the ward patients, and with no violation of the basic claims of childhood, then there must be far greater encouragement generally in our society of a willingness to engage as joint adventurers for medical progress than has been achieved, or believed morally required by the principle of consent, in the past....

NOTES

1 *New York Times,* October 17, 1968.
2 *New York Times,* April 5, 1969, reported that a hundred monks and nuns, from both Anglican and Roman Catholic orders, living in enclosed communities, were the voluntary subjects in testing American, British, and Belgian vaccines against German measles. This project was organized and directed by Dr. J. A. Dudgeon of London's Great Ormond Street Hospital for Sick Children.

Proxy Consent in the Experimentation Situation

Richard A. McCormick

Richard A. McCormick, S.J., a moral theologian, is Rose F. Kennedy Professor of Christian Ethics at the Kennedy Institute, Georgetown University. He is the author of *Ambiguity in Moral Choice* (1973) and *How Brave a New World: Dilemmas in Bioethics* (1981). McCormick's articles include "Fetal Research and Public Policy" and "Transplantation of Organs: A Comment on Paul Ramsey."

McCormick maintains that some cases of nontherapeutic pediatric research are justified even when participation in that research does not benefit the child, despite the fact that the child is incapable of giving informed consent. McCormick first reviews the legal and moral considerations raised by research using children. His discussion of the ethical literature on the topic includes a summary of Paul Ramsey's position. McCormick considers Ramsey to be the strongest proponent of the view that rejects the validity of proxy consent to nonbeneficial pediatric experiments. McCormick argues that parents can give a valid proxy consent to nontherapeutic pediatric research when (1) the risks of such research are minimal and (2) the potential benefits to children as a group may be very great. McCormick's claim is based on his "natural law" ethics. Human beings are, by their very nature, social beings. As social beings, they are mutually interdependent. As mutually interdependent beings, they owe it to each other to perform certain minimal moral duties. Included in these moral duties is the duty to participate in minimally risky nontherapeutic research, whose benefit to society as a whole may be very great. Children as members of society also have these obligations, although they are too young to recognize them. Since children, like adults, should want to promote the greater social good, it is morally acceptable for their parents to consent to their participation in minimally risky experiments.

It is widely admitted within the research community that if there is to be continuing and proportionate progress in pediatric medicine, experimentation is utterly essential. This conviction rests on two closely interrelated facts. First, as Alexander Capron has pointed out [1], "Children cannot be regarded simply as 'little people' pharmacologically. Their metabolism, enzymatic and excretory systems, skeletal development and so forth differ so markedly from adults' that drug tests for the latter provide inadequate information about dosage, efficacy, toxicity, side effects, and contraindications for children." Second, and consequently, there is a limit to the usefulness of prior experimentation with animals and adults. At some point or other, experimentation with children becomes necessary.

LEGAL CONSIDERATION

At this point, however, a severe problem arises. The legal and moral legitimacy of experimentation (understood here as procedures involving no direct benefit to the person participating in the experiment) is founded above all on the informed consent of the subject. But in many instances, the young subject is either legally or factually incapable of consent. Furthermore, it is argued, the parents are neither legally nor morally capable of supplying this consent for the child. As Dr. Donald T. Chalkley of the National Institutes of Health puts it: "A parent has no legal right to give consent for the involvement of his child in an activity not for the benefit of that child. No legal guardian, no person

Reprinted with permission of the author and the publisher from *Perspectives in Biology and Medicine*, vol. 18, no. 1 (Autumn 1974), pp. 2–20. Copyright © 1974 by the University of Chicago.

standing *in loco parentis,* has that right" [2]. It would seem to follow that infants and some minors are simply out of bounds where clinical research is concerned. Indeed, this conclusion has been explicitly drawn by the well-known ethician Paul Ramsey. He notes: "If children are incapable of truly consenting to experiments having unknown hazards for the sake of good to come, and if no one else should consent for them in cases unrelated to their own treatment, then medical research and society in general must choose a perhaps more difficult course of action to gain the benefits we seek from medical investigations" [3, p. 17].

Does the consent requirement taken seriously exclude all experiments on children? If it does, then children themselves will be the ultimate sufferers. If it does not, what is the moral justification for the experimental procedures? The problem is serious, for, as Ramsey notes, an investigation involving children as subjects is "a prismatic case in which to tell whether we mean to take seriously the consent-requirement" [3, p. 28].

Before concluding with Shirkey that those incompetent of consent are "therapeutic orphans" [4], I should like to explore the notion and validity of proxy consent. More specifically, the interest here is in the question, Can and may parents consent, and to what extent, to experiments on their children where the procedures are nonbeneficial for the child involved? Before approaching this question, it is necessary to point out the genuine if restricted input of the ethician in such matters. Ramsey has rightly pointed up the difference between the ethics of consent and ethics in the consent situation. This latter refers to the meaning and practical applications of the requirement of an informed consent. It is the work of prudence and pertains to the competence and responsibility of physicians and investigators. The former, on the other hand, refers to the principle requiring an informed consent, the ethics of consent itself. Such moral principles are elaborated out of competences broader than those associated with the medical community.

A brief review of the literature will reveal that the question raised above remains in something of a legal and moral limbo. The *Nuremburg Code* states only that "the voluntary consent of the human subject is absolutely essential. This means that the person involved should have legal capacity to give consent" [5]. Nothing specific is said about infants or those who are mentally incompetent. Dr. Leon Alexander, who aided

in drafting the first version of the *Nuremberg Code,* explained subsequently that his provision for valid consent from next of kin where mentally ill patients are concerned was dropped by the Nuremberg judges, "probably because they did not apply in the specific cases under trial" [3, p.26; 6]. Be that as it may, it has been pointed out by Beecher [5, p. 231] that a strict observance of Nuremberg's rule 1 would effectively cripple study of mental disease and would simply prohibit all experimentation on children.[1]

The *International Code of Medical Ethics* (General Assembly of the World Medical Association, 1949) states simply: "Under no circumstances is a doctor permitted to do anything that would weaken the physical or mental resistance of a human being except from strictly therapeutic or prophylactic indications imposed in the interest of his patient" [5, p. 236]. This statement is categorical and if taken literally means that "young children and the mentally incompetent are categorically excluded from all investigations except those that directly may benefit the subjects" [7]. However, in 1954 the General Assembly of the World Medical Association (in *Principles for Those in Research and Experimentation*) stated: "It should be required that each person who submits to experimentation be informed of the nature, the reason for, and the risk of the proposed experiment. If the patient is irresponsible, consent should be obtained from the individual who is legally responsible for the individual" [5, p. 240]. In the context it is somewhat ambiguous whether this statement is meant to apply beyond experimental procedures that are performed for the patient's good.

The *Declaration of Helsinki* (1964) is much clearer on the point. After distinguishing "clinical research combined with professional care" and "non-therapeutic clinical research," it states of this latter: "Clinical research on a human being cannot be undertaken without his free consent, after he has been fully informed; if he is legally incompetent the consent of the legal guardian should be procured" [5, p. 278]. In 1966 the American Medical Association, in its *Principles of Medical Ethics,* endorsed the Helsinki statement. It distinguished clinical investigation "primarily for treatment" and clinical investigation "primarily for the accumulation of scientific knowledge." With regard to this latter, it noted that "consent, in writing, should be obtained from the subject, or from his legally authorized representative if the subject lacks the capacity to consent." More specifically, with regard to minors or mentally incompetent persons, the AMA statement reads: "Consent, in writing, is given by a legally authorized representative of the subject under circumstances in which an informed and prudent adult would reasonably be expected to volunteer himself or his child as a subject" [5, p. 223].

In 1963, the Medical Research Council of Great Britain issued its *Responsibility in Investigations on Human Subjects* [5, pp. 262 ff.]. Under title of "Procedures Not of Direct Benefit to the Individual" the Council stated: "The situation in respect of minors and mentally subnormal or mentally disordered persons is of particular difficulty. In the strict view of the law parents and guardians of minors cannot give consent on their behalf to any procedures which are of no particular benefit to them and which may carry some risk of harm." Then, after discussing consent as involving a full understanding of "the implications to himself of the procedures to which he was consenting," the Council concluded: "When true consent in this sense cannot be obtained, procedures which are of no direct benefit and which might carry a risk of harm to the subject should not be undertaken." If it is granted that every experiment involves some risk, then the MRC statement would exclude any experiment on children. Curran and Beecher have pointed out [8] that this strict reading of English law is based on the advice of Sir Harvey Druitt, though there is no statute or case law to support it. Nevertheless, it has gone relatively unchallenged.

Statements of the validity of proxy consent similar to those of the *Declaration of Helsinki* and the American Medical Association have been issued by the American Psychological Association [5, pp. 256 ff.] and the Food and Drug Administration [5, pp. 299 ff.]. The most recent formulation touching on proxy consent is that of the Department of Health, Education, and Welfare in its *Protection of Human Subjects, Policies, and Procedures* [9]. In situations where the subject cannot himself give consent, the document refers to "supplementary judgment." It states: "For the purposes of this document, supplementary judgment will refer to judgments made by local committees in addition to the subject's consent (when possible) and that of the parents or legal guardian (where applicable), as to whether or not a subject may participate in clinical research." The DHEW proposed guidelines admit that the law on parental consent is not clear in all respects. Proxy consent is valid with regard to established and generally accepted therapeutic procedures; it is, in practice, valid for therapeutic research. However, the guidelines state that "when research might expose a subject to risk without defined therapeutic benefit or other positive effect on that subject's well-being, parental or guardian consent appears to be insufficient." These statements about validity concern law, in the sense (I would judge) of what would happen should a case determination be provoked on the basis of existing precedent.

MEDICAL ETHICS

After this review of the legal validity of proxy consent and its limitations, the DHEW guidelines go on to draw two ethical conclusions. First, "When the risk of a proposed study is generally considered not significant, and the potential benefit is explicit, the ethical issues need not preclude the participation of children in biomedical research." Presumably, this means that where there is risk, ethical issues do preclude the use of children. However, the DHEW document did not draw this conclusion. Rather, its second ethical conclusion states: "An investigator proposing research activities which expose children to risk must document, as part of the application for support, that the information to be gained can be obtained in no other way. The investigator must also stipulate either that the risk to the subjects will be insignificant or that, although some risk exists, the potential benefit is significant and far outweighs that risk. In no case will research activities be approved which entail substantial risk except in the cases of clearly therapeutic procedures." These proposed guidelines admit, therefore, three levels of risk within the ethical calculus: insignificant risk, some risk, and substantial risk. Proxy consent is, by inference, ethically acceptable for the first two levels but not for the third.

The documents cited move almost imperceptibly back and forth between legal and moral considerations, so that it is often difficult to know whether the major concern is one or the other, or even how the relationship of the legal and ethical is conceived. Nevertheless, it can be said that there has been a gradual move away from the absolutism represented in the *Nuremberg Code* to the acceptance of proxy consent, possibly because the *Nuremberg Code* is viewed as containing, to some extent, elements of a reaction to the Nazi experiments.

Medical literature of the noncodal variety has revealed this same pattern of ambiguity. For instance, writing in the *Lancet,* Dr. R. E. W. Fisher reacted to the reports of the use of children in research procedures as follows: "No medical procedure involving the slightest risk or accompanied by the slightest physical or mental pain may be inflicted on a child for experimental purposes unless there is a reasonable chance, or at least a hope, that the child may benefit thereby"[10]. On the other hand, Franz J. Ingelfinger, editor of the *New England Journal of Medicine,* contends that the World Medical Association's statement ("Under no circumstances... "[above]) is an extremist position that must be modified [7]. His suggested modification reads: "Only when the risks are small and justifiable is a doctor permitted...." It is difficult to know from Ingelfinger's wording whether he means small and therefore justifiable or whether "justifiable" refers to the hoped-for benefit. Responses to this editorial were contradictory. N. Baumslag and R. W. Yodaiken state: "In our opinion there are no conditions under which any children may be used for experimentation not primarily designed for their benefit" [11]. Ian Shine, John Howieson, and Ward Griffen, Jr., came to the opposite conclusion: "We strongly support his [Ingelfinger's] proposals provided that one criterion of 'small and justifiable risks' is the willingness of the experimentor to be an experimentee, or to offer a spouse or child when appropriate" [12].

Curran and Beecher had earlier disagreed strongly with the rigid interpretation given the statement of the Medical Research Council through Druitt's influence. Their own conclusion was that "children under 14 may participate in clinical investigation which is not for their benefit where the studies are sound, promise important new knowledge for mankind, and there is no discernible risk"[8, p. 81]. The editors of *Archives of Disease in Childhood* recently endorsed this same conclusion, adding only "the necessity of informed parental consent" [13]. Discussing relatively minor procedures such as weighing a baby, skin pricks, venipunctures, etc., they contend that "whether or not these procedures are acceptable must depend, it seems to us, on whether the potential gain to others is commensurate with the discomfort to the individual." They see the Medical Research Council's statement as an understandable but exaggerated reaction to the shocking disclosures of the Nazi era. A new value judgment is required in our time, one based on the low risk/benefit ratio.

This same attitude is proposed by Alan M. W. Porter [14]. He argues that there are grounds "for believing that it may be permissible and reasonable to undertake minor procedures on children for experimental purposes with the permission of the parents." The low risk/benefit ratio is the ultimate justification. Interestingly, Porter reports the reactions of colleagues and the public to a research protocol he had drawn up. He desired to study the siblings of children who had succumbed to "cot death." The research involved venipuncture. A pediatric authority told Porter that venipuncture was inadmissible under the Medical Research Council code. Astonished, Porter showed the protocol to the first 10 colleagues he met. The instinctive reaction of nine out of 10 was "Of course you may." Similarly, a professional market researcher asked (for Porter) 10 laymen about the procedure, and all responded that he could proceed. In other words, Porter argues that public opinion (and therefore, presumably, moral common sense) stands behind the low risk/benefit ratio approach to experimentation on children.

This sampling is sufficient indication of the variety of reactions likely to be encountered when research on children is discussed.

THE VIEWS OF ETHICIANS

The professional ethicians who have written on this subject have also drawn rather different conclusions. John Fletcher argues that a middle path between autonomy (of the physician) and heteronomy (external control) must be discovered [15]. The Nuremberg rule "does not take account of exceptions which can be controlled and makes no allowance whatsoever for the exercise of professional judgment." It is clear that Fletcher would accept proxy consent in some instances, though he has not fully specified what these would be.

Thomas J. O'Donnell, S.J., notes that, besides informed consent, we also speak of three other modalities of consent [16]. First, there is presumed consent. Life-saving measures that are done on an unconscious patient in an emergency room are done with presumed consent. Second, there is implied consent. The various tests done on a person who undergoes a general checkup are done with implied consent, the consent being contained and implied in the very fact of his coming for a checkup. Finally, there is vicarious consent. This is the case of the parent who consents for therapy on an infant. O'Donnell wonders whether these modalities of consent, already accepted in the therapeutic context, can be extended to the context of clinical investigation (and by this he means research not to the direct benefit of the child). It is his conclusion that vicarious consent can be ethically operative "provided it is contained within the strict limits of a presumed consent (on the part of the subject) proper to clinical research and much narrower than the presumptions that might be valid in a therapeutic context." Practically, this means that O'Donnell would accept the validity of vicarious consent only where "danger is so remote and discomfort so minimal that a normal and informed individual would be presupposed to give ready consent." O'Donnell discusses neither the criteria nor the analysis that would set the "strict limits of a presumed consent."

Princeton's Paul Ramsey is the ethician who has discussed this problem at greatest length [3].[2] He is in clear disagreement with the positions of Fletcher and O'Donnell. Ramsey denies the validity of proxy consent in nonbeneficial (to the child) experiments simply and without qualification. Why? We may not, he argues, submit a child either to procedures that involve any measure of risk of harm or to procedures that involve no harm but simply "offensive touching." "A subject can be wronged without being harmed," he writes. This occurs whenever he is used as an object, or as a means only rather than also as an end in himself. Parents cannot consent to this type of thing, regardless of the significance of the experiment. Ramsey sees the morality of experimentation on children to be exactly what Paul Freund has described as the law on the matter: "The law here is that parents may consent for the child if the invasion of the child's body is for the child's welfare or benefit" [17, 18].

In pursuit of his point, Ramsey argues as follows: "To attempt to consent for a child to be made an experimental subject is to treat a child as not a child. It is to treat him as if he were an adult person who has consented to become a joint adventurer in the common cause of medical research. If the grounds for this are alleged to be the presumptive or implied consent of the child, that must simply be characterized as a violent and a false presumption." Thus, he concludes simply that "no parent is morally competent to consent that his child shall be submitted to hazardous *or other experiments* having no diagnostic or therapeutic significance for the child himself" (emphasis added). Though he does not say so, Ramsey would certainly

conclude that a law that tolerates proxy consent to any purely experimental procedure is one without moral warrants, indeed, is immoral because it legitimates (or tries to) treating a human being as a means only.

A careful study, then, of the legal, medical, and ethical literature on proxy consent for nontherapeutic research on children reveals profoundly diverging views. Generally, the pros and cons are spelled out in terms of two important values: individual integrity and societal good through medical benefits. Furthermore, in attempting to balance these two values, this literature by and large either affirms or denies the moral legitimacy of a risk/benefit ratio, what ethicians refer to as a teleological calculus. It seems to me that in doing this, current literature has not faced this tremendously important and paradigmatic issue at its most fundamental level. For instance, Ramsey bases his prohibitive position on the contention that nonbeneficial experimental procedures make an "object" of an individual. In these cases, he contends, parents cannot consent for the individual. Consent is the heart of the matter. If the parents could legitimately consent for the child, then presumably experimental procedures would not make an object of the infant and would be permissible. Therefore, the basic question seems to be, Why cannot the parents provide consent for the child? Why is their consent considered null here while it is accepted when procedures are therapeutic? To say that the child would be treated as an object does not answer this question; it seems that it presupposes the answer and announces it under this formulation.

TRADITIONAL MORAL THEOLOGY

There is in traditional moral theology a handle that may allow us to take hold of this problem at a deeper root and arrive at a principled and consistent position, one that takes account of all the values without arbitrarily softening or suppressing any of them. That handle is the notion of parental consent, particularly the theoretical implications underlying it. If this can be unpacked a bit, perhaps a more satisfying analysis will emerge. Parental consent is required and sufficient for therapy directed at the child's own good. We refer to this as vicarious consent. It is closely related to presumed consent. That is, it is morally valid precisely insofar as it is a reasonable presumption of the child's wishes, a construction of what the child would wish could he consent for himself. But here the notion of "what the child would wish" must be pushed further if we are to avoid a simple imposition of the adult world on the child. Why *would* the child so wish? The answer seems to be that he would choose this if he were capable of choice because he *ought* to do so. This statement roots in a traditional natural-law understanding of human moral obligations and calls for a brief explanation.

Here I shall summarize briefly what has been explained at great length by other authors. The first thing that should be said is that moral convictions do not originate from discursive analyses or arguments. Let us take slavery as an example. We do not hold that slavery is humanly demeaning and immoral chiefly because we have argued to this discursively. Rather, first our sensitivities are sharpened to the meaning and value of human persons. We then experience the out-of-jointness, inequality, and injustice of slavery. We then judge it to be wrong. At this point we develop "arguments" to criticize, modify, and above all communicate this judgment. Reflective analysis or discursive reasoning is an attempt to reinforce rationally, communicably, and from other sources what we grasp at a different level. Discursive reflection does not discover the good but only analyzes it. The good that reason seems to discover is the good that was already hidden in the original intuition.

This calls for explanation. How do we arrive at definite moral obligations, moral prescriptions, and prohibitions? How does the general thrust of our persons toward good and away from evil become concrete, even as concrete as a code of dos and don'ts and caveats? Somewhat as follows—and in this I am following very closely, even verbally at times, the school of J. de Finance, G. de Broglie, G. Grisez, John Finnis, and others who have deep roots in Thomistic philosophy. We proceed by asking what are the goods or values man can seek, the values that define his human opportunity, his flourishing? We can answer this by examining man's basic tendencies, for it is impossible to act without having an interest in the object, and it is impossible to be attracted by, to have interest in, something without some inclination already present. What then are the basic inclinations?

With no pretense at being exhaustive, we could list some of the following as basic inclinations present prior to acculturation: the tendency to preserve life; the tendency to mate and raise children; the tendency to explore and question; the tendency to seek out other men and seek their approval, that is, friendship; the tendency to establish good relations with unknown higher powers; the tendency to use intelligence in guiding action; the tendency to develop skills and exercise them in play and the fine arts. In these inclinations our intelligence spontaneously and without reflection grasps the possibilities or goods to which they point, and prescribes them. Thus, we form naturally and without reflection the basic principles of practical or moral reasoning. Or, as philosopher John Finnis renders it: "What is spontaneously understood when one turns from contemplation to action is not a set of Kantian or neoscholastic 'moral principles' identifying this as right and that as wrong, but a set of values which can be expressed in the form of principles such as 'life is a good-to-be-pursued and realized and what threatens it is to be avoided'" [19, p. 373]....

In summary, then, the natural-law tradition argues that there are certain identifiable values that we *ought* to support, attempt to realize, and never directly suppress because they are definitive of our flourishing and well-being. It further argues that knowledge of these values and of the prescriptions and proscriptions associated with them is, in principle, available to human reason. That is, they require for their discovery no divine revelation.

MORAL LEGITIMACY OF PROXY CONSENT

What does all this have to do with the moral legitimacy of proxy consent? It was noted that parental (proxy, vicarious) consent is required and sufficient for therapy directed to the child's own good. It was further noted that it is morally valid precisely insofar as it is a reasonable presumption of the child's wishes, a construction of what the child would wish could he do so. Finally, it was suggested that the child *would* wish this therapy because he *ought* to do so. In other words, a construction of what the child *would* wish (presumed consent) is not an exercise in adult capriciousness and arbitrariness, subject to an equally capricious denial or challenge when the child comes of age. It is based, rather, on two assertions: *(a)* that there are certain values (in this case life itself) definitive of our good and flourishing, hence values that we *ought* to choose and support if we want to become and stay human, and that therefore these are good also for the child; and *(b)* that these "ought" judgments, at least in their more general formulations, are a common patronage available to all men, and hence form the basis on which policies can be built.

Specifically, then, I would argue that parental consent is morally legitimate where therapy on the child is involved precisely because we know that life and health are goods for the child, that he *would* choose them because he *ought* to choose the good of life, his own self-preservation as long as this life remains, all things considered, a human good. To see whether and to what extent this type of moral analysis applies to experimentation, we must ask, Are there other things that the child *ought,* as a human being, to choose precisely because and insofar as they are goods definitive of his growth and flourishing? Concretely, *ought* he to choose his own involvement in nontherapeutic experimentation, and to what extent? Certainly there are goods or benefits, at least potential, involved. But are they goods that the child *ought* to choose? Or again, if we can argue that a certain level of involvement in nontherapeutic experimentation is good for the child and therefore that he *ought* to choose it, then there are grounds for saying that parental consent for this is morally legitimate and should be recognized as such.

Perhaps a beginning can be made as follows. To pursue the good that is human life means not only to choose and support this value in one's own case, but also in the case of others when the opportunity arises. In other words, the individual *ought* also to take into account, realize, make efforts in behalf of the lives of others also, for we are social beings and the goods that define our growth and invite to it are goods that reside also in others. It can be good for one to pursue and support this good in others. Therefore, when it factually is good, we may say that one *ought* to do so (as opposed to not doing so). If this is true of all of us up to a point and within limits, it is no less true of the infant. He would choose to do so because he *ought* to do so. Now, to support and realize the value that is life means to support and realize health, the cure of disease, and so on. Therefore, up to a point, this support and realization is good for all of us individually. To share in the general effort and burden of health maintenance and disease control is part of our flourishing and growth as humans. To the extent that it is good for all of us to share this burden, we all *ought* to do so. And to the extent that we *ought* to do so, it is a reasonable construction or presumption of our wishes to say that we would do so. The reasonableness of this presumption validates vicarious consent.

It was just noted that sharing in the common burden of progress in medicine constitutes an individual good for all of us *up to a point.* That qualification is crucially important. It suggests that there are limits beyond which sharing is not or might not be a good. What might be the limits of this sharing? When might it no longer be a good for all individuals and therefore something that all need not choose to do? I would develop the matter as follows.

Adults may donate *(inter vivos)* an organ precisely because their personal good is not to be conceived individualistically but socially, that is, there is a natural order to other human persons which is in the very notion of the human personality itself. The personal being and good of an individual do have a relationship to the being and good of others, difficult as it may be to keep this in a balanced perspective. For this reason, an individual can become (in carefully delimited circumstances) more fully a person by donation of an organ, for by communicating to another of his very being he has more fully integrated himself into the mysterious unity between person and person.

Something similar can be said of participation in nontherapeutic experimentation. It can be an affirmation of one's solidarity and Christian concern for others (through advancement of medicine). Becoming an experimental subject can involve any or all of three things: some degree of risk (at least of complications), pain, and associated inconvenience (e.g., prolonging hospital stay, delaying recovery, etc.). To accept these for the good of others could be an act of charitable concern.

There are two qualifications to these general statements that must immediately be made, and these qualifications explain the phrase "up to a point." First, whether it is personally good for an individual to donate an organ or participate in experimentation is a very circumstantial and therefore highly individual affair. For some individuals, these undertakings could be or prove to be humanly destructive. Much depends on their personalities, past family life, maturity, future position in life, etc. The second and more important qualification is that these procedures become human goods for the donor or subject precisely because and therefore only when they are voluntary, for the personal good under discussion is the good of expressed charity. For these two reasons I would conclude that no one else can make such decisions for an individual, that is, reasonably presume his consent. He has a right to make them for himself. In other words, whether a person *ought* to do such things is a highly individual affair and cannot be generalized in the way the good of self-preservation can be. And if we cannot say of an individual that he *ought* to do these things, proxy consent has no reasonable presumptive basis.

But are there situations where such considerations are not involved and where the presumption of consent is reasonable, because we may continue to say of all individuals that (other things being equal) they *ought* to be willing? I believe so. For instance, where organ donation is involved, if the only way a young child could be saved were by a blood transfusion from another child, I suspect that few would find such blood donation an unreasonable presumption on the child's wishes. The reason for the presumption is, I believe, that a great good is provided for another at almost no cost to the child. As the scholastics put it, *parum pro nihilo reputatur* ("very little counts for nothing"). For this reason we may say, lacking countervailing individual evidence, that the individual *ought* to do this.

Could the same reasoning apply to experimentation? Concretely, when a particular experiment would involve no discernible risks, no notable pain, no notable inconvenience, and yet hold promise of considerable benefit, should not the child be constructed to wish this in the same way we presume he chooses his own life, because he *ought* to? I believe so. He *ought* to want this not because it is in any way for his own medical good, but because it is not in any realistic way to his harm, and represents a potentially great benefit for others. He *ought* to want these benefits for others.

WHAT THEY OUGHT TO WANT

If this is a defensible account of the meaning and limits of presumed consent where those incompetent to consent are concerned, it means that proxy consent can be morally legitimate in some experimentations. Which? Those that are scientifically well designed (and therefore offer hope of genuine benefit), that cannot succeed unless children are used (because there are dangers involved in interpreting terms such as "discernible" and "negligible," the child should not unnecessarily be exposed to these even minimal risks), that contain no discernible risk or undue discomfort for the child. Here it must be granted that the notions of "discernible risk" and "undue discomfort" are themselves slippery and difficult, and probably somewhat relative. They certainly involve a value judgment and one that is the heavy responsibility of the medical profession (not the

moral theologian) to make. For example, perhaps it can be debated whether venipuncture involves "discernible risks" or "undue discomfort" or not. But if it can be concluded that, in human terms, the risk involved or the discomfort is negligible or insignificant, then I believe there are sound reasons in moral analysis for saying that parental consent to this type of invasion can be justified.

Practically, then, I think there are good moral warrants for adopting the position espoused by Curran, Beecher, Ingelfinger, the *Helsinki Declaration,* the *Archives of Disease in Childhood,* and others. Some who have adopted this position have argued it in terms of a low risk/benefit ratio. This is acceptable if properly understood, that is, if "low risk" means for all practical purposes and in human judgment "no realistic risk." If it is interpreted in any other way, it opens the door wide to a utilitarian subordination of the individual to the collectivity. It goes beyond what individuals would want because they *ought* to. For instance, in light of the above analysis, I find totally unacceptable the DHEW statement that "the investigator must also stipulate either that the risk to the subjects will be insignificant, or that *although some risk exists, the potential benefit is significant and far outweighs that risk."* This goes beyond what all of us, as members of the community, necessarily *ought* to do. Therefore, it is an invalid basis for proxy consent. For analogous reasons, in light of the foregoing analysis I would conclude that parental consent for a kidney transplant from one noncompetent 3-year-old to another is without moral justification.

In arguing a position that would not allow even that amount of experimentation on children proposed here, Ramsey has stated that this presumptive consent "must simply be characterized as a violent and a false presumption" [3, p. 14]. In developing his thought, he states that "a well child, or a child not suffering from an unrelated disease not being investigated, is not to be compared to an unconscious patient needing specific treatment. To imply the latter's 'constructive' consent is not a violent presumption, it is a life-saving presumption, though it is in some degree 'false'." A careful analysis of this argument will reveal that for Ramsey the presumption is nonviolent precisely because it is life saving for the individual. Furthermore, he would in logic have to argue that whatever invasion is not life saving for the individual concerned is violent if the individual does not consent thereto. I have attempted to show that this is too narrow. Rather, I would suggest that the presumption of consent to this life-saving therapy is nonviolent, not precisely and exclusively because it is life saving but because, being such, it is something the individual would want because he *ought* to want it. I would further propose that there are good warrants for saying that there are other things an individual, as a social being, *ought* to want, and, to the extent that we may say this of him, then presumption of his consent is nonviolent, that is, reasonable.

This point is at the heart of the discussion and calls for a rewording. Ramsey does not believe we may "construct" or presume an infant's consent in non-beneficial experimentation because submission to such experimentation pertains to the realm of charity; and one may not construe that an individual is consenting to works of charity [20].

His argument moves in two steps. First, there is, he notes, "a difference between justice and charity. Charity, of course, is of highest excellence. But the thing one must imply about a child is not that he's charitable. In other words, let's not confuse the realms of nature and grace. You don't imply he's charitable. That comes by grace. That's his moral maturity. Later he can be charitable. Charity is itself not something one can extrapolate and presume to be the good of this child."

Second, to buttress this point, Ramsey attempts to see where such constructive consent would take us if once we allow it for any nonbeneficial experimentation. "Just think of the kind of constructive consents we could imply for children. You can imply, you can construe, that out of all charity this fetus doesn't want to be born because it's the seventeenth. If he's got any sense he doesn't want to fatally increase the poverty of his home....I do not see where one could rationally stop in construing all sorts of works of mercy and self-sacrifice on the part of persons, not themselves capable by nature or grace yet of being the subjects of charity."

This is a very strong argument and deserves to be taken with utmost seriousness. However, I believe some qualification is called for. Does all nonbeneficial experimentation on this infant pertain to what Ramsey calls "charitable works"? By this term, Ramsey obviously refers to works of supererogation, works that not all men just by being members of the human race are held to or *ought* to do. This is the key. It can be argued, and I think successfully, that there are some things that all of us, simply as members of the human community, *ought* to do for others. These are not works of supererogation, nor works of "charity" in this

sense. Here the problem of semantics intrudes. If any involvement in nontherapeutic experimentation must be said to be "charitable" (in the strict sense, i.e., beyond what is required of all of us and supererogatory), then Ramsey is correct. But some of these choices seem to pertain to the area of social justice, one's personal bearing of his share of the burden that all may flourish and prosper. Therefore, they are choices that all *ought* to make. In other words, these choices do not pertain to charity, or not at least to charity in Ramsey's sense, a sense where ordinary, non-heroic responses get collapsed into and identified with heroic and extraordinary responses.

The distinction I am suggesting, therefore, is that between those works that not all of us can be expected to make and those that all of us can be expected to make. To the former category belong choices involving notable risk, discomfort, inconvenience. Whether it is good for one to make these choices, whether therefore he *ought* to make them, is a highly circumstantial affair and cannot be said of all of us in general. These are the works to which, theologically, the particular invitations of the Spirit inspire. They are the works of individual generosity and charity. No presumptive consent is in place here.

But we can establish a baseline and discover other works that involve no notable disadvantages to individuals yet offer genuine hope for general benefit. It is good for all of us to share in these (unless we are by particular and accidental circumstances so weakened that even trivial procedures would constitute a threat to us) and hence we all *ought* to want these benefits for others. And if that is true, a presumption of consent is reasonable and vicarious consent becomes legitimate. In summary, there are some experiments in children that do not pertain to charity in Ramsey's sense— charity as supererogation—and hence do not demand individualization before they can be said to be goods the individual would choose.

Now to Ramsey's second buttressing argument—the slippery slope. "I do not see where one could rationally stop in construing all sorts of works of mercy and self-sacrifice, etc." One stops and should stop precisely at the point where "constructed" consent does indeed involve self-sacrifice or works of mercy, the point beyond which not all of us are called but only individuals inspired by the Spirit to do "the more," the sacrificial thing. This dividing line is reached when experiments involve discernible risk, undue discomfort, or inconvenience.

Ramsey's reluctance or inability to make this distinction is traceable to the fact that he has not analyzed more deeply the validity of proxy consent in therapeutic situations. He states: "An 'implied' or 'constructive' consent—proxy consent—clearly is in order in the case of investigational therapeutic trials (beneficial research) when the patient/subject is incapable for any reason of giving actual consent." True. But why true? If one answers, as Ramsey does, that it is true because where therapeutic research is involved the patient/subject *would* give consent, he has not gone far enough. The patient *would* give consent because therapeutic research is (or can be) something for his own good and to which, therefore, he *ought* to consent. Reasonable presumption or construction of consent is rooted in this. And it suggests immediately the possibility that there may be other procedures which are not necessarily to the individual's therapeutic good but still represent a good to others, a good to which he, like all of us, ought also to consent. Once, therefore, the validity of proxy consent is traced to its deepest roots, we will see both its further legitimate extensions and its limitations.

These considerations do not mean that all noncompetents (where consent is concerned) may be treated in the same way, that the same presumptions are morally legitimate in all cases. For if the circumstances of the infant or child differ markedly, then it is possible that there are appropriate modifications in our construction of what he *ought* to choose. For instance, I believe that institutionalized infants demand special consideration. They are in a situation of peculiar danger for several reasons. First, they are often in a disadvantaged condition physically or mentally so that there is a temptation to regard them as "lesser human beings." Medical history shows our vulnerability to this type of judgment. Second, as institutionalized, they are a controlled group, making them particularly tempting as research subjects. Third, experimentation in such infants is less exposed to public scrutiny. These and other considerations suggest that there is a real danger of overstepping the line between what we all ought to want and what only the individual might want out of heroic, self-sacrificial charity. If such a real danger exists, then what the infant is construed as wanting because he *ought* must be modified. He need not *ought to want* if this involves him in real dangers of going beyond this point....

...[A]n ethics of consent finds its roots in a solid natural-law tradition which maintains that there are basic values that define our potential as human beings; that we ought (within limits and with qualifications) to choose, support, and never directly suppress these values in our conduct; that we can know, therefore, what others would choose (up to a point) because they ought; and that this knowledge is the basis for a soundly grounded and rather precisely limited proxy consent.

NOTES

1 Most of the codal documents subsequently cited can be found in [5].
2 Ramsey has also continued his discussion of this matter in *Biological Revolution: Theological Impact* (p. 51). This title contains the proceedings of a conference held April 6, 1973 (see [20]).

REFERENCES

1 A. Capron. *Clin. Res.*, 21:141, 1973.
2 *Med. World News*, June 8, 1973, p. 41.
3 P. Ramsey. *The patient as person.* New Haven, Conn.: Yale Univ. Press, 1970.
4 H. Shirkey. *J. Pediatr.*, 72:119, 1968.
5 H. K. Beecher, *Research and the individual.* Boston: Little, Brown, 1970.
6 L. Alexander. *Dis. Nerv. Syst.*, 27:62, 1966.
7 F. J. Ingelfinger, *N. Engl. J. Med.*, 288:791, 1973.
8 W. J. Curran and H. K. Beecher. *J. Am. Med. Ass.*, 210:77, 1969.
9 Department of Health, Education, and Welfare. *Federal Register*, 38:31738, 1973.
10 R. E. W. Fisher. *Lancet* (Letters), November 7, 1953, p. 993.
11 N. Baumslag and R. W. Yodaiken, *N. Engl. J. Med.* (Letters), 288:1247, 1973.
12 I. Shine, J. Howieson, and W. Griffen, Jr. *N. Engl. J. Med.* (Letters), 288:1248, 1973.
13 Editorial, *Arch. Dis. Child.*, 48:751, 1973.
14 A. W. Franklin, A. M. Porter, and D. N. Raine. *Br. Med. J.*, May 19, 1973, p. 402.
15 J. Fletcher, *Law Contemp. Probl.*, 32:620, 1967.
16 T. J. O'Donnell, *J. Am. Med. Ass.*, 227:73, 1974.
17 P. Freund, *N. Engl. J. Med.*, 273:691, 1965.
18 ———. *Trial*, 2:48, 1966.
19 J. Finnis. *Heythrop J.*, 11:373, 1970.
20 P. Ramsey. In: *Proceedings of the Institute for Theological Encounter with Science and Technology (ITEST)*, April 1973, n. 27.

Children's Dissent to Research—A Minor Matter?

Gregory E. Pence

Gregory E. Pence is coursemaster, Medical Ethics, School of Medicine, and a member of both the philosophy department and the institutional review board at the University of Alabama in Birmingham. His published articles include "Between Cold Logic and Naive Compassion—On Allowing Defective Babies to Die," and "Towards a Theory of Work."

Pence addresses a number of questions that institutional review boards (IRBs) must face in making judgments about the participation of minors under 18 in research. (An IRB consists of a set of individuals charged with scrutinizing new experimental protocols at hospitals and research centers. IRBs are required to review all research involving human subjects conducted at institutions doing research funded by DHEW under the Public Health Service Act and the Federal Food, Drug, and Cosmetic Act, as well as most research conducted or supported by other DHEW departments and agencies.) Pence identifies and discusses four moral perspectives found in the literature of biomedical ethics regarding minors' participation in research: (1) The Little Adult View, (2) The Ignorance View, (3) The Incompatibility View, and (4) The-Good-of-Others View. Pence then presents his own position, supporting the participation of minors in research but stressing the importance of honoring and safeguarding their dissent.

Research involving minors below the age of 18 presents special problems for institutional review boards. Compared with research, therapeutic procedures involving minors are relatively easy to justify. Parents often overrule children's dissent to therapy. Should parents similarly be able to overrule children's dissent to research? Furthermore, should child-subjects be *told* about participation in research? And, if they are told, should researchers obtain their agreement to participate?

Key concepts need definition before we can understand the real issues. The National Commission for the Protection of Human Subjects of Biomedical and Behavioral Research (the Commission) offered clarifying definitions.[2, at pp. 18-15] The Commission distinguished between (a) *research,* (b) *practice,* and (c) *nonvalidated practices* (innovative therapy). Many commentators have failed to make these distinctions, confusing research (intending no benefit to subjects) with nonvalidated practices (intending benefit to subjects). *Research* is designed to develop generalizable knowledge as illustrated by the cases below. *Practice* intends benefit to patients-subjects, e.g., giving isoniazid for tuberculosis. *Nonvalidated practices* also intend benefit to subject-patients, e.g., the use of a new, potentially superior anesthesia. Researchers commonly call nonvalidated practices "research," but this designation is confusing and leads to overly stringent restrictions on new practices intended to help patients. Henceforth, we will follow the Commission's terminology, using "research" to refer to attempts to obtain generalizable knowledge and not intending direct benefits to subjects. The question is when, if ever, the agreement and objections of subjects matter in research on children.[2]

The following cases illustrate some of the problems of research involving children. We shall refer to these cases to illustrate various points throughout the remainder of this discussion.[3]

Case I—Julian Roy   Julian Roy, a fifteen-year-old, broods restlessly as his mother drives to the county mental health center. At the center, Julian will take psychological tests and provide blood and urine sam-

Reprinted with permission of the author and the publisher from *IRB: A Review of Human Subjects Research,* vol. 2 (December 1980), pp. 1–4.

ples. The tests will provide baseline data for studying causes of schizophrenia in a county with two to three times the national incidence of schizophrenia.

Julian's mother, Sarah, was divorced six years ago. She then began psychotherapy at the center, which she still continues and enjoys. Upon hearing of the study, Mrs. Roy eagerly volunteered her family. When she told Julian, he became upset. Julian associates tests at the center with summer school. During the divorce proceedings, Julian was tested at the center and found to have an above-average I.Q. Because he was behind in school, counselors recommended summer school to ensure that he would not be kept back.

The researchers want Julian's agreement. They explain the study to him, tell him that he may refuse, and that his refusal will not affect his or his mother's relationship with the center. Julian indicates that he would rather go home. Upon hearing of his refusal, Mrs. Roy asks him to take the tests. She explains Julian's association of tests with summer school. The researchers explain that the tests have no relation to summer school. Convinced that Julian understands, a researcher says, "If your mother weren't here and it was just up to you, would you want to participate in this study?" Julian shakes his head negatively.

Case II—Vitamin E Research on Students A shampoo with and without Vitamin E is to be given to adolescents in a large metropolitan high school in grades 9 and 10 to determine whether Vitamin E promotes shinier or faster-growing hair. The department of nutrition and food science at a local university will conduct the research. The research will be a randomized, double-blind trial. Half the students will receive the shampoo with Vitamin E and half will receive a shampoo without the vitamin. No physical risks are foreseen. The shampoo has previously been tested on adults.

Parents will receive a note describing the tests and asked to sign a consent form. The issue is raised whether students should be allowed to decide to participate independently of their parents' consent.

CONSENT, ASSENT, AND DISSENT

It is illuminating to distinguish here between a subject's consent, assent, and dissent in research.[4] *Consent,* short for informed consent, is the legally required agreement of a subject to participate in research. *Assent* is neither legally binding nor legally required: it is a moral

requirement to acquire the closest approximation of consent one can achieve within the child's capacity to understand. Finally, *dissent* is more than lack of assent or consent: it is active disagreement, signified either verbally or nonverbally.[5] Julian dissents in Case I. The assent of the high school students is sought in Case II, but such assent is not consent. (It is unclear, as we shall see, whether it is parents or students who can give consent in such cases.)

The Commission recommended that researchers honor the dissent of minors.[1 at pp. 12–13] It also recommended that researchers obtain the assent of children down to age 7.[1 at pp. 12–13] However, the Department of Health, Education and Welfare (now Health and Human Services, or HHS) did not follow the Commission's recommendations.[6] Instead, it proposes to require each IRB to decide on a case-by-case basis whether the child's assent is necessary. HHS also does not conclude that, as a matter of national policy on research involving children, dissent by a child should preclude the child's participation in research.

HHS in essence puts the burden of judgment on the IRB. IRBs can require assent of children on any (or every) protocol involving research on children. They also can require that dissent in a child must preclude his or her participation in research, either in one case or as institutional policy.

FOUR MORAL PERSPECTIVES

The literature on participation of children in research reflects four distinctive moral perspectives; following is a brief summary of each.

The Little Adult View: Rights of adults should be extended to children insofar as possible. Self-assertion, independence, responsibility, and autonomy should be encouraged in children. Natalie Abrams suggests that denying children such autonomy constitutes the many social, psychological, and physical relationships of child abuse.[7] Following the Little Adult View, a child's assent to participation should be mandatory and such assent should be determinative except in life-or-death decisions. Bersoff, after reviewing the legal and psychological literature on pediatric consent, ends with his personal view, which sums up the Little Adult view:

Only if there is a significant risk of irreversible damage or clear and convincing empirical evidence

that at particular ages children do not have sufficiently developed skills to exercise discretion should
parents and the state have the right to make unilat-
eral decisions that meaningfully affect children. The
burden would fall on those wishing to deny the right
of children to choose; it would not fall to children
and their advocates to show that children are capable.[8]

The Ignorance View: Few adults can give real
informed consent to sophisticated medical and behavioral research. As Franz Ingelfinger wrote, most adult
subjects give "informed (but uneducated) consent."[9]
Since normal adults do not really understand, we can
be certain that minors do not understand. But, since
we allow "ignorant" adults to participate in research,
why should we not allow children? As Norman Fost
concludes, in an admirably clear way:

> If one acknowledges that decisions to use adults are
> ultimately as "coerced" as decisions to use children,
> and if one concludes that the present system is
> justified for adults, there is no reason to exclude
> children from the same benefits.[10]

The Incompatibility View: Most pediatric researchers
simply *assume* that research on children must be ethically justifiable and the problem is to specify how. One
who does not make this assumption is Paul Ramsey, a
theologian who champions an Incompatibility view.
Ramsey systematically attacks the above assumption,
arguing that doing research on a child—without
intending to benefit him or her directly—is always
evil.[11] Ramsey's argument is this: research on a child
can only be justified by intentions to benefit a child
directly and never by intention to benefit other children.
By definition, research is not intended to directly benefit
a child, therefore such research can never be morally
justified.

The Incompatibility view recognizes that it may be
evil at times *not* to do research on children. However
(and perhaps inconsistently) it emphasizes that research
on children is still an "evil." What seems to be meant is
that overall benefits to society are never such that the
evil of using children for research comes out "good"
overall. Also, some people fear a slippery slope: legitimizing any research on children will bring more and
more research.

The Good-of-Others View: It is important to understand that most research involving children is intended

to benefit *other children,* albeit children who may not
yet have been born or children who have no relation to
the subjects. It is misleading to couch the conflict as
one between adult-researchers and child-subjects;
rather, it is a conflict between a minor irritation for a
few child-subjects and a possible very large good for
many children. On this (utilitarian) view, a small risk
to any particular child is justified through its expected
contribution to the good of most children. Cases I and
II may be justified on this view.

LEGAL AND PSYCHOLOGICAL CONSIDERATIONS

Let us now examine some legal and psychological
considerations in order to enhance our capacity to
decide which of the above moral perspectives (or which
combination of them) would be most satisfactory.

Legally, therapeutic procedures may be performed
on children with the consent of the parents (proxy
consent). There is no legal requirement to solicit the
child's assent and the parents may override the child's
dissent. By analogy, proxy consent is generally regarded
as adequate authorization for the performance on
children of therapeutic procedures having "investigational" or "nonvalidated" status. However, the law has
not established the authority of a parent to consent to a
child's participation in research—particularly if the
research presents risk of harm. A California case,
pending for eight years, challenges the validity of proxy
consent for research on infants.[12] There is now no legal
basis to overrule Julian's dissent in Case I.

Psychologists Grisso and Vierling,[13] Bersoff,[8] and
Ferguson[14] conclude that minors 15 years or older can
understand as much about research as adults. They
argue that denial of consent for "minors" 15 years and
older lacks evidence. Ferguson claims that after the
age of 6, minors can understand research—a conclusion
evidently accepted by the Commission as it established
7 as the age of assent. Grisso disputes this conclusion
and draws the line at ages 14 or 15.

Grisso emphasizes that another issue outweighs a
child's understanding in research: a normal child's
deference to authority.[15] Whether because they lack
cognitive understanding or wide human experience,
children before ages 14 or 15 are unlikely to assert
themselves well against "authority figures" like parents,
physicians, and researchers. Adolescents ages 14 or 15
generally have acquired assertive skills and are more
easily able to dissent (inchoate autonomy during such

years is often misleadingly called "rebellion"). When the unusual event occurs that a child under 14 years dissents, he or she is either unusually intelligent, unusually terrified, or unusually hostile. Any one of these possibilities precludes forcing a child to participate.

In sum, not recognizing the dissent of minors 15 years and above is hard to justify according to psychological evidence, e.g., not recognizing Julian Roy's dissent to psychological research is unjustifiable. On the other hand, recognizing only the assent of minors under age 15 is also hard to justify in view of minors' deference to authority. It is unclear whether only the assent of teenagers to the Vitamin E study is sufficient to protect their best interests.

COMMENT ON THE VIEWS

Consideration of the legal and psychological issues deepens our understanding both about the opening cases and about the best overall view among the four moral perspectives. Among these perspectives, there are two sets of polarized extremes. The Good-of-Others view justifies any well-designed research with a good risk/benefit ratio. In contrast, the Incompatibility view sees all research on children as evil. The second set of contrasts reflects opposed judgments about the importance of a child's understanding. The Little Adult view attributes great value to a child's assent, whereas the Ignorance view attributes (at bottom) very little value to such assent.

I suggest that each of the above views contains *part* of the truth (or part of a good, overall policy) and that it is possible to obtain a consistent overall view compatible with the psychological and legal evidence. The Ignorance view is probably correct in that most adults understand little about research. Nevertheless, last year's winner of the Nellie Westerman Prize for medical ethics demonstrated that adult subjects could be brought to a level of understanding about a particular research project better than the average professor teaching in medical school, far better than the average physician, and far, far better than the average medical student.[16] Certainly such understanding is also possible with minors, especially those in their teenage years. Moreover, even though most people may understand little and have no real freedom to dissent, the dissent of those who *are* free and who *do* understand is still very important (at least to them).

The Incompatibility view is peculiar in one way. One interpretation of "It is evil to do research on

children" is that it is *always* (morally) wrong to do research. But to admit there are times when it is evil *not* to do research is equivalent to saying that it is right and good to do research in some cases. Ramsey might reply, "No, it's not good. In this case, the evil of not doing research outweighs the evil of allowing research on children. But it's still evil. It's just a matter of creating the least evil." To which the reply is: yes, of course, one can define morally right either as creating the most good or preventing the most evil. They come to the same. How one describes the procedures here is largely semantic. What is the difference between saying, "In some cases research is right, in others it is not" and "In some cases not doing research creates more evil than the evil of doing research"? Answer: To attempt to burden researchers with a shadow of guilt (because they do evil things)—which researchers will reject—and to set up adversarial relations between researchers and ethicists, all to no avail.

ANOTHER VIEW

One might imagine the "spirits" of future and present children convening to agree on principles of pediatric research. Pursuing this hypothetical thought-experiment, we can imagine them under a veil of ignorance about their real degree of health. The veil of ignorance is used by philosopher John Rawls, in his *A Theory of Justice,* to determine principles of justice.[17] People are assumed to be rational, self-interested, and desirous of acquiring the most in life of health, self-respect, money, and so on. Justice here concerns distributing both benefits and burdens. The relevant burden here is that of participation in scientific research. Under a veil of ignorance, one suddenly knows nothing about one's race, sex, financial status, social class, educational level, profession, or other data that might bias one's choice of principles of justice. One knows only general facts, such as those in science, history, psychology, and the wisdom of common sense. The veil of ignorance strips one of arbitrary biases and forces one to choose as an enlightened, self-interested person who can cooperate with other such persons.

Under the veil or not, each will want to be as healthy as possible. To this end, each child will agree to undergo some research as a normal child in order to better his or her life if he or she unluckily turns out to be an unhealthy child once the veil is removed. We can also imagine such a pediatric social contract *without* a veil of ignorance (if this is too antifactual for some). In this case, unhealthy children might say to normal children, "You have it so good and we have it relatively bad. Don't you owe us some participation in research presenting relatively minor risks that might enormously improve our lives? Try to see participation from our point of view." These two devices of moral philosophers (social contract and veil of ignorance) are in essence formalized methods to force results out of the Golden Rule. Such a rule seems to entail some participation of children in some research.[18]

The above conclusion does not entail the Good-of-Others view, for this latter view needs to be restricted by considerations from the Little Adult view. Perhaps the best way to put the conclusion is that *some* recognition of the Little Adult view, combined with good, well-designed research on children, is indeed the best way to accomplish the most good for the most children. What that "recognition" of the Little Adult view needs to be is that the dissent of a child should be final and that he or she should at least be told about the experiment.[19] The Little Adult view is most plausible with articulate, well-educated children who have been successfully trained to assert themselves. Moreover, such children usually recognize themselves to be potential equals of adults in a pluralistic world. Few children obviously fit this view. Nevertheless, some do. Moreover, some children are extraordinarily terrified of research, tests, or hospitals. It may be impossible for adults to understand such a child's terror and since such children will be rare, there is no reason for not considering their dissent to be final. Other children may be unusually hostile to the researcher, perhaps out of a general hostility toward adults, teachers, or physicians. Again, the rarity of such extreme hostility, and the degree of reluctance to participate expressed by such children, indicates cases where dissent should not be overruled. Finally, the very intelligent child may understand something about himself or herself, about the research, about parents' motivation for agreeing to participate, or even about the researcher, and consequently decide not to participate. Since we recognize similar reasons among adults for declining to participate, we should also recognize such reasons among minors (especially in the teenage years).

Moreover, children are usually deferential to authority, at least as much as the amazing degree of obedience to authority demonstrated by adults in the research of social psychologist Stanley Milgram.[20] Few high school students will even *consider* not going along with the Vitamin E study if their teachers and friends urge their

participation. In view of such great reluctance to disobey authority, if a minor nevertheless does so, we can only infer that something of great importance is happening. The dissent of a minor from research is a very important matter.

This same great deference to authority of minors makes their assent less important as a sufficient condition of participation. It seems nearly impossible for a child to dissent against *both* parents *and* physicians (add nurses, social workers, school teachers, and one has a virtual army against the dissenting child). For any research that presents more than minimal risk (as defined by the Commission) *child advocates* may at times be wisely used to protect children.[21] Such advocates should have status and education equivalent to the researcher.

CONCLUSIONS

The moral and legal ability of parents either to consent for, or overrule the dissent of, their children for research lacks persuasive precedent and justification at this time. Proposed regulations require each IRB to decide whether a child's assent is required for participation and whether his or her dissent precludes participation.

Four moral perspectives are advocated in the literature, consisting of two sets of polarized extremes. Evidence exists both that there is a need for research on children and also that children can understand more than is commonly believed. However, whether a child can *act* on an understanding against authority below age 14 is questionable.

Participation of children in research can be justified, so long as the dissent of children from such research is recognized and safeguarded. Obviously, to be able to dissent, a child-subject must be *told* that he or she is a subject of research. Additionally, there seems to be no evidence for not recognizing the assent of minors above age 14. A cut-off point at age 7 is suggested for telling children that they are participants in research.[22]

REFERENCES

1 National Commission for the Protection of Human Subjects of Biomedical and Behavioral Research: *Report and Recommendations: Research Involving Children.* DHEW Publication No. (OS) 77-0004, Washington, 1977.

2 The definitions, though clarifying in a reforming way, are still not perfect. Many protocols are designed both to help individual subjects and also to obtain generalizable knowledge. One could argue that only by intending and obtaining such knowledge can medicine really help children. This bromide, however, diverts attention from the problems of justifying nonvoluntary participation of children in such research and of deciding whether children should agree to such research.

3 Although the above cases are representative of real cases, neither of them came before the IRB at the author's university.

4 I here follow the Commission, *op. cit.,* p. 13. See also Levine, R. J.: Clarifying the concepts of research ethics. *Hastings Center Report.* 9 (No. 3) 21–26, June, 1979; Levine, R. J.: Research involving children: The National Commission's report. *Clinical Research* 26:61–66, 1978.

5 Dissent may easily be nonverbal in children, e.g., refusing to move.

6 DHEW: Proposed Regulations for Research on Children. *Federal Register.* 43:31786–94, July 21, 1978.

7 Abrams, N.: Problems in defining child abuse and neglect. In *Having Children: Philosophical and Legal Reflections on Parenthood.* Edited by O. O'Neil and W. Ruddick, New York: Oxford University Press, 1979.

8 Bersoff, D.: Legal Issues in Children's Consent to Psychological Research. Presentation at the annual meeting of the American Psychological Association, New York, September, 1979, in a Symposium on Children's Consent to Psychological Research: Problems, Policies, and Principles (copies from author at University of Maryland School of Law and Johns Hopkins University).

9 Ingelfinger, F.: Informed (but uneducated) consent. *New England Journal of Medicine.* 287:465–466, 1972.

10 Fost, N.: Children as renal donors. *New England Journal of Medicine.* 296:363–367, 1977. Also see commentary following the article.

11 Ramsey, P.: The enforcement of morals: Nontherapeutic research on children. *Hastings Center Report.* 6 (No. 4):21–30, August, 1976; Children as research subjects: A reply. *Hastings Center Report* 7 (No. 2): April, 1977.

12 Plaintiff's complaint: Nielsen v. Regents of the University of California et al., case No. 655-049, Superior Court of California, County of San Francisco, as amended Dec. 20, 1973.

13 Grisso, T. and Vierling, L.: Minor's consent to treatment: A developmental perspective. *Professional Psychology.* 412–426, August, 1978.

14 Ferguson, L. R.: The Competence and Freedom of Children to Make Choices Regarding Participation in Biomedical and Behavioral Research. Appendix, *Research on Children.* National Commission for the Protection of Human Subjects of Medical and Behavioral Research. DHEW Publication No. (OS) 77-0005.

15 Grisso, T.: Psychology's Role in Policy on Minors' Informed Consent. Presentation of a Symposium on the Consent of Minors at the annual meeting of the American Psychological Association, New York. September, 1979. Copies from author at the Psychology Department, St. Louis University.

16 Woodward, W. E.: Informed consent of volunteers: A direct measurement of comprehension and retention of information. *Clinical Research* 27:248–252, 1979.

17 This is a key idea behind the theory of justice of John Rawls. Rawls, J.: *A Theory of Justice.* Cambridge: Harvard University Press, 1973.

18 This idea of a spiritual realm and a subsequent social contract based on such conversations is an application of an idea advanced by R. M. Hare. Hare, R. M.: Survival of the weakest. In *Moral Problems in Medicine,* edited by S. Gorovitz et al. Englewood Cliffs: Prentice-Hall Publishing Company, 1978, pp. 364–369.

19 See Bok, S.: Lying to children. *Hastings Center Report* 8 (No. 3): 10–13, June, 1978.

20 Milgram, S.: *Obedience to Authority.* New York: Harper, 1974.

21 I am indebted to Paul Palmisano, M.D., for this idea.

22 I am indebted to the following people for commenting on this article: Gayle Gear, R. J. Levine, William Ruddick, Allen Shealy, Richard Whitley.

Prisoners as Research Subjects

Experiments Behind Bars

Jessica Mitford

Jessica Mitford is the author of several books that critically examine existing American practices and institutions. These include *The Trial of Dr. Spock* (1960), *The American Way of Death* (1963), *The American Prison Business* (1971), *Kind and Usual Punishment* (1973), *A Fine Old Conflict* (1977), and *Poison Penmanship: The Gentle Art of Muckraking* (1979). This selection is excerpted from Mitford's *Kind and Usual Punishment*.

Mitford is opposed to using prisoners as subjects in nontherapeutic medical research. She cites the Nuremberg Code, which states that the voluntary consent of the human subject is absolutely essential before such experimentation can be performed. Mitford questions the capacity of prisoners to give their informed consent to experimentation. She expresses strong doubts about whether the prisoners' consent can be sufficiently free and whether it can be sufficiently informed. If she is correct in her view that prisoners are incapable of exercising freedom of choice, then their consent cannot be free. If she is correct in her view that experimenters will not give prisoners the information required to make "understanding and enlightened decisions," then prisoners' consent will not be informed. Mitford does not argue that prisoners are in principle incapable of the understanding required for informed consent. However, she maintains that the position of prisoners is so vulnerable that we cannot ensure that those who use them as experimental subjects can be trusted to supply them with adequate information.

Before a new drug can be marketed in the United States, it must, according to Food and Drug Administration rules, be tested on human beings. In recent years, most of the early testing of our increasingly exotic drugs has been done in prisons. And prisoners have been the subjects of other medical experiments as well.

For some time, international medical societies have attempted to prohibit the use of prisoners as subjects, but these efforts have been effectively frustrated by American medical experimenters. The World Medical Association proposed in 1961 that prisoners "being captive groups should not be used as the subject of experiments." The recommendation was never formally adopted, largely because of the opposition of American doctors. "Pertinax" writes in the *British Medical Journal* for January, 1963: "I am disturbed that the World Medical Association is now hedging on its clause about using criminals as experimental material. The American influence has been at work on its suspension." He adds wistfully, "One of the nicest American scientists I know was heard to say, 'Criminals in our penitentiaries are fine experimental material—and much cheaper than chimpanzees.' I hope the chimpanzees don't come to hear of this."[1]

Although few involved in prison experiments like to talk openly about them, alarming stories crop up in the press with sufficient regularity to give some indication of the scope and nature of the experiments. In 1963, *Time* magazine reported that the federal government was using prisoner "volunteers" for large-scale research, dispensing rewards ranging from a package of cigarettes to $25 in cash plus reduction of sentence; that prisoners in Ohio and Illinois were injected with live cancer cells and with blood from leukemia patients to determine whether these diseases could be transmitted; that doctors in Oklahoma were grossing an estimated $300,000 a year from deals with pharmaceutical companies to test out new drugs on prisoners; that the same doctors were paying prisoners $5 a quart for blood which they retailed at $15.

In July, 1969, Walter Rugaber of the *New York Times* reported that "the Federal Government has watched without interference while many people sickened and some died in an extended series of drug tests and blood plasma operations...the immediate damage has been done in the penitentiary systems of three states. Hundreds of inmates in voluntary programs have been stricken with serious disease. An undetermined number of the victims have died."

The stakes in prison research are high. The drug companies, usually operating through private physicians with access to the prisons, can obtain healthy human subjects living in controlled conditions that are difficult, if not impossible, to duplicate elsewhere. In addition, the companies can buy these for a fraction—less than one-tenth, according to many medical authorities—of what they would have to pay medical students or other "free-world" volunteers. They can conduct experiments on prisoners that would not be sanctioned for student-subjects at any price because of the degree of risk and pain involved. Guidelines for human experimentation established by HEW and other agencies are easily disregarded behind prison walls.

When the studies are carried out in the privacy of prison, if a volunteer becomes seriously ill, or dies, as a result of the procedures to which he is subjected, the repercussions will likely be smaller than they would be on the outside. As Rugaber discovered when trying to trace deaths resulting from the "voluntary programs," prison medical records that might prove embarrassing to the authorities have a habit of conveniently disappearing. There is minimal risk that subjects disabled by the experiments will bring lawsuits against the drug companies. Prisoners are often required to sign a waiver releasing those responsible from damage claims that may result. Such waivers have been held legally invalid as contrary to public policy and are specifically prohibited by FDA regulations, but the prisoner is unlikely to know this. The psychological effect of signing the waiver, along with the general helplessness of prisoners, make lawsuits a rarity.

For the prisoner, the pittance he gets from the drug company—generally around $1 a day for the more onerous experiments—represents riches when viewed in terms of prison pay scales: $30 a month compared with the $2 to $10 a month he might make in an ordinary prison job.

Dr. Robert Batterman, a clinical pharmacologist, told me, "The prisoner-subject gets virtually nil." He cited an estimate given him for experimenting on prisoners in Vacaville, California: $15 a month for three months to be *lowered* to $12.50 a month should the experiment run for six months. "We would normally do it the other way around with free-world volunteers. We'd give them more money if the experiment ran longer." Dr. Batterman makes considerable use of student-subjects from a nearby Baptist divinity school. For a comparatively undemanding experiment—one requiring a weekly withdrawal of blood—he would pay a student at least $100 a month, he said.

However, the problem as seen by some leaders of the American medical profession is not that the prisoner-subjects are paid too little, but rather that they may be paid too much. That a dollar-a-day stipend to a healthy adult can be so overwhelmingly attractive as to invalidate the results of medical research is a possibility only in the topsy-turvy world of prisons. Yet the fear that this will happen is precisely what is expressed by some spokesmen for the profession. Thus Dr. Herbert L. Ley, Jr., then commissioner of the Food and Drug Administration, testified in 1969 before the Senate Select Committee on Small Business:

"The basic problem here, Mr. Chairman, is that the remuneration to the prisoner was too much. This meant that the prisoner had a very strong pressure not to report and not to withdraw from the study. Therefore he would decline to say that he felt any adverse reactions. This is bad for the prisoner in that it exposes him to unnecessary risk, it is bad for our records in that it does not provide us full information."

Prisoners do indeed view the small sums paid as largesse. In a series of interviews conducted in 1969 at Vacaville prison, California, by Martin Miller, a graduate student at the University of California Department of Criminology, some of the prisoners commented: "Yeah, I was on research but I couldn't keep my chow down. Like I lost about thirty-five pounds my first year in the joint, so I started getting scared. I hated to give it up because it was a good pay test."..."Hey, man, I'm making $30 a month on the DMSO thing [Chronic Topical Application of Dimethylsulfoxide]. I know a couple of guys had to go to the hospital who were on it—and the burns were so bad they had to take *everyone* off it for a while. But who gives a shit about that, man? Thirty is a full canteen draw and I wish the thing would go on for years—I'd be lost without it."..."I was on DMSO last year. It paid real good and it was better than that plague thing [Bubonic Plague Vaccine Immunization Study] that fucked with guys last year. There was a lot of bad reactions to DMSO but I guess that's why it paid so good." Of DMSO Mortin Mintz, staff writer for the *Washington Post,* had written three years earlier: "Human testing has now been severely curbed by FDA because of reports of serious adverse effects" (*Washington Post,* July 24, 1966).

The participating physician cashes in on the programs in various ways. He may make a direct deal with the drug company for financial backing, out of which he pays the expenses of research and pockets the rest as his fee. An individual research grant might run from $5000 to more than $50,000, enabling a doctor with good prison contacts to double or triple his regular income. Or if he is, as many are, a faculty member in a medical school, he can route the grant through his university, to the acclaim of his colleagues. His prestige will be enhanced when the results of his research appear in a professional journal.

Some of the vicissitudes that the medical researcher may expect to encounter in his quest for prisoner-subjects are described by Dr. Robert E. Hodges in the November 6, 1971, issue of the *Journal of the American Medical Associaton.* In the late forties, Dr. Hodges and his colleagues reached a "verbal working arrangement" with Iowa prison officials enabling them to canvass the prison population for volunteers who would submit to prolonged hospitalization in university hospitals as research subjects. "We knew this procedure was not specifically permitted by law," writes Dr. Hodges. "But neither was it specifically prohibited." Eventually the experiments came to the attention of Iowa's Attorney General: "In his judgment, it was not legal for us to accept prison volunteers for medical research." There followed two fallow years in which the experiments were halted, but Dr. Hodges during this time "sought and obtained enactment of a specific law permitting the use of prisoners for medical research at university hospitals." The path thus cleared, a total of 224 convicts were in the course of time delivered over to Dr. Hodges and his colleagues at the university hospitals.

Speculating on the "incentives and motives" that induce prisoners to volunteer for research studies "which are usually somewhat unpleasant and in a few instances involve distinct risks," Dr. Hodges surmises that "for some, it probably represents a new experience which takes them away from the monotony and oppressiveness of prison routine." The relief from monotony: "They have eaten strange diets, swallowed tubes, submitted to repeated venipunctures, and participated in a wide variety of physiological tests...."

For some prisoners, "monetary gain may be the incentive, though inmates are paid only one dollar daily." Iowa prisoners are not supposed to receive reduction of sentence in return for volunteering, but Dr. Hodges routinely sent a thank-you letter to the warden for each subject: "It is possible that this letter in the prisoner's file may favorably influence the parole board." As for the incentives and motives of researchers, Dr. Hodges reports that more than eighty scientific publications resulted from the Iowa studies on prisoners.

Dr. Hodges becomes almost lyrical in his discussion of the moral and ethical aspects of such experimentation. The prisoner-volunteers, he says, are "our companions in medical science and adventure"; the subject "in whatever degree derelict or forlorn has sacred rights which the physician must always put ahead of his burning curiosity." Dr. Hodges, without elaborating on these sacred rights, concludes: "A system of voluntary participation firmly based on legal and ethical standards has provided a rich opportunity for clinical investigators who wish to study metabolic, physiologic, pharmacologic, and medical problems. This has been a rewarding experience both for the physicians and for the subjects."

One such experience is described by Dr. Hodges in one of his papers: "Clinical Manifestations of Ascorbic Acid Deficiency in Man," in the *American Journal of Clinical Nutrition* of April, 1971. The object: "to define the metabolism of this vitamin in the face of severe dietary deficiency." For the study, which consisted of experimentally induced scurvy, five companions in medical science and adventure were recruited from the Iowa State Penitentiary "and their informed consent was obtained." For periods ranging from 84 to 97 days they were fed by stomach tube a liquid formula free of ascorbic acid: "Because of the unpalatability of this formula, the men took it thrice daily via polyethylene gastric tube." They were exposed in a cold-climate "control room" to a temperature of fifty degrees for four hours each day. The volume of blood drawn "for laboratory purposes" was large enough to "cause mild anemia in all the men." In a throwaway line, Dr. Hodges observes that "the mineral supplement [recommended by the National Research Council] was inadvertently omitted from the diets during the first 34 days of the depletion period."

The experiment was a great success. It was the second of its kind, Dr. Hodges having tried it once before with far less favorable results: "Despite a somewhat shorter period of deprivation in the second scurvy study, the subjects in the second study developed a more severe degree of scurvy...although none of the subjects in the first scurvy study developed arthralgia, this was a complaint in four out of five men who participated in the second scurvy study. Joint swelling and pain made themselves evident in Scurvy II, but had not been observed in the subjects participating in Scurvy I."

The gradual onset of scurvy in the five prisoners is traced by Dr. Hodges with some enthusiasm. "The first sign of scurvy to appear in both studies was petechial hemorrhage [hemorrhages in the skin]. Coiled hairs were observed in two of the men and first appeared on the 42nd and 74th days, respectively. The first definite abnormalities of the gums appeared between the 43rd and 84th days of depletion and progressed after the plasma ascorbic acid levels fell....The onset of joint pains began between the 67th and 96th days. ...Beginning on the 88th day of deprivation there was a rapid increase in weight followed by swelling of the legs in the third man, who had the most severe degree of scurvy."

By the time it was all over, Dr. Hodges was able to chalk up these significant accomplishments: all five subjects suffered joint pains, swelling of the legs, dental cavities, recurrent loss of new dental fillings, excessive loss of hair, hemorrhages in the skin and whites of the eyes, excess fluid in the joint spaces, shortness of breath, scaly skin, mental depression, and abnormalities in emotional responses. The youngest, a twenty-six-year-old, "became almost unable to walk as a result of the rapid onset of arthropathy [painful joints] superimposed on bilateral femoral neuropathy [disease in both large nerves to the thighs and legs plus hemorrhage

into nerve sheaths]. The onset of scurvy signaled a period of potentially rapid deterioration." Dr. Hodges' anticlimactic conclusion: "Once again our observations are in accord with those of the British Medical Research Council."

To other doctors, the "Ascorbic Acid Deficiency" study appears as a senseless piece of cruelty visited on the five volunteers. "This study was totally pointless," Dr. Ephraim Kahn of the California Department of Public Health said of Dr. Hodges' publication. "The cause and cure of scurvy have been well known in the medical profession for generations. Some of the side effects he lists may well be irreversible—the young man who had the most severe case of scurvy may never have recovered. There's a clue here to the degree of competence of these so-called 'researchers'—they 'inadvertently' omitted a mineral supplement from the diets. This no doubt weakened the men and exacerbated the other side effects. It might cause them to go into shock, and to suffer severe cardiac abnormalities." Among effects of the experiment recorded in the publication that could be permanent, Dr. Kahn cited heart damage, loss of hair, damage to teeth, hemorrhage into femoral nerve sheaths—the latter is "terribly painful and could lead to permanent nerve damage."

I asked Dr. Hodges, now a professor of internal medicine at the University of California medical school at Davis, how much he had paid the scurvy test volunteers. "I think it was one dollar or maybe two dollars a day," he replied. "Over the years, when I was in Iowa, as the cost of cigarettes and razor blades went up, we increased prisoners' pay somewhat. It's unethical to pay an amount of money that is too attractive. Oh, we had the money, we could have paid much more, of course—but we weren't just being cheap, we were considering the ethics of the situation. The prisoners got a bit extra for really unpleasant things—if we had to put a tube down their throats for several hours, or take a biopsy of the skin the size of a pencil eraser, we'd give them a few dollars more."

Doctors with whom I have discussed the matter agree unanimously that FDA regulations requiring drugs to be tested on humans before being marketed are sound and necessary. But human experimentation, they say, must be conducted within a framework of stringent rules for the protection of the human subject.

Since World War II a number of "guiding principles" and "codes of ethics" have been developed by the medical profession to govern the conduct of experiments. An American Medical Association resolution of 1946 on human research was in turn followed by FDA regulations of 1962 and the Helsinki Declaration of 1966.

These are largely repetitive. All affirm that human experiments must be based on prior laboratory work and research on animals, emphasize the grave responsibility of investigator to subject, and exhort him to avoid experiments that are of no scientific value or that subject humans to unnecessary pain and risk. Above all, the "informed consent" of the subject must be obtained....

In 1947 fifteen German doctors, all distinguished leaders of their profession, were tried and convicted at Nuremberg for their cruel and frequently murderous "medical experiments" performed on concentration camp inmates. The barbarity of these crimes is of course unparalleled, but the Nuremberg tribunal established standards for medical experimentation on humans, which, if observed, would end altogether the practice of using prisoners as subjects: "The voluntary consent of the human subject is absolutely essential. This means the person involved should have legal capacity to give consent; should be so situated as to be able to exercise free power of choice...and should have sufficient knowledge and comprehension of the elements of the subject matter involved as to enable him to make an understanding, enlightened decision." Are prisoners, stripped of their civil rights when they enter the gates, subjected to years or decades of confinement, free agents capable of exercising freedom of choice? Can we trust that they are furnished by the experimenters with "knowledge and comprehension" to enable them to make "understanding and enlightened" decisions? To ask these questions is, I believe, to answer them.

NOTE

1 See M. H. Pappworth, M.D., *Human Guinea Pigs,* Beacon Press, 1967.

Medical Experimentation on Prisoners

Carl Cohen

Carl Cohen is professor of philosophy at the University of Michigan. He specializes in social and political philosophy. Cohen is the author of *Civil Disobedience: Conscience, Tactics, and the Law* (1971) and *Four Systems* (1982), and editor of *Communism, Fascism, and Democracy* (1972) and *Democracy* (1971). He has also published many articles including "Race and the Constitution" and "Genocide and the Nazis: The Case against Group Libel."

Cohen rejects the view that prisoners cannot be used as experimental subjects because they cannot, in their situation, give free and uncoerced consent. He distinguishes two senses of coercion in order to show that Mitford and others who argue against using prisoners as research subjects confuse the two senses. Just because prisoners are in a "coercive" environment it does not follow, according to Cohen, that they are always "coerced" into volunteering for biomedical experiments. Furthermore, Cohen argues, to deny prisoners the right to volunteer, while granting that right to others, is to deny the prisoners' autonomy. If others have the right to participate in such experiments and to be paid for doing so, what justification can we give for denying that right to prisoners? Cohen concludes his article by discussing the great benefits that research in prisons has both for prisoners themselves and for society in general.

Reprinted with permission of the author and the publisher from *Perspectives in Biology and Medicine*, vol. 21, no. 3 (Spring 1978), pp. 357–372. Copyright © 1978 by the University of Chicago.

I PROLOG

Ought we to permit medical experimentation on prisoners? The issue is both practically important and morally complex. Some argue as follows: No human subject may be used in a medical experiment without his informed and freely-given consent. But prisoners, by virtue of their total custody, cannot give free and uncoerced consent. Hence prisoners—no matter how valuable experimentation with their cooperation may prove—must be excluded from all populations of subjects in medical experimentation.

This argument, when expanded and reinforced, is very persuasive, as I shall show. I aim also to show that its key premise is simply mistaken, and the argument unsound.

Government agencies (HEW, NIH, the National Commission for the Protection of Human Subjects) and human subject review committees all provide assorted rules and guidelines for prison experimentation. It is not my aim to report these. My question is this: *Should* we adopt the rule, now proposed by some, excluding all or almost all experimentation involving prison volunteers?[1]

Some clarifications first. The principle that informed consent must be got from every human subject in a medical experiment is well-established. It was eloquently formulated in the Nuremberg Code, and by the World Medical Association in their *Declaration of Helsinki*. It grounds a set of detailed regulations governing the operation of all institutions for medical research in this country funded in whole or in part by any Federal agency. It is the focus of concern for untold numbers of committees, medical practitioners and researchers, lawyers and laymen who deal, day-to-day, with a heavy, valuable, and sometimes threatening stream of research protocols. But "informed consent" involves more than information. Better thought of as "full consent," what is demanded in fact entails three elements: *information*, *competency*, and *voluntariness*. Where the consent received is defective in any one of these respects, we will rightly think the subject to have been improperly used.

Problematic defects of *information* arise when experiments are proposed in which the subjects cannot be told the truth, or the whole truth, about the investigation of which they are part—because their knowing what the investigator is after will have the effect of his not getting it. Deception is not uncommon in behavioral

research, but I bypass the problem here. Problematic defects of *competency* arise when experiments call for subjects who are not (in fact or in law) competent to give their consent—infant children, the mentally disabled, the comatose, and so on. Some experiments with persons in these categories are essential, obviously, if care for them is to be improved; hence principles must be devised for determining who may give third-party consent ("proxy consent") for the incompetent, and under what restrictions it may be given. These issues of competency are sorely vexed, but here I bypass them also. Problematic defects of *voluntariness* arise when potential subjects, although fully informed and competent, are coerced into giving their consent by threat or excessive inducement, or other inappropriate manipulation. This is the more likely where the potential subjects are more vulnerable, more precariously placed. Among these precariously placed potential subjects, the case of prisoners is critical because, on the one hand, their incarceration renders them specially vulnerable, while on the other hand that same incarceration renders them peculiarly well suited for some very valuable long-term experiments. Some resolution of this matter is essential.

II CAN A PRISONER GIVE VOLUNTARY CONSENT?

Voluntariness, the third element of full consent, is most difficult to specify. We insist that a subject's consent be freely given and uncoerced. What does that entail? Clear cases of "volunteers" who did not give their consent freely are not hard to recall or imagine. The archetype—which reality often approximates—is the army platoon, lined up before the First Sergeant who asks sternly for volunteers, and orders those who do not volunteer to take two steps forward. At the other extreme, cases of honest volunteering, genuinely autonomous, are legion. But very many cases fall between the extremes, and that of the prison volunteer is one of these.

It may well seem that, by virtue of the complete custody of their persons, prisoners lack the capacity to act with the kind of uncoerced voluntariness required. If they do lack it, they ought not be subjects. So I want now to put, more carefully than I have found it put anywhere, what precisely it is about the prisoner's condition that might render him or her unfit to be a consenting subject in a medical experiment.

The argument goes like this. The prison environment, both in fact and in principle, is such that consent without coercion is not possible there. This is not because of any defect in prisoners; it flows from the deeply intrusive, literally totalitarian character of prisons. One may take this as a condemnation of prisons, or simply as an unpleasant but unavoidable fact about them. Attitudes about prisons are not in contention here. Prisons being what they are, their inmates are in a state of constant coercion, from which there is no escape within the walls. No matter what the prisoner says, or we say to him, coercion is the essence of his condition. In that condition no consent to put oneself at risk should be accepted as full consent. Hence medical experimentation on prisoners should be forbidden, flatly.

That is the general thrust. Now, more concretely and specifically, see how this coercive spirit permeates the prison environment.

First. The body of the prisoner is simply not under his own control. Orders committing persons to prison are very blunt about this, generally containing the phrase: "the body of the defendant shall be delivered" to the custodial institution appropriately identified. No system of criminal punishment that relies upon prisons, however humane its intent, can evade this fact. The U.S. Solicitor General (in a brief filed with the U.S. Supreme Court, in a 1974 case dealing with the transfer of prisoners from one institution to another) puts the matter brutally but truthfully.

> ...The very fact of his conviction for a crime, and the legitimate placement of his person into the hands of a custodian who will be responsible for his safe-keeping and the supervision of the most intimate details of his life removes from the prisoner any legitimate expectation that he will be able to control the conditions of his confinement. (Brief for the United States, as *Amicus Curiae*, p. 15; *Preiser* v. *Newkirk*, O.T. 1974, no. 74–107)

Second. Not only is the prisoner's person unfree, but the control of that person, and the secure incarceration of his body, are his keepers' chief and overriding concerns. Prisons are closed, tightly guarded places. Anyone who has not visited a medium or maximum security prison can hardly imagine the impact of omnipresent locks, bars and armed guards. Supervision of hour-by-hour conduct is close; inspection is constant; privacy is nil; coercion is the flavor of every moment.

Third. Most prisoners are very poor, and have tightly limited opportunity to earn the most puny wages. Some states pay no wages for prison labor; most states pay less than one dollar per day; only six states pay more than that. And even where wages are paid, not all prisoners have the chance to earn them. From this poverty any decent payment for service is partial rescue.

Fourth. Boredom, killing monotony, is that feature which, next to control, most pervades prison life. The state tells every prisoner when to sleep, when to rise, when to eat and what, when to work and when to play, what to do and how to do it—all with maddening sameness. From this barrenness, any change is relief.

Fifth, and finally. The dominant concern in every prisoner's life is release and the eventual date of it. In this country prison sentences of indeterminate length are very common. That single most important date is therefore subject to the judgment, even to the whim, of administrators whom the prisoner can rarely reach or even address. His behavior in prison—in ways he cannot be sure of—must affect, perhaps determine his date of release. Even for those with determinate sentences, that date remains indeterminate if there is, as usually, a parole board to be pleased. The felt need to please officials—doing what (at least in their own minds) prisoners think might please those who might be in a position to effect a somewhat earlier release—is an unavoidable pressure upon the behavior of prisoners.

It is in this environment that voluntariness of consent to subjection to medical experimentation must be assessed. However freely it appears that he consents, the prisoner is coerced so fully by his circumstances that even asking him must be unfair. His service as subject must be seen by him as a precious opportunity to escape, if only for short or infrequent periods, from the drabness and routine of prison life. He will see new faces, talk to interesting people who are neither inmates nor guards, leave his normal, grim surroundings on occasion for a setting that is lit by freedom and interest. And he is further coerced by the monetary rewards—dollars at a crack, even scores of dollars in a long experiment—promising opportunity for riches not possible otherwise. The risks run are overshadowed by the partial escape from state-imposed penury. Fifty dollars a month, say, for prison subjects in a malaria test—why, that is coercion turned green! And above all, what an opportunity to prove one's good will, one's eagerness to pay his debt to society, one's sincere intention to make up for past evils and be good! Surely they who have power in this sphere will note this evidence of good character. Surely it will not work against the prisoner when parole or release is being considered— and it may, it just *may* do some good. How can the rational prisoner not be coerced by such a concatenation of pressures? He cannot. It is not right (this argument concludes) even to ask the prisoner whether he wishes to put himself at risk when doing so is encouraged by his circumstances so strongly and so perniciously. No matter the circumspection and honest care of the investigator. If, as we have seen, full and uncoerced consent simply cannot be given by prisoners, the request for volunteers, must not, in fairness, be made to them.

The argument has two addenda.

(a) Everything above applies to prison experiments even when delicately and justly supervised. But the *de facto* circumstances in real prisons are such as to make delicacy rare, and justice less than universal. There is enormous potential for abuse in prisons; there *is* a great deal of abuse in prisons. Knowing that, we cannot in good conscience undertake medical experiments that may, in fact, be tainted by that abuse in various ways, but above all in the selection of subjects.

(b) Those who support medical experimentation in prisons quickly point to the great benefits they have yielded for mankind—experiments on polio virus strains, for example, which led directly to the selection of strains now used worldwide in the preparation of polio virus vaccine administered by mouth. Then there is the work on malaria, and dengue fever, and so on. All that is very fine—but if such experiments rely upon the wrongful use of human subjects, they simply shouldn't be done. The critical issues here concern what is right, what is just—not the balancing of benefits. Until the justice of such experimenting on prisoners has been shown, the calculation of benefits simply cannot be reached.

III   A CLOSER LOOK AT COERCION

There is the case, and it is a strong one. But it is not strong enough. The argument is rightly cautionary. Its several considerations show, I submit, that medical experiments using prisoners as subjects must go forward, if at all, under rules more constraining, and supervision more strict, than such experimentation in more ordinary contexts. It has not been shown, I

contend, that a prisoner cannot give full consent in the sense that being a voluntary subject requires full consent.

I begin by granting much of the factual description of the prison environment presented above—although that account was deliberately put in rather purple language. But it is so; prison life is controlled, barren, poor, monotonous. Coercion is the spirit of the prison. Regrettably, however, those who accept the argument above, or some variant of it, are led by their detestation of prisons to equivocate upon the word "coercion." When careful with it we find, reasonably enough, that there are respects in which the prisoner is coerced and respects in which he is not—and, indeed, that the same is true of everyone. We need to identify carefully that sense of coercion employed when we say that coercion vitiates an apparently free consent. Then we must decide whether, when given an opportunity to volunteer as subject, the prisoner is coerced in that sense. We will find upon reflection, I think that another sense of coercion—looser and more suggestive, characterizing the flavor of prison activity—has been drawn upon. To make the argument work a transition is made, perhaps inadvertently, from that broad sense of coercion to a tighter, narrower sense that bears directly upon freedom in making choices.

By "coercion" our common meaning is compulsion by physical or moral pressures. A coerces B when B is compelled or constrained to act as A wishes him to, as a result of measures taken by A to effect just that result. The bandit coerces me, with his revolver, into handing over my wallet. The threat of criminal prosecution if I do not file an income tax return is a coercive instrument designed to constrain my behavior. We are tempted—and too many yield—to leap from this to calling coercive whatever restrains or limits or influences behavior. I may be coerced into giving to the United Fund, say by the threat of discharge or defamation; but I am not coerced into charitable giving by my strong desire to be admired as a public benefactor. Again, if my wealth were unlimited I should sail the seas in splendor; my means being what they are, I cast an admiring glance at every ocean racing yacht, and go on splashing about in my little sailing dinghy. It is an elastic use of English to say I am coerced into doing so. There are, too, desires of the utmost intensity which influence my conduct and with which I must come to terms. But these desires are not imposed (unless one holds a satanic view of the human condition) in order to bend my volition; they are the normal matrix of my life. It is facile or confused to suppose that I am coerced by my own wants. Even my most passionate wants, my sexual desires, cannot be said to coerce me into seduction.

We sometimes think powerful inducements, as well as threats, to be coercive. Sometimes they may be, but only when the subject in question is caused, by an extraordinary and deliberate temptation, to do what should not ever be done. If a poor person is tempted by a huge sum to accept a risk we think it not proper to urge upon anyone, the offer is there coercive. But if the reward be for conduct that is itself reasonable, the fact that one's condition renders that reward exceptionally attractive does not show that coercion has been applied. Professional football players are not coerced by huge salaries into risking their necks, nor are workers coerced into work by their need for earnings.

A definitive account of coercion I do not seek to provide here. No doubt any account, however refined, will leave some rough edges. But moderately thoughtful reflection will show, I believe, that the coercion that full consent precludes is the coercion flowing from the deliberate effort on the part of one who offers the choice (or his agent) to pressure the offeree into a particular decision. The pressure must be such that the offerer could have refrained from exerting it, but deliberately did not refrain.

If I seek admission to a research hospital specializing, say, in eye disease, desperate about my failing sight, and I am admitted upon the condition that I put myself at serious risk in an experiment having nothing to do with my condition, I have indeed been coerced improperly. Even in matters involving minor risks, if I am subjected to a moral barrage regarding the social value of medical research and the importance of the experiment at hand to all mankind, when asked for my consent to serve as subject, I am coerced, if mildly, by the deliberate pressures of the investigator. We do not permit such distortions of potential subjects' volitions, rightly. But if I suffer from a serious disease for which cure is unknown, it is quite reasonable that I should find serving as subject, in an experiment aimed at enlarging knowledge about that disease, attractive in a way that one who does not suffer from that disease does not find attractive. My diseased condition does not coerce me. Or if one insists upon the lingo in which such sickness inevitably renders me "coerced"—then certainly that so-called coercion could not begin to

establish that my freely expressed consent was really involuntary.

Our lives are led, and our decisions made, within a network of needs and wants, some natural, some arising from the acts of others, some aggravated by the acts of the state. We are all bored, or threatened, or tantalized in differing degrees by a perilous world, some hostile people, and a not very sensitive government. Sometimes, within that framework, we are coerced by the design of persons or institutions into choosing X rather than Y. Such design, introduced in order to manipulate our choosing, is the coercion here chiefly of concern to us. The Nuremberg Code, in defining voluntary consent, puts the matter well. It insists that the person involved must in his situation be able to exercise free power of choice "without the intervention of any element of force, fraud, deceit, duress, overreaching, or other ulterior form of constraint or coercion..."

Let's now apply this view of coercion to the case of the prisoner giving informed consent to serve as medical subject. The opportunity is given him, let us suppose, to respond by letter to a notice on a bulletin board, after which, if he proves a suitable subject, he is given full information about procedures, risks, pay and the rest by a research investigator. Is he coerced into giving consent by the fact of his imprisonment? On reflection I think we will see that he is not.

The question is not, "Are prisoners coerced?"—for we agree that, in general, theirs is a condition in which many more choices are foreclosed, and decisions compelled, than in conditions of ordinary life. But the pervasive presence of restraints in the prison leaves open the question of whether, with respect to a particular option put before him, he is coerced. He has a chance, say, to participate as subject in a set of drug tests, requiring intermittent hospital visits, small to moderate risks, occasional days of complete bed rest, and paying twenty dollars per month for the six months of the tests. Most experiments using human subjects involve less time, less money, and less risk. Some involve more. Take this one as a realistic illustration.

It is true that his participation may promise occasional release from boredom. Boredom, however, is not a condition over which the investigator has any control, or in which he has any interest. It is simply the condition that the potential prisoner-subjects (as well as a good many non-prisoner-subjects) were in when the choice of participating or not was encountered by them. They are no more coerced into consenting by their boredom than I am coerced into seducing by my lust. The conditions in which we find ourselves powerfully affect our responses to choices put before us. If the standard of non-coercion be that potential subjects be free of all conditions that may significantly influence their willingness to consent, we will have no subjects and no experiments.

"But," the critic may reply, "although we are, indeed, all in conditions that constrain us in some respects, there remain enormous differences of degree. The prisoner's conditions are unusually severe, and that severity is what we underscore. When, for example, he supposes that giving his consent may help him, somehow, achieve an earlier release, he is in the special condition of desperately wanting release, and blindly hoping that someone up there will be more moved to help him because he did consent. That is what is unusual about his condition."

This reply will not work; it does not serve to distinguish the prisoner's case from the case of others whom we do not regard as improperly coerced. It isn't only prisoners who have desperate desires that they hope may come nearer to fulfillment because of participation in experiment. Indeed, while the prisoner's hopes along that line may be tenuous and largely the result of his own wishful thinking, many non-prisoners are faced with the opportunity to participate in experiments involving considerable risk, which offer more serious hope of fulfilling desperate wants. Consider the person with psoriasis covering much of his body, given the opportunity to participate in an experiment using a new and very powerful ultra-violet light that may increase the likelihood of his developing cancer, and may injure his eyes. No pressure whatever is brought to bear on him by the researcher. But very great pressures he or she must feel from the intense longing to be rid of that disfiguring affliction. Is that potential subject coerced by virtue of the desperation of his desire? Not in any sense that precludes his consent, surely; and if we thought he and others like him were truly coerced, we should have to forbid the experiment. Again, it is not rare for persons suffering from what appear to be terminal cancers to be offered the opportunity to participate in a controlled experiment with a new, highly toxic, chemical therapy that offers only slight hope of remission. All else has failed. Will the patient give consent to be experimental subject? Very probably; he

reaches for every chance to live. Is he coerced into being guinea-pig by the intensity of his desire? Not if the facts are presented to him truly and fairly. Indeed, we are likely to think that, though the new chemotherapy may have dreadful side effects, he is entitled, after being fully informed of the facts, to make up his own mind, and if given his circumstances he thinks it worth the risks, to consent to the desperate try.

If the researcher in this latter case had portrayed the patient's condition more grimly than the facts warranted, in order to get him to consent, we would think the patient to have been coerced, not by the intensity of his desire to live, but by that deceptive account. If the researcher had refrained deliberately from telling the patient of some alternative therapy offering equal hopes, in order to woo his participation, the patient would have been coerced, not by his needs or their grip on him, but by the manipulation of the investigator. Analogously, it is not the degree of boredom, or the passion of the desire for release, or the level of any condition that the prisoner is in, that can coerce him. It is only deliberate conduct, conduct designed to deceive, to pressure, to constrain, that would coerce in the sense required. Therefore the boredom, the desire for early release, the being under constant guard—these cannot in themselves constitute coercion of a potential subject.

The critic may take another tack. "I see now (he may say) that it is not the intensity of desire that marks off the prisoner's case, or renders him coerced. Yet the precariousness of his condition is the key to the immorality I've been driving at. It is the deliberate choosing of prison populations to do experiments we would not do with others, taking advantage of their desperation, that is coercive. This, I now see, is the root of my complaint. By using prisoners the researcher gets away with an exploitation of subjects that would be impossible elsewhere—and that calculated exploitation must not be allowed."

Here the critic gives a caution that deserves to be taken seriously; but its scope must not be overblown. If we do on prisoners experiments we would not do on others, believing that for ordinary persons the risks clearly outweigh the potential benefits, the calculated choice of a precariously placed population enabling us to get away with that would, indeed, be wrongful. What troubles so about it, however, is that experiments would then be done which ought not be done at all. In the same way, where great risk far outweighs potential benefit we would not tolerate huge sums used to inveigle the participation of indigent welfare recipients. To do with some, because we can get away with it, what we ought to do with no one is surely unconscionable. Some experiments in prisons, in the past, have been like that.

But this argument does not have the general force its advocates may suppose. When, for example, subject populations are enlisted both in and out of prisons on the same terms—as is often done—this objection has no place. When the judgment of experimental justifiability is made independently of the special circumstances of possible subject pools, an improper reliance upon those special circumstances cannot be complained of.

Moreover, the special circumstances of subjects may rightly enter when the experiment is of a kind that requires just that kind of subject for scientific reasons. Persons suffering from a given disease are reasonably chosen for experiments dealing with that disease, obviously, and any inclination they have to serve as subjects arising from that circumstance is neither avoidable nor pernicious. Again, some experiments have special requirements for long-term regularity and control, calling for subjects in unusually restricted circumstances. Seeking out those who fit the requirements of the investigation—an investigation whose worthiness is independently established—is equally reasonable, and no less so if those subjects be prisoners. It is a fact that for some scientific purposes prisoners are irreplaceable as subjects. Prisoners constitute extraordinarily stable populations, under constant and detailed observation. Diet, activity, whereabouts, and other factors possibly critical to the experiment are thoroughly known and dependable. And all of this is the case not as an imposed demand of the investigator, but as a consequence of the incarceration with which he had nothing to do. For experiments requiring repeated trials, over long periods, rigorously free of perturbing variables, there are no populations like these. One can imagine the sequestering of a non-prison subject pool for months or years, but there is no practical likelihood of it. Very few other persons, identifiable and accessible, are so situated that the time they must devote as subjects to lengthy experiments does not impose heavy burdens in removing them from what would be their alternate activities. The short of it is that for reasons having nothing to do with manipulative intent, but everything to do with scientific reliability, prison populations serve medicine as no other populations can. The critic rightly

insists that prisoners should not be preyed upon, that we must not do in prisons what should not be done. This is a long way from showing that no experiments ought be conducted in prisons, or that prisoners ought not to be allowed to volunteer as subjects.

What shall we say of payment to prisoners? That, after all, clearly is a factor under the researcher's full control. Moderate remuneration, of course, is widely given to subjects, in and out of prison. Insofar as those sums are deliberately offered to allure and tempt they are, in every case, manipulative. And of course their manipulative force is the greater as the potential subject is the poorer. This argues against payment to subjects in any context, and I think that is an alternative worthy of serious consideration. On the other hand, the prospect of a small money reward (which does serve as a major motivating force in prisons)[2] neither threatens nor pressures nor tempts to do what should not be done. The very moderate sums involved—twenty or forty dollars or so—are also viewed by many not so much as lures as compensation for inconvenience. Some who would be pleased to volunteer cannot otherwise afford the time. In that spirit the sums involved do not coerce anyone. We ought no more permit large sums to tempt prisoners into undue hazards than we ought permit that among non-prisoners. Neither should we withhold from prisoners the minor compensations that serving as subject normally provides. One principle we surely wish to maintain is that prisoners not be in any way special targets for exploitation, and their not being special targets entails their being treated, in the matter of payment, just as non-prisoners are treated. They should be paid no more, no less.

How "more" or "less" ought to be calculated is a nice question. Is it equality of the absolute sum that is required? Or is it the same relative proportion of regular income that is called for? This is arguable. In my judgment it is the same dollar sum that should be used, both to be fair, and to avoid the appearance of unfairness. The sums are in any event small; and adjusting them relatively entails the supposition of an "average regular income" of non-prisoner-subjects that must be wholly arbitrary.

It should be seen that even these small sums will be more alluring to prisoners than to most non-prisoners. If the payment be set at a regular standard, however, its allure is not the result of any deliberate effort by the researcher to twist the volition of the prisoner. Such twisting would be coercive. Given reasonable restrictions, that twisting can be avoided in the case of prisoners as it is in the case of non-prisoners.

I conclude that the argument against permitting prisoners to choose in this sphere, by virtue of their necessarily coerced condition, is simply mistaken. It confuses a wide sense of constraint (rightly characterizing the prison environment) with a different, narrow sense of constraint in the decision at hand—of which the prisoner can, with care, be entirely free. In the sense that one's condition coerces him, we are all coerced, and many of us as severely or more severely than prisoners. In the sense that choices before us, given our condition, may be made by us without ulterior manipulation in view of the merits of the case, the prisoners can, if fairly treated, be as free to choose as the rest of us.

Now it should be emphasized that prisoners and non-prisoners alike must be very carefully protected in making this choice—protected against "force, fraud, deceit, duress, over-reaching, or other ulterior form of constraint." Such protection against unfairness is a delicate and constantly on-going business whose detail I cannot enter here. In the case of potential subjects in prisons, the fact of total custody, the evident potential for the abuses of power, place upon the protecting body stringent demands for caution. Membership of that body, its procedures and powers, reviews and appeals—all are matters requiring utmost circumspection. But seeing to it that the right rules are well enforced is essentially an administrative matter, though a hard one. Mine has been a moral concern, about the rightness of the rule that would forbid all experimentation on prisoners. The common argument supporting that rule, I conclude, is grounded on mistake, on a misunderstanding of what is required for genuinely free consent.

IV PROTECTION OR PATERNALISM?

The argument for that exclusionary rule is bad; the rule itself is worse. Reasons of two different kinds suggest that prisoners should be permitted to volunteer as subjects in medical experiments. Reasons of the first kind arise from the moral importance of protecting, for the prisoners, their right to give or withhold consent. Reasons of the second kind arise from the positive moral worth of the medical experimentation in which prisoners participate of their own volition. I deal briefly with the two categories in turn.

First. Without urging participation in experimentation upon anyone we may insist that prisoners are morally entitled to permission to volunteer. Not to permit them to do so is to deny bluntly the autonomy of the prisoner in this sphere. Persons in full custody need to be protected, not patronized. They need to be guarded from abuse, but not treated as less than the full human beings they are. Prisons are commonly condemned, with much truth, as inhuman environments, demeaning, debasing, decivilizing. Perhaps we ought not have them at all. But since we do have them, and are likely to retain them for a good while into the future, we ought to seek to create within them a spirit in which—so far as is consistent with security and punishment—the humanity of the inmate is respected. One way to register this respect is to give to prisoners, within some feasible contexts, opportunities to make serious decisions about their own lives, just as non-prisoners must. To say of prison inmates that they cannot reach genuine decisions, that they are so cramped in mind that they are not even to be allowed to make effective choices in their personal lives, is to deny them a chunk of that capacity for self-direction that must be as precious to them as to anyone else. Such denial, it seems to me, is not justifiable. It is a usurpation of their self-direction of body and person that prison itself was never intended to effect. I am frankly dismayed by the presumption of well-meaning reformers in this sphere. They will preserve the gentle heifer of freedom in the prisons by shooting it in the head.

The voice of prisoners themselves on this question is not dispositive, but it is worth hearing. Of prisoners who have been subjects, 98% of those interviewed in a University of Michigan study were either very willing or somewhat willing to participate again in a similar project. 87% were very willing.[3] This suggests strongly that they would oppose the denial of the opportunity to do so. I know of no large scale study of prison populations generally on the moral issue itself. But I submit that, were the question we discuss to be put before prisoners for vote: "Should prisoners be permitted to decide for themselves whether they choose to consent to be subjects in medical experiments?" it may be safely predicted that the endorsement of that right by prisoners would be overwhelming.[4] Of course they want the opportunity for relief and earnings, in exchange for discomfort or risk, when they think (based on an honest account of the facts) that they are getting a good deal. Their willingness to make the deal, the critic says, is only a product of their coerced condition. We've looked at that response and, I trust, put it behind us. Beyond any bargain or deal, many prisoners do very genuinely want to be of service to medicine and to fellow human beings. The altruism is genuine for a good number; there is substantial evidence for the seriousness and generality of that motivation.[5] Surely it is presumptuous of the reformer to decide for prisoners that this self-described motivation is not genuine, or is too small a factor in their real set of motivations, to allow them to decide for themselves. That, I submit, is heteronomy on stilts.

V   WHAT COUNTS AS MORAL?

The rule excluding prisoners from experimentation is bad for reasons of a second kind, having to do with the experiments themselves. The advantages accruing to society as a whole (prisoners included, of course) from the medical experiments taking place in prisons are very, very great. I shan't even begin to catalog the benefits that have resulted, and continue to flow, from such programs. "But," says the critic, "such benefits may not be taken as considerations bearing on the proposed exclusionary rule, since they are matters of utilitarian calculation, while the rule is a non-utilitarian protection of justice for prisoners." Allowing that the benefits are real, the critic insists that for judgment on this question the calculation of them cannot even be reached.

Again he errs. For utilitarian moralists his argument is utterly without sense, obviously. For those of us who are not thorough-going utilitarians this argument fails because it treats the process of experimentation, and the effort to acquire knowledge that can alleviate suffering and disease, as being purely non-moral, instruments for the attainment of sheer utilities having nothing to do with justice or duty. Not so. There are strong moral reasons to engage in medical experimentation, to serve the vital interests of persons numerous but unidentified. Reasons supporting such activities may include crass considerations like the reduction of absenteeism in factories, and so on, but also surely include considerations of human pain and longevity that cannot be thought crass. To the extent that there lies upon any of us the obligation to advance inquiry of a beneficent character, a proposed rule that would hinder the fulfillment of that obligation is morally objectionable so far. If we allow that some (and perhaps all) of us have such obligations, the impact of the rule in question here upon the fulfillment of these obligations may certainly be reached in appraising that rule.

Is there a general principle of beneficence that does oblige us to be actively good? If there is, does that principle provide, perhaps, a *prima facie* obligation to advance (or not to obstruct) research aimed at knowledge to be used in healing the sick? I am not sure. It may be so. In any event we will want to insure that our rules do not unduly hinder any of us (including prisoners) who honestly believe that they have that beneficent obligation, or those of us whose special placement yields special duties.

The circumstances of the research investigator are special in this respect. The physician and the physician-researcher do take on, consciously and deliberately, the obligation to do what is reasonably within their power to ease pain, to heal, and to acquire the knowledge needed to promote these ends. The likely long-term consequences of the pursuit of such knowledge must therefore be weighed in the fully moral appraisal of any proposed principle that would restrict such pursuit.

What may mislead the critic here is the fact that while our duties to the subject in an experiment are reasonably precise—we must tell this person these things in this way—our duties to the unidentified beneficiaries of future experimentation are very imprecise. Toward them we have, as Kant would say, "imperfect" duties, because although obliged to serve them, the form of our service is not specifiable in advance. But imperfect duties are as real as those of more perfect form. That understood, we can have little remaining doubt that the results of medical experimentation for which prisoners volunteer is morally relevant in deciding whether they should be permitted to volunteer.

Finally, there are benefits of other kinds, arguably non-moral, that may also be worthy of consideration because they bear directly upon imprisonment, and the well-being of the prisoners concerned. Serving as genuinely voluntary subjects in medical experiments can and often does support the rehabilitative aims of the correctional institution. Studies have shown that such participation adds measureably to the prisoner's sense of self-esteem.[6] This becomes one of the few contexts in which he finds himself able to act purposefully in a larger world of serious affairs. In this role he can be full citizen, participant, taking some risks, gaining some advantages, being of service—in general grappling with serious matters in a way that supposes him to be the rational captain of his own fate. Rehabilitation in our prisons has not generally succeeded, as we know well. This device is no panacea, to be sure. But it does as much, perhaps more, to rehabilitate those it fully involves as any other activity in the prison. To eliminate it, out of regard for the prisoners, is to cut off our noses with theirs.

In sum. The reasons against permitting prisoners to give their consent are not sound. The moral reasons for permitting them to do so are forceful. The consideration of long-term benefits to all, and especially to the prisoners, that flow from the permission merely transforms an argument that is compelling into one that is more so.

VI EPILOG

Two concluding notes. Wherever I refer to the advantages or permissibility of medical experiments with voluntary prison subjects, I suppose that the caution in selecting subjects, in informing them, and in safeguarding their honest volition has been maximal. Horror stories abound; they are instructive in many contexts, but not in this one. Our question concerns the principles that ought to govern experimentation when fairly and honorably conducted.

And lastly. Early on I observed that prisoners are archetypical of persons precariously placed. But there are other categories of persons who, by virtue of their jobs, or custodial status, or the like, are particularly vulnerable to manipulation. The cautions that are rightly introduced in proposing to prisoners that they volunteer as subjects must of course be mirrored, in appropriate form and degree, for others in analogous circumstances: servicemen on military duty; patients in public hospital wards; employees in drug firms and laboratories; even students in school or university classes—all are in need of special protection for reasons like (but of course not identical with) the reasons we are specially concerned [about] with prisoners. By the same token, it is a mistake to assume that persons in such categories are incapable of giving their uncoerced consent, and that they therefore must not be permitted to do so. Of the larger class of the "precariously placed" the category [of] prisoners is the most extreme. Having dealt with it, I take myself—putting aside special

situations—to have dealt, *a fortiori*, with all of the less extreme cases in the same family.

NOTES

1 The report and recommendations of the National Commission for the Protection of Human Subjects of Biomedical and Behavioral Research [*Research Involving Prisoners*, Washington, D.C., Sept. 1976] is an important example. The Commission recommends that "research involving prisoners should not be conducted or supported" unless a lengthy set of detailed conditions in the prison are fully realized. Voluntariness of consent is held to presuppose *grievance procedures* with elected prisoner representatives and prison advocates, and *living conditions* which, in turn, are specified to include such items as: single occupancy cells for all who desire them; arrangements for frequent, private visits; high standards for education, vocational training, health care, and recreation facilities, and so on. Since virtually no prisons are able to meet or approach the standards imposed, the recommendation (if adopted) would have the effect of forbidding almost all experimentation in prisons.

It would appear that the Commission seeks to use permission to experiment in prisons as a social lever for what it views as needed prison reforms. Leaving aside the question of the necessity of the reforms demanded, it is unfortunate that the serious question of whether the consent of prisoners can be truly voluntary is there dealt with as an instrument to influence policy in other spheres rather than on its own merits.

2 See *Research in Prisons*, Survey Research Center, Institute for Social Research, The University of Michigan, Ann Arbor, 1976; pp. 47 ff.

3 Ibid., p. 57.

4 In April of 1973, "96 of the 175 inmates of the Lancaster County, Pa. prison wrote to the local newspaper protesting the state's decision to stop all medical experiments on state prisoners" reads a report in the *Wall Street Journal* of 2 April 1974. Anecdotal evidence only, but not surprising.

5 *Research in Prisons*, op. cit. While this study shows that money is the reason most commonly given by prisoner subjects for volunteering, the second most common reason, cited by 27% of the many subjects

interviewed, was "To help others, help society." (p. 47)

Anecdotal but very persuasive support for this conclusion may be found also in the account of Dr. John C. McDonald, "Why Prisoners Volunteer to Be Experimental Subjects," JAMA, Nov. 6, 1967 (vol. 202, no. 6).

6 See: *Pharmacological Testing in a Correctional Institution*, S. H. Wells, P. Kennedy, et al., Charles C. Thomas, Publisher, Springfield, Ill., 1974. See also: *Proceedings*, Conference on Drug Research in Prisons, National Council on Crime and Delinquency, 1973.

On the Morality of Paying Research Subjects

Due and Undue Inducements: On Paying Money to Research Subjects

Ruth Macklin

A biographical sketch of Ruth Macklin is found on page 162.

Macklin analyzes the concept of undue inducement. She limits her discussion to "normal, healthy" volunteers and to monetary inducements. In her analysis, Macklin attempts to identify criteria that can be used to distinguish due inducements from undue ones. Although it proves impossible to provide a single objective criterion, Macklin presents several examples as paradigms of undue inducement as well as one paradigm of a due inducement. After critically examining these paradigms, Macklin suggests that a practical approach to take in the case of any research project would be to begin by setting payments to normal, healthy volunteers low. If this does not generate enough volunteers, then there might be reason to question the acceptability of the risks, trouble, and time that the project demands of volunteers. In her discussion, Macklin explores some of the moral tensions that arise when payments for research participation are low.

Federal regulations governing the protection of research subjects specify that no "undue inducements" be offered to lure people into volunteering.[1] Two basic assumptions underlie this provision: first, that *some* inducement is necessary to prompt a sufficient number of people to volunteer to serve as research subjects; second, that a theoretically sound and practicably workable distinction can be drawn between inducements that are "undue," and therefore morally unacceptable, and those that are acceptable or "due." The concept of inducement that needs explication has the following characteristics:

• It is weaker than the notion of coercion;

• It allows for a conceptual distinction between due and undue;

• The subcategory of due inducements can be distinguished from other voluntary or uncoerced acts in which the motivation of the agent does not arise out of an offer made by another person (for example, being motivated by altruism, or by the desire to find a cure for the disease that caused a relative's death).

By now it is an unquestioned ethical precept of biomedical and behavioral research practice that subjects should not be coerced into participating. The requirement that people serve as subjects only when

Reprinted with permission of the author and the publisher from *IRB: A Review of Human Subjects Research*, vol. 3 (May 1981), pp. 1–6.

they freely choose to do so is embodied in federally mandated and morally accepted procedures for gaining informed consent. Those who choose to participate in research should be capable of choosing freely; they must do so voluntarily, willingly, without duress, and without being subjected to threats or to a promise of too great a reward.

Worries about the ability of research subjects to consent freely—to be genuine volunteers—have mainly concerned institutionalized populations, especially prisoners, and those debilitated by sickness and prey to its attendant hopes and fears, namely patients. A different range of problems concerning informed consent arises with the institutionalized mentally infirm, incompetent patients, patients who have been medicated beyond their ability to think clearly, to reason, and to judge—the problems of adequately *informed* consent. So as not to complicate the subject of this article by bringing in issues that bear on understanding, memory, cognitive capacities, and other concerns relating to the *informed* part of the doctrine of informed consent, I will focus this discussion on "normal volunteers," or "healthy" research subjects.[2]

My aim will be to examine the distinction between due and undue inducements to serve as a research subject. Can such a distinction be drawn? If so, what criteria are available for making it, and are they practicably workable criteria? Are there *objective* grounds for making a clear and sound distinction between due and undue inducements? Does what counts as undue or due vary from person to person, so that it can only be viewed as a *relative* notion, even though objectively grounded? (In this sense of "objectively grounded," an explanation for which a scientific—biological or psychosocial—basis can be supplied accounts for why some offers are undue inducements for some people, while those same offers do not even tempt others.) Another possibility is, of course, that this situation is entirely *subjective*, meaning that an inducement is due or undue according to each individual's value scheme, and there can be no recourse to objective facts beyond what every person thinks or feels when confronted with the prospect of serving as a research subject.

In addition to limiting the discussion to normal, healthy volunteers who serve as research subjects, I impose a further condition: only monetary inducements will be explored. These restrictions on the topic are not intended to dismiss the wider context in which it is morally significant: clinical trials on patients, research

on sick people unrelated to their disease, and nonmonetary inducements of all sorts to participate in research. In the course of the discussion, examples will be drawn from those other contexts by way of illustration or contrast. But because this entire topic has been given little attention, it seems wise in this beginning effort to limit the scope.

There is no fixed sum of money below which inducements can be judged due and above which they must be deemed undue. Although this point is obvious, it needs to be addressed briefly. Different people attach different values to a monetary sum, so what is for some people an offer they cannot refuse is for others barely tempting. This is so for two reasons. The first, well known from welfare economic theory, is the diminishing marginal utility of a unit of currency. A dollar has more value for the person with low income or wealth than for one who is rich. It is this consideration (rather than intellectual curiosity or altruism) that may account for the large pool of students among normal, healthy volunteers.

A second reason, however, poses a more difficult problem for attempts to arrive at an objective criterion for distinguishing due from undue inducements. Even people having the same general income or wealth attach different values to money. Some shopkeepers stay open seven days a week, fourteen hours each day, in the hopes of raking in a few more dollars. Others, with the same volume of business, value their own time for leisure and recreation more than the additional increment of money, so they close on Sundays and keep a ten-hour daily schedule. Some individuals who work for large companies are constantly seeking new opportunities for employment, in the knowledge that each change of job brings a greater salary increase than would a scheduled raise or promotion at their own institution. Others, who make the same amount of money, place a higher value on not uprooting their families constantly, and are content to remain much longer (for some, their entire working lives) in the same organization, with full knowledge that they could have doubled their annual income by being willing to change jobs frequently.

The difference among people—the value they attach to money that does not derive from its diminishing marginal utility—presents almost insurmountable difficulties for any attempt to find a workable criterion for distinguishing due from undue monetary inducements to serve as a research subject. A still further complicating factor is the difference among people in their willingness to subject themselves to risks. Some who place a high value on money may nonetheless be risk-avoiders, leading them to shun situations they perceive as dangerous even if remuneration is involved. Others, who in general may value money less, will be prepared to place themselves at some risk to gain additional money because of their indifference to taking risks.

These considerations suggest that it will be impossible to arrive at a single, objective criterion serving to mark off due from undue monetary inducements to participate in research. But we should not despair too soon. A fruitful method to use in clarifying a problematic concept is the method of paradigms. This philosophical approach proceeds by identifying clear cases—ones on which virtually universal agreement exists, which then serve as paradigms for judging cases that have some but not all features of the paradigms. This method lacks the precision of a hard-and-fast criterion, which entails stating necessary and sufficient conditions for applying a concept. But what the use of paradigms lacks in precision it gains in greater ease of application. The drawback of this method is, of course, that it leaves a large gray area, an area of uncertainty, requiring that a decision be made in each new case when its features depart sufficiently from those of the paradigm. It is useful to consider briefly some paradigms of due and undue inducements to participate in research.

PARADIGMS OF UNDUE INDUCEMENTS

The following three cases appear to be paradigms of undue inducements. Each one exhibits somewhat different features relevant to drawing the distinction in question. The first case involved the death of a research subject in a sleep experiment at the NIH. Bernadette Gillcrist, a twenty-three-year-old nursing student, died from a cardiac arrest while in the NIH sleep laboratory in April 1980.[3] Although Gillcrist was presumed to be a normal, healthy volunteer, investigations following her death revealed that she had suffered from anorexia nervosa and as a result had engaged in self-induced vomiting, had suffered two previous cardiac arrests, and had concealed all those facts. Participants in the NIH sleep study were paid $100 per day; at the time of her death, Gillcrist had earned $1300. According to one volunteer in this same experiment, "Sure, money was the motivation. Isn't it always?"[4]

Why should the case of Bernadette Gillcrist be considered a paradigm of an undue inducement? Is it because the motivation to participate in the study was undoubtedly money? No, since except in the rare cases of purely altruistic behavior, payment for "services rendered" almost always motivates normal, healthy people to volunteer. If a sufficient number of research subjects could be obtained by appealing to altruistic motives, there would probably be no need to offer money as an inducement in the first place.

Is this case a paradigm because the research subject died in the course of the study? No, for two reasons. First, the experiment itself was not unduly risky for a normal, healthy subject; and it seems clear that Gillcrist's cardiac arrest was not caused by any of the experimental procedures, but rather by a potassium imbalance that resulted from her self-induced vomiting. Second, the death of a research subject cannot *by itself* serve to validate a case as a paradigm of undue inducement, even if the death were a result of procedures undertaken in the course of the experiment. Such an occurrence could serve to validate a claim about the *degree of risk* posed by the experiment, and only then could it be used as evidence that the monetary payment was high enough to induce a person to take what was perhaps an unwarranted risk.

The feature of this case that leads me to treat it as a paradigm of undue inducement is that the subject lied about her past medical history—her previous cardiac arrests, her condition of anorexia nervosa, and the vomiting, which apparently continued right up to the time of her death, since dried vomitus was found in her handbag. She did not tell her psychiatrist that she was participating in the NIH experiment, nor did she inform the NIH researchers that she was seeing a psychiatrist (in fact, she saw her psychiatrist on the night she died). These multiple deceptions and concealments provide reasonably strong evidence that this subject was quite eager to participate in the research. There is little doubt that Gillcrist would have been excluded from participation in the NIH sleep study had any of the facts of her past and continuing medical condition been revealed. However, one important caveat should be issued here. The use of this case as a paradigm is weakened by the factors pointing to the subject's mental illness. The more an individual departs from an ideal of a normal, healthy volunteer, the more questionable a case becomes for the purpose of serving as a paradigm.

The principle emerging from this paradigm is as follows: *Inducements are undue if they prompt subjects to lie, deceive, or conceal information that, if known, would disqualify them as participants in a research project.* The sum of $1300 is a considerable one for a student to receive, especially since the NIH sleep experiment did not involve a large number of waking hours or very much effort on the part of the subjects. But for reasons cited earlier, I think it cannot be the dollar amount alone, in this case or most others, that constitutes a criterion for marking off undue from due inducements. If a potential subject engages in illegal or unethical behavior (in this case, lying) in order to obtain a considerable sum of money, then the offer constitutes an undue inducement.

The second paradigm can only be described briefly, since little information about its details is available. A study was recently reported[5] in which healthy subjects had been recruited to test a vaccine for gonorrhea. The procedure involved infecting male volunteers with the disease, prior to which some subjects received the vaccine and others did not. Since the article gave no information about either the payment or recruitment of these subjects, let us supply those hypothetically. Suppose the monetary sum the volunteers were offered was $1300, the same amount Bernadette Gillcrist received. The main feature of this paradigm that distinguishes it from the first is the risk of harm to the subjects. Unlike the NIH sleep study, which posed little risk to normal, healthy subjects, a study in which subjects deliberately contract venereal disease carries a variety of risks. Beyond the obvious risks of the disease itself (even with the existence of an effective cure), there are psychological risks associated with a disease affecting the sex organs, psychosocial risks of having a stigmatizing disease, social risks of transmitting the disease to others, and possible damage to a marriage if married male volunteers served as subjects.

A paradigm should accord with our presystematic moral intuitions, which is precisely why I find a payment of $1300 for participation in this gonorrhea study a clear case of an undue inducement. We need only ask whether volunteers for this research could be obtained by offering a payment of, say, $5.00 (a standard payment for noninvasive procedures in the course of an experiment) to judge that an inducement of $1300 is undue. What this suggests is that *the nature of the risk* is one of the factors to which the notion of undue inducement must be relativized (other factors will be explored later). Readers who question my use of this case as a paradigm should reflect on what dollar amount they would cite—however high—as constituting a

paradigm of an undue inducement for a study in which volunteers are infected with venereal disease.

The third paradigm may seem a bit tangential, since it is one that did not involve monetary payments, and consent was obtained not from the subjects themselves, but instead, from parents of the research subjects. While not normal volunteers (they were retarded children), the subjects in the Willowbrook hepatitis study were nonetheless healthy at the time their parents volunteered them as participants in an experiment to study the entire course of the disease in persons deliberately infected with hepatitis virus. The ethics of that experiment and the defenses offered by the researchers have been widely discussed,[6] and I will not pursue them here. It is the question of inducements to parents to volunteer their children that I want to explore briefly.

Although Willowbrook was acknowledged even at the time to have one of the more horrendous institutional environments (dirty, understaffed, with disease running rampant), it remained one of the few public institutions in the New York area available for housing retarded children. There was a long waiting list, and parents who lacked the financial resources to place their youngsters in a private facility were desperate to get them in somewhere. The researchers in the Willowbrook hepatitis study were permitted to offer parents who were willing to consent to their retarded-but-healthy children's participation a place in the institution. Furthermore, parents were told that the hygiene, staff attention, and other amenities enjoyed by children who were subjects of this study were superior to conditions in the institution generally. Thus, not only were parents who granted consent for their retarded youngsters to serve as research subjects able to place their children in Willowbrook; they could do so under better conditions than that same institution offered to all other inmates. But they had to be explicitly willing to have their children deliberately infected with hepatitis. That is not merely an undue inducement to grant consent for oneself or one's family member to serve as a research subject. What is worse, it is a "coercive offer."[7] The Willowbrook paradigm is complicated for several reasons: the subjects were not normal; it involved third-party permission, rather than adults granting consent for themselves; and the children would almost surely have contracted hepatitis had they entered Willowbrook as ordinary inmates rather than as experimental subjects (this last consideration was the researchers' main defense of the ethics of their study). Yet the features of the paradigm that make it interesting relate to the motivation of the parents who volunteered their retarded children for the study.

A PARADIGM OF DUE INDUCEMENT

Is there a paradigm of due inducements to serve as a research subject? A recent report of recruitment and payment policies of drug companies that seek volunteers among their own employees is instructive.

> Recruitment and payment policies appear to be quite uniform. There is general agreement that volunteers should be recruited by open, written invitation rather than directly by company personnel. Employees are informed of the program through special brochures and notices placed in in-house publications and posted on bulletin boards. One company, however, encloses solicitation notices in the employees' pay envelopes.
>
> Payment for participation in research is universal. The amount paid is usually an established, reasonable fee-for-service schedule; i.e., the time and procedures and/or inconvenience involved. In most cases the subjects receive the minimum standard hourly wage plus (approximately) $3.00 for a venipuncture, $5.00 for 24-hour urine collection, etc. Some firms offer additional remuneration to employees who volunteer for "unpopular" studies or who take vacation days for studies of longer duration. The objective of most payment policies, however, is to deemphasize the financial inducements.[8]

This report is instructive because of its mention of recruitment practices, as well as payment scales. On the assumption that drug companies are scrupulous in adhering to these procedures, the inducements appear to be due for the following reasons. Dollar amounts are commensurate with what the research subjects might earn if they sought further employment outside their main workplace (moonlighting of some sort); additional increments for specific procedures are modest; increased remuneration for participating during vacation days is entirely reasonable (employees might assess the benefits of additional money against the loss of vacation days by putting that money toward a week in the Caribbean during their remaining vacation time).

Several features of this last paradigm begin to make it clearer what issues are involved in trying to mark off due from undue inducements. Again, it is unlikely that a dollar amount *alone* could serve as a criterion; yet a payment equivalent to, or slightly above, the minimum wage could hardly be charged with constituting an undue inducement. The trouble is, it may be too low to serve even as a due inducement for many people to participate at all. I will return to this point in another connection in the conclusion. A second feature of this paradigm is instructive. It is not only the payment policies, but also the method of recruitment that contributes to an assessment of whether an inducement is due or undue. This point is crucial for the activities of IRBs. Ought IRBs to be informed about the details of payment to research subjects? Is it part of their charge to look at those details? I have no doubt whatever of the relevance of payment scales and policies to the charge of IRBs. Before proceeding with the main inquiry, then, I will digress briefly to elaborate this last point.

In addition to the task of assessing the risks versus benefits of research protocols, IRBs must be concerned with all relevant procedures governing informed consent. The IRB is supposed to determine that subjects of research are genuine volunteers. Federal regulations stipulate that an individual must "be able to exercise free power of choice without undue inducement or any element of force, fraud, deceit, duress, or any other form of constraint or coercion."[9] Obviously, in order to fulfill this charge, IRBs must be informed of recruitment procedures for each protocol, in addition to having a copy of the consent form. How else could an IRB determine whether consent will be obtained freely? The question here is not whether the consent form itself should include the amount of payment subjects will receive; it is with the normative question of whether IRBs *should* concern themselves with the amount of payment. Here the answer seems obvious: IRBs must be aware of both recruitment practices and amounts of monetary payments; otherwise they have insufficient information to fulfill their charge of determining that consent is obtained without force, fraud, deceit, duress, and without undue inducements.

Medical schools, drug companies, and IRBs have all demonstrated concern about whether and how matters relating to payment of subjects constitute an undue inducement. One IRB is careful to strike any reference to payment of subjects from a listing under "benefits" on the consent form. A medical school in a metropolitan area with a large number of urban poor has a policy of not advertising or attempting to recruit subjects from the poor section of town. Its policy is to recruit subjects from among medical students, and there is a general suspicion of efforts to solicit subjects from among community residents because of the fear that monetary payments will serve as an undue inducement. This further complicates the picture of trying to distinguish between due and undue inducements, since medical students, at the time they are students, may well have a lower income than the working poor (or even people receiving welfare payments). Finally, as noted earlier in discussing recruitment and payment policies of drug companies, there is evidence that the objective of such policies is to deemphasize the financial inducements. One can readily believe that drug companies exercise genuine caution in formulating such policies regarding their own employees, without assuming that their motives are entirely those of concern for the subjects' well-being. The motive can be purely one of self-interest on the part of drug companies, in not wanting to be accused of offering undue inducements to their employees. But with drug companies as well as medical schools, a judgment of whether or not their payment and recruitment practices are ethical has nothing to do with their motives.

WHAT ARE NORMAL VOLUNTEERS PAID FOR?

A deeper understanding of the distinction between undue and due inducements might be gained by a brief inquiry into the question of what normal, healthy volunteers are being paid for. One way in which cash payments have been described is as "payment for services rendered."[10] I think that phrase is not quite accurate as a description of what research subjects are being paid for, although the phrase is appropriate to use in distinguishing between money used to induce subjects to participate in research and reimbursements for expenses the subject has incurred.

Are subjects being compensated for the *time* they put in when they participate in a research study? Is the payment being offered for *risks* incurred in the course of the study, or, perhaps, for *pain* or *discomfort* of the procedures involved? Is it for the *trouble* or *inconvenience* subjects are put to when they volunteer for a study? These factors should be distinguished from one another, since a subject may be inconvenienced or even experience pain or discomfort without undergoing any substantial risk; and there may be considerable

inconvenience in a project that takes very little time away from a subject's usual activities during those hours, as in the case of sleep studies conducted at night. Or is the payment an *inducement*, plain and simple (that without which too few subjects could be recruited)?

All these elements are factors used to determine payment scales for normal, healthy volunteers. If *time* alone were the consideration determining the appropriate monetary sum, then subjects should be paid according to one of two payment scales: Method 1, a scale commensurate with what they actually earn in their occupation, adjusted to an hourly wage; or Method 2, a fee roughly equivalent to, or slightly above, the minimum wage. Some studies seeking volunteers use Method 1 to determine pay scales; some use Method 2, usually with additional sums for risky or invasive procedures, in which case the factors are "mixed." Since risky experiments and those involving pain or discomfort usually offer higher payments to volunteers, it cannot be time alone that is used to determine what subjects should be paid. It is likely that volunteers are being paid at least in part for the trouble they are put to by serving as subjects in a research study. It would be virtually impossible, however, to arrive at an objective measure for determining how much people ought to be paid for undergoing what amount of trouble. Since time, risk, pain or discomfort, and trouble all seem to work together, in varying combinations, it may be impossible to factor out any one element in studies that involve all or several of them.

An objective measure can be proposed for the remaining possibility—payment whose purpose is merely to induce subjects to participate in research. This amount would be the lowest sum of money that could be offered to obtain a sufficient number of subjects to carry out the research project. While this amount would no doubt turn out to be a function of the other three factors (time, risk, and trouble) from the subjects' point of view, it would not be based on researchers' antecedent judgments of what those factors are worth. Instead, researchers would have to arrive at the amount empirically, by seeing what the market will bear. After a sufficient amount of data has been gathered to serve as a baseline, payments to subjects in future studies could be determined by those baseline data. One piece of evidence that could be adduced to show that payments offered for a particular study are too high—that they are indeed undue inducements—would be a showing of a significantly larger pool of volunteers than is usually obtained when normal, healthy volunteers are solicited for research. But while this result would count as *evidence* that the amount of money offered was an undue inducement, it could not serve as a *criterion* for undue inducements. This is because other motivating factors might also be present, so that subjects might still have volunteered for the research project even if the payment offered had been lower.

There are three problems with the proposal that monetary payments be set at the lowest amount that would succeed in obtaining a sufficiently large subject pool for the study. The first problem is practical: researchers would have to do a study to determine empirically what that amount of money is before they could embark on their research project. This practical problem could be mitigated somewhat by arriving at a baseline, as mentioned above.

The second problem is one of social justice in distributing the burdens of serving as a research subject.[11] Setting the payment as low as would be necessary to gain a subject pool would virtually ensure that those subjects would all be drawn from lower social and economic classes. This may not be objectionable to some people, but for those whose principles of justice require that society's benefits and burdens be distributed equitably throughout the population, it would be an unacceptable result if the vast majority of normal, healthy research subjects are those who have the lowest income or wealth. A counterclaim to this moral worry is that those who have less money ought to be given the opportunity to earn more, especially in noble pursuits like serving as a research subject, which in most cases do not involve high risks or an inordinate expenditure of time or trouble. The tension between these two moral viewpoints is not easily resolved, especially since people tend to adhere tenaciously to their favored principle of justice.

The third problem with the proposal that monetary payments be set at the lowest amount capable of drawing a sufficient number of volunteers is that it simply fails to guarantee that the payment is not an undue inducement for those who do volunteer. The (hypothetical) $1300 fee offered to those who volunteered for the gonorrhea vaccine study may indeed be the lowest amount that could be paid in order to obtain a pool of subjects. But it remains a paradigm, in my view, of an undue inducement. The difficulty here, as one might have suspected all along, is the relativity of the concept of undue inducements.

To what should the notion of undue inducements be relativized? For reasons noted earlier, it is highly unlikely that we can arrive at a fixed amount of money below which inducements should be considered due and above which undue. We must, therefore, identify factors to which the notion can be relativized, if there is to be an objective measure of any sort. Candidates are as follows:

(1) Prevailing practices in this domain (typical payments offered to research subjects);

(2) A set of facts about each subject who volunteers: financial status; the degree to which the subject values money (the individual's subjective utility scale); whether the subject is a risk taker or a risk avoider; whether the subject has opportunities for obtaining equivalent sums of money by other (legal) means;

(3) A calculation made by the researcher of the time, risks, and trouble involved for subjects in the experiment;

(4) Some combination of (1)–(3).

To use (1) alone is surely unsatisfactory, since payments among the prevailing rates may be undue according to intuitive judgments of that notion (intuitive judgments of the sort used to arrive at the paradigms). To try to secure the information cited in (2) would obviously be practicably unworkable, and would pose some ethical problems as well. To relativize the notion of undue inducements to each volunteer would result in setting a different payment for each individual, or for whole classes of people. In effect, this would be giving unequal pay for equal work (the "work" involved is presumably the same for all subjects in the same experiment). Nothing more need be said here about the ethics of violating the precept of equal pay for equal work.

As discussed in the preceding section, (3) represents virtually the situation we have now. And as for the last alternative, it need only be noted that if (1) and (2) are unsatisfactory when considered alone, they will not be rendered satisfactory by being taken in combination with one another, and with (3).

It is hardly surprising that this analysis has raised more problems than it has resolved. I do think a practical solution is to start with a presumption that payments to normal, healthy volunteers should be set low, rather than high. If the use of this guideline yields an insufficient number of subjects for particular research projects, it may count as evidence that there is something unacceptable about the research—the amount of time it takes, the degree of risk, or the amount of trouble it requires subjects to undergo. Before raising the cash payment, thereby incurring the risk of offering an undue inducement, investigators should rethink the research design to see if alternative methods would be feasible. For example, the researchers engaged in testing the vaccine for gonorrhea might have made an effort to identify by epidemiological means subjects among a pool of applicants at risk for contracting the disease by the usual means. Those subjects would then not be placing themselves at much greater risk than that posed by their everyday life, and they would no doubt enjoy a more pleasurable experience serving as research subjects than those in whose urethras gonococci were implanted.

There is no way, in the end, of circumventing the objection from social justice. A tension exists here, as elsewhere, between two moral precepts. The lower the cash payment, with the aim of avoiding undue inducements, the greater the likelihood that volunteers will be from lower social and economic groups. This arrangement violates the principle of equitable distribution of burdens in society. On the other hand, if an effort is made to adjust payments proportionally to different levels of income of potential pools of volunteers, the result would be a violation of the principle of equal pay for equal work. I believe that the first of these undesirable alternatives is preferable to the second. To adopt a variable payment scale would be to open up a whole new area of abuse. Volunteers would be sorely tempted to lie about their income in order to receive higher pay as a research subject. We should avoid instituting new practices that lend themselves to likely abuse. The steps that would have to be taken to safeguard against such abuses would probably involve invasions of privacy—efforts to discover what a volunteer really earns would be the only way of ascertaining the truth.

THE PROBLEM OF PATERNALISM

There is, finally, the perennial problem of paternalism. So long as the subjects of research are normal, healthy volunteers, some would argue, we should not be overly worried about offering undue inducements. It is one thing if the sick, the disabled, the handicapped, the retarded, the senile, the mentally ill, or children are being recruited as research subjects. They need protection, and are entitled to such protections because of their diminished capacities for rational judgment. But it is yet another instance of unwarranted paternalism, this argument goes, to restrict amounts of money offered to normal, healthy volunteers who are presumably rational enough to determine by their own system of values what tasks to engage in and what risks to undertake. If those who are willing to take the risks involved in skiing, hang gliding, rock climbing, or auto racing choose to incur a different kind of risk by serving as research subjects (perhaps in order to obtain money to pursue their risky recreational ventures), that's their business and their choice to make. After all, if undue inducements are not really instances of coercion, we need only make sure that research subjects are genuine volunteers, that is, that they are not threatened or given coercive offers. Beyond that, the federal regulations should be viewed as lapsing into rhetoric when they caution against undue inducements.

I find the above antipaternalist stance too strong. There are other values besides individual freedom, one of which is respect for persons. One can respect people's liberty, while still recognizing their tendency to succumb to temptations, to fail to recognize their own best interests on occasion, and to undertake what may be irrational risks. Biomedical and behavioral researchers are not being overly paternalistic in guarding against unduly inducing people to take a risk that only a large sum of money would lure them into incurring.

ACKNOWLEDGMENTS

I thank Karin Meyers, Joanne Lynn, Arthur Caplan, Barbara Mishkin, and Robert J. Levine for their help in preparing this article.

REFERENCES

1 45 CFR 46.103.
2 These terms are used to denote research subjects other than patients undergoing clinical trials. I do not mean to beg any questions about the meaning or application of "normal" or "healthy."
3 The information reported below is taken from Kolata, G. B.: NIH shaken by death of research volunteer. *Science* 209:475–479, 1980. See also Kolata, G. B.: The death of a research subject. *Hastings Center Report* 10 (No. 4): 5–6, August 1980.
4 Quoted in Kolata, G. B.: The death of a research subject, p. 6.
5 Vaccine from gonorrhea pili shows up well under challenge. *Medical World News*: October 13, 1980.

6 For details of the research project and discussion of the ethical issues, see the "Willowbrook" articles and letters in *Moral Problems in Medicine*. Edited by S. Gorovitz et al. Englewood Cliffs: Prentice-Hall, Inc., 1976, pp. 123–142.

7 Space does not permit a discussion here of the distinction between undue inducements and coercive offers. Some articles in the philosophical literature that deal with coercion, threats, and coercive offers are as follows: Abrams, N.: Medical experimentation: the consent of prisoners and children. In *Philosophical Medical Ethics: Its Nature and Significance*. Edited by S. F. Spicker and H. T. Engelhardt, Jr., Dordrecht-Holland: D. Reidel Publishing Company, 1977, pp. 111–124. Frankfurt, H.: Coercion and moral responsibility. In *Essays on Freedom of Action*. Edited by T. Honderich, 1973. Lyons, D.: Welcome threats and coercive offers. *Philosophy* 50:425–436, 1975.

Nozick, R.: Coercion. In *Philosophy, Science, and Method*. Edited by S. Morgenbesser, P. Suppes, and Morton White. New York: St. Martin's Press, 1969, pp. 440–472.

8 Meyers, K.: Drug company employees as research subjects: programs, problems, and ethics. *IRB: A Review of Human Subjects Research* 1 (No. 8): 5, December 1979.

9 CFR 46.103, definition of "informed consent."

10 Levine, R. J.: What should consent forms say about cash payments? *IRB: A Review of Human Subjects Research* 1 (No. 6): 7, October 1979.

11 For a discussion of this topic with reference to the work of the National Commission for the Protection of Human Subjects, see Lebacqz, K.: Beyond respect for persons and beneficence: justice in research. *IRB: A Review of Human Subjects Research* 2 (No. 7):1–4, August/September 1980.

Inducement, Due and Otherwise

Lisa Newton

Lisa Newton is professor of philosophy at Fairfield University and adjunct professor at Sacred Heart University. Her areas of specialization are medical ethics, political philosophy, and social philosophy. Newton's published articles include "The Irrelevance of Religion in the Abortion Debate," "Collective Responsibility in Health Care," and "Malpractice from an Ethical Perspective."

Newton criticizes Macklin's analysis of due and undue inducement, rejecting the assumption that paying research subjects "too much" is "somehow coercive." Newton provides a different set of reasons for keeping payments low and for restricting the pool of applicants to volunteers whose primary motivation is not financial. Like Macklin, she rejects the free market approach, but not on the basis of considerations of justice. Rather, Newton maintains, the free market approach is undesirable because it will not produce the kinds of volunteers we want—volunteers who understand the research and its value and are willing to cooperate in carrying it through.

Federal regulations governing the protection of research subjects specify that no "undue inducements" be offered to lure people into volunteering (45 CFR 46.103); if the regulations must use such problematic concepts, I suppose we must try to make sense of them. We are all in Ruth Macklin's debt for her attempt at the thankless task ("On Paying Money to Research Subjects," *IRB: A Review of Human Subjects Research*, May 1981,

Reprinted with permission of the author and the publisher from *IRB: A Review of Human Subjects Research*, vol. 4 (March 1982), pp. 4–6.

pp. 1–6). But the concept of "undue inducement," and its negation, the "due inducement," outrun the resources of sensible analysis.

Considering the origin of the concept of "undue inducement," in the notion of "coercion," Macklin writes:

> By now it is an unquestioned ethical precept of biomedical and behavioral research practice that subjects should not be coerced into participating.... Those who choose to participate in research should be capable of choosing freely; they must do so voluntarily, willingly, without duress and without being subjected to threats or to a promise of too great a reward.

It is the quality of the consent, the "ability of research subjects to consent freely—to be genuine volunteers" that is supposed to be damaged by coercion, including the promise of "too great a reward." If the inducement is too rich my freedom is limited, my capacity to consent destroyed—and any contracts I may sign, presumably, void or voidable at my option. The claim is intuitively implausible. It is as if the University's Chief Financial Officer should argue, during faculty salary negotiations, that an "undue" raise in the salary level would damage the faculty's ability to consent freely, and render the faculty contracts void or voidable. That may be the only argument to that effect that has not yet been advanced by his office; I think I shall not bring it to his attention. The reaction of the Faculty Salary Committee to any such argument can be imagined. For that matter, *any* "normal, healthy" person's reaction can be imagined, to that employerly solicitude for "freedom" that keeps wages conveniently low. No inducement is unduly high from the point of view of the person being induced.

Not until the end of the article does Macklin seem to notice the implausibility, and address directly the "perennial problem of paternalism," as she calls it. In the penultimate paragraph she mentions the possibility that

> it is yet another instance of unwarranted paternalism...to restrict amounts of money offered to normal, healthy volunteers who are presumably rational enough to determine by their own system of values what tasks to engage in and what risks to undertake....

I agree that it is. And in the final paragraph she provides the article's only answer to that argument:

There are other values besides individual freedom, one of which is respect for persons. One can respect people's liberty, while still recognizing the tendency they have to succumb to temptations, to fail to recognize their own best interests on occasion, and to undertake what may be irrational risks...researchers are not being overly paternalistic in guarding against unduly inducing people to take a risk that only a large sum of money would lure them into incurring.

Surely this appeal is unequal to the task assigned to it. Whatever else the principle of "respect for persons" will do in a pinch, it will not justify restricting the range of another person's choices, without consent, in order to protect him or her from weakness of will. To respect a person is to respect moral agency at least. This attempt to justify the paternalism of the restriction of "inducement" to guard against temptation turns the principle of respect inside out.

The justification fails, not because Macklin has failed to discern the proper route to it, but because the assumption underlying the original formulation of the provision, that it is somehow coercive to pay people more than some (undetermined) amount to participate in research—more than you need to pay, more than is somehow appropriate—is simply not justifiable. A fresh start is needed if we are ever to get to the main question Macklin addresses: given that there is some reason (other than avoidance of coercion) not to pay research subjects "too much," how shall we decide in each case how much is too much?

We might well start by inquiring after a plausible reason to keep the payments down, other than the obvious utility of keeping research costs low in an era of diminishing federal support. The selection of a reason is not crucial at this point; all we really need is a cloak of likelihood to cover the regulation's nakedness so that we may proceed with the argument. But it does become crucial later on: as misguided paternalism is ruled out, above, in its role of restricting payments to preserve the volunteer's "freedom," it will also have to be ruled out for the other of Macklin's uses of it, to restrict the pool of subjects.

One very good reason for keeping payments to research subjects low is that, contrary to the implication of the term itself, we do not really want the payments to serve as a sufficient inducement for the subject to volunteer. We acknowledge that some money must be there, or the subject will not be able to justify the loss of time and other "burdens" entailed in the project. But we want the actual decisive motivation to be elsewhere, somewhere in the subcategories of motives ruled out by Macklin in her first paragraph—altruism, for instance, or curiosity, or the desire to find a cure for a specific disease. We want, in short, subjects to volunteer for reasons that entail their willingness to attempt to understand the nature and ends of research generally and the protocol for which they volunteer in particular. There are good reasons that could be advanced for us to want that characteristic—for instance, that the willingness to seek and absorb information is necessary for informed consent—but it suffices for our present purposes that one way to make it more likely that we have it, is to keep monetary inducements down to the point where they will figure in the decision to volunteer but where they alone could not fully explain anyone's participation in the research. And that reasoning brings us to the point where it makes sense to ask: how shall we determine what that point is?

If it is the psychological strength of the motivation we are bound to measure, then, as Macklin points out, we shall never reach a determination. For the power of an inducement (of the offer of a certain amount of money) must vary enormously among people with different life-situations (even among the different points of one person's biography—a point we cannot pursue) depending on present financial status, other commitments, and subjective view of the advantages and disadvantages of participating. So to provide equal "inducement" to different people would require offering a different amount of money to each person, for the same work, a procedure so clearly in conflict with justice as not to merit further consideration, as Macklin points out. We shall simply have to prescind from the psychological fact of differences, and impute identity of reaction to any given sum of money to all "normal, healthy" volunteers, or we shall be able to proceed no further.

But once that assumption is added, we have only allowed the controversy to begin. Two distinct measures for the "due inducement" run through Macklin's piece, not clearly identified until the conclusion. The first measure is the Just Wage for research participation: the subject renders services to the investigator, for which services payment is "due" him, and our only task is to determine what payment justly compensates him for value rendered. Macklin thoroughly covers the determinants of the Just Wage for human subjects

research: compensation shall equal baseline pay (either minimum wage or customary compensation) for time spent, plus a factor or set amount to cover the risks incurred, any pain or discomfort, the trouble and inconvenience the subjects are put to. It is the job of the investigator to evaluate all these factors in advance of recruitment, set the rate of reward, and offer that amount to prospective subjects. (If too few show up, that may mean that he has underestimated some negative factor, should locate it and revalue it upwards.) But a second and totally different measure of the "due inducement" is introduced in subsequent passages: the payment is simply an "inducement" for normal, healthy, subjects to volunteer. It is set as low as it may conceivably be set, well below minimum wage in some instances, and raised only until enough subjects have been recruited. No notion of just wage or compensation is involved; the play of the Free Market determines what level shall be set, and the subject himself decides that the payment is sufficiently just by signing on for the protocol.

If there is a simple and universally acceptable way of deciding whether payments in general should be calculated by a Just Wage determination or left to the play of the Free Market, that way is not known to current political philosophy. One's preference for one method or the other will depend on one's view of history, politics, and human nature, not to mention one's native (or habitual) preference for deontological or teleological reasoning. The settlement of the dispute is not likely to be the by-product of a discussion of human subjects research. As we see, however, the discussion of such research can hardly avoid this longstanding dispute: "due inducement" is a double concept, falling into two parts as soon as the question of its determination arises.

There might, of course, be reasons peculiar to the issue of human research to choose one line of reasoning over the other; Macklin suggests such reasons to support the Just Wage procedure. The most serious of the problems that arise on the Free Market procedure

is one of social justice in distributing the burdens of serving as a research subject. Setting the payment as low as would be necessary [sic: sufficient? or, no higher than necessary?] to gain a subject pool would virtually ensure that these subjects would all be drawn from lower social and economic classes...for those whose principles of justice require that society's benefits and burdens be distributed equitably throughout the population, it would be an unacceptable result if the vast majority of normal, healthy research subjects are those who have the lowest income or wealth...

As she goes on to point out, even if participation in research is regarded as inevitably burdensome, an equally acceptable theory of justice demands that the opportunity to earn money by shouldering such burdens should be extended first to the least advantaged of the society. But the "tension between these two moral viewpoints" on the societal distribution of burdens is quite beside the point if participation in research is not burdensome, and burdensomeness is an empirical concept, the determination of which must be relativized to the situation of the volunteer. Most research carried on indoors over a long period of time will not be burdensome to the homeless and unemployed in the winter; no payment could constitute "undue inducement," for the research conditions themselves are an overwhelming improvement over the baseline life conditions.

If voluntariness, read as entailing the availability of real and attractive alternatives to participation, is a moral necessity for human subjects research, there must then be restrictions on the pool of potential subjects. The possibility that *any* recruitment outside the middle class peers of the investigators may involve "undue inducement" is also advanced; at an earlier point we found that an unidentified

> medical school in a metropolitan area with a large number of urban poor has a policy of not advertising or attempting to recruit subjects from the poor section of town. Their policy is to recruit subjects from among medical students, and there is a general suspicion of efforts to solicit subjects from among community residents because of the fear that monetary payments will serve as undue inducement.

The monetary inducement is not the problem; the problem seems to be that there are no available, attractive alternatives for the commitment of time and energy for the urban poor. (It should be pointed out that the problem of weakness of will imputed to these subject pools is actually a problem of confusion of will for the experimenter: if mere inclusion in the research would substantially benefit some subjects but not others, the researcher's choices during the recruiting process are made that much more difficult.) It would seem, however, that the necessary restricting of the pool of subjects can be accomplished by the same rationale employed above to keep the payments down. We do our recruiting not among the populace at random, but among those populations only that can reasonably be expected to volunteer for certain sorts of motives and with certain expectations concerning the nature of their participation: specifically, we want volunteers who are already interested in research, are capable of understanding the purposes of research in general and, to whatever extent is appropriate, the purpose of the particular investigation. Their participation, motivated at least in part by factors other than the monetary inducement offered, is fruitful for the research precisely because of those factors.

Once we leave the insupportable paternalism of the concern for "undue inducement" behind, then, we find a perfectly coherent justification for keeping payments low and subject pools restrictive. We want volunteers who are aware of the value of the research, able to understand it, willing to cooperate in carrying it through—and the Free Market, extended into the larger community, is not calculated to produce those volunteers. The Just Wage, on the other hand, is totally irrelevant to the transaction. We want only that amount of payment which will serve as recognition for time spent on the cause of research, without elaborate procedures for discovery of the "value" of that time to (presumably) society at large.

So the purpose that the prohibition of "undue inducements" was meant to serve (the moral conduct of human subjects research) can be attained, and attained by the means the prohibition would suggest—limiting payments to volunteers and recruiting only subjects who might be expected to understand what is going on. And if the rationale connecting the means to the end cannot be the paternalism suggested by Macklin, and I think it is clear that it cannot, a plausible candidate for that rationale may be the intellectual and moral partnership of subject and researcher that "induces" the underpaid subjects to volunteer and to carry out their end of the task. In a social climate that is becoming less and less tolerant of paternalism in any form, the latter rationale may prove to be a far steadier and more enduring basis for the suggested restrictions on the conduct of research.

ANNOTATED BIBLIOGRAPHY: CHAPTER 4

Annas, George J., Leonard H. Glantz, and Barbara F. Katz: *Informed Consent to Human Experimentation: The Subject's Dilemma* (Cambridge, Mass.: Ballinger, 1977). Annas, Glantz, and Katz attempt to trace and analyze the legal system's attempt to articulate the law of informed consent to human experimentation, with different types of subjects and different types of research. They show that the research subject is not the only one faced with moral dilemmas. Lawyers and judges, as well as investigators, face numerous and complicated problems in attempting to determine how to implement the ethical and legal requirement of "competent, voluntary, informed, and understanding consent."

Ayd, Frank J., Jr.: "Drug Studies in Prisoner Volunteers," *Southern Medical Journal* 65 (April 1972), pp. 440–44. Ayd argues that research using prisoners is ethically acceptable. He cites the benefits that prisoners gain from their participation in such research.

Beecher, Henry K.: *Research and the Individual* (Boston: Little, Brown, 1970). This is one of the earlier works dealing with the ethical problems raised by research involving human subjects. It includes a collection of codes of ethics for those involved in such research.

Capron, Alexander M.: "Medical Research in Prisons: Should a Moratorium Be Called?" *Hastings Center Report* 3 (June 1973), pp. 4–6. Capron argues that a moratorium should be called on prison research until the problems raised by the current conduct of such research are resolved.

Childress, James F.: "Compensating Injured Research Subjects: I. The Moral Argument," *Hastings Center Report* 6 (December 1976), pp. 21–27. Childress examines the moral arguments for the view that human subjects should be compensated for research-related injuries. He argues that society has a prima facie obligation to compensate human subjects for research-related injuries. This prima facie obligation, however, can be overridden in an actual situation by conflicting obligations.

Daedalus (Spring 1969). This entire issue focuses on the ethical aspects of experimentation with human subjects. Especially useful is David D. Rutstein's article, "The Ethical Design of Human Experiments."

Greenwald, Robert A., Mary Kay Ryan, and James E. Mulvihill: *Human Subjects Research: A Handbook for Institutional Review Boards* (New York: Plenum, 1982). This is a useful, practical handbook for members of Institutional Review Boards as well as for those engaged in research using human subjects who plan to submit a project proposal to an IRB.

IRB: A Review of Human Subjects Research (Hastings-on-Hudson, N.Y.: The Hastings Center). This periodical, published ten times a year, is devoted to articles dealing with the ethical aspects of research using human subjects.

Katz, Jay, with Alexander M. Capron and Eleanor Swift Glass, eds.: *Experimentation with Human Beings: The Authority of the Investigator, Subject, Professions, and State in the Human Experimentation Process* (New York: Russell Sage, 1972). This is an excellent, well-organized collection of edited materials dealing with human experimentation. It includes discussions of the function and limitations of informed consent; discussions of experimentation on specific subject groups, such as dying and uncomprehending subjects; and a wealth of other material on the topic of experimentation.

Macklin, Ruth, and Susan Sherwin: "Experimenting on Human Subjects: Philosophical Perspectives," *Case Western Law Review* 25 (Spring 1975), pp. 434–471. Macklin and Sherwin examine the ethical problems raised by research on human subjects from various philosophical points of view. They are particularly concerned to show the shortcomings of the views of Immanuel Kant and John Stuart Mill. Macklin and Sherwin reject these two views and recommend using John Rawls's theory of social justice as a model for making ethical judgments.

National Commission for the Protection of Human Subjects of Biomedical and Behavioral Research: *The Belmont Report: Ethical Principles and Guidelines for the Protection of Human Subjects of Research.* DHEW (OS) 78-0012. *The Belmont Report. Appendix*, vols. 1, 2. DHEW (OS) 78-0013, 78-0014. (Bethesda, Md., 1978). This report was put out by a Commission established under the National Research Act (P.L. 93-348). The Commission's purpose was to develop ethical guidelines for the conduct of research involving human subjects and to make recommendations for the applications of these guidelines to research conducted or supported by the Department of Health, Education and Welfare. *The Belmont Report* is the Commission's final and most general report. Other reports, listed below, deal with narrower topics. The appendices to this report and to the ones listed below contain many useful papers, reports, and other materials that were reviewed by the Commission prior to formulating its recommendations.

———: *Report and Recommendations: Research Involving Children.* DHEW (OS) 77-0004. *Appendix: Research Involving Children.* DHEW (OS) 77-0005. (Bethesda, Md., 1977).

———: *Report and Recommendations: Research Involving Prisoners.* DHEW (OS) 76-131. *Appendix: Research Involving Prisoners.* DHEW (OS) 76-132. (Bethesda, Md., 1976).

———: *Report and Recommendation: Research Involving Those Institutionalized as Mentally Infirm.* DHEW (OS) 78-0006. *Appendix: Research Involving Those Institutionalized as Mentally Infirm.* DHEW (OS) 78-0007. (Bethesda, Md., 1978).

Robertson, John A.: "Compensating Injured Research Subjects: II. The Law," *Hastings Center Report* 6 (December 1976), pp. 29–31. Robertson first examines the ethical, humanitarian, and economic reasons for compensating persons injured as a result of participating as research subjects. He then points out that at present such compensation is neither given as a rule nor required by law.

Chapter 5

Health, Disease, and Values

INTRODUCTION

The concepts of health and disease are firmly entrenched as fundamental categories in the everyday practice of medicine. Ordinarily we say that the aim of medicine is to foster health. Moreover, aside from preventative measures, it seems clear that the fostering of health is principally accomplished through the diagnosis and treatment of disease. In this chapter, attention is focused on the concepts of health and disease. Certain conceptual issues that have value dimensions are identified and addressed.

The Scope of the Concept of Health

What is the proper scope of the concept of health? The World Health Organization (WHO), in a much discussed and widely criticized formulation that is reprinted in this chapter, defines health as "a state of complete physical, mental and social well-being and not merely the absence of disease or infirmity." It is of some interest to note, in accordance with this definition, that health is construed not merely as the opposite of disease but rather, in a positive vein, as a state of complete well-being. More important to note for present purposes, however, is the fact that the WHO definition of health assigns a most expansive scope to the concept of health. Not only is health applicable to the *physical* domain, not only is it applicable to the *mental* domain, it is also applicable to the *social* domain. Thus we may speak of physical (bodily) health, mental health, and also social health. Presumably, maladies such as unemployment could be construed as incompatible with an individual's social health, although one might wonder exactly how the notion of social health should be explicated.

Should we endorse, in accordance with the WHO definition of health, such an expansive scope for the concept of health? Daniel Callahan, in one of this chapter's selections, argues against the WHO definition, especially against the WHO's incorporation of a social dimension into the scope of the concept of health. In Callahan's view, the WHO definition of health entails a host of problematic implications. With the definition's inclusion of "social well-being," for example, all human problems seem to reduce to health problems, thus quaiifying as problems to be addressed within the province of medicine. In the spirit of Callahan's critique, one wonders what special insight medical professionals might have into social problems such as unemployment.

If the social domain is excluded from the scope of the concept of health, there are still two possible views with regard to its legitimate scope. Should we limit ourselves to speaking only of physical health or should we allow the scope of the concept to extend to mental health as well? Probably the most common view is that the concept of health rightly spans both the physical and the mental domains. Thus, whereas it is recognized that physiological medicine is concerned with physical health and the treatment of physical disease, it is also thought that psychiatry is a legitimate medical specialty concerned with mental health and the treatment of mental disease or illness. Still, many are convinced that the concepts of mental health, disease, and illness are substantially more puzzling than their physical analogs. If it is true, as some so-called radical psychiatrists insist, that mental illness is a myth and psychiatry is a bogus medical specialty, then we ought indeed to exclude the mental domain and restrict the scope of the concept of health to the physical domain.

Lest it be thought that consideration of the scope of the concept of health confronts us with merely a verbal dispute, it is important to insist on the practical consequences of such a discussion. Chapter 11, "Social Justice and Health-Care Policy," features discussion of such topics as a just allocation of the health-care budget and a right to health care. The scope of the concept of health is of no small consequence in such discussions. In allocating the health-care budget, are we to take into account physical health, or also mental health, or perhaps social health as well? In asserting a right to health care, are we asserting only a right to physical health care, or a right to physical and mental health care, or perhaps a right to physical and mental and social health care?

Health and Disease: Value-Laden Concepts?

In recent years, the concepts of health and disease have received much attention in the philosophy of medicine. One area of concern in discussions centering on these concepts seems especially relevant in the context of biomedical ethics. With regard to this area of concern, the following central question may be phrased: Are the concepts of health and disease inherently value-laden? It is widely, though not universally, believed that the concepts of health and disease are inherently value-laden. If this is so, it would seem to be important to specify the exact sense(s) in which it is so. After all, the practice of medicine is normally understood as dedicated to the advancement of health and the eradication of disease. Thus, to the extent that the concepts of health and disease are inherently value-laden, it follows that the practice of medicine is itself a value-laden enterprise.

In considering whether the concepts of health and disease are inherently value-laden, it may be helpful to present examples of purely scientific (descriptive) concepts as contrasted with concepts that are inherently value-laden. The concept of a liquid (or the concept of an acid or the concept of a mammal) is normally understood as a purely scientific concept. In other words, when it is asserted that a certain substance is a liquid, a purely descriptive claim is being made. In saying that a certain substance is a liquid, we imply no approval or disapproval of that substance. The assertion is value-free or value-neutral. In contrast, consider the concept of cruelty, one which is very plausibly construed as inherently value-laden. If I assert that what you did was cruel, it seems that I am not merely describing your action. I am also saying that I disapprove of it. I am saying that I consider your action in some sense undesirable or unjustifiable. If you have disciplined a small child in a certain fashion (e.g., bed without supper), I will identify your disciplinary action as cruel only if I disapprove of it. If I approve of the way in which you have conducted yourself, if I consider it justifiable or appropriate, I will not say that you were cruel. Perhaps I will say that you were firm.

The concept of cruelty, then, may be understood as inherently value-laden. Concepts such as cowardice, pettiness, courage, and graciousness may be construed in similar fashion. The former two necessarily imply a negative evaluation, whereas the latter two necessarily imply a positive evaluation. Such concepts are sometimes labeled "mixed descriptive-normative" concepts. They are said to have both a descriptive component (function) and a normative component (function). It is clear that such concepts have a descriptive function. If I say that you have acted in a cruel fashion, I am describing your action in a certain way. If I say that you have acted in a cowardly fashion, I am describing your action in a different way. If I say that you have acted in a petty fashion, I am describing your action in yet a different way. On the analysis being suggested, of course, in each case I am not merely describing your action. I am also expressing my negative evaluation of it. Mixed descriptive-normative concepts have a descriptive function, but they have a normative function as well. Indeed, it is in virtue of their normative function that they are said to be inherently value-laden.

Are the concepts of health and disease inherently value-laden? If I identify a certain state (condition) as healthy, do I necessarily imply in some sense a positive evaluation of this state? If I identify a certain state (condition) as diseased, do I necessarily imply in some sense a negative evaluation of this state? For expository purposes, the present discussion will be confined to a consideration of *physical* health and disease. Moreover, it is convenient to think primarily about the concept of disease. In modern medicine, numerous physiological states or conditions are identified as pathological. They are said to be states of disease. For example, emphysema, a certain lung condition, is identified as a disease. With such identifications in mind, can the concept of disease be reconstructed as a purely scientific (descriptive) concept? Some answer in the affirmative. They maintain that, when a certain condition is identified as a disease, a purely scientific (descriptive) claim is being made. Although this view is not expressly defended in the readings of this chapter, one of its proponents suggests the following analysis.[1] To say that a certain condition is a disease is simply to say that it constitutes an interference with a function typically performed within the human species. Emphysema, then, counts as a disease because it is a condition that interferes with the species-typical function of breathing. On this view, it is thought possible to ascertain in a purely descriptive way (via biological analysis) a set of functions typically performed within the human species. In one of this chapter's readings, however, Joel Feinberg insists that "the proper working order of the human body" cannot be determined in a purely descriptive fashion. For Feinberg, as for H. Tristram Engelhardt, Jr., in this chapter, the concept of disease (likewise the concept of health) is inherently value-laden. As Engelhardt expresses it, to identify a certain state as a disease is to characterize it "as being in some sense bad." Both Feinberg and Engelhardt insist that varying societal values may lead one society to identify a certain state (condition) as healthy, while another society will identify that same state as a disease. Such disagreements, they maintain, are value-laden.

Is Mental Illness a Myth?

In modern physiological medicine, a patient might be diagnosed as suffering from leukemia. The patient is said to have a certain pathological condition, a physical disease. He or she is physically ill. In modern psychiatry, a patient might be diagnosed as suffering from some type of schizophrenia. The patient is said to have a certain psychopathological condition, a mental disease. He or she is mentally ill.

In our culture, when labels such as "insane" and "sick" are so readily predicated of human behavior, it is difficult not to feel a certain sense of puzzlement in the face of the concepts of mental health and mental illness. Our problem, however, goes deeper than the confusion that is produced by the offhand misuse of such labels. If we had access to a firmly entrenched theory of mental health, we would probably feel ourselves to be on firmer ground. But that is just the problem. Mental health professionals subscribe to widely varying theories of mental health. As if that is not confusing enough, we are also confronted with the fact that psychiatrists in the same school of thought often find it difficult to agree whether or not a certain diagnostic label is applicable to an individual case.

How should we think of mental health and mental illness? From an ethical point of view, we cannot afford to disregard them. The diagnosis of mental illness is a crucial link in justifications advanced for subjecting certain individuals to involuntary civil commitment as well as other kinds of coercive behavior control. The ethical justifiability of involuntary civil commitment is discussed in Chapter 6, but deliberations there are heavily dependent on underlying conceptions of mental illness.

It is sometimes alleged, most prominently in the work of the psychiatrist Thomas S. Szasz, that mental illness is a myth. According to Szasz, as reflected in his selection in this chapter, the concept of mental illness has no scientific or descriptive content whatsoever and thus ought to be abandoned. Although it masquerades as a scientific concept, it functions in an exclusively normative way. When someone is labeled "mentally ill," Szasz holds, it is solely because that individual has deviated from certain ethical, political, or social norms. In answer to a number of Szasz's contentions, Michael S. Moore argues that mental illness is a "cruel and bitter reality" that cannot be simply dismissed as a myth.

T.A.M.

NOTE

1 Christopher Boorse, "On the Distinction between Disease and Illness," *Philosophy and Public Affairs* 5 (Fall 1975), pp. 49–68.

The Scope of the Concept of Health

Preamble to the Constitution of the World Health Organization

In this preamble, a number of principles underlying the foundation of the World Health Organization (WHO) are articulated. The various principles seem to embody a host of ethical and factual claims. However, the first principle is exclusively conceptual, announcing what is now generally referred to as the "WHO Definition of Health."

Reprinted with permission of the World Health Organization from *The First Ten Years of the World Health Organization* (Geneva: World Health Organization, 1958).

The States Parties to this Constitution declare, in conformity with the Charter of the United Nations, that the following principles are basic to the happiness, harmonious relations and security of all peoples:

Health is a state of complete physical, mental and social well-being and not merely the absence of disease or infirmity.

The enjoyment of the highest attainable standard of health is one of the fundamental rights of every human being without distinction of race, religion, political belief, economic or social condition.

The health of all peoples is fundamental to the attainment of peace and security and is dependent upon the fullest co-operation of individuals and States.

The achievement of any State in the promotion and protection of health is of value to all.

Unequal development in different countries in the promotion of health and control of disease, especially communicable disease, is a common danger.

Healthy development of the child is of basic importance; the ability to live harmoniously in a changing total environment is essential to such development.

The extension to all peoples of the benefits of medical, psychological and related knowledge is essential to the fullest attainment of health.

Informed opinion and active co-operation on the part of the public are of the utmost importance in the improvement of the health of the people.

Governments have a responsibility for the health of their peoples which can be fulfilled only by the provision of adequate health and social measures.

Accepting these principles, and for the purpose of co-operation among themselves and with others to promote and protect the health of all peoples, the Contracting Parties agree to the present Constitution and hereby establish the World Health Organization as a specialized agency within the terms of Article 57 of the Charter of the United Nations.

The WHO Definition of Health

Daniel Callahan

Daniel Callahan, a philosopher, has been since 1969 the director of the Institute of Society, Ethics and the Life Sciences, usually called The Hastings Center. He has also been executive editor of *The Commonweal* (1961–1968). In his published articles, Callahan has addressed a wide range of issues in biomedical ethics. In addition, he is the author of such books as *Abortion: Law, Choice and Morality* (1970) and *Ethics and Population Limitation* (1971) and the coeditor of such books as *Ethical Issues in Human Genetics* (1973) and *The Roots of Ethics* (1981).

Callahan undertakes a critical analysis of the WHO definition of health. His principal objection to the WHO definition is that it has undesirable ethical, social, and political implications. He especially finds strongly objectionable the inclusion of "social well-being" within the scope of the concept of health. Such an inclusion leads us to think that all human problems are reducible to matters of health and thus are within the special province of medical professionals. It also leads us to ascribe blamelessness, as one ingredient of the sick role, to the whole range of human behavior. Moreover, it leads us to act in the name of "health" instead of the name of "morality." In order to avoid such undesirable implications, Callahan finds it important to limit the scope of the concept of health. Indeed, his suggestion is that we restrict the concept of health to the *physical* domain.

Reprinted with permission of the author and the publisher from *Hastings Center Studies*, vol. 1, no. 3 (1973), pp. 77–87.

There is not much that can be called fun and games in medicine, perhaps because unlike other sports it is the only one in which everyone, participant and spectator, eventually gets killed playing. In the meantime, one of the grandest games is that version of king-of-the-hill where the aim of all players is to upset the World Health Organization (WHO) definition of "health." That definition, in case anyone could possibly forget it, is "Health is a state of complete physical, mental, and social well-being and not merely the absence of disease or infirmity." Fair game, indeed. Yet somehow, defying all comers, the WHO definition endures, though literally every other aspirant to the crown has managed to knock it off the hill at least once. One possible reason for its presence is that it provides such an irresistible straw man; few there are who can resist attacking it in the opening paragraphs of papers designed to move on to more profound reflections.

But there is another possible reason which deserves some exploration, however unsettling the implications. It may just be that the WHO definition has more than a grain of truth in it, of a kind which is as profoundly frustrating as it is enticingly attractive. At the very least it is a definition which implies that there is some intrinsic relationship between the good of the body and the good of the self. The attractiveness of this relationship is obvious: it thwarts any movement toward a dualism of self and body, a dualism which in any event immediately breaks down when one drops a brick on one's toe; and it impels the analyst to work toward a conception of health which in the end is resistant to clear and distinct categories, closer to the felt experience. All that, naturally, is very frustrating. It seems simply impossible to devise a concept of health which is rich enough to be nutritious and yet not so rich as to be indigestible.

One common objection to the WHO definition is, in effect, an assault upon any and all attempts to specify the meaning of very general concepts. Who can possibly define words as vague as "health," a venture as foolish as trying to define "peace," "justice," "happiness," and other systematically ambiguous notions? To this objection the "pragmatic" clinicians (as they often call themselves) add that, anyway, it is utterly unnecessary to know what "health" means in order to treat a patient running a high temperature. Not only that, it is also a harmful distraction to clutter medical judgment with philosophical puzzles.

Unfortunately for this line of argument, it is impossible to talk or think at all without employing general concepts; without them, cognition and language are impossible. More damagingly, it is rarely difficult to discover, with a bit of probing, that even the most "pragmatic" judgment (whatever *that* is) presupposes some general values and orientations, all of which can be translated into definitions of terms as general as "health" and "happiness." A failure to discern the operative underlying values, the conceptions of reality upon which they are based, and the definitions they entail, sets the stage for unexamined conduct and, beyond that, positive harm both to patients and to medicine in general.

But if these objections to any and all attempts to specify the meaning of "health" are common enough, the most specific complaint about the WHO definition is that its very generality, and particularly its association of health and general well-being as a positive ideal, has given rise to a variety of evils. Among them are the cultural tendency to define all social problems, from war to crime in the streets, as "health" problems; the blurring of lines of responsibility between and among the professions, and between the medical profession and the political order; the implicit denial of human freedom which results when failures to achieve social well-being are defined as forms of "sickness," somehow to be treated by medical means; and the general debasement of language which ensues upon the casual habit of labeling everyone from Adolf Hitler to student radicals to the brat next door as "sick." In short, the problem with the WHO definition is not that it represents an attempt to propose a general definition, but that it is simply a bad one.

That is a valid line of objection, provided one can spell out in some detail just how the definition can or does entail some harmful consequences. Two lines of attack are possible against putatively hazardous social definitions of significant general concepts. One is by pointing out that the definition does not encompass all that a concept has commonly been taken to mean, either historically or at present, that it is a partial definition only. The task then is to come up with a fuller definition, one less subject to misuse. But there is still another way of objecting to socially significant definitions, and that is by pointing out some baneful effects of definitions generally accepted as adequate. Many of the objections to the WHO definition fall in the latter category, building upon the important insight that definitions of crucially important terms with a wide public use have ethical, social, and political implications; defining general terms is not an abstract exercise but a way of shaping the world metaphysically and structuring the world politically.

Wittgenstein's aphorism, "Don't look for the meaning, look for the use," is pertinent here. The ethical problem in defining the concept of "health" is to determine what the implications are of the various uses to which a concept of "health" can be put. We might well agree that there are some uses of "health" which will produce socially harmful results. To carry Wittgenstein a step further, "Don't look for the uses, look for the abuses." We might, then, examine some of the real or possible abuses to which the WHO definition leads, recognizing all the while that what we may term an "abuse" will itself rest upon some perceived *positive* good or value.

HISTORICAL ORIGIN & CONTEXT

Before that task is undertaken, however, it is helpful to understand the historical origin and social context of the WHO definition. If abuses of that definition have developed, their seeds may be looked for in its earliest manifestations.

The World Health Organization came into existence between 1946 and 1948 as one of the first major activities of the United Nations. As an outcome of earlier work, an Interim Commission to establish the WHO sponsored an International Health Conference in New York in June and July of 1946. At that Conference, representatives of 61 nations signed the Constitution of the WHO, the very first clause of which presented the now famous definition of "health." The animating spirit behind the formation of the WHO was the belief that the improvement of world health would make an important contribution to world peace; health and peace were seen as inseparable. Just why this belief gained ground is not clear from the historical record of the WHO. While there have been many historical explanations of the origin of World War II, a lack of world health has not been prominent among them; nor, for that matter, did the early supporters of the WHO claim that the Second World War or any other war might have been averted had there been better health. More to the point, perhaps, was the conviction that health was intimately related to economic and cultural welfare; in turn, that welfare, so it was assumed, had a direct bearing on future peace. No less important was a fervent faith in the possibilities of medical science to achieve world health, enhanced by the development of powerful antibiotics and pesticides during the war.

A number of memorandums submitted to a spring 1946 Technical Preparatory Committee meeting of the WHO capture the flavor of the period. The Yugoslavian memorandum noted that "health is a prerequisite to freedom from want, to social security and happiness." France stated that "there cannot be any material security, social security, or well-being for individuals or nations without health...the full responsibility of a free man can only be assumed by healthy individuals ...the spread of proper notions of hygiene among populations tends to improve the level of health and hence to increase their working power and raise their standard of living...." The United States contended that "international cooperation and joint action in the furtherance of all matters pertaining to health will raise the standards of living, will promote the freedom, the dignity, and the happiness of all peoples of the world."

In addition to those themes, perhaps the most significant initiative taken by the organizers of the WHO was to include mental health as part of its working definition. In its memorandum, Great Britain stated that "it should be clear that health includes mental health," but it was Dr. Brock Chisholm, soon to become the first director of the WHO, who personified what Dr. Chisholm himself called the "visionary" view of health. During the meeting of the Technical Preparatory Committee he argued that: "The world is sick and the ills are due to the perversion of man; his inability to live with himself. The microbe is not the enemy; science is sufficiently advanced to cope with it were it not for the barriers of superstition, ignorance, religious intolerance, misery and poverty.... These psychological evils must be understood in order that a remedy might be prescribed, and the scope of the task before the Committee therefore knows no bounds."

In Dr. Chisholm's statement, put very succinctly, are all of those elements of the WHO definition which led eventually to its criticism: defining all the problems of the world as "sickness," affirming that science would be sufficient to cope with the causes of physical disease, asserting that only anachronistic attitudes stood in the way of a cure of both physical and psychological ills, and declaring that the cause of health can tolerate no limitations. To say that Dr. Chisholm's "vision" was grandiose is to understate the matter. Even allowing for hyperbole, it is clear that the stage was being set for a conception of "health" which would encompass literally every element and item of human happiness. One can hardly be surprised, given such a vision, that our ways of talking about "health" have become all but meaningless. Even though I believe the definition is not without its important insights, it is well to observe why, in part, we are so muddled at present about "health."

HEALTH & HAPPINESS

Let us examine some of the principal objections to the WHO definition in more detail. One of them is that, by including the notion of "social well-being" under its rubric, it turns the enduring problem of human happiness into one more medical problem, to be dealt with by scientific means. That is surely an objectionable feature, if only because there exists no evidence whatever that medicine has anything more than a partial grasp of the sources of human misery. Despite Dr. Chisholm's optimism, medicine has not even found ways of dealing with more than a fraction of the whole range of physical diseases; campaigns, after all, are still being mounted against cancer and heart disease. Nor is there any special reason to think that future forays against those and other common diseases will bear rapid fruits. People will continue to die of disease for a long time to come, probably forever.

But perhaps, then, in the psychological and psychiatric sciences some progress has been made against what Dr. Chisholm called the "psychological ills," which lead to wars, hostility, and aggression? To be sure, there are many interesting psychological theories to be found about these "ills," and a few techniques which can, with some individuals, reduce or eliminate antisocial behavior. But so far as I can see, despite the mental health movement and the rise of the psychological sciences, war and human hostility are as much with us as ever. Quite apart from philosophical objections to the WHO definition, there was no empirical basis for the unbounded optimism which lay behind it at the time of its inception, and little has happened since to lend its limitless aspiration any firm support.

Common sense alone makes evident the fact that the absence of "disease or infirmity" by no means guarantees "social well-being." In one sense, those who drafted the WHO definition seem well aware of that. Isn't the whole point of their definition to show the inadequacy of negative definitions? But in another sense, it may be doubted that they really did grasp that point. For the third principle enunciated in the WHO Constitution says that "the health of all peoples is fundamental to the attainment of peace and security...." Why is it fundamental, at least to peace? The worst wars of the 20th century have been waged by countries with very high standards of health, by nations with superior life-expectancies for individuals and with comparatively low infant mortality rates. The greatest present threats to world peace come in great part (though not entirely) from developed countries, those which have combatted disease and illness most effectively. There seems to be no historical correlation whatever between health and peace, and that is true even if one includes "mental health."

How are human beings to achieve happiness? That is the final and fundamental question. Obviously illness, whether mental or physical, makes happiness less possible in most cases. But that is only because they are only one symptom of a more basic restriction, that of human finitude, which sees infinite human desires constantly thwarted by the limitations of reality. "Complete" well-being might, conceivably, be attainable, but under one condition only: that people ceased expecting much from life. That does not seem about to happen. On the contrary, medical and psychological progress have been more than outstripped by rising demands and expectations. What is so odd about that, if it is indeed true that human desires are infinite? Whatever the answer to the question of human happiness, there is no particular reason to believe that medicine can do anything more than make a modest, finite contribution.

Another objection to the WHO definition is that, by implication, it makes the medical profession the gatekeeper for happiness and social well-being. Or if not exactly the gate-keeper (since political and economic support will be needed from sources other than medical), then the final magic-healer of human misery. Pushed far enough, the whole idea is absurd, and it is not necessary to believe that the organizers of the WHO would, if pressed, have been willing to go quite that far. But even if one pushes the pretension a little way, considerable fantasy results. The mental health movement is the best example, casting the psychological professional in the role of high priest.

At its humble best, that movement can do considerable good; people do suffer from psychological disabilities and there are some effective ways of helping them. But it would be sheer folly to believe that all, or even the most important, social evils stem from bad mental health: political injustice, economic scarcity, food shortages, unfavorable physical environments, have a far greater historical claim as sources of a failure to achieve "social well-being." To retort that all or most of these troubles can, nonetheless, be seen finally as symptoms of bad mental health is, at best, self-serving and, at worst, just plain foolish.

A significant part of the objection that the WHO definition places, at least by implication, too much power and authority in the hands of the medical profession need not be based on a fear of that power as such. There is no reason to think that the world would be any worse off if health professionals made all decisions than if any other group did, and no reason to think it would be any better off. That is not a very important point. More significant is that cultural development which, in its skepticism about "traditional" ways of solving social problems, would seek a technological and specifically a medical solution for human ills of all kinds. There is at least a hint in early WHO discussions that, since politicians and diplomats have failed in maintaining world peace, a more expert group should take over, armed with the scientific skills necessary to set things right; it is science which is best able to vanquish that old Enlightenment bogeyman, "superstition." More concretely, such an ideology has the practical effect of blurring the lines of appropriate authority and responsibility. If all problems—political, economic and social—reduce to matters of "health," then there cease to be any ways to determine who should be responsible for what.

THE TYRANNY OF HEALTH

The problem of responsibility has at least two faces. One is that of a tendency to turn all problems of "social well-being" over to the medical professional, most pronounced in the instance of the incarceration of a large group of criminals in mental institutions rather than prisons. The abuses, both medical and legal, of that practice are, fortunately, now beginning to receive the attention they deserve, even if little corrective action has yet been taken. (Counterbalancing that development, however, are others, where some are seeking more "effective" ways of bringing science to bear on criminal behavior.)

The other face of the problem of responsibility is that of the way in which those who are sick, or purportedly sick, are to be evaluated in terms of their freedom and responsibility. Siegler and Osmond [*Hastings Center Studies*, vol. 1, no. 3, 1973, pp. 41–58] discuss the "sick role," a leading feature of which is the ascription of blamelessness, of non-responsibility, to those who contract illness. There is no reason to object to this kind of ascription in many instances—one can hardly blame someone for contracting kidney disease— but, obviously enough, matters get out of hand when all physical, mental, and communal disorders are put under the heading of "sickness," and all sufferers (all of us, in the end) placed in the blameless "sick role." Not only are the concepts of "sickness" and "illness" drained of all content, it also becomes impossible to ascribe any freedom or responsibility to those caught up in the throes of sickness. The whole world is sick, and no one is responsible any longer for anything. That is determinism gone mad, a rather odd outcome of a development which began with attempts to bring unbenighted "reason" and free self-determination to bear for the release of the helpless captives of superstition and ignorance.

The final and most telling objection to the WHO definition has less to do with the definition itself than with one of its natural historical consequences. Thomas Szasz has seen the most eloquent (and most single-minded) critic of that sleight-of-hand which has seen the concept of health moved from the medical to the moral arena. What can no longer be done in the name of "morality" can now be done in the name of "health": human beings labeled, incarcerated, and dismissed for their failure to toe the line of "normalcy" and "sanity."

At first glance, this analysis of the present situation might seem to be totally at odds with the tendency to put everyone in the blame-free "sick role." Actually, there is a fine, probably indistinguishable, line separating these two positions. For as soon as one treats all human disorders—war, crime, social unrest—as forms of illness, then one turns health into a normative concept, that which human beings must and ought to have if they are to live in peace with themselves and others. Health is no longer an optional matter, but the golden key to the relief of human misery. We *must* be well or we will all perish. "Health" can and must be imposed; there can be no room for the luxury of freedom when so much is at stake. Of course the matter is rarely put so bluntly, but it is to Szasz's great credit that he has discerned what actually happens when "health" is allowed to gain the cultural clout which morality once had. (That he carries the whole business too far in his embracing of the most extreme moral individualism is another story, which cannot be dealt with here.) Something is seriously amiss when the "right" to have healthy children is turned into a further right for children not to be born defective, and from there into an obligation not to bring unhealthy children into the world as a way of respecting the right of those children to health! Nor is everything altogether lucid when abortion decisions are made a matter of "medical judgment" (see *Roe* vs. *Wade*); when decisions to provide psychoactive drugs for the relief of the ordinary stress of living are defined as no less "medical judgment"; when patients are not allowed to die with dignity because of medical indications that they can, come what may, be kept alive; when prisoners, without their consent, are subjected to aversive conditioning to improve their mental health.

ABUSES OF LANGUAGE

In running through the litany of criticisms which have been directed at the WHO definition of "health," and what seem to have been some of its long-term implications and consequences, I might well be accused of beating a dead horse. My only defense is to assert, first, that the spirit of the WHO definition is by no means dead either in medicine or society. In fact, because of the usual cultural lag which requires many years for new ideas to gain wide social currency, it is only now coming into its own on a broad scale. (Everyone now talks about everybody and everything, from Watergate to Billy Graham to trash in the streets, as "sick.") Second, I believe that we are now in the midst of a nascent (if not actual) crisis about how "health" ought properly to be understood, with much dependent upon what conception of health emerges in the near future.

If the ideology which underlies the WHO definition has proved to contain many muddled and hazardous ingredients, it is not at all evident what should take its place. The virtue of the WHO definition is that it tried to place health in the broadest human context. Yet the assumption behind the main criticisms of the WHO definition seem perfectly valid. Those assumptions can be characterized as follows: (1) health is only a part of life, and the achievement of health only a part of the achievement of happiness; (2) medicine's role, however important, is limited; it can neither solve nor even cope with the great majority of social, political, and cultural problems; (3) human freedom and responsibility must be recognized, and any tendency to place all deviant, devilish, or displeasing human beings into the blameless sick-role must be resisted; (4) while it is good for human beings to be healthy, medicine is not morality; except in very limited contexts (plagues and epidemics) "medical judgment" should not be allowed to become moral judgment; to be healthy is not to be righteous; (5) it is important to keep clear and distinct the different roles of different professions, with a clearly circumscribed role for medicine, limited to those domains of life where the contribution of medicine is appropriate. Medicine can save some lives; it cannot save the life of society.

These assumptions, and the criticisms of the WHO definition which spring from them, have some important implications for the use of the words "health," "illness," "sick," and the like. It will be counted an abuse of language if the word "sick" is applied to all individual and communal problems, if all unacceptable conduct is spoken of in the language of medical pathologies, if moral issues and moral judgments are translated into the language of "health," if the lines of authority, responsibility, and expertise are so blurred that the health profession is allowed to pre-empt the rights and responsibilities of others by re-defining them in its own professional language.

Abuses of that kind have no possibility of being curbed in the absence of a definition of health which does not contain some intrinsic elements of limitation— that is, unless there is a definition which, when abused, is self-evidently *seen* as abused by those who know what health means. Unfortunately, it is in the nature of general definitions that they do not circumscribe their own meaning (or even explain it) and contain no built-in safeguards against misuse, e.g., our "peace with honor" in Southeast Asia—"peace," "honor"? Moreover, for a certain class of concepts—peace, honor, happiness, for example—it is difficult to keep them free in ordinary usage from a normative content. In our own usage, it would make no sense to talk of them in a way which implied they are not desirable or are merely neutral: by well-ingrained social custom (resting no doubt on some basic features of human nature) health, peace, and happiness are both desired and desirable—good. For those and other reasons, it is perfectly plausible to say the cultural task of defining terms, and settling on appropriate and inappropriate usages, is far more than a matter of getting our dictionary entries right. It is nothing less than a way of deciding what should be valued, how life should be understood, and what principles should guide individual and social conduct.

Health is not just a term to be defined. Intuitively, if we have lived at all, it is something we seek and value. We may not set the highest value on health—other goods may be valued as well—but it would strike me as incomprehensible should someone say that health was a matter of utter indifference to him; we would well doubt either his sanity or his maturity. The cultural problem, then, may be put this way. The acceptable range of uses of the term "health" should, at the minimum, capture the normative element in the concept as traditionally understood while, at the maximum, incorporate the insight (stemming from criticisms of the WHO definition) that the term "health" is abused if it becomes synonymous with virtue, social tranquility, and ultimate happiness. Since there are no instruction manuals available on how one would go about reaching a goal of that sort, I will offer no advice on the subject. I have the horrible suspicion, as a matter of fact, that people either have a decent intuitive sense on such matters (reflected in the way they use language) or they do not; and if they do not, little can be done to instruct them. One is left with the pious hope that, somehow, over a long period of time, things will change.

IN DEFENSE OF WHO

Now that simply might be the end of the story, assuming some agreement can be reached that the WHO definition of "health" is plainly bad, full of snares, delusions, and false norms. But I am left uncomfortable with such a flat, simple conclusion. The nagging point about the definition is that, in badly put ways, it was probably on to something. It certainly recognized, however inchoately, that it is difficult to talk meaningfully of health solely in terms of "the absence of disease or infirmity." As a purely logical point, one must ask about what positive state of affairs disease and infirmity are an absence of—absent from what? One is left with the tautological proposition that health is the absence of non-health, a less than illuminating revelation. Could it not be said, though, that at least intuitively everyone knows what health is by means of the experiential

contrast posed by states of illness and disease; that is, even if I cannot define health in any positive sense, I can surely know when I am sick (pain, high fever, etc.) and compare that condition with my previous states which contained no such conditions? Thus one could, in some recognizable sense, speak of illness as a deviation from a norm, even if it is not possible to specify that norm with any clarity.

But there are some problems with this approach, for all of its commonsense appeal. Sociologically, it is well known that what may be accounted sickness in one culture may not be so interpreted in another; one culture's (person's) deviation from the norm may not necessarily be another culture's (person's) deviation. In this as in other matters, commonsense intuition may be nothing but a reflection of different cultural and personal evaluations. In addition, there can be and usually are serious disputes about how great a deviation from the (unspecified) norm is necessary before the terms "sickness" and "illness" become appropriate. Am I to be put in the sick role because of my nagging case of itching athlete's foot, or must my toes start dropping off before I can so qualify? All general concepts have their borderline cases, and normally they need pose no real problems for the applicability of the concepts for the run of instances. But where "health" and "illness" are concerned, the number of borderline cases can be enormous, affected by age, attitudinal and cultural factors. Worse still, the fact that people can be afflicted by disease (even fatally afflicted) well before the manifestation of any overt symptoms is enough to discredit the adequacy of intuitions based on how one happens to feel at any given moment.

A number of these problems might be resolved by distinguishing between health as a norm and as an ideal. As a norm, it could be possible to speak in terms of deviation from some statistical standards, particularly if these standards were couched not only in terms of organic function but also in terms of behavioral functioning. Thus someone would be called "healthy" if his heart, lungs, kidneys (etc.) functioned at a certain level of efficiency and efficacy, if he was not suffering physical pain, and if his body was free of those pathological conditions which even if undetected or undetectable could impair organic function and eventually cause pain. There could still be dispute about what should count as a "pathological" condition, but at least it would be possible to draw up a large checklist of items subject to "scientific measurement"; then, having gone through that checklist in a physical exam, and passing all the tests, one could be pronounced "healthy." Neat, clean, simple.

All of this might be possible in a static culture, which ours is not. The problem is that any notion of a statistical norm will be superintended by some kind of ideal. Why, in the first place, should anyone care at all how his organs are functioning, much less how well they do so? There must be some reason for that, a reason which goes beyond theoretical interest in statistical distributions. Could it possibly be because certain departures from the norm carry with them unpleasant states, which few are likely to call "good": pain, discrimination, unhappiness? I would guess so. In the second place, why should society have any interest whatever in the way the organs of its citizens function? There must also be some reason for that, very possibly the insight that the organ functioning of individuals has some aggregate social implications. In our culture at least (and in every other culture I have ever heard of) it is simply impossible, finally, to draw any sharp distinction between conceptions of the human good and what are accounted significant and negatively evaluated deviations from statistical norms.

That is the whole point of saying, in defense of the WHO definition of health, that it discerned the intimate connection between the good of the body and the good of the self, not only the individual self but the social community of selves. No individual and no society would (save for speculative, scientific reasons only) have any interest whatever in the condition of human organs and bodies were it not for the obvious fact that those conditions can have an enormous impact on the whole of human life. People do, it has been noticed, die; and they die because something has gone wrong with their bodies. This can be annoying, especially if one would, at the moment of death, prefer to be busy doing other things. Consider two commonplace occurrences. The first I have alluded to already: dropping a heavy brick on one's foot. So far as I know, there is no culture where the pain which that event occasions is considered a good in itself. Why is that? Because (I presume) the pain which results can not only make it difficult or impossible to walk for a time but also because the pain, if intense enough, makes it impossible to think about anything else (or think at all) or to relate to anything or anyone other than the pain. For a time, I am "not myself" and that simply because my body is making excessive demands on my attention that nothing

is possible to me except to howl. I cannot, in sum, dissociate my "body" from my "self" in that situation; my self is my body and my body is my pain.

The other occurrence is no less commonplace. It is the assertion the old often make to the young, however great the psychological, economic, or other miseries of the latter: "at least you've got your health." They are saying in so many words that, if one is healthy, then there is some room for hope, some possibility of human recovery; and even more they are saying that, without good health, nothing is possible, however favorable the other conditions of life may be. Again, it is impossible to dissociate good of body and good of self. Put more formally, if health is not a sufficient condition for happiness, it is a necessary condition. At that very fundamental level, then, any sharp distinction between the good of bodies and the good of persons dissolves.

Are we not forced, therefore, to say that, if the complete absence of health (i.e., death) means the complete absence of self, then any diminishment of health must represent, correspondingly, a diminishment of self? That does not follow, for unless a disease or infirmity is severe, it may represent only a minor annoyance, diminishing our selfhood not a whit. And while it will not do to be overly sentimental about such things, it is probably the case that disease or infirmity can, in some cases, increase one's sense of selfhood (which is no reason to urge disease upon people for its possibly psychological benefits). The frequent reports of those who have recovered from a serious illness that it made them appreciate life in a far more intense way than they previously had are not to be dismissed (though one wishes an easier way could be found).

MODEST CONCLUSIONS

Two conclusions may be drawn. The first is that some minimal level of health is necessary if there is to be any possibility of human happiness. Only in exceptional circumstances can the good of self be long maintained in the absence of the good of the body. The second conclusion, however, is that one can be healthy without being in a state of "complete physical, mental, and social well-being." That conclusion can be justified in two ways: (a) because some degree of disease and infirmity is perfectly compatible with mental and social well-being; and (b) because it is doubtful that there ever was, or ever could be, more than a transient state of "complete physical, mental, and social well-being," for individuals or societies; that's just not the way life is or could be. Its attractiveness as an ideal is vitiated by its practical impossibility of realization. Worse than that, it positively misleads, for health becomes a goal of such all-consuming importance that it simply begs to be thwarted in its realization. The demands which the word "complete" entail set the stage for the worst false consciousness of all: the demand that life deliver perfection. Practically speaking, this demand has led, in the field of health, to a constant escalation of expectation and requirement, never ending, never satisfied.

What, then, would be a good definition of "health"? I was afraid someone was going to ask me that question. I suggest we settle on the following: "Health is a state of physical well-being." That state need not be "complete," but it must be at least adequate, i.e., without

significant impairment of function. It also need not encompass "mental" well-being; one can be healthy yet anxious, well yet depressed. And it surely ought not to encompass "social well-being," except insofar as that well-being will be impaired by the presence of large-scale, serious physical infirmities. Of course my definition is vague, but it would take some very fancy semantic footwork for it to be socially misused; that brat next door could not be called "sick" except when he is running a fever. This definition would not, though, preclude all social use of the language of "pathology" for other than physical disease. The image of a physically well body is a powerful one and, used carefully, it can be suggestive of the kind of wholeness and adequacy of function one might hope to see in other areas of life.

Health and Disease: Value-Laden Concepts?

Disease and Values

Joel Feinberg

Joel Feinberg is professor of philosophy at the University of Arizona. He has published many articles in the fields of ethics, philosophy of law, and social philosophy. He is also the author of *Doing and Deserving* (1970) and *Social Philosophy* (1973), the editor of *Reason and Responsibility* (1965) and *Moral Concepts* (1969), and the coeditor of *Philosophy of Law* (1975).

After pointing out that the idea of the impairment of a vital function is central to the concept of disease in general, Feinberg contends that the ascription of functions to component parts of a system is not a wholly factual (descriptive) matter. Assigning a particular function to a component part of an organism is a value-laden enterprise, he argues, precisely because it is dependent on the determination (itself value-laden) of the proper function of the organism as a whole. In Feinberg's view, if there is cross-cultural disagreement regarding "the proper working order of the human body," this disagreement is not purely medical (scientific).

Central to the concept of disease in general is the idea of the impairment of a vital function, that is, a function of some organ or faculty upon which the important or proper functioning of the whole organism depends.[1]

To ascribe a function to a component part of an organic system[2]—a liver or a carburetor—is to say that, in virtue of its morphological structure and its place in the general economy of components, it behaves in a certain way and, further, that the macroscopic functioning of the whole system causally depends upon its behaving in this way. It may seem, then, that ascription of functions to component parts or subsystems is a wholly factual matter consisting of, first, a description of a part's effects and, second, a causal judgment that these effects are necessary conditions for the occurrence of some more comprehensive effects. But the illusion of value-neutrality vanishes when we come to ascribe a function to the organic system itself.[3] We do not turn to the medical profession to learn the function of a man.

It follows that even statements ascribing functions to component organs will not be entirely value-neutral, for the macroscopic functions for which their effects are necessary conditions will contain value specifications in *their* descriptions. Thus Carl Hempel interprets the statement that the heartbeat in vertebrates has the function of circulating the blood to mean that "the heartbeat *has the effect* of circulating the blood, and this ensures the satisfaction of certain conditions (supply of nutriment and removal of waste) that are necessary for the *proper working* of the organism."[4] (In another formulation Hempel refers to conditions "necessary for the system's remaining in adequate, or effective, or proper, working order.")[5] Now there is in fact very little disagreement among us over what constitutes the proper working order of the human *body*. We all would agree that a body with paralyzed limbs was no more in "good working order" than a car with flat tires; and, in general, our culture identifies bodily health with vigor and vitality. But we can imagine a society of mystics or ascetics who find vitality a kind of nervous distraction (much as we regard hyperthyroid activity)— a frustrating barrier to contemplation and mystic experience and a source of material needs that make constant and unreasonable demands for gratification. Such a group might regard bodily vitality as a sickness and certain kinds of vapidity and feebleness as exemplary health. Our disagreement with these people clearly would not be a purely medical matter.[6]

NOTES

1 Disease thus differs from local disorders in that its impairments of part-functions lead to a generalized breakdown of the whole organism. One's body as a whole can continue to function more or less efficiently with a cut finger or a broken arm, but not when it is in high fever, nausea, vertigo, or extreme debility.

2 Only living organisms are ever called healthy or sick, though complex machines are often enough honored by these terms through courtesy of metaphor. Machines, of course, are different in many ways from living things. For the most part, only the latter are capable of growth and reproduction, for example. But machines and living bodies are perfectly similar in one important respect: both are *organic systems*, that is, complexes composed of component parts related in such a way that the macroscopic functioning of the whole depends on the microscopic functioning of the parts, and to some extent, at least, vice versa.

3 With a machine or artifact the illusion may persist: the "true function" of a knife or an automobile may be the purpose for which it was designed, or perhaps the task for which it is best suited by its nature. Even a plant or tree might be claimed to have as its "true" or "proper" function the performing of some service for us—yielding fruit or shade. But it becomes quite implausible to interpret judgments about the proper function of an animal—especially a human animal— as pure matters of technological or biological fact.

4 "The Logic of Functional Analysis," in *Symposium on Sociological Theory*, ed. Llewellyn Gross (New York: Harper & Row, 1959); reprinted in *Purpose in Nature*, ed. John V. Canfield (Englewood Cliffs: Prentice-Hall, 1966). The quote is on page 98 of the latter volume. Italics have been added.

5 *Ibid.*, 99.

6 Cf. the following "medical" statement in which a controversial value judgment is hardly disguised at all: "Hormone therapy is based on the theory that the female change of life should be treated as a preventable disease. 'Menopause,' says Dr. Joseph W. Goldzieher...'is one of nature's mistakes.'" *Newsweek*, April 3, 1967, 55.

Steffi Lewis has argued that, if ninety percent of humanity came, through evolution, to be able to digest cellulose, and if, further, this capacity became importantly useful (perhaps through critical shortages of other foods), the remaining ten percent (who are physiologically exactly the same as us, their ancestors) would quite properly be said to be deformed, or sick, or lacking in "basic" human equipment. What is "healthy," then, is relative to our resources, technical capacities, and purposes.

Human Well-Being and Medicine:
Some Basic Value-Judgments in the Biomedical Sciences
H. Tristram Engelhardt, Jr.

H. Tristram Engelhardt, Jr., M.D., Ph.D. (in philosophy), is professor, Center for Ethics, Medicine and Public Issues, Baylor College of Medicine, Texas Medical Center, Houston. He is the author of *Mind-Body: A Categorical Relation* (1973) and has published numerous articles on issues in biomedical ethics and the philosophy of medicine. Engelhardt is associate editor of the *Journal of Medicine and Philosophy* and is coeditor (with Stuart F. Spicker) of a number of volumes called the *Philosophy and Medicine* series.

Engelhardt contends that discussions about what counts as health and disease necessarily involve the *value-laden* consideration of what constitutes human well-being or "what counts as the proper human state." In his view, then, any identification of a state as healthy or diseased is value-laden precisely because such an identification reflects an assessment (evaluation) of what is proper to humans. Engelhardt suggests that, in very general terms, rational free agency is proper to humans. Hence he characterizes health as a state of possessing the physiological and psychological prerequisites of rational free agency. Accordingly, those states which are perceived as restricting the basis of rational free activity are identified as diseases. According to Engelhardt, to identify a certain state as "diseased" is to characterize it "as being in some sense bad." He specifies three criteria as operative in the identification of disease states: (1) the teleological, (2) the algesic, (3) the aesthetic. In his view, each of these criteria reflects a different aspect of human well-being. (1) Some conditions (e.g., blindness) are identified as diseases because they preclude what is taken to be a proper human function. (2) Some conditions (e.g., a migraine headache) are identified as diseases because they occasion pain. (3) Some conditions (e.g., polydactylia, the condition of having more than five fingers or toes) are identified as diseases because they preclude what is taken to be a normal (proper) human form or appearance.

The concepts of well-being and the good life have been of central interest for philosophy. These notions have also been addressed in part by the law and by social institutions. Of the latter, medicine and health care have been engaged in the achievement of the good life, human well-being, in distinctive ways: they have addressed themselves to cure and care. But educators cure ignorance, and congressmen care for their home districts. What then is the special character of the health professions? How is the good of health distinct from the good of an education or that of a just society? Though broken arms are neither vices nor states of ignorance, some states of ill health seem difficult to distinguish from virtue and ignorance. For example, are psychopaths congenitally vicious or are they ill, and how are we to understand the persistent heavy smoker who develops chronic lung disease, or the individual with a phobia whose habits can be corrected by behavior therapy?

These somewhat heterogeneous questions have in common an accent on the ambiguity of both the concept of health and that of disease. Or, to put it another way, the health professions are goal-oriented enterprises focused on the preservation of and/or reestablishment of human well-being, with the nature of that well-being left somewhat vague. But, at least to begin with, one can distinguish the endeavors of the health professions from education and moral discourse in that the former are engaged in explanation, prediction, and control—diagnosis, prognosis, and therapy. The health professions presume that the phenomena they address, whether psychological or somatic, are bound together in nomological regularities. That is, the health professions presuppose at least the possibility of health sciences—that it is possible to study and give scientific accounts in terms of pathology and psychopathology. They deal with empirical regularities, not primarily with blame and praise—with freedom. Thus, the health sciences and professions are not, as such, exercises in applied ethics.

It might seem, then, that biomedical endeavors could be easily distinguished from normative discourse. But both normative ethics and medicine tell one what the good life is (virtue in the one case and health in the other), and how to act so as to maximize the good life (virtue and health) by avoiding or correcting that which mars human life (vice and disease). To say that something is a disease commits one to saying something about human nature and the nature of human well-being. Further, such talk involves choices among human goods. Thus, to characterize polydactylia, for example, as a disease, is to say that six fingers on a hand is profoundly ugly; or to characterize color blindness as a disease, is to say that seeing colors is a human good. The question of the choice among goods is most problematic in the case of mental diseases, in that psychiatry tends to compass a broader range of human life than other medical specialties. Thus, disorders such as homosexuality,[1] masturbation[2] and frigidity[3] have been at times classified as diseases.

In short, discussions about what counts as health and disease involve consideration of what counts as the proper human state, and the latter is caught up with value-judgments which are both explicit and implicit. Insofar as health and disease are concepts that structure the context or life-world not only of health professionals, but of all of us who orient ourselves with regard to our sickness and well-being, value-judgments about human conditions structure reality. In deciding, for example, that sickle cell anemia is a disease, one opens up the possibility of programs for detection and prevention which influence attitudes toward persons with the disease, as well as those who

possess the trait. Being told that one has sickle cell trait may then have impact on one's attitudes toward reproduction, even the choice of one's mate. Health and disease are concepts which direct us and help us in the formation of our life-projects—the goals we set for our lives and the ways in which we pursue them.

The purpose of this paper will be to speak to this issue: the role and nature of value-judgments in defining the realities described by pathology and psychopathology. The paper contains three sections: the first addresses the concepts of well-being and disease; the second focuses on the role of value-judgments in sorting out symptoms and sign complexes (syndromes) and their place in the development of explanatory models in medicine; and the third states a few summary conclusions.

I WELL-BEING AND DISEASE

The concept of health is central to medicine and the conduct of human life but is complex and ambiguous. The ambiguity turns in part on the ambiguity in the concept of human well-being. It turns, too, on the fact that it is not clear what dimensions of human well-being are meant to be encompassed in the concept of health. Consider, for example, the definition of health given by the World Health Organization: "Health is a state of complete physical, mental, and social well-being and not merely the absence of disease or infirmity."[4] This definition, it would seem, is broad enough to encompass both moral and political well-being. Further, on the basis of the concept of complete well-being, few, if any, humans are healthy. Thus, this concept seems to function as an ideal rather than an achievable norm: it indicates how humans *should* live rather than merely indicating how they could, in fact, live.

The relationship between the concepts of health and disease is also unclear. Is there only one concept of health, or are there, on the other hand, numerous concepts of health, each corresponding to a particular concept of disease? The World Health Organization's definition of health as "not merely the absence of disease or infirmity," but "a state of complete physical, mental, and social well-being" addresses this question by suggesting that there is only one standard of health, though there are many ways in which one's health can be deficient, ways in which one can be diseased. In that case, every definition of disease, or of a particular disease, would presuppose a different element of health.

To say that asthma and peptic ulcer are disease states presupposes that ease in breathing and in digestion are elements of health. But those judgments imply that one knows what functions, under what conditions, are proper to human nature. On this issue, for example, turn the questions of the meaning of aging and the significance of widely distributed phenomena such as acne—are they diseases? Do they constitute the absence of "normal" human well-being?

And so the questions seem to multiply without end. One might be tempted to think, then, that such questions are merely academic quibbles to be sorted out at leisure, and that they have little practical significance. But if aging, for example, is considered a disease rather than a normal phenomenon, then one is likely to "treat" aging in a different fashion. The phrase "premature aging" indicates that some aging is proper, other aging is not. If one conceives of menopause as a proper, natural phenomenon, one may, for example, treat changes in the vaginal mucosa of postmenopausal women in a different way than if one regards such changes as diseases to be avoided.[5] That is, if one conceives of postmenopausal women as normally sexually active beings, whose function as such should be preserved as long as possible, one has implicitly made a decision according to a concept of the nature of human well-being.

These issues move into a whole domain and spectrum of states: presbyopia, elevated cholesterol levels, baldness, the morbidity associated with normal teething—the frequent if not usual wear-and-tear and changes associated with living. To some extent, judgments about these states depend on the context: phenylketonuria would never exist as a disease if humans usually ate diets free of phenylalanine. Such considerations suggest that one aspect of health is a successful adaptation to one's environment and that disease is maladaptation. Such judgments are based on the usual state of things, and on what one should be adapted to do or to be. Humans, for example, usually do not eat phenylalanine-free diets. But, again, such judgments cannot merely be made in terms of the usual state as a statistical norm, because even if, for example, presbyopia is the usual state for persons over forty, one may still wish to call such conditions states of disease.

Adaptation is a goal-oriented concept which presupposes that one knows what activities humans should be adapted to engage in and under what conditions. For example, sickle cell trait may be a state of health in an environment where falciparum malaria is endemic and antimalarial drugs are not available; the same trait would be a disease in high mountain villages with low oxygen pressure. Or, to take another example, humans, unlike rats, are not adapted to living on a Vitamin C-free diet, though it does not follow from this fact that all humans are diseased (though a rat which could not synthesize Vitamin C would be considered diseased). What is crucial in understanding adaptation is not the environment or organism as such but the purposes or goals which one holds that the organism should be able to achieve. Human well-being in the sense of health comes to identify a physical or psychological condition of humans that enables them to engage in the activities proper to them as humans. What will count as health, as a result, becomes dependent in part on the range of activity one considers to be a proper element of human life. As a positive concept, the concept of health refers to one's ability to engage in the range of activities or be in the range of states which should be open to other members of one's species, even though, in fact, not all members of the species do engage in such activities. To say that X is healthy is to say that X does not have a physical or psychological inability to do those things that humans should be able to do (or be like—e.g., not have acne).[6]

One must, then, give an account of what is proper to humans in order to give a sketch of the concept of health. The account is circular. One decides what humans should be able to do by deciding what will count as physical and psychological well-being (health) and one decides what should be physical and psychological well-being on the basis of what will count as the projects proper to humans. The nature of health and the scope of human projects are closely bound, for health is a necessary condition for whatever endeavors humans wish to engage in. Painting pictures, building houses, hunting for food, tilling the soil, having sex, bearing children, reading books, conceiving of new ideas—all to varying extents presuppose a state of health. The delineation of the scope of health depends on what one judges to be the elements of normal human life. Moreover, the elements appear not only to be multiple, but diverse. One is forced thus to examine the meaning of a normal human lifestyle in a piecemeal fashion. That is, by seeing what counts as diseases, by seeing what elements of the life process when absent would not support well-being, we might be able to understand what is meant by health. Even if health may not be merely the absence of disease, what we take to be diseases can help us to understand the scope of the concept of health. By recognizing what is not health, we can sketch in the boundaries or limits of health. We will move, thus, to consider the concept of health in a "backwards" fashion—through the concept of disease.

What will count as a proper human goal is openended and turns on a decision concerning what humans should be, as well as what they are. Even if 95 percent of the human population developed juvenile diabetes, and the "normals" were thus statistically deviant, one could still decide that diabetes is a disease. Similarly, aging can be seen as a disease if one wants to decide that a particular life-span, free of certain limitations upon action, should exist. The less pain is involved, and the less widely distributed the limitation on action, then the more the judgment that a particular condition (a particular limitation on free, rational action) is a disease is open to cultural variability. Thus, whether or not color blindness, or the inability to roll the sides of one's tongue inwards, will count as diseases will depend upon what a group of people decide should be the goals of man.

The decision is a group decision. To call someone ill is a social judgment involving particular social roles. But how do groups decide upon the proper goals of humans (and thus upon the geography of health and disease), and are there ways in which one might say a group decided wrongly (or rightly)? The last question is fundamental to the issue of the nature of disease. At least two general types of answers are forthcoming. First, proper human goals can be defined in terms of what is conducive to the long-range survival of the species.[7] This has the advantage of giving an evolutionary aura to the criterion—health is that which is conducive to the long-range adaptability and success of the species.

There are difficulties with such an answer, however. For example, given such an interpretation, persons with sickle cell disease could not be said to be diseased; in the absence of antimalarial drugs and the presence of falciparum malaria (sickle cell trait appears to give adaptive advantage to individuals in environments where there is a great deal of falciparum malaria and thus to be an element of normal function).[8] Their discomfort, and even death, would simply be the price of group survival and a part of the adaptability of the species. Such an analysis presupposes, of course, that long-term survival of the species is a fundamental or

overriding goal—a goal that may or may not be accepted by individual humans or even the community of humans. In fact, one might somewhat perversely turn this naturalistic argument around and point out that it is natural for species to die out. For example, merely possible future humans, as not actually humans, would not be treated as means merely if we decided not to bring them into existence and, instead, consume for ourselves the resources available which they could have claimed, had they come into existence, become actual persons.

Further, human nature is not necessarily adapted to human goals. Or, to quote Sir Peter Medawar, "...nature does *not* know best,"[9] but creates a "...tale of woe [including] anaphylactic shock, allergy, and hypersensitivity,"[10] due to the character of human nature. What nature imposes often is not at all what reasonable humans would choose as goals. The proper or essential human goals to which healthy human processes contribute are those in accord with human judgments about what should be the case, which obliquely makes a Kantian point: the truly human is rational free agency and what contributes to that is healthy and what does not is diseased. But, of course, there are a great number of ways to be rational and free, and hence the ambiguity with respect to specifying essential or proper human goals in this fashion.

This brings us to the second method of deciding what counts as essential or proper human goals. Humans are distinguished from other species in being rational free agents. Rational free action is *the* proper human goal, in terms of which all other human purposes are best pursued, including moments of impetuous abandon. In such terms, those states that augment rational free action would count as health and those that restrict the basis of such activity would be diseases. This answer has both advantages and disadvantages. On the one hand, it helps explain the plasticity of the definition of health and disease: the goal of rational free agency is abstract and can be specified in many fashions. Thus, though anything that impeded intelligence (such as schizophrenia) or limited action (such as paralysis) would, *prima facie*, count as a disease state, the diseases of homosexuality or color blindness would remain moot. Decisions as to what would be a disease would then to a great extent hinge on the finitude which humans as finite agents would accept and the character of the life they wished to live. Thus one sees, for example, discussions of aging which really amount to considerations of the amount of aging one will accept and what amount one will treat as a disease.

The second answer also forces a clearer delineation of medical problems from political or moral problems which might circumscribe free agency as well. That is, if medical problems are not problems for which one is responsible as one is for one's moral problems, how are the lines to be drawn? Siegler and Osmond give a summary of Talcott Parsons' sketch of the sick role that highlights the fact that though being sick is not a state of affairs for which one is immediately responsible, it is a state for which one is responsible for seeking treatment. "First, depending on the nature and severity of the illness, the sick person is exempted from some or all of his normal social role responsibilities. Second, the sick person cannot help being ill, and cannot get well by an act of decision or will. Third, the sick person is expected to want to get well as soon as possible. Fourth, he is expected to seek appropriate help, usually that of a physician, and cooperate with that help toward the end of getting well."[11] The division between lack of responsibility for having the disease and responsibility for treating the disease is not as clear-cut as this sketch may suggest. One is also responsible for not having prevented the diseases one has, insofar as such prevention was possible. In short, it is hard to sift out the elements of moral responsibility with respect to disease.

On the one hand, having a disease cannot be an immediate result of an act of the will, like stealing a car or telling a lie. Otherwise, it would be appropriate to say to the diseased person, "Stop that at once!" Yet, one can be responsible for one's disease, as a smoker can be responsible for having bronchogenic carcinoma, or a person with angina can be responsible for an attack if he imprudently runs up a flight of stairs. Such responsibility for one's illness is liable to increase as it becomes easier to predict what available actions will lead to or prevent illness. Thus, a smoker can be properly blamed for getting cancer. Further, if he or she requires treatment that is a burden on the general community, one has a basis for saying that he or she acted immorally with respect to the responsibility to avoid cancer and its public costs. One can imagine increasing the tax on cigarettes specifically to pay for the cost of treating the diseases of smokers. They have a special duty to pay for the costs that have resulted from their acquiring a disease they could have avoided. They are to blame. The same conclusions can be made with respect to drug addicts. One can blame them for

becoming addicted, though one could not blame them for *being* addicted.

In short, with respect to disease, one wishes both to blame and not to blame. The distinctions turn on the fact that diseases, mental and physical, are as such held to be due to a fabric of causal events imposed upon the person afflicted, even if that person may have initiated the causal sequence (the smoking which led to the disease). Thus, to say that someone is responsible for having a disease is to say that one has a condition (mental or physical) at time t_0, which is causally imposed independently of one's volition at t_0, though at a previous time, t_{-1}, one could have avoided initiating the causal sequence that led to the disease. As a result, it makes sense to blame a person with angina for developing the disease if a different diet would have prevented it, and for blaming the anginal patient for a present attack if more prudent behavior would have avoided it. But one cannot hold him responsible for having angina (in the sense of "keeping" the angina) with respect to any of his or her choices at that present time at which he or she already has the disease.

Judgments concerning disease states thus have complex social implications. They are the basis for both excusing and for blaming, for saying that having a disease is not dependent upon human volition, though acquiring a disease may be the result of human negligence. The problem of defining the scope of the groups which share common judgments about the proper goals of humans is a task for medical sociologists. It is a task of describing social groups that share a lifeworld in which certain abilities and human activities are seen as essential to the human condition. But cross-cultural criticism is still possible when and if concepts of disease fail to distinguish political and moral judgments from medical judgments. Criticism would, for example, be possible if a group held that exceptionally high intelligence or clarity in making decisions were diseases. Such judgments would fly in the face of the nature of being human, of being a rational agent.[12] Finally, expectations with respect to health that did not recognize the limits of human life (those who might want to speak of death itself as something to be overcome by medicine) could be judged as mistaken. Death itself should, for example, never count as a disease.[13]

One is thus confronted with a spectrum of diseases ranging from those which obviously limit humans in some essential fashion in their capacity as agents (coronary artery disease, carcinoma) to those states which may or may not be seen as limitations (homosexuality, color blindness). Norms as far as they can be had are thus somewhat abstract: the proper goal of humans is to act freely and rationally. But there are many ways to achieve that goal, and so only the more severe limitations on its pursuit show themselves unambiguously to be diseases. In other cases, the choice is open to variations, such as those with respect to whether alcoholism or drug addiction or obesity should count as diseases. This is not to say that choices of whether or not such states should be considered diseases are arbitrary, but only that they are much less clear-cut.

Medicine is thus involved in deciding the nature and geography of human well-being. The geography is, as the above attests, heterogeneous. Many things are gathered under the rubric disease and for diverse reasons: considerations of teleology, pain, and aesthetics. Beyond that, there is a whole clan of loosely related usages: "He has a disease," "He has a congenital deformity," "He has a birth defect," "He has a deformity of his hand due to an auto accident...due to surgery ...due to an infection." Are all these conditions to be spoken of as disease states in some extended sense? Is an amputee to be said to be suffering from a disease (the absence of a leg), and does it matter whether the amputation resulted from the injury of an accident or was performed because of osteogenic carcinoma?

Dorland's Dictionary defines disease as "a definite morbid process having a characteristic train of symptoms," and a syndrome as "a set of symptoms which occur together."[14] Thus, there may be a point in saying that the person who has a gunshot wound has a syndrome, though not a disease—the process that caused the damage was not immediately part of a physiological or psychological train of causality (though that may incidentally be the case—the person who did the shooting may have been psychotic). The gunshot wound, though, constitutes a syndrome, a collect of morbid symptoms and signs which are the business of medicine to address. The amputee may or may not be in a similar circumstance, depending on the extent to which he or she is still crippled or rehabilitated by a prosthesis. Syndromes, the patterns of observables which medicine addresses with treatment, are patterns of physical and/or mental limitations accountable (or at least held theoretically to be accountable) in terms of physiological and/or psychological laws—even the state of affairs treated for other than a pathological process (loss of a limb from shark bite).

In short, the language of medicine is complex and exceeds the language of its nosologies. "He is crippled because he lost his right leg in an auto accident," and "He is crippled because his right leg was amputated because of osteogenic carcinoma" identify states of non-health illness so that it is possible to recognize both individuals as being in a state properly the object of medical concern, even if the individuals are not diseased in the sense of still being subject to a "morbid process." One can be sick (fulfill Talcott Parsons' criteria for the sick role) without being diseased, if one uses the term "disease" in the restricted fashion prominent in some of the ordinary usages of "disease" ("He is crippled but he is not diseased," or "He is crippled but does not have a disease"). Finally, at this juncture one more qualification or reminder is perhaps needed: not all morbid states are the results of presently active morbid processes. Morbid states can be the end stages of long-ceased morbid processes (the scars of smallpox), or of nondisease processes (the scars of a burn). Consequently, one can say of someone, "He is not in perfect health; after all, he is a paraplegic because of his accident, but he does not have any diseases."

The concepts of health and illness are more ample than the concept of disease. Disease language involves a move to generate scientific explanations of syndromes by reference to some ongoing processes leading to those syndromes. In contrast, some people are ill, not healthy, because of diseases long ended or because of accidents. But the disorders, disabilities, and syndromes to which medicine does turn its attention define by contrast the geography of health and indicate the various groups of evaluations which identify the elements of human well-being. This geography is a heterogeneous domain of concerns, presupposing variously related judgments about human well-being and its absence.

II   DISCOVERING THE PATHOLOGICAL

But how does one recognize a particular state as a state of illness, open to being explained as a disease, given the general conditions outlined above? To begin with, in recognizing clusters of phenomena as syndromes, one engages in evaluation, not description alone. One identifies a complex of signs and symptoms, a constellation of complaints and associated physical findings, as morbid—that is, as constituting a recognizable pattern that should be treated. The pattern is not merely recognized as a pattern, but as one which is in some way wrong and which should, if possible, be corrected. Syndromes are, as I will consider them, collections of observables considered apart from any explicit theoretical account of their nature and composition. They are identified through collections of reports of pain and discomfort, as well as observations of dysfunction and deformity. At the level of syndrome identification, there are important evaluative judgments as to what is unpleasant, dysfunctional, or deforming. The judgment as to what should be brought within the scope of a syndrome turns on what coheres as a pattern of signs and symptoms, as well as whether the pattern is an illness, a disagreeable state attributable to somatic or psychological dysfunction rather than to willful obstinancy (a common fit of anger), or a planned deception (a case of malingering), or the action of supernatural powers (a demonic possession). Syndromes are thus observable patterns in search of a medical explanation. They presuppose that the cluster of observables constitutes a pattern which can be explained in terms of the laws of pathology and/or psychology. As a consequence, a subset of the universe of observation statements is mapped onto the universe of explanations insofar as a cluster of observables is identified as morbid (as an illness) and is then given a disease explanation.[15]

To call a state of affairs an illness is not simply to identify the state, but also to characterize it as being in some sense bad. The types of evaluative judgments involved in such selections of clusters of phenomena as syndromes (illnesses) are diverse. They can, however, be arrayed into at least three groups: the teleological, the algesic, the aesthetic—each concerned with a different aspect of human well-being. The first, the teleological, speak to the issue of those functions proper to humans; they concern the goals humans should be adapted to achieve. In this first group one might, for example, place toxic amaurosis, blindness following exposure to such agents as wood alcohol. One presumes seeing to be a proper function of humans, and the blindness to be caused, not feigned. But specifying the scope of that natural function brings one to borderline cases which emphasize the role of evaluative judgments concerning the proper range of human abilities. There is thus the question of whether color blindness is a disease: is seeing colors an ability the lack of which would count as a disease? That judgment seems in part to turn on the fact that most humans can see color. Because no humans are adapted (able) to see ultraviolet, "blindness" to ultraviolet is not a disease (and is thus,

in a sense, not blindness at all). Whether color blindness is a disease thus depends on what we hold are the proper goals of humans.

Such teleological judgments also play a role in deciding whether aging is a disease, whether the pain of normal childbirth is pathological, whether respiratory distress when climbing a mountain is normal or an indication of disease. In each case, one is deciding whether the discomfort is to be accepted or to be treated as abnormal. Judgments of these sorts are complex, but can be put this way: X is (under these criteria) a disease state, (1) if and only if it is a state arising out of physiological and/or psychological processes of an individual beyond the direct control at that time of the person afflicted; and (2) if that state precludes a proper or essential human goal.[16] Thus, if seeing color is part of being a human, color blindness is a disease. If being able to see colors is not an essential or proper function, then being able to see colors turns out to be merely an ability which enhances, but is not central to, human well-being.

The use of terms such as "function" or "dysfunction" indicates that such judgments concerning what will count as a disease presuppose judgments concerning goals to be served. Thus, the fact that a large number of individuals cannot taste phenylthiocarbamide is, most likely, not going to cause anyone to call them diseased.[17] Tasting phenylthiocarbamide is just not important to any human goals in the same way that seeing colors is. The same can be said with regard to the genetic trait of being able to roll the edges of one's tongue inwards.[18] Whether or not such functions are important enough so that their absence would constitute a disease depends on what one considers to be proper human goals and abilities. In short, judgments concerning disease states involve a whole range of more or less subtle judgments concerning the activities humans should be able to perform, the goals they should be able to achieve. Humans should be able to walk up five flights of stairs if they are not ninety; they should be able to make precise movements with their hands; they should be able to balance themselves with great precision; they should be able to taste and enjoy their food, enjoy sex, see the world, and hear a certain range of sounds.

For example, if, as Dr. Robert Heath maintains, marijuana is pathogenic because it causes a decrease in interest and drive, then there is a presupposition that humans should be able to accomplish a certain quantity or quality of things in order to be healthy, to realize the proper goals of humans.[19] Or, to place the issue in a different perspective, if it is important to have a natural resistance to many of the effects of the falciparum malaria, sickle cell trait becomes a state of health, and sickle cell disease becomes the cost to a population of being healthy.

One should also notice that the pattern of a syndrome can be such as to collect mental as well as physical signs and symptoms. Behavior patterns can be judged to be pathological as, for example, are schizophrenia and obsessive-compulsive neuroses, even though there are not well-established causal accounts of these phenomena. They count as diseases (at least as syndromes), not only because they are dysfunctional (untreated schizophrenics cannot do abstract thinking well, or participate well in the affairs of life; obsessive-compulsive neurotics find their compulsions interfering with their activities, goals, and projects), but also because people with these states find them unpleasant (painful in an extended sense).

The notorious difficulties in deciding with regard to the character of natural teleology should also be noted here. The nosologic standing of homosexuality is a good example. The judgment that homosexuality is a disease was made in part on the basis of an alleged dysteleological character of such sexuality (it is not natural), and in part on its compulsive character.[20] Yet, on the second point, heterosexuals seem as compelled in their behavior as do homosexuals. Again, these difficulties in specifying what is normal with regard to psychological syndromes are, it should be added, not unknown with regard to somatic conditions. Persons who are color-blind tend to discriminate differences in intensity much better than those who see colors, and thus, among other things, are good at detecting camouflage.[21] The noncolor-blind thus have a disadvantage as well. In short, the difficulty of specifying goals is widespread.

The second type of judgments made with regard to disease states are made in terms of their being painful. A migraine headache counts as an illness in terms of pain alone, independently of any regard to loss of function. One might term these algesic criteria. These can be overridden in the case of painful activities held to be essential to proper goals of humans: childbirth, teething, pain after unaccustomed exercise. Here the judgment appears to be that X is a disease (under these criteria) (1) if and only if the state (here that of pain) arises out of a physiological and/or psychological process beyond the direct control at that time of the person afflicted; and (2) if the state of pain is not part of a process conducive to a proper or essential human goal. Of the three factors used in sorting out clusters of phenomena as diseases, the algesic appear to be the least variant: a pain is a pain even if cultural circumstances influence its evaluation. Moreover, as a relatively simple reaction to stimuli, there has been fair success in identifying its physiological substrata. Thus, broken legs, angina, and colitis show themselves relatively unproblematically to be disease states: they are appreciated as collections of phenomena which involve pain held to be due to physiological processes beyond the direct control of the persons affected (and the same could be said with regard to pain associated with similarly uncontrollable psychological processes).

The third set of criteria is aesthetic. Some states of affairs are taken to be disease states because of aesthetic judgments like "Polydactylia is a disease," or "Supernumerary breasts is a deformity." A woman and her society might very well consider alopecia areata a disease since women in our culture, even more than men, seem to be perturbed by becoming bald, even if only partially. Further, as David Mechanic points out, one South American tribe considers anyone not marked by the colored spots of dyschromic spirochetosis to be diseased and excludes the person from marriage.[22] The aesthetic is the most evasive of the criteria. It is very difficult (if not impossible) to specify what counts as a human deformity or, to reverse the statement, what counts as physical well-being with respect to human form and appearance. Are achondroplastic dwarfs diseased because they are dwarfs? What are proper human proportions? In any event, the judgment here again requires that the state of affairs held to be a disease or pathologic deformity not be under the direct control of the person afflicted and that the state of affairs be appreciated as abnormal, as a deviant form.

As heterogeneous as these judgments may appear, they draw the line between physiology and pathology; they isolate and associate clusters of phenomena for medicine and the biomedical sciences to explain. They define implicitly what *pathos*, suffering, is.

III SOME CONCLUSIONS

This series of considerations of the concept of human well-being and medicine leads to at best a very general concept of health, namely, a state of possessing the physiological and psychological prerequisites (or substrata) of rational free agency. But one can be free in so many ways and rationally pursue so many goals that only very general things can be said beyond the judgment that rational free agency, and, *a fortiori*, its physical and mental preconditions, are the cardinal goods for the health of any person. Thus any physiological or psychological processes or states not under the immediate control of a person which (1) preclude the goals chosen as integral to the general life of humans (inability to engage in the range of physical activity held integral to human life); (2) cause pain (if that pain is not integral to a process leading to goals held to be integral to human life); (3) preclude a physical form that other humans would hold to be normal (not deformed)—will count as diseases. One should notice that much of the ambiguity of the concepts of health and disease stems from the fact that what is said about human well-being would be true of embodied persons generally, not just human persons. This essay has given an account of the well-being of embodied persons insofar as that well-being can be considered by medicine. Anything more concrete will have to be provided by a medical-sociological and anthropological study of the goals humans accept as integral to their physiological and psychological well-being. Surely much awaits an interdisciplinary effort by philosophers, medical sociologists, and anthropologists. Humans are animals which make their own nature, set their own standards of health and disease, and thus raise core issues concerning the directions and goods of life. They raise issues which are ineluctably both philosophical and scientific.

NOTES

This paper is drawn in part from a lecture given in the Matchette Lecture Series, Southern Methodist University, Dallas, Texas, December 9, 1974. I am in many respects in the debt of recent publications concerning the concept of health and disease: Lester S. King, "What is Disease?" *Philosophy of Science* 21 (July 1954), 193–203; Horocio Fabrega, "Concepts of Disease: Logical Features and Social Implications," *Perspectives in Biology and Medicine* 15 (Summer 1972), 583–616; Robert P. Hudson, "The Concept of Disease," *Annals of Internal Medicine* 65 (September 1966), 595–601; *Hastings Center Studies* 1:3 (1973), "The Concept of Health"; Ruth Macklin, "Mental Health and Mental Illness; Some Problems of Definition and Concept Formation," *Philosophy of Science*

39 (September 1972), 341–65; Owsei Temkin, "The Scientific Approach to Disease: Specific Entity and Individual Sickness," in *Scientific Changes*, A. C. Crombie, ed. (London: Heinemann, 1961), pp. 629–47; Henry Cohen, *Concepts of Medicine* (Oxford: Pergamon Press, 1960), p. 160; and Stewart Wolf, "Disease as a Way of Life: Neural Integration in Systematic Pathology," *Perspectives in Biology and Medicine* 4 (Spring 1961), 288–305. I am particularly in debt to Lester King and Laurence B. McCullough for their suggestions concerning this paper.

1 American Psychiatric Association, "Sexual Deviation," *Diagnostic and Statistical Manual: Mental Disorders* (Washington, D.C.: American Psychiatric Association, 1952), pp. 38–39.

2 H. Tristram Engelhardt, Jr., "The Disease of Masturbation: Values and the Concept of Disease," *Bulletin of the History of Medicine* 48 (Summer 1974), 234–48.

3 *American Handbook of Psychiatry*, Silvano Arieti, ed. (New York: Basic Books, 1959), I, 719.

4 Constitution of the World Health Organization (preamble). *The First Ten Years of the World Health Organization* (Geneva: World Health Organization, 1958), p. 459.

5 Robert W. Kistner, "The Menopause," *Clinical Obstetrics and Gynecology* 16 (December 1973), 107–29; Robert A. Wilson, Raimondo E. Brevetti, and Thelma A. Wilson, "Specific Procedures for the Elimination of the Menopause," *Western Journal of Surgery, Obstetrics, and Gynecology* 71 (May–June 1963), 110–21.

6 The accent must fall on one's physical or psychological state, rather than on one's moral state, with the presumption that the first, unlike the second, is properly described in terms of psychological and physiological regularities and nomological structures; and the second is described in terms of one's free actions or states open to alterations immediately through one's exercise of free choice. For example, one's ability to survive under physical stress may be a sign of health, even though that condition is the result of free action, such as being in good physical condition due to frequent exercise. That state of good health, though, is only mediately the result of one's free choice—namely, the choice is mediated by the physical exercise. A moral resolution, though, is immediately connected to one's free choice.

7 Chauncey D. Leake and Patrick Romanell, *Can*

We Agree? (Austin: University of Texas Press, 1950).

8 F. B. Livingstone, "The Distributions of the Abnormal Hemoglobin Genes and Their Significance for Human Evolution," *Evolution* 18 (1964), 685.

9 Peter Brian Medawar, *The Future of Man* (London: Methuen and Company, 1960), p. 100.

10 *Ibid.*, p. 101.

11 Miriam Siegler and Humphry Osmond, "The 'Sick Role' Revisited," *Hastings Center Studies* 1:3 (1973), 41.

12 It should be noted that these boundaries of the natural for humans as free agents are the boundaries for persons as such, not only human persons. That is, they would apply to all persons, whether human or not. This implies that what is important here is not human nature, but the nature of persons. In particular, human persons can for good reasons change human nature as, for example, is done with birth control, which divorces the social and biological dimensions of sexuality. Human nature becomes something for human persons to modify and change.

13 To fail to recognize death as a natural limit would be to fail to recognize the necessary contingency of human life. It would thus, in a sense, be irrational. See H. Tristram Engelhardt, Jr., "The Counsels of Finitude," *Hastings Center Report* 5:2 (April 1975), 29–35.

14 *Dorland's Illustrated Medical Dictionary*, 24th ed., s.v. "disease."

15 One could thus distinguish illness and disease as *explanandum* and *explanans*, the first belonging to the universe of observation statement, the second belonging to the universe of explanatory statements. A suggestion in this vein is made by Alvan Feinstein. *Clinical Judgment* (Huntington, N.Y.: Robert E. Krieger Publishing Co., 1967). In this paper I will somewhat loosely use the terms "illness," "disease state," and "syndrome" as equivalent statements identifying a complex of phenomena recognized as morbid. In fact, syndromes will often simply be called "diseases" to indicate that they are illnesses subject to a disease explanation.

16 The reference to the state of disease being beyond direct control of the individual rules out calling states such as not being able to see because one's eyes are closed, diseases.

17 This condition may, though, be correlated with diseases. H. Harris, H. Kalmus, and W. R. Trotter, "Taste Sensitivity to Phenylthiourea in Goitre and Diabetes," *Lancet* 2 (1949), 1038.

18 Amram Scheinfeld, *Your Heredity and Environment* (Philadelphia: J. B. Lippincott, 1965), pp. 480–81.

19 *People* 2 (December 9, 1974), 12–13.

20 Morton Prince, "Sexual Perversion or Vice? A Pathological and Therapeutic Inquiry," *Journal of Nervous and Mental Disease* 25 (1898); 237–65.

21 Richard H. Post, "Population Differences in Red and Green Color Vision Deficiency: A Review, and a Query on Selection Relaxation," *Eugenics Quarterly* 9 (March 1962), 131–46.

22 David Mechanic, *Medical Sociology* (New York: The Free Press, 1968), p. 16.

Is Mental Illness a Myth?

The Myth of Mental Illness

Thomas S. Szasz

Thomas S. Szasz, M.D., is professor of psychiatry at the State University of New York, Upstate Medical Center in Syracuse. A cofounder of the American Association for the Abolition of Involuntary Mental Hospitalization, he has long been an outspoken critic of contemporary psychiatric practice. Among his numerous published works are *The Myth of Mental Illness* (1961), *The Ethics of Psychoanalysis* (1965), *The Manufacture of Madness* (1970), and *Heresies* (1976).

Szasz contends that there is no such thing as mental illness. In his view, the concept of mental illness has no cognitive (descriptive) content, functioning instead as a myth. Although he maintains that the term "mental illness" is unnecessary and misleading when used to refer to brain diseases, he especially objects to employing the term "mental illness" to refer to alleged deformities of personality. Szasz maintains that, whereas physical illness may be ascribed on the basis of deviation from the norm of structural and functional integrity of the body, mental illness is ascribed solely on the basis that there is deviation (of personal behavior) from certain ethical, political, or social norms. According to Szasz, psychiatrists are mistaken in thinking that they are engaged in diagnosing and treating medical illness. Their patients do not have mental diseases but rather are experiencing "problems in living."

I

At the core of virtually all contemporary psychiatric theories and practices lies the concept of mental illness. A critical examination of this concept is therefore indispensable for understanding the ideas, institutions, and interventions of psychiatrists.

My aim in this essay is to ask if there is such a thing as mental illness and to argue that there is not. Of course, mental illness is not a thing or physical object; hence it can exist only in the same sort of way as do other theoretical concepts. Yet, to those who believe in them, familiar theories are likely to appear, sooner or later, as "objective truths" or "facts." During certain historical periods, explanatory concepts such as deities, witches, and instincts appeared not only as theories but as *self-evident causes* of a vast number of events. Today mental illness is widely regarded in a similar fashion, that is, as the cause of innumerable diverse happenings.

As an antidote to the complacent use of the notion of mental illness—as a self-evident phenomenon, theory, or cause—let us ask: What is meant when it is asserted that someone is mentally ill? In this essay I shall describe the main uses of the concept of mental illness, and I shall argue that this notion has outlived whatever cognitive usefulness it might have had and that it now functions as a myth.

II

The notion of mental illness derives its main support from such phenomena as syphilis of the brain or delirious conditions—intoxications, for instance—in which persons may manifest certain disorders of thinking and behavior. Correctly speaking, however, these are diseases of the brain, not of the mind. According to one school of thought, *all* so-called mental illness is of this type. The assumption is made that some neurological defect, perhaps a very subtle one, will ultimately be found to explain all the disorders of thinking and behavior. Many contemporary physicians, psychiatrists, and other scientists hold this view, which implies that people's troubles cannot be caused by conflicting personal needs, opinions, social aspirations, values, and so forth. These difficulties—which I think we may simply call *problems in living*—are thus attributed to physico-chemical processes that in due time will be discovered (and no doubt corrected) by medical research.

Mental illnesses are thus regarded as basically similar to other diseases. The only difference, in this view, between mental and bodily disease is that the former, affecting the brain, manifests itself by means of mental symptoms; whereas the latter, affecting other organ systems—for example, the skin, liver, and so on—manifests itself by means of symptoms referable to those parts of the body.

In my opinion, this view is based on two fundamental errors. In the first place, a disease of the brain, analogous to a disease of the skin or bone, is a neurological defect, not a problem in living. For example, a *defect* in a person's visual field may be explained by correlating it with certain lesions in the nervous system. On the other hand, a person's *belief*—whether it be in Christianity, in Communism, or in the idea that his internal organs are rotting and that his body is already dead—cannot be explained by a defect or disease of the nervous system. Explanations of this sort of occurrence—assuming that one is interested in the belief itself and does not regard it simply as a symptom or expression of something else that is more interesting—must be sought along different lines.

The second error is epistemological. It consists of interpreting communications about ourselves and the world around us as symptoms of neurological functioning. This is an error not in observation or reasoning, but rather in the organization and expression of knowledge. In the present case, the error lies in making a dualism between mental and physical symptoms, a dualism that is a habit of speech and not the result of known observations. Let us see if this is so.

In medical practice, when we speak of physical disturbances we mean either signs (for example, fever) or symptoms (for example, pain). We speak of mental symptoms, on the other hand, when we refer to a patient's communications about himself, others, and the world about him. The patient might assert that he is Napoleon or that he is being persecuted by the Communists. These would be considered mental symptoms only if the observer believed that the patient was *not* Napoleon or that he was *not* being persecuted by the Communists. This makes it apparent that the statement "*X* is a mental symptom" involves rendering a judgment that entails a covert comparison between the patient's ideas, concepts, or beliefs and those of the observer and the society in which they live. The notion of mental symptom is therefore inextricably tied to the social, and particularly the ethical, context in which it is made, just as the notion of bodily symptom is tied to an anatomical and genetic context.[1]

To sum up: For those who regard mental symptoms as signs of brain disease, the concept of mental illness is unnecessary and misleading. If they mean that people so labeled suffer from diseases of the brain, it would seem better, for the sake of clarity, to say that and not something else.

III

The term "mental illness" is also widely used to describe something quite different from a disease of the brain. Many people today take it for granted that living is an arduous affair. Its hardship for modern man derives, moreover, not so much from a struggle for biological survival as from the stresses and strains inherent in the social intercourse of complex human personalities. In this context, the notion of mental illness is used to identify or describe some features of an individual's so-called personality. Mental illness—as a deformity

of the personality, so to speak—is then regarded as the cause of human disharmony. It is implicit in this view that social intercourse between people is regarded as something inherently harmonious, its disturbance being due solely to the presence of "mental illness" in many people. Clearly, this is faulty reasoning, for it makes the abstraction "mental illness" into a cause of, even though this abstraction was originally created to serve only as a shorthand expression for, certain types of human behavior. It now becomes necessary to ask: What kinds of behavior are regarded as indicative of mental illness, and by whom?

The concept of illness, whether bodily or mental, implies deviation from some clearly defined norm. In the case of physical illness, the norm is the structural and functional integrity of the human body. Thus, although the desirability of physical health, as such, is an ethical value, what health is can be stated in anatomical and physiological terms. What is the norm, deviation from which is regarded as mental illness? This question cannot be easily answered. But whatever this norm may be, we can be certain of only one thing: namely, that it must be stated in terms of psychosocial, ethical, and legal concepts. For example, notions such as "excessive repression" and "acting out an unconscious impulse" illustrate the use of psychological concepts for judging so-called mental health and illness. The idea that chronic hostility, vengefulness, or divorce are indicative of mental illness is an illustration of the use of ethical norms (that is, the desirability of love, kindness, and a stable marriage relationship). Finally, the widespread psychiatric opinion that only a mentally ill person would commit homicide illustrates the use of a legal concept as a norm of mental health. In short, when one speaks of mental illness, the norm from which deviation is measured is a *psychosocial and ethical* standard. Yet, the remedy is sought in terms of *medical* measures that—it is hoped and assumed—are free from wide differences of ethical value. The definition of the disorder and the terms in which its remedy are sought are therefore at serious odds with one another. The practical significance of this covert conflict between the alleged nature of the defect and the actual remedy can hardly be exaggerated.

Having identified the norms used for measuring deviations in cases of mental illness, we shall now turn to the question, Who defines the norms and hence the deviation? Two basic answers may be offered: First, it may be the person himself—that is, the patient—who decides that he deviates from a norm; for example, an artist may believe that he suffers from a work inhibition; and he may implement this conclusion by seeking help *for himself* from a psychotherapist. Second, it may be someone other than the "patient" who decides that the latter is deviant—for example, relatives, physicians, legal authorities, society generally; a psychiatrist may then be hired by persons other than the "patient" to do something *to him* in order to correct the deviation.

These considerations underscore the importance of asking the question, Whose agent is the psychiatrist? and of giving a candid answer to it. The psychiatrist (or non-medical mental health worker) may be the agent of the patient, the relatives, the school, the military services, a business organization, a court of law, and so forth. In speaking of the psychiatrist as the agent of these persons or organizations, it is not implied that his moral values, or his ideas and aims concerning the proper nature of remedial action, must coincide exactly with those of his employer. For example, a patient in individual psychotherapy may believe that his salvation lies in a new marriage; his psychotherapist need not share this hypothesis. As the patient's agent, however, he must not resort to social or legal force to prevent the patient from putting his beliefs into action. If his *contract* is with the patient, the psychiatrist (psychotherapist) may disagree with him or stop his treatment, but he cannot engage others to obstruct the patient's aspirations.[2] Similarly, if a psychiatrist is retained by a court to determine the sanity of an offender, he need not fully share the legal authorities' values and intentions in regard to the criminal, nor the means deemed appropriate for dealing with him; such a psychiatrist cannot testify, however, that the accused is not insane, but that the legislators are—for passing the law that decrees the offender's actions illegal.[3] This sort of opinion could be voiced, of course—but not in a courtroom, and not by a psychiatrist who is there to assist the court in performing its daily work.

To recapitulate: In contemporary social usage, the finding of mental illness is made by establishing a deviance in behavior from certain psychosocial, ethical, or legal norms. The judgment may be made, as in medicine, by the patient, the physician (psychiatrist), or others. Remedial action, finally, tends to be sought in a therapeutic—or covertly medical—framework. This creates a situation in which it is claimed that psychosocial, ethical, and legal deviations can be corrected by medical action. Since medical interven-

tions are designed to remedy only medical problems, it is logically absurd to expect that they will help solve problems whose very existence have been defined and established on non-medical grounds.

IV

Anything that people *do*—in contrast to things that *happen* to them[4]—takes place in a context of value. Hence, no human activity is devoid of moral implications. When the values underlying certain activities are widely shared, those who participate in their pursuit often lose sight of them altogether. The discipline of medicine—both as a pure science (for example, research) and as an applied science or technology (for example, therapy)—contains many ethical considerations and judgments. Unfortunately, these are often denied, minimized, or obscured, for the ideal of the medical profession as well as of the people whom it serves is to have an ostensibly value-free system of medical care. This sentimental notion is expressed by such things as the doctor's willingness to treat patients regardless of their religious or political beliefs. But such claims only serve to obscure the fact that ethical considerations encompass a vast range of human affairs. Making medical practice neutral with respect to some specific issues of moral value (such as race or sex) need not mean, and indeed does not mean, that it can be kept free from others (such as control over pregnancy or regulation of sex relations). Thus, birth control, abortion, homosexuality, suicide, and euthanasia continue to pose major problems in medical ethics.

Psychiatry is much more intimately related to problems of ethics than is medicine in general. I use the word "psychiatry" here to refer to the contemporary discipline concerned with problems in living, and not with diseases of the brain, which belong to neurology. Difficulties in human relations can be analyzed, interpreted, and given meaning only within specific social and ethical contexts. Accordingly, the psychiatrist's socioethical orientations will influence his ideas on what is wrong with the patient, on what deserves comment or interpretation, in what directions change might be desirable, and so forth. Even in medicine proper, these factors play a role, as illustrated by the divergent orientations that physicians, depending on their religious affiliations, have toward such things as birth control and therapeutic abortion.

Can anyone really believe that a psychotherapist's ideas on religion, politics, and related issues play no role in his practical work? If, on the other hand, they do matter, what are we to infer from it? Does it not seem reasonable that perhaps we ought to have different psychiatric therapies—each recognized for the ethical positions that it embodies—for, say, Catholics and Jews, religious persons and atheists, democrats and Communists, white supremacists and Negroes, and so on? Indeed, if we look at the way psychiatry is actually practiced today, especially in the United States, we find that the psychiatric interventions people seek and receive depend more on their socioeconomic status and moral beliefs than on the "mental illnesses" from which they ostensibly suffer.[5] This fact should occasion no greater surprise than that practicing Catholics rarely frequent birth-control clinics, or that Christian Scientists rarely consult psychoanalysts.

V

The position outlined above, according to which contemporary psychotherapists deal with problems in living, not with mental illnesses and their cures, stands in sharp opposition to the currently prevalent position, according to which psychiatrists treat mental diseases, which are just as "real" and "objective" as bodily diseases. I submit that the holders of the latter view have no evidence whatever to justify their claim, which is actually a kind of psychiatric propaganda: their aim is to create in the popular mind a confident belief that mental illness is some sort of disease entity, like an infection or a malignancy. If this were true, one could *catch* or *get* a mental illness, one might *have* or *harbor* it, one might *transmit* it to others, and finally one could *get rid* of it. Not only is there not a shred of evidence to support this idea, but, on the contrary, all the evidence is the other way and supports the view that what people now call mental illnesses are, for the most part, *communications* expressing unacceptable ideas, often framed in an unusual idiom.

This is not the place to consider in detail the similarities and differences between bodily and mental illnesses. It should suffice to emphasize that whereas the term "bodily illness" refers to physicochemical occurrences that are not affected by being made public, the term "mental illness" refers to sociopsychological events that are crucially affected by being

made public. The psychiatrist thus cannot, and does not, stand apart from the person he observes, as the pathologist can and often does. The psychiatrist is committed to some picture of what he considers reality, and to what he thinks society considers reality, and he observes and judges the patient's behavior in the light of these beliefs. The very notion of "mental symptom" or "mental illness" thus implies a covert comparison, and often conflict, between observer and observed, psychiatrist and patient. Though obvious, this fact needs to be re-emphasized, if one wishes, as I do here, to counter the prevailing tendency to deny the moral aspects of psychiatry and to substitute for them allegedly value-free medical concepts and interventions.

Psychotherapy is thus widely practiced as though it entailed nothing other than restoring the patient from a state of mental sickness to one of mental health. While it is generally accepted that mental illness has something to do with man's social or interpersonal relations, it is paradoxically maintained that problems of values—that is, of ethics—do not arise in this process. Freud himself went so far as to assert: "I consider ethics to be taken for granted. Actually I have never done a mean thing."[6] This is an astounding thing to say, especially for someone who had studied man as a social being as deeply as Freud had. I mention it here to show how the notion of "illness"—in the case of psychoanalysis, "psychopathology," or "mental illness"—was used by Freud, and by most of his followers, as a means of classifying certain types of human behavior as falling within the scope of medicine, and hence, by fiat, outside that of ethics. Nevertheless, the stubborn fact remains that, in a sense, much of psychotherapy revolves around nothing other than the elucidation and weighing of goals and values—many of which may be mutually contradictory—and the means whereby they might best be harmonized, realized, or relinquished.

Because the range of human values and of the methods by which they may be attained is so vast, and because many such ends and means are persistently unacknowledged, conflicts among values are the main source of conflicts in human relations. Indeed, to say that human relations at all levels—from mother to child, through husband and wife, to nation and nation—are fraught with stress, strain, and disharmony is, once again, to make the obvious explicit. Yet, what may be obvious may be also poorly understood. This, I think, is the case here. For it seems to me that in our scientific theories of behavior we have failed to accept the simple fact that human relations are inherently fraught with difficulties, and to make them even relatively harmonious requires much patience and hard work. I submit that the idea of mental illness is now being put to work to obscure certain difficulties that at present may be inherent—not that they need to be unmodifiable—in the social intercourse of persons. If this is true, the concept functions as a disguise: Instead of calling attention to conflicting human needs, aspirations, and values, the concept of mental illness provides an amoral and impersonal "thing"—an "illness"—as an explanation for problems in living. We may recall in this connection that not so long ago it was devils and witches that were held responsible for man's problems of living. The belief in mental illness, as something other than man's trouble in getting along with his fellow man, is the proper heir to the belief in demonology and witchcraft. Mental illness thus exists or is "real" in exactly the same sense in which witches existed or were "real."

VI

While I maintain that mental illnesses do not exist, I obviously do not imply or mean that the social and psychological occurrences to which this label is attached also do not exist. Like the personal and social troubles that people had in the Middle Ages, contemporary human problems are real enough. It is the labels we give them that concern me, and, having labeled them, what we do about them. The demonologic concept of problems in living gave rise to therapy along theological lines. Today, a belief in mental illness implies—nay, requires—therapy along medical or psychotherapeutic lines.

I do not here propose to offer a new conception of "psychiatric illness" or a new form of "therapy." My aim is more modest and yet also more ambitious. It is to suggest that the phenomena now called mental illnesses be looked at afresh and more simply, that they be removed from the category of illnesses, and that they be regarded as the expressions of man's struggle with *the problem of how he should live.* This problem is obviously a vast one, its enormity reflecting not only man's inability to cope with his environment, but even more his increasing self-reflectiveness.

By problems in living, then, I refer to that explosive chain reaction that began with man's fall from divine grace by partaking of the fruit of the tree of knowledge. Man's awareness of himself and of the world about him seems to be a steadily expanding one, bringing in its wake an even larger *burden of understanding*.[7] This burden is to be expected and must not be misinterpreted. Our only rational means for easing it is more understanding, and appropriate action based on such understanding. The main alternative lies in acting as though the burden were not what in fact we perceive it to be, and taking refuge in an outmoded theological view of man. In such a view, man does not fashion his life and much of his world about him, but merely lives out his fate in a world created by superior beings. This may logically lead to pleading non-responsibility in the face of seemingly unfathomable problems and insurmountable difficulties. Yet, if man fails to take increasing responsibility for his actions, individually as well as collectively, it seems unlikely that some higher power or being would assume this task and carry this burden for him. Moreover, this seems hardly a propitious time in human history for obscuring the issue of man's responsibility for his actions by hiding it behind the skirt of an all-explaining conception of mental illness.

VII

I have tried to show that the notion of mental illness has outlived whatever usefulness it may have had and that it now functions as a myth. As such, it is a true heir to religious myths in general, and to the belief in witchcraft in particular. It was the function of these belief-systems to act as social tranquilizers, fostering hope that mastery of certain problems may be achieved by means of substitutive, symbolic-magical, operations. The concept of mental illness thus serves mainly to obscure the everyday fact that life for most people is a continuous struggle, not for biological survival, but for a "place in the sun," "peace of mind," or some other meaning or value. Once the needs of preserving the body, and perhaps of the race, are satisfied, man faces the problem of personal significance: What should he do with himself? For what should he live? Sustained adherence to the myth of mental illness allows people to avoid facing this problem, believing that mental health, conceived as the absence of mental illness, automatically insures the making of right and safe choices in the conduct of life. But the facts are all the other way. It is the making of wise choices in life that people regard, retrospectively, as evidence of good mental health!

When I assert that mental illness is a myth, I am not saying that personal unhappiness and socially deviant behavior do not exist; what I am saying is that we categorize them as diseases at our own peril.

The expression "mental illness" is a metaphor that we have come to mistake for a fact. We call people physically ill when their body-functioning violates certain anatomical and physiological norms; similarly, we call people mentally ill when their personal conduct violates certain ethical, political, and social norms. This explains why many historical figures, from Jesus to Castro, and from Job to Hitler, have been diagnosed as suffering from this or that psychiatric malady.

Finally, the myth of mental illness encourages us to believe in its logical corollary: that social intercourse would be harmonious, satisfying, and the secure basis of a good life were it not for the disrupting influences of mental illness, or psychopathology. However, universal human happiness, in this form at least, is but another example of a wishful fantasy. I believe that human happiness, or well-being, is possible—not just for a select few, but on a scale hitherto unimaginable. But this can be achieved only if many men, not just a few, are willing and able to confront frankly, and tackle courageously, their ethical, personal, and social conflicts. This means having the courage and integrity to forego waging battles on false fronts, finding solutions for substitute problems—for instance, fighting the battle of stomach acid and chronic fatigue instead of facing up to a marital conflict.

Our adversaries are not demons, witches, fate, or mental illness. We have no enemy that we can fight, exorcise, or dispel by "cure." What we do have are problems in living—whether these be biologic, economic, political, or socio-psychological. In this essay I was concerned only with problems belonging in the last-mentioned category, and within this group mainly with those pertaining to moral values. The field to which modern psychiatry addresses itself is vast, and I made no effort to encompass it all. My argument was limited to the proposition that mental illness is a myth, whose function it is to disguise and thus render more palatable the bitter pill of moral conflicts in human relations.

NOTES

1 See Szasz, T. S.: *Pain and Pleasure: A Study of Bodily Feelings* (New York: Basic Books, 1957), especially pp. 70–81; "The problem of psychiatric nosology." *Amer. J. Psychiatry*, 114:405–13 (Nov.), 1957.

2 See Szasz, T. S.: *The Ethics of Psychoanalysis: The Theory and Method of Autonomous Psychotherapy* (New York: Basic Books, 1965).

3 See Szasz, T. S.: *Law, Liberty, and Psychiatry: An Inquiry into the Social Uses of Mental Health Practices* (New York: Macmillan, 1963).

4 Peters, R. S.: *The Concept of Motivation* (London: Routledge & Kegan Paul, 1958), especially pp. 12–15.

5 Hollingshead, A. B., and Redlich, F. C.: *Social Class and Mental Illness* (New York: Wiley, 1958).

6 Quoted in Jones, E.: *The Life and Work of Sigmund Freud* (New York: Basic Books, 1957), Vol. III, p. 247.

7 In this connection, see Langer, S. K.: *Philosophy in a New Key* [1942] (New York: Mentor Books, 1953), especially Chaps. 5 and 10.

Some Myths about "Mental Illness"

Michael S. Moore

Michael S. Moore is Robert Kingsley Professor of Law at the University of Southern California. He is the author of *Law and Psychiatry: Rethinking the Relationship* (1984), and his published articles include "Responsibility and the Unconscious" and "Semantics of Judging."

Reprinted with permission of the publisher (Universitetsforlaget: Oslo, Norway) from *Inquiry*, vol. 18, no. 3 (Autumn 1975), pp. 233–265.

Moore, committed to the view that mental illness is not a myth, sets out to identify and attack various versions of the myth argument. First of all, he rejects the argument that since there is no referent of the phrase "mental illness," there is no such thing as mental illness. Secondly, he rejects the "empirical version" of the myth argument, the contention that those called "mentally ill" are really as rational as everyone else. Finally, he rejects the argument that mental illness is a myth simply because the language of "mental illness" can be and is used (abused) for the purpose of condemning behavior thought to be undesirable.

I INTRODUCTION

The concept of mental illness has had a long and interesting history in man's thoughts about himself, his nature, and his responsibility. It stands at one junction of law, morals, and medicine, with the result that lawyers, psychiatrists, and philosophers have long shared a concern for the nature of the concept. This shared concern has not given rise to any consensus, however, and the debates, particularly between lawyers and psychiatrists, have often been acrimonious and unfruitful. Since the advent of 'radical psychiatry,' the theoretical justification of which is to be found notably in the works of Thomas Szasz, the battle lines have been to some extent redrawn across professional boundaries, but the result has not been added clarity about the nature of the concept of mental disease or its moral and legal relevance.

Indeed, quite the reverse. Increasingly answers to essentially ethical and political questions about psychiatric practices or legal doctrines with regard to the mentally ill are being given by trundling out the contemporary shibboleth that mental illness is a myth, rather than in terms of the ethical and political arguments necessary for such answers. There is a disturbing tendency to regard complicated legal issues, notably the proper place of mental illness in various legal tests (of insanity in criminal trials, of incompetency to perform various legal acts or to stand trial, the tests for civil commitments), as solved by the new truth that mental illness is but a myth anyway. Equally disturbing is the apparent belief that problems of social policy and social justice, such as what in fact society should do with dangerous persons who have not committed any criminal acts, can be satisfactorily resolved if legislatures will but recognize mental illness for the sham that it is.

If mental illness were a myth, acceptance of such a truth would provide straightforward answers to such

legal, ethical, and political questions. One would not have to muddle along in the grubby details of comparing awful prisons with almost as awful hospitals for the criminally insane. One would not have to grapple with difficult policy issues such as the rationale for punishment generally and its relation to those found not guilty by reasons of insanity. For it would be instantly clear that those we call 'mentally ill' should be punished just like anyone else if they commit a criminal act; that they should have all the rights of an accused criminal if society should seek to deprive them of their liberty no matter how the proceeding or the place of confinement might be named; that legal tests should abolish the phrase; and, easiest of all, that psychiatrists should mind their own business and leave the law to the lawyers.

The problem is that mental illness is not a myth. It is not some palpable falsehood propagated amongst the populace by power-mad psychiatrists, but a cruel and bitter reality that has been with the human race since antiquity. This is such an obvious truism that to have stated it twenty years ago would have been an embarrassment. Since the advent of radical psychiatry and its legal entourage, however, such truths need restatement. Even more, they need restatement in a form specifically addressed to the various senses in which mental illness has been thought to be a myth....

II THE MYTHOLOGY OF RADICAL PSYCHIATRY

(A) The Myth as a Question of Ontological Status: There Is No Such Thing as Mental Illness because There Is No Referent of the Phrase

Mental illness is a myth because, stated popularly, 'there is neither such a thing as "insanity" nor such a thing as "mental disease." These terms do not identify entities having separate existence.'[1]

Less popularly:

> It is a term without ostensive referent [*sic*] and lacking any, it cannot even be said to have outlived its usefulness, because there is no reason to think that it ever had any.[2]

Szasz and his psychiatric and legal followers are suspicious of mental illness as an entity or thing; when looking into their ontology they see no such thing. Three points require discussion here:

(1) If the argument is that entity-thinking *as such* is to be regarded with suspicion, as Szasz at times suggests, then the critique is radical indeed. As Quine has noted, 'we talk so inveterately of objects that to say we do so seems almost to say nothing at all; for how else is there to talk?'[3] 'Thing-theory' is implicit throughout our ordinary and scientific speech, and it is simply wrong to regard it as some primitive form of speech that is replaced with a more sophisticated mode of talk with the maturity of a science. Thus, Szasz's statement that 'Entity thinking has always preceded process-thinking'[4] is not an accurate characterization of the development of modern science. In fact, higher order theoretical statements characteristic of advancing science *increase* the number of entities we admit into our ontology, not decrease it. Forces, fields, and electrons are obvious examples.

(2) If the argument is that entity thinking is scientifically legitimate, but only about those entities referred to by terms capable of ostensive reference, such as 'Nixon,' or 'St. Elizabeth's Hospital,' the radical psychiatrists have a radically impoverished ontology—a nominalist ontology that would not admit the thinghood of abstract entities such as the number 2, squareness, shape, zoological species, or, more to the point perhaps, psychological states. Such a restricted ontology is characteristic neither of science nor of common understanding.

Indeed, in such a restrictive ontological system physical illnesses would not exist either. For the names of physical illnesses do not refer to concrete entities: 'Diseases are not things in the same sense as rocks, or trees, or rivers. Diseases...are not material.'[5] Although diseases might be *caused* by the presence in the body of some such entity (as a cold may be caused by a virus), and although they might be associated with *symptoms* that are concrete entities (e.g. the fluid present in the sinuses), a physical illness is not (identical with) either its causes or its symptoms. The only thing one can fix as the referent of the names of various physical illnesses are states the ill are in, abstract entities incapable of being pointed at in some ostensive definition.

(3) In any case, most of the things people have wanted to say about mental illness can be said without making ontological commitments to any entity, concrete or abstract, referred to by the phrase, and thus any criticism of its use based on its lack of a referent, ostensive or otherwise, is misconceived. In his essay on 'Sense and Reference' Frege made famous the distinction between the sense of a term and its reference.[6] The important corollary for our purpose is that words may be used significantly (make good sense) and yet *not refer*. As Quine has elaborated: 'Being a name of something is a much more special feature than being meaningful.' Even 'a singular term need not name to be significant.'[7]

This is particularly evident in our use of predicates. We can say 'some dogs are white' or 'some houses are red,' without making ontological commitments to (without presupposing there are such things as) whiteness or redness. Similarly, we can say that 'some persons are mentally ill' without making ontological commitments to any *thing* referred to by 'illness.' More colloquially: denial of the existence of anything called 'mental illness' hardly entails a denial of the existence of *persons* who are mentally ill.

In addition to describing people as being mentally ill, we also often wish to explain their behavior as being due to their mental illness. While such statements as 'He did it because of his mental illness' appear to require an entity referred to by the phrase 'mental illness,' in fact such explanations mean nothing more than is conveyed by: 'He did it because he is mentally ill'—another use of the predicate, 'is mentally ill' that does not require a reference to be significant.

To the extent that common and psychiatric discourse about mental illness can be paraphrased so as to avoid the hypostasis of an entity named by the phrase, then any criticism that complains that there is no such thing as mental illness is beside the point; for orthodox psychiatry and common understanding can happily agree, but still use the phrase to make significant (albeit non-referring) statements. We often make use of the names of states, attributes, properties, and traits as if they named some things in our ontology, for economy of speech is often gained by so doing.[8]

To be sure, if someone (such as Szasz) makes an issue of the ontological commitments involved in our uses of 'redness,' or 'illness,' 'the burden is of course on us to paraphrase or retract.'[9] But if we can paraphrase the usage into the non-committing use of 'ill,' then the phraseology is a harmless but convenient mode of speaking against which the 'ontological discovery' of radical psychiatry is irrelevant.

For my own part I think this detour into ontology is a red herring. The lack of any thing one can point to as the referent of the phrase 'mental illness' does not do orthodox psychiatry the damage Szasz *et al.* suppose; if mental illness is a myth in this sense, it is in the good company of many other words and phrases useful in science and everyday life which have either no reference or a reference only to abstract entities. That this herring is constantly being dragged across our path is doubtless due to the immense popular appeal of the denial-of-existence idiom in the hands of a skillful polemicist. It makes the study of mental illness *sound* about as useful as the study of unicorns.[10]

Once one perceives that ontological status is not really at issue here, then other types of arguments must be marshaled in favor of eliminating 'mental illness' from our vocabulary.

(B) The Myth as an Empirical Discovery: No One is in Fact Mentally Ill

Often mental illness is said to be a myth, not just in the sense that it doesn't exist, but also in the sense that no one is in fact mentally ill. The claim, in other words, denies not just that 'mental illness' is a name of some thing, but that 'mentally ill' is ever truly predicable of a person. The claim is that no one is really mentally ill.

This claim that mental illness is a myth is put forward as an empirical discovery: all of those people that have been thought to be mentally ill (i.e. irrational) are in fact just as rational as you and I. Szasz makes this claim when he argues that 'insane behavior no less than sane, is goal-directed and motivated . . . ,' and concludes from this that we should regard 'the behavior of the madman as perfectly rational from the point of view of the actor.'[11] Braginsky, Braginsky, and Ring purport to have made the same 'discovery' regarding schizophrenics:

the residents who remain in 'mental hospitals' are behaving in a perfectly rational manner to achieve

a personally satisfying way of life—often the most satisfying of which they are capable . . . in a certain sense an individual *chooses* his career as a mental patient; it is not thrust upon him as a consequence of his somehow becoming 'mentally ill.' But in just what sense does the individual 'choose' his career? In our view, having and maintaining the status of a mental patient is the outcome of *purposive* behavior. Furthermore, given the life circumstances of most of the persons who become and remain residents of mental hospitals, their doing so evinces a realistic appraisal of their available alternatives; it is, in short, a *rational* choice.[12]

The central thrust of this form of the argument is not to claim that 'mental illness' or 'mentally ill' are meaningless—their meaning is assumed to be closely connected with that of 'irrational'—but to dispute as a factual matter that there are persons who fit the agreed-upon definition of mental illness (irrationality). In fact, however, what has been done here is not to present a discovery of new facts, overlooked by orthodox psychiatrists because of their own self-interest or whatever, but rather to stretch our concepts of 'rationality' and 'purposive behavior' to accommodate within their criteria facts well known to orthodox, as well as to radical, psychiatrists. The facts—the behavior of patients—are often undisputed. What is disputed is the precise nature of the criterion to be applied in judging the behavior as rational or not.

As the above quotations from Szasz and Braginsky *et al.* make clear, the notion of rationality relevant here is linked to the actor's having reasons (purposes, motives) for his actions. A more precise account of the relationship between an agent's being thought to be rational and his acting for reasons may perhaps best be brought out by the following schema of reason-giving explanations. When we explain an action by giving the actor's motive, the following premises are involved:

1 Agent X wants result R to obtain.
2 X believes that in situation S action A will cause R to obtain.
3 X believes that he is in situation S.
4 If X believes that he is in situation S and believes that in S action A will cause R to obtain, and if X wants R to obtain, then, *ceteris paribus*, X will do A.
5 *Ceteris paribus.*

With these premises, it follows that X will do A.

In ordinary English, in order to make out a motivational explanation we need to know: what the agent wanted and what he believed about the situation and about his abilities to achieve through action what he wanted. In addition, we need to know that he is a rational creature in the fundamental sense of 'rational' defined by the fourth premise, that is, one who, other things being equal, will act so as to further his desires in light of his beliefs; and we need to know that other things are in fact equal, namely, that the agent does not have desires and beliefs that conflict with the desires and beliefs on which he is about to act.

The actions of the mentally ill may be nonrational or irrational in any of five corresponding senses: *R* may be an unintelligible thing to want, such as soaking one's elbow in the mud for its own sake; the belief that *A* will lead to *R* may be an irrational belief (e.g. a belief that saying 'storks' instead of 'stocks' will make one a mother); the belief that one is in situation *S* may also be irrational (e.g. a belief that one is being persecuted by spirits); there may be no set of beliefs and desires, no matter how bizarre, by virtue of which one can make out the action as the rational thing to do; or the beliefs and desires of the particular practical syllogism may be inconsistent with other standing beliefs and desires.

The rationality of an *agent* is a function of the rationality of his actions over time. The greater amount of irrational behavior we observe in an individual in any of these five senses, the less rational we will judge him as an agent to be.

By and large the empirical version of the myth argument is only intended to show that the behavior of the mentally ill is rational in the fundamental sense defined by the fourth premise above, i.e. there is *some* set of beliefs and desires (no matter how bizarre) furthered by the act in question. The crunch for even this limited attempt at making out the behavior of the mentally ill as rational, comes in making more precise the nature of the beliefs and desires of mental patients in terms of which their actions are to be so adjudged. More specifically, the fudge occurs with the use of *unconscious* beliefs and desires to fill in where we all know that mental patients did not consciously guide their actions to achieve such goals in light of such beliefs. Braginsky, Braginsky, and Ring are explicit about this:

> It is obvious that rational goal-directed behavior does not guarantee that the individual appreciates what he is up to.[13]

Szasz's glossing over of this distinction is particularly transparent:

> In describing this contrast between lying and erring, I have deliberately avoided the concept of consciousness. It seems to me that when the adjectives 'consciously' and 'unconsciously' are used as explanations, they complicate and obscure the problem. The traditional psychoanalytic idea that so-called conscious imitation of illness is 'malingering' and hence 'not illness,' whereas its allegedly unconscious simulation is itself 'illness' ('hysteria'), creates more problems than it solves. It would seem more useful to *distinguish between goal-directed and rule-following behavior on the one hand, and indifferent mistakes on the other*...In brief, *it is more accurate to regard hysteria as a lie than as a mistake*. People caught in a lie usually maintain that they were merely mistaken. The difference between mistakes and lies, when discovered, is chiefly pragmatic. From a purely cognitive point of view, both are simply falsehoods.[14]

The fudge occurs in the shift from our judgments of rationality being based on the agent's conscious beliefs and objectives, to a notion of rationality by virtue of which we adjudge an action at least minimally rational if we can posit any set of beliefs or objectives with which we can explain the action. The problem is that it is notoriously easy to posit beliefs and desires to explain any finite sequence of the behavior of anything. Simply pick a consequence of the behavior and label it the objective, pick a set of beliefs by virtue of which it would appear likely that such a consequence would indeed ensue as a result of the behavior, and one is then in a position to adjudge the behavior as rational, relative to that objective and that set of beliefs. The shedding of leaves by a tree, the falling of stones, the pumping of blood by the heart, and the most chaotic word salad of a schizophrenic, are all 'rational' activities judged by such a standard. The 'action' of a tree in shedding its leaves is rational if we suppose that it desires to survive the coming winter, and believes that the only way to do this is to lower its sap level thereby killing off its leaves. Similarly for stones, hearts, and schizophrenics.

The reason why such explanations are so easy to manufacture is that without the requirement that an agent be conscious of the beliefs and the desires by which we (and he) judge his action as rational, there is no means of fixing the nature of such beliefs or wants independently of the behavior to be explained and adjudged.[15] Behavior is by itself inherently ambiguous as a criterion for such matters. If we know by some independent means that an agent believes that action A will lead to result R, and he does A, we have good grounds for attributing to him a desire for R; if we know that he desires R, and does A, we have equally good grounds for supposing that he believes that A will lead to R. But if we know neither his beliefs nor his desires, but only that he does A and that A does result in R being the case, we have no means of singling out R as his motive, for any other consequence of A would do as well. 'There is nothing in a pure behaviorist theory to prevent us from regarding each piece of behavior as a desire for whatever happens next.'[16]

Thus Szasz can ignore the conscious/unconscious distinction only at the price of significance. What he fails to realize is that any behavior can be seen as rational (or as in accordance with rules of a game, or as furthering certain goals—Szasz's substitute criteria for consciousness), if one allows oneself the freedom to *invent* the beliefs and desires in terms of which the behavior is to be so viewed.[17]

On occasion the empirical version of the myth claim is put forward without any extensive reliance on some supposed unconscious beliefs or desires of the mentally ill. R. D. Laing in particular explicitly disavows use of unconscious beliefs or desires in reaching his well known conclusion that '*without exception* the experience and behavior that gets labelled schizophrenic is *a special strategy that a person invents in order to live in an unlivable situation.*'[18] Nonetheless such studies do not show schizophrenics to be as rational as everyone else, for the conscious beliefs such patients admittedly do have are themselves irrational beliefs; and actions that are predicated on irrational beliefs, and actors who hold them, are, in common understanding, irrational.

This is quite clear with regard to many of Laing's reported patients. The woman who avoids crowds may be rational in so doing, *given* her belief that 'when she was in a crowd she felt the ground would open up under her feet.' Similarly, many of the peculiar actions of one who believes that 'she had an atom bomb inside her'[19] may be rational, *given* such a belief. But the beliefs themselves are irrational, with the result that neither the agent nor the action they explain can be said to be rational. To be sure, Laing's studies of the 'social intelligibility' of schizophrenic symptoms do not end with the discovery of such obvious beliefs; Laing often attempts to go further and explain how

such beliefs could be formed by an individual in the patient's situation. Yet the explanation Laing typically gives—the patient 'adopts' the symptom as the only response to an intolerable situation—involves reference to further beliefs that are also irrational.

A convenient example is the case of 'Joan,' a catatonic who was not one of Laing's patients but whose case Laing believed to afford 'striking confirmation' of his views regarding schizophrenia. Joan's own subsequent avowals were used by Laing in attributing to her catatonic withdrawal a rational basis. She recalled that when she was catatonic, she 'tried to be dead and grey and motionless.' She thought that her mother 'would like that: 'She could carry me around like a doll.' She also felt that she 'had to die to keep from dying. I know that sounds crazy but one time a boy hurt my feelings very much and I wanted to jump in front of a subway. Instead I went a little catatonic so I wouldn't feel anything.'

Laing finds in such statements the two typical motives for catatonic withdrawal. First, 'there is the primary guilt of having no right to life…and hence of being entitled at most only to a dead life.' Since Joan's parents had wanted a boy, and since 'she could not be anything other than what her parents wanted her to be,' she sought to be 'nothing,' i.e. a passive catatonic. Secondly, Joan's withdrawal was viewed by Laing as a defensive mechanism to avoid the loss of identity (Joan's metaphorical 'dying') with which she was threatened by any normal relationship with others:

> One no longer fears being crushed, engulfed, overwhelmed by realness and aliveness…since one is already dead [by the catatonic withdrawal]. Being dead, one cannot die, and one cannot kill. The anxieties attendant on the schizophrenic's phantastic omnipotence are undercut by living in a condition of phantastic impotence.[20]

None of this would convince us that Joan or others like her were rational in effecting catatonic withdrawal (even if we were convinced that at least in her case the withdrawal was an *action* she performed for reasons at all). Her action (or non-action) is based on a series of beliefs that are irrational, including her belief in a disembodied self, a belief in her parents' complete determination of her worth, and a belief in her own omnipotence and impotence.

It is sometimes thought that the rationality of beliefs is not a matter that can be objectively judged and that calling them 'irrational' is simply a pejorative way of saying that they are false. The conclusion in the present context would be that people like Joan are thus as rational as the rest of us, only mistaken about certain facts. While the topic of rational belief is a difficult one, prima facie the most obvious way to differentiate beliefs that are irrational from those that are merely false is by looking at the influence relevant evidence would have on the holder of the belief. It is characteristic of irrational beliefs that their holder maintains them despite countervailing evidence, or despite inconsistencies with other beliefs he has. There is a 'fixed' or 'frozen' nature about such beliefs, in the sense that they are not corrigible by relevant evidence. Irrational beliefs are held with a strength (relative to other beliefs the actor has) disproportionate to the evidence known to the actor. Thus the man 'who believes very strongly that his brother is trying to poison him (in spite of appearances) and who believes, rather weakly by comparison, that Boston is north of New York, is likely to be flying in the face of the evidence and the claims that the evidence renders likely'[21]—he is likely, in other words, to be irrational in his belief of his imminent poisoning.

The empirical version of the myth argument fails because it is, empirically, false. By our shared concept of what it is to be rational, the mentally ill are not as rational as the rest of the population. Only by muddling the concept of rationality have the radical psychiatrists appeared to call into question this obvious truth. Only by attributing unconscious beliefs and desires to the mentally ill for which there is no evidence, or only by referring to beliefs that are themselves irrational, can motives be found for the peculiar behavior symptomatic of mental illness. Neither of these moves satisfies what we usually mean by 'rational' as applied to actions and agents. One may, of course, like Humpty Dumpty, choose to make a word like 'rationality' mean what he pleases, but surely it is unhelpful when one does so to then present the manufactured match between the facts and the new criteria for the word as a discovery of new facts, previously overlooked because of the willful blindness of self-interested psychiatrists or whatever. To do so is to create one's own myths....

(C) The Myth as an Evaluation Masquerading as an Explanation: The Abuse of the Normative Connotations of 'Mental Illness' by Orthodox Psychiatry

Sensitivity to the normative connotations of the concepts of 'mental health' and 'mental illness' is, I suspect, rather widespread. When one of the psychiatrists at the annual meeting of the American Psychiatric Association some years ago loudly diagnosed a women's libber who was disrupting the meeting as a 'stupid, paranoid bitch,' something other than a value-neutral explanation of her behavior was intended. The same suspicions are engendered when psychiatrists label homosexuals as mentally ill, or when 'mental health' is used as a synonym for whatever way of life is adjudged good. The radical psychiatrists build on these kinds of examples to argue that 'mental illness' and the predicate 'mentally ill' are used *only* to make evaluations of others' behavior, and that these terms are particularly effective as evaluations because they are paraded as value-neutral, scientific explanations: 'while allegedly describing conduct, psychiatrists often prescribe it.'[22]

> The masquerading of promotive assertions in the guise of indicative sentences is of great practical significance in psychiatry. Statements concerning 'psychosis' or 'insanity'...almost always revolve around unclarified equations of these two linguistic forms. For example, the statement 'John Doe is psychotic' is ostensibly indicative and informative. Usually, however, it is promotive rather than informative...[23]

It may seem curious to claim that 'mental illness' is used like 'bad' or 'wrong' or 'ug'—that is, used to pass moral evaluations—when by our shared notions for moral responsibility we use the same phrase to *excuse* those who are mentally ill. To attribute a harmful action to the actor's mental illness, then, cannot always be exactly the same as attributing it, say, to his 'murderous personality.' What Szasz *sometimes* has in mind in saying that 'mental illness' is used prescriptively or promotively is not that moral judgments are made with such use; rather, psychiatric usage of the phrase is often promotive, etc. in the quite different sense that the capability of being morally responsible is denied. 'Mental illness' for Szasz is evaluative often only in the sense that it denies the 'personhood' of those to whom it is applied:

> What better way is there...for degrading the culprit than to declare him incapable of knowing what he is doing.... This is the general formula for the dehumanization and degradation of all those persons

whose conduct psychiatrists now deem to be 'caused' by mental illness.[24]

Although needlessly stated in inflammatory terms (as if orthodox psychiatry were universally motivated by a desire to degrade the mentally ill), Szasz here suggests a very important feature of mental illness. 'Insanity' and 'mental illness' mean, and historically have meant, 'irrational'; to be insane, or to be mentally ill, is to fail to act rationally often enough to have the same assumption of rationality made about one as is made of most of humanity. And without that assumption being made, one cannot be fully regarded as a person, for our concept of what it is to be a person is centered on the notions of rationality introduced earlier. Unless we can perceive another being as acting for intelligible ends in light of rational beliefs, we cannot understand that being in the same fundamental way that we understand each other's actions in daily life. Such beings lack an essential attribute of our humanity.[25] It is thus easy to appreciate that historically the insane have been likened to young children, the intoxicated, and wild beasts.[26] For lacking rationality, the mentally ill are, as Bleuler said of his schizophrenic patients, stranger to us than the birds in our gardens.

Such statements are of course offensive to the ears of those concerned about the moral claims and legal rights of mental patients. Yet unless radical psychiatry and its lawyerly following can show, as I have argued earlier in this paper it has not, that those we label mentally ill are just as rational as everyone else, part of our fundamental explanatory scheme and part of our fundamental notion of personhood are not applicable to the mentally ill. This includes notions about their lack of responsibility and inability to choose and act upon their own conception of their good. If one believes (*contra* Szasz *et al.*) that there are in fact people who do not act rationally often enough for us to make the same assumption of rationality for them as we do for most of our fellows, then this 'evaluative' feature of the phrase 'mental illness' is accurate enough in its reflection of how the mentally ill fit into our fundamental conceptual scheme.

Szasz at other times seems to have in mind a second kind of normative use which we do on occasion make of 'mentally ill,' in everyday expressions such as 'That was an insane thing to do' or 'That's crazy!' In such usages we do seem to be expressing disapproval of the agent's ends and his actions, recommending that one ought not to do such things or seek such ends, etc. Thus Szasz is also right to note that at times 'mentally ill' or 'insane' can be used as terms of general disapproval:

> The difference between saying 'He is wrong' and 'He is mentally ill' is not factual but psychological.[27]

Other examples with which we began this section were the diagnosis of the women's libber and the use of 'mental health' by some psychoanalysts, e.g. Erich Fromm, as if it were synonymous with 'good.'

To the extent that orthodox psychiatry uses these words in this way it is plainly abusing them. The phrase 'mental illness' and its companions are so abused not by being applied to those who are in fact irrational, but by being applied to persons whose actions are often rational but of whose ends prevailing psychiatric opinion does not approve. An action that is fully rational in each of the senses examined earlier cannot, without ignoring the meaning of the words, be said to be insane or due to mental illness, no matter how deviant may be the end pursued. The fact that homosexuals have a preference for a sexual relationship not shared by most of the populace is hardly a ground (as the APA with strong dissent implicitly recognized recently in its deletion of homosexuality as an illness) for labeling that preference irrational (ill). Homosexuals may (sometimes, often, or always) be mentally ill, if their capacity for rational action is significantly diminished below our expectations; such irrationality is hardly shown, however, by their unpopular sexual desires alone if those ends are pursued on the basis of rational and consistent beliefs, without conflict with other strong desires, and by relatively efficient means.

The mistake of radical psychiatry is to assume that mental illness is a myth just because the phrase can be so abused. The mistake is to assume that because words such as 'murder,' 'greediness,' 'mental illness,' or even 'good' can be used to express attitudes, kindle emotions, pass evaluations and the like, they cannot also be used at the same time as a legitimate form of explanation and/or description, or at different times only as a description/explanation. Those moral philosophers who have raised another logical gulf between evaluative and descriptive statements insufficiently stress the fact that words used in evaluations can also be used to express descriptions. Merely because a woman may call the doctor who through surgical error kills her husband a murderer, despite the fact that one of the main criteria for that term's proper use is not met (viz. *intentional* killing), is not sufficient to show that the term 'murderer' cannot have legitimate descriptive and explanatory uses.

To the extent that one views mental illness as a myth solely because of its evaluative connotations, one makes the same mistake. I don't think Szasz himself can be accused of this error, because he conjoins this point with one of the preceding [two] points; mental illness is a myth because it has no descriptive meaning [cf. (A) and (B) above] *and* because it can be and is sometimes used to pass moral judgment on those so labeled. If, however, one rejects the first part of this thesis, the second is an insufficient basis on which to label mental illness a myth. 'Mental illness' is perhaps a dangerous term because its normative connotations make possible the kind of abuse mentioned earlier; but then the same can be said of many of the terms with which we describe and explain human action, such as 'greedy,' 'stupid,' 'murder,' 'manipulative,' etc....

NOTES

1 *Blocker v. United States*, 229 F.2nd 853, 859 (D.C. Cir. 1961) (Concurring opinion of Warren Burger, present Chief Justice of the United States Supreme Court, quoting Philip Roche).

2 B. M. Braginsky, O. D. Braginsky and K. Ring, *Methods of Madness: The Mental Hospital as Last Resort*, Holt, Rinehart & Winston, New York 1969, p. 164 (the authors are here speaking of schizophrenia).

3 W. V. Quine, 'Speaking of Objects,' in *Ontological Relativity and Other Essays*, Columbia University Press, New York 1969, p. 1.

4 T. Szasz, *The Myth of Mental Illness*, Harper & Row, New York 1961, p. 1.

5 L. S. King, 'What is Disease?' *Philosophy of Science*, Vol. 21 (1954), p. 199. King recognizes that 'the problem... is the ontological status of a relationship,' *not* the existence of concrete objects such as witches. Thus Szasz's scornful, 'Mental illness thus exists or is "real" in exactly the same sense in which witches existed or were "real"' (*Ideology and Insanity. Essays on the Psychiatric Dehumanization*

of Man, Doubleday, New York 1970, p. 21), completely misses the only ontological point at issue.

6 G. Frege, 'Über Sinn und Bedeutung,' *Zeitschrift für Philosophie und Philosophische Kritik*, Vol. 100 (1892), trans. and reprinted in H. Feigl and W. Sellars (Eds.), *Readings in Philosophical Analysis*, New York 1949, and in P. T. Geach and M. Black (Eds.), *The Philosophical Writings of Gottlob Frege*, Basil Blackwell, Oxford 1960.

7 W. V. Quine, 'On What There Is,' in *From a Logical Point of View*, Harvard University Press, Cambridge, Mass. 1953, pp. 9 and 11.

8 See the examples by Quine in his 'Speaking of Objects,' in *Ontological Relativity and Other Essays*, op. cit., pp. 14–15; see also his *Philosophy of Logic*, Prentice-Hall, Englewood Cliffs, N.J. 1970, pp. 68–69.

9 Quine, 'Existence and Quantification,' in *Ontological Relativity and Other Essays*, op. cit., p. 100. Quine goes on to observe that 'many of our casual remarks in the "there are" form would want dusting up when our thoughts turn seriously ontological.'

10 Szasz expressly uses the argument this way; see pp. 1–2 of *The Myth of Mental Illness*, where he likens psychiatry to alchemy and astrology:

> Psychiatry is said to be a medical specialty concerned with the study and treatment of mental illness. Similarly, astrology was the study of the influence of planetary movements and positions on human behavior and destiny. These are typical instances of defining a science by specifying the subject matter of study. These definitions completely disregard method and are based instead on false substantives.... But suppose, for a moment, that there is no such thing as mental illness and health. Suppose, further, that these words refer to nothing more substantial or real than the astrological conception of planetary influences on human conduct. What then?

11 *The Manufacture of Madness*, Harper & Row, New York 1970, p. 123.

12 *Methods of Madness: The Mental Hospital as Last Resort*, op. cit., p. 171 (emphasis in original).

13 Ibid., p. 171.

14 *The Myth of Mental Illness*, pp. 142–43 (emphasis in original). Alan Stone has some fun exposing other aspects of the illogic of this passage in 'Psy-

chiatry Kills: A Critical Evaluation of Dr. Thomas Szasz,' *Journal of Psychiatry and Law*, Vol. 1 (1973), pp. 23–37.

15 This does not mean that good sense cannot be made of the idea of unconscious beliefs, desires, motives, etc. Such sense can be made of these ideas if, as in psychoanalytic therapy, the agent's first-person statements of his *memory* of his motives, etc. are accorded the same authority as are his normal, first-person, present tense reports of them. See Stuart Hampshire, 'Disposition and Memory,' *International Journal of Psychoanalysis*, Vol. 43 (1962), pp. 59–68; and I. Dilman, 'Is the Unconscious a Theoretical Construct?' *Monist*, Vol. 56 (1972), pp. 313–42. Yet Szasz abandons even this limitation in attempting to find strategies or goals pursued by hysterics. In addition, it is worth pointing out that such unconscious motive explanations as do satisfy this limitation do not typically render the behavior which they explain fully rational. See P. Alexander, 'Rational Behaviour and Psychoanalytic Explanation,' *Mind*, Vol. LXXI (1962), pp. 326–41; T. Mischel, 'Concerning Rational Behaviour and Psychoanalytic Explanation,' *Mind*, Vol. LXXIV (1965), pp. 71–78; H. Mullane, 'Psychoanalytic Explanation and Rationality,' *Journal of Philosophy*, Vol. 68 (1971), pp. 413–26.

16 A. Kenny, *Action, Emotion, and Will*, Routledge & Kegan Paul, London 1963, p. 108. A more complete discussion of the 'epistemic interdependence of belief attributions and goal attributions' will be found in Carl Hempel's 'Rational Action,' *Proceedings and Addresses of the American Philosophical Association*, Vol. 35 (1962), reprinted in Care and Landesman, *Readings in the Theory of Action*, Indiana University Press, Bloomington 1968.

17 In the text I have avoided dealing directly with Szasz's 'etiotic, rule-following, game-playing' theory of human behavior. Szasz's extension of these notions to cover all actions of the mentally ill is no more legitimate than his extension of 'rationality,' and indeed, fails for the same reason. See A. R. Louch, *Explanation and Human Action*, University of California Press, Berkeley 1969, Ch. 9.

18 R. D. Laing, *The Politics of Experience*, Ballantine Books, New York 1967, pp. 114–15 (emphasis in original). Laing here relies on his own and Esterson's *Sanity, Madness and the Family*, Penguin Books, Baltimore 1970, where on p. 26 he disavows any use of unconscious motives or beliefs to make out his thesis.

19 *Sanity, Madness and the Family*, op. cit., pp. 75, 131.

20 R. D. Laing, *The Divided Self*, Penguin Books, Baltimore 1965, Ch. 10. The case was originally reported in M. Hayward and J. E. Taylor, 'A Schizophrenic Patient Describes the Action of Intensive Psychotherapy,' *Psychiatric Quarterly*, Vol. 30 (1956), pp. 211–48.

21 R. J. Ackermann, *Belief and Knowledge*, Doubleday, New York 1972, p. 33. See generally Ch. 3, 'Rational Belief.'

22 Szasz, *Law, Liberty, and Psychiatry*, Collier Books ed., the Macmillan Co., New York 1968, p. 18.

23 *The Myth of Mental Illness*, op. cit., p. 131.

24 *The Manufacture of Madness*, pp. 122–23. See also *Ideology and Insanity*, op. cit., p. 204: 'Most psychiatric diagnoses may be used, and are used, as invectives: their aim is to degrade—and, hence, socially constrain—the person diagnosed.' Laing makes the same objection in numerous places in his work. E.g. *The Politics of Experience*, op. cit., pp. 121–22.

25 The capability for rational action in the sense of motivated action is an essential condition for our regarding another as a person. See D. Dennett, 'Mechanism and Responsibility,' in T. Honderich (Ed.), *Essays on Freedom of Action*, Routledge & Kegan Paul, London 1973.

26 For a history of the concept in legal contexts that emphasizes these features, see A. Platt and B. Diamond, 'The Origin and the Development of the "Wild Beast" Concept of Mental Illness and Its Relation to Theories of Criminal Responsibility,' *Journal of the History of the Behavioral Sciences*, Vol. 1 (1965), p. 355.

27 *Law, Liberty, and Psychiatry*, op. cit., p. 205. See also ibid., p. 19: 'The new label "mental illness" (and its variants) became only a substitute for the abandoned words of denigration.'

ANNOTATED BIBLIOGRAPHY: CHAPTER 5

Boorse, Christopher: "On the Distinction between Disease and Illness," *Philosophy and Public Affairs* 5 (Fall 1975), pp. 49–68. Boorse contends that the concepts of health and disease are not inherently value-laden. He distinguishes health as a theoretical notion (whose opposite is disease) from health as a practical notion (whose opposite is illness). In his view, an organism is healthy in the theoretical sense inasmuch as its mode of functioning conforms to the natural design of its species. However, he argues, in contrast to ascriptions of disease (and health in the theoretical sense), ascriptions of illness (and health in the practical sense) are inherently value-laden.

————: "What a Theory of Mental Health Should Be," *Journal for the Theory of Social Behavior* 6 (April 1976), pp. 61–84. Insisting on the need to develop a theory of mental health predicated upon an analogy between mental health and physical health, Boorse argues that the practice of clinical psychology and psychiatry may rightly be founded on the model of health and disease.

Caplan, Arthur L., H. Tristram Engelhardt, Jr., and James J. McCartney, eds.: *Concepts of Health and Disease: Interdisciplinary Perspectives* (Reading, Mass.: Addison-Wesley, 1981). This volume provides an extensive collection of material on the concepts of health and disease. Especially noteworthy are the selections included in Part Six, under the heading of "New Directions."

"Changing Social and Psychological Concepts of Mental Illness," *Journal of Contemporary Issues* 1 (August 1973), pp. 31–56. This excellent review article examines a number of efforts to reevaluate both the nature of mental illness and the practice of psychiatry. A long and useful bibliography is also provided.

Culver, Charles M., and Bernard Gert: *Philosophy in Medicine* (New York: Oxford, 1982). In Chapter 4 of this book, Culver and Gert present a conceptual analysis of "malady" (understood as a general category including disease, illness, injury, etc.). They maintain that "objective definitional criteria do exist." In Chapter 5, the authors consider the nature of mental maladies.

Engelhardt, H. Tristram, Jr.: "The Disease of Masturbation: Values and the Concept of Disease," *Bulletin of the History of Medicine* 48 (Summer 1974), pp. 234–248. Engelhardt presents an historical account of the way in which the putative moral offense of masturbation was transformed into a disease with both physical and psychological dimensions. In his view, the disease of masturbation is an "eloquent example of the value-laden nature" of medicine.

————: "Health and Disease: Philosophical Perspectives," *Encyclopedia of Bioethics* (1978), vol. 2, pp. 599–606. In this survey article, Engelhardt identifies and examines five philosophical questions that bear on the concepts of health and disease.

Hasker, William: "The Critique of 'Mental Illness': Conceptual and/or Ethical Crisis?" *Journal of Psychology and Theology* 5 (Spring 1977), pp. 110–124. After analyzing Szasz's attack on the concept of mental illness, Hasker argues that Szasz's critique has not as yet received a satisfactory response. Hasker contends that the most promising strategy of response is to try to define "a limited concept of mental illness."

Hastings Center Studies 1 (no. 3, 1973). This issue, entitled "The Concept of Health," features five major articles related to this theme. Of special interest is an article by Peter Sedgwick, "Illness—Mental and Otherwise" (pp. 19–40). Sedgwick contends that all ascriptions of illness and disease, both mental and physical, are inherently value-laden.

Journal of Medicine and Philosophy 1 (September 1976). This issue is entitled "Concepts of Health and Disease." Of special interest is an article by Joseph Margolis, "The

Concept of Disease" (pp. 238–255), and a response by H. Tristram Engelhardt, Jr., "Ideology and Etiology" (pp. 256–268).

Kass, Leon R.: "Regarding the End of Medicine and the Pursuit of Health," *The Public Interest* 40 (Summer 1975), pp. 11–42. The first two sections of this rather long article are especially noteworthy. In these sections, after arguing that health is the only legitimate goal of medicine, Kass contends that physical health is rightly construed as a positive state, "the well-working of the organism as a whole."

Lappé, Marc: "Genetic Knowledge and the Concept of Health," *Hastings Center Report* 3 (September 1973), pp. 1–3. Lappé discusses some of the difficulties involved in arriving at an adequate definition of "genetic health."

Macklin, Ruth: "Mental Health and Mental Illness: Some Problems of Definition and Concept Formation," *Philosophy of Science* 39 (September 1972), pp. 341–365. Macklin examines a number of difficulties associated with attempts to define mental health and mental illness. In part 5 of this article, she directly addresses the views of Szasz, concluding that there is no compelling reason to adopt his view that mental illness is a myth.

Rosenhan, D. L.: "On Being Sane in Insane Places," *Science* 179 (January 19, 1973), pp. 250–258. This much discussed article describes the results of an experiment in which sane people gained admittance to mental hospitals. Once inside the hospital, they were perceived as insane, leading Rosenhan to conclude that in psychiatric hospitals we cannot distinguish sane from insane.

Szasz, Thomas S.: *Ideology and Insanity: Essays on the Psychiatric Dehumanization of Man* (New York: Doubleday, 1970). In this collection of essays, Szasz advances a multifaceted critique of contemporary psychiatric practice.

Temkin, Owsei: "Health and Disease," *Dictionary of the History of Ideas,* vol. II, pp. 395–407. Temkin briefly surveys the history of the ideas of health and disease.

Chapter 6

Involuntary Civil Commitment, Sterilization, and the Rights of the Mentally Retarded

INTRODUCTION

As numerous readings in the previous chapters illustrate, issues surrounding autonomy are central in biomedical ethics. Related questions about the rights of self-determination, informed consent, justified paternalism, and conceptions of competency are explored in most of these chapters. The primary focus in many of these readings, however, is on individual relationships in therapeutic and research contexts. Yet some of the most difficult questions regarding the requirements of autonomy arise when social policies are at issue. Consider this question, for example: What social policies should we adopt in regard to persons whose autonomy is diminished due to internal factors such as mental illness or mental retardation?[1] The policies we adopt largely determine the roles played by professionals in the lives of mentally ill and mentally retarded individuals. This chapter focuses first on moral issues raised regarding some social policies dealing with the mentally ill, and then on moral issues raised regarding some social policies dealing with the mentally retarded.

Involuntary Civil Commitment and the Mentally Ill

Mental illness poses both personal and social problems. On the personal level, mental illness often disrupts family relationships, severely incapacitates individuals, and makes everyday living a hazardous, torturous affair. Mentally ill individuals who are severely disoriented or deluded may be unable to care for their routine needs and may thus pose a serious risk to their own well-being. Those who are sufficiently depressed may run the risk of committing suicide. Those who are extremely agitated or confused may pose a threat of serious harm not just to themselves but to their families as well. On a wider social level, the mentally ill may be nuisances, may disrupt social activities, and may engage in serious antisocial behavior. In light of all this, questions arise concerning the state's legitimate role regarding those classified as mentally ill. Does morality permit or, perhaps, even require laws that give representatives of the state, such as judges and psychiatrists, the power to control the lives of those diagnosed as mentally ill? This power is exercised when patients are committed to mental institutions against their "will" or when they are subjected to some form of therapy either without their consent or with "consent" that is given only because acceptance of therapy is a necessary condition for release.

Disputes about the correct answer to this question incorporate conceptual, empirical, and ethical considerations. The articles in Chapter 5 illustrate the conceptual issue— disputants disagree about the definition of mental illness. This disagreement is evidenced in their positions on involuntary civil commitment. Szasz, for example, whose social deviance model of mental illness is presented in Chapter 5, attacks involuntary civil commitment as a crime against humanity. Disputants also disagree on empirical issues, such as the "dangerousness" of the mentally ill or the extent of their competency. The bearing of these empirical disagreements on the moral positions taken regarding involuntary civil commitment emerges in the discussion below concerning the kinds of moral justifications that are advanced for the practice.

Explorations of the morality of involuntary civil commitment procedures usually involve implicit or explicit discussion of the liberty-limiting principles presented in Chapter 1. Should those classified as mentally ill be committed on any of the following grounds?

1 To keep them from seriously harming others (the harm principle);
2 To prevent them from offending others (the offense principle);
3 To keep them from harming themselves (the principle of paternalism);
4 To benefit them (the principle of extreme paternalism).

In assessing attempted justifications of involuntary civil commitment practices, we must keep two other questions in mind: (*a*) which of the above principles are morally acceptable liberty-limiting principles? (*b*) Which principle is actually being used (explicitly or implicitly) to justify commitment? In regard to (*a*), for example, if the principles of paternalism are *not* acceptable liberty-limiting principles, involuntary civil commitment cannot be justified on paternalistic grounds. In regard to (*b*), critics of involuntary civil commitment often argue as follows: It is not uncommon to commit individuals to institutions simply because their behavior is offensive; but the attempt to justify their commitment is made on other inapplicable grounds, such as their supposed dangerousness. Much of the behavior that earns the mentally ill the label of "dangerous" is at most offensive to others. Shouting harangues on street corners and other bizarre behaviors, although offensive to some, pose no threat of serious harm. If offensive behavior is the real basis for committing someone to a mental institution, then the justifying ground would have to be provided by the offense principle and not the harm principle. But few of us would hold that offensive behavior alone is a sufficient ground for the deprivation of liberty. Therefore, exposing the actual reasons for commitment in certain cases may lead to the conclusion that interference in these cases is not justified.

Dangerousness and the Harm Principle   Since the harm principle is a widely accepted liberty-limiting principle, that principle alone would provide a strong ground for the involuntary civil commitment of mentally ill individuals *if* the mentally ill pose a serious threat of harm to others. It is not surprising, therefore, that the harm principle is often invoked, implicitly or explicitly, to justify involuntary civil commitment procedures. But are the mentally ill so dangerous that their commitment is necessary to protect others from harm? To answer this question it is necessary to distinguish between different kinds of cases.

In some cases there is very little doubt that those labeled "mentally ill" are dangerous and pose a *serious threat of physical harm to others.* One example is an individual, classified as schizophrenic perhaps, who attempts to carry out the commands of a disembodied voice ordering the execution of parents or siblings. Persons of this sort certainly pose a serious imminent threat to others. Or another example is the individual, labeled paranoid perhaps, who has a history of violent and apparently irrational acts and who gives every indication of repeating such acts. Persons of this sort might also be correctly perceived as dangerous. Thus, in cases involving either imminent potential physical violence or actual physical violence, involuntary civil commitment would certainly seem to be justified by the harm principle. Not everyone would agree with this conclusion. Thomas S. Szasz, for example, wants no special treatment for those considered mentally ill. If they perform acts forbidden by law, they should be subject to the same legal sanctions as anyone else, Szasz argues. But if they break no laws, the state has no moral right to interfere with their freedom.

Even if Szasz is wrong, however, and the harm principle is correctly invoked in justifying *some* involuntary civil commitments, it does not follow that it justifies the commitment of everyone who is labeled both "mentally ill and dangerous." Mental health workers often diagnose individuals as mentally ill when their behavior seems inexplicable, bizarre, or threatening. They then make predictions about their dangerousness. The purported dangerousness of *most of those* diagnosed as mentally ill, however, is unsupported by actual evidence. Studies have shown either that mental patients as a group are no more dangerous than others[2] or that, if they are, the differences are so small that they allow very little success in prediction.[3] If a psychiatrist's prediction of dangerousness is accepted as sufficient justification for involuntary commitment, the uncertainty of those predictions would result in the commitment of a very large number of nondangerous people. As Livermore, Malmquist, and Meehl bring out in this chapter, for every actually dangerous person detained, many innocent, nondangerous people, who had committed no violent acts and broken no laws, would also be deprived of their freedom. This certainly seems morally unacceptable.

Paternalism and Autonomy   As we saw in Chapter 1, taking decisions out of people's hands for their own good is paternalistic. When individuals are incapable temporarily or permanently of making decisions about their own well-being, there is no usurpation of autonomy, since the conditions for acting autonomously are absent. In these sorts of cases it would be incorrect to hold that the individual's autonomy has been infringed, interfered with, or limited. The problematic cases arise, however, when an individual's abilities to effectively deliberate and make decisions are diminished by delusions, compulsions, and other internal factors associated with mental illness; and yet the person is an adult capable of understanding enough about his or her situation to refuse to assent to commitment. When the organ responsible for the cognitive functions required for informed consent is itself considered to be malfunctioning, how much weight should be given to a person's refusal? Proponents of paternalistic interventions in such cases sometimes argue as follows. Suppose individuals reject commitment or psychiatric help because their present condition renders them incapable of realizing that these are in their own long-term interest. If they were thinking more clearly, if they were not confused or severely depressed by their illnesses, would they not want the benefits involved? Would they not want others to keep them from running the risks to their physical and mental well-being that they will continue to run if they are not committed? Would they not want the treatment that would restore their competency for rational decision making—a competency that is presently limited by internal factors? Those who argue in this way believe that the autonomy of those diagnosed as mentally ill is sometimes sufficiently diminished to justify their involuntary commitment not only to keep them from harming themselves but to help them in regaining lost autonomy. In this chapter, Livermore, Malmquist, and Meehl analyze some of the conceptual and empirical difficulties implicit in paternalistic arguments for involuntary civil commitment.

The Mentally Retarded—Sterilization and Rights

The mentally ill are not the only group whose members have often been almost routinely institutionalized in the past or whose freedoms have been limited because of their presumed incompetency in decision making. Many mentally retarded persons have spent their lives in institutions. Many have been denied educational and other opportunities. Some have been sterilized without their consent. In many states today, even the mildly retarded, if considered legally incompetent, cannot decide to marry, have children, live alone, or enter into any contractual relations without the consent of a guardian. As in the case of the mentally ill, the usual reason given for denying even those who are mildly retarded the freedom of decision possessed by other adults is the purported danger posed by those with cognitive deficiencies to themselves and others. As some of the readings in previous chapters bring out, however, competency is not "all or nothing." Individuals may lack the cognitive skills to solve a geometric problem and yet have sufficient cognitive ability to make everyday decisions about housing, meals, and other practical affairs. As Rosalind Pollack Petchesky notes in a reading in this chapter, over three-quarters of those considered retarded in our society are classified as "mildly retarded." Those who fit this classification have an I.Q. range of 68 to 52 as measured on the Stanford-Binet Scale; and their ability to function on a day-to-day level differs widely, depending on their education, training, and experience.[4]

The routine paternalistic treatment of the mentally retarded, especially of the mildly retarded, has been increasingly challenged. One issue around which challenges have centered is involuntary sterilization. Robert Neville and Petchesky, in this chapter, offer arguments respectively for and against sterilizing the mentally retarded without their consent. Neville sees involuntary sterilization as morally justified when it is in the best interests of mildly retarded persons who lack the capacity to give or withhold informed consent because they do not understand the issues involved. Petchesky disagrees, seeing involuntary sterilization as an unjustified infringement on the reproductive freedom of the mildly retarded, performed not in their interests but to serve the needs of others. Both Petchesky and Neville agree, however, that many empirical questions about the competency of mentally retarded individuals remain to be answered.

Questions about the morally correct treatment of the retarded are not easily resolved, however, simply by a rejection of paternalism on their behalf or by showing that they are often capable of becoming functionally much more competent than was believed in the past. The retarded do have problems, which require special attention if they are to develop and exercise their autonomy to the fullest extent possible. Yet advocates for the retarded sometimes argue that those who are intellectually disadvantaged should be treated just like everyone else, with the same basic rights as all other citizens. This point of view is expressed in a code of rights proclaimed at a 1981 conference on mental retardation. The code demands "the closing of all institutions for intellectually disadvantaged persons."[5] While this statement was not the first articulated demand for a shift from custodialism to community care for the mentally retarded, it was the first code incorporating such demands written by "intellectually handicapped" representatives. In asserting their right to make their own choices about employment, housing, and so forth, the delegates argued, "We are humans first and disadvantaged second."[6] Another code, proclaimed by the International League of Societies for the Mentally Handicapped and reprinted in this chapter, asserts both the same basic rights for the mentally retarded as those held by other citizens of the same country and age and a set of special rights. In this chapter, Barry Hoffmaster discusses some of the problems raised when "rights" are asserted for the mentally retarded that, on the one hand, involve a rejection of any "special classification" status to the retarded and, on the other hand, call for a special status. Hoffmaster's article also examines a number of other problems raised by attempts to (1) provide moral justifications for social practices dealing with the mentally retarded and (2) develop appropriate policies.

J.S.Z.

NOTES

1 For the sake of simplicity, the expressions "mental illness" and "mentally ill" will be used throughout this introduction. This usage is not intended, however, to prejudge questions about the correct use of such expressions.

2 Jonas R. Rappeport, ed., *The Clinical Evaluation of the Dangerousness of the Mentally Ill* (Springfield, Ill.: Charles C Thomas, 1967), pp. 72–80.

3 Alan A. Stone, *Mental Health and Law: A System in Transition* (Rockville, Md.: Center for Studies of Crime and Delinquency, National Institute of Mental Health, DHEW Publication No. [ADM] 75-176, 1975).

4 The figures used in classifying the mentally retarded vary. One classification made on the basis of I.Q. and social adaptation tests classifies retardation as mild, moderate, severe, or profound as follows: *Mild*—I.Q. 50–70. The mildly retarded are often indistinguishable from other children until they show difficulty learning conceptual subjects. (About 80 percent of those classified as mentally retarded in the United States fall into this category.) *Moderate*—I.Q. 35–50. The moderately retarded do have the capacity to develop self-supportive and self-protective skills if they are given the proper training. *Severe*—I.Q. 20–35. The severely mentally retarded are often, but not always, physically handicapped. They show motor, speech, and language retardation and require custodial care. *Profound*—I.Q. less than 20. The profoundly retarded are often physically handicapped and need constant care or supervision if they are to survive. From David F. Allen and Victoria S. Allen, *Ethical Issues in Mental Retardation: Tragic Choices—Living Hope* (Nashville, Tenn.: Abingdon Press, 1979), pp. 19–20.

5 The Australian Voice of Intellectually Disadvantaged Citizens, "Code of Rights" (Resolutions of the Second South Pacific Conference on Mental Retardation, Melbourne, Australia, presented by members of the Fifth Strand to Senator Fred Chaney, Federal Social Security Minister, August 28, 1981).

6 Stanley S. Herr, *Rights and Advocacy for Retarded People* (Lexington, Mass.: Lexington Books, 1983), p. 37.

Involuntary Civil Commitment

Majority Opinion in *O'Connor v. Donaldson*

Justice Potter Stewart

Justice Potter Stewart served as an associate justice of the Supreme Court of the United States from 1958 until 1981. Prior to that appointment, he practiced law (1941–1954) and served as a judge on the United States Circuit Court of Appeals for the 6th District (1954–1958).

In 1943, Kenneth Donaldson's parents asked a judge to commit their 34-year-old son to a mental institution for treatment. They did this after Donaldson's fellow workers apparently knocked him unconscious after he made a political comment. Once Donaldson was institutionalized and his reactions to what he perceived as injustices were diagnosed as pathological, he was given electroconvulsive therapy. After eleven weeks of ECT, he was released. In 1956, Donaldson visited his parents in Florida. During his visit, he made some complaints, which led his father to request a sanity hearing for his son. The senior Donaldson argued that his son was suffering from a "persecution complex." As a result of this complaint, Donaldson was arrested, jailed, and diagnosed as "paranoid schizophrenic" by a sheriff and two physicians. The physicians, each of whom spoke to Donaldson for less than two minutes, were not psychiatrists. Later a judge visited him and informed him that he would be sent to Florida State Hospital. This decision was based on the physicians' conclusions. Donaldson's requests for a judicial hearing and a lawyer were granted; but the hearing was held in jail, the physicians did not attend, and Donaldson's lawyer left while Donaldson was still testifying. Donaldson was sent to the hospital for a "few weeks rest." He remained there for fifteen years, never seeing a judge and seeing a psychiatrist only a few times a year. During those fifteen years, Donaldson petitioned various courts eighteen times, asking for a hearing. All but one of these requests were dismissed on the basis of physicians' reports and his previous institutionalization. When his case was finally going to be heard in 1971, Donaldson was released and certified as "no longer incompetent." However, he continued his suit asking $100,000 in damages for the fifteen years he had been committed without treatment. He won his case against J. B. O'Connor, the superintendent of the institution, and a codefendant physician, although only $38,500 was granted in damages.

The case was ultimately appealed to the United States Supreme Court. In handing down its 1975 landmark decision, the court ruled that a finding of mental illness alone is insufficient grounds for confining a nondangerous individual who has the capacity to survive safely in freedom, either by himself or with the help of responsible and willing relatives or friends. Justice Potter Stewart wrote the majority opinion, which is partially reprinted here.

United States Supreme Court; June 26, 1975, 422 U.S. 563. 95 S.Ct. 2486.

I

Donaldson's commitment was initiated by his father, who thought that his son was suffering from "delusions." After hearings before a county judge of Pinellas County, Fla., Donaldson was found to be suffering from "paranoid schizophrenia" and was commited for "care, maintenance, and treatment" pursuant to Florida statutory provisions that have since been repealed. The state law was less than clear in specifying the grounds necessary for commitment, and the record is scanty as to Donaldson's condition at the time of the judicial hearing. These matters are, however, irrelevant, for this case involves no challenge to the initial commitment, but is focused, instead, upon the nearly 15 years of confinement that followed.

The evidence at the trial showed that the hospital staff had the power to release a patient, not dangerous to himself or others, even if he remained mentally ill and had been lawfully committed. Despite many requests, O'Connor refused to allow that power to be exercised in Donaldson's case. At the trial, O'Connor indicated that he had believed that Donaldson would have been unable to make a "successful adjustment outside the institution," but could not recall the basis for that conclusion. O'Connor retired as superintendent shortly before the suit was filed. A few months thereafter, and before the trial, Donaldson secured his release and a judicial restoration of competency, with the support of the hospital staff.

The testimony at the trial demonstrated, without contradiction, that Donaldson had posed no danger to others during his long confinement, or indeed at any point in his life. O'Connor himself conceded that he had no personal or secondhand knowledge that Donaldson had ever committed a dangerous act. There was no evidence that Donaldson had ever been suicidal or been thought likely to inflict injury upon himself. One of O'Connor's codefendants acknowledged that Donaldson could have earned his own living outside the hospital. He had done so for some 14 years before his commitment, and immediately upon his release he secured a responsible job in hotel administration.

Furthermore, Donaldson's frequent requests for release had been supported by responsible persons willing to provide him any care he might need on release. In 1963, for example, a representative of Helping Hands, Inc., a halfway house for mental patients, wrote O'Connor asking him to release Donaldson to its care. The request was accompanied by a supporting letter from the Minneapolis Clinic of Psychiatry and Neurology, which a codefendant conceded was a "good clinic." O'Connor rejected the offer, replying that Donaldson could be released only to his parents. That rule was apparently of O'Connor's own making. At the time, Donaldson was 55 years old, and, as O'Connor knew, Donaldson's parents were too elderly and infirm to take responsibility for him. Moreover, in his continuing correspondence with Donaldson's parents, O'Connor never informed them of the Helping Hands offer. In addition, on four separate occasions between 1964 and 1968, John Lembcke, a college classmate of Donaldson's and a longtime family friend, asked O'Connor to release Donaldson to his care. On each occasion O'Connor refused. The record shows that Lembcke was a serious and responsible person, who was willing and able to assume responsibility for Donaldson's welfare.

The evidence showed that Donaldson's confinement was a simple regime of enforced custodial care, not a program designed to alleviate or cure his supposed illness. Numerous witnesses, including one of O'Connor's codefendants, testified that Donaldson had received nothing but custodial care while at the hospital. O'Connor described Donaldson's treatment as "milieu therapy." But witnesses from the hospital staff conceded that, in the context of this case, "milieu therapy" was a euphemism for confinement in the "milieu" of a mental hospital. For substantial periods, Donaldson was simply kept in a large room that housed 60 patients, many of whom were under criminal commitment. Donaldson's requests for ground privileges, occupational training, and an opportunity to discuss his case with O'Connor or other staff members were repeatedly denied.

At the trial, O'Connor's principal defense was that he had acted in good faith and was therefore immune from any liability for monetary damages. His position, in short, was that state law, which he had believed valid, had authorized indefinite custodial confinement of the "sick," even if they were not given treatment and their release could harm no one.

The trial judge instructed the members of the jury that they should find that O'Connor had violated Donaldson's constitutional right to liberty if they found that he had confined [Donaldson] against his will, knowing that he was not mentally ill or dangerous or knowing that if mentally ill he was not receiving treatment for his alleged mental illness....

Now, the purpose of involuntary hospitalization is treatment and not mere custodial care or punishment if a patient is not a danger to himself or others. Without such treatment there is no justification from a constitutional stand-point for continued confinement unless you should also find that [Donaldson] was dangerous to either himself or others.

The trial judge further instructed the jury that O'Connor was immune from damages if he

reasonably believed in good faith that detention of [Donaldson] was proper for the length of time he was so confined....

However, mere good intentions which do not give rise to a reasonable belief that detention is lawfully required cannot justify [Donaldson's] confinement in the Florida State Hospital.

The jury returned a verdict for Donaldson against O'Connor and a codefendant, and awarded damages of $38,500, including $10,000 in punitive damages.

The Court of Appeals affirmed the judgment of the District Court in a broad opinion dealing with "the far-reaching question whether the Fourteenth Amendment guarantees a right to treatment to persons involuntarily civilly committed to state mental hospitals." The appellate court held that when, as in Donaldson's case, the rationale for confinement is that the patient is in need of treatment, the Constitution requires that minimally adequate treatment in fact be provided. The court further expressed the view that, regardless of the grounds for involuntary civil commitment, a person confined against his will at a state mental institution has "a constitutional right to receive such individual treatment as will give him a reasonable opportunity to be cured or to improve his mental condition." Conversely, the court's opinion implied that it is constitutionally permissible for a State to confine a mentally ill person against his will in order to treat his illness, regardless of whether his illness renders him dangerous to himself or others.

II

We have concluded that the difficult issues of constitu-

tional law dealt with by the Court of Appeals are not presented by this case in its present posture. Specifically, there is no reason now to decide whether mentally ill persons dangerous to themselves or to others have a right to treatment upon compulsory confinement by the State, or whether the State may compulsorily confine a nondangerous, mentally ill individual for the purpose of treatment. As we view it, this case raises a single, relatively simple, but nonetheless important question concerning every man's constitutional right to liberty.

The jury found that Donaldson was neither dangerous to himself nor dangerous to others, and also found that, if mentally ill, Donaldson had not received treatment. That verdict, based on abundant evidence, makes the issue before the Court a narrow one. We need not decide whether, when, or by what procedures, a mentally ill person may be confined by the State on any of the grounds which, under contemporary statutes, are generally advanced to justify involuntary confinement of such a person—to prevent injury to the public, to ensure his own survival or safety,[1] or to alleviate or cure his illness. For the jury found that none of the above grounds for continued confinement was present in Donaldson's case.

Given the jury's findings, what was left as justification for keeping Donaldson in continued confinement? The fact that state law may have authorized confinement of the harmless mentally ill does not itself establish a constitutionally adequate purpose for the confinement. Nor is it enough that Donaldson's original confinement was founded upon a constitutionally adequate basis, if in fact it was, because even if his involuntary confinement was initially permissible, it could not constitutionally continue after that basis no longer existed.

A finding of "mental illness" alone cannot justify a State's locking a person up against his will and keeping him indefinitely in simple custodial confinement. Assuming that that term can be given a reasonably precise content and that the "mentally ill" can be identified with reasonable accuracy, there is still no constitutional basis for confining such persons involuntarily if they are dangerous to no one and can live safely in freedom.

May the State confine the mentally ill merely to ensure them a living standard superior to that which they enjoy in the private community? That the State has a proper interest in providing care and assistance to the unfortunate goes without saying. But the mere presence of mental illness does not disqualify a person from preferring his home to the comforts of an institution. Moreover, while the State may arguably confine a person to save him from harm, incarceration is rarely if ever a necessary condition for raising the living standards of those capable of surviving safely in freedom, on their own or with the help of family or friends.

May the State fence in the harmless mentally ill solely to save its citizens from exposure to those whose ways are different? One might as well ask if the State, to avoid public unease, could incarcerate all who are physically unattractive or socially eccentric. Mere public intolerance or animosity cannot constitutionally justify the deprivation of a person's physical liberty.

In short, a State cannot constitutionally confine without more evidence a nondangerous individual who is capable of surviving safely in freedom by himself or with the help of willing and responsible family members or friends. Since the jury found, upon ample evidence, that O'Connor, as an agent of the State, knowingly did so confine Donaldson, it properly concluded that O'Connor violated Donaldson's constitutional right to freedom.

III

O'Connor contends that in any event he should not be held personally liable for monetary damages because his decisions were made in "good faith." Specifically, O'Connor argues that he was acting pursuant to state law which, he believed, authorized confinement of the mentally ill even when their release would not compromise their safety or constitute a danger to others, and that he could not reasonably have been expected to know that the state law as he understood it was constitutionally invalid. A proposed instruction to this effect was rejected by the District Court.

The District Court did instruct the jury, without objection, that monetary damages could not be assessed against O'Connor if he had believed reasonably and in good faith that Donaldson's continued confinement was "proper," and that punitive damages could be awarded only if O'Connor had acted "maliciously or wantonly or oppressively." The Court of Appeals approved those instructions. But that court did not consider whether it was error for the trial judge to refuse the additional instruction concerning O'Connor's claimed reliance on state law as authorization for

Donaldson's continued confinement. Further, neither the District Court nor the Court of Appeals acted with the benefit of this Court's most recent decision on the scope of the qualified immunity possessed by state officials.... [*Wood v. Strickland* (1975)]

Under that decision, the relevant question for the jury is whether O'Connor "knew or reasonably should have known that the action he took within his sphere of official responsibility would violate the constitutional rights of [Donaldson], or if he took the action with the malicious intention to cause a deprivation of constitutional rights or other injury to [Donaldson]." For the purposes of this question, an official has, of course, no duty to anticipate unforeseeable constitutional developments.

Accordingly, we vacate the judgment of the Court of Appeals and remand the case to enable that court to consider, in light of *Wood v. Strickland,* whether the District Judge's failure to instruct with regard to the effect of O'Connor's claimed reliance on state law rendered inadequate the instructions as to O'Connor's liability for compensatory and punitive damages.[2]

It is so ordered.

Vacated and remanded.

NOTES

1 The judge's instructions used the phrase "dangerous to himself." Of course, even if there is no foreseeable risk of self-injury or suicide, a person is literally "dangerous to himself" if for physical or other reasons he is helpless to avoid the hazards of freedom either through his own efforts or with the aid of willing family members or friends. While it might be argued that the judge's instructions could have been more detailed on this point, O'Connor raised no objection to them, presumably because the evidence clearly showed that Donaldson was not "dangerous to himself" however broadly that phrase might be defined.

2 Upon remand, the Court of Appeals is to consider only the question whether O'Connor is to be held liable for monetary damages for violating Donaldson's constitutional right to liberty. The jury found, on substantial evidence and under adequate instructions, that O'Connor deprived Donaldson, who was dangerous neither to himself nor to others and was provided no treatment, of the constitutional right to liberty. That finding needs no further consideration.

If the Court of Appeals holds that a remand to the District Court is necessary, the only issue to be determined in that court will be whether O'Connor is immune from liability for monetary damages.

Of necessity our decision vacating the judgment of the Court of Appeals deprives that court's opinion of precedential effect, leaving this Court's opinion and judgment as the sole law of the case.

Involuntary Mental Hospitalization: A Crime Against Humanity

Thomas S. Szasz

A biographical sketch of Thomas S. Szasz is found on page 263.

Szasz attacks the practice of committing persons to mental institutions against their will. He calls such commitments "a crime against humanity" and condemns the use of coercive state power against the "mentally ill." Szasz criticizes those who maintain that such commitments (1) *benefit* the mentally ill and/or (2) *protect* the mentally healthy members of society. Against (1), Szasz cites medical, moral, historical, and literary "evidence" to support his view that commitment does not serve the patient's interests; rather it serves the interests of others. Against (2), Szasz again cites the same sorts of evidence to show that the "danger posed by mental patients" is usually vaguely defined (e.g., their behavior may merely be offensive to some). Underlying Szasz's arguments here is the conception of mental illness presented in his article in the preceding chapter.

I

For some time now I have maintained that commitment—that is, the detention of persons in mental institutions against their will—is a form of imprisonment;[1] that such deprivation of liberty is contrary to the moral principles embodied in the Declaration of Independence and the Constitution of the United States;[2] and that it is a crass violation of contemporary concepts of fundamental human rights.[3] The practice of "sane" men incarcerating their "insane" fellow men in "mental hospitals" can be compared to that of white men enslaving black men. In short, I consider commitment a crime against humanity.

Existing social institutions and practices, especially if honored by prolonged usage, are generally experienced and accepted as good and valuable. For thousands of years slavery was considered a "natural" social arrangement for the securing of human labor; it

was sanctioned by public opinion, religious dogma, church, and state;[4] it was abolished a mere one hundred years ago in the United States; and it is still a prevalent social practice in some parts of the world, notably in Africa.[5] Since its origin, approximately three centuries ago, commitment of the insane has enjoyed equally widespread support; physicians, lawyers, and the laity have asserted, as if with a single voice, the therapeutic desirability and social necessity of institutional psychiatry. My claim that commitment is a crime against humanity may thus be countered—as indeed it has been—by maintaining, first, that the practice is beneficial for the mentally ill, and second, that it is necessary for the protection of the mentally healthy members of society.

Illustrative of the first argument is Slovenko's assertion that "Reliance solely on voluntary hospital admission procedures ignores the fact that some persons may desire care and custody but cannot communicate their desire directly."[6] Imprisonment in mental hospitals is here portrayed—by a professor of law!—as a service provided to persons by the state because they "desire" it but do not know how to ask for it. Felix defends involuntary mental hospitalization by asserting simply, "We *do* [his italics] deal with illnesses of the mind."[7]

Illustrative of the second argument is Guttmacher's characterization of my book *Law, Liberty, and Psychiatry* as "...a pernicious book...certain to produce intolerable and unwarranted anxiety in the families of psychiatric patients."[8] This is an admission of the fact that the families of "psychiatric patients" frequently resort to the use of force in order to control their "loved ones," and that when attention is directed to this practice it creates embarrassment and guilt. On the other hand, Felix simply defines the psychiatrist's duty as the protection of society: "Tommorrow's psychiatrist will be, as is his counterpart today, one of the gate-keepers of his community."[9]

These conventional explanations of the nature and uses of commitment are, however, but culturally accepted justifications for certain quasi-medical forms of social control, exercised especially against individuals and groups whose behavior does not violate criminal laws but threatens established social values.

II

What is the evidence that commitment does not serve the purpose of helping or treating people whose behavior deviates from or threatens prevailing social norms or moral standards; and who, because they inconvenience their families, neighbors, or superiors, may be incriminated as "mentally ill"?

1. *The medical evidence.* Mental illness is a metaphor. If by "disease" we mean a disorder of the physiochemical machinery of the human body, then we can assert that what we call functional mental diseases are not diseases at all.[10] Persons said to be suffering from such disorders are socially deviant or inept, or in conflict with individuals, groups, or institutions. Since they do not suffer from disease, it is impossible to "treat" them for any sickness.

Although the term "mentally ill" is usually applied to persons who do not suffer from bodily disease, it is sometimes applied also to persons who do (for example, to individuals intoxicated with alcohol or other drugs, or to elderly people suffering from degenerative disease of the brain). However, when patients with demon-strable diseases of the brain are involuntarily hospitalized, the primary purpose is to exercise social control over their behavior,[11] treatment of the disease is, at best, a secondary consideration. Frequently, therapy is non-existent, and custodial care is dubbed "treatment."

In short, the commitment of persons suffering from "functional psychoses" serves moral and social, rather than medical and therapeutic, purposes. Hence, even if, as a result of future research, certain conditions now believed to be "functional" mental illnesses were to be shown to be "organic," my argument against involuntary mental hospitalization would remain unaffected.

2. *The moral evidence.* In free societies, the relationship between physician and patient is predicated on the legal presumption that the individual "owns" his body and his personality.[12] The physician can examine and treat a patient only with his consent; the latter is free to reject treatment (for example, an operation for cancer).[13] After death, "ownership" of the person's body is transferred to his heirs; the physician must obtain permission from the patient's relatives for postmortem examination. John Stuart Mill explicitly affirmed that "...each person is the proper guardian of his own health, whether bodily, or mental and spiritual."[14] Commitment is incompatible with this moral principle.

3. *The historical evidence.* Commitment practices flourished long before there were any mental or psychiatric "treatments" of "mental diseases." Indeed, madness or mental illness was not always a necessary condition for commitment. For example, in the seventeenth century, "children of artisans and other poor inhabitants of Paris up to the age of 25,...girls who were debauched or in evident danger of being debauched,..."and other "misérables" of the community, such as epileptics, people with venereal diseases, and poor people with chronic diseases of all sorts, were all considered fit subjects for confinement in the Hôpital Général.[15] And, in 1860, when Mrs. Packard was incarcerated for disagreeing with her minister-husband,[16] the commitment laws of the State of Illinois explicitly proclaimed that "...married women... may be entered or detained in the hospital at the request of the husband of the woman or the guardian..., without the evidence of insanity required in other cases."[17] It is surely no coincidence that this piece of legislation was enacted and enforced at about the same time that Mill published his essay *The Subjection of Women.*[18]

4. *The literary evidence.* Involuntary mental hospitalization plays a significant part in numerous short

stories and novels from many countries. In none that I have encountered is commitment portrayed as helpful to the hospitalized person; instead, it is always depicted as an arrangement serving interests antagonistic to those of the so-called patient.[19]

III

The claim that commitment of the "mentally ill" is necessary for the protection of the "mentally healthy" is more difficult to refute, not because it is valid, but because the danger that "mental patients" supposedly pose is of such an extremely vague nature.

1. *The medical evidence.* The same reasoning applies as earlier: If "mental illness" is not a disease, there is no medical justification for protection from disease. Hence, the analogy between mental illness and contagious disease falls to the ground: The justification for isolating or otherwise constraining patients with tuberculosis or typhoid fever cannot be extended to patients with "mental illness."

Moreover, because the accepted contemporary psychiatric view of mental illness fails to distinguish between illness as a biological condition and as a social role,[20] it is not only false, but also dangerously misleading, especially if used to justify social action. In this view, regardless of its "causes"—anatomical, genetic, chemical, psychological, or social—mental illness has "objective existence." A person either has or has not a mental illness; he is either mentally sick or mentally healthy. Even if a person is cast in the role of mental patient against his will, his "mental illness" exists "objectively"; and even if, as in the case of the Very Important Person, he is never treated as a mental patient, his "mental illness" still exists "objectively"— apart from the activities of the psychiatrist.[21]

The upshot is that the term "mental illness" is perfectly suited for mystification: It disregards the crucial question of whether the individual assumes the role of mental patient voluntarily, and hence wishes to engage in some sort of interaction with a psychiatrist; or whether he is cast in that role against his will, and hence is opposed to such a relationship. This obscurity is then usually employed strategically, either by the subject himself to advance *his* interests, or by the subject's adversaries to advance *their* interests.

In contrast to this view, I maintain, first, that the involuntarily hospitalized mental patient is, by defini-

tion, the occupant of an ascribed role; and, second, that the "mental disease" of such a person—unless the use of this term is restricted to demonstrable lesions or malfunctions of the brain—is always the product of interaction between psychiatrist and patient.

2. *The moral evidence.* The crucial ingredient in involuntary mental hospitalization is coercion. Since coercion is the exercise of power, it is always a moral and political act. Accordingly, regardless of its medical justification, commitment is primarily a moral and political phenomenon—just as, regardless of its anthropological and economic justifications, slavery was primarily a moral and political phenomenon.

Although psychiatric methods of coercion are indisputably useful for those who employ them, they are clearly not indispensable for dealing with the problems that so-called mental patients pose for those about them. If an individual threatens others by virtue of his beliefs or actions, he could be dealt with by methods other than "medical": if his conduct is ethically offensive, moral sanctions against him might be appropriate; if forbidden by law, legal sanctions might be appropriate. In my opinion, both informal, moral sanctions, such as social ostracism or divorce, and formal, judicial sanctions, such as fine and imprisonment, are more dignified and less injurious to the human spirit than the quasi-medical psychiatric sanction of involuntary mental hospitalization.[22]

3. *The historical evidence.* To be sure, confinement of so-called mentally ill persons does protect the community from certain problems. If it didn't, the arrangement would not have come into being and would not have persisted. However, the question we ought to ask is not *whether* commitment protects the community from "dangerous mental patients," but rather from precisely *what danger* it protects and by *what means?* In what way were prostitutes or vagrants dangerous in seventeenth century Paris? Or married women in nineteenth century Illinois?

It is significant, moreover, that there is hardly a prominent person who, during the past fifty years or so, has not been diagnosed by a psychiatrist as suffering from some type of "mental illness." Barry Goldwater was called a "paranoid schizophrenic";[23] Whittaker Chambers, a "psychopathic personality";[24] Woodrow Wilson, a "neurotic" frequently "very close to psychosis";[25] and Jesus, "a born degenerate" with a "fixed delusional system," and a "paranoid" with a "clinical picture [so typical] that it is hardly conceivable that people can even question the accuracy of the diagnosis."[26] The list is endless.

Sometimes, psychiatrists declare the same person sane *and* insane, depending on the political dictates of their superiors and the social demand of the moment. Before his trial and execution, Adolph Eichmann was examined by several psychiatrists, all of whom declared him to be normal; after he was put to death, "medical evidence" of his insanity was released and widely circulated.

According to Hannah Arendt, "Half a dozen psychiatrists had certified him [Eichmann] as 'normal.'" One psychiatrist asserted, "...his whole psychological outlook, his attitude toward his wife and children, mother and father, sisters and friends, was 'not only normal but most desirable.'..." And the minister who regularly visited him in prison declared that Eichmann was "a man with very positive ideas."[27] After Eichmann was executed, Gideon Hausner, the Attorney General of Israel, who had prosecuted him, disclosed in an article in *The Saturday Evening Post* that psychiatrists diagnosed Eichmann as "'a man obsessed with a dangerous and insatiable urge to kill,' 'a perverted, sadistic personality.'"[28]

Whether or not men like those mentioned above are considered "dangerous" depends on the observer's religious beliefs, political convictions, and social situation. Furthermore, the "dangerousness" of such persons—whatever we may think of them—is not analogous to that of a person with tuberculosis or typhoid fever; nor would rendering such a person "nondangerous" be comparable to rendering a patient with a contagious disease non-infectious.

In short, I hold—and I submit that the historical evidence bears me out—that people are committed to mental hospitals neither because they are "dangerous," nor because they are "mentally ill," but rather because they are society's scapegoats, whose persecution is justified by psychiatric propaganda and rhetoric.[29]

4. *The literary evidence.* No one contests that involuntary mental hospitalization of the so-called dangerously insane "protects" the community. Disagreement centers on the nature of the threat facing society, and on the methods and legitimacy of the protection it employs. In this connection, we may recall that slavery, too, "protected" the community: it freed the slaveowners from manual labor. Commitment likewise shields the non-hospitalized members of society: first, from having to accommodate themselves to the annoying or idiosyncratic demands of certain members of the community who have not violated any criminal statues; and, second, from having to prosecute, try, convict, and punish members of the community who have broken the law but who either might not be convicted in court, or, if they would be, might not be restrained as effectively or as long in prison as in a mental hospital. The literary evidence cited earlier fully supports this interpretation of the function of involuntary mental hospitalization.

IV

I have suggested that commitment constitutes a social arrangement whereby one part of society secures certain advantages for itself at the expense of another part. To do so, the oppressors must possess an ideology to justify their aims and actions; and they must be able to enlist the police power of the state to impose their will on the oppressed members. What makes such an arrangement a "crime against humanity"? It may be argued that the use of state power is legitimate when law-abiding citizens punish lawbreakers. What is the difference between this use of state power and its use in commitment?

In the first place, the difference between committing the "insane" and imprisoning the "criminal" is the same as that between the rule of man and the rule of law:[30] whereas the "insane" are subjected to the coercive controls of the state because persons more powerful than they have labeled them as "psychotic," "criminals" are subjected to such controls because they have violated rules applicable equally to all.

The second difference between these two proceedings lies in their professed aims. The principal purpose of imprisoning criminals is to protect the liberties of the law-abiding members of society.[31] Since the individual subject to commitment is not considered a threat to liberty in the same way as the accused criminal is (if he were, he would be prosecuted), his removal from society cannot be justified on the same grounds. Justification for commitment must thus rest on its therapeutic promise and potential: it will help restore the "patient" to "mental health." But if this can be accomplished only at the the cost of robbing the individual of liberty, "involuntary mental hospitalization" becomes only a verbal camouflage for what is, in effect, punishment. This "therapeutic" punishment differs, however, from traditional judicial punishment, in that the accused criminal enjoys a rich panoply of constitutional protections against false accusations and oppressive prosecution, whereas the accused mental patient is deprived of these protections.[32]...

V

A basic assumption of American slavery was that the Negro was racially inferior to the Caucasian. "There is no malice toward the Negro in Ulrich Phillips' work," wrote Stanley Elkins about the author's book *American Negro Slavery,* a work sympathetic with the Southern position. "Phillips was deeply fond of the Negroes as a people; it was just that he could not take them seriously as men and women; they were children."[33]

Similarly, the basic assumption of institutional psychiatry is that the mentally ill person is psychologically and socially inferior to the mentally healthy. He is like a child: he does not know what is in his best interests and therefore needs others to control and protect him.[34] Psychiatrists often care deeply for their involuntary patients, whom they consider—in contrast with the merely "neurotic" persons—"psychotic," which is to say, "very sick." Hence, such patients must be cared for as the "irresponsible children" they are considered to be.

The perspective of paternalism has played an exceedingly important part in justifying both slavery and involuntary mental hospitalization. Aristotle defined slavery as "an essentially domestic relationship"; in so doing, wrote Davis, he "endowed it with the sanction of paternal authority, and helped to establish a precedent that would govern discussions of political philosophers as late as the eighteenth century."[35] The relationship between psychiatrists and mental patients has been and continues to be viewed in the same way. "If a man brings his daughter to me from California," declares Braceland, "because she is in manifest danger of falling into vice or in some way disgracing herself, he doesn't expect me to let her loose in my hometown for that same thing to happen."[36] Indeed, almost any article or book dealing with the "care" of involuntary mental patients may be cited to illustrate the contention that physicians fall back on paternalism to justify their coercive control over the unco-operative patient. "Certain cases" [not individuals!]—writes Solomon in an article on suicide—"...must be considered irresponsible, not only with respect to violent impulses, but also in all medical matters." In this class, which he labels "The Irresponsible," he places "Children," "The Men-

tally Retarded," "The Psychotic," and "The Severely or Terminally Ill." Solomon's conclusion is that "Repugnant though it may be, he [the physician] may have to act against the patient's wishes in order to protect the patient's life and that of others."[37] The fact that, as in the case of slavery, the physician needs the police power of the state to maintain his relationship with his involuntary patient does not alter this self-serving image of institutional psychiatry.

Paternalism is the crucial explanation for the stubborn contradiction and conflict about whether the practices employed by slaveholders and institutional psychiatrists are "therapeutic" or "noxious." Masters and psychiatrists profess their benevolence; their slaves and involuntary patients protest against their malevolence. As Seymour Halleck puts it: "...the psychiatrist experiences himself as a helping person, but his patient may see him as a jailer. Both views are partially correct."[38] Not so. Both views are completely correct. Each is a proposition about a different subject: the former, about the psychiatrist's self-image; the latter, about the involuntary mental patient's image of his captor. In *Ward 7,* Valeriy Tarsis presents the following dialogue between his protagonist-patient and the mental-hospital physician: "This is the position. I don't regard you as a doctor. You call this a hospital. I call it a prison....So now, let's get everything straight. I am your prisoner, you are my jailer, and there isn't going to be any nonsense about my health...or treatment."[39]

This is the characteristic dialogue of oppression and liberation. The ruler looks in the mirror and sees a liberator; the ruled looks at the ruler and sees a tyrant. If the physician has the power to incarcerate the patient and uses it, their relationship will inevitably fit into this mold. If one cannot ask the subject whether he likes being enslaved or committed, whipped or electroshocked—because he is not a fit judge of his own "best interests"—then one is left with the contending opinions of the practitioners and their critics. The practitioners insist that their coercive measures are beneficial; the critics, that they are harmful.

The defenders of slavery thus claimed that the Negro "is happier...as a slave, than he could be as a free man; this is the result of the peculiarities of his character,"[40] that "...it was actually an act of liberation to remove Negroes from their harsh world of sin and dark superstition"[41] and that "...Negroes were better off in a Christian land, even as slaves, than living like beasts in Africa."[42]

Similarly, the defenders of involuntary mental hospitalization claim that the mental patient is healthier—the twentieth-century synonym for the nineteenth-century term "happier"—as a psychiatric prisoner than he would be as a free citizen; that "[t]he basic purpose [of commitment] is to make sure that sick human beings get the care that is appropriate to their needs...,"[43] and that "[i]t is a feature of some illnesses that people do not have insight into the fact that they are sick. In short, sometimes it is necessary to protect them [the mentally ill] for a while from themselves...."[44] It requires no great feat of imagination to see how comforting—indeed, how absolutely necessary—these views are to the advocates of slavery and involuntary mental hospitalization, even when they are contradicted by facts.

For example, although it was held that "a merrier being does not exist on the face of the globe than the Negro slave of the United States,"[45] there was an ever-lurking fear of Negro violence and revolt. As Elkins put it, "the failure of any free workers to present themselves for enslavement can serve as one test of how much the analysis of the 'happy slave' may have added to Americans' understanding of themselves."[46]

The same views and the same inconsistencies apply to involuntary psychiatric hospitalization. Defenders of this system maintain that committed patients are better off in hospitals, where they are contented and harmless; "most patients," declares Guttmacher, "when they get in a [mental] hospital are quite content to be there...."[47] At the same time, such patients are feared for their potential violence, their escapes from captivity occasion intense manhunts, and their crimes are prominently featured in the newspapers. Moreover, as with slavery, the failure of citizens to present themselves for involuntary psychiatric hospitalization can serve as a test of how much the currently popular analysis of mental health problems has added to Americans' understanding of themselves.

The social necessity, and hence the basic value, of involuntary mental hospitalization, at least for some people, is not seriously questioned today. There is massive consensus in the United States that, properly used, such hospitalization is a good thing. It is thus possible to debate *who* should be hospitalized, or *how,* or for *how long*—but not whether *anyone should* be. I submit, however, that just as it is improper to enslave anyone—whether he is black or white, Moslem or Christian—so it is improper to hospitalize anyone without his consent—whether he is depressed or paranoid, hysterical or schizophrenic....

NOTES

1 Szasz, T. S.: "Commitment of the mentally ill: Treatment or social restraint?" *J. Nerv. & Ment. Dis.* 125:293–307 (Apr.-June) 1957.

2 Szasz, T. S.: *Law, Liberty, and Psychiatry: An Inquiry into the Social Uses of Mental Health Practices* (New York: Macmillan, 1963), pp. 149–90.

3 Ibid., pp. 223–55.

4 Davis, D. B.: *The Problem of Slavery in Western Culture* (Ithaca, N. Y.: Cornell University Press, 1966).

5 See Cohen, R.: "Slavery in Africa." *Trans-Action* 4:44–56 (Jan.-Feb.), 1967; Tobin, R. L.: "Slavery still plagues the earth." *Saturday Review,* May 6, 1967, pp. 24–25.

6 Slovenko, R.: "The psychiatric patient, liberty, and the law." *Amer. J. Psychiatry,* 121:534–39 (Dec.), 1964, p. 536.

7 Felix, R. H.: "The image of the psychiatrist: Past, present, and future." *Amer. J. Psychiatry,* 121:318–22 (Oct.), 1964, p. 320.

8 Guttmacher, M. S.: "Critique of views of Thomas Szasz on legal psychiatry." *AMA Arch. Gen. Psychiatry,* 10:238–45 (March), 1964, p. 244.

9 Felix, op. cit., p. 231.

10 See Szasz, T. S.: "The myth of mental illness." This volume [*Ideology and Insanity*] pp. 12–24; *The Myth of Mental Illness: Foundations of a Theory of Personal Conduct* (New York: Hoeber-Harper, 1961); "Mental illness is a myth." *The New York Times Magazine,* June 12, 1966, pp. 30 and 90–92.

11 See, for example, Noyes, A. P.: *Modern Clinical Psychiatry,* 4th ed. (Philadelphia: Saunders, 1956), p. 278.

12 Szasz, T. S.: "The ethics of birth control; or, who owns your body?" *The Humanist,* 20:332–36 (Nov.-Dec.) 1960.

13 Hirsch, B. D.: "Informed consent to treatment," in Averbach, A. and Belli, M. M., eds., *Tort and Medical Yearbook* (Indianapolis: Bobbs-Merrill, 1961), Vol. I, pp. 631–38.

14 Mill, J. S.: *On Liberty* [1859] (Chicago: Regnery, 1955), p. 18.

15 Rosen, G.: "Social attitudes to irrationality and madness in 17th and 18th century Europe." *J. Hist. Med. & Allied Sciences,* 18:220–40 (1963), p. 223.

16 Packard, E. W. P.: *Modern Persecution, or Insane Asylums Unveiled,* 2 Vols. (Hartford: Case, Lockwood, and Brainard, 1873).

17 Illinois Statute Book, Sessions Laws 15, Section 10, 1851. Quoted in Packard, E. P. W.: *The Prisoner's Hidden Life* (Chicago: published by the author, 1868), p. 37.

18 Mill, J. S.: *The Subjection of Women* [1869] (London: Dent, 1965).

19 See, for example, Chekhov, A. P.: *Ward No. 6,* [1892], in *Seven Short Novels by Chekhov* (New York: Bantam Books, 1963), pp. 106–57; De Assis, M.: *The Psychiatrist* [1881–82], in De Assis, M., *The Psychiatrist and Other Stories* (Berkeley and Los Angeles: University of California Press, 1963), pp. 1–45; London, J.: *The Iron Heel* [1907] (New York: Sagamore Press, 1957); Porter, K. A.: *Noon Wine* [1937], in Porter, K. A., *Pale Horse, Pale Rider: Three Short Novels* (New York: Signet, 1965), pp. 62–112; Kesey, K.: *One Flew Over the Cuckoo's Nest* (New York: Viking, 1962); Tarsis, V.: *Ward 7: An Autobiographical Novel* (London and Glasgow: Collins and Harvill, 1965).

20 See Szasz, T. S.: "Alcoholism: A socio-ethical perspective," *Western Medicine,* 7:15–21 (Dec.) 1966.

21 See, for example, Rogow, A. A.: *James Forrestal: A Study of Personality, Politics, and Policy* (New York: Macmillan, 1964); for a detailed criticism of this view, see Szasz, T. S.: "Psychiatric classification as a strategy of personal constraint." This volume [*Ideology and Insanity*] pp. 190–217.

22 Szasz, T. S.: *Psychiatric Justice* (New York: Macmillan, 1965).

23 "The Unconscious of a Conservative: A Special Issue on the Mind of Barry Goldwater." *Fact,* Sept.-Oct. 1964.

24 Zeligs, M. A.: *Friendship and Fratricide: An Analysis of Whittaker Chambers and Alger Hiss* (New York: Viking, 1967).

25 Freud, S. and Bullitt, W. C.: *Thomas Woodrow Wilson: A Psychological Study* (Boston: Houghton Mifflin, 1967).

26 Quoted in Schweitzer, A.: *The Psychiatric Study of Jesus* [1913] transl. by Charles R. Joy (Boston: Beacon Press, 1956) pp. 37, 40–41.

27 Arendt, H.: *Eichmann in Jerusalem: A Report on the Banality of Evil* (New York: Viking, 1963), p. 22.

28 Ibid., pp. 22–23.

29 For a full articulation and documentation of this thesis, see Szasz, T. S.: *The Manufacture of Madness: A Comparative Study of the Inquisition and the Mental Health Movement* (New York: Harper & Row, 1970).

30 Hayek, F. A.: *The Constitution of Liberty* (Chicago: University of Chicago Press, 1960), especially pp. 162–92.

31 Mabbott, J. D.: "Punishment" [1939], in Olafson, F. A., ed., *Justice and Social Policy: A Collection of Essays* (Englewood Cliffs, N.J.: Prentice-Hall, 1961), pp. 39–54.

32 For documentation, see Szasz, T. S.: *Law, Liberty, and Psychiatry: An Inquiry into the Social Uses of Mental Health Practices* (New York: Macmillan, 1963); *Psychiatric Justice* (New York: Macmillan, 1965).

33 Elkins, S. M.: *Slavery: A Problem in American Institutional and Intellectual Life* [1959] (New York: Universal Library, 1963), p. 10.

34 See, for example, Linn, L.: *A Handbook of Hospital Psychiatry* (New York: International Universities Press, 1955), pp. 420–22; Braceland, F. J.: Statement, in *Constitutional Rights of the Mentally Ill* (Washington, D. C.: U. S. Government Printing Office, 1961), pp. 63–74; Rankin, R. S. and Dallmayr, W. B.: "Rights of Patients in Mental Hospitals," in *Constitutional Rights of the Mentally Ill, supra,* pp. 329–70.

35 Davis, op. cit., p. 69.

36 Braceland, op. cit., p. 71.

37 Solomon, P.: "The burden of responsibility in suicide." *JAMA,* 199:321–24 (Jan. 30), 1967.

38 Halleck, S. L.: *Psychiatry and the Dilemmas of Crime* (New York: Harper & Row, 1967), p. 230.

39 Tarsis, V.: *Ward 7: An Autobiographical Novel* (London and Glasgow: Collins and Harvill, 1965), p. 62.

40 Elkins, op. cit., p. 190.

41 Davis, op. cit., p. 186.

42 Ibid., p. 190.

43 Ewalt, J.: Statement, in *Constitutional Rights of the Mentally Ill, supra,* pp. 74–89, p. 75.

44 Braceland, op. cit., p. 64.

45 Elkins, op. cit., p. 216.

46 Ibid.

47 Guttmacher, M.: Statement, in *Constitutional Rights of the Mentally Ill, supra,* pp. 143–60, 156.

On the Justifications for Civil Commitment

Joseph M. Livermore, Carl P. Malmquist, and Paul E. Meehl

Joseph M. Livermore is professor of law at the University of Arizona College of Law. He is the author of *Minnesota Evidence* (1968) and of articles such as "On Uses of a Competitor's Trademark." Carl P. Malmquist is associate professor of psychology and child development at the University of Minnesota. He is also the psychiatric consultant for Hennepin County (Minnesota) District Courts. Malmquist is the author of *Youth: Development and Delinquency* (1977) and "Can the Committed Patient Refuse Psychotherapy?" Paul E. Meehl is professor of psychology in the college of liberal arts and professor of clinical psychology in the department of psychiatry in the medical school at the University of Minnesota. He is the author of *Clinical vs. Statistical Prediction: A Theoretical Analysis and a Review of the Evidence* (1954) and *Psychodiagnosis: Selected Papers* (1973).

Livermore, Malmquist, and Meehl explore the possible philosophical justifications for civil commitment procedures, which deprive the mentally ill of liberty. Noting the elasticity of the concept of mental illness, the authors argue that mental illness should at best be a necessary rather than a sufficient condition for civil commitment. Livermore, Malmquist, and Meehl discuss the problems raised by attempts to justify such commitments on the basis of (1) dangerousness to others, (2) dangerousness to self, and (3) the need for care, custody, or treatment. They reject the usual justifications given because these rest on premises which are either false or too broad to support *existing* procedures. Unlike Szasz, they do not reject all involuntary civil commitments. Rather, they present a range of cases to bring out the kinds of situations where civil commitment might be justified.

Involuntary confinement is the most serious deprivation of individual liberty that a society may impose. The philosophical justifications for such a deprivation by means of the criminal process have been thoroughly explored. No such intellectual effort has been directed at providing justifications for societal use of civil commitment procedures.

When certain acts are forbidden by the criminal law, we are relatively comfortable in imprisoning those who have engaged in such acts. We say that the imprisonment of the offender will serve as an example to others and thus deter them from violating the law. If we even stop to consider the morality of depriving one man of his liberty in order to serve other social ends, we usually are able to allay anxiety by referring to the need to incarcerate to protect society from further criminal acts or the need to reform the criminal. When driven to it, at last, we admit that our willingness to permit such confinement rests on the notion that the criminal has justified it by his crime. Eligibility for social tinkering based on guilt, retributive though it may be, has so far satisfied our moral sensibilities.

It is, we believe, reasonably clear that the system could not be justified were the concept of guilt not part of our moral equipment. Would we be comfortable with a system in which any man could go to jail if by so doing he would serve an overriding social purpose? The normal aversion to punishment by example, with its affront to the principle of equality, suggests that we would not. Conversely, could we abide a rule that only those men would be punished whose imprisonment would further important social ends? Again, the thought of vastly different treatment for those equally culpable would make us uneasy.

Similarly, if we chose to justify incarceration as a means of isolating a group quite likely to engage in acts dangerous to others, we would, without the justification of guilt, have difficulty explaining why other groups, equally or more dangerous in terms of actuarial data, are left free. By combining background environmental data, we can identify categories of persons in which we can say that fifty to eighty per cent will engage in criminal activity within a short period of time. If social protection is a sufficient justification for incarceration, this group should be confined as are those criminals who are likely to sin again.

The same argument applies when rehabilitative considerations are taken into account. Most, if not all of us could probably benefit from some understanding of psychological rewiring. Even on the assumption that confinement should be required only in those cases where antisocial acts may thereby be averted, it is not at all clear that criminals are the most eligible for such treatment. In addition, most people would bridle at the proposition that the state could tamper with their minds whenever it seemed actuarially sound to do so.

Fortunately, we can by reason of his guilt distinguish the criminal from others whom we are loathe to confine. He voluntarily flouted society's commands with an awareness of the consequences. Consequently, he may serve utilitarian purposes without causing his imprisoners any moral twinge.

This same sort of analysis is not available once we move beyond the arena of the criminal law. When people are confined by civil process, we cannot point to their guilt as a basis for differentiating them from others. What can we point to?

The common distinguishing factor in civil commitment is aberrance. Before we commit a person we demand either that he act or think differently than we believe he should. Whether our label be inebriate, addict, psychopath, delinquent, or mentally diseased, the core concept is deviation from norms.[1] Our frequently expressed value of individual autonomy, however, renders us unable to express those norms, however deeply they may be felt, in criminal proscriptions. We could not bring ourselves to outlaw senility, or manic behavior, or strange desires. Not only would this violate the common feeling that one is not a criminal if he is powerless to avoid the crime, but it might also reach conduct that most of us feel we have a right to engage in. When a man squanders his savings in a hypomanic

episode, we may say, because of our own beliefs, that he is "crazy," but we will not say that only reasonable purchases are allowed on pain of criminal punishment. We are not yet willing to legislate directly the Calvinist ideal.

What we are not willing to legislate, however, we have been willing to practice through the commitment process. That process has been used to reach two classes of persons, those who are mentally ill and dangerous to themselves or others and those who are mentally ill and in need of care, custody or treatment. While those terms seem reasonably clear, on analysis that clarity evaporates.

One need only glance at the diagnostic manual of the American Psychiatric Association to learn what an elastic concept mental illness is. It ranges from the massive functional inhibition characteristic of one form of catatonic schizophrenia to those seemingly slight aberrancies associated with an emotionally unstable personality, but which are so close to conduct in which we all engage as to define the entire continuum involved. Obviously, the definition of mental illness is left largely to the user and is dependent upon the norms of adjustment that he employs. Usually the use of the phrase "mental illness" effectively masks the actual norms being applied. And, because of the unavoidably ambiguous generalities in which the American Psychiatric Association describes its diagnostic categories, the diagnostician has the ability to shoehorn into the mentally diseased class almost any person he wishes, for whatever reason, to put there.

All this suggests that the concept of mental illness must be limited in the field of civil commitment to a necessary rather than a sufficient condition for commitment. While the term has its uses, it is devoid of that purposive content that a touchstone in the law ought to have. Its breadth of meaning makes for such difficulty of analysis that it answers no question that the law might wish to ask.

DANGEROUSNESS TO OTHERS

The element of dangerousness to others has, at least in practice, been similarly illusive. As Professors Goldstein and Katz have observed, such a test, at a minimum, calls for a determination both of what acts are dangerous and how probable it is that such acts will occur. The first question suggests to a criminal lawyer the answer: crimes involving a serious risk of physical or psychical harm to another. Murder, arson and rape are the obvious examples. Even in criminal law, however, the notion of dangerousness can be much broader. If one believes that acts that have adverse effects on social interests are dangerous, and if one accepts as a generality that the criminal law is devoted to such acts, any crime can be considered dangerous. For example, speeding in a motor vehicle, although traditionally regarded as a minor crime, bears great risk to life and property, and thus may be viewed as a dangerous act. Dangerousness can bear an even more extensive definition as well. An act may be considered dangerous if it is offensive or disquieting to others. Thus, the man who walks the street repeating, in a loud monotone, "fuck, fuck, fuck," is going to wound many sensibilities even if he does not violate the criminal law. Other examples would be the man, found in most cities, striding about town lecturing at the top of his lungs, or the similar character in San Francisco who spends his time shadow boxing in public. If such people are dangerous, it is not because they threaten physical harm but because we are made uncomfortable when we see aberrancies. And, of course, if dangerousness is so defined, it is at least as broad a concept as mental illness. The cases are unfortunately silent about what meaning the concept of danger bears in the commitment process.

Assuming that dangerousness can be defined, the problem of predictability still remains. For the man who can find sexual release only in setting fires, one may confidently predict that dangerous acts will occur. For the typical mentally aberrant individual, though, the matter of prediction is not susceptible of answer. However nervous a full-blown paranoiac may make us, there are no actuarial data indicating that he is more likely to commit a crime than any normal person. Should he engage in criminal activity, his paranoia would almost certainly be part of the etiology. But on a predictive basis we have, as yet, nothing substantial to rely on.

Even if such information were available, it is improbable that it would indicate that the likelihood of crime within a group of individuals with any particular psychosis would be any greater than that to be expected in a normal community cross-section. Surely the degree of probability would not be as high as that in certain classes of convicted criminals after their release from prison or that in certain classes of persons having particular sociological or psychological characteristics.

DANGEROUSNESS TO SELF

The concept of "dangerousness to self" raises similar problems. The initial thought suggested by the phrase is the risk of suicide. But again it can be broadened to include physical or mental harm from an inability to take care of one's self, loss of assets from foolish expenditures, or even loss of social standing or reputation from behaving peculiarly in the presence of others. Again, if read very broadly this concept becomes synonymous with that of mental illness. And, of course, reliable prediction is equally impossible.

IN NEED OF CARE, CUSTODY, OR TREATMENT

The notion of necessity of care or treatment provides no additional limitation beyond those imposed by the concepts already discussed. One who is diagnosably mentally ill is, almost by definition, in need of care or treatment. Surely the diagnostician reaching the first conclusion would reach the second as well. And, if a man is dangerous, then presumably he is in need of custody. The problem, of course, lies with the word "need." If it is defined strictly as, for example, "cannot live without," then a real limitation on involuntary commitment is created. In normal usage, however, it is usually equated with "desirable," and the only boundary on loss of freedom is the value structure of the expert witness.

It is difficult to identify the reasons that lie behind incarceration of the mentally ill. Three seem to be paramount:

1 It is thought desirable to restrain those people who may be dangerous;

2 It is thought desirable to banish those who are a nuisance to others;

3. It is thought humanitarian to attempt to restore to normality and productivity those who are not now normal and productive.

Each of these goals has social appeal, but each also creates analytic difficulty.

As already mentioned, in order to understand the concept of danger one must determine what acts are dangerous and how likely is it that they will occur. There is a ready inclination to believe that experts in the behavioral sciences will be able to identify those members of society who will kill, rape, or burn. The fact is, however, that such identification cannot presently be accomplished. First, our growing insistence on privacy will, in all but a few cases, deny the expert access to the data necessary to the task of finding potential killers. Second, and of much greater importance, even if the data were available it is unlikely that a test could be devised that would be precise enough to identify only those individuals who are dangerous. Since serious criminal conduct has a low incidence in society, and since any test must be applied to a very large group of people, the necessary result is that in order to isolate those who will kill it is also necessary to incarcerate many who will not. Assume that one person out of a thousand will kill. Assume also that an exceptionally accurate test is created which differentiates with ninety-five percent effectiveness those who will kill from those who will not. If 100,000 people were tested, out of the 100 who would kill 95 would be isolated. Unfortunately, out of the 99,900 who would not kill, 4,995 people would also be isolated as potential killers.[2] In these circumstances, it is clear that we could not justify incarcerating all 5,090 people. If, in the criminal law, it is better that ten guilty men go free than that one innocent man suffer, how can we say in the civil commitment area that it is better that fifty-four harmless people be incarcerated lest one dangerous man be free?

The fact is that without any attempt at justification we have been willing to do just this to one disadvantaged class, the mentally ill. This practice must rest on the common supposition that mental illness makes a man more likely to commit a crime. While there may be some truth in this, there is much more error. Any phrase that encompasses as many diverse concepts as does the term "mental illness" is necessarily imprecise. While the fact of paranoid personality might be of significance in determining a heightened probability of killing, the fact of hebephrenic schizophrenia probably would not. Yet both fit under the umbrella of mental illness.

Even worse, we have been making assessments of potential danger on the basis of nothing as precise as the psychometric test hypothesized. Were we to ignore the fact that no definition of dangerous acts has been agreed upon, our standards of prediction have still been horribly imprecise. On the armchair assumption

that paranoids are dangerous, we have tended to play safe and incarcerate them all. Assume that the incidence of killing among paranoids is five times as great as among the normal population. If we use paranoia as a basis for incarceration we would commit 199 non-killers in order to protect ourselves from one killer. It is simply impossible to justify any commitment scheme so premised. And the fact that assessments of dangerousness are often made clinically by a psychiatrist, rather than psychometrically and statistically, adds little if anything to their accuracy.

We do not mean to suggest that dangerousness is not a proper matter of legal concern. We do suggest, however, that limiting its application to the mentally ill is both factually and philosophically unjustifiable. As we have tried to demonstrate, the presence of mental illness is of limited use in determining potentially dangerous individuals. Even when it is of evidentiary value, it serves to isolate too many harmless people. What is of greatest concern, however, is that the tools of prediction are used with only an isolated class of people. We have alluded before to the fact that it is possible to identify, on the basis of sociological data, groups of people wherein it is possible to predict that fifty to eighty per cent will engage in criminal or delinquent conduct. And, it is probable that more such classes could be identified if we were willing to subject the whole population to the various tests and clinical examinations that we now impose only on those asserted to be mentally ill. Since it is perfectly obvious that society would not consent to a wholesale invasion of privacy of this sort and would not act on the data if they were available, we can conceive of no satisfactory justification for this treatment of the mentally ill.

One possible argument for different treatment can be made in terms of the concept of responsibility. We demonstrate our belief in individual responsibility by refusing to incarcerate save for failure to make a responsible decision. Thus, we do not incarcerate a group, eighty per cent of whom will engage in criminal conduct, until those eighty per cent have demonstrated their lack of responsibility—and even then, the rest of the group remains free. The mentally diseased, so the argument would run, may be viewed prospectively rather than retrospectively because for them responsibility is an illusory concept. We do not promote responsibility by allowing the dangerous act to occur since, when it does, we will not treat the actor as responsible. One way of responding to this is to observe that criminal responsibility and mental illness are not synonymous, and that if incarceration is to be justified on the basis of irresponsibility, only those mentally ill who will probably, as a matter of prediction, commit a crime for which they will not be held responsible should be committed. A more fundamental response is to inquire whether susceptibility to criminal punishment is reasonably related to any social purpose. Granted that there is a gain in social awareness of individual responsibility by not incarcerating the responsible in advance of their crime, it does not necessarily follow that it is sufficiently great to warrant the markedly different treatment of the responsible and the irresponsible.

The other possible justification for the existing differential is that the mentally diseased are amenable to treatment. We shall explore the ramifications of this at a later point. It is sufficient now to observe that there is no reason to believe that the mentally well, but statistically dangerous, individual is any less amenable to treatment, though that treatment would undoubtedly take a different form.

Another basis probably underlying our commitment laws is the notion that it is necessary to segregate the unduly burdensome and the social nuisance. Two cases typify this situation. This first is the senile patient whose family asserts inability to provide suitable care. At this juncture, assuming that the family could put the person on the street where he would be unable to fend for himself, society must act to avoid the unpleasantness associated with public disregard of helplessness. This caretaking function cannot be avoided. Its performance, however, is a demonstration of the psychological truth that we can bear that which is kept from our attention. Most of us profess to believe that there is an individual moral duty to take care of a senile parent, a paranoid wife, or a disturbed child. Most of us also resent the bother such care creates. By allowing society to perform this duty, masked in medical terminology, but frequently amounting in fact to what one court has described as "warehousing," we can avoid facing painful issues.

The second case is the one in which the mentally ill individual is simply a nuisance, as when he insists on sharing his paranoid delusions or hallucinations with us. For reasons that are unclear, most of us are extremely uncomfortable in the presence of an aberrant individual, whether or not we owe him any duty, and whether or not he is in fact a danger to us in any defensible use of that concept. Our comfort, in short,

depends on his banishment, and yet that comfort is equally dependent on a repression of any consciousness of the reason for his banishment. It is possible, of course, to put this in utilitarian terms. Given our disquietude, is not the utility of confinement greater than the utility of liberty? Perhaps so, but the assertions either that we will act most reasonably if we repress thinking about why we are acting or, worse yet, that our legislators will bear this knowledge for us in order to preserve our psychic ease make us even more uncomfortable than the thought that we may have to look mental aberrance in the eye.

Again, we do not wish to suggest that either burden or bother is an inappropriate consideration in the commitment process. What we do want to make clear is that when it is a consideration it ought to be advertently so. Only in that way can intelligent decisions about care, custody, and treatment be made.

The final probable basis for civil commitment has both humanitarian and utilitarian overtones. When faced with an obviously aberrant person, we know, or we think we know, that he would be "happier" if he were as we are. We believe that no one would want to be a misfit in society. From the very best of motives, then, we wish to fix him. It is difficult to deal with this feeling since it rests on the unverifiable assumption that the aberrant person, if he saw himself as we see him, would choose to be different than he is. But since he cannot be as we, and we cannot be as he, there is simply no way to judge the predicate for the assertion.

Our libertarian views usually lead us to assert that treatment cannot be forced on anyone unless the alternative is very great social harm. Thus while we will require smallpox vaccinations and the segregation of contagious tuberculars, we will not ordinarily require bed rest for the common cold, or a coronary, or even require a pregnant woman to eat in accordance with a medically approved diet. Requiring treatment whenever it seemed medically sound to do so would have utilitarian virtues. Presumably, if death or serious incapacitation could thereby be avoided society would have less worry about unsupported families, motherless children, or individuals no longer able to support themselves. Similarly, if the reasoning were pursued, we could insure that the exceptionally able, such as concert violinists, distinguished scholars, and inspiring leaders would continue to benefit society. Nonetheless, only rarely does society require such treatment. Not only does it offend common notions of bodily integrity and individual autonomy, but it also raises those issues of value judgment which, if not insoluble, are at least discomforting. For example, is the treatment and cure of the mentally ill individual of more benefit to society than the liberty of which he is deprived and the principle (lost, or tarnished) that no one should assert the right to control another's beliefs and responses absent compelling social danger?

The reason traditionally assigned for forcing treatment on the mentally ill while making it voluntary for other afflicted persons is that the mentally ill are incapable of making a rational judgment whether they need or desire such help. As with every similar statement, this depends on what kind of mental illness is present. It is likely that a pederast understands that society views him as sick, that certain kinds of psychiatric treatment may "cure" him, and that such treatment is available in certain mental institutions. It is also not unlikely that he will, in these circumstances, decide to forego treatment, at least if such treatment requires incarceration. To say that the pederast lacks insight into his condition and therefore is unable to intelligently decide whether or not to seek treatment is to hide our real judgment that he ought to be fixed, like it or not. It is true that some mentally ill people may be unable to comprehend a diagnosis and, in these instances, forced treatment may be more appropriate. But this group is a small proportion of the total committable population. Most understand what the clinician is saying though they often disagree with his view.

We have tried to show that the common justifications for the commitment process rest on premises that are either false or too broad to support present practices. This obviously raises the question of alternatives. Professor Ehrenzweig has suggested in another context that the definition of mental illness ought to be tailored to the specific social purpose to be furthered in the context in question. That is what we propose here.

Returning to the first of our considerations supporting commitment, we suggest that before a man can be committed as dangerous it must be shown that the probabilities are very great that he will commit a dangerous act. Just how great the probabilities need be will depend on two things: how serious the probable dangerous act is and how likely it is that the mental condition can be changed by treatment. A series of hypotheticals will indicate how we believe this calculus ought to be applied.

Case 1: A man with classic paranoia exhibits in clinical interview a fixed belief that his wife is attempting to poison him. He calmly states that on release he will be forced to kill her in self-defense. The experts agree that his condition is untreatable. Assume that statistical data indicate an eighty per cent probability that homicide will occur. If society will accept as a general rule of commitment, whether or not mental illness is present, that an eighty per cent probability of homicide is sufficient to incarcerate, then this man may be incarcerated. In order to do this, of course, we must be willing to lock up twenty people out of 100 who will not commit homicide.

Case 2: Assume the same condition with only a forty per cent probability of homicide. We do not know whether, if the condition is untreatable, commitment is justified in these circumstances. If lifetime commitment is required because the probabilities are constant, we doubt that the justification would exist. Our own value structure would not allow us to permanently incarcerate sixty harmless individuals in order to prevent forty homicides. On the other hand, if incarceration for a year would reduce the probability to ten per cent, then perhaps it is justified. Similarly, if treatment over the course of two or three years would substantially reduce the probability, then commitment might be thought proper.

Case 3: A man who compulsively engages in acts of indecent exposure has been diagnosed as having a sociopathic personality disturbance. The probability is eighty per cent that he will again expose himself. Even if this condition is untreatable, we would be disinclined to commit. In our view, this conduct is not sufficiently serious to warrant extended confinement. For that reason, we would allow confinement only if "cure" were relatively quick and certain.

The last case probably is more properly one of nuisance than of danger. The effects of such conduct are offensive and irritating but it is unlikely that they include long-term physical or psychical harm. That does not mean, however, that society has no interest in protecting its members from such upset. Again, the question is one of alternatives. Much nuisance behavior is subject to the control of the criminal law or of less formal social restraints. In mental institutions patients learn that certain behavior or the recounting of delusions or hallucinations will be met with disapproval. Accordingly, they refrain from such behavior or conversation. There is no reason to believe that societal disapproval in the form of criminal proscriptions or of less formal sanctions will be less effective as a deterrent. And, from our standpoint, the liberty of many mentally ill individuals is worth far more than the avoidance of minor nuisances in society.

Case 4: A person afflicted with schizophrenia walks about town making wild gestures and talking incessantly. Those who view him are uncomfortable but not endangered. We doubt that commitment is appropriate even though it would promote the psychic ease of many people. Arguably we would all be happier if our favorite bogey man, whether James Hoffa, Rap Brown, Mario Savio, or some other, were incarcerated. Most of us would be outraged if any of these men were committed on such a theory. If we cannot justify such a commitment in these cases, we doubt that it is any more justifiable when social anxiety is a consequence of seeing mentally ill individuals. While it might be proper to commit if speedy cure were possible, such cures are, as a matter of fact, unavailable. Moreover, we have some difficulty distinguishing the prevention of psychic upset based on cure of the mentally ill and prevention based on neutralizing other upsetting behavior.

The next justification of commitment is more solid, though it too presents the question of the necessity of utilizing less burdensome alternatives. This is the rationale of care for the person who is unable to care for himself and who has no one else to provide care for him. As we suggested earlier, such care must be provided if we are unwilling to allow people to die in the streets.

Case 5: An elderly woman with cerebro-vascular disease and accompanying cerebral impairment has the tendency to leave her home, to become lost, and then to wander helplessly about until someone aids her. At other times she is perfectly able to go shopping or visit friends. She has no relatives who will care for her in the sense that they will prevent her from wandering or will find her when she has become lost. In some ways, this is another case of a public

nuisance and it may well be that it is impossible to find a justification for incarcerating this woman. On the other hand, to allow this woman to die from exposure on one of her forays is as disquieting as the loss of her freedom. Since her condition is untreatable, provision of treatment offers no justification for confinement. It might be justifiable to exercise some supervision over her, but surely that justification will not support total incarceration. In these circumstances, we believe that if the state wishes to intervene it must do so in some way that does not result in a total loss of freedom. The desire to help ought not to take the form of simple jailing.

Case 6: A schizophrenic woman is causing such an upset in her family that her husband petitions for commitment. It is clear that the presence of this woman in the family is having an adverse effect on the children. Her husband is simply unwilling to allow the situation to continue. The alternatives here are all unpleasant to contemplate. If the husband gets a divorce and custody, he may accomplish his end. But the social opprobrium attaching to that solution makes it unlikely. The question, then, is whether the state should provide a socially acceptable alternative. If that alternative is her loss of freedom, we find it hard to justify. Assuming that the condition is untreatable, that the woman is not dangerous, and that her real sin is her capacity to disrupt, it is almost incomprehensible that she should be subject to a substantial period of incarceration. Yet that is what it has meant. Presumably, in order to isolate the woman from her family, it is necessary to transport her to a location where she will no longer bother her family. Then, if she is able to support herself she could have complete freedom. If she is not able, the state will have to provide care. That care, of course, need not involve a total deprivation of freedom.

The final justification for commitment—the need to treat—is in many ways the most difficult to deal with. As we have said before, society has not traditionally required treatment of treatable diseases even though most people would agree that it was "crazy" for the diseased person not to seek treatment. The problem has been complicated by the fact that religious beliefs against certain forms of treatment often are present and by the fact that most cases of stubborn refusal to accept treatment never come into public view. There is, however, a competing analogy that suggests that mandatory treatment may sometimes be appropriate.

Without going into unnecessary detail, we think it can be said that one of the reasons society requires compulsory education is that it believes a certain minimum amount of socialization is necessary for everyone lest they be an economic burden or a personal nuisance. That principle can also be used to support mandatory psychiatric rewiring if the individual to be refurbished is in fact a burden or nuisance and can be fixed. The difficulty, of course, lies in the extent to which the principle can be carried. To take a mild example outside the field of mental disease, assume an unemployable individual who is unable to support his large and growing family. Could society incarcerate him until he had satisfactorily acquired an employable skill? In the context of mental disease, then, can society demand that an individual obtain an employable psyche?

Case 7: An individual has been suffering from paranoid schizophrenia for several years without remission and has lost his job because of his behavior. He is divorced, but he is able to support himself from prior savings. He is not dangerous, and if he is committed it is unlikely that he will be cured since the recovery rates from such long-term schizophrenia are very low. In addition, the availability of treatment in a state mental institution is problematic. We doubt that he can justifiably be committed. If treatment is an adequate basis for confinement, it surely ceases to be so either when the illness is untreatable or when treatment is in fact not given or given in grossly insufficient amounts. No other basis for commitment being present, it is unjustifiable.

Case 8: A distinguished law school professor, known for a series of brilliant articles, is suffering from an involutional depression. His scholarship has dried up, and, while he is still able to teach, the spark is gone and his classes have become extremely depressing. There is a chance, though probably not more than twenty-five per cent, that he will commit suicide. He has been told that he would recover his old élan if he were subjected to a series of electroshock treatments but this he has refused to do. In fact, in years past when he was teaching a course in law and psychology, he stated that if he ever became depressed he wanted it known that before the onset of depression he explicitly rejected such treatment.

Should he be compelled to undergo treatment? The arguments of social utility would suggest that he should. Yet we are unable to dislodge the notion that potential added productivity is not a license for tampering.

Case 9: A woman suffers from a severe psychotic depression resulting in an ability to do little more than weep. Again shock treatment is recommended with a reasonable prospect of a rapid recovery. The woman rejects the suggestion saying that nothing can make her a worthy member of society. She is, she claims, beyond help or salvation. It is possible to distinguish this from the preceding case on the ground that her delusional thought processes prevent her from recognizing the desirability of treatment. But any distinction based on a proposed patient's insight into her condition will probably be administered on the assumption that any time desirable treatment is refused, insight is necessarily lacking. And that, of course, would destroy the distinction.

These cases suggest that the power to compel treatment is one that rarely ought to be exercised. We are unable to construct a rationale that will not as well justify remolding too many people to match predominant ideas of the shape of the ideal psyche. We recognize, of course, that we are exhibiting a parade of horrors. In this instance, however, we believe such reference justified. The ease with which one can be classified as less than mentally healthy, and the difficulty in distinguishing degrees of sickness, make us doubt the ability of anyone to judge when the line between minimum socialization and aesthetically pleasing acculturation has been passed. Regardless of our views, however, it seems clear that if society chooses to continue to exercise the power to compel treatment, it ought to do so with constant awareness of the threat to autonomy thus posed.

Different considerations are present when commitment is not based on the need to treat. If one is committed as dangerous, or as a nuisance, or as unable to care for oneself, and treatment can cure this condition, then it is easier to strike the balance between deprivation of liberty and the right to refuse treatment in favor of compulsory treatment. If told that this is the price of freedom, the patient may accede; if he prefers confinement to treatment, perhaps the state ought not to override his wishes. But at least in this situation the question is ethically a close one.

The difficulty with present commitment procedures is that they tend to justify all commitments in terms that are appropriate only to some, and to prescribe forms of treatment that are necessary in only some cases. Thus, while danger stemming from mental illness may be a proper basis for commitment, it does not follow that all mentally ill are dangerous, or that the standards of danger should be markedly less rigid in cases of mental illness. Similarly, because mentally ill people may be a nuisance and some means of preventing such nuisance must be found, it does not follow that nuisance commitments ought to involve the same restraints as commitments based upon potential danger. Finally, because treatment is humanitarian when applied to those confined for danger, nuisance, or care, does not in itself suggest that treatment can be applied whenever administrators believe it proper or humane to do so.

We recognize that many people will not agree with the manner in which we have drawn the balance in individual cases. We hope that few will disagree that the balance must be drawn. We suggest, therefore, that in each case of proposed commitment, the following questions be asked:

I What social purpose will be served by commitment?

  A If protection from potential danger, what dangerous acts are threatened? How likely are they to occur? How long will the individual have to be confined before time or treatment will eliminate or reduce the danger so that he may be released?

  B If protection from nuisance, how onerous is the nuisance in fact? Ought that to justify loss of freedom? If it should, how long will confinement last before time or treatment will eliminate or reduce the risk of nuisance so that release may occur?

  C If the need for care, is care in fact necessary? If so, how long will confinement last before time or treatment will eliminate the need for care so that release may occur?

II Can the social interest be served by means less restrictive than total confinement?

III Whatever standard is applied, is it one that can comfortably be applied to all members of society, mentally ill or healthy?

IV If confinement is justified only because it is believed that it will be of short term for treatment, is the illness in fact treatable? If it is, will appropriate treatment in fact be given?

If these questions are asked—and we view it as the duty of the attorney for the potential patient to insure that they are—then more intelligent commitment practices may follow.

NOTES

1 The concept "abnormal" or "aberrant" is sorely in need of more thorough logical analysis than it has, to our knowledge, as yet received. It seems fairly clear that several components—perhaps even utterly distinct kinds of meaning—can be discerned in the current usage of medicine and social science. The most objective meaning is the purely statistical one, in which "abnormal" designates deviation from the (statistical) "norm" of a specified biological or social population of organisms. Whether an individual specimen, or bit of behavior, is abnormal in this sense is readily ascertained by adequate sampling methods plus a more or less arbitrary choice of cutting score (*e.g.,* found in less than 1 in 100 cases). But for legal purposes this purely statistical criterion does not suffice, because the *kind* and *direction* of statistical deviation from population norms, as well as the *amount* of deviation which threatens a protected social interest sufficiently to justify legal coercion, are questions not answerable by statistics alone. Thus, anyone who has an IQ of 180, or possesses absolute pitch, or is color-blind, is statistically abnormal but hardly rendered thereby a candidate for incarceration, mandatory treatment, or deprivation of the usual rights and powers of a "normal" individual. A second component in the concept of normality relies upon our (usually inchoate or implicit) notions of biological health, of a kind of proper functioning of the organism conceived as a teleological system of organs and capacities. From a biological viewpoint, it is not inconsistent to assert that a sizable proportion—conceivably a majority—of persons in a given population are abnormal or aberrant. Thus, if an epidemiologist found that 60% of the persons in a society were afflicted with

plague or avitaminosis, he would (quite correctly) reject an argument that "Since most of them have it, they are okay, *i.e.,* not pathological and not in need of treatment." It is admittedly easier to defend this non-statistical, biological-fitness approach in the domain of physical disease, but its application in the domain of behavior is fraught with difficulties. *See* W. SCHOFIELD, PSYCHOTHERAPY: THE PURCHASE OF FRIENDSHIP 12 (1964). Yet even here there is surely something to be said for it in extreme cases, as, for example, the statistically "normal" frigidity of middle-class Victorian women, which any modern sexologist would confidently consider a biological maladaptation in need of repair, induced by "unhealthy" social learnings. A third component invokes some sort of subjective norm, such as an aesthetic, religious, ethical, or political ideal or rule. Finally, whether an a priori concept of "optimal psychological adjustment" should be considered as yet a fourth meaning of normality, or instead subsumed under one or more of the preceding, is a difficult question. In any event, it is important to keep alert to hidden fallacies in legal and policy arguments that rely upon the notion of abnormality or aberration, such as subtle transitions from one of these criteria to another. It is especially tempting to the psychiatrist or clinical psychologist, given his usual clinical orientation, to slip unconsciously from the idea of "sickness," where treatment of a so-called "patient" is the model, to an application that justifies at most a statistical or ideological or psychological-adjustment usage of the word "norm." Probably the most pernicious error is committed by those who classify as "sick" behavior that is aberrant in *neither* a statistical sense *nor* in terms of any defensible biological or medical criterion, but solely on the basis of the clinician's personal ideology of mental health and interpersonal relationships. Examples might be the current psychiatric stereotype of what a good mother or a healthy family must be like, or the rejection as "perverse" of forms of sexual behavior that are not biologically harmful, are found in many infra-human mammals and in diverse human cultures, and have a high statistical frequency in our own society. *See generally* F. BEACH, SEXUAL BEHAVIOR IN ANIMALS AND MEN (1950); H. ELLIS, STUDIES IN THE PSYCHOLOGY OF SEX (1936); C. FORD & F. BEACH, PATTERNS OF SEXUAL BEHAVIOR (1951); A. KINSEY, W. POMEROY & C. MARTIN, SEXUAL BEHAVIOR IN THE HUMAN MALE (1948); A. KINSEY, W. POMEROY, C. MARTIN & P. GEBHARD, SEXUAL BEHAVIOR IN THE HUMAN FEMALE (1953); W. MASTERS & V. JOHNSON, HUMAN SEXUAL RESPONSE (1966); ELLIS, *What is "Normal" Sexual Behavior,* 28 SEXOLOGY 364 (1962); S. FREUD, *Three Essays on the Theory of Sexuality,* in 7 COMPLETE PSYCHOLOGICAL WORKS 123 (J. Strachey ed. 1962).

2 See Meehl & Rosen, *Antecedent Probability and the Efficiency of Psychometric Signs, Patterns, or Cutting Scores,* 52 PSYCHOLOGICAL BULL. 194 (1955); Rosen, *Detection of Suicidal Patients: An Example of Some Limitations in the Prediction of Infrequent Events,* 18 J. CONSULTING PSYCHOLOGY 397 (1954).

Sterilization and the Rights of the Mentally Retarded

Sterilizing the Mildly Mentally Retarded Without Their Consent

Robert Neville

Robert Neville is professor of philosophy and religious studies at the State University of New York at Stonybrook. His published articles include "Behavior Control: Ethical Analysis," "On the National Commission: A Puritan Critique of Consensus Ethics," "Philosophical Perspectives on Freedom of Inquiry," and "Pots and Black Kettles: A Philosopher's Perspective on Psychosurgery."

Neville maintains that it is sometimes morally permissible to sterilize mildly retarded individuals without their consent. He advances, and argues for, two claims: (1) Involuntary sterilization is in the best interests of some mildly mentally retarded persons because it will maximize their freedom to enjoy heterosexual activity; (2) Involuntary sterilization enhances the dignity of the mildly mentally retarded's position in the moral community insofar as it fosters and encourages their capacity for moral behavior.

Under certain specific circumstances it is morally permissible to sterilize some mildly mentally retarded people without their consent. At the outset of my argument I want to acknowledge that there is a grave difficulty, conceptually and empirically, in identifying which individuals belong to the relevant class of the mentally retarded. If that class is either conceptually so vague or empirically so confused that individuals who do not belong in it are inadvertently placed there, then it would be ethically impermissible to subject the class to involuntary sterilization. But let me put that difficulty aside until the end, and proceed with the argument as if we knew with acceptable exactness who the mildly mentally retarded are and which of them meet the specified requirements for sterilization.

THE HUMBLE ARGUMENT

My argument is really two arguments, one nested in the other. The first can be called the "humble argument" for involuntary sterilization, and it attempts to make the case that involuntary sterilization is in the best interest of certain mildly mentally retarded people. The second can be called the "philosophical argument," and it interprets the "humble argument" as a problem of rights and responsibilities, and attempts to show that involuntary sterilization in the right cases fosters rather than denies the membership of the mildly mentally retarded in the moral community.

The humble argument begins with certain observations. First, at least some mildly mentally retarded people are capable of engaging in and taking pleasure in heterosexual intercourse. My following remarks concern only this group; presumably those incapable of such intercourse would not need sterilization; those who, because of inexperience, do not know their capacities for pleasure should be viewed as capable of engaging in and taking pleasure from sexual activity until proved otherwise.

Second, for some mildly retarded people sexual activity is capable of being integrated into emotional aspects of affection, which can in turn contribute to positive, rewarding fulfillments of personal and social life. Freed from pregnancy, childbearing, and child rearing, an active heterosexual life can enrich the existence of some mildly mentally retarded people in much the way it can that of so-called "normals." Other things being equal, mildly mentally retarded people can benefit from and have a right to sexual activity and the social forms sexual relationships can involve, such as marriage. Capacities for marriage and long-lasting affection do not have to be clearly present, however, for the retarded to have a claim on sexual activity for purposes of pleasure alone.

Third, what begins to make the situation for the retarded "not equal" to that for "normals"? For mildly mentally retarded women the physiological and emotional changes that take place during pregnancy, and the violence of childbirth, are often experienced as disorienting and terrifying traumata. To the extent that a retarded man participates in the process, he too can be disoriented and lose his personal equilibrium.

Fourth, child rearing is sometimes beyond the capacities of mildly mentally retarded people precisely because of the characteristics of their retardation. The fact that child rearing is in practice also beyond the emotional capacities of many normal people should not obscure the overwhelming difficulty that it often poses for the retarded. Now it seems a prima facie argument that children ought not be conceived if there is not some reasonable expectation that they will receive minimal care. (Note that this is not an argument that conceived children should be aborted, which is more difficult to sustain.)

Fifth, mildly mentally retarded people have very great difficulty in managing impermanent forms of contraception. I am assuming that sterilization is the only permanent contraceptive; at least it cannot be reversed without medical help. Therefore, if these mildly mentally retarded people are to engage in sexual intercourse, which is otherwise desirable, without fear of the woman becoming pregnant, sterilization seems the only responsible contraceptive choice.

The humble argument, then, puts together these observations and says that the mildly mentally retarded people to whom these conditions apply should be sterilized so that they may enjoy heterosexual activity if they are so inclined. If they were not sterilized they would have to be prevented from engaging in sexual activity, or conditioned to homosexual or autoerotic sexual activity exclusively, which would be hard to guarantee. If their sex lives were not so controlled, they would run the risk of pregnancy with likely trauma for themselves and improper care for their child. If the retarded people do not or cannot give consent, then someone should have the standing to insist that the retarded be sterilized involuntarily.

An added consideration may be raised at the level of the humble argument. Who is to be sterilized, men, women, or both? The answer to that question clearly depends on the circumstances—whether the candidates are living in an institution, whether that institution is highly regulated or more informal in its management of personal associations; or, if the candidates are living outside institutions, in what kinds of settings. But generally the point of sterilization is to maximize the freedom of the mildly mentally retarded in sexual matters, and it is relevant to administer the procedure to any candidate meeting the conditions who stands to suffer harm or loss of freedom without it.

THE PHILOSOPHICAL ARGUMENT

The humble argument is a fairly straightforward, prudential argument operating within the limits and categories generally taken for granted when dealing with the mildly mentally retarded. The philosophical argument differs by calling into question the limits and categories otherwise taken for granted.

My philosophical argument consists of two main parts. The first considers the objection that sterilization of the mildly mentally retarded is wrong if done involuntarily because it would thereby deny the subjects their proper place in the moral community, treating them as means only and not ends in themselves. I shall argue on the contrary that the procedure enhances the dignity of their position in the moral community. The second part raises the very large problem of who decides about sterilization in the context of the mildly mentally retarded. Whereas some people might argue that no third party has sufficient standing in the matter to warrant doing violence to the candidate, I shall argue that it is the responsibility (a) of the moral community to establish policy creating such standing, and (b) of its properly delegated representatives to carry out the policy subject to a variety of checks.

Membership in the Moral Community

In that tradition of Western theory which takes most seriously the dignity of the human individual, the Kantian, one of the central concepts is that of the moral community. The dignity that should be accorded to each person as a human being consists in being regarded as a member of the moral community. Membership in that community means that a person is held to be morally responsible for his or her actions and life, and is to be held responsible by the rest of the community for assuming that responsibility.

With respect to human dignity, the grave danger is that a person will be treated as a thing rather than a responsible agent. This may happen when someone or some group treats a person merely as a means toward their own ends; this was Immanuel Kant's particular worry. It may also happen when the community simply fails to recognize the person as a moral agent, which happens most often when people's behavior is explained in such a way as to shift responsibility onto causes other than themselves. This objectification or alienation has been a primary worry of existentialists and many other social critics. In a strict philosophical sense (deriving from Aristotle), violence is done to people when they are prevented by external forces from fulfilling their basic or natural goals; one form of violence is to prevent someone from exercising membership in the moral community.

The mildly retarded suffer enough from their incapacities that special care should be taken to ensure them as full a membership in the moral community as possible. To sterilize them involuntarily, some people argue, is to do them unnecessary and dehumanizing violence. It is to regard them first of all as incapable of making a responsible decision about sterilization, thus ruling them out of membership in this respect; no defender of involuntary sterilization could deny this fact. It is, second, to regard their sex lives and childbearing and child rearing lives as so controlled by irresponsible impulses that the people may just as well be managed like objects in those areas of life. Third, it is quite possible and indeed likely, according to this position, that sterilization is sought for the mildly mentally retarded in order to make their custody easier, in which cases the people are treated in that respect as means only, not as ends in themselves.

In answer to these arguments let me point out three characteristics of the moral community. First, membership in the moral community is relative to the capacity for taking moral responsibility; there is no membership in the moral community under ordinary circumstances in the respects in which there is no capacity for taking responsibility. Second, most capacities for taking moral responsibility need to be developed; ordinary socialization develops most of them. The state of moral adulthood can be defined as being in possession of the capacity to take responsibility for developing the other capacities for responsible action that might be called upon. Third, a general moral imperative for any community is that its structures and practices foster the development of the capacities for responsible behavior wherever possible, and avoid hindering that development.

The idea of a moral community is an ideal that exists in pure form only in the imagination. When the ideal is applied to actual communities, it must be tailored to the fact that some people can have only partial memberships because of limited capacity for morally responsible behavior. Children, for example, only slowly take on the capacities for full membership in the moral community, and come to be treated as full members by degrees. Ordinarily we think of young children as full human beings because of their potential to develop into adults with full capacity for responsible action; when the coherence of their lives is extended over a reasonable life span, they can be expected to have moral capacities in due season.

Other people have other sorts of limited capacities for responsible behavior, such as those resulting from mental illness or senility, in which certain areas of life may involve severe incapacities for responsible behavior whereas others do not. In these cases, we usually regard people as fully human members of the moral community by according them the rights of responsibility where they do in fact have the capacity and by assigning to other people the responsibilities of proxy in areas of incapacity. The concept of a proxy, in the restrictive use of my distinction, is that of an agent who fits into the patient's overall moral responsibility as a sub-stitute in a certain area or under certain circumstances; the concept of proxy is used to maintain and support the notion that a person is a member of the moral community in circumstances where the direct capacity for that is lacking.

The case of the mildly mentally retarded is somewhat different from that of children and from the limited capacity of the mentally ill or senile. Like children, their capacities for development may be far greater than would have been imagined a few years ago. But unlike children, the pacing and sequencing of their development does not lead to emotional maturity at the same time they reach bodily maturity. For instance, the emotional and intellectual capacities to manage conventional birth control methods, to adjust to pregnancy, or to raise children do not develop by the time their physical development and their social peers among nonretarded people are ready for sexual activity.

Neither, sometimes, does the capacity to make informed decisions about sterilization. Indeed, if one were to say that heterosexual activity should be prevented among certain mildly mentally retarded people until such time as they develop the capacities for responsible behavior regarding pregnancy, or for consenting to surgical sterilization, the result is very likely to be the prevention of heterosexual activity altogether. As the humble argument says, this approach would amount to preventing the development of an important capacity for responsible behavior in areas that would be possible if an active sex life were possible, and would therefore be contrary to the imperative that the moral community foster such capacities.

Mildly mentally retarded people are like certain kinds of mentally ill people in that, from the adult perspective, there are certain areas of life in which they may lack capacities for responsible behavior and other areas where they may have them. But they are unlike mentally ill people in an important respect. A mentally ill person is conceived to be a member of the moral community because even though a proxy might exercise some of his or her responsibilities, he or she is believed to have the structure of a person who possesses the capacities for those responsibilities.

This belief is based on the fact, for instance, that the person once exercised those responsibilities before becoming ill. With the help of a proxy, almost as a prosthetic device, a mentally ill person can be presented to the moral community as a fully responsible moral agent. A mildly mentally retarded person, however, lacks the full personality structure that would come from having had the capacities for morally responsible behavior in the past. Although another person might make decisions in areas in which the retarded person is incapacitated, that would not strictly speaking be a case of proxy because the retarded person does not have a personality structured around the capacity for which a proxy might have to substitute.

Paternalism and proxy are models for enabling persons—children and the mentally ill, respectively—to enjoy membership in the moral community when they themselves have capacities for only partial membership. Another model is needed for the limited capacity of mildly mentally retarded people, one which I propose to call the model of "involuntary restrictive conditions." The model depicts mildly mentally retarded people as members of the moral community on the condition that they meet certain restrictions. Just as people with bad eyesight may be licensed to drive with the restriction that they wear glasses, so mildly mentally retarded people may be required to meet certain restrictions in order to be members of the moral community.

The analogy with driver's licenses is imperfect, however, because a person with bad eyesight can always choose not to drive and thereby not to need to wear glasses. But a person cannot choose to be in or out of the moral community; one is either in the position to be held responsible or one is not. Mildly mentally retarded people, and perhaps other groups, must meet the restrictions as conditions for being in the community. Therefore, from the standpoint of mildly mentally retarded people, the restrictive conditions are involuntary.

In a moment I shall urge that sterilization may be a proper involuntary restrictive condition for membership in the moral community for mildly mentally retarded people, subject to the limitations mentioned in connection with the humble argument. Before that, however, I want to address the question of who decides about involuntary restrictive conditions.

Who Should Decide?

Whether a certain restrictive condition does indeed foster the capacity for responsible moral behavior is an empirical question. The suggestion has been made that, with sterilization, mildly mentally retarded people will be able to engage in the kind of sex life that can develop their capacities for responsible behavior in various human relationships. Without sterilization they either would be prevented from having sex, and there-

fore would not develop those capacities for sexual affection and comradeship, or they would have sex and find themselves in such trouble that sexual affection and companionship would again be beyond them.

Furthermore, this empirical argument suggests that behavior having to do with sexual affection and companionship is more important than what mildly mentally retarded people might gain from opportunities for pregnancy, childbirth, and child rearing. The first "who decides" question is: Who decides whether that empirical argument is right? I suggest that this decision is a broad social one, which should be as informed as possible by experts in all the relevant fields, including both mental retardation and ethics. Clearly that argument will always be under redefinition and refinement.

But the next "who decides" question is: Who sets the policies regarding the treatment of the mildly mentally retarded? The answer is that the decision must come from the political process (again informed by relevant experts, and formulated by broad intellectual dialogue). The reason for locating the decision in the political process is that that is the only legitimate way by which individuals can be dealt with against their wills by due process. But there are two normative factors within the political process. One is that the process should conform to whatever political norm structures it—for instance, that of a representative democracy. According to this factor, what the political process decides about mildly mentally retarded people is legitimate if due political procedures have been followed. The other normative factor, however, is the demands of being a moral community, since the political process is the vehicle for actualizing those demands. A political decision is moral if it accords with what is required as a minimum for a moral community.

If the sterilization of mildly mentally retarded people, subject to appropriate limitations, does indeed foster important capacities for morally responsible behavior, and if a moral community ought to foster such capacities where possible, the warrant for politically deciding to sterilize certain mildly mentally retarded people is a moral one, not merely one of political legitimacy. There is a prima facie obligation to foster people's capacity for responsibility, since this capacity is the basis of their membership in the moral community. Paradoxically, to refrain from sterilization is to do them the violence of preventing them from participating in the moral community in one of the important respects of which they are capable.

Assuming that the political process results in a sterilization policy, by what procedures and what officers should decisions be made about particular candidates? That is a prudential political question that I shall not attempt to address. It is necessary at this point, however, to refer to what Hastings Center lore calls the "klutz factor," namely, that translating a theoretical moral argument into a public policy with significant effects is likely to lead to blunders and abuse. Because of the "klutz factor," prudence may very well dictate that policies should be far more conservative than morality otherwise would dictate.

For instance, as I stated in the "humble argument," the candidates for involuntary sterilization should include those who are capable of engaging in and taking pleasure in heterosexual activity, and yet who are incapable of taking responsibility for this activity in regards to pregnancy and the rest. This is a positive argument for sterilizing a class of people. In light of the "klutz factor," according to which the wrong people might be sent to the surgeon, perhaps it would be a prudent extra restriction to insist that candidates have demonstrated their need for sterilization by having already gotten into trouble by their sexual activity. I am not sure how to prevent such a restriction from being turned into a punitive measure against the retarded, however.

In general, with regard to all the "who decides" questions, it is important to make sure that the process of decision is self-critical and that opposition to any point of view is always funded as a corrective support.

UNIFYING THE ARGUMENTS

The philosophical side of the argument has intended to show that, contrary to the beliefs of some, involuntary sterilization does not involve treating the mildly mentally retarded as if they were not members of the moral community; rather, it acknowledges real incapacities and neutralizes their effects, thereby enabling other capacities to be realized. Furthermore, if sterilization does in some important ways lead to the development of greater capacities for responsibility, then it is part of the obligation a society owes to its potential members to provide it, subject to appropriate protections against abuse. If a mildly mentally retarded person lacks the capacity to give or withhold informed consent because he or she does not understand the subtle issues involved, then having the decision made by the society's agents is one of the involuntary restrictive conditions that might help place the person in the community. The society has the prima facie obligation to make that decision and should do so unless other considerations prevail.

The basic philosophical principle involved in this argument is that a moral community has the social responsibility to foster capacities for morally responsible behavior. It should do so paternalistically in the case of children; it should do so with appropriate proxies in the case of impaired capacities; and it should do so through the institution of involuntary restrictive conditions in the case of basic human capacities that are undevelopable only in a future that is too late for other valuable capacities to be developed that otherwise would have been possible.

This reasoning brings us back to the "humble argument." From a philosophical point of view, the humble argument might well be valid. At least it is not wrong by virtue of violating the canons of membership in the moral community; it does not deny human dignity. Indeed, the structure of the humble argument is to provide for the dignity of humane heterosexual relations by removing the unbearable complications of potential pregnancy. Whether its premises are valid is an empirical matter.

Let me close by dealing with the question of adequate diagnosis of the appropriate conditions for involuntary sterilization. Some structure must be worked out to determine appropriate subjects. We have seen that to do so requires two sorts of determinations. The first is whether informed and emotionally balanced decisions regarding sterilization are within the capacities of the candidates; if they are, then the candidates' word should be decisive, and if they prefer nonsterilization then society should respect that choice, whatever other compensatory restrictions it requires (such as no sexual activity). The second is whether the candidates are capable of heterosexual intercourse but not capable of coping adequately with pregnancy, childbirth, and child rearing. Not all mentally retarded people would fall into this category, and specific empirical criteria would have to be developed before a program of involuntary sterilization could be instituted.

If no mildly mentally retarded people can be found who fall into this category, then none of them should be involuntarily sterilized. The consequence of this requirement is that the validity of involuntary-sterilization programs depends upon the development of criteria and diagnostic skills sufficient to discriminate the proper category of people. There have been dis-agreements concerning whether the definitions of rele-vant characteristics, and diagnostic skills for discerning them, are sufficiently developed to provide a capacity for responsible programs. In the face of excessive modesty and caution it should be pointed out that people are now classified as mildly mentally retarded and subjected to programs intended to help them.

There is one final point. It is sometimes believed that there is a totalitarian impetus lurking in any social policy that might require people to be good—in this case, to submit to involuntary restrictive conditions in order to develop the amiable responsibilities of a decent sex life. I admit that there is a danger, but urge that it be guarded against by specific safeguards and internal critical mechanisms rather than by a blanket rejection. If people could be whole and fully responsible by themselves, society would have no positive responsibil-ities, only negative, peace-keeping ones. But because people become responsible through the grace of social life, and because some people need special help in exercising responsibility, society does have positive duties in developing the capacity for responsible moral behavior.

Reproductive Freedom and the Mentally Retarded

Rosalind Pollack Petchesky

Rosalind Pollack Petchesky is associate professor of political theory and women's studies at Ramapo College of New Jersey. Petchesky is the author of *Abortion and Woman's Choice: The State, Sexuality, and Reproductive Freedom (*1984). Her published articles include "Antiabortion, Antifeminism, and the Rise of the New Right."

Petchesky maintains that involuntary sterilization is morally wrong because it violates autonomy insofar as it robs individuals of reproductive freedom. She rejects Neville's contention that involuntary sterilization is in the best interests of some mildly retarded people. In her arguments, Petchesky challenges some of the empirical assumptions that supporters of involuntary sterilization make about the capacities of the retarded.

On March 8, 1979, the Department of Health, Educa-tion, and Welfare's rules governing federal financial participation in sterilization programs went into effect....[1] The regulations attempt to formulate a government policy for some difficult ethical questions: the meaning of "voluntary consent," the boundary between justifiable protection from abuse and unjustifi-able paternalism, and the rights of those judged "incompetent to decide...."

Surgical sterilization is a procedure that renders a person permanently unable to bear children. While the ethics of a biomedical procedure are never determined by technology alone, the virtually irreversible nature of surgical sterilization makes the choice a more drastic one than it might be otherwise. The question of "voluntariness" becomes more problematic and the conditions under which the decision is made—including the social, economic, institutional, and sexual con-ditions—require critical scrutiny.

A. WHAT IS REPRODUCTIVE FREEDOM?

Whether sterilization is moral or immoral in itself may be debated among theologians and ethicists. For the purposes of public policy and of this article, however, it is the *social arrangements* in which the procedure is embedded—the degree to which those arrangements allow for full participation and consciousness of the person being sterilized, and respond to that person's concrete social and biological needs—that are critical.

Reprinted with permission of the author and the publisher from *Hastings Center Report*, vol. 9 (October 1979), pp. 37–39.

The value of any method of contraception must be determined not only with regard to effectiveness and safety for the user (risks), but also with regard to *reproductive freedom* (autonomy). This means the degree to which the form and the social relations implied by a particular birth control method allow the user fully to understand its medical consequences, actively to control its use and nonuse, and consciously to integrate its use with thoughtful decisions about the meaning of sexuality and childbearing in her or his own life and in society. In this view, *sterilization abuse* (or any form of involuntary sterilization) is wrong because it subverts the need of a person to control her or his own body and to decide, in a fully informed and conscious way, what sort of interventions may be made into bodily processes, including the biological capacity to procreate....

Involuntary sterilization is an invasion of a woman's bodily integrity and identity for ends that usually accommodate the needs of others in disregard of her own needs, and that pre-empt her bodily self-determination. This is not to say that the need for control over one's body and reproductive capacities is absolute or exists in isolation from one's connections to other people. Individuals exist as social beings whose needs are defined by family, class, and racial as well as gender identities. Individual women exercise, limit, or lose their capacity to bear children in relation to others to whom they are responsible and who are responsible for them—sexual partners, parents, children, and wider communities beyond the family. But in the last analysis these social connections and responsibilities do not abrogate the necessity, in any morally acceptable system of "fertility control," to maximize the consciousness and participation of the individuals whose fertility is directly involved....

B. UNDER WHAT CONDITIONS IS VOLUNTARY CONSENT UNOBTAINABLE?

The DHEW has continued its moratorium on sterilizations of certain groups for whom voluntary consent may be problematic. These include minors (under age twenty-one), institutionalized persons, and persons declared mentally incompetent....

The moratorium on the mentally incompetent is based on two considerations. As with the moratorium on minors, the intention is to avoid *prima facie* judgments about the inherent capacities of mentally incompetent persons as a category and instead to assess the concrete conditions under which such persons live either in existing institutional or "deinstitutionalized" settings. First, the comments oppose sterilization of mentally incompetent persons on the ground that such persons may be "only temporarily incompetent," and that medical and legal judgments about the permanence of incompetence are susceptible to error and difficult to monitor. The "normalization," or "developmental," view of retardation as an often changeable, ameliorable, rather than a fixed, condition is implicit in this view. Second, and most important, the Department recognizes the danger that caretakers, including parents, may "be tempted to consent to sterilization" as a way of avoiding the more difficult responsibilities of sex education, training in other forms of birth control, or alternatives to sterilization, "irrespective of the 'best interests' of the individual," and that this "could lead to abuse."[2] While parents have tended to consider this conclusion a dismissal of their needs and concerns, it could be seen as an acknowledgment of existing social realities—for example, the lack of sufficient training and community support services for mentally incompetent individuals, which increases the burden on parents and pressures them to seek sterilization for their retarded child.

There is, however, a loophole in the prohibition on federally funded sterilizations of the mentally incompetent. According to the regulations, a mentally incompetent person could seek a court judgment and be separately "readjudicated competent for the purposes which include the ability to consent to sterilization."[3] (This, of course, does not apply to institutionalized persons under any circumstances.) In addition, the informed consent provisions require that the person securing consent and the physician performing the sterilization certify that "the individual to be sterilized appear mentally competent." After such certification and with court approval, a mentally incompetent person could be sterilized under federally funded programs without violating the regulations, since the sterilization would be legally voluntary....

C. CAPACITIES AND THE LIMITS OF VOLUNTARISM

Proposals for involuntary sterilization, particularly of the mentally incompetent, rest on the premise that such persons lack a capacity to exercise voluntary consent. For those who oppose the federal regulations, especially the moratorium, claims on behalf of the mentally incompetent have tended to dominate those on behalf of interested others, such as parents and potential children of the retarded. Clearly, the courts have been more favorably disposed to benevolent-protective arguments than to utilitarian ones where involuntary sterilization is concerned.[4] In both cases, however, the claims are supported by assumptions or assertions about the inherent characteristics of mentally incompetent persons as a group—their capacity to use alternative forms of birth control and to exercise consent, as well as their capacity to bear and raise children (these issues are often and unjustly conflated).

What are the real limits on the capacity of retarded persons to participate in their own reproductive and sexual decisions, and how should these limits be determined? A full discussion of this question lies outside the bounds of this article, but certain general issues may be considered without venturing into debates about the etiology of retardation. Two main points, widely accepted by specialists in developmental disabilities, need emphasis: first, the tremendous range in both functional and cognitive abilities represented by different degrees of retardation, and particularly within the largest classification, the "mildly retarded"; and, second, the necessity of taking "each case on its own merits rather than on generalized emotion or blanket legal solution."[5] While the American Association on Mental Deficiency's classifications of mental retardation into "mild," "moderate," "severe," and "profound" are based primarily on IQ levels, it is important to remember that IQ—for "retarded" as for "normal" persons—is only a crude measure at best; that the functional capacities of persons with similar IQ levels may differ greatly depending on the quality of training, services, and care to which they have had access; and that IQ levels themselves may be increased through environmental ameliorations. Indeed, as one geneticist of retardation points out, the retarded are in fact "simply those individuals at the tail end of the normal distribution of intelligence and differ quantitatively rather than qualitatively from the remainder of the population."[6] Functional variation is particularly broad among those approximately 5.25 million persons classified as "mildly retarded" (indicating an IQ range of 68 to 52 on the Stanford-Binet Scale), who in fact represent well over three-fourths of all the retarded. But even among those whose disabilities place them in the "moderate" or "severe" category, counselors working in the field attest that there are some who develop an ability not only to function sexually and to use contraceptives but to understand what they are doing.[7]

In contrast, state involuntary sterilization laws and opponents of the moratorium rely on a set of assumptions about the origins of retardation and the inherent incapacities of retarded persons as an abstract category. These assumptions commonly include the following: (1) that retardation is in most cases genetically determined;[8] (2) that most *mildly* retarded persons are "incapable of managing temporary forms of birth control,"[9] (3) that most mildly retarded persons are incapable of raising children, although they may be capable of marrying or otherwise engaging in sexual activity,[10] and (4) that the capacity of retarded persons to understand and consent freely to contraceptive planning, including sterilization, is negligible or nonexistent. The logical conclusion to such views was unceremoniously drawn in a recent newspaper column by George Will: "It is arguable that the right of the retarded to procreate...is problematic. And it is arguable that the state should—let us speak bluntly—license procreation."[11]

Leaving aside for a moment the issue of parenting capacity (and Will's "blunt" proposal), all of these assumptions are highly questionable, particularly when applied to the mildly retarded. First, there is little scientific basis for assuming a strict genetic determinism in most cases of mental disability, or that its incidence in the population could be "significantly" affected by preventing the retarded themselves from propagating. There are a few disorders that are known to be genetically transmitted, such as Down Syndrome and Tay-Sachs disease. In such cases, it is possible to use genetic counseling and diagnosis to prevent unwanted births. For the most part, however, it would seem truer to view mental disability as simply one tail of a bell-shaped curve. Like all variations in intelligence, its sources represent a complex set of interactions between genetic and environmental determinants; the genetic determinants of intellectual abilities cannot be isolated, since these are themselves affected by environmental conditions.[12] The evidence suggests, moreover, that a large proportion of mental deficiencies are associated with environmental conditions such as poverty, malnutrition, low birth weight, poor health care, or exposure to toxic substances such as lead or radiation, usually experienced prenatally and leading to permanent brain or central nervous system damage.[13] And these are the conditions, of course, that characterize the lives of lower-class and minority people, and many people working in hazardous occupations. Clearly it is cheaper and more politically expedient—particularly in a period of economic crisis and neoconservatism—to sterilize retarded persons rather than dealing with the economic, nutritional, medical, and environmental conditions that are known threats to healthy mental development. But such eugenics programs, based on totally faulty scientific premises, can never work even on their own terms; and their "blame-the-victim" connotations are morally obnoxious.

While little is known about the ability of mildly retarded persons to use alternative forms of birth control, much is taken for granted rather than empirically verified. As one rather cautious authority points out, in this as in any other area of functional behavior, the "capacity" of mildly retarded persons will vary greatly depending on the individual user's level of cognitive and functional ability; the presence of necessary counseling and education programs, including clinicians, parents, and personnel trained and sensitive in this particular area; and a cooperative state social service agency.[14] In the absence of such clinical and social conditions, we have little basis for assuming anything about the potential capacity of "many" or "most" retarded persons to adjust to temporary forms of birth control. On the other hand, there are reports of experimental programs that are attempting to provide retarded persons in group homes with sexual counseling services, birth control counseling and methods, and regular opportunities for a variety of sexual experiences (homosexual and auto-erotic as well as heterosexual). These pilot projects indicate that such programs, when offered seriously and with sensitivity and follow-up, may be quite successful (result in a high degree of self-regulation, low pregnancy rates, and satisfying social and sexual lives). Retarded persons involved in such programs, when given the necessary training and supervision, have been able to manage nonpermanent forms of birth control.[15] The point is not that other forms of birth control are always "better" for retarded persons than is sterilization (the pill, for example, has been associated with far more serious risks to health), or that they will always work. Rather, it is that access to a variety of options and services to enhance their reproductive and sexual experience is a necessary condition for retarded persons (or any persons) to develop the capacity to engage actively and voluntarily in such

experience. Until programs of this kind are widely available and taken seriously, we will not really know much about the potential capacity of the mildly retarded either for sexuality or for self-administered birth control.

The assumption that many mildly retarded persons will be incapable of exercising sufficient foresight and responsibility to raise children independently may well be valid under existing social conditions. Yet even here it is important to point out the absence of empirical data. There are no studies reported that compare the behavior and effectiveness of retarded and nonretarded parents. Moreover, the argument voiced by advocates of the retarded is persuasive: that summary denial of the childbearing rights of retarded persons is discriminatory. What about other categories of "social deviants" whose behavior or condition may be detrimental to their children but whose legal right to raise their children is not challenged *a priori* (alcoholics, neurotics, emotionally disturbed persons)? Why are the issues any different in these cases?[16] Again, it would seem necessary to deal with the question of childbearing capacity in terms of an individual situation rather than on a wholesale basis through procedures that provide adequate guarantees of due process and effective advocacy.

This discussion might be clarified if we could separate the issue of child-rearing capacity from that of capacity to give informed consent. Social welfare workers and mentally disabled persons themselves have convincingly argued that many, perhaps most, persons classified as "mildly retarded" are capable of understanding the issues involved in decisions about sterilization and birth control, and at the same time may feel undesirous or incapable of raising a child.[17] In fact, the federal regulations do allow for such a possibility by leaving it open to the courts and clinicians to determine whether a particular mentally incompetent individual may be competent to exercise informed consent in reproductive matters and thus to become voluntarily sterilized under federally funded programs. How this will work out in practice, and whether the courts can be relied upon to assure that the "voluntary consent" of retarded persons is genuine and not manipulated, remains to be seen. Presumably, the "readjudication of capacity to consent" would *not* mean third-party consent, and would require that the retarded person herself or himself be adequately represented by an independent counsel or advocate.

The issue that remains, and to which the moratorium allows no exceptions, is that of profoundly or severely

severely an profoundly

retarded persons who are not capable of voluntary consent, who may be unable to use temporary forms of birth control, who are at risk of pregnancy, and for whom such a pregnancy would by all objective standards present a real hardship. It seems altogether likely that, given both the sexual underdevelopment of such persons and their vulnerability, the vast majority of such pregnancies are the result of rape or incest.[18] This raises, once again, the point made earlier—the danger that introducing sterilization as a "solution" in such cases may encourage neglect of adequate staffing, services, and other protections to guard against incidents of sexual assault. I know of no study that systematically documents pregnancy rates among populations of retarded women, institutionalized as well as deinstitutionalized, much less the circumstances in which those pregnancies arise (which are often not known, since the victims usually do not know how to report). One might agree that, for certain severely retarded persons, sterilization would be a better alternative for the individual involved than anything else available, and therefore not be morally objectionable. However, under existing conditions the position of the federal regulations seems reasonable: that lifting the moratorium even in these cases would create a greater danger, since it would allow sterilization as an alternative to the development of decent care and social programs that maximize the potentialities of *all* persons, even the most disabled.

NOTES

1 *Federal Register* 43:217 (Nov. 8, 1978), 52146–175. The applicability of the federal regulations is limited to programs or projects funded in whole or in part through federal grants (through the Title XX Social Services Program or the Public Health Service), or to individuals receiving Medicaid. Thus sterilization programs not funded through federal monies, including many done through private hospitals and clinics, are under no obligation to comply with the regulations, except with regard to their Medicaid patients.

2 *Federal Register* 43:217, p. 52154.

3 Ibid., p. 52155.

4 *Wyatt v. Aderholt,* 368 F. Supp. 1383 (M.D. Ala., 1974); *In re Sterilization of Moore,* 289 N.C. 95 (Sup. Ct., N.C., 1976); *North Carolina Assoc. for Retarded Children v. State of N.C.,* 420 F. Supp. 451 (M.D.N.C., 1976); *Cook v. State of Oregon,* 9 Ore. App. 1972.

5 On this point, see Isabel P. Robinault, *Sex, Society, and the Disabled* (Hagerstown, MD.: Harper & Row, 1978), p. 67; Paul Friedman, *The Rights of Mentally Retarded Persons* (New York: Avon, 1976), *passim;* President's Committee on Mental Retardation, *Mental Retardation: Century of Decision,* Report to the President (U.S. Government Printing Office, Washington, D.C., 1976), pp. 58–59; and Patricia M. Wald, "Basic Personal and Civil Rights," in Michael Kindred *et al., The Mentally Retarded Citizen and the Law* (New York: The Free Press, 1976), p. 5.

6 Irving I. Gottesman, "An Introduction to Behavioral Genetics of Mental Retardation," in Robert M. Allen *et al., The Role of Genetics in Mental Retardation* (Coral Gables, Fla.: University of Miami Press, 1971), pp. 50 and 62.

7 Oral interviews with I. Lipner, Developmental Center, Maimonides Hospital, and Karen Wolf, Garfield Manor Group Residence, Brooklyn, New York, January and February 1979. The views stated are based on the clinical experience of those interviewed and do not necessarily reflect agency or professional policy. See also, Winifred Kempton, "Sexual Rights and Responsibilities of the Retarded Person," *Social Welfare Forum, 1976* (New York: Columbia University Press, 1977).

8 George F. Will, "Sterilization and the Retarded," *Washington Post,* Dec. 3, 1978, p. C7; Medora S. Bass, "Surgical Contraception: A Key to Normalization and Prevention," *Journal of Mental Retardation* (December 1978); *Cook v. Oregon;* and *North Carolina Assoc. for Retarded Children.*

9 Robert Neville, "Sterilizing the Mildly Mentally Retarded Without Their Consent," *Hastings Center Report* 8:3 (June 1978), p. 33; Bass, pp. 399–400; *Ruby v. Massey* (D.C. Conn., 1978); *North Carolina Assoc. for Retarded Children.*

10 Neville, pp. 33 and 35; Bass, pp. 401–402; *Cook v. Oregon;* cf. President's Committee on Mental Retardation, p. 63.

11 Will, "Sterilization and the Retarded." I am grateful to Dr. Irvin Cushner for calling my attention to Will's article. Will approvingly summarizes the articles by Neville and Travis Thompson ("Sterilization of the Retarded: In Whose Interests?") in the June 1978 *Hastings Center Report,* using these as the basis of his argument.

12 See, for example, Irving I. Gottesman, "An Introduction to Behavioral Genetics of Mental Retardation," in Robert M. Allen *et al., The Role of
Genetics in Mental Retardation* (Coral Gables,
Fla.: University of Miami Press, 1971), p. 50, who
in the earlier part of his article presents this complex,
multi-dimensional view of "causality" quite clearly,
even though he later draws conclusions that are
completely inconsonant with it (e.g., "that the
voluntary restriction of fertility by retarded individuals would have a marked effect on reducing
their own and society's burdens").

13 For a particularly thorough treatment of the existing
empirical data in this area and its legal and social
implications, see John R. Kramer, "The Right Not
to Be Mentally Retarded," in Kindred *et al.,* pp.
31–59.

14 Robinault, pp. 63–64.

15 *Ibid.,* reporting on programs in Eastern Pennsyl-
vania and Washington, D.C.; Kempton, "Sexuality
and the Mentally Retarded," *Hospital Tribune,*
February 1979, pp. 3–6; Winifred Kempton,
Medora S. Bass, and Sol Gordon, *Love, Sex and
Birth Control for the Mentally Retarded: A Guide
for Parents* (Philadelphia: Planned Parenthood
Association, 1971); and interviews cited in n. 7.

16 This argument is made strongly by S. John Vitello,
"Involuntary Sterilization: Recent Developments,"
Journal of Mental Retardation (December 1978),
p. 406; and Friedman, *op. cit.,* p. 122, who concludes: "Although we lack adequate predictive tools
to distinguish beforehand between suitable and
unsuitable parents, the absence of such refined
techniques does not justify discriminating against
mentally retarded parents in custody matters."

17 Opposition to involuntary sterilization of the mentally handicapped was expressed unanimously by a
group of retarded persons attending a workshop
on the "Childbearing Rights of the Mentally Handicapped" at a Conference on Childbearing Rights,
sponsored by Low-Income Planning Aid, in Wor-
cester, Mass., November 18–19, 1978, and attended
by the author. Some among the group were parents,
some had been voluntarily sterilized, and at least
one woman reported having been molested by her
father. Their strong consensus was that, while they
themselves might individually prefer sterilization or
decide that raising children would be too burdensome, they and most mildly retarded persons are
competent to participate fully in making this decision.

18 Ibid. and sources cited in note 7; of necessity, the
evidence here is anecdotal rather than documented.

Declaration of General and Special Rights of the Mentally Retarded

International League of Societies for the Mentally Handicapped

The International League of Societies for the Mentally Handicapped, now known
as the International League of Societies for Persons with Mental Handicap, was
founded in 1960. Its founders included representatives of parent organizations
and professional groups as well as individuals concerned with the interests of the
mentally handicapped. The current chairperson of the League is Stanley S. Herr of
Columbia University, who recently published *Rights and Advocacy for Retarded
People* (1983). The current president of the League is Peter Mittler, professor of
special education at the University of Manchester. Since proclaiming the rights
below, the League has published *Step by Step: Implementation of the Rights of
Mentally Retarded Persons*.

Reprinted with the permission of the International League of Societies for Persons with Mental Handicap.

This declaration of rights was officially proclaimed in 1968 at a meeting of the League. In 1971 it was adopted almost word for word by the United Nations General Assembly. Among the positive rights it asserts are the rights to economic security, a decent standard of living, and the education, training, habilitation, and guidance requisite to develop abilities and potentials to the fullest possible extent.

Whereas the universal declaration of human rights, adopted by the United Nations, proclaims that all of the human family, without distinction of any kind, have equal and inalienable rights of human dignity and freedom;

Whereas the declaration of the rights of the child, adopted by the United Nations, proclaims the rights of the physically, mentally or socially handicapped child to special treatment, education and care required by his particular condition.

Now therefore, The International League of Societies for the Mentally Handicapped expresses the general and special rights of the mentally retarded as follows:

Article I.

The mentally retarded person has the same basic rights as other citizens of the same country and same age.

Article II.

The mentally retarded person has a right to proper medical care and physical restoration and to such education, training, habilitation and guidance as will enable him to develop his ability and potential to the fullest possible extent, no matter how severe his degree of disability. No mentally handicapped person should be deprived of such services by reason of the costs involved.

Article III.

The mentally retarded person has a right to economic security and to a decent standard of living. He has a right to productive work or to other meaningful occupation.

Article IV.

The mentally retarded person has a right to live with his own family or with fosterparents; to participate in all aspects of community life, and to be provided with appropriate leisure time activities. If care in an institution becomes necessary it should be in surroundings and under circumstances as close to normal living as possible.

Article V.

The mentally retarded person has a right to a qualified guardian when this is required to protect his personal wellbeing and interest. No person rendering direct services to the mentally retarded should also serve as his guardian.

Article VI.

The mentally retarded person has a right to protection from exploitation, abuse and degrading treatment. If accused, he has a right to a fair trial with full recognition being given to his degree of responsibility.

Article VII.

Some mentally retarded persons may be unable, due to the severity of their handicap, to exercise for themselves all their rights in a meaningful way. For others, modification of some or all of these rights is appropriate. The procedure used for modification or denial of rights must contain proper legal safeguards against every form of abuse, must be based on an evaluation of the social capability of the mentally retarded person by qualified experts and must be subject to periodic reviews and to the right of appeal to higher authorities.

Above all—The mentally retarded person has the right to respect.

Caring for Retarded Persons—Ethical Ideals and Practical Choices

Barry Hoffmaster

Barry Hoffmaster is associate professor of philosophy at the University of Western Ontario. His areas of specialization are philosophy of law, ethics, and medical ethics. Hoffmaster is the coeditor of *Contemporary Issues in Biomedical Ethics* (1979) as well as the coauthor of "Physicians, Patients, and Paternalism" and "Ethical Issues in Family Medicine."

Hoffmaster explores some of the difficulties faced by attempts to develop a set of consistent and defensible positions on ethical issues involving retarded persons. He addresses five questions: (1) Is mental retardation in and of itself a morally relevant characteristic? (2) Is a rights-based approach to ethical issues involving retarded persons adequate? (3) Do general principles such as the principle of normalization and the principle of the least restrictive alternative provide any help in resolving moral issues? (*The principle of normalization* states that the retarded have the right to a range of goods and services that make their lives as normal as possible. *The principle of the least restrictive alternative* can be understood as requiring that the care, treatment, and habilitation provided to the mentally retarded, as well as the setting in which it is provided, be the least restrictive of the person's personal liberty.) (4) How should problems involving the allocations of resources be handled? (5) Does the degree of mental handicap make a difference from a moral point of view?

The question with which I would like to begin is "Why is it important to discuss moral issues involving retarded persons?" There are two answers to the question: one that is obvious and one that is not so obvious. People who work with retarded persons constantly encounter situations in which they must make moral decisions. These decisions frequently are difficult; they may involve genuine moral dilemmas. Discussion of these moral issues perhaps can remove some of the moral perplexity. It may reveal what the correct course of action is and lead people to adopt that course of action. In this respect, discussion of moral issues involving retarded persons has intrinsic value—that is, it is valuable in and of itself. This is the obvious answer.

Discussion of these issues also has instrumental value, however. This instrumental value derives from the advocacy role that many organizations are now playing on behalf of retarded persons. The question that needs to be asked, though, is, "What is the proper role for an advocacy group?" The natural response is that a group advocating for retarded persons should function just as any other self-interested pressure group does. It should lobby for programs and benefits for retarded persons. Unfortunately, there are two problems with this answer. One is that if an advocacy group for the retarded is simply a self-interested pressure group competing with other pressure groups for society's scarce resources, it most likely will lose in this general war of self-interest. Consider, for example, the situation in which an advocacy group is trying to get a group home for retarded people in an area zoned for single-family dwelling. There simply are more property owners who would fight a group home than there are people who would argue on behalf of retarded persons. When it comes to a pure numbers game, those who

From Stanley Hauerwas, editor, *Responsibility for Devalued Persons* (1982), pp. 28–41. Courtesy of Charles C Thomas, Publisher, Springfield, Illinois.

advocate on behalf of retarded persons are going to be outnumbered, and for this reason they will lose their fights. A second reason is that a kind of argument open to other self-interested pressure groups is not available to those who engage in advocacy for the retarded. For example, Chrysler Corporation can argue that giving special privileges to it will in the long run benefit all of society. If Chrysler Corporation remains viable, competition will continue to exist in the auto industry and this, in the long run, will benefit all of society. This kind of argument, however, is not available to those who advocate on behalf of the retarded. The special benefits that they are after go directly to retarded persons and do not have any substantial spin-offs for the rest of society. Given these problems, what is the alternative? What kind of foundation should an advocacy group for the retarded have for its positions? The answer is that these positions should be founded on what is ethically required. What gives claims for special privileges and programs for the retarded their force or their bite and what makes them persuasive is that these claims are based on what is ethically required. This, then, is the less obvious reason for discussing moral issues. An advocacy group on behalf of retarded persons needs to develop a consistent, coherent, defensible set of positions, and this requires an overall ethical framework on which those positions can rest.

What I want to do is outline the lay of the land in this area, that is, sketch the moral landscape and point out the obstacles that one encounters in trying to develop a set of consistent, defensible positions on ethical issues involving retarded persons. I will provide no map and compass; each person must chart his own course through the obstacles. Moreover, to continue the metaphor, one is in virgin territory here for two reasons. One is that standard moral philosophy is of no help when one begins talking about ethical issues involving retarded persons. Moral philosophers rarely, if ever, talk about ethical issues involving retarded persons, and when they do, they often come up with answers that many people who advocate on behalf of retarded persons would not be able to accept.[2] Thus one cannot turn to prevailing traditions in moral philosophy for help. The second reason is that the example of other groups who have been victims of discrimination in society is of no help either. Take, for example, blacks, who have made people realize that being black is not a feature that should be disvalued, and, furthermore, that skin color is not a morally relevant charac-

teristic. They have taught society that being black cannot be used as a reason for discriminating against people. They have gone even further, however, and turned being black from a disvalued characteristic into a valued characteristic. The slogan, "black is beautiful," helped to develop this pride. This kind of strategy unfortunately will not work for mentally retarded persons. Being mentally retarded is not like being black. Being retarded is, in and of itself, a disvalued characteristic. If one had a choice, no one would choose to have a retarded child rather than a nonretarded child. And no one would dream up a slogan extolling the virtues of being retarded. In addition, being retarded does seem to be a relevant characteristic in certain circumstances. Consider, for example, the question of employment. Recent proposed legislation to prohibit discrimination against the handicapped in Ontario would allow exceptions when a handicap renders a person incapable of performing essential tasks.[3] In this respect, being retarded does seem to be a morally relevant characteristic, unlike being black. I will soon return to the question of whether being retarded is a morally relevant characteristic. For these two reasons, however, the ethical problems that arise with respect to retarded persons appear to be novel and unique.

I will now raise five more specific issues. First, is mental retardation in and of itself a morally relevant characteristic? Second, is a rights-based approach to ethical issues involving retarded persons adequate? Third, do general principles such as the principle of normalization and the principle of the least restrictive alternative provide any help in resolving moral issues? Fourth, how should problems involving the allocation of resources be handled? Fifth, does the degree of mental handicap make a difference from a moral point of view?

Let me turn to the first issue. Is mental retardation in and of itself morally relevant? To illustrate this problem, consider some of the statements made about the rights of retarded persons. If one looks at the rights of the retarded as delineated by the International League of Societies for the Mentally Handicapped, one sees the following in Article I: "The mentally retarded person has the same basic rights as other citizens of the same country and same age."[4] If one looks at the United Nations Declaration on the Rights of Mentally Retarded Persons, one sees a similar statement: "The mentally retarded person has, to the maximum degree of feasibility, the same rights as other human beings."[5] These statements suggest that mental retardation *is not* an ethically relevant characteristic. Mentally retarded persons should not be discriminated against *because* they are mentally retarded. The phrase, "because they are mentally retarded," does not count here; it is not a relevant reason. Mentally retarded persons cannot be discriminated against because they are mentally retarded, just as blacks cannot be discriminated against because they are black. If one reads on, though, and looks at Articles II and III in the Rights of the Retarded from the International League, one sees the following kinds of statements: a retarded person has a right to [such] education, training, habilitation, and guidance as will enable him to develop his ability and potential *to the fullest possible extent,* and a retarded person has a right to productive work or to other *meaningful* occupation.[6] Similarly, in the United Nations Declaration, one finds the claim that a retarded person has a right to medical care, physical therapy, and to [such] education, training, rehabilitation, and guidance as would enable him to develop his ability and *maximum potential.*[7] The United Nations Declaration also says that a retarded person has a right to perform productive work or to engage in any other *meaningful* occupation to the *fullest extent of his capabilities.*[8] The difficulty is that non-retarded people do not have these kinds of rights. A non-retarded person does not have a right to develop his ability and potential to the fullest possible extent or to engage in a meaningful occupation. One does not have a right to pursue an education through a Ph.D. degree even if that is required to develop one's potential to the fullest possible extent. Society guarantees a minimum level of education, but it does not guarantee an education that will develop one's potential to the fullest possible extent. These claims, these statements of rights, therefore, suggest that mental retardation *is* an ethically relevant characteristic. Mentally retarded people are entitled to special considerations, special programs, and special privileges *because* they are retarded. Here the phrase "because they are retarded" does count; here it is taken to be a relevant reason. Mentally retarded persons are entitled to special considerations because they are mentally retarded, unlike blacks who are not entitled to special considerations because they are black. The situation is even more dramatic in the position papers of the American Association on Mental Deficiency, where the following sentences occur: "Mentally retarded citizens are entitled to enjoy and exercise the same rights as are available to non-retarded citizens, to the limits of their ability to do so. As handicapped citizens, they are also entitled to specific extensions of, and additions to, these basic rights, in order to allow their free exercise and enjoyment."[9] The first sentence seems to state that mental retardation is not an ethically relevant characteristic in that it cannot be used as a basis for denying people rights. Again, the claim is that mentally retarded people have the same rights as everybody else because being mentally retarded cannot be used as a reason to justify discrimination. But in the sentence that immediately follows, mental retardation seems to be regarded as an ethically relevant characteristic that entitles mentally retarded persons to special considerations others do not receive. The claim is that mentally retarded persons are entitled to specific extensions of and additions to certain rights *because* they are mentally retarded. This makes mental retardation a morally relevant characteristic. The problem is, how can one have it both ways? It is inconsistent to hold that mental retardation is not a morally relevant characteristic and that mental retardation is a morally relevant characteristic. This is a serious problem for those who advocate on behalf of the retarded because their opponents, I believe, perceive this inconsistency. How can advocates for the retarded hold two inconsistent views about the moral relevance of mental retardation? And there is a genuine dilemma here. If one opts for one horn of the dilemma and holds that mental retardation is not morally relevant, how can one argue for special services, programs or considerations for retarded persons? If one takes the other horn of the dilemma and holds that mental retardation is morally relevant, opponents of retarded persons can argue that if mental retardation is a relevant reason for providing a service or benefit, it also can be a relevant reason for denying rights or benefits to retarded persons. This is a serious, underlying moral problem that must be addressed.

The second issue I want to discuss is the adequacy of a rights-based approach for dealing with moral problems involving mentally retarded persons. I should point out immediately that I am talking about moral rights, not legal rights. The question to ask is whether a rights-based approach can handle the problem of the moral relevance of mental retardation. The answer, as one might guess, is that it depends. It depends on the kind of right one is talking about. There is a distinction between a right to an opportunity and a right to an outcome. Think, for example, about the rights to life, liberty, and the pursuit of happiness. The right to life is a right to an outcome. The right does not mandate merely the opportunity to pursue those things necessary for the maintenance of life, but rather requires that everyone be provided with those necessities. The right to happiness, on the other hand, is a right to an opportunity. The right does not protect happiness per se and thus guarantee that everyone as a matter of fact will be happy. This obviously is impossible. The right protects only one's pursuit of happiness: no one is allowed to interfere with the attempts of others to be happy. So there is a fundamental difference between a right to an opportunity and a right to an outcome. This distinction arises with respect to the rights of mentally retarded persons as well. Some of these rights are rights to outcomes, for example, the rights to food, clothing, shelter, and health care. With rights to outcomes there is no problem with the moral relevance of mental retardation. Take, for example, the right to adequate psychiatric care for mentally retarded persons. If guaranteeing the right to adequate psychiatric care requires special training for psychiatrists, psychiatric nurses, or psychiatric social workers, there is no difficulty justifying that special training. Mentally retarded persons have the same right to basic psychiatric care that everyone else has. The special training is required to insure that mentally retarded persons have the same outcome (that is, an adequate level of psychiatric care) as everyone else. To deny them this outcome would be to discriminate against them. Because this is a right to an outcome, the special training required can be justified without admitting that mental retardation is a morally relevant characteristic. With rights to opportunities, however, there is a problem. An example of a right to an opportunity with respect to mentally retarded persons is the right to sexual activity. No one guarantees sexual partners for mentally retarded persons, so this is not a right to an outcome. It is only a right to an opportunity to engage in sexual activity. But with rights to opportunities, it is difficult to see how they can be meaningful without conceding the moral relevance of mental retardation. A right to an opportunity insures the right to compete with others. Think, for example, about the right to a job. If this is understood as a right to an opportunity, it means only that mentally retarded persons have an opportunity to compete with everyone else. Or think about the right to participate in a Little League baseball team. This guarantees mentally retarded children the right to try out for a team; it does

not guarantee them membership on a team. The obvious difficulty is that if mentally retarded persons are given only the right to compete, they generally will not be successful. Special training therefore is required to enable them to compete meaningfully. But what is the justification for this special training? Why would not everyone else be entitled to special training as well? For example, unemployed but nonmentally retarded persons might argue that if they were given special training, they would be able to compete more successfully in the job market. Why should special training go only to mentally retarded persons and not to everyone else? An attempt to answer this question raises another dilemma. The dilemma is that one either must admit that mental retardation is a morally relevant characteristic or convert all rights to rights to outcomes. If one argues that only mentally retarded persons are entitled to special training programs, then one is conceding the moral relevance of mental retardation. If one argues that everyone who could benefit is entitled to a special training program, then one converts the right from a right to an opportunity into a right to an outcome. Pursuing this line consistently would destroy the fundamental distinction that society recognizes between rights to outcomes and rights to opportunities. Thus, a rights-based approach does not seem to be able to deal with the problem of the moral relevance of mental retardation.

The third issue is the role of the principles of normalization and the least restrictive alternative in moral decision making. I take these principles to be mid-level principles—that is, they fall somewhere between more abstract, general statements of the rights of mentally retarded persons and more concrete, specific judgments about particular moral problems. If this interpretation is correct, a general problem is how these principles are connected to statements of the rights of mentally retarded persons. How are these principles to be derived from claims about the rights that mentally retarded persons have? That is a problem for both the principle of normalization and the principle of the least restrictive alternative. There are additional problems with both principles, however.

I will consider the principle of normalization first. Here there are two main problems. One is how to interpret the principle and the other is how to apply the principle. With respect to interpretation, is the principle to be understood as an end or a means? If normalization sets out an end or a goal to be achieved, is that end in fact desirable? It is, I think, "culturally normative" for people to sit around watching television for hours on end. If one adopts normalization as an end and holds that the appropriate goal for mentally retarded people is to engage in activities that are culturally normative, does this mean that retarded persons also should sit around watching television for hours on end? Is it really plausible to claim that mentally retarded persons should engage in culturally normative activities simply because they are culturally normative?

A second objection to the principle, understood as setting out a desirable end, comes from Stanley Hauerwas. Hauerwas says:

> The great temptation in caring for the retarded, as for any child, is to make them conform to what we think they should want to be—namely, that they should wish to be 'normal.' We thus often care for the retarded on the assumption that our task is to make them as much like the rest of us as we can... We must... be very careful that we do not impose on them a form of life born from our frustration because they are not and cannot be like us. For example, the so-called 'principle of normalization' is a valuable check against the sentimental and often cruel care of the retarded that tries to spare them the pain of learning basic skills of living. But, as an ideology, it tends to suggest that our aim is to make the retarded 'normal.' This, of course, ignores entirely the fact that we have no clear idea of what it means to be 'normal.' Thus in the name of 'normalcy,' we stand the risk of making the retarded conform to convention because they lack the power to resist.[10]

The principle of normalization, on the other hand, may be understood as specifying a means. That is, engaging in culturally normative activities may be seen as a way of achieving certain other ends such as attaining independence or fulfilling to the maximum extent possible the potential of a mentally retarded person. The difficulty with this interpretation is that engaging in culturally normative activities may not always be the most effective and efficient means to achieving such ends. Roos raises this problem in connection with behavior modification techniques.[11] Roos points out that whether normalization techniques or behavior modification techniques are more effective in achieving a given goal, say, independence for severely or profoundly retarded persons, remains an open question.

This is, in fact, an empirical or factual question for which one needs evidence. One cannot know a priori that normalization techniques will be more effective than behavior modification techniques in leading to any given end.

The overall danger here is that the principle of normalization seems to have acquired the status of dogma. The kinds of difficulties and questions just raised are not being addressed because of the dogmatic status of the principle. More important, other value questions are being obscured by a dogmatic allegiance to the principle. Consider, for example, the issue of mainstreaming. Maloney and Ward, the authors of a recent textbook on mental retardation, point out that research suggests that retarded students in regular classes perform at a higher academic level than their peers in special classes, but that retarded students in special classes do better in terms of social competence, adjustment, and self-concept.[12] Thus, there is an important value judgment to be made here, a value judgment that is obscured by a slavish attachment to the principle of normalization. The principle of normalization dictates that mentally retarded students be put into regular classes. That, however, chooses the value of academic performance over the value of social competence, social adjustment, and self-concept. Is it so obvious that academic performance is to be preferred in this kind of competition? Such a value judgment should not be obscured by a strict adherence to the principle of normalization.

The second problem concerns the application of the principle of normalization to concrete problems. The difficulty is that the principle is too general or too vague to handle concrete problems, and in some cases it may come up with an intuitively incorrect answer. One actual example that I know of concerns a decision about community living for a retarded person. A retarded person had found an apartment that overlooked a cemetery. But an objection, founded on the principle of normalization, was raised to allowing this person to live in the apartment. The argument was that it was not culturally normative to live in an apartment that overlooked a cemetery. Since most people do not live in places that overlook cemeteries, mentally retarded people should not be allowed to have such accommodations. This example illustrates both problems with the principle. Does such a specific conclusion actually follow from the principle, and if it does, is it a conclusion that is acceptable?

The principle of the least restrictive alternative is primarily a principle of United States constitutional law, although there is a common sense moral idea behind it. This common sense notion is that a person is entitled to the maximum degree of freedom of liberty possible. Since there are many different kinds of freedom, however, the possibility of trade-offs among these different freedoms arises, and the principle of the least restrictive alternative says nothing about how these trade-offs are to be made. In addition, there are problems with the application of the principle. Consider, for example, various forms of treatment decisions. How does one decide whether medication is less restrictive than seclusion, whether seclusion is less restrictive than restraint, whether restraint is less restrictive than sedation, and whether sedation is less restrictive than electro convulsive therapy?[13] Does it even make sense to talk about the notion of "less restrictive" with respect to these kinds of treatment modalities? Since the principle places a high premium on freedom, another problem is how to handle situations where the exercise of this freedom is likely to jeopardize the welfare of a mentally retarded person. For example, does one allow a mentally retarded person the freedom to refuse routine dental checkups or inoculations? The principle of the least restrictive alternative does not seem to be able to answer these kinds of questions.

The fourth issue concerns the allocation of resources. This is, I think, the most serious and most pervasive moral problem that must be faced in this area. Consider the following kind of situation.[14] A treatment commitment in the form of a crisis team, that is four staff members for one client, has brought about rather spectacular treatment results in a short period of time in the case of a young profoundly retarded, multiply handicapped boy. This boy, unfortunately, is so impaired that no matter how much progress he makes, he never will get beyond the stage of "surviving" within some sort of treatment setting, whether it is an institution or at home. Now, however, a decision has to be made about continuation of treatment. A number of alternatives are possible. One is a minimal treatment commitment that would allow the behavioral results achieved so far to be maintained. This would require one person to continue programming in the home on a basis of forty hours per week. A second option is a more concentrated treatment commitment that would utilize two staff members doing programming in the home. With this approach there would be the possibility of improving behavior in areas that so far have been untapped. A third possibility is to continue the present crisis team approach. With this alternative it is reasonable to expect a rate of continued behavioral acquisition comparable to that achieved in the previous months. This decision raises a fundamental moral dilemma. How much does society owe to a child in this situation? Should scarce resources be devoted to one individual when using these resources for, say, four other retarded children who are not as severely handicapped might enable them to live relatively independent lives in the community? The professional in this kind of situation might feel that resources would be misallocated if the present crisis team approach were continued. If one were the parent of this boy, however, he or she most likely would fight vigorously to get everything possible for the boy. How should society reconcile these competing claims?

The final issue concerns whether the degree of mental retardation makes a difference. Should the severity of a person's retardation ethically be ignored? Advocates for retarded persons have in the past been correct in pointing out the wide variety that exists in the degree of handicap and the level of functioning. This has been necessary to counter the assumption—one that perhaps still prevails in society—that most mentally retarded people are severely or profoundly retarded and therefore without any hope for improvement. But it seems now that the same mistake is being committed in reverse by advocates for the retarded. When it comes to moral issues, all mentally retarded persons seem to be lumped together and treated as if they were only mildly retarded. Is this correct? Is an approach that is in the best interest of a person who is mildly or moderately retarded always going to be in the best interest of a person who is severely or profoundly retarded? In some situations, the degree of mental retardation does seem to make an important difference. Elizabeth Boggs raises this issue in her discussion of why she rejects normalization as the appropriate goal for her profoundly retarded and multiply handicapped son. Boggs says:

> There are some parents who like the idea of normalization because it is useful in glossing over the realities of difference. I sometimes think there are profes-

sionals who like it for the same reason. Rather than trying to create a 'normal' environment for my son, I try to think of how the world must look from his point of view, and what kind of an environment would not only minimize his boredom and loneliness but enhance his sense of dominance.[15]

The important question that Boggs raises is when do the "realities of difference" make a difference from a moral point of view?

In conclusion, I should emphasize that I do not wish to deny the significant progress that has been made on behalf of retarded persons through principles such as normalization and the least restrictive alternative. These principles have been needed correctives to the abuse, degradation, and exploitation of the retarded that have existed for so long. What I have tried to do is rather to point out the limitations of these principles. I think they are essentially backward-looking principles. An emphasis on rights and normalization looks to the past and tries to rectify the abuses and injustices that have been heaped upon mentally retarded persons; certainly much work remains to be done along these lines. It is not clear, however, that principles such as normalization and the least restrictive alternative are desirable forward-looking approaches. That is, it is not clear that they specify goals that are intrinsically desirable in caring for retarded persons. At a minimum, these principles should not be accepted as dogma but rather should be scrutinized critically, and alternative approaches which may be better should be explored.

Finally, a word of caution. It is important in moral decision making, especially with respect to retarded persons I think, not to ignore the role of emotions and feelings. It is easy to discuss these problems on a rational, intellectual level, and this in fact is an approach that is quite conducive to a philosopher. But I would like to remind you of a quotation from George Bateson. Bateson says, "For the attainment of grace, the reasons of the heart must be integrated with the reasons of the reason." I do not think this quotation has to be understood literally. Rather than talking about the attainment of grace, one can talk about leading a good life or making the right decisions. To do this, one needs to integrate the reasons of the heart and the reasons of the reason. A purely rational, intellectual approach will not work, and a purely emotional approach will not work. I think this is true in any area of moral decision making, but it is especially so when one is dealing with mentally retarded persons.

NOTES

1 Much of this paper is taken from a report, "Ethical Foundations of OAMR Position Statements," written by Michael D. Bayles and C. Barry Hoffmaster under the auspices of the Westminster Institute for Ethics and Human Values for the Ontario Association for the Mentally Retarded (1980).

2 See Daniel Wikler, "Moral Theory and Mental Retardation," a paper presented to the Fifth Congress, International Association for the Scientific Study of Mental Retardation, Jerusalem, 3 August 1979.

3 "Change to Protect Disabled Planned for Fall, Elgie Says," *Globe and Mail* (Toronto), 20 June 1980, p. 5.

4 "Declaration of General and Special Rights of the Mentally Retarded," International League of Societies for the Mentally Handicapped, 1969.

5 "The United Nations Declaration on the Rights of Mentally Retarded Persons," 1971.

6 *Supra,* note 4.

7 *Supra,* note 5, article 2.

8 *Ibid.,* article 3.

9 *Position Papers of the American Association on Mental Deficiency 1975* (Washington, D.C.: American Association on Mental Deficiency, n.d.), p. 1.

10 Stanley Hauerwas, "Having and Learning How to Care for Retarded Children: Some Reflections," *Catholic Mind,* April, 1976, pp. 24–33. Reprinted in Stanley Reiser, *et al.,* eds., *Ethics in Medicine* (Cambridge: MIT Press, 1977), pp. 631–635. The quotation is on p. 635 in the Reiser volume.

11 See Philip Roos, "Reconciling Behavior Modification Procedures with the Normalization Principle," in Wolf Wolfensberger, *The Principle of Normalization in Human Services* (Toronto: National Institute on Mental Retardation, 1972), p. 146 and Philip Roos, "Normalization, De-Humanization, and Conditioning—Conflict or Harmony," *Mental Retardation,* August, 1970, pp. 12–14.

12 Michael P. Maloney and Michael P. Ward, *Mental Retardation and Modern Society* (New York: Oxford University Press, 1979), p. 81.

13 Benjamin Goldberg, "Ethics of Mental Health Administration," paper presented to Workshop on Bioethics, Westminster Institute for Ethics and Human Values, London, Ontario, July 1980, p. 7.

14 I am indebted to Dieter Blindert for this example.

15 Elizabeth Boggs, "Who is Putting Whose Head in the Sand Or in the Clouds As the Case May Be?" in Ann Turnbull and H. Rutherford Turnbull, III, eds., *Parents Speak Out* (Columbus: Charles E. Merrill Pub. Co., 1978), p. 62.

ANNOTATED BIBLIOGRAPHY: CHAPTER 6

Ackerman, Susan Rose: "Mental Retardation and Society: The Ethics and Politics of Normalization," *Ethics* 93 (October 1982), pp. 81–101. In this survey article, Ackerman examines several general normative political theories and their implications for the treatment of the mentally retarded. She brings out some of the premises underlying the normalization movement and the different policy implications of various basic principles.

Chodoff, Paul: "The Case for Involuntary Hospitalization of the Mentally Ill," *American Journal of Psychiatry* 133 (May 1976), pp. 496–501. Chodoff presents a number of cases to bring out the conditions under which society has the right to commit individuals to mental institutions against their will.

Edwards, Rem B., Ed.: *Psychiatry and Ethics: Insanity, Autonomy, and Mental Health Care* (Buffalo, N.Y.: Prometheus Books, 1982). This well organized collection of articles includes chapters on the concept of mental illness, the therapist-patient relationship and rights, the informed consent requirement, coercion in commitment and therapy, controversial behavioral control therapies, the insanity defense, and deinstitutionalization. The authors include psychologists, psychiatrists, sociologists, lawyers, surgeons, medical directors, and political scientists.

Forst, Martin L.: *Civil Commitment and Social Control* (Lexington, Mass.: Lexington Books, 1978). Forst offers an empirical investigation of the operation and functioning of one civil commitment statute (California's "Mentally Disordered Sex Offender [MDSO] Statute") and its relation to the criminal justice system. He does a comparative study of the relationship between the civil and criminal commitment systems.

Goffman, Erving: *Asylums* (New York: Doubleday Anchor, 1961). Goffman provides an analysis of life in total institutions in general and in mental institutions in particular.

Hauerwas, Stanley: *Responsibility for Devalued Persons* (Springfield, Ill.: Charles C Thomas, 1982). The papers in this collection were delivered in 1980 at a Conference on Responsibility for Devalued Persons: Ethical Interactions Between Society, the Family, and the Retarded. The authors, who come from a wide variety of disciplines, include Stanley Hauerwas, David Rothman, Bonita Raine, Josh Greenfeld, and Evelyn Messer as well as Barry Hoffmaster, whose paper is included in this chapter. The primary thrust of the articles is to present the kinds of ethical issues raised by the care of the retarded.

Herr, Stanley S.: *Rights and Advocacy for Retarded People* (Lexington, Mass.: Lexington Books, 1983). This is a comprehensive, coherent review of the legal and judicial processes that have shaped the field of mental retardation. Herr provides an historical background, brings out the assumptions that underlie our treatment of the mentally retarded, and suggests a future agenda for those who serve as advocates for the mentally retarded.

Macklin, Ruth, and Willard Gaylin, eds.: *Mental Retardation and Sterilization: A Problem of Competency and Paternalism* (New York: Plenum Press, 1981). In 1976–1977, the Hastings Center conducted a project titled "Ethical Issues in the Care and Treatment of the Mildly Mentally Retarded." This book is the result of the interdisciplinary meetings held as part of that project. Participants included philosophers, psychiatrists, psychologists, social scientists, and lawyers. The book has two parts and an appendix. Part I is a report of the outcome of the deliberations. Part II contains several articles written by seminar participants. The appendix contains excerpts from five court cases involving the sterilization of mentally retarded persons.

Rouse v. Cameron. 373 F 2d 451 (1966). In deciding this case, the District of Columbia Circuit Court of Appeals ruled that an involuntarily committed patient has a right to treatment. Furthermore, it held that the Court has a responsibility to determine whether the patient is receiving the treatment, and if he or she is not receiving it, why.

Wikler, Daniel: "Paternalism and the Mildly Retarded," *Philosophy and Public Affairs* 8 (Summer 1979), pp. 377–392. Wikler examines the paternalistic argument frequently advanced to justify limitations on the civil liberties of the mildly mentally retarded. He criticizes the argument and concludes that the fairness of denying civil liberties to the mildly retarded depends on the legitimacy of giving a higher priority to the general social welfare than to equalizing liberties.

Suicide and the Refusal of Lifesaving Treatment

INTRODUCTION

This chapter is designed to address the most prominent ethical questions about suicide and a closely related topic, the refusal of lifesaving treatment. The occurrence of a suicide is, in typical cases, a rather grim reminder of the possibility of human despair. The suicide of a friend or relative usually occasions shock and almost always occasions sadness. However, many people are inclined to say not only that suicide is tragic but also that it is immoral. Accordingly, one focal point of discussion in this chapter is the morality of suicide. Two other focal points of discussion share a common thread. In both cases, questions are raised about the justifiability of state intervention. At issue in one case is the justifiability of state intervention for the purpose of coercively preventing a person from committing suicide. At issue in the other, closely related case is the justifiability of state intervention for the purpose of compelling a person to accept lifesaving treatment. One final pocket of ethical concern in this chapter can be identified—the refusal of lifesaving treatment by patients who are in the process of dying.

What Is Suicide?

It is unwise to attempt to discuss the moral dimensions of suicide without paying some attention to the concept of suicide itself. Consider two people, one saying that suicide is always immoral and the other saying that suicide is sometimes morally acceptable. It is possible that these two people are in substantive moral agreement and differ only with regard to an operating definition of suicide. One of them may hold that suicide is immoral but say that a certain action is not suicide and is therefore morally acceptable, whereas the other may call the same action suicide but consider it a morally acceptable form of suicide. The following cases and the accompanying analysis are presented in order to shed some measure of light on the concept of suicide.

(1) A woman, having despaired of achieving a satisfying life, leaps to her death from the top of a city skyscraper. (2) An elderly man dies from a massive overdose of sleeping pills, leaving behind a note explaining that he is not bitter but that life seems to have passed him by. He has outlived his friends, he has no employment, he finds no enjoyment in his pastimes, etc. (1) and (2) provide us with clear cases of suicide. In accordance with what might be called the standard definition of suicide, each of these cases is a suicide precisely because it features the *intentional termination of one's own life*. Consider a third case. (3) In time of war, a soldier is captured and subjected to torture. Feeling unable to resist any longer, but determined not to yield any information that would endanger the lives of his comrades, he hangs himself. This third case is noteworthy, in contrast to (1) and (2), in that it features an other-directed rather than a self-directed motivation. Still, it seems to be a clear case of the intentional termination of one's own life. It is sometimes said that the self-killing in such cases is sacrificial rather than suicidal, but to deny that (3) is a case of suicide is surely to abandon the standard definition of suicide.

(4) A truckdriver, foreseeing his own death, nevertheless steers his runaway truck into a concrete abutment in order to avoid hitting a schoolbus that has stopped on the roadway to discharge children. (5) In a somewhat similar and much discussed actual case, a certain Captain Oates fell ill and found himself physically unable to continue on with a party of explorers in the Antarctic. The explorers were struggling to find their way out of a blizzard. Captain Oates, determined not to further endanger his colleagues by hindering their progress, but unable to convince them to leave him to die, simply walked off to meet his death in the blizzard. One may feel some puzzlement as to whether (4) and (5) are to be identified as cases of suicide. As in (3), the notion of sacrificial death may come to mind. Presumably neither the truckdriver nor Captain Oates wanted to die; each sacrificed his own life so that the lives of others might be protected. In contrast to (3), however, it is plausible to say, in accordance with the standard definition, that (4) and (5) are not cases of suicide. On this view, it would be said that neither the truckdriver nor Captain Oates *intentionally terminated* his life. While each initiated a chain of events that was foreseen as leading to his own death, neither initiated the chain of events because he desired to die, but quite the contrary, because he desired to attain some other objective, that is, the protection of others. Thus the primary intention of the basic action (redirecting the truck, walking away from camp) was to protect others; one's own death, it is said, is foreseen but not intended. Still, many would insist, contrary to the line of thought just developed, that both the truckdriver and Captain Oates did *intentionally terminate* their lives, since it was in their power to avoid their deaths but they chose (seemingly in noble fashion) not to do so.

One final case must be introduced. (6) A Jehovah's Witness, as a matter of religious principle, refuses to consent to a blood transfusion and dies. Is (6) a case of suicide? This judgment turns, as does our judgment regarding (4) and (5), on the interpretation of the phrase "intentional termination." The Jehovah's Witness, in many ways similar to the traditional Christian martyr, refuses to sacrifice religious principle and thereby brings about his or her own death. Those who say that (6) is not a case of suicide point out that the Jehovah's Witness typically does not want to die. The Jehovah's Witness foresees but does not intend his or her own death. Those who say that (6) is a case of suicide point out that, in effect, the avoidance of death is within the power of the Jehovah's Witness. Thus choosing to refuse the blood transfusion constitutes an intentional termination of life.

Notice, under certain circumstances, that refusal of lifesaving treatment is undeniably suicide. Suppose a person in good health is accidently injured and needs a routine blood transfusion in order to recover. Suppose further that this person refuses lifesaving treatment simply because he or she wants to die. In such a case, refusing lifesaving treatment is simply a convenient way of committing suicide. The phrase "intentional termination," however it is to be finally analyzed, clearly incorporates passive as well as active means. A person can commit suicide just as effectively by (passively) refusing to eat as by (actively) taking an overdose of drugs.

The Morality of Suicide

The preceding discussion of the concept of suicide has been presented as a necessary prelude to a consideration of ethical questions about suicide. As previously indicated, the first focal point of discussion in this chapter is the question: Under what circumstances, if at all, is suicide morally acceptable? Classical literature on the morality of suicide provides a number of sources who issue a strong moral condemnation of suicide. St. Augustine, St. Thomas Aquinas, and Immanuel Kant are prominent examples. Augustine's arguments are dominantly theological in character, but Aquinas and Kant advance philosophical as well as religiously based arguments against suicide. According to Aquinas, suicide is to be condemned not only because it violates our duty to God but also because it violates the natural law, and, moreover, because it injures the community. Kant, in the first selection of this chapter, argues that suicide degrades human worth and is therefore always immoral. R. B. Brandt, in this chapter's second selection, critically analyzes the most influential of the classical arguments against suicide. Brandt also forcefully defends the view that suicide is not necessarily immoral. This more liberal viewpoint, it is important to note, is not unprecedented in the classical literature on suicide. The Roman Stoic Seneca and the eighteenth-century Scottish philosopher David Hume are quite notable in their explication and defense of such a view.

The more liberal view on the morality of suicide might be explicated in general terms as follows. Suicide, to the extent that it does no substantial damage to the interests of other individuals, is morally acceptable. Moreover, even in cases where suicide has some impact on others, no person is morally obliged to undergo extreme distress to save others some smaller measure of sadness, and so forth. In accordance with this line of thought, it can be argued that suicide is morally acceptable even in some cases where a person has some rather significant social obligations, such as the duty to care for minor children. Suppose that a person has fallen unaccountably into a profound and inescapable depression. Suppose further that psychiatric counseling provides no relief. If the person becomes so undermined as to be incapable of caring for the minor children anyway, the argument goes, then suicide is morally acceptable.

Suicide Intervention

The second focal point of discussion in this chapter is the question: Is it justifiable for some agent of the state, acting in the name of society, to intervene and coercively prevent a person from committing suicide? Consider first the case of a competent adult with a reasoned and settled intention to commit suicide. In such a case, state intervention for the purpose of coercively preventing suicide would seem to present a significant ethical difficulty. The libertarian,[1] committed to the rejection of paternalistic interferences with individual liberty, argues that a competent adult's self-determination must be respected, even if his or her decision to commit suicide is considered unwise by others. In contrast, those who are more sympathetic to the legitimacy of paternalism are likely to argue that it is justifiable for society to interfere paternalistically with an individual's liberty (even a competent adult's) in order to protect that person from *serious and irrevocable* kinds of harm. One other line of argument deserves mention in the context of paternalism. In order to undermine the force of the libertarian contention that a competent adult's decision to commit suicide must be respected, it is sometimes asserted that a suicidal intention is necessarily irrational, thus a symptom of mental illness and incompetence. In other words, on this line of thought, it is impossible for a competent adult to have a suicidal intention. Although this point seems to be built into some psychiatric theories, it is considered by many philosophers to be an implausible contention. Brandt, in his discussion of the rationality of suicide, argues that suicide is surely a rational choice under certain kinds of circumstances.

Two other arguments may be presented in defense of societal intervention to prevent competent adults from committing suicide. First, it might be said that intervention is necessary in order to protect society's general interest in the sanctity of human life. The libertarian usually responds that such a vague interest cannot override individual self-determination. Second, it might be said that suicide is rightly prevented because it is immoral. Clearly, this second argument is asserted only by those who believe the law may rightly function to enforce morality. Needless to say, libertarians argue forcefully against this general principle.

In discussing the justifiability of state intervention for the purpose of coercively preventing a person from committing suicide, we should keep in mind that suicide attempts are very frequently not the result of a reasoned and settled intention. A humane social policy would certainly allow state intervention in cases where *temporary* disordering factors such as drugs, alcohol, or extreme (but fleeting) depression are operative. Indeed, libertarian principles are no more incompatible with intervention in the case of a temporarily disordered person than they are with intervention in the case of children or incompetent adults. In the case of a temporarily disordered person threatening suicide, intervention constitutes no substantive deprivation of liberty. The person involved, by hypothesis, is not acting in character; he or she does not really want to commit suicide. In typical cases, after the temporary crisis period, the individual is grateful for the (paternalistic) intervention. In one of this chapter's readings, David F. Greenberg argues in support of a suicide prevention policy that would allow temporary but not permanent intervention.

The Refusal of Lifesaving Treatment

The third focal point of discussion in this chapter is the question: Is it justifiable for some agent of the state, acting in the name of society, to compel a *competent* adult to accept lifesaving medical treatment? Discussions here largely parallel discussions of suicide intervention.

Some of the most dramatic cases involving the rejection of lifesaving treatment feature Jehovah's Witnesses who refuse to accept blood transfusions for religious reasons. It is important to remember, however, that reasons other than religious principle can motivate the refusal of lifesaving treatment. A terminally ill person may reject lifesaving treatment in order to shorten the agony of dying. Or, as indicated earlier, a person may reject lifesaving treatment simply because this possibility has presented itself as a convenient way of terminating an unsatisfying life. Libertarians argue, primarily on grounds of self-determination, that it is unjustifiable for society to interfere with the decision of a competent adult to refuse lifesaving treatment, except perhaps where such a decision causes substantial harm to other people, such as minor children. In the case of Jehovah's Witnesses, considerations of religious freedom are conjoined with considerations of self-determination to further strengthen the libertarian position.

Both Ruth Macklin and Norman L. Cantor, in this chapter's selections, reflect the libertarian perspective on the refusal of lifesaving treatment. Kenney F. Hegland provides a vivid contrast. He asserts a valid state interest in the life of every individual and holds that society's interest in the sanctity of human life is incompatible with allowing an individual, however competent, to choose to die. (Cantor responds rather directly to Hegland's contentions.) Aside from appeals to the sanctity of human life, and parallel to discussions of suicide intervention, arguments in support of compelling lifesaving treatment are also based on (1) the alleged right of society to enforce its conventional morality and (2) the alleged right of society to act (paternalistically) to protect an individual from the harmful exercise of his or her own volition.

The Dying Patient and the Refusal of Treatment

In considering the refusal of lifesaving treatment, there seem to be important differences between the following: (1) cases in which a patient will return to a state of health by accepting lifesaving treatment, and (2) cases in which a terminally ill patient, by accepting "lifesaving" treatment, will in essence *prolong the dying process*. Surely "suicide" is a label that seems inappropriate for (2), even if it is not inappropriate for (1). In dealing with the issue of the legitimacy of compelling a competent adult to accept lifesaving treatment, discussion in this chapter tends to emphasize (1), the more dramatic cases—especially the case of the Jehovah's Witness who refuses to accept a routine blood transfusion. But there is also much to be gained by focusing attention exclusively on (2), the less dramatic but pervasive cases. In part, this more narrow focus, which is reflected in this chapter's last two selections, effectively serves to pave the way for the introduction of a complex set of issues under the heading of "euthanasia" in Chapter 8.

In many cases of terminal illness, "aggressive" treatment is capable of warding off death—for a time. Cardiopulmonary resuscitation is especially notable in this regard. When a terminally ill patient undergoes cardiac arrest, resuscitation techniques can sometimes restore heartbeat and thus prolong life. Yet, in many cases, the patient does not desire and cannot benefit from resuscitation. Of course, in other cases, the patient does desire and can benefit from resuscitation. In still other cases, the appropriateness of resuscitation is more in doubt. Perhaps the patient has been ambivalent in expressing a preference about resuscitation. Perhaps the physician is uncertain whether or not resuscitation would be of genuine benefit to the patient. Perhaps the physician believes that resuscitation is in the patient's best interest, but the patient has expressed a preference not to be resuscitated. Or perhaps the physician believes that resuscitation is not in the patient's best interest, but the patient has expressed a preference to be resuscitated. In this chapter's final selection, the President's Commission for the Study of Ethical Problems in Medicine and Biomedical and Behavioral Research provides an extensive analysis of the ethical considerations relevant to resuscitation decisions—decisions that are ordinarily made within the framework of the physician-patient relationship. According to the Commission, patient self-determination is the single most important ethical consideration in resuscitation decisions, although the physician's assessment of benefit to the patient, which is sometimes in conflict with patient preference, is also relevant. In proposing an overall scheme to guide decision making, the Commission attempts to come to grips not only with the conflicts that may arise between patient preference and physician's assessment of benefit but also with the uncertainties that may arise from either perspective.

Some terminally ill patients willingly submit to any medical intervention thought to be capable of extending their lives. Many others, in the light of the seriously compromised character of their present existence, are more concerned to achieve what M. Pabst Battin in this chapter calls "the least worst death." Battin's principal point is that a patient, with the advice of a physician, has the best chance of achieving "the least worst death" by the *selective* refusal of treatment.

T.A.M.

NOTE

1 The label "libertarian," in this context, refers to a person who asserts the primacy of individual liberty. In particular, a libertarian is reluctant to accept the principles of paternalism and the principle of legal moralism as legitimate liberty-limiting principles. (These principles are discussed in Chapter 1.)

The Morality of Suicide

Suicide

Immanuel Kant

Immanuel Kant (1724–1804), widely acknowledged to be one of the most influential figures in the history of Western philosophy, was a native of East Prussia. Kant largely dedicated his life to academic philosophy and was eventually appointed to the chair of logic and metaphysics at the University of Königsberg. His works are voluminous and address a very wide range of philosophical issues. Kant's ethical theory, discussed in Chapter 1, is a landmark of deontological thought. The *Groundwork of the Metaphysic of Morals* (1785) and *The Critique of Practical Reason* (1788) are two of his most notable works in ethics.

Kant issues a blanket moral condemnation of suicide: "Suicide is in no circumstances permissible." In his view, suicide is characterized by the intention to destroy oneself. Thus neither the "victim of fate" nor the person whose intemperance leads to a shortened life is guilty of suicide. Kant insists that suicide is self-contradictory, in the sense that the power of free will is used for its own destruction. In a related consideration, suicide is said to be a moral abomination because it degrades human worth. Kant also claims that suicide is rightly condemned on religious grounds.

DUTIES TOWARDS THE BODY IN REGARD TO LIFE

What are our powers of disposal over our life? Have we any authority of disposal over it in any shape or form? How far is it incumbent upon us to take care of it? These are questions which fail to be considered in connexion with our duties towards the body in regard to life. We must, however, by way of introduction, make the following observations. If the body were

From Immanuel Kant, *Lecture on Ethics,* translated by Louis Infield (New York: Harper & Row, 1963), pp. 147–154. Reprinted by permission of Methuen & Co. Ltd.

related to life not as a condition but as an accident or circumstance so that we could at will divest ourselves of it; if we could slip out of it and slip into another just as we leave one country for another, then the body would be subject to our free will and we could rightly have the disposal of it. This, however, would not imply that we could similarly dispose of our life, but only of our circumstances, of the movable goods, the furniture of life. In fact, however, our life is entirely conditioned by our body, so that we cannot conceive of a life not mediated by the body and we cannot make use of our freedom except through the body. It is, therefore, obvious that the body constitutes a part of ourselves. If a man destroys his body, and so his life, he does it by the use of his will, which is itself destroyed in the process. But to use the power of a free will for its own destruction is self-contradictory. If freedom is the condition of life it cannot be employed to abolish life and so to destroy and abolish itself. To use life for its own destruction, to use life for producing lifelessness, is self-contradictory. These preliminary remarks are sufficient to show that man cannot rightly have any power of disposal in regard to himself and his life, but only in regard to his circumstances. His body gives man power over his life; were he a spirit he could not destroy his life; life in the absolute has been invested by nature with indestructibility and is an end in itself; hence it follows that man cannot have the power to dispose of his life.

SUICIDE

Suicide can be regarded in various lights; it might be held to be reprehensible, or permissible, or even heroic. In the first place we have the specious view that suicide can be allowed and tolerated. Its advocates argue thus. So long as he does not violate the proprietary rights of others, man is a free agent. With regard to his body there are various things he can properly do; he can have a boil lanced or a limb amputated, and disregard a scar; he is, in fact, free to do whatever he may consider useful and advisable. If then he comes to the conclusion that the most useful and advisable thing that he can do is to put an end to his life, why should he not be entitled to do so? Why not, if he sees that he can no longer go on living and that he will be ridding himself of misfortune, torment and disgrace? To be sure he robs himself of a full life, but he escapes once and for all from calamity and misfortune. The argument

sounds most plausible. But let us, leaving aside religious considerations, examine the act itself. We may treat our body as we please, provided our motives are those of self-preservation. If, for instance, his foot is a hindrance to life, a man might have it amputated. To preserve his person he has the right of disposal over his body. But in taking his life he does not preserve his person; he disposes of his person and not of its attendant circumstances; he robs himself of his person. This is contrary to the highest duty we have towards ourselves, for it annuls the condition of all other duties; it goes beyond the limits of the use of free will, for this use is possible only through the existence of the Subject.

There is another set of considerations which make suicide seem plausible. A man might find himself so placed that he can continue living only under circumstances which deprive life of all value; in which he can no longer live comfortably to virtue and prudence, so that he must from noble motives put an end to his life. The advocates of this view quote in support of it the example of Cato. Cato knew that the entire Roman nation relied upon him in their resistance to Caesar, but he found that he could not prevent himself from falling into Caeser's hands. What was he to do? If he, the champion of freedom, submitted, every one would say, "If Cato himself submits, what else can we do?" If, on the other hand, he killed himself, his death might spur on the Romans to fight to the bitter end in defence of their freedom. So he killed himself. He thought that it was necessary for him to die. He thought that if he could not go on living as Cato, he could not go on living at all. It must certainly be admitted that in a case such as this, where suicide is a virtue, appearances are in its favour. But this is the only example which has given the world the opportunity of defending suicide. It is the only example of its kind and there has been no similar case since. Lucretia also killed herself, but on grounds of modesty and in a fury of vengeance. It is obviously our duty to preserve our honour, particularly in relation to the opposite sex, for whom it is a merit; but we must endeavour to save our honour only to this extent, that we ought not to surrender it for selfish and lustful purposes. To do what Lucretia did is to adopt a remedy which is not at our disposal; it would have been better had she defended her honour unto death; that would not have been suicide and would have been right; for it is no suicide to risk one's life against one's enemies, and even to sacrifice it, in order to observe one's duties towards oneself.

No one under the sun can bind me to commit suicide; no sovereign can do so. The sovereign can call upon his subjects to fight to the death for their country, and those who fall on the field of battle are not suicides, but the victims of fate. Not only is this not suicide, but the opposite; a faint heart and fear of the death which threatens by the necessity of fate, is no true self-preservation; for he who runs away to save his own life, and leaves his comrades in the lurch, is a coward; but he who defends himself and his fellows even unto death is no suicide, but noble and high-minded; for life is not to be highly regarded for its own sake. I should endeavour to preserve my own life only so far as I am worthy to live. We must draw a distinction between the suicide and the victim of fate. A man who shortens his life by intemperance is guilty of imprudence and indirectly of his own death; but his guilt is not direct; he did not intend to kill himself; his death was not premeditated. For all our offences are either *culpa* or *dolus*. There is certainly no *dolus* here, but there is *culpa;* and we can say of such a man that he was guilty of his own death, but we cannot say of him that he is a suicide. What constitutes suicide is the intention to destroy oneself. Intemperance and excess which shorten life ought not, therefore, to be called suicide; for if we raise intemperance to the level of suicide, we lower suicide to the level of intemperance. Imprudence, which does not imply a desire to cease to live, must, therefore, be distinguished from the intention to murder oneself. Serious violations of our duty towards ourselves produce an aversion accompanied either by horror or by disgust; suicide is of the horrible kind, *crimina carnis* of the disgusting. We shrink in horror from suicide because all nature seeks its own preservation; an injured tree, a living body, an animal does so; how then could man make of his freedom, which is the acme of life and constitutes its worth, a principle for his own destruction? Nothing more terrible can be imagined; for if man were on every occasion master of his own life, he would be master of the lives of others; and being ready to sacrifice his life at any and every time rather than be captured, he could perpetrate every conceivable crime and vice. We are, therefore, horrified at the very thought of suicide; by it man sinks lower than the beasts; we look upon a suicide as carrion, whilst our sympathy goes forth to the victim of fate.

Those who advocate suicide seek to give the widest interpretation to freedom. There is something flattering in the thought that we can take our own life if we are so minded; and so we find even right-thinking persons defining suicide in this respect. There are many circumstances under which life ought to be sacrificed. If I cannot preserve my life except by violating my duties towards myself, I am bound to sacrifice my life rather than violate these duties. But suicide is in no circumstances permissible. Humanity in one's own person is something inviolable; it is a holy trust; man is master of all else, but he must not lay hands upon himself. A being who existed of his own necessity could not possibly destroy himself; a being whose existence is not necessary must regard life as the condition of everything else, and in the consciousness that life is a trust reposed in him, such a being recoils at the thought of committing a breach of his holy trust by turning his life against himself. Man can only dispose over things; beasts are things in this sense; but man is not a thing, not a beast. If he disposes over himself, he treats his value as that of a beast. He who so behaves, who has no respect for human nature and makes a thing of himself, becomes for everyone an Object of freewill. We are free to treat him as a beast, as a thing, and to use him for our sport as we do a horse or a dog, for he is no longer a human being; he has made a thing of himself, and, having himself discarded his humanity, he cannot expect that others should respect humanity in him. Yet humanity is worthy of esteem. Even when a man is a bad man, humanity in his person is worthy of esteem. Suicide is not abominable and inadmissible because life should be highly prized; were it so, we could each have our own opinion of how highly we should prize it, and the rule of prudence would often indicate suicide as the best means. But the rule of morality does not admit of it under any condition because it degrades human nature below the level of animal nature and so destroys it. Yet there is much in the world far more important than life. To observe morality is far more important. It is better to sacrifice one's life than one's morality. To live is not a necessity; but to live honourably while life lasts is a necessity. We can at all times go on living and doing our duty towards ourselves without having to do violence to ourselves. But he who is prepared to take his own life is no longer worthy to live at all. The pragmatic ground of impulse to live is happiness. Can I then take my own life because I cannot live happily? No! It is not necessary that whilst I live I should live happily; but it is necessary that so long as I live I should live honourably. Misery gives no right to any man to take his own life, for then we should all be entitled to take our lives for lack of pleasure. All our duties towards ourselves would then be directed towards pleasure; but the fulfillment of those duties may demand that we should even sacrifice our life.

Is suicide heroic or cowardly? Sophistication, even though well meant, is not a good thing. It is not good to defend either virtue or vice by splitting hairs. Even right-thinking people declaim against suicide on wrong lines. They say that it is arrant cowardice. But instances of suicide of great heroism exist. We cannot, for example, regard the suicides of Cato and Atticus as cowardly. Rage, passion and insanity are the most frequent causes of suicide, and that is why persons who attempt suicide and are saved from it are so terrified at their own act that they do not dare to repeat the attempt. There was a time in Roman and in Greek history when suicide was regarded as honourable, so much so that the Romans forbade their slaves to commit suicide because they did not belong to themselves but to their masters and so were regarded as things, like all other animals. The Stoics said that suicide is the sage's peaceful death; he leaves the world as he might leave a smoky room for another, because it no longer pleases him; he leaves the world, not because he is no longer happy in it, but because he disdains it. It has already been mentioned that man is greatly flattered by the idea that he is free to remove himself from this world, if he so wishes. He may not make use of this freedom, but the thought of possessing it pleases him. It seems even to have a moral aspect, for if man is capable of removing himself from the world at his own will, he need not submit to any one; he can retain his independence and tell the rudest truths to the cruellest of tyrants. Torture cannot bring him to heel, because he can leave the world at a moment's notice as a free man can leave the country, if and when he wills it. But this semblance of morality vanishes as soon as we see that man's freedom cannot subsist except on a condition which is immutable. This condition is that man may not use his freedom against himself to his own destruction, but that, on the contrary, he should allow nothing external to limit it. Freedom thus conditioned is noble. No chance or misfortune ought to make us afraid to live; we ought to go on living as long as we can do so as

human beings and honourably. To bewail one's fate and misfortune is in itself dishonourable. Had Cato faced any torments which Caesar might have inflicted upon him with a resolute mind and remained steadfast, it would have been noble of him; to violate himself was not so. Those who advocate suicide and teach that there is authority for it necessarily do much harm in a republic of free men. Let us imagine a state in which men held as a general opinion that they were entitled to commit suicide, and that there was even merit and honour in so doing. How dreadful everyone would find them. For he who does not respect his life even in principle cannot be restrained from the most dreadful vices; he recks neither king nor torments.

But as soon as we examine suicide from the standpoint of religion we immediately see it in its true light. We have been placed in this world under certain conditions and for specific purposes. But a suicide opposes the purpose of his Creator; he arrives in the other world as one who has deserted his post; he must be looked upon as a rebel against God. So long as we remember the truth that it is God's intention to preserve life, we are bound to regulate our activities in conformity with it. We have no right to offer violence to our nature's powers of self-preservation and to upset the wisdom of her arrangements. This duty is upon us until the time comes when God expressly commands us to leave this life. Human beings are sentinels on earth and may not leave their posts until relieved by another beneficent hand. God is our owner; we are His property; His providence works for our good. A bondman in the care of a beneficent master deserves punishment if he opposes his master's wishes.

But suicide is not inadmissible and abominable because God has forbidden it; God has forbidden it because it is abominable in that it degrades man's inner worth below that of the animal creation. Moral philosophers must, therefore, first and foremost show that suicide is abominable. We find, as a rule, that those who labour for their happiness are more liable to suicide; having tasted the refinements of pleasure, and being deprived of them, they give way to grief, sorrow, and melancholy.

The Morality and Rationality of Suicide

R. B. Brandt

R. B. Brandt is professor of philosophy at the University of Michigan. He is the author of *Ethical Theory* (1959) and *A Theory of the Good and the Right* (1979), and he is the coeditor of *Meaning and Knowledge* (1965) and *The Problems of Philosophy* (2d ed., 1974). Brandt's article "Toward a Credible Form of Utilitarianism" is one prominent example of his many contributions to contemporary discussions of utilitarian theory.

Operating on the assumption that suicide is to be understood as the intentional termination of one's own life, Brandt sets himself firmly against the view that suicide is always immoral. He critically analyzes, and finds wanting, various classes of arguments that have been advanced to support the alleged immorality of suicide: (1) theological arguments, (2) arguments from natural law, and (3) arguments to the effect that suicide necessarily does harm to other persons or to society in general. Brandt does acknowledge that there is some obligation to refrain from committing suicide when that act would be injurious to others, but he insists that this obligation may often be overridden by other morally relevant considerations. Clearly, for Brandt, suicide is sometimes morally acceptable. He also insists that a person's decision to commit suicide may be quite rational, although he is careful to warn of potential errors in judgment. He concludes by analyzing the various factors that are relevant in establishing the moral obligation of other persons toward those who are contemplating suicide.

THE MORAL REASONS FOR AND AGAINST SUICIDE

[Assuming that there is suicide if and only if there is intentional termination of one's own life,] persons who say suicide is morally wrong must be asked which of two positions they are affirming: Are they saying that *every* act of suicide is wrong, *everything considered;* or are they merely saying that there is always *some* moral obligation—doubtless of serious weight—not to commit suicide, so that very often suicide is wrong, although it is possible that there are *countervailing considerations* which in particular situations make it right or even a moral duty? It is quite evident that the first position is absurd; only the second has a chance of being defensible.

In order to make clear what is wrong with the first view, we may begin with an example. Suppose an army pilot's single-seater plane goes out of control over a heavily populated area; he has the choice of staying in the plane and bringing it down where it will do little damage but at the cost of certain death for himself, and of bailing out and letting the plane fall where it will, very possibly killing a good many civilians. Suppose he chooses to do the former, and so, by our definition, commits suicide. Does anyone want to say that his action is morally wrong? Even Immanuel Kant, who opposed suicide in all circumstances, apparently would not wish to say that it is; he would, in fact, judge that this act is not one of suicide, for he says, "It is no suicide to risk one's life against one's enemies, and even to sacrifice it, in order to preserve one's duties toward oneself."[1] St. Thomas Aquinas, in his discussion of suicide, may seem to take the position that such an act would be wrong, for he says, "It is altogether unlawful to kill oneself," admitting as an exception only the case of being under special command of God. But I believe St. Thomas would, in fact, have concluded that the act is right because the basic intention of the pilot was to save the lives of civilians, and whether an act is right or wrong is a matter of basic intention.[2]

In general, we have to admit that there are things with some moral obligation to avoid which, on account of other morally relevant considerations, it is sometimes right or even morally obligatory to do. There may be some obligation to tell the truth on every occasion, but surely in many cases the consequences of telling the truth would be so dire that one is obligated to lie. The same goes for promises. There is some moral obligation to do what one has promised (with a few exceptions); but, if one can keep a trivial promise only at serious cost to another person (i.e., keep an appointment only by failing to give aid to someone injured in an accident), it is surely obligatory to break the promise.

The most that the moral critic of suicide could hold, then, is that there is *some* moral obligation not to do what one knows will cause one's death; but he surely cannot deny that circumstances exist in which there are obligations to do things which, in fact, will result in one's death. If so, then in principle it would be possible to argue, for instance, that in order to meet my obligation to my family, it might be right for me to take my own life as the only way to avoid catastrophic hospital expenses in a terminal illness. Possibly the main point that critics of suicide on moral grounds would wish to make is that it is never right to take one's own life *for reasons of one's own personal welfare,* of any kind whatsoever. Some of the arguments used to support the immorality of suicide, however, are so framed that if they were supportable at all, they would prove that suicide is *never* moral.

One well-known type of argument against suicide may be classified as *theological.* St. Augustine and others urged that the Sixth Commandment ("Thou shalt not kill") prohibits suicide, and that we are bound to obey a divine commandment. To this reasoning one might first reply that it is arbitrary exegesis of the Sixth Commandment to assert that it was intended to prohibit suicide. The second reply is that if there is not some consideration which shows on the merits of the case that suicide is morally wrong, God had no business prohibiting it. It is true that some will object to this point, and I must refer them elsewhere for my detailed comments on the divine-will theory of morality.[3]

Another theological argument with wide support was accepted by John Locke, who wrote:"... Men being all the workmanship of one omnipotent and infinitely wise Maker; all the servants of one sovereign Master,

sent into the world by His order and about His business; they are His property, whose workmanship they are made to last during His, not one another's pleasure ... Every one ... is bound to preserve himself, and not to quit his station wilfully.... "[4] And Kant: "We have been placed in this world under certain conditions and for specific purposes. But a suicide opposes the purpose of his Creator; he arrives in the other world as one who has deserted his post; he must be looked upon as a rebel against God. So long as we remember the truth that it is God's intention to preserve life, we are bound to regulate our activities in conformity with it. This duty is upon us until the time comes when God expressly commands us to leave this life. Human beings are sentinels on earth and may not leave their posts until relieved by another beneficent hand."[5] Unfortunately, however, even if we grant that it is the duty of human beings to do what God commands or intends them to do, more argument is required to show that God does *not* permit human beings to quit this life when their own personal welfare would be maximized by so doing. How does one draw the requisite inference about the intentions of God? The difficulties and contradictions in arguments to reach such a conclusion are discussed at length and perspicaciously by David Hume in his essay "On Suicide," and in view of the unlikelihood that readers will need to be persuaded about these, I shall merely refer those interested to that essay.[6]

A second group of arguments may be classed as arguments *from natural law.* St. Thomas says: "It is altogether unlawful to kill oneself, for three reasons. First, because everything naturally loves itself, the result being that everything naturally keeps itself in being, and resists corruptions so far as it can. Wherefore suicide is contrary to the inclination of nature, and to charity whereby every man should love himself. Hence suicide is always a mortal sin, as being contrary to the natural law and to charity."[7] Here St. Thomas ignores two obvious points. First, it is not obvious why a human being is morally bound to do what he or she has some inclination to do. (St. Thomas did not criticize chastity.) Second, while it is true that most human beings do feel a strong urge to live, the human being who commits suicide obviously feels a stronger inclination to do something else. It is as natural for a human being to dislike, and to take steps to avoid, say, great pain, as it is to cling to life.

A somewhat similar argument by Immanuel Kant may seem better. In a famous passage Kant writes that the maxim of a person who commits suicide is "From self-love I make it my principle to shorten my life if its continuance threatens more evil than it promises pleasure. The only further question to ask is whether this principle of self-love can become a universal law of nature. It is then seen at once that a system of nature by whose law the very same feeling whose function is to stimulate the furtherance of life should actually destroy life would contradict itself and consequently could not subsist as a system of nature. Hence this maxim cannot possibly hold as a universal law of nature and is therefore entirely opposed to the supreme principle of all duty."[8] What Kant finds contradictory is that the motive of self-love (interest in one's own long-range welfare) should sometimes lead one to struggle to preserve one's life, but at other times to end it. But where is the contradiction? One's circumstances change, and, if the argument of the following section in this [paper] is correct, one sometimes maximizes one's own long-range welfare by trying to stay alive, but at other times by bringing about one's demise.

A third group of arguments, a form of which goes back at least to Aristotle, has a more modern and convincing ring. These are arguments to show that, in one way or another, a suicide necessarily does harm to other persons, or to society at large. Aristotle says that the suicide treats the *state* unjustly.[9] Partly following Aristotle, St. Thomas says: "Every man is part of the community, and so, as such, he belongs to the community. Hence by killing himself he injures the community."[10] Blackstone held that a suicide is an offense against the king "who hath an interest in the preservation of all his subjects," perhaps following Judge Brown in 1563, who argued that suicide cost the king a subject—"he being the head has lost one of his mystical members."[11] The premise of such arguments is, as Hume pointed out, obviously mistaken in many instances. It is true that Freud would perhaps have injured society had he, instead of finishing his last book, committed suicide to escape the pain of throat cancer. But surely there have been many suicides whose demise was not a noticeable loss to society; an honest man could only say that in some instances society was better off without them.

It need not be denied that suicide is often injurious to other persons, especially the family of a suicide. Clearly it sometimes is. But, we should notice what this fact establishes. Suppose we admit, as generally would be done, that there is some obligation not to perform any action which will probably or certainly be injurious to other people, the strength of the obligation being dependent on various factors, notably the seriousness of the expected injury. Then there is *some* obligation not to commit suicide, when that act would probably or certainly be injurious to other people. But, as we have already seen, many cases of *some* obligation to do something nevertheless are *not* cases of a duty to do that thing, *everything considered.* So it could sometimes be morally justified to commit suicide, even if the act will harm someone. Must a man with a terminal illness undergo excruciating pain because his death will cause his wife sorrow—when she will be caused sorrow a month later anyway, when he is dead of natural causes? Moreover, to repeat, the fact that an individual has some obligation not to commit suicide when that act will probably injure other persons does not imply that, everything considered, it is wrong for him to do it, namely, that in all circumstances suicide *as such* is something there is some obligation to avoid.

Is there any sound argument, convincing to the modern mind, to establish that there is (or is not) *some moral obligation* to avoid suicide *as such,* an obligation, of course, which might be overridden by other obligations in some or many cases? (Captain Oates may have had a moral obligation not to commit suicide as such, but his obligation not to stand in the way of his comrades getting to safety might have been so strong that, everything considered, he was justified in leaving the polar camp and allowing himself to freeze to death.)

To present all the arguments necessary to answer this question convincingly would take a great deal of space. I shall, therefore, simply state one answer to it which seems plausible to some contemporary philosophers. Suppose it could be shown that it would maximize the long-run welfare of everybody affected if people were taught that there is a moral obligation to avoid suicide—so that people would be motivated to avoid suicide just because they thought it wrong (would have anticipatory guilt feelings at the very idea), and so that other people would be inclined to disapprove of persons who commit suicide unless there were some excuse.... One might ask: how could it maximize utility to mold the conceptual and motivational structure of persons in this way? To which the answer might be: feeling in this way might make persons who are impulsively inclined to commit suicide in a bad mood, or a fit of anger or jealousy, take more time to deliberate; hence, some suicides that have bad effects generally might be prevented. In other words, it might be a good thing in its effects for people to feel about suicide in the way they feel about breach of promise or injuring others, just as it might be a good thing for people to feel a moral obligation not to smoke, or to wear seat belts. However, it might be that negative moral feelings about suicide as such would stand in the way of action by those persons whose welfare really is best served by suicide and whose suicide is the best thing for everybody concerned.

WHEN A DECISION TO COMMIT SUICIDE IS RATIONAL FROM THE PERSON'S POINT OF VIEW

The person who is contemplating suicide is obviously making a choice between future world-courses; the world-course that includes his demise, say, an hour from now, and several possible ones that contain his demise at a later point. One cannot have precise knowledge about many features of the latter group of world-courses, but it is certain that they will all end with death some (possibly short) finite time from now.

Why do I say the choice is between *world*-courses and not just a choice between future life-courses of the prospective suicide, the one shorter than the other? The reason is that one's suicide has some impact on the world (and one's continued life has some impact on the world), and that conditions in the rest of the world will often make a difference in one's evaluation of the possibilities. One *is* interested in things in the world other than just oneself and one's own happiness.

The basic question a person must answer, in order to determine which world-course is best or rational for him to choose, is which he *would* choose under conditions of optimal use of information, when *all* of his desires are taken into account. It is not just a question of what we prefer *now,* with some clarification of all the possibilities being considered. Our preferences change, and the preferences of tomorrow (assuming we can know something about them) are just as legitimately taken into account in deciding what to do now as the preferences of today. Since any reason that can be given today for weighting heavily today's preference can be given tomorrow for weighting heavily tomorrow's preference, the preferences of any time-stretch have a rational claim to an equal vote. Now the importance of that fact is this: we often know quite well that our desires, aversions, and preferences may change after a short while. When a person is in a state of despair—perhaps brought about by a rejection in love or discharge from a long-held position—nothing but

the thing he cannot have seems desirable; everything else is turned to ashes. Yet we know quite well that the passage of time is likely to reverse all this; replacements may be found or other types of things that are available to us may begin to look attractive. So, if we were to act on the preferences of today alone, when the emotion of despair seems more than we can stand, we might find death preferable to life; but, if we allow for the preferences of the weeks and years ahead, when many goals will be enjoyable and attractive, we might find life much preferable to death. So, if a choice of what is best is to be determined by what we want not only now but later (and later desires on an equal basis with the present ones)—as it should be—then what is the best or preferable world-course will often be quite different from what it would be if the choice, or what is best for one, were fixed by one's desires and preferences now.

Of course, if one commits suicide there are no future desires or aversions that may be compared with present ones and that should be allowed an equal vote in deciding what is best. In that respect the course of action that results in death is different from any other course of action we may undertake. I do not wish to suggest the rosy possibility that it is often or always reasonable to believe that next week "I shall be more interested in living than I am today, if today I take a dim view of continued existence." On the contrary, when a person is seriously ill, for instance, he may have no reason to think that the preference-order will be reversed—it may be that tomorrow he will prefer death to life more strongly.

The argument is often used that one can never be *certain* what is going to happen, and hence one is never rationally justified in doing anything as drastic as committing suicide. But we always have to live by probabilities and make our estimates as best we can. As soon as it is clear beyond reasonable doubt not only that death is now preferable to life, but also that it will be every day from now until the end, the rational thing is to act promptly.

Let us not pursue the question of whether it is rational for a person with a painful terminal illness to commit suicide; it is. However, the issue seldom arises, and few terminally ill patients do commit suicide. With such patients matters usually get worse slowly so that no particular time seems to call for action. They are often so heavily sedated that it is impossible for the mental processes of decision leading to action to occur; or else they are incapacitated in a hospital and the very physical possibility of ending their lives is not available.

Let us leave this grim topic and turn to a practically more important problem: whether it is rational for persons to commit suicide for some reason other than painful terminal physical illness. Most persons who commit suicide do so, apparently, because they face a nonphysical problem that depresses them beyond their ability to bear.

Among the problems that have been regarded as good and sufficient reasons for ending life, we find (in addition to serious illness) the following: some event that has made a person feel ashamed or lose his prestige and status; reduction from affluence to poverty; the loss of a limb or of physical beauty; the loss of sexual capacity; some event that makes it seem impossible to achieve things by which one sets store; loss of a loved one; disappointment in love; the infirmities of increasing age. It is not to be denied that such things can be serious blows to a person's prospects of happiness.

Whatever the nature of an individual's problem, there are various plain errors to be avoided—errors to which a person is especially prone when he is depressed—in deciding whether, everything considered, he prefers a world-course containing his early demise to one in which his life continues to its natural terminus. Let us forget for a moment the relevance to the decision of preferences that he may have tomorrow, and concentrate on some errors that may infect his preference as of today, and for which correction or allowance must be made.

In the first place, depression, like any severe emotional experience, tends to primitivize one's intellectual processes. It restricts the range of one's survey of the possibilities. One thing that a rational person would do is compare the world-course containing his suicide with his *best* alternative. But his best alternative is precisely a possibility he may overlook if, in a depressed mood, he thinks only of how badly off he is and cannot imagine any way of improving his situation. If a person is disappointed in love, it is possible to adopt a vigorous plan of action that carries a good chance of acquainting him with someone he likes at least as well; and if old age prevents a person from continuing the tennis game with his favorite partner, it is possible to learn some other game that provides the joys of competition without the physical demands.

Depression has another insidious influence on one's planning; it seriously affects one's judgment about probabilities. A person disappointed in love is very likely to take a dim view of himself, his prospects, and his attractiveness; he thinks that because he has been

rejected by one person he will probably be rejected by anyone who looks desirable to him. In a less gloomy frame of mind he would make different estimates. Part of the reason for such gloomy probability estimates is that depression tends to repress one's memory of evidence that supports a nongloomy prediction. Thus, a rejected lover tends to forget any cases in which he has elicited enthusiastic response from ladies in relation to whom he has been the one who has done the rejecting. Thus his pessimistic self-image is based upon a highly selected, and pessimistically selected, set of data. Even when he is reminded of the data, moreover, he is apt to resist an optimistic inference.

Another kind of distortion of the look of future prospects is not a result of depression, but is quite normal. Events distant in the future feel small, just as objects distant in space look small. Their prospect does not have the effect on motivational processes that it would have if it were of an event in the immediate future. Psychologists call this the "goal-gradient" phenomenon; a rat, for instance, will run faster toward a perceived food box than a distant unseen one. In the case of a person who has suffered some misfortune, and whose situation now is an unpleasant one, this reduction of the motivational influence of events distant in time has the effect that present unpleasant states weigh far more heavily than probable future pleasant ones in any choice of world-courses.

If we are trying to determine whether we now prefer, or shall later prefer, the outcome of one world-course to that of another (and this is leaving aside the questions of the weight of the votes of preferences at a later date), we must take into account these and other infirmities of our "sensing" machinery. Since knowing that the machinery is out of order will not tell us what results it would give if it were working, the best recourse might be to refrain from making any decision in a stressful frame of mind. If decisions have to be made, one must recall past reactions, in a normal frame of mind, to outcomes like those under assessment. But many suicides seem to occur in moments of despair. What should be clear from the above is that a moment of despair, if one is seriously contemplating suicide, ought to be a moment of reassessment of one's goals and values, a reassessment which the individual must realize is very difficult to make objectively, because of the very quality of his depressed frame of mind.

A decision to commit suicide may in certain circumstances be a rational one. But a person who wants to act rationally must take into account the various possible "errors" and make appropriate rectification of his initial evaluations.

THE ROLE OF OTHER PERSONS

What is the moral obligation of other persons toward those who are contemplating suicide? The question of their moral blameworthiness may be ignored and what is rational for them to do from the point of view of personal welfare may be considered as being of secondary concern. Laws make it dangerous to aid or encourage a suicide. The risk of running afoul of the law may partly determine moral obligation, since moral obligation to do something may be reduced by the fact that it is personally dangerous.

The moral obligation of other persons toward one who is contemplating suicide is an instance of a general obligation to render aid to those in serious distress, at least when this can be done at no great cost to one's self. I do not think this general principle is seriously questioned by anyone, whatever his moral theory; so I feel free to assume it as a premise. Obviously the person contemplating suicide is in great distress of some sort; if he were not, he would not be seriously considering terminating his life.

How great a person's obligation is to one in distress depends on a number of factors. Obviously family and friends have special obligations to devote time to helping the prospective suicide—which others do not have. But anyone in this kind of distress has a moral claim on the time of any person who knows the situation (unless there are others more responsible who are already doing what should be done).

What is the obligation? It depends, of course, on the situation, and how much the second person knows about the situation. If the individual has decided to terminate his life if he can, and it is clear that he is right in this decision, then, if he needs help in executing the decision, there is a moral obligation to give him help. On this matter a patient's physician has a special obligation, from which any talk about the Hippocratic oath does not absolve him. It is true that there are some damages one cannot be expected to absorb, and some risks which one cannot be expected to take, on account of the obligation to render aid.

On the other hand, if it is clear that the individual should not commit suicide, from the point of view of his own welfare, or if there is a presumption that he should not (when the only evidence is that a person is discovered unconscious, with the gas turned on), it would seem to be the individual's obligation to intervene, prevent the successful execution of the decision, and see to the availability of competent psychiatric advice and temporary hospitalization, if necessary. Whether one has a right to take such steps when a clearly sane person, after careful reflection over a period of time, comes to the conclusion that an end to his life is what is best for him and what he wants, is very doubtful, even when one thinks his conclusion a mistaken one; it would seem that a man's own considered decision about whether he wants to live must command respect, although one must concede that this could be debated.

The more interesting role in which a person may be cast, however, is that of adviser. It is often important to one who is contemplating suicide to go over his thinking with another, and to feel that a conclusion, one way or the other, has the support of a respected mind. One thing one can obviously do, in rendering the service of advice, is to discuss with the person the various types of issues discussed above, made more specific by the concrete circumstances of his case, and help him find whether, in view, say, of the damage his suicide would do to others, he has a moral obligation to refrain, and whether it is rational or best for him, from the point of view of his own welfare, to take this step or adopt some other plan instead.

To get a person to see what is the rational thing to do is no small job. Even to get a person, in a frame of mind when he is seriously contemplating (or perhaps has already unsuccessfully attempted) suicide, to recognize a plain truth of fact may be a major operation. If a man insists, "I am a complete failure," when it is obvious that by any reasonable standard he is far from that, it may be tremendously difficult to get him to see the fact. But there is another job beyond that of getting a person to see what is the rational thing to do; that is to help him *act* rationally, or *be* rational, when he has conceded what would be the rational thing.

How either of these tasks may be accomplished effectively may be discussed more competently by an experienced psychiatrist than by a philosopher. Loneliness and the absence of human affection are states which exacerbate any other problems; disappointment, reduction to poverty, and so forth, seem less impossible to bear in the presence of the affection of another. Hence simply to be a friend, or to find someone a friend, may be the largest contribution one can make either to helping a person be rational or see clearly what is rational for him to do; this service may make one who was contemplating suicide feel that there is a future for him which it is possible to face.

NOTES

1 Immanuel Kant, *Lectures on Ethics,* New York: Harper Torchbook (1963), p. 150.

2 See St. Thomas Aquinas, *Summa Theologica,* Second Part of the Second Part, Q. 64, Art. 5. In Article 7, he says: "Nothing hinders one act from having two effects, only one of which is intended, while the other is beside the intention. Now moral acts take their species according to what is intended, and not according to what is beside the intention, since this is accidental as explained above" (Q. 43, Art. 3: I-II, Q. 1, Art. 3, as 3). Mr. Norman St. John-Stevas, the most articulate contemporary defender of the Catholic view, writes as follows: "Christian thought allows certain exceptions to its general condemnation of suicide. That covered by a particular divine inspiration has already been noted. Another exception arises where suicide is the method imposed by the state for the execution of a just death penalty. A third exception is *altruistic* suicide, of which the best known example is Captain Oates. Such suicides are justified by invoking the principles of double effect. The act from which death results must be good or at least morally indifferent; some other good effect must result: The death must not be directly intended or the real means to the good effect, and a grave reason must exist for adopting the course of action"[*Life, Death and the Law,* Bloomington, Ind.: Indiana University Press (1961), pp. 250–51]. Presumably the Catholic doctrine is intended to allow suicide when this is required for meeting strong moral obligations; whether it can do so consistently depends partly on the interpretation given to "real means to the good effect." Readers interested in pursuing further the Catholic doctrine of double effect and its implications for our problem should read Philippa Foot, "The Problem of Abortion and the Doctrine of Double Effect," *The Oxford Review,* 5:5–15 (Trinity 1967).

3 R. B. Brandt, *Ethical Theory,* Englewood Cliffs, N.J.: Prentice Hall (1959), pp. 61–82.

4 John Locke, *Two Treatises of Government,* Ch. 2.

5 Kant, *Lectures on Ethics,* p. 154.

6 This essay appears in collections of Hume's works.

7 For an argument similar to Kant's, see also St. Thomas Aquinas, *Summa Theologica,* II, II, Q. 64, Art. 5.

8 Immanuel Kant, *The Fundamental Principles of the Metaphysic of Morals,* trans H. J. Paton, London: The Hutchinson Group (1948), Ch. 2.

9 Aristotle, *Nicomachaean Ethics,* Bk. 5, Ch. 10., p. 1138a.

10 St. Thomas Aquinas, *Summa Theologica,* II, II, Q. 64, Art. 5.

11 Sir William Blackstone, *Commentaries,* 4:189; Brown in Hales v. Petit, I Plow. 253, 75 E.R. 387 (C. B. 1563). Both cited by Norman St. John-Stevas, *Life, Death and the Law,* p. 235.

Suicide Intervention

Interference with a Suicide Attempt

David F. Greenberg

David F. Greenberg, after receiving a Ph.D. in physics and serving as senior fellow, Committee for the Study of Incarceration (Washington, D.C.), is presently associate professor of sociology at New York University. He is the author, coauthor, or editor of *University of Chicago Graduate Problems in Physics* (1965), *Struggle for Justice* (1971), *Corrections and Punishment* (1977), *Mathematical Criminology* (1979), and *Crime and Capitalism: Essays in Marxist Criminology* (1981).

Reprinted with permission of the author and the publisher from *New York University Law Review,* 49 (May-June 1974), pp. 227–269.

Greenberg sets out to design an appropriate suicide prevention policy. He suggests, as an aid to impartial thinking, that we consider this matter from behind a "veil of ignorance," in accordance with the theory of John Rawls. We would be willing, he argues, to authorize some measure of interference, yet would also insist that such interference not be unlimited. After identifying the main objectives of an ideal suicide prevention policy, he argues in support of a policy that would allow temporary intervention.

REFORMULATING THE SUICIDE DEBATE

... The advocate of intervention typically assumes that the individual under consideration *is* suicidal, not someone mistakenly thought to be suicidal or maliciously and wrongfully accused of being suicidal. Consequently, he may pay insufficient attention to the problem of screening. In addition, he is likely to assume that intervention motivated by the goal of preventing suicides will, at least some of the time, attain its goal. Yet this need not be the case. The effectiveness of any given measure in preventing suicides is an empirical question the answer to which may not simply be assumed. The libertarian, on the other hand, assumes, perhaps with no greater justification, that suicide attempters want to die, so that abstaining from interference conforms to their wishes. This assumption, too, may be wide of the mark. These hidden assumptions require careful examination before an objective look at the suicide prevention debate may be had.

A   Do Suicide Attempters Want to Die?

Unlike early research on suicide, recent studies have considered the conscious, self-perceived motivations of suicide attempters to be worthy of study, and have attempted to situate these motivations in the life experiences and circumstances of the attempters. Researchers are in agreement that most attempters do not unequivocally want to die. For example, sociologist Jack Douglas concludes:

> In the vast majority of cases, ... individuals committing dangerous acts against themselves do have what they themselves see as some degree of intention to die. ... But there is also every indication that in the great majority of cases where there is such an intention to die, there is also an intention to use suicide, through the construction of certain meanings for others involved, so that they can live better either in this world or the next. Suicide, then, is generally a

highly ambivalent action. Even those individuals with very serious intentions of dying by suicide rarely give up hope of living. After taking pills, they call for help or move toward others; when cutting their throats they make "hesitation" cuts; and most individuals who attempt or commit suicide have given their friends and relations serious warnings of their intentions to kill themselves.[1]

In accord with the foregoing observations is the report of a team of psychiatrists: "[W]e have come to regard attempted suicide not as an effort to die but rather as a communication to others in an effort to improve one's life."[2] Although a suicide attempt may seem like a peculiar way to improve one's life, we should not assume without further investigation that a suicide attempt is irrational or foolish. For adults, at least, a suicide attempt frequently is successful in bringing about an improved relationship with significant others. According to one psychiatrist, "[t]he suicidal act ... usually arouses sufficient sympathy to bring about some change in the circumstances surrounding the person who makes the attempt."[3] Similarly, the authors of another study made the following observation: "We regard these 34 attempts as successful in the sense that desired changes in the life situation of the patient occurred as a consequence of the attempt."[4]

The foregoing research findings as to the motivation of suicide attempts and the responses which these attempts often elicit suggest the relevance of a game theory perspective. From this angle the suicide attempter is a player in a game, so desperate as to be willing to risk a highly unfavorable outcome (death) in order to obtain a favorable outcome (survival and transformed relationships with others, or solved problems). It becomes easier, then, to understand the efforts of so many attempters to bring about lifesaving intervention as well as the high survival rate among attempters. It is estimated that only about one of every eight or ten suicide attempts results in death.

Studies of the subsequent mortality rate among survivors of suicide attempts tend to confirm the view of attempters as persons who, for the most part, are not intent on dying. Only about 1% of all surviving attempters kill themselves within a year of the attempt. This is still quite a bit higher than the suicide rate in the general population, but far lower than would be anticipated if most attempters unambivalently wanted to die.

The long-range suicide rate among surviving attempters is somewhat higher. Follow-up studies lasting as long as 15 years suggest that eventually somewhere between five and 15 percent of surviving attempters will kill themselves. Not surprisingly, subsequent suicide may depend on the response to the initial attempt. Thus, the authors of one study "found consistently that recovery requires a major change in the life situation."[5] This, of course, is just what we would expect if most attempters prefer to live, and, at least in part, have used the suicide attempt in order to manipulate a relationship to better advantage. Those who are successful in doing this, and they seem to be the majority, do not attempt suicide again. Others, discovering after a period of time has elapsed that their lives have not improved or have deteriorated, may well attempt suicide again, perhaps with greater definiteness of purpose in bringing about death.

B   Suicide Prevention behind the Veil of Ignorance

If most suicide attempters either do not want to die or change their minds within a very short time after an attempt, a posited "right to commit suicide" may be a weak basis for defending a policy of non-interference with suicide attempts. Were there no other pertinent considerations, the saving of the lives of the high proportion of attempters who, having been restrained, would then want to live and who would be grateful for having been saved[6] would seem to constitute adequate grounds for authorizing interference.[7] As is often the case, however, there are other considerations, such as our desire to remain free from erroneous or unnecessary interference. The attempt, then, must be to find a suicide prevention policy that will reconcile our goal of saving lives with the preservation of values we consider it important not to jeopardize.

Let us imagine that we are asked to agree upon a suicide prevention policy, given what is known about suicide but prevented by a "veil of ignorance"[8] from knowing who among us will attempt or commit suicide, who may mistakenly be identified or vindictively accused of being suicidal, who will have easy access to top-quality legal representation, and so on. We insist upon the presence of the veil to prevent persons from demanding conditions or provisions tailored in advance to meet their own individual contingencies. Thus, a man who is fairly certain that he never would be falsely identified as suicidal and therefore wrongly threatened with deprivation of liberty might be willing to sacrifice the interests of others in not being misidentified. Such a person, therefore, should not be allowed to formulate a policy taking that knowledge into account.

It seems clear that behind the veil of ignorance we would be willing to tolerate some degree of interference with suicide attempts. We would want to save the lives of those among us who would attempt suicide, but who research indicated did not desire the outcome of death, and who later would be grateful for having been rescued. Moreover, there often are times when we decide to do something on the spur of the moment that we later regret. When the consequences of impulsive action are as extreme as they are in the case of suicide, we might well want some form of intervention to compel us to reflect on whether we really want the choice we have made. Here the motivation for intervention is not that the attempter does not at the moment of the attempt want to die, but that after some consideration he may not want to do so. This later, more considered judgment is preferred over the impulsive one, perhaps because we think it more accurately represents his "true" wishes.

We might also reasonably want to be restrained against committing suicide when our judgment is clouded or distorted, as it might be through chemical processes affecting the functioning of the brain (toxic psychosis) or when a highly upsetting event (such as a death in the family) occurs.

While rationally we would be willing to authorize some measure of interference to prevent us from committing suicide under circumstances such as those mentioned above, we also would insist that a number of limitations on the extent and methods of interference with suicidal individuals be imposed, lest other values be jeopardized. Central among these would be the retention of the ultimate right to commit suicide for those who found the pain or distress of living intolerable, and for whom the desire to end life represented something more than momentary dejection or discouragement. This ultimate control over the decision whether to continue living is something we would be extremely loath to give up, lest we be forced to live in misery for a long time. Moreover, since we would recognize that distress is subjective, we would be reluctant, in making provision for the right to die, to permit others to pass on the rationality of our decision to end life.

As a further requirement, we unquestionably would insist on procedural and substantive safeguards designed to protect nonsuicidal individuals from wrongful intervention, mistaken or deliberate.[9] The more extensive the intervention, the more safeguards we would require. When the intervention is so drastic as to entail loss of liberty for an extended period, loss of some civil rights, loss of earnings, separation from family and friends and serious stigmatization, we would want to be careful indeed that only those who were actually suicidal should be the subjects of intervention.

A third concern would be that the intervention not be excessively painful, unpleasant or protracted, for, if it were, the human costs of prevention might well be thought to exceed its benefits.

This analysis suggests that the ideal suicide prevention policy is one that would: (1) save, through methods entailing minimal unpleasantness, the lives of as many as possible of those who do not wish to die; (2) interfere as little as possible with those who after some chance for consideration persist in wanting to die; and (3) afford maximum protection against interference with the liberty of those who pose no threat of suicide. This suggested policy goes very far toward respecting individual choice, but, on the basis of a principle of retrospective gratitude, departs from the most extreme libertarian position to allow very limited paternalistic intervention....

INTERFERENCE WITH A SUICIDE ATTEMPT

[We now consider a suicide prevention policy specified as] the "minimal" policy of interfering with a suicide attempt in progress or about to begin and providing medical assistance, where needed, to the attempter. The degree of interference here is quite minor; it might include, for example, removing a person from a building ledge from which he was about to leap, giving artificial respiration to a person found unconscious from gas inhalation, or lavaging the stomach of someone who has taken sleeping pills. Where necessary, because of medical considerations or for purposes of restraint, transportation to a hospital emergency room or de-

tention facility would be authorized. The duration of intervention, however, would be limited; the time span required for the kind of intervention we have in mind would not exceed 24 hours, and might frequently be less.[10]

At the end of this brief period, restraint would no longer be authorized; persons wishing to go about their business would be free to do so. In particular, they would be free to resume their suicidal behavior. To prevent the minimal policy from escalating into more protracted restraint, it would be necessary to require a waiting period before intervention could be repeated.

The foregoing policy confers benefits and also entails costs. The major benefit is that it would save the lives of almost all suicide attempters. There is abundant testimony from psychiatrists experienced in the treatment of suicide attempters that survivors of an attempt rarely pose a danger of immediate suicide, even when opportunities for further attempts are not lacking. For this reason, the stringent time limit on intervention would entail a sacrifice of very few lives. This feature makes the policy especially attractive. Moreover, even the small number of subsequent suicides that will continue to occur need not necessarily be considered failures of the policy, since those persons will at least have been provided a chance for reconsideration.[11]

There are several disadvantages to this policy. Some small number of individuals will die who would have changed their minds had they been held for a longer period. Others, firmly committed to suicide, will be detained for a period of some hours. This may be annoying, perhaps extremely distressing. Nevertheless, there are reasons for not being too concerned with this small number of individuals. First, their distress will come to an end in a few hours; secondly, those concerned with avoiding this delay could simply choose a time, place and method unlikely to attract attention.[12]

To reduce some of this imposition, the state might even accommodate determined attempters by granting immunity from any interference to those who register their intention to commit suicide in advance, or by providing resources for painless suicide following a short waiting period so as to be confident that only those who wish to die kill themselves. Despite these provisions, however, some genuinely suicidal persons are likely to be subjected to distress, embarrassment and inconvenience because, contrary to plans, their suicide attempt has been interrupted.

A third class of individuals who may suffer from the

minimal policy consists of those who are falsely identified as having been engaged in a suicide attempt or whose attempt would have had no serious consequences and who would not have gone on to a more serious attempt in the absence of intervention. These persons may incur inconvenience and some degree of stigmatization as the result of having been considered suicidal.

Nevertheless, the negative consequences of mistaken identification do not seem serious enough to constitute fatal objections to this proposal. An analogy to arrests for criminal law violations is instructive. Under the "probable cause" standard some innocent persons undoubtedly are wrongly arrested and charged. Though regrettable, the undeserved inconvenience and stigmatization are thought to be unavoidable consequences of law enforcement practices believed to be necessary to the public welfare. Our desire to minimize the unavoidable evil might, for example, lead to protection of the confidentiality of arrest records, but not to outright elimination of the power to arrest, absent an alternative procedure to handle the charging of individuals with crimes and the production of them at trial. The judgment is made that our interest in safety from crime is sufficient to warrant risking some interference with our activities through wrongful arrest.[13] On the other side of the coin, a person suspected of criminal activity cannot lawfully be taken into custody unless there is at least "probable cause" to believe that he committed the crime. Relaxation of this restriction might result in the taking into custody of some criminals who at present are free to continue preying on innocent victims, but we forfeit this potential benefit in order to remain free from arrest based on mere suspicion of involvement in criminal activity.

It is doubtful that coercive suicide prevention is as justifiable as coercive crime prevention; the social consequences of unpunished serious crime probably are much greater than those of unprevented suicide. Failing to attach legal sanctions to acts seriously harmful to the life of another, for example, may lead to vigilantism. Nevertheless, the considerable benefits to be obtained from minimal restraint of suicide attempters seem to us sufficient to justify the limited degree of interference proposed here, notwithstanding its costs for "truly" suicidal persons and for those who are not suicidal at all....

NOTES

1 Douglas, "The Absurd in Suicide," in *On the Nature of Suicide* 111, 117–18 (E. Shneidman ed. 1969).

2 Rubinstein, Moses & Lidz, "On Attempted Suicide, 79 *A.M.A. Archives of Neurology & Psychiatry* 103, 111(1958). Characteristically, the authors of this study found:

> The patient was involved in a struggle with the persons important to him and sought a modification of their attitudes or a specific change in his relationships with them. After a crisis was reached in this struggle, the patient sought to effect these changes through a suicide attempt.... Patients sometimes told of seeking such changes prior to their suicide attempt, of seeking them through the attempt, and by still other means afterward....

Id. at 109.

3 Weiss, "The Suicidal Patient," in *American Handbook of Psychiatry* 115, 121 (S. Arieto ed. 1966).

4 Rubinstein, Moses & Lidz, *supra,* at 105.

5 Moss & Hamilton, "Psychotherapy of the Suicidal Patient," in *Clues to Suicide* 99, 107 (E. Shneidman & N. Farberow eds. 1957).

6 J. Choron, *Suicide* 50 (1972), cites several studies from different countries in which 90% to 100% of rescued suicide attempters reported they were glad they had been saved.

7 Alan Dershowitz has called this line of reasoning the "Thank you, doctor" doctrine (private conversation with the author). The concept also is employed under the label "future-oriented consent" in Wexler, "Therapeutic Justice," 57 *Minn. L. Rev.* 289, 330–32 (1972). We shall refer to the concept in this article as the principle of retrospective gratitude.

8 J. Rawls, *A Theory of Justice* 136–42 (1971).

9 Thus, in Litman & Farberow, "Emergency Evaluation of Suicidal Potential," in *The Psychology of Suicide* 259, 268 (E. Shneidman, N. Farberow, & R. Litman eds. 1970), an example is given of a woman who claimed that her husband was living "in a dream world" and wanted him committed on grounds that he was likely to kill himself. Upon investigation it turned out that he frequently lost much of his wages gambling. The woman wanted him committed so that she could use his money to straighten out their financial affairs. Sympathetic as we might be with her plight, we would want to provide protection against the use of suicide prevention commitment proceedings to advance goals having nothing to do with suicide prevention. Even where there is no deliberate attempt to deceive or

to misuse statutory provisions, we still would need to be on guard against family members who are sincere but mistaken in their belief that a suicide attempt may be imminent.

10 As defined here, then, minimal interference includes simple restraint at the scene, arrest and removal from the scene and very short-term detainment. Although we consider these together as "minimal," it ultimately might prove useful to distinguish among them and perhaps permit only the least restrictive. These distinctions need not be discussed here.

11 This need not mean that we should be complacent about suicides, only that this particular coercive policy cannot be made to shoulder the burden of suicide prevention.

12 Ordinarily this should not be too difficult. A major exception might be individuals incarcerated in total institutions where suicide, though certainly not impossible, can be made much more difficult by intensive surveillance and deprivation of materials from which weapons can be constructed. I am indebted to Andrew von Hirsch for this observation.

13 On the other hand, we become much more alarmed at more extended pretrial detention, as its disruptive effects mount rapidly when its duration begins to exceed 24 hours. It is clear that, behind the veil of ignorance, we would never accept the class bias built into current pretrial release procedures.

The Refusal of Lifesaving Treatment

Consent, Coercion, and Conflicts of Rights

Ruth Macklin

A biographical sketch of Ruth Macklin is found on page 162.

Macklin focuses attention on the moral issues raised by the case of the Jehovah's Witness who desires to refuse a blood transfusion for religious reasons. In her analysis, the right to refuse blood transfusions may be defended not only by appeal to the right to exercise one's religious beliefs but also by appeal to the autonomy of the patient *qua* person, that is, to the individual's right to decide matters affecting his or her own life and death. In direct conflict with these rights, however, is the right of the doctor to do what correct medical practice dictates. Macklin argues that it is morally justifiable to administer blood transfusions to minor children against the religious objections of parents. It is also morally justifiable to administer blood transfusions to *incompetent* adult patients. However, she insists, the only justification for compelling a competent adult Jehovah's Witness to accept blood transfusions is a paternalistic one, and such a paternalistic intervention is morally unjustified. Still, the doctor's right to do what correct medical practice dictates must be respected. "A patient can knowingly refuse treatment, but he cannot demand mistreatment."

Cases of conflict of rights are not infrequent in law and morality. A range of cases that has gained increasing prominence recently centers around the autonomy of persons and their right to make decisions in matters affecting their own life and death. This paper will focus on a particular case of conflict of rights: the case of

Reprinted with permission of the author and the publisher from *Perspectives in Biology and Medicine*, vol. 20, no. 3 (Spring 1977), pp. 360–371. Copyright © 1977 by the University of Chicago.

Jehovah's Witnesses who refuse blood transfusions for religious reasons and the question of whether or not there exists a right to compel medical treatment. The Jehovah's Witnesses who refuse blood transfusions do not do so because they want to die: in most cases, however, they appear to believe that they will die if their blood is not transfused. Members of this sect are acting on what is generally believed to be a constitutionally guaranteed right: freedom of religion, which is said to include not only freedom of religious belief, but also the right to act on such beliefs.

This study will examine a cluster of moral issues surrounding the Jehovah's Witness case. Some pertain to minor children of Jehovah's Witness parents, while others concern adult Witnesses who refuse treatment for themselves. The focus will be on the case as a moral one rather than a legal one, although arguments employed in some of the legal cases will be invoked. This is an issue at the intersection of law and morality—one in which the courts themselves have rendered conflicting decisions and have looked to moral principles for guidance. As is usually the case in ethics, whatever the courts may have decided does not settle the moral dispute, but the arguments and issues invoked in legal disputes often mirror the ethical dimensions of the case. The conflict—in both law and morals—arises out of a religious prohibition against blood transfusions, a prohibition that rests on an interpretation of certain scriptural passages by the Jehovah's Witness sect.

THE RELIGIOUS BASIS FOR THE PROHIBITION OF BLOOD TRANSFUSIONS

The Witnesses' prohibition of blood transfusions derives from an interpretation of several Old Testament passages, chief among which is the following from Lev. 17:10–14:

> And whatsoever man there be of the house of Israel, or of the strangers that sojourn among you, that eateth any manner of blood: I will even set my face against that soul that eateth blood, and will cut him off from among his people....

The question immediately arises, On what basis do the Jehovah's Witnesses construe intravenous blood transfusions as an instance of eating blood? Witnesses sometimes claim that the prohibition against transfusions arises out of a literal interpretation of the relevant biblical passages, but the interpretation in question seems anything but "literal." One explanation for this

is as follows: "Since they have been prohibited by the Bible from eating blood, they steadfastly proclaim that intravenous transfusion has no bearing on the matter, as it basically makes no difference whether the blood enters by the vein or by the alimentary tract. In their widely quoted reference *Blood, Medicine, and the Law of God* they constantly refer to the medical printed matter which early in the 20th century declared that blood transfusions are nothing more than a source of nutrition by a shorter route than ordinary" [1, p. 539]. Whether based on a literal interpretation of the Bible or not, the Witnesses' prohibition against transfusions extends not only to whole blood, but also to any blood derivative, such as plasma and albumin (blood substitutes are, however, quite acceptable) [1, p.539].

This brief account of the basis of the religious prohibition has not yet addressed the moral issues involved: but for the sake of completeness, let us note two additional features of the Jehovah's Witness view—features that bear directly on the moral conflict.

The first point concerns the Witnesses' belief about the consequences of violating the prohibition: Receiving blood transfusions is an unpardonable sin resulting in withdrawal of the opportunity to attain eternal life [2]. In particular, the transgression is punishable by being "cut off": "Since the Witnesses do not believe in eternal damnation, to be 'cut off' signifies losing one's opportunity to qualify for resurrection" [3, p. 75]. A second, related feature of the Witnesses' belief system is their view that man's life on earth is not important: "They fervently believe that they are only passing through and that the faithful who have not been corrupted nor polluted will attain eternal life in Heaven" [1, p. 539]. This belief is important in the structure of a moral argument that pits the value of preservation of life on earth against other values, for example, presumed eternal life in Heaven. Put another way, the Witnesses can argue that the duty to preserve or prolong human life is always overridden by their perceived duty to God, so in a case of conflict, duty to God dictates the right course of action.

THE ADULT JEHOVAH'S WITNESS PATIENT

Freedom to exercise one's religious beliefs is one important aspect of the moral and legal issues involved in these cases. But in addition to this specific constitutionally guaranteed right, there are other rights and moral values that would be relevant even if religious freedom were not at issue. Even in cases that do not involve religious freedom at all, the question of the right to compel medical treatment against a patient's wishes raises some knotty moral problems. The Jehovah's Witness case may prove instructive for the range of cases in which religious freedom is not at issue.

Just which rights or values are involved in the adult Jehovah's Witness case, and how do they conflict? We shall return later to the right to act on one's religious beliefs, but first let us look at other moral concepts that enter into Witnesses' moral defense. Chief among these is the notion of autonomy. Does the patient in a medical setting have the autonomy that we normally accord persons simply by virtue of their being human? Or does one's status as a *patient* deprive him of a measure of autonomy normally accorded him as a nonpatient *person*? Many medical practitioners tend to argue for decreased autonomy of patients, while some religious ethicists, a number of moral philosophers, and a small number of physicians defend autonomous decision making on the part of patients. So one clearly identifiable moral issue concerns the autonomy of a person who becomes a patient. Does he or she have the right to make decisions about the details of medical treatment and about whether some treatments are to be undertaken at all? One may defend the Witnesses' right to refuse blood transfusions by appealing to the autonomy of the patient *qua* person solely on moral grounds, without even invoking First Amendment freedoms (i.e., freedom of religion).

The right of autonomous decision making on the part of the patient is in direct conflict with a right claimed on behalf of the treating physician: the "professional" right (duty, perhaps) of a doctor to do what correct medical practice dictates. As one writer notes: "In our society, medical treatment is a right which is guaranteed to every citizen, regardless of his religious tenets. But it is also the physician's inherent, albeit uncodified, right not to have constraints applied to a therapeutic program, which he regards as necessary for the patient's welfare or survival" [3, p. 73]. Unlike other sorts of cases involving refusal of medical treatment on religious grounds (notably, Christian Scientists' refusal to accept any medical treatment), Jehovah's Witnesses are opposed only to one specific treatment regimen: transfusion of whole blood or blood fractions. As a result, Witnesses visit doctors, voluntarily enter hospitals, and submit themselves to the usual range of treatments, with the singular exception of accepting transfusions. The question arises, then, Does the physician have a duty to do everything for a patient that is dictated by accepted medical practice? In a court case in 1965 *(United States v. George,* 33 LW 2518), the court argued that "the patient voluntarily submitted himself to and insisted on medical treatment. At the same time, he sought to dictate a course of treatment to his physician which amounted to malpractice. The court held that under these circumstances, a physician cannot be required to ignore the mandates of his own conscience, even in the name of the exercise of religious freedom. A patient can knowingly refuse treatment, but he cannot demand mistreatment" [3, p. 78].

The right or duty of a physician, as described here, does seem to be in direct conflict with both (1) the religious freedom of the Jehovah's Witness patient and (2) the autonomy of the patient as a person, or his right to decide on matters affecting his own life and death. The worth of human life and the duty to preserve it are usually viewed as paramount moral values in our culture. Since those arguing in favor of the right to compel medical treatment will invoke this important value in their defense, the moral dilemma has no clear solution.

It is worth noting briefly several additional moral issues involved in the adult Jehovah's Witness case. One is the issue of informed consent. Because of the refusal of Jehovah's Witnesses to grant consent to transfuse themselves or their relatives (including minor children), physicians may not (morally or legally) act contrary to the patient's wishes. But a court order may be obtained authorizing the physician to transfuse the patient. What, then, is the status of the requirement for "informed consent" in medical matters if the patient's publicly expressed wishes can be overridden by a doctor who obtains a court order? A second relevant moral issue concerns the competency of the Jehovah's Witness patient to make the decision about transfusion at the time that decision needs to be made. Is a semicomatose person competent to make decisions? Is a person in excruciating pain competent? A person suffering from mild shock? Surely, an unconscious person is not. In this last case, and perhaps the preceding ones as well, someone other than the patient must make the decision to refuse transfusion for him. Perhaps the patient, with death as the consequence of refusing treatment, would abandon his religious tenet in favor of the desire to live. Ought a family member decide for the patient, when the patient is unable to decide for himself? There is, obviously, no easy solution to these moral dilemmas. Arguments that rest on sound moral principles can be constructed to support either view, and such arguments have been embodied in several legal cases in the past few years. We shall return to these considerations in the final section, but first we turn to the overlapping, yet somewhat different set of issues concerning minor children of Jehovah's Witnesses.

TRANSFUSING MINOR CHILDREN OF JEHOVAH'S WITNESSES

The moral principles involved in the case of minor children of Jehovah's Witnesses differ in some important respects from principles that enter into the case of adult Witnesses who refuse transfusions for themselves. It is worth noting that all legal cases in which the transfusion of minor children was at issue were decided in favor of transfusing the child, against the religious objections of the parents. In these cases, the arguments given by the courts are a mixture of citation of legal statutes and precedents and appeal to moral principles. In one case in Ohio the court argued as follows: "...While [parents] may, under certain circumstances, deprive [their child] of his liberty or his property, under no circumstances, with or without religious sanction, may they deprive him of his life!" [4, p. 131]. In this and other legal decisions, the religious right of the parents is seen as secondary to the right to life and health on the part of the child....

It might be argued that Jehovah's Witness parents, in refusing permission for blood to be given to their child, are acting in accordance with their perceived duty to God, as dictated by their religion, and that this duty to God overrides whatever secular duties they may have to preserve the life and health of their child. Here it can only be replied that when an action done in accordance with perceived duties to God results in the likelihood of harm or death to another person (whether child or adult), then the duties to preserve life here on earth take precedence. The duties of a physician are to preserve and prolong life and to alleviate suffering. These duties are not in the least mitigated by considerations of God's will, the possibility of life after death, or a view that God at some later time rewards those who suffer here on earth. Freedom of religion does not include the right to act in a manner that will result in harm or death to others.

If the parents refuse to grant permission for blood to be given to their child when failure to give blood will result in death or severe harm to the child, their *prima facie* right to retain control over their child no longer exists. Whatever the parents' reasons for refusing to allow blood to be given, and whether the parents believe that the child will survive or not, the case sufficiently resembles that of child neglect (in respect to harm to the child): in the absence of fulfillment of their primary duties, it is morally justifiable to take control of the child away from parents and administer blood transfusions against the parents' wishes and contrary to their religious convictions.

RIGHTS AND THE CONFLICT OF RIGHTS

It is evident that the case of the adult Jehovah's Witness who refuses blood transfusions for himself is a good deal more complicated than that of minor children of Jehovah's Witness parents. The arguments—both moral and legal—in the case of children rest largely on the moral belief that no one has the right or authority to make life-threatening decisions for persons unable to make those decisions for themselves. If this analysis is sound, it supplies a principle for dealing with the case of the adult patient who is not in a position to state his wishes at the time the treatment is medically required. This principle is avowedly paternalistic but is intended to be applied in those cases where a measure of paternalism seems morally justifiable. To the extent that a person is unable or not fully competent to decide for himself at the time transfusion is needed, it seems appropriate for medical personnel to decide in favor of life-saving treatment. Whatever a person may have claimed prior to an emergency in which death is imminent, and regardless of what relatives may claim on his behalf, it is morally wrong for others to act in a manner that will probably result in his death.

The task of ascertaining a person's competence to make decisions for himself presents a myriad of problems, some of them moral, some epistemological, and some conceptual. These problems are no different, in principle, from the difficulty of ascertaining the competency of retarded persons, the mentally ill, aged senile persons, and others. This is not to suggest that no difficulty exists but, rather, that similar problems arise in many other sorts of cases where competency needs to be ascertained for moral or legal or practical reasons.

There are several recent court cases dealing with adult Jehovah's Witness patients. In some of these cases the court refused the request to transfuse the patient: in others, the court decided that transfusion was warranted, despite the religious objections. The case of *John F. Kennedy Memorial Hospital v. Heston* was one of those in which transfusion was ordered, contrary to the patient's religious convictions. But it is important to note that the patient was deemed incompetent to make the decision for herself at the time transfusion was needed. The judge who delivered the court's opinion stated:

> Delores Heston, age 22 and unmarried, was severely injured in an automobile accident. She was taken to the plaintiff hospital where it was determined that she would expire unless operated upon for a ruptured spleen and that if operated upon she would expire unless whole blood was administered.... Miss Heston insists she expressed her refusal to accept blood, but the evidence indicated she was in shock on admittance to the hospital and in the judgment of the attending physicians and nurses was then or soon became disoriented and incoherent. Her mother remained adamant in her opposition to a transfusion, and signed a release of liability for the hospital and medical personnel. Miss Heston did not execute a release; presumably she could not. Her father could not be located. [5, p. 671]

This case, then, fits the principle suggested above: To the extent that a person is unable or not fully competent to decide for himself at the time transfusion is needed, it seems appropriate for medical personnel to decide in favor of life-saving treatment.

In another case, *In re Osborne,* the court decided against transfusion. But here it was ascertained that the patient was not impaired in his ability to make judgments, that he "understood the consequences of his decision, and had with full understanding executed a statement refusing the recommended transfusion and releasing the hospital from liability" [6, p. 373]. This decision might be defended, in a moral argument, by appealing to the notion of the autonomy of persons; the legal defense rests, however, on the constitutionally guaranteed freedom of religion. A footnote in the court's opinion in *Osborne* says: "No case has come to light where refusal of medical care was based on individual choice absent religious convictions." But whether based on the moral concept of autonomy, or on the legal and moral right to act on one's religious beliefs, the right of a person (whose competency has been ascertained) to refuse medical treatment must be viewed as a viable moral alternative. Such a right rests on the precept of individual liberty that protects persons of sound mind against paternalistic interference by others.

CONCLUSION

It seems apparent that the only justification that can be offered for the coercive act of administering a blood transfusion without a person's consent and against his will is a paternalistic one. I follow that characterization of paternalism put forth by Gerald Dworkin: "the interference with a person's liberty of action justified by reasons referring exclusively to the welfare, good, happiness, needs, interests or values of the person being coerced" [7, p. 65]. Now a person's life is involved in his welfare or good in the extreme—so much so, it might be argued, that it is not on a par with other things that contribute to one's welfare. Indeed, the existence of life is a necessary condition for there being any welfare, happiness, needs, interests, or values at all. Still, interference with a person's (presumably rational) decision to end his life or allow it to end presupposes a belief on the part of the interferer that he knows what is best for the person. This would, in fact, be the case if a Jehovah's Witness patient believed that he would not die if he were not transfused in cases where informed medical opinion predicts the reverse. But the Witness who accepts the high probability of his own death and still refuses transfusion does not disagree concerning matters of empirical fact with those who wish to interfere on his behalf. Dworkin identifies this as a value conflict, a case in which "a value such as health—or indeed life—may be overridden by competing values. Thus the problem with the [Jehovah's Witness] and blood transfusions. It may be more important for him to reject 'impure substances' than to go on living" [7, p. 78]. But Dworkin is wrong if he construes this as solely a question of conflict in values, and he is also mistaken in identifying one of the competing values as rejection of "impure substances." It is, rather, eternal life over against mortal life that the Jehovah's Witness is weighing, and rather than risk being "cut off" he opts to allow his mortal life to terminate.

It would appear, then, that beliefs about metaphysical matters of fact—as well as competing values—are involved in the Jehovah's Witness's decision. That such beliefs may be mistaken or ill founded is not sufficient warrant for paternalistic interference, unless it can be shown that persons who entertain such beliefs are irrational. But it would fly in the face of long-standing traditions and practices—especially in America—to deem persons irrational solely on the basis of religious convictions that differ from our own. If, however, the Witnesses are not to be judged irrational by virtue of their religious belief system, then the one clearly acceptable ground for paternalistic intervention is pulled out from under. Medical practitioners are sometimes criticized for acting in a paternalistic manner toward patients, so it is not surprising to see physicians advocate a course of action that overrides a patient's expressed wishes. But if the patient is deemed competent or rational (by whatever practical criteria are employed or ought to be adopted), then there is no warrant for interfering with his decisions, even those that affect his continued existence. Unless all decisions to end one's life (or allow it to terminate) are viewed as *ex hypothesi* irrational, interference with a person's liberty to choose in favor of what he believes to take precedence over continued mortal existence is an act of unjustified paternalism. Paternalism may be considered justifiable in cases where the agent is incompetent to make informed or rational judgments about his own welfare. The Jehovah's Witness who refuses a blood transfusion may be *mistaken* about what is in his long-range welfare, but he is not incompetent to make judgments based on his belief system. It is only if we decide that his particular set of religious beliefs constitutes good evidence for his overall irrationality that we are justified in interfering paternalistically with his liberty. While I am personally inclined to view such religious belief systems as irrational (because they are not warranted on the evidence), I do not thereby deem their proponents irrational *in a general sense* for holding such beliefs. And this, it seems, is the correct way of looking at the case of adult Jehovah's Witnesses who are deemed mentally competent (according to the usual medical criteria) and yet who refuse blood transfusions. Only if we are prepared to accept paternalistic interference with the liberty of (otherwise) rational or competent adults in similar cases are we justified in transfusing these patients against their expressed wishes.

We cannot let the matter rest here, however, because of the problems this solution would pose for medical practice. It has been argued above that the physician has a "right not to have constraints applied to a therapeutic program, which he regards as necessary for the patient's welfare or survival"; and one court opinion stated that "a physician cannot be required to ignore the mandates of his own conscience, even in the name of the exercise of religious freedom. A patient can knowingly refuse treatment, but he cannot demand mistreatment." Jehovah's Witnesses who present themselves for treatment and who are judged rational or competent to give or withhold consent should be given

the option of either *(a)* being treated in accordance with the dictates of accepted medical practice, including blood transfusion if necessary; or *(b)* refusing in advance any treatment in which transfusion is normally a necessary component or is likely to be required in the case at hand. Presenting these options to the patient preserves his decision-making autonomy while not requiring the physician to embark on a treatment that amounts to malpractice.

If it is objected that this proposed solution violates the precepts of accepted medical practice, I can only reply that those precepts embody a measure of paternalism that is unjustifiable when judged against a principle of individual liberty that mandates autonomy of decision making for rational adult persons. Moreover, the precepts of accepted medical practice have been known to change, varying with the introduction of new medical technology, transformations in social consciousness, and other alterations in the status quo. Not all patients who can be treated vigorously are so treated; one aspect of current debates focuses on the moral dilemmas surrounding patient autonomy—the sorts of problems addressed in this paper. Consistent with the decision-making autonomy accorded a patient who is deemed rational enough to offer informed consent is the right of a physician to refuse to be dictated to in matters of medical competence. Once treatment is undertaken, the judgment that a blood transfusion is necessary would seem to be a judgment requiring medical competence. The decision to undertake treatment at all in such cases is not a purely medical matter but might well be decided by a patient who has full knowledge of the consequences yet who insists nonetheless on what amounts to partial treatment or mistreatment by attending physicians.

I have argued that the autonomy of patients, as rational persons, ought to be respected. But this autonomy implies a responsibility for one's decision—a responsibility that entails acceptance of the consequences. And these consequences include the right of physicians to reject a treatment regimen proposed by the patient, which is contrary to sound medical practice. If, faced with this consequence, some Jehovah's Witnesses opt for treatment with transfusion rather than no treatment at all, so much the better for such cases of conflict of rights. Those Witnesses who remain steadfast in their refusal to accept transfusions are exercising their right of autonomous decision making in matters concerning their own welfare—in the words of Justice Louis Brandeis, "the right to be let alone." In a judicial opinion rendered in a case involving a Jehovah's Witness who refused transfusion, Justice Warren Burger recalled Brandeis's view as follows: "Nothing in [his] utterance suggests that Justice Brandeis thought an individual possessed these rights only as to *sensible* beliefs, *valid* thoughts, *reasonable* emotions, or *well-founded* sensations. I suggest he intended to include a great many foolish, unreasonable, and even absurd ideas which do not conform, such as refusing medical treatment even at great risk"[8]. The risks are indeed great in the cases we have been discussing. But the sorts of risks to health or life a person may take, in the interest of something he considers worth the risk, appear to know no bounds. If an adult agent is rational and competent to make decisions, the risks are his to take.

REFERENCES

1 I. G. Thomas, R. W. Edmark, and T. W. Jones. *Am. Surg.,* 34:538, 1968.
2 W. T. Fitts, Jr., and M. J. Orloff. *Surg. Gynecol. Obstet.,* 180:502, 1959.
3 D. C. Schechter. *Am. J. Surg.,* 116:73, 1968.
4 *In re* Clark, 185 N.E. 2d 128, 1962.
5 John F. Kennedy Memorial Hospital *v* Heston, 279 A. 2d 670, 1971.
6 *In re* Osborne, 294 A. 2d 372, 1972.
7 G. Dworkin. *Monist,* 56:64, 1972.
8 Application of President and Directors of Georgetown College, 331 F. 2n 1010 (D.C. Cir.), 1964.

Unauthorized Rendition of Lifesaving Medical Treatment

Kenney F. Hegland

Kenney F. Hegland is professor of law at the University of Arizona. He has written a book for laypeople on common legal problems, *The Trouble Book* (1974), and is the author of a book on lawyering skills, *Trial and Practice Skills in a Nutshell* (1978). His other publications include "Moral Dilemmas in Teaching Trial Advocacy" and *Introduction to the Study and Practice of Law* (1983).

Hegland identifies his thesis in this way: "The rendition of emergency lifesaving medical treatment on the person of the objecting adult patient is proper." He apparently means to argue not only the legal point that the current state of the law allows such coercion but also the ethical point that the law *justifiably* does so. Thus, according to Hegland, there is no legally enforceable right to reject lifesaving medical treatment and no such right *should* be recognized. After arguing that neither the common law nor the first amendment affords the individual the right to reject lifesaving treatment, Hegland expands upon his central point: There is a valid public interest in the individual's life. This interest is recognized in three analogous areas of law: euthanasia, the "snake cases," and suicide. To refuse lifesaving treatment is tantamount to consenting to one's own death, but the law, in keeping with its traditional commitment to the sanctity of human life, cannot allow an individual to consent to his or her own death.

Anglo-American law starts with the premise of thorough-going self determination. It follows that each man is considered to be master of his own body, and he may, if he be of sound mind, ex-

From *California Law Review*, 53 (August 1965), pp. 860–877. Copyright © 1965, California Law Review, Inc. Reprinted by permission.

pressly prohibit the performance of lifesaving surgery.... [1]

Do our humane laws make it the duty of a physician to leave the bedside of a dying man, because he demands it, and, if he remains and relieves him by physical touch, hold him guilty of assault? [2]

An adult hospital patient refuses to consent to lifesaving medical treatment, such as a blood transfusion: The individual's right to determine what shall be done with his own body and the sanctity of life come into direct conflict. Should a court order that the treatment be given, or should it respect the individual's commands and let him die? The few courts which have faced this problem are divided as to the proper course.

In September 1963 the mother of a seven-month-old baby entered the Georgetown College Hospital. Massive internal bleeding, caused by a ruptured ulcer, necessitated an immediate transfusion. Due to religious conviction, both the patient and her husband refused to authorize the transfusion. Hospital officials sought a court order authorizing the transfusion. After a district judge had refused the order, Circuit Judge Wright was contacted and after conferring with the patient, her husband, and attending physicians, signed an order authorizing the administration of "such transfusions as are in the opinion of the physicians in attendance necessary to save...[her] life." Transfusions were given and the patient recovered.

Application of the President of Georgetown College, Inc. [3] is one of several cases in which a court has authorized lifesaving treatment on the adult patient who has refused to consent. The Illinois Supreme Court, however, has recently held that where the refusal of treatment was due to religious conviction, such action constituted an unconstitutional infringement of religious liberty. [4]

The thesis of this Comment is that the rendition of emergency lifesaving medical treatment on the person of the objecting adult patient is proper. It will be seen that neither the common law nor the "free exercise" clause of the first amendment of the United States Constitution gives the individual a right to reject lifesaving treatment. The law's traditional view of the sanctity of human life and the importance of the individual's life to the welfare of society, deny the individual a right to, in effect, consent to his own death....

RIGHT TO REFUSE MEDICAL TREATMENT

In most circumstances the individual is afforded the right to reject medical treatment. Both the common law and the first amendment afford protection of the individual's right to determine what shall be done with his own body. However, an examination of these two sources of protection indicates that they do not give the individual the right to reject lifesaving treatment in the emergency situation.

A Common Law Protection: Unauthorized Medical Treatment As Battery

Common law recognizes the right to refuse medical treatment at least in the non-emergency situation. Tort liability is imposed on the physician who renders treatment without his patient's authorization, or, having once obtained it, goes beyond it by rendering treatment different from, or more extensive than that authorized. The plaintiff suing for an intentional, as opposed to a negligent, tort need only show that the treatment was given without authorization; he need not rely on the expert witnesses generally required in a malpractice action. Since the heart of the battery action is the absence of legal consent, it is no defense that the unauthorized treatment was given with a high degree of skill or that it actually benefitted the patient.

The common law does not, however, afford an absolute right to reject medical treatment, at least under certain circumstances. An exception to the requirement of prior consent is recognized in the emergency situation where the patient is in a condition, such as unconsciousness, which renders him incapable of either giving or withholding his consent. The physician is then privileged to give the emergency aid. The privilege is supported on two grounds. First, it is assumed that the patient, if capable, would consent to the treatment and hence its rendition does not conflict with his right to determine what shall be done with his own body. Second, although the particular patient might reject the treatment were he able to do so, the lives of other patients in like circumstances would be lost if the physician were held to act at his peril, *i.e.,* if the physician were held liable for battery if it developed that the patient would have refused consent. Thus, without yet reaching the question of whether there is ever a right to reject lifesaving treatment, it appears proper in many emergencies to ignore the patient's refusal. Certainly the physician may ignore the refusal to consent of an insane or delirious patient.

Where the patient is neither insane nor delirious, it would be proper in many cases to render the treatment over the patient's commands when failure to do so would mean the patient's death. Assuming that the individual has, in effect, a right to choose death, the law should require a high degree of certainty that he really desires to exercise this prerogative before giving it operative significance. In many emergency situations, such certainty is not possible.

Assume that an individual's leg has been crushed in an automobile accident. Without immediate amputation he will die of blood poisoning. Stating that he would rather die than live with one leg, the patient refuses to consent. Just as it is assumed that an unconscious patient, if capable, would consent to emergency treatment, it seems justified to assume that this refusal of lifesaving aid is due to weakness, confusion, and pain rather than deliberation.

Such an assumption could, of course, be overcome if the refusal had been confirmed by a course of conduct antedating the emergency. For example, refusal by a Jehovah's Witness to consent to a blood transfusion is probably an expression of true preference. Yet, in a case like *Georgetown,* where the patient is suddenly seized by a condition requiring a transfusion, his refusal may be due to his physically weakened condition. Even here there may be insufficient certainty to allow the patient to die.

In many cases involving the refusal of lifesaving aid, the physician should, therefore, be allowed to proceed, either by prior judicial order or by holding him privileged in a subsequent battery action, because of the inherent difficulties in distinguishing the rash refusal from that representing true choice. Whether the refusal was in fact rash should not be determinative, for to require the physician to act at his peril would tend to deter all action, thus costing the lives of those whose refusal was due to confusion and weakened physical condition.

This rationale, however, cannot be applied where it is clear that the patient's true desire is to refuse consent. For example, physicians inform a pregnant woman that blood transfusions will be necessary to save her life after the delivery of her child. While in perfect health, before any loss of blood, she refuses to consent. Here the issue is clearly raised: Does the individual have a legally protected right to reject lifesaving treat-

ment? The few cases which have faced the issue in the battery context have given no clear answer. Does the Constitution afford such a right?

B Constitutional Protection: Freedom of Religion

If the refusal of required treatment is due to religious belief, to ignore it might violate the free exercise of religion clause of the first amendment to the United States Constitution. Yet reliance on the first amendment raises rather than answers the question because that amendment has not been held to give absolute freedom to religious practice.

In the early case of *Reynolds v. United States,*[5] the private secretary of Brigham Young appealed his conviction for bigamy, arguing that the statute was unconstitutional as applied to him because his religion required its violation. The United States Supreme Court, affirming, held that whereas freedom of conscience was absolute, the right to free exercise of religion could not justify acts against the public well being.

In the cases since *Reynolds,* the question has been whether a religious practice is sufficiently detrimental to the public good to justify its curtailment: Courts have held that the practice must present an immediate threat to a valid public interest. Whether a religiously motivated refusal of lifesaving medical treatment is constitutionally protected turns on whether there is a valid public interest in the individual's life. In many analogous areas of the law, courts have recognized this interest.

PUBLIC INTEREST IN THE LIFE OF THE INDIVIDUAL

Refusal of lifesaving treatment does not constitute an immediate and direct threat to the well being of others; however, several areas of the law recognize the propriety of curtailing activities which do not directly endanger others. Certain activities, because they adversely affect the participants and thus indirectly affect the welfare of society, have fallen under legal proscription. Polygamy, for example, does not present an immediate and direct threat to the welfare of other individuals but this practice may be made criminal even for those whose religion dictates it. It is likewise arguable that much of modern narcotics legislation is designed primarily to protect users. The use of narcotics presents primarily an indirect threat to society by harming the individual user.

Similarly, this Comment argues that refusal of lifesaving treatment constitutes an activity which should be curtailed despite the fact that it does not endanger others. Such a refusal is tantamount to consenting to death. In the analogous areas of euthanasia, the "snake cases" and suicide, the law has uniformly denied operative significance to the individual's consent to his own death and consequently it should be expected that the same result will follow in the case of the refusal of lifesaving treatment.

A Euthanasia

It is no defense to homicide prosecution that the decedent desired to die. In effect, the individual cannot consent to his own death at the hands of a second party. The primary concern of the law in condemning "mercy killing" is apparently not with the difficult proof problems in the prosecution of homicide that the defense of consent would generate; hence, the case of taking life cannot be distinguished from that of saving it by unauthorized treatment. First, there is society's interest in the life of the individual. If this is the reason why the individual has no right to consent to his own death in the euthanasia situation, then he would have no right to prohibit lifesaving medical treatment. Second, there is the fear that any exception to the sanctity of life cannot but cheapen it. The same fear would lead to hesitation before condemning any act which saves life, e.g., the rendition of lifesaving aid. If the individual has the right to command his own death, the form of the command should not be determinative: that is, whether it commands another individual to do something, as in the case of euthanasia, or whether it commands him not to do something, as in the case of the refusal of required medical treatment.

B Poisonous Snake Rituals

The "snake cases" provide additional precedent for the proposition that the state may act to prevent the individual from consenting to his own death. A small religious sect, known as the Holiness Church, believes that the true test of faith is the handling of poisonous snakes: The true believer will not be harmed. Several state legislatures made this practice criminal. Several state courts, upholding the constitutionality of the statutes, iterated the traditional language about the safety of onlookers, but a close reading of the cases indicates that the concern was with the individuals who handled the snakes.

It is difficult to find a meaningful distinction between an individual who handles a poisonous snake and one who refuses required medical treatment. A distinction between misfeasance and nonfeasance is nonsense; each individual is making basically the same decision. Walking into a burning house is tantamount to refusing to walk out. In terms of the danger to others presented by the two acts, there is little distinction. The ceremonies of the Holiness Church create a slight public danger in that the poisonous snake might escape. If minor considerations are determinative, then it could be argued that the hospital patient, in refusing lifesaving treatment, creates a danger to others by bringing otherwise unneeded physicians to his bedside and by generally interrupting the smooth operation of the hospital.

A stronger argument for curtailing religious practice can be made in the case of the hospital patient than in the case of the snake handler. First, the extent of social harm presented by the practice is greater because death from the refusal of lifesaving treatment is as certain as medical knowledge can be, whereas death from the handling of snakes is a mere possibility. Second, the extent that religious practice must be curtailed is less in the case of the hospital patient. Handling snakes is essential to the ritual of the Holiness Church; the proscription of a given form of medical treatment is generally just one of many proscriptions found in religious doctrines. In addition, while the members of the Holiness Church are forever barred from practicing the dictates of their religion, the members of a sect which prohibits a given form of treatment are free to follow their religious dictates in all but the most limited of situations: the life and death situation. As to the manner of curtailment, criminal sanctions are imposed on the individual who handles snakes due to his religion, while in the case of the individual who refuses a form of medical treatment due to his religion, no such sanctions are imposed. When a patient refuses lifesaving treatment, the propriety of his decision is not at issue: The only question is whether a physician's act in violation of that decision is proper.

C Analogy to Prevention of Suicide

It is obviously proper for a physician to save his patient's life by unauthorized treatment if the physician in doing so is in the same position as the individual who has prevented a suicide. It is not a legal wrong to prevent suicide. To hold the physician liable and the rescuer from suicide privileged, a distinction must be found either in their respective actions or in the actions of the person saved.

There are two possible ways to distinguish the acts of the suicide from that of the patient who refuses lifesaving treatment: first, by the misfeasance-nonfeasance analysis, and second, in terms of the motivation of the person saved. Neither, however, appear to justify intervention in one case but not in the other.

The misfeasance-nonfeasance analysis would be misapplied in this context because the concern is not with whether the individual is "guilty" of his own death but rather with the preservation of his life. The misfeasance-nonfeasance analysis is employed to determine an individual's culpability in relation to a given result which society has condemned, and not to reassess the social disutility of that result. For example, a defendant drowns another by pushing him in a lake. He is guilty of homicide. A second defendant refuses to take affirmative action which would effectuate an easy rescue. He is guilty of nothing. In both cases, however, the man is dead, and the loss to society is equally great. Similarly, the result of the suicide's "misfeasance" and the patient's "nonfeasance" is the same.

The second ground for a possible distinction between the suicide and the hospital patient lies in their respective motivations. The suicide wishes to die, whereas the patient who declines treatment for religious reasons wishes to live, but prefers death to a breach of religious commandment. The act of the patient does not "seem" like suicide. It may well be that society's condemnation of suicide is directed at the motivation behind the act and not the act itself because, as one author explains:

> Suicide shows contempt for society. It is rude.... This most individualistic of all actions disturbs society profoundly. Seeing a man who appears not to care for the things it prizes, society is compelled to question all it has thought desirable. The things which make its own life worth living, the suicide boldly jettisons. Society is troubled, and its natural and nervous reaction is to condemn the suicide. Thus it bolsters up again its own values.[6]

This may be good psychology but to use motivation as a basis of legal distinction in this context would be absurd. Take, for example, two hospital patients both in dire need of blood transfusions. One rejects them because of a desire to die, the other because of religious conviction. Should the law allow the patient wishing

to live but preferring death to breach of religious faith, to die, while forcing the one wishing to die, to live? To ask the question is to answer it.

In *Reynolds v. United States,* the Court stated in a dictum that it is within the power of government to prevent a religious suicide. The dictum makes sense. If the non-religious suicide may be prevented, so may the religious suicide. If judicial response were to vary in the two situations, it would be the sheerest of hypocrisies: Life may be saved, not because it is valuable, but rather because suicide is "rude."

Failure to find a meaningful distinction between the refusal of lifesaving treatment and suicide, either in their respective motivations or in the misfeasance-nonfeasance analysis, leads to the conclusion that, based on the quality of their respective conduct, neither the patient nor the suicide can demand legal protection from lifesaving touching. Consequently, if the physician who renders unauthorized treatment is to be held liable while the individual who prevents suicide is held privileged, a distinction must be found in the respective acts of the rescuers. It may be that the latter would be held privileged because he was justified in assuming that the would-be suicide was acting rashly. However, it is apparent that not all suicide attempts are rash. If the rescuer knew that the would-be suicide was not acting rashly, would he commit a legal wrong if he prevented the suicide? If he would not be, then neither would the physician.

D Is There a Right to Choose Death?

To hold that a court order which allows the physician to proceed with lifesaving treatment over the religious objections of the patient is an unconstitutional infringement of religious liberty, or to hold that the physician who has rendered the treatment is liable for battery, is to hold that the individual has a legally enforceable right to choose death. Because of society's interest in the life of the individual, because of the law's traditional view of the sanctity of human life, and because life can be saved without too great a curtailment of the religious liberty of those patients who refuse treatment on religious grounds, the law should not give its protection to the individual's decision to choose death.

Society has an interest in the life of the individual. In the *Georgetown* case, the patient was the mother of a seven-month-old child and it is apparent that others than herself would have suffered had she died. Once it is admitted that there is sufficient interest in the life of a particular patient to deny him a legal right to refuse lifesaving treatment, then the decision must be the same for all patients. That is, the criterion of the "social worth" of the patient would lead the courts into insolvable problems. Any distinction based on "social worth" in this area is repugnant to the basic ideal of equality: If the mother of several children is to be saved, then so must the childless individual.

It would be out of line with the law's traditional affirmation of life were it to label the saving of life as either unconstitutional or as a civil wrong. To bring the issue into focus, take the case of a Buddhist monk's attempt to burn himself. Does the individual commit battery if he prevents the attempted suicide? Does a court unconstitutionally deny the free exercise of religion if it acts to prevent the suicide? There seems but one answer.

To deny the individual a legally enforceable right to reject lifesaving treatment for religious reasons does not greatly curtail his religious freedom, where objection to treatment is on this ground. First, no criminal sanctions are imposed on him. Second, he is allowed to practice the dictates of his religion in all but the most limited of circumstances: the life and death situation. Third, neither he nor his religion, at least in the case of the Jehovah's Witnesses, will deem him to have sinned. He did not voluntarily breach religious dictates....

CONCLUSION

The *Georgetown* case, in ordering that lifesaving treatment may be given to the objecting adult patient, seems to be in accord with the traditional legal view of the sanctity of human life and the interest society has in the life of the individual. To hold otherwise is to hold that the individual has a legally enforceable right, in effect, to choose death, and that the saving of human life, under these circumstances, is a legal wrong....

NOTES

1 Natanson v. Kline, 186 Kan. 393, 406–07, 350 P. 2d 1093, 1104 (1960) (dictum).

2 Meyer v. Knights of Pythias, 178 N.Y. 63, 67, 70 N.E. 111, 112 (1904) (dictum).

3 331 F. 2d 1000 (D.C.Cir.), *cert. denied.* 377 U.S. 978 (1964).

4 *In re* Estate of Brooks, 32 Ill. 2d 361, 205 N.E. 2d 435 (1965); *accord,* Erickson v. Dilgard, 44 Misc. 2d 27, 252 N.Y.S. 2d 705 (Sup. Ct. 1962).

5 98 U.S. 145 (1878).

6 Feeden, *Suicide* 42 (1938), as quoted in Williams, *The Sanctity of Life and the Criminal Law* 267 (1957).

A Patient's Decision to Decline Lifesaving Medical Treatment: Bodily Integrity Versus the Preservation of Life

Norman L. Cantor

Norman L. Cantor is professor of law at Rutgers Law School. He is the author of "Strikes over Non-Arbitrable Labor Disputes" and "Uses and Abuses of the Agency Shop." He is also the author of several articles relating to legal aspects of handling dying medical patients, including "Quinlan, Privacy, and the Handling of Incompetent Dying Patients."

In contrast to the views of Hegland, Cantor defends a rather comprehensive right to decline lifesaving treatment. He argues that a patient's decision to refuse lifesaving treatment must be respected, no matter what the reason for refusal. Cantor reaches this conclusion after an exhaustive analysis of the various interests

Reprinted with permission of the publisher from *Rutgers Law Review,* vol. 26, no. 2 (Winter 1973), pp. 228–264.

that might be claimed in support of judicial intervention to compel lifesaving treatment. He holds that asserted state interests in the preservation of society and the sanctity of life are not sufficient to override the individual's serious interests in religious freedom, bodily integrity, and self-determination. He also rejects rationales based on the effort to enforce public morality and the effort to paternalistically save an individual from harm. Turning to an analysis of the interests of third parties, Cantor concludes that only the interests of surviving minors may be sufficient to limit an individual's right to reject lifesaving treatment.

The scene is a local community hospital. The patient is a 25-year-old man or woman suffering from a perforated ulcer, potentially fatal but curable by a simple operation. The patient is unmarried, childless, and fully coherent. With the threat of death looming, physicians request that the patient consent to surgery and an accompanying blood transfusion. The patient refuses because: *(a)* religious convictions forbid either the surgery or the blood transfusion; *(b)* the patient wants to die because of shame and anxiety over recent financial or romantic setbacks; *(c)* the patient wants to die because he or she is also the victim of a terminal illness which will inevitably entail considerable pain and gradual bodily degeneration; or *(d)* the patient is refusing treatment as a symbolic protest against a governmental policy, such as Viet Nam, and will only submit to surgery when that policy is officially changed. The hospital administrator, acting on the principle that a hospital's paramount mission is to preserve life, seeks a judicial order appointing himself temporary guardian for purposes of consenting to the necessary lifesaving medical treatment.

Can or should a judge grant the relief requested? Does refusal to intervene entail acceptance of a "right to die" in the context of suicide and euthanasia? Does it matter whether the patient is motivated by reasons of conscience or simply by the will to die? Does it matter that the patient has dependents who will be disadvantaged by his or her death? The strong temptation is to respond positively to the opportunity to preserve life. Judges have been anguished by the knowledge that failure to order treatment would likely mean the patient's death, particularly where the patient did not really wish to die but was only following religious dictates. Religious freedom, bodily integrity, or individual self-determination appear as evanescent or ephemeral principles in the face of an immediate threat to life. Yet, both religious freedom and control of one's body are cherished values in our society, and both are

of constitutional dimension when threatened by governmental invasion....

ANALYSIS OF INTERESTS

A variety of public interests have been arrayed both by courts and commentators in support of judicial intervention to order lifesaving medical treatment for a reluctant patient. These interests run the gamut from a noble reference to the sanctity of life to a banal concern for the economic burden left by a patient who dies after refusing treatment.... All deserve careful scrutiny.

A   Preservation of Society

One writer has argued that the "importance of the individual's life to the welfare of society" precludes allowing a patient to spurn lifesaving treatment.[1] This is an appealing notion, but it cannot withstand critical examination. Certainly, a society and its duly constituted institutions have a strong and legitimate interest in their own preservation. Any significant diminution in population might be a matter of real concern, but no one has ever suggested that the volume of persons declining medical treatment constitutes a threat to the maintenance of population levels. Nor is the refusal of treatment an act likely to be widely imitated or duplicated if openly allowed; it is unlike narcotics addiction in that respect. In short, society's existence is by no means threatened by patients' refusals of treatment.

The state also has a legitimate interest in promoting a thriving and productive population. Compulsory education laws are one manifestation of such an interest, yielding both economic and political benefits to society as a whole. In this context, the state might assert an interest in the productivity of an individual—talents, skills, taxpaying potential, military service potential—justifying compelled treatment to keep the individual alive. It is submitted, however, that this concern with productivity cannot override the competing interests in bodily integrity or religious liberty. In the first place, the marginal social utility involved is generally outweighed by the direct and immediate invasion of the patient's personal privacy, both because of the small numbers involved and the attenuated impact on the economy. Secondly, in each instance of refusal, the societal interest would vary according to the individual patient's attributes. In terms of productivity, for example, an industrialist or nuclear physicist has more "social worth" than a vagrant. The problem here is obvious. It is both unseemly and unrealistic to measure the social worth of each patient who declines medical treatment. One solution would be to assume the high value of every patient.[2] But this approach exalts the interest of government, the state, or society over individual self-determination. It is also a fictive approach since in reality the vast majority of us do not contribute so much to the social fabric as to enable the state to claim a paramount interest in our preservation.

B   Sanctity of Life

The state has an indisputable interest in the preservation of life. The criminal law and police power are focused on the protection of public safety. But this use of governmental authority is grounded on the assumption that citizens invariably want to enjoy bodily safety and uninterrupted life. Where a competent individual chooses to decline lifesaving treatment, the normal congruity of interest between individual welfare and state protection against death is disrupted. Entirely new interests, self-determination and privacy from state intrusions, are asserted. The assumption that the citizen demands self-preservation can no longer be operative.

Some writers have nonetheless argued that preservation of a resisting patient's life is relevant to the lives and safety of the general public. The theory is that by denying the patient an opportunity to choose death, a court promotes general respect for life. If a court acquiesced in a patient's rejection of treatment and consequent death, the value of life would be degraded since "any exception to the sanctity of life cannot but cheapen it."[3]

This argument cannot be taken lightly. Sanctity of life is not just a vague theological precept. It is the foundation of a free society. Indeed, libertarians recently campaigned against capital punishment on a similar theory that destruction of life (even the life of a convicted malefactor) degrades the value of life and under-

mines a society's regard for its sanctity. The countervailing consideration, of course, is the dignity tied up with bodily control and self-determination.

> Control by men over their circumstances of action is, along with knowledge of their circumstances, an indispensable part of their personal integrity. Knowledge and control are what make the difference between puppets and people.[4]

It is true that non-interference in an individual's decision to refuse treatment may mean that the patient dies for a reason which may appear silly or inconsequential to most observers. But the rejection of lifesaving medical treatment normally represents a principled invocation of personal or religious convictions, not a deprecation of life. Restraint by courts would be impelled by profound respect for the individual's bodily integrity and religious freedom, not by disregard or disdain for the sanctity of life. Human dignity is enhanced by permitting the individual to determine for himself what beliefs are worth dying for. Through the ages, a multitude of noble causes, religious and secular, have been regarded as worthy of self-sacrifice. Certainly, most governments and societies, our own included, do not consider the sanctity of life to be the supreme value. Nations still insist on the prerogative to engage in mass killing for furtherance of the "national interest," "wars of liberation," or the "defense of democracy." Bodily control, self-determination, and religious freedom are beneficial both to the individual and to the society whose atmosphere and tone are determined by the human values which it respects.

C   Public Morals

As the debate over so-called victimless crimes illustrates, the use of law to reinforce a dominant morality without tangible benefit to public health, safety, and welfare is fraught with difficulties. This is particularly true where the moral underpinnings of laws no longer enjoy a wide community consensus. Many laws aimed primarily at morality nonetheless have been enacted and we must acknowledge that all law is infused with some moral view.

These factors are relevant here because the rejection of lifesaving treatment is a form of suicide—in that it is a voluntary act undertaken with knowledge that death will likely result.[5] Suicide, in turn, has traditionally been anathema in a Judaeo-Christian culture. In the religious sphere, the revulsion toward suicide is grounded primarily on the sixth commandment and the belief that only a divinity can control the withdrawal of life. Antipathy toward suicide, however, extends well beyond the theological realm and public attitudes have sometimes mirrored religious ones. The English common law attached both criminal and civil penalties to suicide or attempted suicide. Suicide was viewed as an offense against nature, violating instincts of self-preservation, as well as an offense against God, the society, and the king. The common revulsion of western culture toward self-imposed death has, then, an ethical or moral base as well as a religious one. Self-destruction in considered to be contrary to man's natural inclinations, a deprivation of a person's productive capacity, an evil example to others and even a rude expression of contempt for society. "Public morals," specifically the "immorality" of self-destruction, cannot provide a legitimate basis for intervention in the patient's decision, however. Contemporary condemnation of suicide as "immoral" is largely clerical in nature and public attitudes toward suicide have markedly changed. While embarrassment about the subject persists, the individual is no longer generally regarded as a sinner or crazed demon. Changes in law have accompanied changes in public opinion. In the vast majority of states, attempted suicide is no longer covered by the criminal law. To the extent that anti-suicide laws remain on the books, they are directed toward authorizing officials to take temporary custody of the individual to prevent the immediate infliction of harm and to render psychological assistance. Suicide is no longer considered, either legally or popularly, as inherently immoral. A morality grounded on an individual's service to the state would be threatened by a patient's conduct in refusing treatment. However, that moral scheme is not widely accepted within a democratic society which stresses maximum individual liberty compatible with the comfort and welfare of others.

D   Protection of the Individual against Himself

Normally, the state's police power is exercised for the general public's health, safety, or welfare. This is so even in the case of certain ostensibly individual invasions, such as compulsory immunizations or blood tests. There are a few areas of law, however, where the state apparently undertakes to protect the individual against his own imprudence. . . .

There is [one] area of paternalistic state conduct which has universally been upheld despite its ostensible interference with individual freedom of choice. A plethora of pure food and drug laws, licensure schemes, and regulations controlling noxious substances exists which incidentally prevents consumers from injuring themselves. Even where the restrictions apply to sellers or distributors, the objective is to prevent the buyer from subjecting himself to risks which the government deems unadvisable. Some observers have articulated concern about the legal implications of this interference with individual self-determination, but these protective health measures nonetheless proliferate. They are generally salutary and are seldom challenged. Yet they may occasionally prevent consumer access to an enjoyable food (for example, swordfish, cyclamate-containing beverages) or to an experimental drug which might be highly beneficial. The individual is effectively precluded from selecting his own risks. Because such protective laws remain judicially inviolate, the question arises whether they provide an effective precedent for governmental prevention of individual risk-taking which might be extended to the lifesaving medical treatment problem.

Most protective legislation is clearly warranted because it guards against abuses which individual consumers are generally helpless to detect or control. For example, most consumers cannot determine the minimum competency of a physician, the iodine content of a food, or the spoilage of meat without regulatory controls. Furthermore consumers alone may be impotent to eliminate the dangerous products of an entire industry (for example, flammable fabrics or unsafe cars). The regulated items also have such wide potential distribution that the public safety and welfare is actually promoted by the protective legislation. These observations about regulatory schemes, however, in no way apply to refusal of medical treatment, since judicial intervention to compel treatment is a very different matter than common regulatory controls. Although both forms of governmental action interfere with individual choice, the regulatory schemes are generally impelled by conditions which preclude real individual choice. The elimination of dangerous products also constitutes, in most instances, a lesser deprivation than interference with religious liberty or bodily integrity. Thus, while precedents may be cited for governmental efforts to preclude individual risk-taking, none sanction judicial intervention to protect a patient against his own decision to decline treatment. Clearly, there are limitations on attempts to guarantee the individual's safety, for otherwise an individual's personal habits, including eating and sleeping, would be potentially subject to governmental dictates. The rights to freedom of religion and personal privacy circumscribe paternalistic impulses in the context of compelled medical treatment.

E Protection of Third Parties

The patient's important interests in religious freedom or bodily integrity could be overridden if refusal of medical treatment were shown to inflict legally cognizable harm on persons other than the patient. Various third party injuries have been suggested by courts and commentators discussing compelled treatment. They all warrant consideration.

1 Surviving Adults The death of a relative or close friend may provoke grief, despair, or other emotional harm in the surviving person. This phenomenon will undoubtedly be present in cases of compelled treatment, and may be urged as a ground for judicial intervention. It is submitted, however, that this factor cannot justify a court in overriding a patient's determination. A variety of conduct by an individual may inflict emotional harm upon his loved ones. The dissolution of a marriage by separation or divorce, or simply abusive conduct toward loved ones can cause emotional wounds, yet no court would contemplate a judicial order to force an adult to be considerate or kind to adult relatives. A similar independence of conduct must be accorded to the patient who may be asserting religious or personal principles in his refusal of treatment. The emotional consequences to survivors will likely be temporary, should be tempered by respect for the patient's principled decision, and, in any event, do not outweigh the patient's interests at stake.

2 Fellow Patients One source has argued that a patient's rejection of lifesaving treatment will distract physicians, provoke turmoil in the hospital staff, and generally disrupt hospital procedure to the detriment of other patients.[6] This argument is speculative and seems rather farfetched. If the patient's choice is honored, precisely the converse of the predicted result should follow. That is, by declining treatment, medical care may well be reduced to the administration of analgesics, freeing staff to attend to other functions. Once a policy of judicial nonintervention is established and publicized, the hospital staff will not expend futile effort in seeking court orders. Although there may be

occasions when the rejection of therapy engenders medical complications which necessitate diverting hospital staff to the patient, this situation is more likely to be the exception than the rule and cannot operate as a general justification for judicial interference with patients' decisions.

3 Physicians Several courts have noted the interests of physicians in compelling lifesaving treatment. One concern is that the physician, if required to respect the patient's choice to decline treatment, must act against his best professional judgment. It is difficult for a physician, trained and dedicated to preservation of life, to allow a salvageable patient to die. In addition, by withholding therapy, the physician may theoretically risk subsequent civil or criminal liability, particularly if the physician were found to have honored an incompetent patient's choice.

While a physician's interest in proper practice of medicine is both valid and legally cognizable, the above concerns do not justify judicial intervention to compel lifesaving treatment. Unfettered exercise of medical judgment has never been a sacrosanct value. The doctrine of informed consent is grounded on the premise that a physician's judgment is subservient to the patient's right to self-determination. Further, other situations exist where a physician's professional judgment is legally restricted or precluded. Laws governing contraception, narcotics, experimental drugs, and compulsory reporting demonstrate that professional judgment is not always a paramount consideration. The assertion of constitutional interests in bodily integrity and free exercise of religion in the context of refusal of care deserve no less deference, even in derogation of a physican's best judgment. While it may be harrowing for a physician to determine whether a patient is voluntarily and competently declining lifesaving treatment, difficult medical decisions must inevitably be made. This is so, for example, whenever a patient is certified as mentally ill for purposes of civil commitment or when a patient ostensibly consents to medical operations which entail substantial risks.

4 Surviving Minors Both courts and commentators have supported judicial intervention to compel medical treatment where the patient is the parent of a minor child, based on an extension of the *parens patriae* doctrine. Since the state can generally act to safeguard a child's welfare, it can act to prevent "ultimate abandonment" of a child by the parent's self-destruction.

By keeping the parent alive, the child presumably benefits emotionally, by continued love and reassurance from the parent, and economically, by continued financial support.

The argument that a court should act to preserve the emotional well-being of children is an appealing one. The legitimacy of the state's interest can be sustained on either of two grounds: there may be altruistic concern with providing each child with a healthful environment, or, development of stable children may be viewed as promoting the political and social well-being of the country. Of course, the loss of a parent will not always produce emotional harm in a child. Not all parents are loving and supportive of their children. It is conceivable that in some instances the surviving child would benefit emotionally from a court's acquiescence in the parent's decision to decline lifesaving treatment. But judicial inquiry, on a case by case basis, into the complex emotional relationships among parents and children might well be too time-consuming and unpleasant to be undertaken. Assuming that the death of a parent will likely provoke some emotional harm to a surviving child, the question becomes whether that harm justifies exercise of the state's *parens patriae* authority to compel a patient to undergo unwanted treatment.

There are numerous situations where a child may be left alone by a parent with consequent emotional upheaval in the child. Death of a parent from natural causes, service in the armed forces, divorce, or even extended travel might cause some emotional wounds. Yet these unintended inflictions of emotional harm are never the source of state intervention; to suggest such intervention would undoubtedly provoke indignant cries of interference with personal liberty. Indeed, an infinite variety of parental conduct could be regulated if prevention of the infliction of emotional harm upon children were accepted as an unlimited basis for interference with parental conduct not intended to harm the child. The state could, under such a theory, compel medical checkups or dictate diets in order to preserve the health of parents.

Some interference with parental conduct is not only justified, but necessary, as the existence of "neglect" statutes demonstrates. Nevertheless, the loss of one of two parents because of the parent's adherence to religious or personal convictions in declining treatment is, arguably, too remote from the state's interest in a child's emotional well being to support judicial intervention. Perhaps a legislature could make a contrary judgment and dictate intervention, but a court operating without such authorization must hesitate to intervene on the basis of protecting children's psychic well being.

A second, less speculative basis exists for judicial intervention to preserve parent's lives—the economic interest of the state in avoiding the burden of supporting surviving children. In many contexts, protection of the public fisc has served as a justification for state conduct or regulations which otherwise would be considered to infringe upon fundamental personal rights.... It must be conceded, then, that some judicial concern with the financial plight of a patient's survivors is both understandable and proper....

Despite this concession, an important caveat should be considered before a court intervenes to compel treatment on an "avoidance of public wards" theory. The economic factors justifying intervention are not present in every case of a parent's refusal of treatment. The surviving spouse, accumulated savings, or other sources may be available to avoid penury even if the patient dies. Thus, the problem would have to be approached on a case by case basis and the economic circumstances sifted in each instance. This type of judicial inquiry is neither difficult nor unseemly; courts commonly examine financial status with regard to support payments, bankruptcy, and enforcement of judgments, to cite a few examples. However, tying the question of judicial intervention to financial circumstances of the patient may prove distasteful to the judiciary. The effect is to tell the patient that his convictions will not be respected because he does not have enough money. It is at least arguable that this de facto wealth discrimination would violate the equal protection clause. In any event, it appears rather mercenary to hinge exercise of rights of privacy and free exercise upon wealth. Perhaps the public should be expected to absorb the economic burden when the refusal of medical treatment leaves indigent survivors. Courts might well take this approach. In light of the relatively small number of people who can be expected to spurn medical treatment when they know their family will be left impecunious, the overall economic burden shifted to the public can be expected to be slight. Judges who rely on the public ward theory to compel lifesaving medical treatment will likely be impelled not by real concern for the public coffers, but by their personal distaste for the patient's decision....

CONCLUSION

As to an independent adult who genuinely objects to treatment, the patient's decision to refuse lifesaving treatment must be respected by the judiciary no matter what the reason for refusal. Respect for bodily integrity, as dictated by constitutional rights of personal privacy, mandates this result in light of the inadequacy or inapplicability of asserted governmental interests in compelling treatment. Even where familial circumstances would constitutionally permit judicial intervention, a judge should normally respect the patient's decision. Intervention to protect survivors' emotional or economic interests, with concomitant government avoidance of fiscal burdens, would too often reflect judicial distaste for a decision to accept death rather than recognition of compelling state interests sufficient to override a patient's decision.

Acceptance of a patient's right to decline lifesaving treatment will mean emotional strain for both physicians and judges. On occasion, it will even be difficult to determine whether the patient's decision is the product of a sound mind. Yet deference to the patient's refusal of treatment reflects sensitivity toward personal interests in bodily integrity and self-determination, not callousness toward life.

NOTES

1 Hegland, *Unauthorized Rendition of Lifesaving Medical Treatment,* 53 Calif. L. Rev. 860 (1965) [hereinafter cited as *Unauthorized Rendition*], at 862. [This volume, p. 355.]
2 This is the approach urged in *Unauthorized Rendition,* at 872. [This volume, pp. 358–359.]
3 *Unauthorized Rendition,* at 867. [This volume, p. 357.]
4 Fletcher, Morals and Medicine 66 (1954).
5 This is not to say that it falls within the legal definition of suicide. Indeed, refusal of treatment is not suicide since the patient, unlike the genuine suicide, does not normally wish to die.
6 *Unauthorized Rendition,* at 868. [This volume, p. 357.]

The Dying Patient and the Refusal of Treatment

The Least Worst Death

M. Pabst Battin

M. Pabst Battin is associate professor of philosophy at the University of Utah. She is the author of *Ethical Issues in Suicide* (1982) and the coeditor of *Suicide: The Philosophical Issues* (1980). Her published articles include "Manipulated Suicide" and "Exact Replication in the Visual Arts."

Battin analyzes the notion of a "natural death" and its relationship to the refusal of medical treatment. On her analysis, a dying patient who chooses to embrace a "natural death" usually has in mind "a painless, conscious, dignified, culminative slipping-away." Such a patient will then typically assert his or her right to refuse medical treatment, since this is the only legally protected mechanism available for a patient trying to achieve a "natural death." But often, Battin maintains, refusal of treatment brings about a sort of death very far from what the patient had in mind. In her view, the key to this dilemma is the *selective* refusal of treatment. With a physician in the role of "strategist of natural death," Battin argues, a patient can effectively achieve "the least worst death among those that could naturally occur."

Reprinted with permission of the author and the publisher from *Hastings Center Report*, vol. 13 (April 1983), pp. 13–16.

In recent years "right-to-die" movements have brought into the public consciousness something most physicians have long known: that in some hopeless medical conditions, heroic efforts to extend life may no longer be humane, and the physician must be prepared to allow the patient to die. Physician responses to patients' request for "natural death" or "death with dignity" have been, in general, sensitive and compassionate. But the successes of the right-to-die movement have had a bitterly ironic result: institutional and legal protections for "natural death" have, in some cases, actually made it more painful to die.

There is just one legally protected mechanism for achieving natural death: refusal of medical treatment. It is available to both competent and incompetent patients. In the United States, the competent patient is legally entitled to refuse medical treatment of any sort on any personal or religious grounds, except perhaps where the interests of minor children are involved. A number of court cases, including *Quinlan*, *Saikewicz*, *Spring*, and *Eichner*,[1] have established precedent in the treatment of an incompetent patient for a proxy refusal by a family member or guardian. In addition, eleven states now have specific legislation protecting the physician from legal action for failure to render treatment when a competent patient has executed a directive to be followed after he is no longer competent. A durable power of attorney, executed by the competent patient in favor of a trusted relative or friend, is also used to determine treatment choices after incompetence occurs.

AN EARLIER BUT NOT EASIER DEATH

In the face of irreversible, terminal illness, a patient may wish to die sooner but "naturally," without artificial prolongation of any kind. By doing so, the patient may believe he is choosing a death that is, as a contributor to the *New England Journal of Medicine* has put it, "comfortable, decent, and peaceful";[2] "natural death," the patient may assume, means a death that is easier than a medically prolonged one.[3] That is why he is willing to undergo death earlier and that is why, he assumes, natural death is legally protected. But the patient may conceive of "natural death" as more than pain-free; he may assume that it will allow time for reviewing life and saying farewell to family and loved ones, for last rites or final words, for passing on hopes, wisdom, confessions, and blessings to the next genera-

tion. These ideas are of course heavily stereotyped; they are the product of literary and cultural traditions associated with conventional death-bed scenes, reinforced by movies, books, and news stories, religious models, and just plain wishful thinking. Even the very term "natural" may have stereotyped connotations for the patient: something close to nature, uncontrived, and appropriate. As a result of these notions, the patient often takes "natural death" to be a painless, conscious, dignified, culminative slipping-away.

Now consider what sorts of death actually occur under the rubric of "natural death." A patient suffers a cardiac arrest and is not resuscitated. Result: sudden unconsciousness, without pain, and death within a number of seconds. Or a patient has an infection that is not treated. Result: the unrestrained multiplication of micro-organisms, the production of toxins, interference with organ function, hypotension, and death. On the way there may be fever, delirium, rigor or shaking, and light-headedness; death usually takes one or two days, depending on the organism involved. If the kidneys fail and dialysis or transplant is not undertaken, the patient is generally more conscious, but experiences nausea, vomiting, gastrointestinal hemorrhage (evident in vomiting blood), inability to concentrate, neuromuscular irritability or twitching, and eventually convulsions. Dying may take from days to weeks, unless such circumstances as high potassium levels intervene. Refusal of amputation, although painless, is characterized by fever, chills, and foul-smelling tissues. Hypotension, characteristic of dehydration and many other states, is not painful but also not pleasant: the patient cannot sit up or get out of bed, has a dry mouth and thick tongue, and may find it difficult to talk. An untreated respiratory death involves conscious air hunger. This means gasping, an increased breathing rate, a panicked feeling of inability to get air in or out. Respiratory deaths may take only minutes; on the other hand, they may last for hours. If the patient refuses intravenous fluids, he may become dehydrated. If he refuses surgery for cancer, an organ may rupture. Refusal of treatment does not simply bring about death in a vacuum, so to speak; death always occurs from some specific cause.

Many patients who are dying in these ways are either comatose or heavily sedated. Such deaths do not allow for a period of conscious reflection at the end of life, nor do they permit farewell-saying, last rites, final words, or other features of the stereotypically "dignified" death.

Even less likely to match the patient's conception of natural death are those cases in which the patient is still conscious and competent, but meets a death that is quite different than he had bargained for. Consider the bowel cancer patient with widespread metastases and a very poor prognosis who—perhaps partly out of consideration for the emotional and financial resources of his family—refuses surgery to reduce or bypass the tumor. How, exactly, will he die? This patient is clearly within his legal rights in refusing surgery, but the physician knows what the outcome is very likely to be: obstruction of the intestinal tract will occur, the bowel wall will perforate, the abdomen will become distended, there will be intractible vomiting (perhaps with a fecal character to the emesis), and the tumor will erode into adjacent areas, causing increased pain, hemorrhage, and sepsis. Narcotic sedation and companion drugs may be partially effective in controlling pain, nausea, and vomiting, but this patient will *not* get the kind of death he thought he had bargained for. Yet, he was willing to shorten his life, to use the single legally protected mechanism—refusal of treatment—to achieve that "natural" death. Small wonder that many physicians are skeptical of the "gains" made by the popular movements supporting the right to die.

WHEN THE RIGHT TO DIE GOES WRONG

Several distinct factors contribute to the backfiring of the right-to-die cause. First, and perhaps the most obvious, the patient may misjudge his own situation in refusing treatment or in executing a natural-death directive: his refusal may be precipitous and ill informed, based more on fear than on a settled desire to die. Second, the physician's response to the patient's request for "death with dignity" may be insensitive, rigid, or even punitive (though in my experience most physicians respond with compassion and wisdom). Legal constraints may also make natural death more difficult than might be hoped: safeguards often render natural-death requests and directives cumbersome to execute, and in any case, in a litigation-conscious society, the physician will often take the most cautious route.

But most important in the apparent backfiring of the right-to-die movement is the underlying ambiguity in the very concept of "natural death." Patients tend to think of the character of the experience they expect to undergo—a death that is "comfortable, decent, peaceful"—but all the law protects is the refusal of medical procedures. Even lawmakers sometimes confuse the two. The California and Kansas natural-death laws claim to protect what they romantically describe as "the natural process of dying." North Carolina's statute says it protects the right to a "peaceful and natural" death. But since these laws actually protect only refusal of treatment, they can hardly guarantee a peaceful, easy death. Thus, we see a widening gulf between the intent of the law to protect the patient's final desires, and the outcomes if the law is actually followed. The physician is caught in between: he recognizes his patient's right to die peacefully, naturally, and with whatever dignity is possible, but foresees the unfortunate results that may come about when the patient exercises this right as the law permits.

Of course, if the symptoms or pain become unbearable the patient may change his mind. The patient who earlier wished not to be "hooked up on tubes" now begins to experience difficulty in breathing or swallowing, and finds that a tracheotomy will relieve his distress. The bowel cancer patient experiences severe discomfort from obstruction, and gives permission for decompression or reductive surgery after all. In some cases, the family may engineer the change of heart because they find dying too hard to watch. Health care personnel may view these reversals with satisfaction: "See," they may say, "he really wants to live after all." But such reversals cannot always be interpreted as a triumph of the will to live; they may also be an indication that refusing treatment makes dying too hard.

OPTIONS FOR AN EASIER DEATH

How can the physician honor the dying patient's wish for a peaceful, conscious, and culminative death? There is more than one option.

Such a death can come about whenever the patient is conscious and pain-free; he can reflect and, if family, clergy, or friends are summoned at the time, he will be able to communicate as he wishes. Given these conditions, death can be brought on in various direct ways. For instance, the physician can administer a lethal quantity of an appropriate drug. Or the patient on severe dietary restrictions can violate his diet: the kidney-failure patient, for instance, for whom high potassium levels are fatal, can simply overeat on avocados. These ways of producing death are, of course, active euthanasia, or assisted or unassisted suicide.

For many patients, such a death would count as "natural" and would satisfy the expectations under which they had chosen to die rather than to continue an intolerable existence. But for many patients (and for many physicians as well) a death that involves deliberate killing is morally wrong. Such a patient could never assent to an actively caused death, and even though it might be physically calm, it could hardly be emotionally or psychologically peaceful. This is not to say that active euthanasia or assisted suicide are morally wrong, but rather that the force of some patients' moral views about them precludes using such practices to achieve the kind of death they want. Furthermore, many physicians are unwilling to shoulder the legal risk such practices may seem to involve.

But active killing aside, the physician can do much to grant the dying patient the humane death he has chosen by using the sole legally protected mechanism that safeguards the right to die: refusal of treatment. This mechanism need not always backfire. For in almost any terminal condition, death can occur in various ways, and there are many possible outcomes of the patient's present condition. The patient who is dying of emphysema could die of respiratory failure, but could also die of cardiac arrest or untreated pulmonary infection. The patient who is suffering from bowel cancer could die of peritonitis following rupture of the bowel, but could also die of dehydration, of pulmonary infection, of acid-base imbalance, of electrolyte deficiency, or of an arrhythmia.

As the poet Rilke observes, we have a tendency to associate a certain sort of end with a specific disease: it is the "official death" for that sort of illness. But there are many other ways of dying than the official death, and the physician can take advantage of these. Infection and cancer, for instance, are old friends: there is increased frequency of infection in the immuno-compromised host. Other secondary conditions, like dehydration or metabolic derangement, may set in. Of course certain conditions typically occur a little earlier, others a little later, in the ordinary course of a terminal disease, and some are a matter of chance. The crucial point is that certain conditions will produce a death that is more comfortable, more decent, more predictable, and more permitting of conscious and peaceful experience than others. Some are better, if the patient has to die at all, and some are worse. Which mode of death claims the patient depends in part on circumstance and in part on the physician's response to conditions that occur. What the patient who rejects active euthanasia or assisted suicide may realistically hope for is this: the least worst death among those that could naturally occur. Not all unavoidable surrenders need involve rout; in the face of inevitable death, the physician becomes strategist, the deviser of plans for how to meet death most favorably.

He does so, of course, at the request of the patient, or, if the patient is not competent, the patient's guardian or kin. Patient autonomy is crucial in the notion of natural death. The physician could of course produce death by simply failing to offer a particular treatment to the patient. But to fail to *offer* treatment that might prolong life, at least when this does not compromise limited or very expensive resources to which other patients have claims, would violate the most fundamental principles of medical practice; some patients do not want "natural death," regardless of the physical suffering or dependency that prolongation of life may entail.

A scenario in which natural death is accomplished by the patient's selective refusal of treatment has one major advantage over active euthanasia and assisted suicide: refusal of treatment is clearly permitted and protected by law. Unfortunately, however, most patients do not have the specialized medical knowledge to use this self-protective mechanism intelligently. Few are aware that some kinds of refusal of treatment will better serve their desires for a "natural death" than others. And few patients realize that refusal of treatment can be selective. Although many patients with life-threatening illness are receiving multiple kinds of therapy, from surgery to nutritional support, most assume that it is only the major procedures (like surgery) that can be refused. (This misconception is perhaps perpetuated by the standard practice of obtaining specific consent for major procedures, like surgery, but not for minor, ongoing ones.) Then, too, patients may be unable to distinguish therapeutic from palliative procedures. And they may not understand the interaction between one therapy and another. In short, most patients do not have enough medical knowledge to foresee the consequences of refusing treatment on a selective basis; it is this that the physician must supply.

It is already morally and legally recognized that informed consent to a procedure involves explicit disclosure, both about the risks and outcomes of the proposed procedure and about the risks and outcomes of alternative possible procedures. Some courts, as in

Quackenbush,[4] have also recognized the patient's right to explicit disclosure about the outcomes of refusing the proposed treatment. But though it is crucial in making a genuinely informed decision, the patient's right to information about the risks and outcomes of alternative kinds of refusal has not yet been recognized. So, for instance, in order to make a genuinely informed choice, the bowel cancer patient with concomitant infection will need to know about the outcomes of each of the principal options: accepting both bowel surgery and antibiotics; accepting antibiotics but not surgery; accepting surgery but not antibiotics; or accepting neither. The case may of course be more complex, but the principle remains: To recognize the patient's right to autonomous choice in matters concerning the treatment of his own body, the physician must provide information about all the legal options open to him, not just information sufficient to choose between accepting or rejecting a single proposed procedure.

One caveat: It sometimes occurs that physicians disclose the dismal probable consequences of refusing treatment in order to coerce patients into accepting the treatment they propose. This may be particularly common in surgery that will result in ostomy of the bowel. The patient is given a graphic description of the impending abdominal catastrophe—impaction, rupture, distention, hemorrhage, sepsis, and death. He thus consents readily to the surgery proposed. The paternalistic physician may find this maneuver appropriate, particularly since ostomy surgery is often refused out of vanity, depression, or on fatalistic grounds. But the physician who frightens a patient into accepting a procedure by describing the awful consequences of refusal is not honoring the patient's right to informed, autonomous choice: he has not described the various choices the patient could make, but only the worst.

Supplying the knowledge a patient needs in order to choose the least worst death need not require enormous amounts of additional energy or time on the part of the physician; it can be incorporated into the usual informed consent disclosures. If the patient is unable to accommodate the medical details, or instructs the physician to do what he thinks is best, the physician may use his own judgment in ordering and refraining from ordering treatment. If the patient clearly prefers to accept less life in hopes of an easy death, the physician should act in a way that will allow the least worst death to occur. In principle, however, the competent patient, and the proxy deciders for an incompetent patient, are entitled to explicit disclosure about all the alternatives for medical care. Physicians in burn units are already experienced in telling patients with very severe burns, where survival is unprecedented, what the outcome is likely to be if aggressive treatment is undertaken or if it is not—death in both cases, but under quite different conditions. Their expertise in these delicate matters might be most useful here. Informed refusal is just as much the patient's right as informed consent.

The role of the physician as strategist of natural death may be even more crucial in longer-term degenerative illnesses, where both physician and patient have far more advance warning that the patient's condition will deteriorate, and far more opportunity to work together in determining the conditions of the ultimate death. Of course, the first interest in both physician and patient will be strategies for maximizing the good life left. Nevertheless, many patients with long-term, eventually terminal illnesses, like multiple sclerosis, Huntington's chorea, diabetes, or chronic renal failure, may educate themselves considerably about the expected courses of their illnesses, and may display a good deal of anxiety about the end stages. This is particularly true in hereditary conditions where the patient may have watched a parent or relative die of the disease. But it is precisely in these conditions that the physician's opportunity may be greatest for humane guidance in the unavoidable matter of dying. He can help the patient to understand what the long-term options are in refusing treatment while he is competent, or help him to execute a natural-death directive or durable power of attorney that spells out the particulars of treatment refusal after he becomes incompetent.

Of course, some diseases are complex and not easy to explain. Patients are not always capable of listening very well, especially to unattractive possibilities concerning their own ends. And physicians are sometimes reluctant to acknowledge that their efforts to sustain life will eventually fail. Providing such information may also seem to undermine whatever hope the physician can nourish in the patient. But the very fact that the patient's demise is still far in the future makes it possible for the physician to describe various scenarios of how that death could occur, and at the same time give the *patient* control over which of them will actually happen. Not all patients will choose the same strategies of ending, nor is there any reason that they should. What may count as the "least worst" death to one person may be the most feared form of death to another.

The physician may be able to increase the patient's psychological comfort immensely by giving him a way of meeting an unavoidable death on his own terms.

In both acute and long-term terminal illnesses, the key to good strategy is flexibility in considering *all* the possibilities at hand. These alternatives need not include active euthanasia or suicide measures of any kind, direct or indirect. To take advantage of the best of the naturally occurring alternatives is not to cause the patient's death, which will happen anyway, but to guide him away from the usual, frequently worst, end.

In the current enthusiasm for "natural death" it is not patient autonomy that dismays physicians. What does dismay them is the way in which respect for patient autonomy can lead to cruel results. The cure for that dismay lies in the realization that the physician can contribute to the *genuine* honoring of the patient's autonomy and rights, assuring him of "natural death" in the way in which the patient understands it, and still remain within the confines of good medical practice and the law.

REFERENCES

1 *In re Quinlan*, 355 A. 2d 647 (N.J. 1976); *Superintendent of Belchertown v. Saikewicz*, 370 N.E. 2d 417 (Mass. 1977); *In re Spring*, Mass. App., 399 N.E. 2d 493; *In re Eichner*, 73 A.D. 2d 431 (2nd Dept. 1980).
2 S. S. Spencer, "'Code' or 'No Code': A Nonlegal Opinion," *New England Journal of Medicine* 300 (1979), 138–140.
3 See Dallas M. High's analysis of the various senses of the term "natural death" in ordinary language, in "Is 'Natural Death' an Illusion?" *Hastings Center Report*, August 1978, pp. 37–42.
4 *In re Quackenbush*, 156 N.J. Super. 282, 353 A. 2d 785 (1978).

Resuscitation Decisions for Hospitalized Patients

President's Commission for the Study of Ethical Problems in Medicine and Biomedical and Behavioral Research

A descriptive account of the President's Commission is found on page 103.

Emphasizing the importance of advance deliberation, the Commission provides an extensive analysis of the ethical considerations relevant to resuscitation decisions. In the view of the Commission, patient self-determination is the most important ethical consideration. Accordingly, the decision of a competent patient should ordinarily be accepted. But the Commission also recognizes another important ethical consideration—patient well-being. Will resuscitation, in the judgment of the physician, promote patient welfare? After rejecting the idea that it is also appropriate to consider the costs of resuscitation in arriving at resuscitation decisions, the Commission proposes an overall scheme to guide decision making, taking into account both the competent and the incompetent patient.

Resuscitation after a cardiac arrest involves a series of steps directed toward sustaining adequate circulation of oxygenated blood to vital organs while heartbeat is restored.

Efforts typically involve the use of cardiac massage or chest compression and the delivery of oxygen under compression through an endo-tracheal tube into the lungs. An electrocardiogram is connected

Reprinted from President's Commission for the Study of Ethical Problems in Medicine and Biomedical and Behavioral Research, *Deciding to Forego Life-Sustaining Treatment* (1983), chapter 7, pp. 234–236, 239–248.

to guide the resuscitation team.... Various plastic tubes are usually inserted intravenously to supply medications or stimulants directly to the heart. Such medications can also be supplied by direct injection into the heart.... A defibrillator may be used, applying electric shock to the heart to induce contractions. A pacemaker... may be fed through a large blood vessel directly to the heart's surface.... These procedures, to be effective, must be initiated with a minimum of delay.... Many of the procedures are obviously highly intrusive, and some are violent in nature. The defibrillator, for example, causes violent (and painful) muscle contractions which... may cause fracture of vertebrae or other bones.[1]

Though initially developed for otherwise healthy persons whose heartbeat and breathing failed following surgery or near-drowning, resuscitation procedures are now used with virtually everyone who has a cardiac arrest in a hospital. The initial success rate for in-hospital resuscitation is about one in three for all victims and two in three for patients hospitalized with irregularities of heart rhythm. Among patients who are successfully resuscitated, about one in three recovers enough to be discharged from the hospital eventually. Especially when used on the general hospital population, long-term success is fairly rare. In the past decade, health care providers have begun to express concern that resuscitation is being used too frequently and sometimes on patients it harms rather than benefits.

Special Characteristics of CPR

Cardiopulmonary resuscitation of hospitalized patients has certain special features that must be taken into account in both individual and institutional decision-making:

- Cardiac arrest occurs at some point in the dying process of every person, whatever the underlying cause of death. Hence the decision whether or not to attempt resuscitation is potentially relevant for all patients.
- Without a heartbeat, a person will die within a very few minutes (that is, heartbeat and breathing will both irreversibly cease).
- Once a patient's heart has stopped, any delay in resuscitation greatly reduces the efficacy of the effort. Hence a decision about whether to resuscitate ought to be made in advance.
- Although resuscitation grants a small number of patients both survival and recovery, attempts at it

usually fail; even when they reestablish heartbeat, they can cause substantial morbidity.

- Clinical signs during resuscitation efforts do not reliably predict functional recovery of a patient. Thus it is difficult to apply the sorts of adjustment and reconsideration that other interventions receive to a decision to resuscitate. Usually, the full range of efforts has to be applied until it is clear whether heartbeat can be restored.
- The conjectural nature of advance deliberations about whether or not to resuscitate may make the discussions difficult for the patient, family, and health care professionals.

Policies on Order Not to Resuscitate

Pioneering policies on "No Code" orders ("code" being the shorthand term for the emergency summoning of a "resuscitation team" by the announcement of "Code Blue" over a hospital's public address system) or "DNR orders" (for "Do Not Resuscitate") were published by several hospitals in 1976.[2] The policies followed the recognition by professional organizations that non-resuscitation was appropriate when well-being would not be served by an attempt to reverse cardiac arrest....

ETHICAL CONSIDERATIONS

The Presumption Favoring Resuscitation

Resuscitation must be instituted immediately after cardiac arrest to have the best chance of success. Because its omission or delayed application is a grievous error when it should have been used to attempt to save a life, most hospitals now provide for the rapid assembling of a team of skilled resuscitation professionals at the bedside of any patient whose heart stops.

When there has been no advance deliberation, this presumption in favor of resuscitation is justified. Although the concern a few years ago was about overtreatment, some health care professionals are now worried about unwarranted undertreatment—a weakening of the presumption in favor of resuscitation. Very different presuppositions are involved when a physician feels a need to justify resuscitating as opposed to not resuscitating someone. In either case, however, the risks of an inappropriate decision with grave consequences for a patient are great if the issues are not properly addressed according to well-developed criteria. In order to avoid using resuscitation in circumstances when it would be appropriate to omit it, advance deliberation on the subject is indicated in most cases. As in all decisions in medicine, the basic issue should be what medical interventions, if any, serve a particular patient's interests and preferences best. When a person's interests or preferences cannot be known under the circumstances, a presumption to sustain the patient's life is warranted.

The Values at Stake

In considering the relative merits of a decision to resuscitate a patient, concerns arise from each of three value considerations—self-determination, well-being, and equity.

Self-determination   Patient self-determination is especially important in decisions for or against resuscitation. Such decisions require that the value of extending life—usually for brief periods and commonly under conditions of substantial disability and suffering—be weighed against that of an earlier death. Different patients will have markedly different needs and concerns at the end of their lives; having a few more hours, days, or even weeks of life under constrained conditions can be much less important to some people than to others. In decisions concerning competent patients, therefore, first importance should be accorded to patient self-determination, and the patient's own decision should be accepted.

This great weight accorded to competent patients' self-determination means that attending physicians have a duty to ascertain patients' preferences,[3] which involves informing each patient of the possible need for CPR and of the likely consequences (both beneficial and harmful) of either employing or foregoing it if the need arises. When cardiac arrest is considered a significant possibility for a competent patient, a DNR order should be entered in the patient's hospital chart only after the patient has decided that is what he or she wants. When resuscitation is a remote prospect, however, the physician need not raise the issue unless CPR is known to be a subject of particular concern to the patient or to be against the patient's wishes. Some patients in the final stages of a terminal illness would experience needless harm in a detailed discussion of resuscitation procedures and consequences.[4] In such cases, the physician might discuss the situation in more general terms, seeking to elicit the individual's general preferences concerning

"vigorous" or "extraordinary" efforts and inviting any further questions he or she may have.[5]

Well-being   A second important ethical consideration is whether resuscitation will promote a patient's welfare. A physician's assessment of "benefit" to a patient incorporates both objective facts, based on the physician's evaluation of the patient's physical status before and following resuscitation, and subjective values, in considering whether resuscitation or non-resuscitation best serves the patient's own values and goals. In virtually all cases the attending physician is in a better position to evaluate the former, while a competent patient is best able to determine the relative value of alternative outcomes.

Even though decisions about resuscitation should recognize the importance of patients' self-determination it may sometimes be necessary to question patients' choices on the grounds of protecting well-being. First, a patient may be mistaken about the course of treatment that will actually achieve the end he or she desires. Even a competent patient may initially misunderstand the nature of alternative outcomes or their relationship to his or her values because of the complexity of the alternatives, the psychological barriers to understanding information, and so forth. Dissonance between the physician's and the patient's assessments of benefit point to the need for such steps as further discussion, reexamination of the patient's decisionmaking capacity, and reassessment of the physician's understanding of patient's goals and values; indeed, in some cases patients may even wish to evaluate their values and goals.

Second, decisions may have to be based on "well-being" because "self-determination" is not possible under the circumstances. Many patients for whom a decision not to resuscitate is indicated have inadequate decisional capacity, often due to their underlying illnesses. In these cases, providers and surrogates must assess whether resuscitation—like any other medical intervention—is or is not likely to benefit the patient. Of course, physicians face many of the same difficulties in deciding that patients do, and their attempts to assess "benefit" will not always lead to clear conclusions.

Equity   The Commission has concluded previously that "society has an ethical obligation to ensure equitable access to...an adequate level of care without excessive burdens."[6] Should resuscitation always be considered part of the "adequate level"? Resuscitation decisions are currently made with little regard to the costs incurred or to the manner in which costs are distributed, except when competent patients decide to include such considerations as a reflection of their own concern for family well-being or for distributional justice. The Commission heard from a number of people, however, who wondered if providers and others should consider whether the costs of resuscitation are warranted for those patients for whom survival is very unlikely and who would, in any case, suffer overwhelming disabilities and diseases.

To determine whether cardiac resuscitation is a component of care that all hospitalized patients should have access to, the predicted value of this procedure would have to be compared with other medical procedures that generate comparable expenses and burdens. It is the Commission's sense that, at the moment, resuscitation efforts usually provide benefits that justify their cost, and thus resuscitation services generally should continue to be provided when desired by a patient or an appropriate surrogate. When, in a particular case, an attempt to resuscitate would clearly be against the patient's stated wishes or best interests, then the reason for not resuscitating does not arise from concerns for equitable use of societal resources, though it may incidentally help conserve them.

Of course, a more refined analysis of whether particular cases or categories of cases should be excluded under the definition of "adequate care" might be attempted. A controversial step would be to attempt to eliminate resuscitations that, while advancing a patient's interests or in accord with a patient's preferences, sustained a very marginal existence at a very high cost.[7]

However, the negative consequences of trying to discern such categories in a workable way provide strong arguments against adopting such policies. Explicitly precluding resuscitation for some categories of patients would almost certainly be insensitive to their values, denigrating to their self-esteem, and distressing to health care professionals. Also, the uncertainties over prognosis with resuscitation for each individual patient would make it very difficult to write clear and workable categories. It is unlikely that the costs incurred by marginally beneficial resuscitation are so substantial that their reduction should be a higher priority than the reduction of other well-documented kinds of wasteful or expensive and marginally beneficial care.

GUIDANCE FOR DECISIONMAKING

Competent Patients

When a competent patient's preference about resuscitation and a physician's assessment of its probable benefits coincide, the decision should simply be in accord with that agreement (see Table 1). When a physician is unclear whether resuscitation would benefit a patient but a competent patient has a clear preference on the subject, the moral claim of autonomy supports acting in accord with the patient's preference. Self-determination also supports honoring a previously competent patient's instructions.

Some patients, although apparently competent, do not express a preference for one course over another. Such patients may not have reached a judgment in their own minds (saying, for example, merely, "whatever you think, Doc") or they may simply be unwilling to articulate a view one way or the other. Provided that the patient's unwillingness to declare a view at the

Table 1   Resuscitation (CPR) of Competent Patients—Physician's Assessment in Relation to Patient's Preference

Physician's assessment	Patient favors CPR*	No preference	Patient opposes CPR*
CPR would benefit patient	Try CPR	Try CPR	Do not try CPR; review decision**
Benefit of CPR unclear	Try CPR	Try CPR	Do not try CPR
CPR would not benefit patient	Try CPR; review decision**	Do not try CPR	Do not try CPR

*Based on an adequate understanding of the relevant information.

**Such a conflict calls for careful reexamination by both patient and physician. If neither the physician's assessment nor the patient's preference changes, then the competent patient's decision should be honored.

moment does not reflect incompetence, the physician should not immediately ask family members to substitute their views for those of the patient, but should instead seek to involve family members in other useful ways (assuming that the patient does not object to their participation), comparable to the roles sometimes played by clergy, nurses, and other professionals. First, the family may be able to facilitate communication between the hospital staff and the patient, making sure that the issues to be addressed have been understood and helping to overcome any barriers to understanding. Second, they may be able to help the patient to make his or her preferences known to the care giving professionals. Ideally, these efforts will lead the patient to express a preference for or against resuscitation.

Of course, it is necessary to have some operative policy while a patient is being encouraged to make a choice, and patients should be informed about what that will be. Until the person expresses a clear preference, the policy in effect should be based on the physician's assessment of benefit to the patient; when it is unclear whether an attempt at CPR would be beneficial, there should be a presumption in favor of trying resuscitation.

When physicians and patients disagree about resuscitation, further discussion is warranted. Each can explain the basis of his or her position and why the other person's judgment seems unwarranted or mistaken. In some cases, consultation with experts may be helpful to resolve doubts about the facts of the case. Together, such steps often produce agreement.

Although disagreement in no way implies that a patient is incompetent, it will often be appropriate for the physician, and perhaps consultants or an advisory committee, to reexamine this issue if discussion does not lead to agreement between patient and physician—and also for the physician to reexamine his or her own thinking and to talk with advisors about it. The serious consequences of the patient's choice—which may include severe disability if resuscitation is tried or death if it is foregone—demand that this process be carried out with care. Once the adequacy of the patient's decisionmaking capacity is confirmed, then the patient's preference should be honored on grounds of self-determination, especially since the choice touches such important subjective values.

If a physician finds the course of action preferred by a competent patient to be medically or morally unacceptable and is unwilling to participate in carrying out the choice, he or she should help the patient find another physician. Indeed, such a change should be explored even when the physician is prepared to carry out the patient's wishes despite an initial disagreement if the difference of opinion created barriers to a good relationship.

Incompetent Patients

Decisionmaking for incompetent patients parallels that for competent ones except that when a physician or surrogate decisionmaker believes that resuscitation is not likely to benefit the patient, there are some additional constraints (see Table 2). Whenever a surrogate and physician disagree, as when only one thinks that resuscitation is warranted, the case should receive careful review, initially through intrainstitutional consultation or ethics committees. Urgent situations, however, or disagreements that are not resolved in this way should go to court. During such proceedings, resuscitation should be attempted if cardiac arrest occurs.

The review entailed will vary. When a physician feels that there is no benefit, a surrogate may either concur after additional consultations or may find another physician, especially if a consulting physician disagrees with the doctor who initially attended the patient. When a surrogate opposes resuscitation that a physician feels is beneficial, discussing the reasons in an impartial setting may uncover erroneous presuppositions, misunderstandings, or self-interested motives and allow for a resolution that is in the patient's best interests. When a surrogate is ambivalent, confirmation of the expected value of resuscitation by a consultant may be persuasive; continued ambivalence may signal the need for a new surrogate. The hospital will have to be able to ensure that helpful and effective responses are provided for these various situations.

If a patient has no surrogate and orders against resuscitation are contemplated, at least a *de facto* surrogate should be designated. When the physician feels that the decision against resuscitation is quite uncontroversial, a consultation with another physician, professional staff consensus, or agreement from an institutionally designated patient advocate can provide suitable confirmation of the initial judgment. Decisions like these are made commonly and should be within the scope of medical practice rather than requiring judicial proceedings. Decisions that are more complex or uncertain should occasion more formal intrainstitutional review and sometimes judicial appointment of a guardian.

Table 2 Resuscitation (CPR) of Incompetent Patients—Physician's Assessment in Relation to Surrogate's Preference

Physician's assessment	Surrogate favors CPR*	No preference	Surrogate opposes CPR*
CPR would benefit patient	Try CPR	Try CPR	Try CPR until review of decision
Benefit of CPR unclear	Try CPR	Try CPR	Try CPR until review of decision
CPR would not benefit patient	Try CPR until review of decision	Try CPR until review of decision	Do not try CPR

*Based on an adequate understanding of the relevant information.

Judicial Oversight

As made clear throughout this Report, the Commission believes that decisionmaking about life-sustaining care is rarely improved by resort to courts. Although physicians might want court adjudication when they believe that a patient's decision against resuscitation is clearly and substantially against his or her interests, courts are unlikely to require people to submit to such an intrusive and painful therapy unless they conclude that the patient is incompetent. Some form of review mechanism within a hospital is generally more appropriate and desirable for such disagreements. The courts are sometimes the appropriate forum for serious, intractable disagreements between a patient's surrogate and physician, however. When intrainstitutional procedures have not led to agreement in such cases, judges may well have to decide between two differing accounts of a patient's interests.

NOTES

1 *In re Dinnerstein*, 380 N.E.2d 134, 135–36 (Mass. App. 1978).

2 Mitchell T. Rabkin, Gerald Gillerman, and Nancy R. Rice, *Orders Not to Resuscitate*, 295 NEW ENG. J MED. 364 (1976); Optimum Care for Hopelessly Ill Patients: A Report of the Critical Care Committee of the Massachusetts General Hospital, 295 NEW ENG. J. MED. 362 (1976)....

3 Although the attending physician bears the responsibility, often others among the care giving professionals, religious advisors, or family members are in a good or better position to discuss the issues and convey the information. This is to be encouraged, but the physician is still obliged to see that it is done well.

4 *See, e.g.*, "Such explanations to the patient, on the other hand, are thoughtless to the point of being cruel, unless the patient inquires, which he is extremely unlikely to do." Steven S. Spencer, *"Code" or "No Code": A Non Legal Opinion*, 300 NEW ENG J. MED. 138, 139 (1979). *But see* "The physician and family often underestimate the patient's ability to handle this issue and participate in the decision." Steven H. Miles, Ronald E. Cranford, and Alvin L. Schultz, *The Do-Not-Resuscitate Order in a Teaching Hospital*, 96 ANNALS INT. MED. 660, 661 (1982).

5 Sometimes it seems cruel and unnecessary. Other times it is just difficult, in the midst of what is usually a very emotional and difficult time, to get around to the question of whether you want us pumping on your chest when you die.... Having taken care of someone for some period of time has usually generated prior tacit, if not overt, understanding between the patient and me on these issues.

Michael Van Scoy-Mosher, *An Oncologist's Case for No-Code Orders*, in A. Edward Doudera and J. Douglas Peters, eds., LEGAL AND ETHICAL ASPECTS OF TREATING CRITICALLY AND TERMINALLY ILL PATIENTS., AUPHA Press, Ann Arbor, Mich. (1982) at 16....

6 President's Commission for the Study of Ethical Problems in Medicine and Biomedical and Behavioral Research, SECURING ACCESS TO HEALTH CARE, U.S. Government Printing Office, Washington (1983) at 4.

7 Resuscitation efforts themselves commonly cost over $1000 and usually entail substantial derivative costs in caring for the surviving patients who suffer side effects.

ANNOTATED BIBLIOGRAPHY: CHAPTER 7

Battin, M. Pabst: *Ethical Issues in Suicide* (Englewood Cliffs, N.J.: Prentice-Hall, 1982). In this very useful book, Battin provides a comprehensive discussion of the traditional arguments concerning suicide. She also suggests an analysis of the concept of rational suicide, discusses suicide intervention as well as suicide facilitation, and considers the notion of suicide as a right.

———, and David J. Mayo, eds.: *Suicide: The Philosophical Issues* (New York: St. Martin's Press, 1980). This valuable collection of articles includes material on the concept of suicide, the morality of suicide, and the rationality of suicide. There are also subsections entitled "Suicide and Psychiatry" and "Suicide, Law, and Rights."

Beauchamp, Tom L.: "Suicide and the Value of Life." in Tom Regan, ed., *Matters of Life and Death* (New York: Random House, 1980), pp. 67–108. In this long essay on the philosophical aspects of suicide, Beauchamp provides both a conceptual analysis of suicide and an evaluation of various moral views.

Beck, Robert N., and John B. Orr, eds.: *Ethical Choice: A Case Study Approach* (New York: Free Press, 1970). Section 2 of this work is entitled "Suicide" and conveniently reprints several classical sources on suicide: Seneca, St. Augustine, St. Thomas Aquinas, Hume, and Schopenhauer.

Byrn, Robert M.: "Compulsory Lifesaving Treatment for the Competent Adult," *Fordham Law Review* 44 (October 1975), pp. 1–36. In an effort to elucidate the state of the law, Byrn examines a large number of cases involving the rejection of lifesaving treatment. He concludes that, apart from cases that feature governmental interests in preventing the spread of communicable disease or protecting the welfare of minor children, competent adults do have a legal right to reject lifesaving treatment.

Frey, R. G.: "Suicide and Self-Inflicted Death," *Philosophy* 56 (April 1981), pp. 193–202. In presenting an analysis of the concept of suicide, Frey emphasizes that a person's death may be "self-inflicted" (and thus a suicide) in a broad as well as a narrow sense. He also contends that a person can commit suicide by planning his or her own death in such a way that he or she is killed by another person.

Greenberg, David F.: "Involuntary Psychiatric Commitments to Prevent Suicide," *New York University Law Review* 49 (May-June 1974), pp. 227–269. Although a short excerpt from this article is reprinted in the present chapter, the article as a whole is noteworthy. Greenberg provides an intensive and broad-based discussion of considerations relevant to establishing what overall suicide prevention policy we ought to adopt. He would restrict coercive intervention to an extremely short period and reject what he calls the more drastic forms of suicide prevention policy, principally involuntary psychiatric commitment.

Holland, R. F.: "Suicide." As reprinted in James Rachels, ed., *Moral Problems*, 2d ed. (New York: Harper & Row, 1975), pp. 388–400. In conjunction with an effort to discuss suicide as an ethico-religious problem, Holland insists on the importance of the question "What is suicide?" He introduces a number of very helpful examples calculated to shed light on the concept of suicide.

Hume, David: "On Suicide." Widely reprinted; for example, in David Hume, *Of the Standard of Taste and Other Essays* (New York: Bobbs-Merrill, 1965), pp. 151–160. In this classic work on the morality of suicide, Hume argues that suicide is morally acceptable inasmuch as it involves no "transgression of our duty either to God, our neighbor, or ourselves."

Jackson, David L., and Stuart Youngner: "Patient Autonomy and 'Death with Dignity':

Some Clinical Caveats," *New England Journal of Medicine* 301 (August 23, 1979), pp. 404–408. The authors introduce a number of clinical case reports from a medical intensive care unit. Their principal point is that "superficial and automatic acquiescence to the concepts of patient autonomy and death with dignity" can lead to clinically inappropriate decisions.

Miller, Bruce L.: "Autonomy and the Refusal of Lifesaving Treatment," *Hastings Center Report* 11 (August 1981), pp. 22–28. Miller distinguishes four senses of autonomy in an effort to deal with refusal of lifesaving treatment cases that feature at least an apparent conflict between medical judgment and patient autonomy.

Paris, John J.: "Compulsory Medical Treatment and Religious Freedom: Whose Law Shall Prevail?" *University of San Francisco Law Review* 10 (Summer 1975), pp. 1–35. Paris holds that the fundamental issue in all blood transfusion cases is the conflict between religious freedom and an alleged "compelling state interest." After an extensive review of relevant cases and arguments, he concludes that decisions to require such transfusions are constitutionally unsound in the case of competent adult patients.

Szasz, Thomas S.: "The Ethics of Suicide," *The Antioch Review* 31 (Spring 1971), pp. 7–17. Intent on developing a strong anti-paternalistic view, Szasz argues that unwanted psychiatric intervention, for the purpose of suicide intervention, constitutes an unjustifiable abridgement of individual liberty.

Wanzer, Sidney H., et al.: "The Physician's Responsibility toward Hopelessly Ill Patients," *New England Journal of Medicine* 310 (April 12, 1984), pp. 955–959. A group of ten physicians suggests a set of guidelines for the treatment of hopelessly ill (adult) patients. The patient's role in decision making is asserted as paramount, and aggressive treatment of the hopelessly ill patient is identified as inappropriate when it would "only prolong a difficult and uncomfortable process of dying." It is also claimed that withholding nutrition and hydration is morally justified in certain cases.

Chapter 8

Euthanasia: The Dying Adult and the Defective Newborn

INTRODUCTION

The moral justifiability of euthanasia is not a newly emerging issue, but it is an issue that is debated with a new intensity in contemporary times. Recent advances in biomedical technology have made it possible to prolong human life in ways undreamed of by past generations of medical practitioners. As a result, it is not unusual to find a person who has lived a long and useful life now permanently incapable of functioning in any recognizably human fashion. Biological life continues; but some find it tempting to say that human life, in any meaningful sense, has ceased. In one case the patient is in an irreversible coma, reduced to a vegetative existence. In another case the patient's personality has completely deteriorated. In still another case the patient alternates inescapably between excruciating pain and drug-induced stupor. In each of these cases, the quality of human life has deteriorated. There is no longer any capacity for creative employment, intellectual pursuit, or the cultivation of interpersonal relationships. In short, in each of these three cases life seems to have been rendered meaningless in the sense that the individual has lost all capacity for normal human satisfactions. In the first case there is simply no consciousness, which is a necessary condition for deriving satisfaction. In the second case consciousness has been dulled to such an extent that there is no longer any capacity for satisfaction. In the third case excruciating pain and sedation combine to undercut the possibility of satisfaction.

At the other end of the spectrum of life, we are confronted with the severely defective newborn child. In some tragic cases, a child seems to have no significant potential for meaningful human life. For example, an anencephalic child, one born with a partial or total absence of the brain, has no prospect for human life as we know it. Biomedical technology is sometimes sufficient to sustain or at least temporarily prolong the life of a severely defective newborn, depending on the particular nature of the child's medical condition, but one question commands attention. Is the child better off dead?

Religious people pray and nonreligious people hope that death will come quickly to themselves or to loved ones who are in the midst of terminal illnesses and forced to endure pain and/or indignity. The same attitudes often prevail in the face of tragically defective newborns. The prevalence of these attitudes seems to confirm the truth, however sad, that some human beings, by virtue of their medical condition, are better off dead. But if it is true that someone is better off dead, then mercy is on the side of death, and the issue of euthanasia comes to the fore. Euthanasia, in its various forms, is the focal point of discussion in this chapter.

The Moral Justifiability of Euthanasia

Discussions of the moral justifiability of euthanasia often involve reference to distinctions that are themselves controversial. Such distinctions include that between ordinary and extraordinary means of prolonging life, that between killing and allowing to die, and that between active and passive euthanasia. Indeed, the very concept of euthanasia is controversial. In accordance with what might be called the "narrow construal of euthanasia," euthanasia is equivalent to mercy *killing*. In this view, if a physician administers a lethal dose of a drug to a terminally ill patient (on grounds of mercy), this act is a paradigm of euthanasia. If, on the other hand, a physician *allows the patient to die* by ceasing to employ "extraordinary means" (such as a respirator), this does not count as euthanasia. In accordance with what might be called the "broad construal of euthanasia," the category of euthanasia encompasses both killing and allowing to die (on grounds of mercy). Those who adopt the broad construal of euthanasia often distinguish between active euthanasia (i.e., killing) and passive euthanasia (i.e., allowing to die). Although there seem to be clear cases of killing (e.g., the lethal dose) and clear cases of allowing to die (e.g., withdrawing a respirator), there are more troublesome cases as well. Suppose a physician administers pain medication with the knowledge that the patient's life will be shortened as a result. A case of killing? Suppose a physician withholds "ordinary means" of life support, whatever that might be. A case of allowing to die? Sometimes it is even said that *withdrawing* extraordinary means of life support is active ("pulling the plug!") in a way that *withholding* extraordinary means is not. And at a time when coronary bypass surgery and hemodialysis treatments are almost routine medical procedures, just what distinguishes ordinary means from extraordinary ones? Cost? Availability? The age of the patient? The condition of the patient?

There is one further distinction, itself relatively uncontroversial, that plays an important role in discussions of euthanasia. *Voluntary euthanasia* proceeds with the (informed) consent of the person involved. *Involuntary euthanasia* proceeds without the consent of the person involved, that is, the person involved is *incapable* of (informed) consent. The possibility of involuntary euthanasia might arise, for example, in the case of a comatose adult.[1] The much discussed case of Karen Ann Quinlan is a case of this sort.[2] The possibility of involuntary euthanasia might also arise with regard to incompetent adults and children. Indeed, the most prominent variety of involuntary euthanasia involves severely defective newborns. When the voluntary/involuntary distinction is combined with the active/passive distinction, it is clear that four types of euthanasia can be generated: (1) active voluntary euthanasia, (2) passive voluntary euthanasia, (3) active involuntary euthanasia, and (4) passive involuntary euthanasia.

A very common view on the morality of euthanasia, so common that it might justifiably be termed the "standard view," may be explicated as follows: Withholding or withdrawing extraordinary means of life support is morally acceptable (under certain specifiable conditions), but mercy killing is never morally acceptable. Those who operate in accordance with the narrow conception of euthanasia would express the standard view by saying that withholding or withdrawing extraordinary means of life support is morally acceptable, but *euthanasia* is never morally acceptable. Those who operate in accordance with the broad conception of euthanasia would express the standard view by saying that *passive euthanasia* is morally acceptable (under certain specifiable conditions), but *active euthanasia* is never morally acceptable. The standard view, as officially endorsed by the American Medical Association (AMA), is vigorously attacked by James Rachels in one of this chapter's readings. Thomas D. Sullivan accuses Rachels of misconstruing the sense behind the standard view. Sullivan offers a defense of the standard view. Rachels, in turn, criticizes Sullivan's reliance on the distinction between intentional and nonintentional terminations of life and the distinction between ordinary and extraordinary means of life support.

The withholding or withdrawing of extraordinary means of life support in the case of terminally ill patients is surely an established part of medical practice, as reflected in the AMA's official endorsement of the standard view. Moreover, several religious traditions explicitly acknowledge the morality of this practice. In addition, it is widely believed that a patient has the moral (and legal) right to refuse treatment, a right that would encompass the refusal of extraordinary means of life support. Thus, despite any difficulties that might be involved in specifying what counts as "extraordinary means" of life support, there is a substantial body of opinion, perhaps something close to a consensus view, maintaining the moral legitimacy of withholding or withdrawing extraordinary means of life support in the case of terminally ill patients. There is no such consensus view on the morality of *mercy killing*, which will be referred to here as "active euthanasia."

Those who argue for the moral legitimacy of active euthanasia emphasize considerations of humaneness. In the case of *voluntary* active euthanasia, the humanitarian appeal is often conjoined with an appeal to the primacy of individual freedom. Thus the case for the morality of voluntary active euthanasia incorporates two basic arguments: (1) It is cruel and inhumane to refuse the plea of a terminally ill person that his or her life be mercifully ended in order to avoid future suffering and indignity. (2) Individuals should be free to do as they choose as long as their actions do not result in harm to others. Since no one is harmed by terminally ill patients undergoing active euthanasia, their freedom to have their lives ended in this fashion should not be infringed.

Typically, those who argue against the moral legitimacy of voluntary active euthanasia rest their case on one or both of the following strategies of argument: (1) They appeal to some "sanctity of life" principle to the effect that the intentional termination of (innocent) human life is always immoral. Sullivan advances this sort of argument in his defense of the standard view. (2) They advance a rule-utilitarian argument to the effect that any systematic acceptance of active euthanasia would lead to damaging consequences for society (e.g., via a lessening of respect for human life). This second sort of argument recurs in discussions of the legalization of voluntary active euthanasia.

Euthanasia and the Definition of Death

Two groups of patients are at the center of controversy in contemporary discussions of "the definition of death." In the first group are patients whose *entire* brain has irreversibly ceased functioning. They are irreversibly comatose, but cardiopulmonary function (heartbeat and respiration) is successfully maintained by a respirator and concomitant life-support systems. These patients are frequently identified as "brain-dead" or "whole-brain-dead." They will be referred to here as "brain-dead." In a second group of patients, brainstem function is sufficient to sustain heartbeat and respiration, but irreversible damage to "the higher brain," the cerebral cortex, is so severe that these patients are suspended in what is called a "persistent vegetative state." Consciousness, and thus cognition, has been irreversibly lost. Are the patients in each of these groups alive or dead? In any case, what treatment is morally appropriate for patients in each group?

The traditional standard for the determination of death is the permanent absence of respiration and pulsation. According to this standard, "brain-dead" patients are alive so long as artificial life-support systems sustain cardiopulmonary functioning. In 1968, an ad hoc committee of the Harvard Medical School issued a report that is a frequent reference point in contemporary discussions of "the definition of death." In this report, the Ad Hoc Committee specified a set of tests for the identification of a permanently nonfunctioning (whole) brain—the condition of "brain-death." In the view of the Ad Hoc Committee, when this condition has been diagnosed, "death is to be declared and *then* the respirator turned off."[3] Thus, in essence, the Ad Hoc Committee advanced a new standard for the determination of death. A "brain-dead" patient is a dead patient, despite the fact that cardiopulmonary functioning is artificially sustained.

It is a matter of substantial import whether "brain-dead" patients are alive or dead. Taking the vital organs of these patients for transplantation purposes is morally unproblematic if they are dead, presuming of course that appropriate consent procedures have been followed. If they are alive, however, taking their vital organs could well be the cause of their death. There are also important implications in the context of passive euthanasia discussions. When a respirator is withdrawn from a "brain-dead" patient, how are we to conceptualize this action? If the patient is alive, then it is sensible to describe withdrawing the respirator as an act of passive euthanasia. But if the patient is already dead, we cannot say, in withdrawing the respirator, that we are allowing the patient to die; hence we cannot say that we are dealing with an act of passive euthanasia.

In one of this chapter's selections, David J. Mayo and Daniel I. Wikler argue against contemporary proposals to "redefine death." They take issue in particular with the proposal of the Harvard Ad Hoc Committee. Mayo and Wikler deny that a "brain-dead" patient whose cardiopulmonary function is being maintained by artificial life-support is dead. It is nevertheless true that the substance of the Harvard proposal has achieved a significant measure of public acceptance. For example, the President's Commission for the Study of Ethical Problems in Medicine and Biomedical and Behavioral Research in its 1981 report, *Defining Death*, recommends the adoption by all states of the Uniform Determination of Death Act:

An individual who has sustained either (1) irreversible cessation of circulatory and respiratory functions, or (2) irreversible cessation of all functions of the entire brain, including the brain stem, is dead. A determination of death must be made in accordance with accepted medical standards.

Charles M. Culver and Bernard Gert, in another of this chapter's selections, define death as the permanent cessation of functioning of the *organism as a whole*. In their view, which is compatible with the substance of the Harvard proposal, a patient who has undergone a permanent loss of functioning of the entire brain is dead, but a patient in a "persistent vegetative state" is not dead, even though, as they say, the organism has ceased to be a person. Indeed, Culver and Gert explicitly argue against a competing definition of death, according to which the permanent loss of consciousness and cognition is sufficient for death. They insist that "we must not confuse the death of an organism which was a person with an organism's ceasing to be a person." Culver and Gert also consider in some detail the morally appropriate treatment for patients who are in a "persistent vegetative state." Though they reject the notion of killing such a patient, they endorse allowing the patient to die by discontinuing all care, even "ordinary and routine care." Presumably the discontinuance of "ordinary and routine care" would include the withdrawing of nutrition and hydration—"food and water"—from the patient. But at this point we are confronted with a question that has relevance to other sorts of patients as well (e.g., severely defective newborns). Is it ever morally appropriate to withhold nutrition and hydration from a patient? Those who systematically oppose withholding nutrition and hydration often call attention to the symbolic significance of food and water—their intimate connection with notions of care and concern.

The Legalization of Euthanasia

In recent years a mass of so-called euthanasia legislation has been proposed in the various state legislatures. Most of these legislative proposals have been advanced to establish an individual's right to some form of passive rather than active euthanasia, but even this apparently undramatic sort of legislation has met with much opposition. Some people oppose passive euthanasia legislation because of the difficulties inherent in trying to define crucial phrases such as "meaningless life," "natural death," "extraordinary means," "heroic measures," and so forth. Others, although supporting the spirit of the proposed legislation, nevertheless argue that it is unnecessary because there is already a generally recognized right to refuse even lifesaving treatment. (Cf. Chapter 7.) Still others are worried that the legalization of passive euthanasia would lead to the legalization of active euthanasia.

Active euthanasia is illegal in all fifty states, yet the more dramatic euthanasia proposals would seek to legalize active euthanasia, specifically in its *voluntary* form. The debate between Yale Kamisar and Glanville Williams, featured in the readings of this chapter, centers on the legalization of voluntary active euthanasia.

There are some who consider active euthanasia in any form intrinsically immoral (sometimes on overtly religious grounds) and thus are opposed to the legalization of voluntary active euthanasia. Others, however, like Kamisar, see nothing intrinsically wrong with individual acts of voluntary active euthanasia, but still stand opposed to any systematic social policy that would permit voluntary active euthanasia. Arguments made in this vein have a rule-utilitarian character, emphasizing the undesirable consequences that might attend the legalization of voluntary active euthanasia. It is said that the law will be commonly abused and that patients will needlessly die when mistakingly thought to be incurably ill. Most importantly, it is said, the legalization of voluntary active euthanasia will lead to disrespect for the sanctity of human life. This latter argument, usually identified as a "wedge argument," has several versions. Kamisar's version runs like this: The legalization of voluntary active euthanasia will lead to the legalization of *involuntary* active euthanasia and thus the "mercy killing" not only of irreversibly comatose patients but also of the senile, the deformed, and perhaps eventually the politically undesirable.

Those, like Williams, who support the legalization of voluntary active euthanasia argue that prohibitive laws are cruel and inhumane. Moreover, they typically conjoin this consideration with an appeal to personal liberty. Since persons who voluntarily choose to undergo active euthanasia harm no one, it is argued, prohibitive laws unjustifiably deprive individuals of liberty. Those who support the legalization of voluntary active euthanasia recognize that some bad consequences may result from such legislation. However, they seek to establish that potential dangers are minimal.

The Treatment of Defective Newborns

The well-established medical practice of allowing (selected) severely defective newborns to die, often identified as the practice of passive (involuntary) euthanasia, has recently made its way into the public consciousness. Media attention has been focused on a rash of "Baby Doe" cases, and the Reagan administration has been conspicuous in its effort to activate the machinery of government via the introduction of "Baby Doe" regulations. As a result, the practice of allowing (selected) severely defective newborns to die has been subjected to intense scrutiny, with regard to both its legality and its morality. It is perhaps important to notice that "allowing to die," in this context, apparently includes the withholding of *ordinary,* not just extraordinary medical treatment. At any rate, a severely defective newborn might be denied the antibiotics necessary to fight pneumonia, although the pneumonia is totally unrelated to the condition that renders the child severely defective.

The central moral question with regard to the treatment of defective newborns may be identified as follows: Under what conditions, if any, is it morally acceptable to allow a severely defective newborn to die? Two other closely related issues are also worthy of mention. The first has to do with the procedural question: Who should make the decision to treat or not treat? It has sometimes been argued that the decision is a medical one, to be made by physicians. But the more common view is that the parents are the appropriate decision makers, as informed by consultation with physicians and (perhaps) as limited by boundaries set by society at large. In this regard, it is often suggested that hospital ethics committees be assigned the responsibility of reviewing decisions to treat or not treat severely defective newborns. The second issue worthy of mention has to do with the moral legitimacy of active euthanasia. If it is morally acceptable to allow a severely defective newborn to die, on grounds that the child is better off dead, then is it not also morally acceptable (perhaps morally preferable) to kill the child as painlessly as possible?

Broadly speaking, there are three different views on the moral acceptability of allowing severely defective newborns to die.

(1) It is morally acceptable to allow a severely defective newborn to die if and only if there is no significant potential for a meaningful human existence. Defenders of this view, such as Richard A. McCormick in one of this chapter's selections, are firmly committed to so-called quality-of-life judgments. Importantly, in this view, the cost of caring for severely defective newborns is considered an irrelevant factor in the decision to treat or not treat. (A very similar but somewhat more restrictive view would endorse allowing a severely defective newborn to die if and only if death would be in the infant's best interests, that is, if and only if the infant would be better off dead.)

(2) It is morally acceptable to allow a severely defective newborn to die if at least one of the following conditions is satisfied: (*a*) There is no significant potential for a meaningful human existence; (*b*) The emotional and/or financial hardship of caring for the severely defective newborn child would constitute a grave burden for the family. It is the introduction of the cost factor that distinguishes view (2) from view (1). Defenders of this second view, such as H. Tristram Engelhardt, Jr., often emphasize that the newborn child does not have the status of personhood, thereby defending the legitimacy of the cost factor.

(3) It is never morally acceptable to allow a severely defective newborn to die. Or, to put it more exactly, it would never be morally acceptable to withhold treatment from a severely defective newborn unless it would be morally acceptable to withhold such treatment from a normal infant. Although there is no requirement to prolong the life of a *dying* infant, whatever medical treatment is considered appropriate for an otherwise normal infant must be provided for the seriously defective newborn as well. For example, if antibiotics are indicated for an otherwise normal infant with pneumonia, then antibiotics may not be

withheld in a case where pneumonia arises for an infant whose central nervous system is severely compromised. In this view, it is usually presumed that a newborn child has the status of personhood and, however severely defective, has a right to life. Defenders of this view, such as John A. Robertson in one of this chapter's selections, often make arguments against the validity of quality-of-life judgments (as featured in both of the aforementioned views) as well as the validity of the cost factor (as featured exclusively in the second view).

T. A. M.

NOTES

1 It is often suggested that competent adults make "a living will" in order to express their wishes with regard to the treatment they would desire, should they become incompetent. In this way, it is thought, individual autonomy is fostered, and others (e.g., physicians and family) can be relieved of the responsibility for making involuntary euthanasia decisions. One well-known example of "a living will" has been promulgated by the Euthanasia Educational Council. Addressed to all those who may be concerned, the statement reads as follows:

> Death is as much a reality as birth, growth, maturity and old age—it is the one certainty of life. If the time comes when I, _____ , can no longer take part in decisions for my own future, let this statement stand as an expression of my wishes, while I am still of sound mind.
>
> If the situation should arise in which there is no reasonable expectation of my recovery from physical or mental disability, I request that I be allowed to die and not be kept alive by artificial means or "heroic measures." I do not fear death itself as much as the indignities of deterioration, dependence and hopeless pain. I, therefore, ask that medication be mercifully administered to me to alleviate suffering even though this may hasten the moment of death.
>
> This request is made after careful consideration. I hope you who care for me will fell morally bound to follow its mandate. I recognize that this appears to place a heavy responsibility upon you, but it is with the intention of relieving you of such responsibility and of placing it upon myself in accordance with my strong convictions, that this statement is made.

2 In the Quinlan case, Joseph Quinlan, the father of comatose 21-year-old Karen Ann Quinlan, sought to be appointed guardian of the person and property of his daughter. As guardian, he would then authorize the discontinuance of the mechanical respirator that was thought to be sustaining the vital life processes of his daughter. Judge Muir of the Superior Court of New Jersey decided against the request of Joseph Quinlan. *In re Quinlan*, 137 N. J. Super 227 (1975). Justice Hughes of the Supreme Court of New Jersey overturned the lower-court decision. *In re Quinlan*, 70 N. J. 10, 335 A. 2d 647 (1976). When the respirator was finally withdrawn, Karen Ann Quinlan proved capable of breathing on her own. She remained alive in a "persistent vegetative state" for a period of about ten years.

3 The Ad Hoc Committee of the Harvard Medical School to Examine the Definition of Brain Death, "A Definition of Irreversible Coma," *Journal of the American Medical Association* 205 (August 6, 1968), p. 338.

General Conceptual and Ethical Issues

Active and Passive Euthanasia

James Rachels

James Rachels is professor of philosophy at the University of Alabama in Birmingham. Specializing in ethics, he is the author of such articles as "Why Privacy is Important," "On Moral Absolutism," and "Can Ethics Provide Answers?" He is also the editor of *Moral Problems: A Collection of Philosophical Essays* (1971, 3d ed., 1979) and *Understanding Moral Philosophy* (1976).

Rachels identifies the standard (conventional) view on the morality of euthanasia as the doctrine that permits passive euthanasia but rejects active euthanasia. He then argues that the conventional doctrine may be challenged for four reasons. First of all, active euthanasia is in many cases more humane than passive euthanasia. Second, the conventional doctrine leads to decisions concerning life and death on irrelevant grounds. Third, the doctrine rests on a distinction between killing and letting die that itself has no moral importance. Fourth, the most common arguments in favor of the doctrine are invalid.

The distinction between active and passive euthanasia is thought to be crucial for medical ethics. The idea is that it is permissible, at least in some cases, to withhold treatment and allow a patient to die, but it is never permissible to take any direct action designed to kill the patient. This doctrine seems to be accepted by most doctors, and it is endorsed in a statement adopted by the House of Delegates of the American Medical Association on December 4, 1973:

> The intentional termination of the life of one human being by another—mercy killing—is contrary to that for which the medical profession stands and is contrary to the policy of the American Medical Association.
>
> The cessation of the employment of extraordinary means to prolong the life of the body when there is irrefutable evidence that biological death is imminent is the decision of the patient and/or his immediate family. The advice and judgment of the physician should be freely available to the patient and/or his immediate family.

However, a strong case can be made against this doctrine. In what follows I will set out some of the relevant arguments, and urge doctors to reconsider their views on this matter.

To begin with a familiar type of situation, a patient who is dying of incurable cancer of the throat is in terrible pain, which can no longer be satisfactorily alleviated. He is certain to die within a few days, even if present treatment is continued, but he does not want to go on living for those days since the pain is unbearable. So he asks the doctor for an end to it, and his family joins in the request.

Suppose the doctor agrees to withhold treatment, as the conventional doctrine says he may. The justification for his doing so is that the patient is in terrible agony, and since he is going to die anyway, it would be wrong to prolong his suffering needlessly. But now notice this. If one simply withholds treatment, it may take the patient longer to die, and so he may suffer more than he would if more direct action were taken and a lethal injection given. This fact provides strong reason for thinking that, once the initial decision not to prolong his agony has been made, active euthanasia is actually preferable to passive euthanasia, rather than the reverse. To say otherwise is to endorse the option that leads to more suffering rather than less, and is contrary to the humanitarian impulse that prompts the decision not to prolong his life in the first place.

Part of my point is that the process of being "allowed to die" can be relatively slow and painful, whereas

Reprinted by permission from the *New England Journal of Medicine*, vol. 292, no. 2 (January 9, 1975), pp. 78–80.

being given a lethal injection is relatively quick and painless. Let me give a different sort of example. In the United States about one in 600 babies is born with Down's syndrome. Most of these babies are otherwise healthy—that is, with only the usual pediatric care, they will proceed to an otherwise normal infancy. Some, however, are born with congenital defects such as intestinal obstructions that require operations if they are to live. Sometimes, the parents and the doctor will decide not to operate, and let the infant die. Anthony Shaw describes what happens then:

> ... When surgery is denied [the doctor] must try to keep the infant from suffering while natural forces sap the baby's life away. As a surgeon whose natural inclination is to use the scalpel to fight off death, standing by and watching a salvageable baby die is the most emotionally exhausting experience I know. It is easy at a conference, in a theoretical discussion, to decide that such infants should be allowed to die. It is altogether different to stand by in the nursery and watch as dehydration and infection wither a tiny being over hours and days. This is a terrible ordeal for me and the hospital staff—much more so than for the parents who never set foot in the nursery.[1]

I can understand why some people are opposed to all euthanasia, and insist that such infants must be allowed to live. I think I can also understand why other people favor destroying these babies quickly and painlessly. But why should anyone favor letting "dehydration and infection wither a tiny being over hours and days"? The doctrine that says that a baby may be allowed to dehydrate and wither, but may not be given an injection that would end its life without suffering, seems so patently cruel as to require no further refutation. The strong language is not intended to offend, but only to put the point in the clearest possible way.

My second argument is that the conventional doctrine leads to decisions concerning life and death made on irrelevant grounds.

Consider again the case of the infants with Down's syndrome who need operations for congenital defects unrelated to the syndrome to live. Sometimes, there is no operation, and the baby dies, but when there is no such defect, the baby lives on. Now, an operation such as that to remove an intestinal obstruction is not prohibitively difficult. The reason why such operations are not performed in these cases is, clearly, that the child has Down's syndrome and the parents and doctor judge that because of that fact it is better for the child to die.

But notice that this situation is absurd, no matter what view one takes of the lives and potentials of such babies. If the life of such an infant is worth preserving, what does it matter if it needs a simple operation? Or, if one thinks it better that such a baby should not live on, what difference does it make that it happens to have an unobstructed intestinal tract? In either case, the matter of life and death is being decided on irrelevant grounds. It is the Down's syndrome, and not the intestines, that is the issue. The matter should be decided, if at all, on that basis, and not be allowed to depend on the essentially irrelevant question of whether the intestinal tract is blocked.

What makes this situation possible, of course, is the idea that when there is an intestinal blockage, one can "let the baby die," but when there is no such defect there is nothing that can be done, for one must not "kill" it. The fact that this idea leads to such results as deciding life or death on irrelevant grounds is another good reason why the doctrine should be rejected.

One reason why so many people think that there is an important moral difference between active and passive euthanasia is that they think killing someone is morally worse than letting someone die. But is it? Is killing, in itself, worse than letting die? To investigate this issue, two cases may be considered that are exactly alike except that one involves killing whereas the other involves letting someone die. Then, it can be asked whether this difference makes any difference to the moral assessments. It is important that the cases be exactly alike, except for this one difference, since otherwise one cannot be confident that it is this difference and not some other that accounts for any variation in the assessments of the two cases. So, let us consider this pair of cases:

In the first, Smith stands to gain a large inheritance if anything should happen to his six-year-old cousin. One evening while the child is taking his bath, Smith sneaks into the bathroom and drowns the child, and then arranges things so that it will look like an accident.

In the second, Jones also stands to gain if anything should happen to his six-year-old cousin. Like Smith, Jones sneaks in planning to drown the child in his bath. However, just as he enters the bathroom Jones sees the child slip and hit his head, and fall face down in the water. Jones is delighted; he stands by, ready to push the child's head back under if it is necessary, but it

Sullivan, responding directly to Rachels, offers a defense of the standard (traditional) view on the morality of euthanasia. Sullivan charges Rachels with misconstruing the sense behind the traditional view. On Sullivan's analysis, the traditional view is not dependent on the distinction between killing and letting die. Rather, it simply forbids the *intentional* termination of life, whether by killing or letting die. The cessation of *extraordinary* means, he maintains, is morally permissible because, although death is foreseen, it need not be intended.

Because of recent advances in medical technology, it is today possible to save or prolong the lives of many persons who in an earlier era would have quickly perished. Unhappily, however, it often is impossible to do so without commiting the patient and his or her family to a future filled with sorrows. Modern methods of neurosurgery can successfully close the opening at the base of the spine of a baby born with severe myelomeningocoele, but do nothing to relieve the paralysis that afflicts it from the waist down or to remedy the patient's incontinence of stool and urine. Antibiotics and skin grafts can spare the life of a victim of severe and massive burns, but fail to eliminate the immobilizing contractions of arms and legs, the extreme pain, and the hideous disfigurement of the face. It is not surprising, therefore, that physicians and moralists in increasing number recommend that assistance should not be given to such patients, and that some have even begun to advocate the deliberate hastening of death by medical means, provided informed consent has been given by the appropriate parties.

The latter recommendation consciously and directly conflicts with what might be called the "traditional" view of the physician's role. The traditional view, as articulated, for example, by the House of Delegates of the American Medical Association in 1973, declared:

The intentional termination of the life of one human being by another—mercy killing—is contrary to that for which the medical profession stands and is contrary to the policy of the American Medical Association.

The cessation of the employment of extra-ordinary means to prolong the life of the body when there is irrefutable evidence that biological death is imminent is the decision of the patient and/or his immediate family. The advice and judgment of the physician should be freely available to the patient and/or his immediate family.

Basically this view involves two points: (1) that it is impermissible for the doctor or anyone else to terminate intentionally the life of a patient, but (2) that it is permissible in some cases to cease the employment of "extraordinary means" of preserving life, even though the death of the patient is a foreseeable consequence.

Does this position really make sense? Recent criticism charges that it does not. The heart of the complaint is that the traditional view arbitrarily rules out all cases of intentionally acting to terminate life, but permits what is in fact the moral equivalent, letting patients die. This accusation has been clearly articulated by James Rachels in a widely-read article that appeared in a recent issue of the *New England Journal of Medicine,* entitled "Active and Passive Euthanasia."[1] By "active euthanasia" Rachels seems to mean *doing something* to bring about a patient's death, and by "passive euthanasia," not doing anything, i.e., just letting the patient die. Referring to the A.M.A. statement, Rachels sees the traditional position as always forbidding active euthanasia, but permitting passive euthanasia. Yet, he argues, passive euthanasia may be in some cases morally indistinguishable from active euthanasia, and in other cases even worse. To make his point he asks his readers to consider the case of a Down's syndrome baby with an intestinal obstruction that easily could be remedied through routine surgery. Rachels comments:

I can understand why some people are opposed to all euthanasia and insist that such infants must be allowed to live. I think I can also understand why other people favor destroying these babies quickly and painlessly. But why should anyone favor letting 'dehydration and infection wither a tiny being over hours and days'? The doctrine that says that a baby may be allowed to dehydrate and wither, but may not be given an injection that would end its life without suffering, seems so patently cruel as to require no further refutation.[2]

Rachels' point is that decisions such as the one he describes as "patently cruel" arise out of a misconceived moral distinction between active and passive euthanasia, which in turn rests upon a distinction between killing and letting die that itself has no moral importance.

One reason why so many people think that there is an important difference between active and passive euthanasia is that they think killing someone is morally worse than letting someone die. But is it?... To investigate this issue two cases may be considered that are exactly alike except that one involves killing whereas the other involves letting someone die. Then, it can be asked whether this difference makes any difference to the moral assessments....

In the first, Smith stands to gain a large inheritance if anything should happen to his six-year-old cousin. One evening while the child is taking his bath, Smith sneaks into the bathroom and drowns the child, and then arranges things so that it will look like an accident.

In the second, Jones also stands to gain if anything should happen to his six-year-old cousin. Like Smith, Jones sneaks in planning to drown the child in his bath. However, just as he enters the bathroom Jones sees the child slip and hit his head, and fall face down in the water. Jones is delighted; he stands by, ready to push the child's head back under if it is necessary, but it is not necessary. With only a little thrashing about, the child drowns all by himself, "accidentally," as Jones watches and does nothing.[3]

Rachels observes that Smith killed the child, whereas Jones "merely" let the child die. If there's an important moral distinction between killing and letting die, then, we should say that Jones' behavior from a moral point of view is less reprehensible than Smith's. But while the law might draw some distinctions here, it seems clear that the acts of Jones and Smith are not different in any important way, or, if there is a difference, Jones' action is even worse.

In essence, then, the objection to the position adopted by the A.M.A. of Rachels and those who argue like him is that it endorses a highly questionable moral distinction between killing and letting die, which, if accepted, leads to indefensible medical decisions. Nowhere does Rachels quite come out and say that he favors active euthanasia in some cases, but the implication is clear. Nearly everyone holds that it is sometimes pointless to prolong the process of dying and that in those cases it is morally permissible to let a patient die even though a few hours or days could be salvaged by procedures that would also increase the agonies of the dying. But if it is impossible to defend a general distinction between letting people die and acting to terminate their lives directly, then it would seem that active euthanasia also may be morally permissible.

Now what shall we make of all this? It *is* cruel to stand by and watch a Down's baby die an agonizing death when a simple operation would remove the intestinal obstruction, but to offer the excuse that in failing to operate we didn't *do* anything to bring about death is an example of moral evasiveness comparable to the excuse Jones would offer for his action of "merely" letting his cousin die. Furthermore, it is true that if someone is trying to bring about the death of another human being, then it makes little difference from the moral point of view if his purpose is achieved by action or by malevolent omission, as in the cases of Jones and Smith.

But if we acknowledge this, are we obliged to give up the traditional view expressed by the A.M.A. statement? Of course not. To begin with, we are hardly obliged to assume the Jones-like role Rachels assigns the defender of the traditional view. We have the option of operating on the Down's baby and saving its life. Rachels mentions that possibility only to hurry past it as if that is not what his opposition would do. But, of course, that is precisely the course of action most defenders of the traditional position would choose.

Secondly, while it may be that the reason some rather confused people give for upholding the traditional view is that they think killing someone is always worse than letting them die, nobody who gives the matter much thought puts it that way. Rather they say that killing someone is clearly morally worse than not killing them, and killing them can be done by acting to bring about their death or by refusing ordinary means to keep them alive in order to bring about the same goal.

What I am suggesting is that Rachels' objections leave the position he sets out to criticize untouched. It is worth noting that the jargon of active and passive euthanasia—and it is jargon—does not appear in the resolution. Nor does the resolution state or imply the distinction Rachels attacks, a distinction that puts a moral premium on overt behavior—moving or not moving one's parts—while totally ignoring the intentions of the agent. That no such distinction is being drawn seems clear from the fact that the A.M.A. resolution speaks approvingly of ceasing to use extraordinary means in certain cases, and such withdrawals might easily involve bodily movement, for example unplugging an oxygen machine.

In addition to saddling his opposition with an indefensible distinction it doesn't make, Rachels proceeds to ignore one that it does make—one that is crucial to a just interpretation of the view. Recall the A.M.A. allows the withdrawal of what it calls extra-ordinary means of preserving life; clearly the contrast here is with ordinary means. Though in its short statement those expressions are not defined, the definition Paul Ramsey refers to as standard in his book, *The Patient as Person*, seems to fit.

Ordinary means of preserving life are all medicines, treatments, and operations, which offer a reasonable hope of benefit for the patient and which can be obtained and used without excessive expense, pain, and other inconveniences.

Extra-ordinary means of preserving life are all those medicines, treatments, and operations which cannot be obtained without excessive expense, pain, or other inconvenience, or which, if used, would not offer a reasonable hope of benefit.[4]

Now with this distinction in mind, we can see how the traditional view differs from the position Rachels mistakes for it. The traditional view is that the intentional termination of human life is impermissible, irrespective of whether this goal is brought about by action or inaction. Is the action or refraining *aimed at* producing a death? Is the termination of life *sought, chosen or planned?* Is the intention deadly? If so, the act or omission is wrong.

But we all know it is entirely possible that the unwillingness of a physician to use extra-ordinary means for preserving life may be prompted not by a determination to bring about death, but by other motives. For example, he may realize that further treatment may offer little hope of reversing the dying process and/or be excruciating, as in the case when a massively necrotic bowel condition in a neonate is out of control. The doctor who does what he can to comfort the infant but does not submit it to further treatment or surgery may foresee that the decision will hasten death, but it certainly doesn't follow from that fact that he intends to bring about its death. It is, after all, entirely possible to foresee that something will come about as a result of one's conduct without intending the consequence or side effect. If I drive downtown, I can foresee that I'll wear out my tires a little, but I don't drive downtown

with the intention of wearing out my tires. And if I choose to forego my exercises for a few days, I may think that as a result my physical condition will deteriorate a little, but I don't omit my exercise with a view to running myself down. And if you have to fill a position and select Green, who is better qualified for the post than her rival Brown, you needn't appoint Mrs. Green with the intention of hurting Mr. Brown, though you may foresee that Mr. Brown will feel hurt. And if a country extends its general education programs to its illiterate masses, it is predictable the suicide rate will go up, but even if the public officials are aware of this fact, it doesn't follow that they initiate the program with a view to making the suicide rate go up. In general, then, it is not the case that all the foreseeable consequences and side effects of our conduct are necessarily intended. And it is because the physician's withdrawal of extra-ordinary means can be otherwise motivated than by a desire to bring about the predictable death of the patient that such action cannot categorically be ruled out as wrong.

But the refusal to use ordinary means is an altogether different matter. After all, what is the point of refusing assistance which offers reasonable hope of benefit to the patient without involving excessive pain or other inconvenience? How could it be plausibly maintained that the refusal is not motivated by a desire to bring about the death of the patient? The traditional position, therefore, rules out not only direct actions to bring about death, such as giving a patient a lethal injection, but malevolent omissions as well, such as not providing minimum care for the newborn.

The reason the A.M.A. position sounds so silly when one listens to arguments such as Rachels' is that he slights the distinction between ordinary and extra-ordinary means and then drums on cases where *ordinary* means are refused. The impression is thereby conveyed that the traditional doctrine sanctions omissions that are morally indistinguishable in a substantive way from direct killings, but then incomprehensively refuses to permit quick and painless termination of life. If the traditional doctrine would approve of Jones' standing by with a grin on his face while his young cousin drowned in a tub, or letting a Down's baby wither and die when ordinary means are available to preserve its life, it would indeed be difficult to see how anyone could defend it. But so to conceive the traditional doctrine is simply to misunderstand it. It is not a doctrine that rests on some supposed distinction between "active" and "passive euthanasia," whatever those words are supposed to mean, nor on a distinction between moving and not moving our bodies. It is simply a prohibition against intentional killing, which includes both direct actions and malevolent omissions.

To summarize—the traditional position represented by the A.M.A. statement is not incoherent. It acknowledges, or more accurately, insists upon the fact that withholding ordinary means to sustain life may be tantamount to killing. The traditional position can be made to appear incoherent only by imposing upon it a crude idea of killing held by none of its more articulate advocates.

Thus the criticism of Rachels and other reformers, misapprehending its target, leaves the traditional position untouched. That position is simply a prohibition of murder. And it is good to remember, as C. S. Lewis once pointed out:

> No man, perhaps, ever at first described to himself the act he was about to do as Murder, or Adultery, or Fraud, or Treachery.... And when he hears it so described by other men he is (in a way) sincerely shocked and surprised. Those others 'don't understand.' If they knew what it had really been like for him, they would not use those crude 'stock' names. With a wink or a titter, or a cloud of muddy emotion, the thing has slipped into his will as something not very extraordinary, something of which, rightly

understood in all of his peculiar circumstances, he may even feel proud.[5]

I fully realize that there are times when those who have the noble duty to tend the sick and the dying are deeply moved by the sufferings of their patients, especially of the very young and the very old, and desperately wish they could do more than comfort and companion them. Then, perhaps, it seems that universal moral principles are mere abstractions having little to do with the agony of the dying. But of course we do not see best when our eyes are filled with tears.

NOTES

1 *New England Journal of Medicine*, 292; 78–80, Jan. 9, 1975. [Reprinted, this volume, pp. 385–388.]
2 Ibid., pp. 78–79. [This volume, p. 386.]
3 Ibid., p. 79. [This volume, pp. 386–387.]
4 Paul Ramsey, *The Patient As Person* (New Haven and London: Yale University Press, 1970), p.122. Ramsey abbreviates the definition first given by Gerald Kelly, S.J., *Medico-Moral Problems* (St. Louis, Missouri: The Catholic Hospital Association, 1958), p. 129.
5 C. S. Lewis, *A Preface to Paradise Lost* (London and New York: Oxford University Press, 1970), p. 126.

More Impertinent Distinctions

James Rachels

A biographical sketch of James Rachels is found on page 385.

Rachels makes a new departure in responding to Sullivan. He presents two further arguments against the standard (traditional) view on the morality of euthanasia. Rachels contends, first, that the traditional view is mistaken because it is dependent on an indefensible distinction between intentional and nonintentional terminations of life. Second, he contends, the traditional view is mistaken because it is dependent on an indefensible distinction between ordinary and extraordinary means of treatment.

Many thinkers, including almost all orthodox Catholics, believe that euthanasia is immoral. They oppose

killing patients in any circumstances whatever. However, they think it is all right, in some special circumstances, to allow patients to die by withholding treatment. The American Medical Association's policy statement on mercy killing supports this traditional view. In my paper "Active and Passive Euthanasia"[1] I argued, against the traditional view, that there is in fact no moral difference between killing and letting die—if one is permissible, then so is the other.

Professor Sullivan[2] does not dispute my argument; instead he dismisses it as irrelevant. The traditional doctrine, he says, does not appeal to or depend on the distinction between killing and letting die. Therefore, arguments against that distinction "leave the traditional position untouched."

Is my argument really irrelevant? I don't see how it can be. As Sullivan himself points out,

> Nearly everyone holds that it is sometimes pointless to prolong the process of dying and that in those cases it is morally permissible to let a patient die even though a few more hours or days could be salvaged by procedures that would also increase the agonies of the dying. But if it is impossible to defend a general distinction between letting people die and acting to terminate their lives directly, then it would seem that active euthanasia also may be morally permissible. (390)

But traditionalists like Professor Sullivan hold that active euthanasia—the direct killing of patients—is *not* morally permissible; so, if my argument is sound, their view must be mistaken. I cannot agree, then, that my argument "leaves the traditional position untouched."

However, I shall not press this point. Instead I shall present some further arguments against the traditional position, concentrating on those elements of the position which Professor Sullivan himself thinks most important. According to him, what is important is, first, that we should never *intentionally* terminate the life of a patient, either by action or omission, and second, that we may cease or omit treatment of a patient, knowing that this will result in death, only if the means of treatment involved are *extraordinary*.

INTENTIONAL AND NONINTENTIONAL TERMINATION OF LIFE

We can, of course, distinguish between what a person does and the intention with which he does it. But what is the significance of this distinction for ethics?

> The traditional view [says Sullivan] is that the intentional termination of human life is impermissible,

irrespective of whether this goal is brought about by action or inaction. Is the action or refraining *aimed at* producing a death? Is the termination of life *sought, chosen or planned?* Is the intention deadly? If so, the act or omission is wrong. (391)

Thus on the traditional view there is a very definite sort of moral relation between act and intention. An act which is otherwise permissible may become impermissible if it is accompanied by a bad intention. The intention makes the act wrong.

There is reason to think that this view of the relation between act and intention is mistaken. Consider the following example. Jack visits his sick and lonely grandmother, and entertains her for the afternoon. He loves her and his only intention is to cheer her up. Jill also visits the grandmother, and provides an afternoon's cheer. But Jill's concern is that the old lady will soon be making her will; Jill wants to be included among the heirs. Jack also knows that his visit might influence the making of the will, in his favor, but that is no part of his plan. Thus Jack and Jill do the very same thing—they both spend an afternoon cheering up their sick grandmother—and what they do may lead to the same consequences, namely influencing the will. But their intentions are quite different.

Jack's intention was honorable and Jill's was not. Could we say on that account that what Jack did was right, but what Jill did was wrong? No; for Jack and Jill did the very same thing, and if they did the same thing, we cannot say that one acted rightly and the other wrongly.[3] Consistency requires that we assess similar actions similarly. Thus if we are trying to evaluate their *actions,* we must say about one what we say about the other.

However, if we are trying to assess Jack's *character,* or Jill's, things are very different. Even though their actions were similar, Jack seems admirable for what he did, while Jill does not. What Jill did—comforting an elderly sick relative—was a morally good thing, but we would not think well of her for it since she was only scheming after the old lady's money. Jack, on the other hand, did a good thing *and* he did it with an admirable intention. Thus we think well, not only of what Jack did, but of Jack.

The traditional view, as presented by Professor Sullivan, says that the intention with which an act is done is relevant to determining whether the act is right. The example of Jack and Jill suggests that, on the contrary, the intention is not relevant to deciding whether the *act* is right or wrong, but instead it is relevant to assessing the character of the person who does the act, which is very different.

Now let us turn to an example that concerns more important matters of life and death. This example is adapted from one used by Sullivan himself.(391) A massively necrotic bowel condition in a neonate is out of control. Dr. White realizes that further treatment offers little hope of reversing the dying process and will only increase the suffering; so, he does not submit the infant to further treatment—even though he knows that this decision will hasten death. However, Dr. White does not seek, choose, or plan that death, so it is not part of his intention that the baby dies.

Dr. Black is faced with a similar case. A massively necrotic bowel condition in a neonate is out of control. He realizes that further treatment offers little hope of saving the baby and will only increase its suffering. He decides that it is better for the baby to die a bit sooner than to go on suffering pointlessly; so, with the intention of letting the baby die, he ceases treatment.

According to the traditional position, Dr. White's action was acceptable, but Dr. Black acted wrongly. However, this assessment faces the same problem we encountered before. Dr. White and Dr. Black did *the very same thing:* their handling of the cases was identical. Both doctors ceased treatment, knowing that the baby would die sooner, and both did so because they regarded continued treatment as pointless, given the infants' prospects. So how could one's action be acceptable and the other's not? There was, of course, a subtle difference in their *attitudes* toward what they did. Dr. Black said to himself, "I want this baby to die now, rather than later, so that it won't suffer more; so I won't continue the treatment." A defender of the traditional view might choose to condemn Dr. Black for this, and say that his character is defective (although I would not say that); but the traditionalist should not say that Dr. Black's *action* was wrong on that account, at least not if he wants to go on saying that Dr. White's action was right. A pure heart cannot make a wrong act right; neither can an impure heart make a right act wrong. As in the case of Jack and Jill, the intention is relevant, not to determining the rightness of actions, but to assessing the character of the people who act.

There is a general lesson to be learned here. The rightness or wrongness of an act is determined by the reasons for or against it. Suppose you are trying to decide, in this example, whether treatment should be continued. What are the reasons for and against this course of action? On the one hand, if treatment is ceased the baby will die very soon. On the other hand, the baby will die eventually anyway, even if treatment is continued. It has no chance of growing up. Moreover, if its life is prolonged, its suffering will be prolonged as well, and the medical resources used will be unavailable to others who would have a better chance of a satisfactory cure. In light of all this, you may well decide against continued treatment. But notice that is no mention here of anybody's intentions. The intention you would have, if you decided to cease treatment, is not one of the things you need to consider. It is not among the reasons either for or against the action. That is why it is irrelevant to determining whether the action is right.

In short, a person's intention is relevant to an assessment of his character. The fact that a person intended so-and-so by his action may be a reason for thinking him a good or a bad person. But the intention is not relevant to determining whether the act itself is morally right. The rightness of the act must be decided on the basis of the objective reasons for or against it. It is permissible to let the baby die, in Sullivan's example, because of the facts about the baby's condition and its prospects—not because of anything having to do with anyone's intentions. Thus the traditional view is mistaken on this point.

ORDINARY AND EXTRAORDINARY MEANS OF TREATMENT

The American Medical Association policy statement says that life-sustaining treatment may sometimes be stopped if the means of treatment are "extraordinary": the implication is that "ordinary" means of treatment may not be withheld. The distinction between ordinary and extraordinary treatments is crucial to orthodox Catholic thought in this area, and Professor Sullivan reemphasizes its importance: he says that, while a physician may sometimes rightly refuse to use extraordinary means to prolong life, "the refusal to use ordinary means is an altogether different matter."(391)

However, upon reflection it is clear that it is sometimes permissible to omit even very ordinary sorts of treatment.

Suppose that a diabetic patient long accustomed to self-administration of insulin falls victim to terminal cancer, or suppose that a terminal cancer patient suddenly develops diabetes. Is he in the first case obliged to continue, and in the second case obliged to begin, insulin treatment and die painfully of cancer, or in either or both cases may the patient choose rather to pass into diabetic coma and an earlier death?... What of the conscious patient suffering from painful incurable disease who suddenly gets pneumonia? Or an old man slowly deteriorating who from simply being inactive and recumbent gets pneumonia: Are we to use antibiotics in a likely successful attack upon this disease which from time immemorial has been called "the old man's friend"?[4]

These examples are provided by Paul Ramsey, a leading theological ethicist. Even so conservative a thinker as Ramsey is sympathetic with the idea that, in such cases, life-prolonging treatment is not mandatory: the insulin and the antibiotics need not be used. Yet surely insulin and antibiotics are "ordinary" treatments by today's medical standards. They are common, easily administered, and cheap. There is nothing exotic about them. So it appears that the distinction between ordinary and extraordinary means does not have the significance traditionally attributed to it.

But what of the *definitions* of "ordinary" and "extraordinary" means which Sullivan provides? Quoting Ramsey, he says that

> Ordinary means of preserving life are all medicines, treatments, and operations, which offer a reasonable hope of benefit for the patient and which can be obtained and used without excessive expense, pain, and other inconveniences.
>
> Extra-ordinary means of preserving life are all those medicines, treatments, and operations which cannot be obtained without excessive expense, pain, or other inconvenience, or which, if used, would not offer a reasonable hope of benefit. (391)

Do these definitions provide us with a useful distinction— one that can be used in determining when a treatment is mandatory and when is it not?

The first thing to notice is the way the word "excessive" functions in these definitions. It is said that a treatment is extraordinary if it cannot be obtained without *excessive* expense or pain. But when is an expense "excessive"? Is a cost of $10,000 excessive? If it would save the life of a young woman and restore her to perfect health, $10,000 does not seem excessive. But if it would only prolong the life of Ramsey's cancer-stricken diabetic a short while, perhaps $10,000 is

excessive. The point is not merely that what is excessive changes from case to case. The point is that what is excessive *depends on* whether it would be a good thing for the life in question to be prolonged.

Second, we should notice the use of the word "benefit" in the definitions. It is said that ordinary treatments offer a reasonable hope of *benefit* for the patient; and that treatments are extraordinary if they will not benefit the patient. But how do we tell if a treatment will benefit the patient? Remember that we are talking about life-prolonging treatments; the "benefit," if any, is the continuation of life. Whether continued life is a benefit depends on the details of the particular case. For a person with a painful terminal illness, a temporarily continued life may not be a benefit. For a person in irreversible coma, such as Karen Quinlan, continued biological existence is almost certainly not a benefit. On the other hand, for a person who can be cured and resume a normal life, life-sustaining treatment definitely is a benefit. Again, the point is that in order to decide whether life-sustaining treatment is a benefit we must *first* decide whether it would be a good thing for the life in question to be prolonged.

Therefore, these definitions do not mark out a distinction that can be used to help us decide when treatment may be omitted. We cannot by using the definitions identify which treatments are extraordinary, and then use that information to determine whether the treatment may be omitted. For the definitions require that we must *already* have decided the moral questions of life and death *before* we can answer the question of which treatments are extraordinary!

We are brought, then, to this conclusion about the distinction between ordinary and extraordinary means. If we apply the distinction in a straightforward, commonsense way, the traditional doctrine is false, for it is clear that it is sometimes permissible to omit ordinary treatments. On the other hand, if we define the terms as suggested by Ramsey and Sullivan, the distinction is useless in practical decision-making. In either case, the distinction provides no help in formulating an acceptable ethic of letting die.

SUMMARY

The distinction between killing and letting die has no moral importance; on that Professor Sullivan and I agree. He, however, contends that the distinctions between intentional and nonintentional termination of life, and ordinary and extraordinary means, must be at the heart of a correct moral view. I believe that the arguments given above refute this view. Those distinctions are no better than the first one. The traditional view is mistaken.

In my original paper I did not argue in favor of active euthanasia. I merely argued that active and passive euthanasia are equivalent: *if* one is acceptable, so is the other. However, Professor Sullivan correctly inferred that I do endorse active euthanasia: I believe that it is in some instances morally justified, and that it ought to be made legal.[5] This he believes to be pernicious. In his penultimate paragraph he says that the traditional doctrine is "simply a prohibition of murder," and that those of us who think otherwise are confused, teary-eyed sentimentalists. But the traditional doctrine is not that. It is a muddle of indefensible claims, backed by tradition but not by reason.

NOTES

1 James Rachels, "Active and Passive Euthanasia," *The New England Journal of Medicine,* vol. 292 (Jan. 9, 1975), pp. 78–80. [Reprinted, this volume, pp. 385–388.]

2 Thomas D. Sullivan, "Active and Passive Euthanasia: An Impertinent Distinction?" *The Human Life Review,* vol. III (1977), pp. 40–46. Parenthetical references in the text are to this article [as reprinted in this volume, pp. 388–392.]

3 It might be objected that they did not "do the same thing," for Jill manipulated and deceived her grandmother, while Jack did not. If their actions are described in this way, then it may seem that "what Jill did" was wrong, while "what Jack did" was not. However, this description of what Jill did incorporates her intention into the description of the act. In the present context we must keep the act and the intention separate, in order to discuss the relation between them. If they *cannot* be held separate, then the traditional view makes no sense.

4 Paul Ramsey, *The Patient as Person* (New Haven: Yale University Press, 1970), pp. 115–116.

5 For arguments in support of this position, see J. Rachels, "Euthanasia," in *Matters of Life and Death,* edited by Tom Regan (New York: Random House, 1980).

Euthanasia and the Definition of Death

Why "Update" Death?

President's Commission for the Study of Ethical Problems in Medicine and Biomedical and Behavioral Research

A descriptive account of the President's Commission is found on page 103.

In this selection, taken from the first chapter of its report, *Defining Death*, the Commission provides a compact account of both (1) the interrelationships of brain, heart, and lung functions and (2) the loss of brain functions. Emphasis is placed on the difference between "whole brain death" and a "persistent vegetative state" in which brainstem function persists. Although reference is made to the Commission's view that "the cessation of the vital functions of the entire brain [is] the only proper neurologic basis for declaring death," the analysis and argumentation the Commission presents in support of this view is found only in subsequent chapters of the report.

Reprinted from President's Commission for the Study of Ethical Problems in Medicine and Biomedical and Behavioral Research, *Defining Death* (1981), pp. 13–20.

For most of the past several centuries, the medical determination of death was very close to the popular one. If a person fell unconscious or was found so, someone (often but not always a physician) would feel for the pulse, listen for breathing, hold a mirror before the nose to test for condensation, and look to see if the pupils were fixed. Although these criteria have been used to determine death since antiquity, they have not always been universally accepted.

DEVELOPING CONFIDENCE IN THE HEART-LUNG CRITERIA

In the eighteenth century, macabre tales of "corpses" reviving during funerals and exhumed skeletons found to have clawed at coffin lids led to widespread fear of premature burial. Coffins were developed with elaborate escape mechanisms and speaking tubes to the world above, mortuaries employed guards to monitor the newly dead for signs of life, and legislatures passed laws requiring a delay before burial....

...The invention of the stethoscope in the mid-nineteenth century enabled physicians to detect heartbeat with heightened sensitivity. The use of this instrument by a well-trained physician, together with other clinical measures, laid to rest public fears of premature burial. The twentieth century brought even more sophisticated technological means to determine death, particularly the electrocardiograph (EKG), which is more sensitive than the stethoscope in detecting cardiac functioning.

THE INTERRELATIONSHIPS OF BRAIN, HEART, AND LUNG FUNCTIONS

The brain has three general anatomic divisions: the cerebrum, with its outer shell called the cortex; the cerebellum; and the brainstem, composed of the midbrain, the pons, and the medulla oblongata. Traditionally, the cerebrum has been referred to as the "higher brain" because it has primary control of consciousness, thought, memory and feeling. The brainstem has been called the "lower brain," since it controls spontaneous, vegetative functions such as swallowing, yawning and sleep-wake cycles. It is important to note that these generalizations are not entirely accurate. Neuroscientists generally agree that such "higher brain" functions as cognition or consciousness probably are not mediated strictly by the cerebral cortex; rather, they probably

result from complex interrelations between brainstem and cortex.

Respiration is controlled in the brainstem, particularly the medulla. Neural impulses originating in the respiratory centers of the medulla stimulate the diaphragm and intercostal muscles, which cause the lungs to fill with air. Ordinarily, these respiratory centers adjust the rate of breathing to maintain the correct levels of carbon dioxide and oxygen. In certain circumstances, such as heavy exercise, sighing, coughing or sneezing, other areas of the brain modulate the activities of the respiratory centers or even briefly take direct control of respiration.

Destruction of the brain's respiratory center stops respiration, which in turn deprives the heart of needed oxygen, causing it too to cease functioning. The traditional signs of life—respiration and heartbeat—disappear: the person is dead. The "vital signs" traditionally used in diagnosing death thus reflect the direct interdependence of respiration, circulation and the brain.

The artificial respirator and concomitant life-support systems have changed this simple picture. Normally, respiration ceases when the functions of the diaphragm and intercostal muscles are impaired. This results from direct injury to the muscles or (more commonly) because the neural impulses between the brain and these muscles are interrupted. However, an artificial respirator (also called a ventilator) can be used to compensate for the inability of the thoracic muscles to fill the lungs with air. Some of these machines use negative pressure to expand the chest wall (in which case they are called "iron lungs"); others use positive pressure to push air into the lungs. The respirators are equipped with devices to regulate the rate and depth of "breathing," which are normally controlled by the respiratory centers in the medulla. The machines cannot compensate entirely for the defective neural connections since they cannot regulate blood gas levels precisely. But, provided that the lungs themselves have not been extensively damaged, gas exchange can continue and appropriate levels of oxygen and carbon dioxide can be maintained in the circulating blood.

Unlike the respiratory system, which depends on the neural impulses from the brain, the heart can pump blood without external control. Impulses from brain centers modulate the inherent rate and force of the heartbeat but are not required for the heart to contract at a level of function that is ordinarily adequate. Thus, when artificial respiration provides adequate oxygenation and associated medical treatments regulate essential plasma components and blood pressure, an intact heart will continue to beat, despite loss of brain functions. At present, however, no machine can take over the functions of the heart except for a very limited time and in limited circumstances (e.g., a heart-lung machine used during surgery). Therefore, when a severe injury to the heart or major blood vessels prevents the circulation of the crucial blood supply to the brain, the loss of brain functioning is inevitable because no oxygen reaches the brain.

LOSS OF VARIOUS BRAIN FUNCTIONS

The most frequent causes of irreversible loss of functions of the whole brain are: (1) direct trauma to the head, such as from a motor vehicle accident or a gunshot wound, (2) massive spontaneous hemorrhage into the brain as a result of ruptured aneurysm or complications of high blood pressure, and (3) anoxic damage from cardiac or respiratory arrest or severely reduced blood pressure.

Many of these severe injuries to the brain cause an accumulation of fluid and swelling in the brain tissue, a condition called cerebral edema. In severe cases of edema, the pressure within the closed cavity increases until it exceeds the systolic blood pressure, resulting in a total loss of blood flow to both the upper and lower portions of the brain. If deprived of blood flow for at least 10–15 minutes, the brain, including the brainstem, will completely cease functioning. Other pathophysiologic mechanisms also result in a progressive and, ultimately, complete cessation of intracranial circulation.

Once deprived of adequate supplies of oxygen and glucose, brain neurons will irreversibly lose all activity and ability to function. In adults, oxygen and/or glucose deprivation for more than a few minutes causes some neuron loss. Thus, even in the absence of direct trauma and edema, brain functions can be lost if circulation to the brain is impaired. If blood flow is cut off, brain tissues completely self-digest (autolyze) over the ensuing days.

When the brain lacks all functions, consciousness is, of course, lost. While some spinal reflexes often persist in such bodies (since circulation to the spine is separate from that of the brain), all reflexes controlled by the brainstem as well as cognitive, affective and integrating functions are absent. Respiration and circulation in these bodies may be generated by a ventilator together with intensive medical management. In adults who have experienced irreversible cessation of the functions of the entire brain, this mechanically generated functioning can continue only a limited time because the heart usually stops beating within two to ten days. (An infant or small child who has lost all brain functions will typically suffer cardiac arrest within several weeks, although respiration and heartbeat can sometimes be maintained even longer.)

Less severe injury to the brain can cause mild to profound damage to the cortex, lower cerebral structures, cerebellum, brainstem, or some combination thereof. The cerebrum, especially the cerebral cortex, is more easily injured by loss of blood flow or oxygen than is the brainstem. A 4–6 minute loss of blood flow—caused by, for example, cardiac arrest—typically damages the cerebral cortex permanently, while the relatively more resistant brainstem may continue to function.

When brainstem functions remain, but the major components of the cerebrum are irreversibly destroyed, the patient is in what is usually called a "persistent vegetative state" or "persistent noncognitive state." Such persons may exhibit spontaneous, involuntary movements such as yawns or facial grimaces, their eyes may be open and they may be capable of breathing without assistance. Without higher brain functions, however, any apparent wakefulness does not represent awareness of self or environment (thus, the condition is often described as "awake but unaware"). The case of Karen Ann Quinlan has made this condition familiar to the general public. With necessary medical and nursing care—including feeding through intravenous or nasogastric tubes, and antibiotics for recurrent pulmonary infections—such patients can survive months or years, often without a respirator. (The longest survival exceeded 37 years.)

CONCLUSION: THE NEED FOR RELIABLE POLICY

Medical interventions can often provide great benefit in avoiding *irreversible* harm to a patient's injured heart, lungs, or brain by carrying a patient through a period of acute need. These techniques have, however, thrown new light on the interrelationship of these crucial organ systems. This has created complex issues for public policy as well.

For medical and legal purposes, partial brain impairment must be distinguished from complete and irreversible loss of brain functions or "whole brain death." The President's Commission, as subsequent chapters explain more fully, regards the cessation of the vital functions of the entire brain—and not merely portions thereof, such as those responsible for cognitive functions—as the only proper neurologic basis for declaring death. This conclusion accords with the overwhelming consensus of medical and legal experts and the public.

Present attention to the "definition" of death is part of a process of development in social attitudes and legal rules stimulated by the unfolding of biomedical knowledge. In the nineteenth century increasing knowledge and practical skill made the public confident that death could be diagnosed reliably using cardiopulmonary criteria. The question now is whether, when medical intervention may be responsible for a patient's respiration and circulation, there are other equally reliable ways to diagnose death....

Euthanasia and the Transition from Life to Death

David J. Mayo and Daniel I. Wikler

David J. Mayo is associate professor of philosophy at the University of Minnesota, Duluth. He is coeditor of *Suicide: The Philosophical Issues* (1980) and the author of "Contemporary Philosophical Literature on Suicide: A Review," and "Confidentiality in Crisis Counseling: A Philosophical Perspective." Daniel I. Wikler is associate professor of philosophy at the University of Wisconsin, Madison. Wikler has also served on the staff of the President's Commission for the Study of Ethical Problems in Medicine and Biomedical and Behavioral Research. His many articles in biomedical ethics include "Paternalism and the Mildly Retarded," "Ought We to Try to Save Aborted Fetuses?" and "The Central Ethical Problem in Human Experimentation and Three Solutions."

Mayo and Wikler begin their discussion by distinguishing four possible states of the human organism. In stage 4, most or all principal life functions have irreversibly ceased functioning. In stage 3, a patient is irreversibly comatose because the *entire brain* has irreversibly ceased functioning, but cardiovascular and pulmonary function is maintained by artificial life-support. In stage 2, a patient is irreversibly comatose because the *cortex* has irreversibly ceased functioning, but brainstem activity is sufficient to sustain continued cardiovascular and pulmonary function. In stage 1, a dying patient is conscious and in pain and desires to be in stage 4. In conjunction with their systematic effort to assess the moral appropriateness of "acquiescing" to transitions to stage 4 from each of the other stages, Mayo and Wikler identify three relevant principles: the Principle of Autonomy, the Principle of Beneficence, and the Preservation of Life Principle. This last principle, however, is introduced only after reasons are given for rejecting a somewhat similar but more radical principle—the Primacy of Life Principle. Mayo and Wikler conclude their expansive discussion by taking issue with contemporary proposals to "redefine death." They insist that death is properly understood only as stage 4; patients in stage 2 and stage 3 are *not* dead.

Reprinted with permission of the authors and the publisher from *Medical Responsibility*, edited by Wade L. Robison and Michael S. Pritchard (Clifton, N.J.: Humana Press, 1979).

In discussions of medical ethics, euthanasia is sometimes referred to as if it involved a single issue. But the problems involved are numerous: Must any attempt to justify euthanasia refer exclusively to the interests of the patient? Must death be requested by the patient? Who has the right to make the decision? Is there a moral difference between killing and letting die?[1] The list goes on. One difficulty facing anyone who is discussing euthanasia generally is that of finding a way to relate all of these questions, particularly since their answers may be interdependent.

The advent of modern life-saving technology has made the situation even more complex. Previously, the issue concerned the propriety of acquiescing to a clear and unmistakable transition from life to death. That transition is no longer so clear, and we must now consider transitions from and to various states. The moral acceptability of any position on euthanasia may vary, depending on whether the transition under consideration involves full consciousness, coma independent of life support systems, coma dependent on life-support systems, or functional decomposition. Since medicine now has the ability to sustain patients in many cases in any of these states, it must develop moral policies which are appropriate to each. Extant views of euthanasia which were conceived with only the transition from the first to the last of these states in mind may fail for lack of specificity. The problem must be addressed anew.

In Part I of this essay, we will give brief descriptions of the four states just mentioned, and we will proceed to examine some aspects of the euthanasia question as they apply to transitions from each of the first three to the fourth. Part II is concerned with the matter of the definition of death itself. The definition of death has been regarded as having significant logical and moral relationships to the question we are considering. By labeling these states neutrally in Part I, we postpone any discussion on this matter until Part II. Since the disposition of a body after death is not considered to be as serious a moral issue in medical ethics as that of euthanasia, the claim that any one of the states we define is death would imply that any transitions to subsequent states were not really matters of major moral importance. We will argue, however, that death is properly construed as the last of these states only, and hence that it is appropriate to regard the acquiescence to any transition to the final state as euthanasia. And we find fault with recent "redefinitions" of death, in part because they seem to be motivated by the mistaken notion that substantive moral issues can be side-stepped by simply clarifying or reinterpreting our concept of "death."

I TRANSITIONS

This section highlights some of the moral considerations which are relevant to assessing the moral desirability of transitions between various states occurring near the end of human life. We begin with rough and ready descriptions of four possible states of a human organism, which are described in terms which do not presuppose an answer to the question, to be explored in Part II, of how death is to be defined.

State 4: Most or all principal life systems—cardiovascular, central-nervous, and pulmonary—have irreversibly ceased functioning.

State 3: The cortex and brain stem have ceased functioning irreversibly; the patient is irreversibly comatose. Metabolic processes in the patient's body continue only because cardiovascular and pulmonary functions are sustained by artificial life-support systems.

State 2: The cortex has permanently ceased functioning, and the patient is irreversibly comatose; but principal life functions continue without artificial support due to brain stem activity.

State 1: The patient is moving quickly and inexorably to subsequent states; however, the patient is conscious and suffering pain, and wishes to be in state 4, rather than in pain.

For patients in any of the first three states, the transition to state 4 is usually more or less imminent, with no significant chance of transition in the direction of regained health. There are three fundamental moral principles which usually bear on the question of whether the inevitable transition to state 4 should always be resisted as long as possible, at whatever cost, or whether there may be circumstances under which one should acquiesce to such a transition:

The Primacy of Life Principle: The preservation of human life is not only valuable, but something the value of which so exceeds any other values we may have that it must never be subordinated to them.

The Principle of Beneficence: A doctor ought to do what is in the best interests of the patient's well-being.

The Principle of Autonomy: Whenever possible, individuals should themselves be the ones to make decisions in matters which involve primarily their own welfare (unless of course their proposed courses of action might infringe on the rights of others).

The fact that each of these principles has an air of plausibility to it, combined with the fact that any two of them may come into conflict, accounts in large measure for the moral difficulty of decisions which confront modern medicine in the treatment of persons in states 1, 2 or 3, and it is to specific consideration of these cases that we now turn.

Patients in State 1

The conflict of principles is straightforward enough in the case of patients in state 1: the Principle of Autonomy supports the view that patients' wishes to acquiesce to the transition to state 4 should be respected. Similarly, the Principle of Beneficence would dictate that patients should be spared unnecessary suffering, and the terminal nature of their condition suggests their suffering may be useless and hence unnecessary. However, the Primacy of Life Principle would dictate that patients' lives must be preserved as long as possible, since the value of life overrides competing values, including the values we place on beneficence and autonomy.

Since the Primacy of Life Principle figures prominently in much popular thinking about these issues, it is worth taking time here to scrutinize this principle carefully. Specifically, we argue against this principle by pointing out that anyone who consistently acted on it would lead an outrageously eccentric and unattractive life. We then deal with the question of what might have seduced anyone in the first place into thinking they should accept a principle, the implications of which are so obviously objectionable.

The Primacy of Life Principle claims that the value of preserving human life is so great that it should never be subordinated to competing values. Reflection suggests that this is a very strong principle, for the force of the word "never" precludes the possibility of compromise, or of weighing life-sustaining considerations against other pressing concerns we may have. In this it differs, for instance, from the much weaker but ultimately more defensible principle that human life has *some* value. Adherence to the Primacy of Life Principle would require that people never do anything which involved risking their lives in any way if they could avoid doing so, however valuable the risk-taking activity might be in other respects. But everyone takes avoidable risks with their lives. Nearly all of us ride in cars and planes and cross streets when we could avoid doing so, and pursue careers in fields in spite of actuarial evidence indicating other vocations would be safer from the point of view of longevity. Many of us live in polluted metropolitan areas, smoke, keep ourselves in less than peak physical shape, and indulge in cuisine proscribed by considerations of taste as well as by considerations of diet. Some people even seek out risks by mountain climbing, sky diving, motorcycling or space exploration. Nor is such behavior universally regarded as irrational; while different people draw the line between courage and foolhardiness at different points, most of us tend to admire certain persons precisely because they do take such risks. Conversely, people who consistently opted only for behavior which involved no avoidable risk to life would be viewed as terribly odd, and rightly so, for they would lead very dull and eccentric lives. Such persons would have to forgo not only aspiration to high public office, but even passionate, emotional involvements with other human beings, since both increase the risk of being murdered. And any woman who accepted the principle with respect to her own life or even all existing lives would have to forgo childbearing.

We believe these considerations show the Primacy of Life Principle is unacceptable. But if this is so, the question arises of how sensible people could ever have come to espouse it? The most obvious answer is that usually we place a very high value on preserving lives, and in the absence of critical scrutiny this *high* value might mistakenly be thought to be an *absolute* one. Some, doubtless, have accepted it on religious grounds. Religious dispute is well beyond the scope of this essay, but it is perhaps relevant to note that many contemporary Western religious authorities in fact endorse acquiescence to death under certain circumstances, and hence do not accept the Primacy of Life Principle. Anyone who did endorse the Primacy of Life Principle on religious grounds, it seems, would also be obliged to lead the very bizarre risk-free life we have sketched previously in our critique of the principle.

A somewhat subtler argument is sometimes given for the Primacy of Life Principle: people value many things, including being alive. But since people must be alive before they can pursue any of their other values, and before they can experience any of the experiences they value, the value on life assumes a special significance. Pursuing the value one places on being alive is a prerequisite for pursuing any other values one may hold. This tempting argument seems to yield the Primacy of Life Principle, which in effect holds that preserving life is to be valued above all other things. But this argument embodies two confusions: the first identifies valuing something with valuing the experience of that something. This mistaken identification may go undetected because *many* of the things we value *are* experiences. But this is not always the case. People may have values which can be satisfied without their experiencing these values being satisfied, and, indeed, which can be satisfied only without their lives being preserved; the most obvious case of this sort may be the value terminally ill patients in state 1 place on the end of their suffering. (Others would be the value people place on having their estates distributed as they wished after their death, or of being fondly remembered, or of being buried in such-and-such a place.)

The second confusion identifies the requirement that one be alive at one time in order to experience something one values experiencing, with a requirement that one be alive as long as possible afterwards. Even though one may value some kind of experience, it does not follow that that value could not lead the person to act in a way which would ultimately speed death. There would be no logical blunder, nor indeed even any irrationality, in people placing such a high value on the cultural advantages of a big city that they opt to live in cities, even though they realized that they would probably die a few years earlier because of their accompanying tensions and pollution.

The Primacy of Life Principle must be rejected as too strong, and it is clear that some weaker principle must be substituted. Even though we do not place an *uncompromisable* value on preserving human life, we still place a *very high* value on doing so as a rule. A reasonable alternative to the Primacy of Life Principle is this weaker, but more realistic one:

The Preservation of Life Principle: Unless there are overriding considerations to the contrary, human life should be preserved whenever possible.

We suggest there are such considerations in the medical context. The first has to do with the fact that while human life is generally of value, some lives are of greater value than others, and just how valuable a particular life may be depends on a number of things. That different lives are of different values *to others,* or

to society at large, is evidenced by some of the considerations that go into triage policies. That different lives are of different value to the persons whose lives they are, is evidenced by the fact that some persons wish their lives would end as soon as possible. Thus lives of unmitigated suffering which are the lot of persons in state 1 are reasonably held to be of less value than healthy lives. That some such persons wish to die because of the pain and hopelessness of their situation certainly shows that their lives are held *by them* to have negative value *for them,* all things considered.

We feel this consideration significantly strengthens the case in favor of acquiescing to the transition from state 1 to state 4, particularly in light of the relatively high value we place on treating others beneficently and on respecting personal autonomy. In our view, these considerations add up to a strong *prima facie* case in favor of respecting the wishes of an individual to acquiesce to the transition from state 1 to state 4, in many cases.

However, this is only a *prima facie* case, for in certain situations, the relevance of beneficence and respect for autonomy may not be so straightforward. For instance, imagine persons whose conditions are terminal and who are suffering greatly at the moment, but for whom the best prognosis is that they will have some relatively pain-free months ahead before they finally succumb. Here, one may feel the Principle of Beneficence requires that such persons be kept alive through the passing period of pain, and even in spite of their present pleas for the release death would bring. A more general doubt may be raised about the relevance of the Principle of Autonomy. All but the most ardent libertarians, for instance, concede that a person's autonomy should not be absolute, and that if people are "not in control of themselves"—whether from fear, anger, depression, pain or some other form of stress—it may be right to intervene to prevent them from doing significant and irreparable harm to themselves. Of course, persons who are in pain and who are told their condition is terminal may very well "lose control" in this sense—or else be so drugged as to be unable to appraise their situation realistically or reasonably. In such cases, the Principle of Autonomy hardly requires that we respect their stated wishes. Indeed, their stated wishes may even fluctuate wildly from one moment to the next.

The seriousness of this problem should not be underestimated; virtually all serious euthanasia legislation has been sensitive to it. Legislation considered in Great Britain involved a provision whereby persons in state 1 who requested active euthanasia would be given a "cooling off" period during which they could reconsider their request before being killed. The Euthanasia Educational Council's "Living Will" is a document which they urge people to consider and discuss with those who will be involved in decision-making, *prior* to finding themselves in the grips of a terminal illness.

On the basis of such considerations, some have argued that the wishes of a person in state 1 should *never* be respected. It is the feeling of the present authors, however, that no such simplistic conclusion is legitimate. Rather, we believe the conclusion to be drawn is that these matters must be considered on a case-by-case basis, in light of the three principles that we have been discussing, along with any others which may apply in particular cases—for instance, those which may involve rights or special interests of other parties. It is our suspicion that in many cases the difficulties cited above are not sufficient to warrant paternalistic intervention, and that to some extent wholesale resistance to respecting the wishes of patients in such situations stems more from an uncritical commitment to the Primacy of Life Principle than it does from any legitimate appeal to considerations which would justify overriding beneficence and the autonomy of the individual.[2]

The conclusion which emerges regarding persons in state 1 is that there is no general reason why all should be denied the transition they wish for to state 4, and that in cases where their wishes are denied, the burden of proof should be on those who feel such paternalistic intervention is warranted. Viewed in this light, the problem of persons in state 1 comes to be seen as a special case of the problem of determining the conditions under which it is proper to intervene paternalistically at the expense of someone else's autonomy. A more general point also emerges, however, and that is that any simple principle which would stipulate a standard handling of all cases is highly suspect, for the considerations which are relevant to such cases are moral considerations, the proper weighing of which depends upon the specifics of individual cases.

Patients in State 2

State 2 is the state in which the cessation of cortex function results in irreversible coma, but life functions

continue without the aid of artificial support due to brain stem activity. What considerations are relevant in this case to the morality of acquiescing to a transition to state 4?

It seems clear enough that here the Principle of Beneficence is irrelevant. The comatose experience no pleasure or pain, and hence the question of what is conducive to their well-being is moot; in an important sense, such individuals really have no "well-being."

The relevance of the Principle of Autonomy may at first seem likewise negated. In a very straightforward sense, persons in state 2 have and will continue to have no decision-making capacity, and to that extent they lack autonomy. (This is surely one consideration behind the frequently made claim that such individuals are no longer "persons.") Thus on first blush it seems that neither acquiescing nor refusing to acquiesce to the death of such patients could constitute a violation of their autonomy.

By the same token, irreversible coma may well be the most straightforward case of a special circumstance which absolves us from the general obligation imposed by the Preservation of Life Principle, since the factors which normally prompt us to attribute value to human life are completely absent. Surely, it would be wrong to claim that a person's continued existence in state 2 has value from *that person's* point of view; in fact, it seems difficult to make sense of the claim that that person even continues to embody a "point of view." At the very least, the obligation imposed by the Preservation of Life Principle seems drastically weakened.

Within the Hippocratic tradition, it is generally held that peoples' medical care should be dictated by considerations having to do with their well-being, the value their life has for them, their wishes and their autonomy. If, however, all of these considerations become moot at the onset of irreversible coma, medicine then seems justified in departing from the traditional Hippocratic orientation which focuses on these patient-oriented considerations, and in turning instead to considerations having to do with the welfare or well-being of others. While one can imagine circumstances in which the continued maintenance of a person in state 2 is most desirable from the point of view of the welfare of others, this surely is not the standard case. Normally there are various stiff costs involved in maintaining individuals in state 2, as well as important benefits which are lost. The most obvious are the actual costs of the medical care. Next may be the "emotional costs" to relatives. Then come the indirect "costs" or loss of benefits which others might have received if scarce medical resources had been used on them instead of being tied up in the maintenance of "hopelessly" comatose patients. The final indirect cost—and surely an underlying consideration behind certain proposed redefinitions of death—is the cost in lives which could have been saved if organs of individuals in state 2 had been available for transplant. With the advent of transplant technology, parts of the comatose individuals themselves come to be regarded as "scarce medical resources" just as legitimately as the hospital beds and medical attention which are required to sustain them in state 2.

In our view, these considerations add up to an impressive case in favor of acquiescing to a transition from state 2 to state 4, unless there are special considerations to the contrary. Unfortunately, however, the matter is not quite this simple. Considerable philosophical complexity is injected into the above analysis, by the fact noted previously, that a person's interests may post-date that person's being interested in them, and even that person's death. Persons may have interests in events, and indeed are routinely granted decision-making autonomy over matters, which they themselves will never experience, because these events occur after their deaths. The most obvious example of this is found in the institution of wills. It is generally recognized the people are entitled to stipulate what is to be done with their property following their death, and that these stipulations will be respected. Similarly, organs to be used for transplant purposes must be donated, not just in the trivial sense that they were previously part of some other body, but in the stronger sense that someone—ideally the person they previously belonged to—must agree to their use by another.

This difficulty is compounded by the fact the survivors frequently invoke not only the expressed wishes of deceased persons in these matters, but also hypothetical wishes. Thus the claim that someone would have wanted his or her organs made available for transplant (had he or she gotten around to considering the matter) might well figure in the proxy decision by a relative to authorize the harvesting of organs and transplant.

There are a number of philosophical complexities surrounding the issue of posthumous interests. Is our respect for wills to be justified in terms of autonomy and posthumous interests, as we suggest above, or is it rather to be justified in terms of the comfort and security the living find in the belief that their wills will in turn be respected? Does the Principle of Autonomy really have any bearing on what becomes of one's kidneys, once one is dead? It is obviously not an issue which bears on the *life* of the deceased person. At what point do appeals to what a dead person wanted, or would have wanted, rely on sentimentality rather than on legitimate respect for the dead person's autonomy? These are all difficult issues, which have received little attention in the literature, and they will not be resolved here. Suffice to say at this point that in any event, unless we are particularly wealthy or particularly sentimental, most of us place some limits on the extent to which we feel the lives of the living are determined by the wishes of the dead, and we do so for the very sound reason that what we do is of no consequence to the dead, in the sense that it does not alter their experience in any way. Because the irreversibly comatose (even if they are alive) at least resemble the dead in this respect, it seems appropriate, in determining whether to acquiesce to the transition to state 4 of a patient in state 2, to at least weigh alongside any actual or hypothetical interest of the comatose patient those considerations having to do with the interests and welfare of others which were mentioned earlier.

As this is done in individual cases, the outcome may be far from clear. At one extreme, it would seem completely unreasonable to sustain a patient in state 2 who had never considered the possibility of being in that condition, if by doing so severe financial hardship were imposed on the family, and scarce medical resources were tied up which otherwise might make an important difference for other patients. At the other extreme, it might seem quite reasonable to sustain in state 2 a patient who had expressed a clear desire to be maintained in the event of having become irreversibly comatose, if the family had sufficient funds, and if doing so did not require scarce medical resources which would be readily available for others if they were not being used in maintaining the comatose patient. Although the vast majority of actual cases doubtless lie closer to the former of these cases than to the latter, difficult intermediate cases exist, and that is in part responsible for the fact that present medical practice is by no means consistent in handling cases of this type. Perhaps philosophical analysis might clear away some of the present confusion, with the result that increasing numbers of persons will clearly assert their own wishes in the matter—hopefully in the direction of acquiescing, in light of the stiff social costs which others must bear if a person is to be maintained in state 2.

Patients in State 3

The state of these patients differs from state 2 in that these patients have suffered irreversible loss of function of the entire brain, with the result that they are not only irreversibly comatose, but in addition they require artificial life-support systems to be maintained. Virtually all of the considerations relevant to the previous case derived from the fact that the patients were in irreversible coma, and hence apply to patients in state 3 as well. The only additional consideration which is relevant to patients in state 3 is that such persons require more in the way of scarce medical resources— the artificial life-support systems and the supervision required for their operation—and this, of course, becomes an additional reason for acquiescing to the transition to state 4. Even here, however, this does not strike us as absolutely decisive; there still remains the possibility that the various social costs might be small or could be easily met, and also that the patient might have expressed vigorous interest in being sustained in the event of irreversible coma. We feel that such cases would be rare, however, and that in the absence of such special circumstances, it would be morally desirable to acquiesce to the transition to state 4.

Mention should be given to a final consideration in favor of maintaining patients in either stages 2 or 3, which is quite different from any of the previous ones. When organs are transplanted, there is frequently some lapse of time between the time a person is selected as a suitable donor, and the time the donated organ is harvested for transplant. During this time, the individual is maintained in state 2 or 3, not for any of the reasons mentioned above, but simply in order to maintain the organ so it will be suitable when it is time to transplant. Of course, the need to preserve an organ for transplant would justify maintaining a patient for the brief period of time in question. However, it is important to note that in this case, the decision to "maintain" a patient in state 2 or 3 until the organ is needed for transplant already presupposes a decision to acquiesce to the transition to state 4 at the moment

when the organ finally is needed, so this is a case of a "decision to maintain" only in the most trivial sense.

II   THE REDEFINITION OF DEATH

Throughout the previous discussion we have spoken in the clumsy idiom of "transitions betweens states" in order to avoid prejudging the question of which state(s) constitute death. It is to this question which we now must turn. To begin, it should be noted that the above discussion would not have strained common sense if it had been conducted in the language of euthanasia. Bearing in mind the literal meaning of the term "euthanasia"—"good death"—the discussion would then have been presented as dealing with the circumstances under which the transition from life to death would be a good thing rather than a bad one, and hence of the circumstances under which moral agents might acquiesce to death.

That issue, of course, is not an academic one. At this moment, there are in this country alone literally thousands of persons in state 3, as well as some in state 2, and thousand more—friends, relatives, and medical staff—who are presently agonizing over the questions of when these patients will undergo the transition to state 4, and what role, if any, they should play in speeding or delaying that transition. Some of these people (the medical staff) will continue to charge substantial fees for their services until that transition is complete, while others (the friends, relatives, and insurance companies) will doubtless pay those bills, firm in the belief that they are making payment for services rendered to someone who was dying. This belief is obviously shared by the medical staff, who do not as a rule knowingly minister and devote their closest attentions to the dead.

Dying is a process engaged in by the living. Death marks the end of the dying process, not the beginning or middle of it. Just as it is clear to all that someone in state 4 is dead, so it is clear to the vast majority of us that persons who are in states 2 and 3 are dying, and hence not yet dead. The transitions to state 4 from 2 and 3 constitute dying just as clearly as the transition to state 4 from state 1. Although different moral considerations are relevant to acquiescing to death depending on whether the patient is in state 1, or 2 or 3, it seems indisputable that the considerations which are relevant are moral ones in the latter cases just as clearly as in the first. In fact, while in practice it may be psychologically less trying to opt for death in the case of the irreversibly comatose than in the case of the terminal patient who is suffering and wants to die, the case of the comatose is perhaps the more difficult in theory, precisely because it involves the extremely subtle and difficult issues of the limits of a person's autonomy, as well as the shift from the Hippocratic mode of decision-making focusing on patient-related considerations, to a perspective which includes appeals to the welfare of others as well.

Nevertheless, there are those who insist that we are simply wasting our moral energy if we construe the problem of continued treatment of comatose patients as a moral issue. Their view is that it is not really a moral issue at all, but rather a conceptual or scientific one, having to do with the definition of death. If this view is sound, it is certainly of central significance, for it promises a way out of moral choices which are difficult by almost anyone's reckoning. It is to an examination of this strategy, then, that we must now turn our attention.

Several different definitions of death have recently been proposed, calculated to pluck us from the grips of a difficult moral decision to acquiesce to death, by the easy mechanism of redefinition of death. Although the so-called "Harvard definition" of death is only one such definition, it is the one which has presently received the widest attention and acceptance. Accordingly, it will be our central focus here, although one other redefinition of death which has similar objectives will be mentioned in passing.

The substance of the Harvard proposal is well known.[3] The report spells out tests designed to tell whether the patient's cortex and brain stem have irreversibly ceased to function; the tests range from reflex-tests to examination by EEG. It is an empirical claim that a patient who meets these criteria is in fact in state 3 and irreversibly comatose, and medical scientists are obviously qualified to make such a claim if anyone is.

The crux of the Harvard proposal is that persons who meet these conditions should be considered (and pronounced) dead.[4] Thus, for those who accept the proposal, the question of acquiescing to the death of a comatose patient in state 3 is not *answered*, but rather *dismissed* as a logically mistaken question, with no need for any moral deliberation at all. According to the proposal, there really is no question here of "acquiescing to the death" of such patients, for one can only acquiesce to the death of someone who is living, and to accept the Harvard proposal is to accept the claim that patients in state 3 are already dead—and hence, presumably, that they are *not* dying. What has previously struck doctors, concerned relatives, and moral philosophers as a grim and weighty moral issue is in effect made to vanish.

We believe, however, that this is only conceptual sleight of hand, which obscures the inevitable moral component of the problem of the continued maintenance of the irreversibly comatose. The most that can be claimed in the name of cold, hard science is that certain conditions inevitably indicate irreversible coma and loss of brain function. The additional step of claiming that patients in state 3 are dead (and hence of course can be treated as dead people) is surely not cold, hard fact at all. It seems, rather, to be a claim which grows out of conceptual confusion, and which appears plausible only because it seduces with a promise of deliverance from the clutches of difficult moral decisions.

The conceptual confusion implicit in the Harvard proposal grows out of confusing value judgments with biological ones. It is enormously plausible to suggest that one of the conditions for a human life *having value* is the possibility of consciousness. But, while the possibility of consciousness seems quite clearly to be a condition of human life *having value,* that is not to say that it is a condition of a human being *having life.*

This might be illustrated by a somewhat facetious analogy. Imagine oil shortages reaching the point where neither heating oil nor synthetics for clothing are available, as a result of which we turn again to animal furs for clothing. Suppose further that rabbits come to be especially valued both because of their warm fur and because of their legendary breeding habits. If, for some reason, a rabbit should have the misfortune of being both bald and sterile, he would *not* be a valuable rabbit. But that is of course not to say that he would be a dead rabbit. In the case of both rabbits and persons, a creature having life is one matter, and that life having value is quite another. "Death" is not a value notion, but a biological notion, to be made sense of in terms of the absence of life, not in terms of the absence of value.

A similar confusion has prompted even more radical proposals for redefining death. While the Harvard proposal focuses on state 3, Robert Veatch[5] notes that state 2 is also an identifiable state: a person may suffer irreversible coma (through the death of the neo-cortex of the brain) even though lower brain stem activity makes spontaneous breathing and heartbeat possible. Such people are not in state 3 and do not meet the Harvard criteria for death, but Veatch argues that this is a defect of the Harvard proposal. The rationale Veatch provides for this is as follows: first, that death is the "irreversible loss of that which is essentially significant to the nature of man," and second, that what is essentially significant to the nature of man is the capacity for experience and social interaction. When these are lost, Veatch argues the person should be regarded as dead. An integral part of Veatch's position is the identification of what is essential to being human, with what is essential to a human being being alive. But of course this too is a confusion, for those are two very different things. Humans are only one kind of living thing: what is essential to being human is something that *differentiates* us from other living things, something which we *do not* share with dogs or trees or mosquitoes. Being alive, on the other hand, is something we *do* share with other living things. To extend our rabbit analogy, suppose we singled out as particularly valuable those rabbits which were especially fertile and whose offspring were particularly furry, and labeled them "schmabbits." Then, a rabbit who first made the status of schmabbit and then became sterile would no longer manifest what was "essentially significant to the nature of schmabbits"—that is, it would not longer be a schmabbit. But that, again, does not mean that it would properly be considered a dead schmabbit, much less that it would be dead *simpliciter.*

More generally, the death of a rabbit, a schmabbit, or of a human being has nothing to do with the loss of those characteristics which differentiate each of them from other kinds of living things, but rather with loss of what they have in common with other living things. Biologists have a concept of life, or of when an organism is alive, that does not appeal to what is unique to some particular living species, but which appeals instead to features common to all living things. It is only because biology has some notion of what life is, apart from the specifics of any species, that it was possible to ask meaningfully "Is there life on Mars, and if so, what is it like?" Being alive is something we have in common with our pets and the lawns and trees in front of our houses; we are all living things. The proper place to

turn for a definition of death is not to the kinds of considerations which make this or that life valuable, or which make it different from other forms of life, but rather to the kinds of general biological considerations which justify saying that something is alive.

An adequate definition of life is beyond the scope of this essay, but a few preliminary remarks may be in order. Since life is a process, or rather a structured group of processes, an adequate definition of life will presumably be in terms of the occurrence of life processes, and the definition of death will then be in terms of the cessation of these processes. The matter is not simple, for these processes go on at different levels, and, of course, do not stop all at once. Specifically, being alive cannot mean that all parts are functioning normally (they don't in a deaf, sterile or blind person), or that no parts are machine- or drug-dependent (the diabetic and pacemaker patients are alive). When a biologist says an organism is dead, he or she surely means something like "principal life systems have irreversibly ceased to function." Of course, this raises a series of difficult issues, including the questions of which life systems are the principal ones, how many of them have shut down, and how completely. No biological sophistication is required to realize that they may shut down by degrees—this strikes us as obvious in the case of large plants such as trees, because the processes shut down over long periods of time. Unfortunately, for many purposes we need—or at least presently feel we need—to be be able to speak of the "moment of death," and if modern medicine continues to refine its techniques for prolonging the process of dying, it is possible that our present notion of death will prove to be inadequate. Our thesis is not that a redefinition of death will never be needed. Our only concern is to argue that when and if such a time arrives, two very different questions must be kept distinct. The question of when the life of an organism has ended is a conceptual question—one focusing on the central concept in biology—and it obviously must be answered in terms of our biological concepts and theory, for that theory embodies our understanding of what life *is.*

The question of when an organism's life *ought* to be terminated, on the other hand, is not a scientific question, nor a conceptual one, but a moral one. Unless these are seen to be very different questions, decisions about whether or not to acquiesce to a person's death— tough and important moral decisions which deserve all the honesty and precision our moral thinking can give them—will come to be regarded as "purely medical judgments," or "purely scientific" judgments, and moral debate and argument will be dismissed as irrelevant to them.

In the course of the Harvard proposal, it is urged that once it has been established that the patient is in an irreversible coma, the patient should be pronounced dead, and then the respirator turned off. It goes on to say:

> The decision to do this and the responsibility for it are to be taken by the physician-in-charge, in consultation with one or more physicians who have been directly involved in the case. It is unsound and undesirable to force the family to make the decision.[6]

While this eagerness to exclude non-professionals spares relatives from having to make a morally difficult decision, it also denies them their rightful role in such decision-making. But even more troubling is the fact that the Harvard proposal would spare even the doctors the realization that they are in fact deciding that someone should die. Some such decisions are correct ones we believe, but all ought to be faced honestly for what they are—decisions to end someone's life.

NOTES

1 The killing/letting die distinction is a very difficult issue, one which we wish to avoid here. In order to keep our language neutral with respect to this issue, we will speak about the moral desirability of "acquiescing" to certain transitions from one state to another, and thereby leave open for further discussion the question of whether the moral acceptability of "acquiescing" might depend on whether, in a particular case, it was a matter of accelerating the transition, or of merely not acting to decelerate it.

2 The medical context generates some curious paradoxes with respect to our usual thinking about autonomy. Many of our decisions in life—whom to marry, whether to go mountain climbing—are made on impulse, even in confusion. They may have irreversible consequences. But no one makes us prove that we are in a rational frame of mind before we are allowed to act in these matters. Similarly, sick persons may decide not to see doctors, and that, too, is their privilege. Once the patient is in the doctor's care, however, the requirements for free action are made more stringent. Patients must show that they are rational before their wish to die is respected—and it may not be respected even then. The patient, who may be suffering from cancer or other physical disease, is treated as a psychiatric patient. We do not want to claim that obviously confused or irrationally depressed patients should be allowed to order their own deaths. The issue is much subtler, and our own intuitions are mixed. Yet, we wish to point out the inconsistency: perhaps physicians' fealty to the principle that they must do all they can for their patients should not lead them to forget that this principle merely sets the limit on what may be asked of them by their patients. If the patients' autonomy is strictly respected, perhaps they must be free to ask for less.

3 Ad Hoc Committee of the Harvard Medical School to Examine the Definition of Brain Death, "A Definition of Irreversible Coma," *J.A.M.A.* 205, No. 6, pp. 337–340, 1968.

4 It is not entirely clear whether the Ad Hoc Committee proposed its tests as new tests for the same condition tested for by previous criteria, or whether a new condition was being defined; we will assume the latter here.

5 Robert M. Veatch, "The Whole-Brain-Oriented Concept of Death: An Outmoded Philosophical Formulation," *J. Thanat.* 3, pp. 13–30, No. 1 for 1975.

6 Ad Hoc Committee, *op. cit,* p. 338.

The Definition and Criterion of Death

Charles M. Culver and Bernard Gert

Charles M. Culver is professor of psychiatry, Dartmouth Medical School, and adjunct professor of philosophy, Dartmouth College. Bernard Gert is Stone Professor of Intellectual and Moral Philosophy, Dartmouth College, and adjunct professor of psychiatry, Dartmouth Medical School. Frequent collaborators, Culver and Gert are the coauthors of *Philosophy in Medicine: Conceptual and Ethical Issues in Medicine and Psychiatry* (1982) and of such articles as the "The Justification of Paternalism" and "The Morality of Involuntary Hospitalization." Very prominent among Gert's other philosophical works is *The Moral Rules* (1970).

Culver and Gert consider it essential to distinguish among the *definition* of death, the *criterion* of death, and the *tests* of death. In discussing the definition of death, they begin by giving reasons why death must be considered an event rather than a process. They define death as the permanent cessation of functioning of the *organism as a whole*, and they argue against a competing definition according to which the permanent loss of consciousness and cognition is sufficient for death. In their view, patients who are in a chronic vegetative state are alive but are no longer persons, and it is morally justifiable to allow them to die by discontinuing even "ordinary and routine care." With regard to the *criterion* of death, Culver and Gert maintain that the correct criterion is the permanent loss of functioning of the entire brain, *not* the permanent loss of cardiopulmonary function. They conclude with a brief discussion of the appropriate *tests* of death.

Much of the confusion arising from the current brain death controversy is due to the failure to distinguish three distinct elements: (1) the definition of death; (2) the medical criterion for determining that death has occurred; and (3) the tests to prove that the criterion has been satisfied. We shall first define death in a way which makes its ordinary meaning explicit, then provide a criterion of death which fulfills this definition, and finally, indicate which tests have demonstrated perfect validity in determining that the criterion of death is satisfied.[1]

The definitions of death which appear in legal dictionaries and the new statutory definitions of death do not say what the layman actually means by death but merely set out the criteria by which physicians legally determine when death has occurred. *Death*, however, is not a technical term but a common term in everyday use. We believe that a proper understanding of the ordinary meaning of this word or concept must be developed before a medical criterion is chosen. We

must decide what is ordinarily meant by death before physicians can decide how to measure it.

Agreement on the definition and criterion of death is literally a life-and-death matter. Whether a spontaneously breathing patient in a chronic vegetative state is classified as dead or alive depends on our understanding of the definition of death. Even given the definition, the status of a patient with a totally and permanently nonfunctioning brain who is being maintained on a ventilator depends on the criterion of death employed. Defining death is primarily a philosophical task; providing the criterion of death is primarily medical; and choosing the tests to prove that the criterion is satisfied is solely a medical matter.

THE DEFINITION OF DEATH

Death as a Process or an Event

It has been claimed that death is a process rather than an event (Morison, 1971). This claim is supported by the fact that a standard series of degenerative and destructive changes occurs in the tissues of an organism, usually following but sometimes preceding the irreversible cessation of spontaneous ventilation and circulation. These changes include: necrosis of brain cells, necrosis of other vital organ cells, cooling, rigor mortis, dependent lividity, and putrefaction. This process actually persists for years, even centuries, until the skeletal remains have disintegrated, and could even be viewed as beginning with the failure of certain organ systems during life. Because these changes occur in a fairly regular and ineluctable fashion, it is claimed that the stipulation of any particular point in this process as the moment of death is arbitrary.

The following argument, however, shows the theoretical inadequacy of any definition which makes death a process. If we regard death as a process, then either (1) the process starts when the person is still living, which confuses the process of death with the process of dying, for we all regard someone who is dying as not yet dead, or (2) the process of death starts when the person is no longer alive, which confuses the process of death with the process of disintegration. Death should be viewed not as a process but as the event that separates the process of dying from the process of disintegration.

On a practical level, regarding death as a process makes it impossible to declare the time of death with any precision. This is not a trivial issue. There are pressing medical, legal, social, and religious reasons to declare the time of death with some precision, including the interpretation of wills, burial times and procedures, mourning times, and decisions regarding the aggressiveness of medical support. There are no countervailing practical or theoretical reasons for regarding death as a process rather than an event in formulating a definition of death. We shall say that death occurs at some definite time, although this time may not always be specifiable with complete precision.

Choices for a Definition of Death

The definition of death must capture our ordinary use of the term, for *death*, as noted earlier, is a word used by everyone and is not primarily a medical or legal term. In this ordinary use, certain facts are assumed, and we shall assume them as well. Therefore we shall not apply our analysis to science fiction speculations, for example, about brains continuing to function independently of the rest of the organism (Gert, 1967,

1971). Thus we shall assume that all and only living organisms can die, that the living can be distinguished from the dead with very good reliability, and that the moment when an organism leaves the former state and enters the latter can be determined with a fairly high degree of precision. We shall regard death as permanent. We know that some people claim to have been dead for several minutes and then to have returned to life, but we regard this as only a dramatic way of saying that consciousness was temporarily lost (for example, because of a brief episode of cardiac arrest).

Although there are religious theories that death involves the soul leaving the body, we know that religious persons and secularists do not disagree in their ordinary application of the term *dead*. We acknowledge that the body can remain physically intact for some time after death and that some isolated parts of the organism may continue to function (for example, it is commonly believed that hair and nails continue to grow after death). We shall now present our definition of death and contrast it to a proposed alternative.

We define death as the permanent cessation of functioning of the organism as a whole. By the organism as a whole, we do not mean the whole organism, that is, the sum of its tissue and organ parts, but rather the highly complex interaction of its organ subsystems. The organism need not be whole or complete—it may have lost a limb or an organ (such as the spleen)—but it still remains an organism.

By the functioning of the organism as a whole, we mean the spontaneous and innate activities of integration of all or most subsystems (for example, neuroendocrine control) and at least limited response to the environment (for example, temperature change). However, it is not necessary that all of the subsystems be integrated. Individual subsystems may be replaced (for example, by pacemakers, ventilators, or pressors) without changing the status of the organism as a whole.

It is possible for individual subsystems to function for a time after the organism as a whole has permanently ceased to function. Spontaneous ventilation ceases either immediately after or just before the permanent cessation of functioning of the organism as a whole, but spontaneous circulation, with artificial ventilation, may persist for up to two weeks after the organism as a whole has ceased to function.

An example of an activity of the organism as a whole is temperature regulation. The control of this complex process is located in the hypothalamus and is important for normal maintenance of all cellular processes. It is lost when the organism as a whole has ceased to function.

Consciousness and cognition are sufficient to show the functioning of the organism as a whole in higher animals, but they are not necessary. Lower organisms never have consciousness and even when a higher organism is comatose, evidence of the functioning of the organism as a whole may still be evident, for example, in temperature regulation.

We believe that the permanent cessation of the functioning of the organism as a whole is what has traditionally been meant by death. This definition retains death as a biological occurrence which is not unique to human beings; the same definition applies to other higher animals. We believe that death is a biological phenomenon and should apply equally to related species. When we talk of the death of a human being, we mean the same thing as we do when we talk of the death of a dog or a cat. This is supported by our ordinary use of the term *death*, and by law and tradition. It is also in accord with social and religious practices and is not likely to be affected by future changes in technology.

An alternative definition of death as the irreversible loss of that which is essentially significant to the nature of man has been proposed by Veatch (1976). Though this definition initially seems very attractive, it does not state what we ordinarily mean when we speak of death. It is not regarded as self-contradictory to say that a person has lost that which is essentially significant to the nature of man, but is still alive. For example, we all acknowledge that permanently comatose patients in chronic vegetative states are sufficiently brain-damaged that they have irreversibly lost all that is essentially significant to the nature of man but we still consider them to be living (for example, Karen Ann Quinlan; see Beresford, 1977).

The patients described by Brierley and associates (1971) are also in this category. These patients had complete neocortical destruction with preservation of the brainstem and diencephalic (posterior brain) structures. They had isoelectric (flat) electroencephalograms (EEGs) (indicating neocortical death) and were permanently comatose, although they had normal spontaneous breathing and brainstem reflexes; they were essentially in a permanent, severe, chronic vegetative state (Jennett and Plum, 1972). They retained many of the vital functions of the organism as a whole, including

neuroendocrine control (that is, homeostatic interrelationships between the brain and various hormonal glands) and spontaneous circulation and breathing.

This alternative definition actually states what it means to cease to be a person rather than what it means for that person to die. *Person* is not a biological concept but rather a concept defined in terms of certain kinds of abilities and qualities of awareness. It is inherently vague. Death is a biological concept. Thus in a literal sense, death can be applied directly only to biological organisms and not to persons. We do not object to the phrase "death of a person," but the phrase in common usage actually means the death of the organism which was the person. For example, one might overhear in the hospital wards, "The person in room 612 died last night." In this common usage, one is referring to the death of the organism which was a person. By our analysis, Veatch (1976) and others have used the phrase "death of a person" metaphorically, applying it to an organism which has ceased to be a person but has not died.

Without question, consciousness and cognition are essential human attributes. If they are lost, life has lost its meaning. A patient in a chronic vegetative state is usually regarded as living in only the most basic biological sense. But it is just this basic biological sense that we want to capture in our definition of death. We must not confuse the death of an organism which was a person with an organism's ceasing to be a person. We are immediately aware of the loss of personhood in these patients and are repulsed by the idea of continuing to treat them as if they were persons. But were we to consider these chronic vegetative patients as actually dead, serious problems would arise. First, a slippery slope condition would be introduced wherein the question could be asked: How much neocortical damage is necessary before we declare a patient dead? Surely patients in a chronic vegetative state, although usually not totally satisfying the tests for neocortical destruction, have permanently lost their consciousness and cognition. Then what about the somewhat less severely brain-damaged patient?

By considering permanent loss of consciousness and cognition as a criterion for ceasing to be a person and not for death of the organism as a whole, the slippery slope phenomenon is put where it belongs: not in the definition of death, but in the determination of possible grounds for nonvoluntary euthanasia, that is, providing possible grounds for killing the organism, or allowing it to die, in those instances in which the organism is no longer a person. The justification of nonvoluntary euthanasia must be kept strictly separate from the definition of death. Most of us would like our organism to die when we cease to be persons, but this should not be accomplished by blurring the distinctions between biological death and the loss of personhood.

When an organism ceases to be a person, that is, when it permanently loses all consciousness and cognition, then practical problems arise. How are we to treat this organism? (1) Should we treat it just as we treat a person, making every effort to keep it alive? (2) Should we cease caring for it, either in part or at all, and allow it to die? (3) Should we kill it?

In our view, an organism that is no longer a person has no claim to be treated as a person. But just as one treats a corpse with respect, even more so would one expect that such a living organism be treated with respect. This does not mean, however, that one should strive to keep the organism alive. No one benefits by doing this; on the contrary, given the care needed to keep such an organism alive, it seems an extravagant waste of both economic and human resources to attempt to do so. On the other hand, it seems unjustified to require anyone to actively kill it. Even though the organism is no longer a person, it still looks like a person, and unless there are overwhelming reasons for killing it, it seems best not to do anything that might weaken the prohibition against killing. This leaves the second alternative, discontinuing all care and allowing the patient to die. This can take either of two forms: discontinuing medical treatment or discontinuing all ordinary and routine care. The latter is the position we favor.

It is important to note that the patient will not suffer from lack of care, for since the patient is no longer a person this means that it has permanently lost all consciousness and cognition. Any patient who retains even the slightest capacity to suffer pain or discomfort of any kind remains a person and must be treated as such. We make this point to emphasize our position that only patients who have completely and permanently lost all consciousness and cognition should have all care discontinued. We believe that discontinuing all care and allowing the patient who is no longer a person to die is the preferred alternative, and the one that should be recommended to the legal guardian or next of kin as the course of action to be followed.

THE CRITERION OF DEATH

We have argued that the correct definition of death is permanent cessation of functioning of the organism as a whole. We will now inspect the two competing criteria of death: (1) the permanent loss of cardiopulmonary functioning and (2) the total and irreversible loss of functioning of the whole brain.

Characteristics of Optimum Criteria and Tests

Given that death is the permanent cessation of functioning of the organism as a whole, a criterion will yield a false-positive if it is satisfied, and yet it would still be possible for that organism to function as a whole. By far the most important requirement for a criterion of death is that it yield no false-positives.

A criterion of death, however, cannot have any exceptions; this is what enables it to serve as a legal definition of death. It is not sufficient that the criterion be correct 99.99 percent of the time. This means that not only can the criterion yield no false-positives, it can also yield no false-negatives. A criterion of death yields a false-negative if it is not satisfied and yet the organism as a whole has irreversibly ceased to function. Of course, one may sometimes determine death without using the criterion, but it can never be that the criterion satisfied and yet the person is not dead, or that the criterion is not satisfied and the person is dead. This is why it is so easy to mistake a criterion for an ordinary definition; it is rather a kind of operational definition, and serves as part of the legal definition, but the real operational definition is provided by the tests which show whether or not the criterion is satisfied.

Permanent Loss of Cardiopulmonary Functioning

Permanent termination of heart and lung function has been used as a criterion of death throughout history. The ancients observed that all other bodily functions ceased shortly after cessation of these vital functions, and the irreversible process of bodily disintegration inevitably followed. Thus permanent loss of spontaneous cardiopulmonary function was found to predict permanent nonfunctioning of the organism as a whole. Further, if there were no permanent loss of spontaneous cardiopulmonary function, then the organism as a whole continued to function. Therefore permanent loss of cardiopulmonary function served as an adequate criterion of death.

Because of current ventilation/circulation technology, permanent loss of spontaneous cardiopulmonary functioning is no longer necessarily predictive of permanent nonfunctioning of the organism as a whole. Consider a conscious, talking patient who is unable to breathe because of suffering from poliomyelitis and who requires an iron lung (thus having permanent loss of spontaneous pulmonary function), who has also developed asystole (loss of spontaneous heartbeat) requiring a permanent pacemaker (thus having permanent loss of spontaneous cardiac function). It would be absurd to regard such a person as dead.

It might be proposed that it is not the permanent loss of *spontaneous* cardiopulmonary function that is the criterion of death, but rather the permanent loss of all cardiopulmonary function, whether spontaneous or artificially supported. But now that ventilation and circulation can be mechanically maintained, an organism with permanent loss of whole brain functioning can have permanently ceased to function as a whole days to weeks before the heart and lungs cease to function with artificial support. Thus this supposed criterion would not be satisfied, yet the person would be dead. The heart and lungs now seem to have no unique relationship to the functioning of the organism as a whole. Continued artificially supported cardiopulmonary function is no longer perfectly correlated with life, and permanent loss of spontaneous cardiopulmonary functioning is no longer perfectly correlated with death.

Total and Irreversible Loss of Whole Brain Functioning

The criterion for the cessation of functioning of the organism as a whole is the permanent loss of functioning of the entire brain. This criterion is perfectly correlated with the permanent cessation of functioning of the organism as a whole because it is the brain that is necessary for the functioning of the organism as a whole. It integrates, generates, interrelates, and controls complex bodily activities. A patient on a ventilator with a totally destroyed brain is merely a preparation of artificially maintained subsystems since the organism as a whole has ceased to function.

The brain generates the signal for breathing through brainstem ventilatory centers and aids in the control of circulation through brainstem blood pressure control centers. Destruction of the brain produces apnea

(inability to breath) and generalized vasodilatation (opening of the peripheral blood vessels); in all cases, despite the most aggressive support, the adult heart stops within a week and that of the child within two weeks (Ingvar et al., 1978). Thus when the organism as a whole has ceased to function, the artificially supported vital subsystems quickly fail. Many other functions of the organism as a whole, including neuroendocrine control, temperature control, food-searching behaviors, and sexual activity, reside in the more primitive regions (hypothalamus, brainstem) of the brain. Thus total and irreversible loss of functioning of the whole brain and not merely the neocortex is required as the criterion for the permanent loss of the functioning of the organism as a whole.

Using permanent loss of functioning of the whole brain as the criterion for death of the organism as a whole is also consistent with tradition. Throughout history, whenever a physician was called to ascertain the occurrence of death, his examination included the following important signs indicative of permanent loss of functioning of the whole brain: unresponsivity, lack of spontaneous movements including breathing; and absence of pupillary light response. Only one important sign, lack of heartbeat, was not directly indicative of whole brain destruction. But since the heartbeat stops within several minutes of apnea, permanent absence of the vital signs is an important sign of permanent loss of whole brain functioning. Thus, in an important sense, permanent loss of whole brain functioning has always been the underlying criterion of death.

THE TESTS OF DEATH

Given the definition of death as the permanent cessation of functioning of the organism as a whole, and the criterion of death as the total and irreversible cessation of functioning of the whole brain, the next step is the examination of the available tests of death. The tests must be such that they will never yield a false-positive result. Of secondary importance, they should produce few and relatively brief false-negatives.

Cessation of Heartbeat and Ventilation

The physical findings of permanent absence of heartbeat and respiration are the traditional tests of death. In the vast majority of deaths not complicated by artificial ventilation, these classic tests are still applicable. They show that the criterion of death has been satisfied since they always quickly produce permanent loss of functioning of the whole brain. However, when mechanical ventilation is being used, these tests lose most of their utility due to the production of numerous false-negatives for as long a time as one to two weeks, that is, death of the organism as a whole with still intact circulatory-ventilatory subsystems. Thus though the circulation-ventilation tests will suffice in most instances of death, if there is artificial maintenance of circulation or ventilation the special tests for permanent cessation of whole brain functioning will be needed.

Irreversible Cessation of Whole Brain Functioning

Numerous formalized sets of tests have been established to determine that the criterion of permanent loss of whole brain functioning has been met. These include, among others, tests described by the Harvard Medical School Ad Hoc Committee (Beecher, 1968) and the National Institutes of Health Collaborative Study of Cerebral Survival (1977). They have all been recently reviewed (Black, 1978; Molinari, 1978). What we call tests have sometimes been called "criteria," but it is important to distinguish these second-level criteria from the first-level criteria. While the first-level criteria must be for the death of the organism and must be understandable by the layman, the second-level criteria (tests) determine the permanent loss of functioning of the whole brain and need not be understandable by anyone except qualified clinicians. To avoid confusion, we prefer to use the designation "tests" for the second-level criteria.

All the proposed tests require total and permanent absence of all functioning of the brainstem and both hemispheres. They vary slightly from one set to another, but all require unresponsivity (deep coma), absent pupillary light reflexes, apnea (inability to breathe), and absent brainstem relfexes. They also require the absence of drug intoxication and low body temperature, and the newer sets require the demonstration that a lesion of the brain exists. Isoelectric (flat) EEGs are generally required, and tests disclosing the absence of cerebral blood flow are of confirmatory value (NIH Collaborative Study, 1977). All tests require the given loss of function to be present for a particular time interval, which in the case of the absence of cerebral blood flow may be as short as thirty minutes.

Current tests of irreversible loss of whole brain function may produce many false-negatives of a sort during the thirty-minute to twenty-four-hour interval between the successive neurologic examinations which the tests require. Certain sets of tests, particularly those requiring electrocerebral silence by EEG, may produce false-negatives if an EEG artifact is present and cannot confidently be distinguished from brain wave activity. Generally, a few brief false-negatives are tolerable and even inevitable, since tests must be delineated conservatively in order to eliminate any possibility of false-positives.

There are many studies which show perfect correlation between the loss of whole brain function tests of the Ad Hoc Committee of the Harvard Medical School and total brain necrosis at postmortem examination. Veith et al. (1977a) conclude that "the validity of the criteria [tests] must be considered to be established with as much certainty as is possible in biology or medicine" (p. 1652). Thus, when a physician ascertains that a patient satisfies the validated loss of whole brain function tests, he can be confident that the loss of whole brain functioning is permanent. Physicians should apply only tests which have been completely validated....

NOTE

1 This chapter is adapted in part from Bernat, Culver, and Gert (1981).

REFERENCES

American Bar Association. House of Delegates redefines death, urges redefinition of rape, and undoes the Houston amendments. *American Bar Association Journal*, 1975, *61*, 463–464.

Beecher, Henry K. A definition of irreversible coma: report of the Ad Hoc Committee of the Harvard Medical School to examine the definition of brain death. *Journal of the American Medical Association*, 1968, *205*, 337–340.

Beresford, H. Richard. The Quinlan decision: problems and legislative alternatives. *Annals of Neurology*, 1977, *2,* 74–81.

Bernat, James L., Culver, Charles M., and Gert, Bernard. On the definition and criterion of death. *Annals of Internal Medicine*, 1981, *94*, 389–394.

Black, Peter M. Brain death. *New England Journal of Medicine*, 1978, *299*, 338–344, 393–401.

Brierley, J.B., Adams, J.H., Graham, D.I., and Simpson, J.A. Neocortical death after cardiac arrest. *Lancet*, 1971, *2*, 560–565.

Capron, Alexander M., and Kass, Leon R. A statutory definition of the standards for determining human death: an appraisal and a proposal. *University of Pennsylvania Law Review*, 1972, *121*, 87–118.

Gert, Bernard. Can the brain have a pain? *Philosophy and Phenomenological Research*, 1967, *27*, 432–436.

Gert, Bernard. Personal identity and the body. *Dialogue*, 1971, *10*, 458–478.

Hastings Center Task Force on Death and Dying. Refinements in criteria for the determination of death: an appraisal. *Journal of the American Medical Association*, 1972, *221*, 48–53.

Ingvar, David H., Brun, Arne, Johansson, Lars, and Sammuelsson, Sven M. Survival after severe cerebral anoxia with destruction of the cerebral cortex: the apallic syndrome. *Annals of the New York Academy of Science*, 1978, *315*, 184–214.

Jennett, B., and Plum, F. Persistent vegetative state after brain damage. A syndrome in search of a name. *Lancet*, 1972, *1*, 734–737.

Jonas, Hans. *Philosophical Essays: From Ancient Creed to Technological Man*. Englewood Cliffs, N.J.: Prentice-Hall, 1974, pp. 134–140.

Law Reform Commission of Canada. *Criteria for the Determination of Death*. Ottawa: Law Reform Commission of Canada, 1979.

Molinari, Gaetano F. Review of clinical criteria of brain death. *Annals of the New York Academy of Science*, 1978, *315*, 62–69.

Morison, Robert S. Death: process or event? *Science* 1971, *173*, 694–698.

NIH Collaborative Study of Cerebral Survival. An appraisal of the criteria of cerebral death: a summary statement. *Journal of the American Medical Association*, 1977, *237*, 982–986.

President's Commission for the Study of Ethical Problems in Medicine and Biomedical and Behavioral Research. *"Defining Death,"a Report on the Medical, Legal and Ethical Issues in the Determination of Death*. Washington, D.C., 1981.

Veatch, Robert M. *Death, Dying and the Biological Revolution: Our Last Quest for Responsibility*. New Haven, Conn.: Yale University Press, 1976.

Veith, Frank J., Fein, Jack M., Tendler, Moses D., Veatch, Robert M., Kleiman, Marc A., and Kalkines, George. Brain death I. A status report of medical and ethical considerations. *Journal of the American Medical Association*, 1977a, *238*, 1651–1655.

Veith, Frank J., Fein, Jack M., Tendler, Moses D., Veatch, Robert M., Kleiman, Marc A., and Kalkines, George. Brain death II. A status report of legal considerations. *Journal of the American Medical Association*, 1977b, *238*, 1744–1748.

The Legalization of Voluntary (Active) Euthanasia

Euthanasia Legislation: Some Nonreligious Objections

Yale Kamisar

Yale Kamisar is professor of law at the University of Michigan Law School. He has served on several national commissions and has published numerous articles in legal journals. He is the coauthor of such books as *Criminal Justice in Our Time* (1965), *Modern Criminal Procedure: Cases and Commentaries* (5th ed., 1980), and *Constitutional Law: Cases, Comments, and Questions* (5th ed., 1980).

Kamisar, in a debate with Glanville Williams, argues against the legalization of voluntary euthanasia, especially against the specific proposal advanced by Williams for its legalization. In the context of their discussion, "euthanasia" is equated with

Reprinted with permission of the author and the publisher from *Minnesota Law Review*, vol. 42, no. 6 (1958).

"mercy killing." Thus Kamisar and Williams are concerned with voluntary *active* (as opposed to passive) euthanasia. Kamisar holds that voluntary euthanasia may be acceptable on pure philosophical (ethical) grounds, yet he argues that it ought not to be legalized. He advances three major lines of argument, all focusing on alleged bad effects that will attend the legalization of voluntary euthanasia. (1) It is difficult to ascertain whether consent is voluntary. Thus there is substantial danger that the law will be abused. (2) The judgment that a person is *incurably ill* may be wrong on two counts: *(a)* The diagnostic judgment may be in error. *(b)* The judgment that no cure will be available within the life expectancy of the patient may be in error. Thus there is substantial risk that some will die unnecessarily. (3) To legalize voluntary euthanasia is to accept the "thin edge of the wedge," thus preparing the way for the legalization of *involuntary* euthanasia.

A book by Glanville Williams, *The Sanctity of Life and the Criminal Law*,[1] once again brought to the fore the controversial topic of euthanasia, more popularly known as 'mercy-killing'. In keeping with the trend of the euthanasia movement over the past generation, Williams concentrates his efforts for reform on the *voluntary* type of euthanasia, for example the cancer victim begging for death, as opposed to the *involuntary* variety—that is, the case of the congenital idiot, the permanently insane or the senile....

The existing law on euthanasia is hardly perfect. But if it is not too good, neither, as I have suggested, is it much worse than the rest of the criminal law. At any rate, the imperfections of existing law are not cured by Williams' proposal. Indeed, I believe adoption of his views would add more difficulties than it would remove.

Williams strongly suggests that 'euthanasia can be condemned only according to a religious opinion'.[2] He tends to view the opposing camps as Roman Catholics versus Liberals. Although this has a certain initial appeal to me, a non-Catholic and self-styled liberal, I deny that this is the only way the battle lines can, or should, be drawn. I leave the religious arguments to the theologians. I share the view that 'those who hold the faith may follow its precepts without requiring those who do not hold it to act as if they did'.[3] But I do not find substantial utilitarian obstacles on the high road to euthanasia. I am not enamoured of the *status quo* on mercy-killing. But while I am not prepared to defend it against all comers, I am prepared to defend it against the proposals for change which have come forth to date.

As an ultimate philosophical proposition, the case for voluntary euthanasia is strong. Whatever may be said for and against suicide generally, the appeal of death is immeasurably greater when it is sought not for a poor reason or just any reason, but for 'good cause', so to speak; when it is invoked not on behalf of a 'socially useful' person, but on behalf of, for example, the painracked 'hopelessly incurable' cancer victim. *If* a person is *in fact* (1) presently incurable, (2) beyond the aid of any respite which may come along in his life expectancy, suffering (3) intolerable and (4) unmitigable pain and of a (5) fixed and (6) rational desire to die, I would hate to have to argue that the hand of death should be stayed. But abstract propositions and carefully formed hypotheticals are one thing; specific proposals designed to cover everyday situations are something else again.

In essence, Williams's specific proposal is that death be authorized for a person in the above situation 'by giving the medical practitioner a wide discretion and trusting to his good sense'.[4] This, I submit, raises too great a risk of abuse and mistake to warrant a change in the existing law. That a proposal entails risk of mistake is hardly a conclusive reason against it. But neither is it irrelevant. Under any euthanasia programme the consequences of mistake, of course, are always fatal. As I shall endeavour to show, the incidence of mistake of one kind or another is likely to be quite appreciable. If this indeed be the case, unless the need for the authorized conduct is compelling enough to override it, I take it the risk of mistake *is* a conclusive reason against such authorization. I submit, too, that the possible radiations from the proposed legislation— for example, involuntary euthanasia of idiots and imbeciles (the typical 'mercy-killings' reported by the press)—and the emergence of the legal precedent that there are lives not 'worth living,' give additional cause for reflection.

I see the issue, then, as the need for voluntary euthanasia versus (1) the incidence of mistake and abuse; and (2) the danger that legal machinery initially designed to kill those who are a nuisance to themselves may some day engulf those who are a nuisance to others....

THE "CHOICE"

Under current proposals to establish legal machinery, elaborate or otherwise, for the administration of a quick and easy death, it is not enough that those authorized to pass on the question decide that the patient, in effect, is 'better off dead'. The patient must concur in this opinion. Much of the appeal in the current proposal lies in this so-called 'voluntary' attribute.

But is the adult patient really in a position to concur? Is he truly able to make euthanasia a 'voluntary' act? There is a good deal to be said, is there not, for Dr. Frohman's pithy comment that the 'voluntary' plan is supposed to be carried out 'only if the victim is both sane and crazed by pain'.[5]

By hypothesis, voluntary euthanasia is not to be resorted to until narcotics have long since been administered and the patient has developed a tolerance to them. *When*, then, does the patient make the choice? While heavily drugged? Or is narcotic relief to be withdrawn for the time of decision? But if heavy dosage no longer deadens pain, indeed, no longer makes it bearable, how overwhelming is it when whatever relief narcotics offer is taken away too?

'Hypersensitivity to pain after analgesia has worn off is nearly always noted'.[6] Moreover, 'the mental side-effects of narcotics, unfortunately for anyone wishing to suspend them temporarily without unduly tormenting the patient, appear to outlast the analgesic effect' and 'by many hours'.[7] The situation is further complicated by the fact that 'a person in terminal stages of cancer who had been given morphine steadily for a matter of weeks would certainly be dependent upon it physically and would probably be addicted to it and react with the addict's response'.[8]

The narcotics problem aside, Dr Benjamin Miller, who probably has personally experienced more pain than any other commentator on the euthanasia scene, observes:

Anyone who has been severely ill knows how distorted his judgment became during the worst moments of the illness. Pain and the toxic effect of disease, or the violent reaction to certain surgical procedures may change our capacity for rational and courageous thought.[9]

Undoubtedly, some euthanasia candidates will have their lucid moments. How they are to be distinguished from fellow-sufferers who do not, or how these instances are to be distinguished from others when the patient is exercising an irrational judgment, is not an easy matter. Particularly is this so under Williams' proposal, where no specially qualified persons, psychiatrically trained or otherwise, are to assist in the process.

Assuming, for purposes of argument, that the occasion when a euthanasia candidate possesses a sufficiently clear mind can be ascertained and that a request for euthanasia is then made, there remain other problems. The mind of the painracked may occasionally be clear, but is it not also likely to be uncertain and variable? This point was pressed hard by the great physician, Lord Horder, in the House of Lords debates:

During the morning depression he [the patient] will be found to favour the application under this Bill, later in the day he will think quite differently, or will have forgotten all about it. The mental clarity with which noble Lords who present this Bill are able to think and to speak must not be thought to have any counterpart in the alternating moods and confused judgments of the sick man.[10]

The concept of 'voluntary' in voluntary euthanasia would have a great deal more substance to it if, as is the case with voluntary admission statutes for the mentally ill, the patient retained the right to reverse the process within a specified number of days after he gives written notice of his desire to do so—but unfortunately this cannot be. The choice here, of course, is an irrevocable one.

The likelihood of confusion, distortion or vacillation would appear to be serious drawbacks to any voluntary plan. Moreover, Williams' proposal is particularly vulnerable in this regard, since as he admits, by eliminating the fairly elaborate procedure of the American and British Societies' plans, he also eliminates a time period which would furnish substantial evidence of the patient's settled intention to avail himself of euthanasia.[11] But if Williams does not always choose to slug it out, he can box neatly and parry gingerly:

[T]he problem can be exaggerated. Every law has to face difficulties in application, and these difficulties are not a conclusive argument against a law if it has a beneficial operation. The measure here proposed is designed to meet the situation where the patient's consent to euthanasia is clear and incontrovertible. The physician, conscious of the need to protect himself against malicious accusations, can devise his own safeguards appropriate to the circumstances; he would normally be well advised to get the patient's consent in writing, just as is now the practice before operations. Sometimes the patient's consent will be particularly clear because he will have expressed a desire for ultimate euthanasia while he is still clear-headed and before he comes to be racked by pain; if the expression of desire is never revoked, but rather is reaffirmed under the pain, there is the best possible proof of full consent. If, on the other hand, there is no such settled frame of mind, and if the physician chooses to administer euthanasia when the patient's mind is in a variable state, he will be walking in the margin of the law and may find himself unprotect-ed.[12]

If consent is given at a time when the patient's condition has so degenerated that he has become a fit candidate for euthanasia, when, if ever, will it be 'clear and incontrovertible'? Is the suggested alternative of consent in advance a satisfactory solution? Can such a consent be deemed an informed one? Is this much different from holding a man to a prior statement of intent that if such and such an employment opportunity would present itself he would accept it, or if such and such a young woman were to come along he would marry her? Need one marshal authority for the proposition that many an 'iffy' inclination is disregarded when the actual facts are at hand?

Professor Williams states that where a pre-pain desire for 'ultimate euthanasia' is 'reaffirmed' under pain, 'there is the best possible proof of full consent'. Perhaps. But what if it is alternately renounced and reaffirmed under pain? What if it is neither affirmed or renounced? What if it is only renounced? Will a physician be free to go ahead on the ground that the prior desire was 'rational', but the present desire 'irrational'? Under Williams' plan, will not the physician frequently 'be walking in the margin of the law'—just as he is now? Do we really accomplish much more under this pro-posal than to put the euthanasia principle on the books?

Even if the patient's choice could be said to be 'clear

and incontrovertible', do not other difficulties remain? Is this the kind of choice, assuming that it can be made in a fixed and rational manner, that we want to offer a gravely ill person? Will we not sweep up, in the process, some who are not really tired of life, but think others are tired of them; some who do not really want to die, but who feel they should not live on, because to do so when there looms the legal alternative of euthanasia is to do a selfish or a cowardly act? Will not some feel an obligation to have themselves 'eliminated' in order that funds allocated for their terminal care might be better used by their families or, financial worries aside, in order to relieve their families of the emotional strain involved?

It would not be surprising for the gravely ill person to seek to inquire of those close to him whether he should avail himself of the legal alternative of euthana-sia. Certainly, he is likely to wonder about their attitude in the matter. It is quite possible, is it not, that he will not exactly be gratified by any inclination on their part—however noble their motives may be in fact—that he resort to the new procedure? At this stage, the patient-family relationship may well be a good deal less than it ought to be.

And what of the relatives? If their views will not always influence the patient, will they not at least influence the attending physician? Will a physician assume the risks to his reputation, if not his pocketbook, by administering the *coup de grâce* over the objection—however irrational—of a close relative? Do not the relatives, then, also have a 'choice'? Is not the decision on their part to do nothing and say nothing *itself* a 'choice'? In many families there will be some, will there not, who will consider a stand against euthanasia the only proof of love, devotion and gratitude for past events? What of the stress and strife if close relatives differ over the desirability of euthanatizing the patient?

At such a time, members of the family are not likely to be in the best state of mind, either, to make this kind of decision. Financial stress and conscious or uncon-scious competition for the family's estate aside,

The chronic illness and persistent pain in terminal carcinoma may place strong and excessive stresses upon the family's emotional ties with the patient. The family members who have strong emotional attachment to start with are most likely to take the patient's fears, pains and fate personally. Panic often strikes them. Whatever guilt feelings they may have toward the patient emerge to plague them.

If the patient is maintained at home, many frustrations and physical demands may be imposed on the family by the advanced illness. There may develop extreme weakness, incontinence and bad odors. The pressure of caring for the individual under these circumstances is likely to arouse a resentment and, in turn, guilt feelings on the part of those who have to do the nursing.[13]

Nor should it be overlooked that while Professor Williams would remove the various procedural steps and personnel contemplated in the British and American Bills and bank his all on the 'good sense' of the general practitioner, no man is immune to the fear, anxieties and frustrations engendered by the apparently helpless, hopeless patient. Not even the general practitioner....

THE "HOPELESSLY INCURABLE" PATIENT AND THE FALLIBLE DOCTOR

Professor Williams notes as 'standard argument' the plea that 'no sufferer from an apparently fatal illness should be deprived of his life because there is always the possibility that the diagnosis is wrong, or else that some remarkable cure will be discovered in time'.[14]...

Until the Euthanasia Societies of Great Britain and America had been organized and a party decision reached, shall we say, to advocate euthanasia only for incurables on their request, Dr Abraham L. Wolbarst, one of the most ardent supporters of the movement, was less troubled about putting away 'insane or defective people [who] have suffered mental incapacity and tortures of the mind for many years' than he was about the 'incurables'.[15] He recognized the 'difficulty involved in the decision as to incurability' as one of the 'doubtful aspects of euthanasia': 'Doctors are only human beings, with few if any supermen among them. They make honest mistakes, like other men, because of the limitations of the human mind'.[16]

He noted further that 'it goes without saying that, in recently developed cases with a possibility of cure, euthanasia should not even be considered', that 'the law might establish a limit of, say, ten years in which there is a chance of the patient's recovery'.[17]

Dr Benjamin Miller is another who is unlikely to harbour an ulterior theological motive. His interest is more personal. He himself was left to die the death of a 'hopeless' tuberculosis victim, only to discover that he was suffering from a rare malady which affects the lungs in much the same manner but seldom kills. Five years and sixteen hospitalizations later, Dr Miller dramatized his point by recalling the last diagnostic clinic of the brilliant Richard Cabot, on the occasion of his official retirement:

He was given the case records [complete medical histories and results of careful examinations] of two patients and asked to diagnose their illnesses.... The patients had died and only the hospital pathologist knew the exact diagnosis beyond doubt, for he had seen the descriptions of the post-mortem findings. Dr Cabot, usually very accurate in his diagnosis, that day missed both.

The chief pathologist who had selected the cases was a wise person. He had purposely chosen two of the most deceptive to remind the medical students and young physicians that even at the end of a long and rich experience one of the greatest diagnosticians of our time was still not infallible.[18]

Richard Cabot was the John W. Davis, the John Lord O'Brian, of his profession. When one reads the account of his last clinic, one cannot help but think how fallible the *average* general practitioner must be, how fallible the *young doctor just starting practice* must be—and this, of course, is all that some small communities have in the way of medical care—how fallible the *worst* practitioner, young or old, must be. If the range of skill and judgment among licensed physicians approaches the wide gap between the very best and the very worst members of the bar—and I have no reason to think it does not—then the minimally competent physician is hardly the man to be given the responsibility for ending another's life. Yet, under Williams' proposal at least, the marginal physician, as well as his more distinguished brethren, would have legal authorization to make just such decisions. Under Williams' proposal, euthanatizing a patient or two would all be part of the routine day's work....

Faulty diagnosis is only one ground for error. Even if the diagnosis is correct, a second ground for error lies in the possibility that some measure of relief, if not a full cure, may come to the fore within the life expectancy of the patient. Since Glanville Williams does not deign this objection to euthanasia worth more than a passing reference,[19] it is necessary to turn elsewhere to ascertain how it has been met. One answer is: 'It must be little comfort to a man slowly coming apart from multiple sclerosis to think that fifteen years from now, death might not be his only hope'.[20]

To state the problem this way is, of course, to avoid it entirely. How do we know that fifteen *days* or fifteen *hours* from now, 'death might not be [the incurable's] only hope'?

A second answer is: '[N]o cure for cancer which might be found "tomorrow" would be of any value to a man or woman "so far advanced in cancerous toxemia as to be an applicant for euthanasia".'[21]

As I shall endeavour to show, this approach is a good deal easier to formulate than it is to apply. For one thing, it presumes that we know today *what* cures will be found tomorrow. For another, it overlooks that if such cases can be said to exist, the patient is likely to be *so far* advanced in cancerous toxemia as to be no longer capable of understanding the step he is taking and hence *beyond* the stage when euthanasia ought to be administered.

Thirty-six years ago, Dr Haven Emerson, then President of the American Public Health Association, made the point that 'no one can say today what will be incurable tomorrow. No one can predict what disease will be fatal or permanently incurable until medicine becomes stationary and sterile'.[22]...

VOLUNTARY VERSUS INVOLUNTARY EUTHANASIA

Ever since the 1870s, when what was probably the first euthanasia debate of the modern era took place, most proponents of the movement—at least when they are pressed—have taken considerable pains to restrict the question to the plight of the unbearably suffering incurable who *voluntarily seeks* death, while most of their opponents have striven equally hard to frame the issue in terms which would encompass certain involuntary situations as well, e.g. the 'congenital idiots', the 'permanently insane', and the senile.

Glanville Williams reflects the outward mood of many euthanasiasts when he scores those who insist on considering the question from a broader angle:

The [British Society's] bill [debated in the House of Lords in 1936 and 1950] excluded any question of compulsory euthanasia, even for hopelessly defective infants. Unfortunately, a legislative proposal is not assured of success merely because it is worded in a studiously moderate and restrictive form. The

method of attack, by those who dislike the proposal, is to use the 'thin end of the wedge' argument.... There is no proposal for reform on any topic, however conciliatory and moderate, that cannot be opposed by this dialectic.[23]

Why was the bill 'worded in a studiously moderate and restrictive form'? If it were done as a matter of principle, if it were done in recognition of the ethico-moral-legal 'wall of separation' which stands between voluntary and compulsory 'mercy-killings', much can be said for the euthanasiasts' lament about the methods employed by the opposition. But if it were done as a matter of political expediency—with great hopes and expectations of pushing through a second and somewhat less restrictive bill as soon as the first one had sufficiently 'educated' public opinion and next a third, still less restrictive bill—what standing do the euthanasiasts then have to attack the methods of the opposition? No cry of righteous indignation could ring more hollow, I would think, than the protest from those utilizing the 'wedge' principle themselves that their opponents are making the wedge objection....

The boldness and daring which characterize most of Glanville Williams' book dim perceptibly when he comes to involuntary euthanasia proposals. As to the senile, he states:

At present the problem has certainly not reached the degree of seriousness that would warrant an effort being made to change traditional attitudes towards the sanctity of life of the aged. Only the grimmest necessity could bring about a change that, however cautious in its approach, would probably cause apprehension and deep distress to many people, and inflict a traumatic injury upon the accepted code of behaviour built up by two thousand years of the Christian religion. It may be, however, that as the problem becomes more acute it will itself cause a reversal of generally accepted values.[24]

To me, this passage is the most startling one in the book. On page 310 Williams invokes 'traditional attitudes towards the sanctity of life' and 'the accepted code of behaviour built up by two thousand years of the Christian religion' to check the extension of euthanasia to the senile, but for 309 pages he had been merrily rolling along debunking both. Substitute 'cancer victim' for 'the aged' and Williams' passage is essentially the argument of many of his *opponents* on the voluntary euthanasia question.

The unsupported comment that 'the problem [of senility] has certainly not reached the degree of seriousness' to warrant euthanasia is also rather puzzling, particularly coming as it does after an observation by Williams on the immediately preceding page that 'it is increasingly common for men and women to reach an age of "second childishness and mere oblivion," with a loss of almost all adult faculties except that of digestion'.[25]

How 'serious' does a problem have to be to warrant a change in these 'traditional attitudes'? If, as the statement seems to indicate, 'seriousness' of the problem is to be determined numerically, the problem of the cancer victim does not appear to be as substantial as the problem of the senile. For example, taking just the 95,837 first admissions to 'public prolonged-care hospitals' for mental diseases in the United States in 1955, 23,561—or one-fourth—were cerebral arteriosclerosis or senile brain disease cases. I am not at all sure that there are twenty thousand cancer victims per year who die *unbearably painful* deaths. Even if there were, I cannot believe that among their ranks are some twenty thousand per year who, when still in a rational state, so long for a quick and easy death that they would avail themselves of legal machinery for euthanasia.

If the problem of the incurable cancer victim has reached 'the degree of seriousness that would warrant an effort being made to change traditional attitudes towards the sanctity of life', as Williams obviously thinks it has, then so has the problem of senility. In any event, the senility problem will undoubtedly soon reach even Williams' requisite degree of seriousness:

A decision concerning the senile may have to be taken within the next twenty years. The number of old people are increasing by leaps and bounds. Pneumonia, 'the old man's friend', is now checked by antibiotics. The effects of hardship, exposure, starvation and accident are now minimized. Where is this leading us? . . . What of the drooling, helpless, disorientated old man or the doubly incontinent old woman lying log-like in bed? Is it here that the real need for euthanasia exists?[26]

If, as Williams indicates, 'seriousness' of the problem is a major criterion for euthanatizing a category of unfortunates, the sum total of mentally deficient persons would appear to warrant high priority, indeed.

When Williams turns to the plight of the 'hopelessly defective infants', his characteristic vim and vigour are, as in the senility discussion, conspicuously absent:

While the Euthanasia Society of England has never advocated this, the Euthanasia Society of America did include it in its original programme. The proposal certainly escapes the chief objection to the similar proposal for senile dementia: it does not create a sense of insecurity in society, because infants cannot, like adults, feel anticipatory dread of being done to death if their condition should worsen. Moreover, the proposal receives some support on eugenic grounds, and more importantly on humanitarian grounds— both on account of the parents, to whom the child will be a burden all their lives, and on account of the handicapped child itself. (It is not, however, proposed that any child should be destroyed against the wishes of its parents.) Finally, the legalization of euthanasia for handicapped children would bring the law into closer relation to its practical administration, because juries do not regard parental mercy-killing as murder. For these various reasons the proposal to legalize humanitarian infanticide is put forward from time to time by individuals. They remain in a very small minority, and the proposal may at present be dismissed as politically insignificant.[27]

It is understandable for a reformer to limit his present proposals for change to those with a real prospect of success. But it is hardly reassuring for Williams to cite the fact that only 'a very small minority' has urged euthanasia for 'hopelessly defective infants' as the *only* reason for not pressing for such legislation now. If, as Williams sees it, the only advantage voluntary euthanasia has over the involuntary variety lies in the organized movements on its behalf, that advantage can readily be wiped out.

In any event, I do not think that such 'a very small minority' has advocated 'humanitarian infanticide'. Until the organization of the British and American societies led to a concentration on the voluntary type, and until the by-products of the Nazi euthanasia programme somewhat embarrassed, if only temporarily, most proponents of involuntary euthanasia, about as many writers urged one type as another. Indeed, some euthanasiasts have taken considerable pains to demonstrate the superiority of defective infant euthanasia over incurably ill euthanasia.

As for dismissing euthanasia of defective infants as 'politically insignificant', the only poll that I know of which measured the public response to both types of euthanasia revealed that *45 per cent favoured euthanasia for defective infants under certain conditions while only 37.3 per cent approved euthanasia for the incurably and painfully ill under any conditions.*[28] Furthermore, of those who favoured the mercy-killing cure for incurable adults, some 40 percent would require only family permission or medical board approval, but not the patient's permission.

Nor do I think it irrelevant that while public resistance caused Hitler to yield on the adult euthanasia front, the killing of malformed and idiot children continued unhindered to the end of the war, the definition of 'children' expanding all the while. Is it the embarrassing experience of the Nazi euthanasia programme which has rendered destruction of defective infants presently 'politically insignificant'? If so, is it any more of a jump from the incurably and painfully ill to the unorthodox political thinker than it is from the hopelessly defective infant to the same 'unsavoury character'? Or is it not so much that the euthanasiasts are troubled by the Nazi experience as it is that they are troubled that the public is troubled by the Nazi experience?

I read Williams' comments on defective infants for the proposition that there are some very good reasons for euthanatizing defective infants, but the time is not yet ripe. When will it be? When will the proposal become politically significant? After a voluntary euthanasia law is on the books and public opinion is sufficiently 'educated'?

Williams's reasons for not extending euthanasia— once we legalize it in the narrow 'voluntary' area—to the senile and the defective are much less forceful and much less persuasive than his arguments for legalizing voluntary euthanasia in the first place. I regard this as another reason for not legalizing voluntary euthanasia in the first place.

NOTES

1 First published in the U.S. in 1957, by arrangement with the Columbia Law School. Page references in the notes following relate to the British edition (Faber & Faber, 1958).

2 Williams, p. 278.

3 Wechsler and Michael, 'A Rationale of the Law of Homicide', *Columbia Law Review*, 37 (1937).

4 Williams, p. 302.

5 Frohman, 'Vexing Problems in Forensic Medicine: A Physician's View', *New York Univ. Law Review*, 31 (1956), 1215, 1222.

6 Goodman and Gilman, *The Pharmacological Basis of Therapeutics* (2nd edn. 1955), p. 235.

7 Sharpe, 'Medication as a Threat to Testamentary Capacity', *N. Carolina Law Review*, 35 (1957), 380, 392, and medical authorities cited therein.

8 Sharpe, op. cit., 384.

9 'Why I Oppose Mercy Killings', *Woman's Home Companion* (June 1950), pp. 38, 103.

10 *House of Lords Debates*, 103, 5th series (1936), cols 466, 492–3.

11 Williams, pp. 306–7.

12 Ibid., p. 307.

13 Zarling, 'Psychological Aspects of Pain in Terminal Malignancies', *Management of Pain in Cancer* (Schiffrin edn., 1956), pp. 211–12.

14 Williams, p. 283.

15 Wolbarst, 'Legalize Euthanasia!', *The Forum*, 94 (1935), 330, 332. But see Wolbarst, 'The Doctor Looks at Euthanasia', *Medical Record*, 149 (1939), 354.

16 Wolbarst, 'Legalize Euthanasia!', loc. cit.

17 Ibid., 332.

18 Op. cit. (n. 9 above), p. 39.

19 See Williams, p. 283.

20 'Pro & Con: Shall We Legalize "Mercy Killing"?', *Reader's Digest* (Nov. 1938), pp. 94, 96.

21 James, 'Euthanasia—Right or Wrong?', *Survey Graphic* (May 1948), pp. 241, 243; Wolbarst, 'The Doctor Looks at Euthanasia', *Medical Record*, 149 (1939), 354, 355.

22 Emerson, 'Who Is Incurable? A Query and a Reply,' *New York Times* (Oct. 22, 1933), § 8, p. 5 col. 1.

23 Williams, pp. 297–8.

24 Williams, p. 310.

25 Ibid.

26 Banks, 'Euthanasia', *Bulletin of the New York Academy of Medicine*, 26 (1950), 297, 305.

27 Williams, pp. 311–12.

28 The Fortune Quarterly Survey: IX, *Fortune Magazine* (July 1937), pp. 96, 106.

Euthanasia Legislation: A Rejoinder to the Nonreligious Objections

Glanville Williams

Glanville Williams is a fellow of Jesus College and Rouse Ball Professor of the Laws of England at the University of Cambridge. Since 1959 he has been a member of the Standing Committee on Criminal Law Revision. Williams is a prominent spokesperson for the movement to legalize voluntary euthanasia, and his primary work in this regard is *The Sanctity of Life and the Criminal Law* (U.S. ed., 1957; British ed., 1958). Among his other works are *The Proof of Guilt* (1955; 3d ed., 1963) and *The Mental Element in Crime* (1965).

Before beginning his direct reply to the arguments raised by Kamisar in the previous selection, Williams reiterates the basic case for the legalization of voluntary euthanasia. In his view there are two principal arguments: (1) It is simply cruel to refuse an agonized and incurably ill person's request for "merciful release." (2) There is no demonstrable social interest sufficient to warrant the infringement of liberty (the patient's and the doctor's) that accompanies the legal prohibition of voluntary euthanasia.

In response to Kamisar's arguments against the legalization of voluntary euthanasia, Williams acknowledges that there is the possibility of abuse (concerning the ascertaining of consent), the possibility of mistaken diagnoses, and the possibility of dramatic medical discoveries. But he plays down the force of such factors and argues that they do not warrant the continued legal prohibition of voluntary euthanasia. In response to Kamisar's claim that the legalization of euthanasia is the thin edge of the wedge that will open the door to legalized involuntary euthanasia, Williams argues that this claim is without foundation.

I welcome Professor Kamisar's reply to my argument for voluntary euthanasia, because it is on the whole a careful, scholarly work, keeping to knowable facts and accepted human values. It is, therefore, the sort of reply that can be rationally considered and dealt with. In this short rejoinder I shall accept most of Professor Kamisar's valuable notes, and merely submit that they do not bear out his conclusion.

The argument in favour of voluntary euthanasia in the terminal stages of painful diseases is a quite simple one, and is an application of two values that are widely recognized. The first value is the prevention of cruelty. Much as men differ in their ethical assessments, all agree that cruelty is an evil—the only difference of opinion residing in what is meant by cruelty. Those who plead for the legalization of euthanasia think that it is cruel to allow a human being to linger for months in the last stages of agony, weakness and decay, and to refuse him his demand for merciful release. There is also a second cruelty involved—not perhaps quite so compelling, but still worth consideration: the agony of the relatives in seeing their loved one in his desperate plight. Opponents of euthanasia are apt to take a cynical view of the desires of relatives, and this may sometimes be justified. But it cannot be denied that a wife who has to nurse her husband through the last stages of some terrible disease may herself be so deeply affected by the experience that her health is ruined, either mentally or physically. Whether the situation can be eased for such a person by voluntary euthanasia

Reprinted with permission of the author and the publisher from *Minnesota Law Review*, vol. 43, no. 1 (1958).

I do not know; probably it depends very much upon the individuals concerned, which is as much as to say that no solution in terms of a general regulatory law can be satisfactory. The conclusion should be in favour of individual discretion.

The second value involved is that of liberty. The criminal law should not be invoked to repress conduct unless this is demonstrably necessary on social grounds. What social interest is there in preventing the sufferer from choosing to accelerate his death by a few months? What positive value does his life still possess for society, that he is to be retained in it by the terrors of the criminal law?

And, of course, the liberty involved is that of the doctor as well as that of the patient. It is the doctor's responsibility to do all he can to prolong worth-while life, or, in the last resort, to ease his patient's passage. If the doctor honestly and sincerely believes that the best service he can perform for his suffering patient is to accede to his request for euthanasia, it is a grave thing that the law should forbid him to do so.

This is the short and simple case for voluntary euthanasia, and, as Kamisar admits, it cannot be attacked directly on utilitarian grounds. Such an attack can only be by finding possible evils of an indirect nature. These evils, in the view of Professor Kamisar, are (1) the difficulty of ascertaining consent, and arising out of that the danger of abuse; (2) the risk of an incorrect diagnosis; (3) the risk of administering euthanasia to a person who could later have been cured by developments in medical knowledge; (4) the 'wedge' argument....

Kamisar's first objection, under the heading 'The Choice', is that there can be no such thing as truly voluntary euthanasia in painful and killing diseases. He seeks to impale the advocates of euthanasia on an old dilemma. Either the victim is not yet suffering pain, in which case his consent is merely an uninformed and anticipatory one—and he cannot bind himself by contract to be killed in the future—or he is crazed by pain and stupefied by drugs, in which case he is not of sound mind. I have dealt with this problem in my book; Kamisar has quoted generously from it, and I leave the reader to decide. As I understand Kamisar's position, he does not really persist in the objection. With the laconic 'perhaps', he seems to grant me, though unwillingly, that there are cases where one can be sure of the patient's consent. But having thus abandoned his own point, he then goes off to a different horror, that the patient may give his consent only in order to relieve his relatives of the trouble of looking after him.

On this new issue, I will return Kamisar the compliment and say: 'Perhaps'. We are certainly in an area where no solution is going to make things quite easy and happy for everybody, and all sorts of embarrassments may be conjectured. But these embarrassments are not avoided by keeping to the present law: we suffer from them already. If a patient, suffering pain in a terminal illness, wishes for euthanasia partly because of his pain and partly because he sees his beloved ones breaking under the strain of caring for him, I do not see how this decision on his part, agonizing though it may be, is necessarily a matter of discredit either to the patient himself or to his relatives. The fact is that, whether we are considering the patient or his relatives, there are limits to human endurance.

Kamisar's next objection rests on the possibility of mistaken diagnosis.... I agree with him that, before deciding on euthanasia in any particular case, the risk of mistaken diagnosis would have to be considered. Everything that is said in the essay would, therefore, be most relevant when the two doctors whom I propose in my suggested measure come to consult on the question of euthanasia; and the possibility of mistake might most forcefully be brought before the patient himself. But have these medical questions any true relevance to the legal discussion?

Kamisar, I take it, notwithstanding his wide reading in medical literature, is by training a lawyer. He has consulted much medical opinion in order to find arguments against changing the law. I ought not to object to this, since I have consulted the same opinion for the opposite purpose. But what we may well ask ourselves is this: is it not a trifle bizarre that we should be doing so at all? Our profession is the law, not medicine. How does it come about that lawyers have to examine medical literature to assess the advantages and disadvantages of a medical practice?

If the import of this question is not immediately clear, let me return to my imaginary state of Ruritania. Many years ago, in Ruritania as elsewhere, surgical operations were attended with great risk. Lister had not discovered antisepsis, and surgeons killed as often as they cured. In this state of things, the legislature of Ruritania passed a law declaring all surgical operations to be unlawful in principle, but providing that each specific type of operation might be legalized by a statute specially passed for the purpose. The result is that, in Ruritania, as expert medical opinion sees the possibility of some new medical advance, a pressure group has to be formed in order to obtain legislative approval for it. Since there is little public interest in these technical questions, and since, moreover, surgical operations are thought in general to be inimical to the established religion, the pressure group has to work for many years before it gets a hearing. When at last a proposal for legalization is seriously mooted, the lawyers and politicians get to work upon it, considering what possible dangers are inherent in the new operation. Lawyers and politicians are careful people, and they are perhaps more prone to see the dangers than the advantages in a new departure. Naturally they find allies among some of the more timid or traditional or less knowledgeable members of the medical profession, as well as among the priesthood and the faithful. Thus it is small wonder that whereas appendicectomy has been practised in civilized countries since the beginning of the present century, a proposal to legalize it has still not passed the legislative assembly of Ruritania.

It must be confessed that on this particular matter the legal prohibition has not been an unmixed evil for the Ruritanians. During the great popularity of the appendix operation in much of the civilized world during the 'twenties and 'thirties of this century, large numbers of these organs were removed without adequate cause, and the citizens of Ruritania have been spared this inconvenience. On the other hand, many citizens of that country have died of appendicitis, who would have been saved if they had lived elsewhere. And whereas in other countries the medical profession has now learned enough to be able to perform this operation with wisdom and restraint, in Ruritania it is still not being performed at all. Moreover, the law has destroyed scientific inventiveness in that country in the forbidden fields.

Now, in the United States and England we have no such absurd general law on the subject of surgical operations as they have in Ruritania. In principle, medical men are left free to exercise their best judgment, and the result has been a brilliant advance in knowledge and technique. But there are just two—or possibly three—'operations' which are subject to the Ruritanian principle. These are abortion, euthanasia, and possibly sterilization of convenience. In these fields we, too, must have pressure groups, with lawyers and politicians warning us of the possibility of inexpert practitioners and mistaken diagnosis, and canvassing medical opin-

ion on the risk of an operation not yielding the expected results in terms of human happiness and the health of the body politic. In these fields we, too, are forbidden to experiment to see if the foretold dangers actually come to pass. Instead of that, we are required to make a social judgment on the probabilities of good and evil before the medical profession is allowed to start on its empirical tests.

This anomaly is perhaps more obvious with abortion than it is with euthanasia. Indeed, I am prepared for ridicule when I describe euthanasia as a medical operation. Regarded as surgery it is unique, since its object is not to save or prolong life but the reverse. But euthanasia has another object which it shares with many surgical operations—the saving of pain. And it is now widely recognized, as Lord Dawson said in the debate in the House of Lords, that the saving of pain is a legitimate aim of medical practice. The question whether euthanasia will effect a net saving of pain and distress is, perhaps, one that we can attempt to answer only by trying it. But it is obscurantist to forbid the experiment on the ground that until it is performed we cannot certainly know its results. Such an attitude, in any other field of medical endeavour, would have inhibited progress.

The argument based on mistaken diagnosis leads into the argument based on the possibility of dramatic medical discoveries. Of course, a new medical discovery which gives the opportunity of remission or cure will almost at once put an end to mercy-killings in the particular group of cases for which the discovery is made. On the other hand, the discovery cannot affect patients who have already died from their disease. The argument based on mistaken diagnosis is therefore concerned only with those patients who have been mercifully killed just before the discovery becomes available for use. The argument is that such persons may turn out to have been 'mercy-killed' unnecessarily, because if the physician had waited a bit longer they would have been cured. Because of this risk for this tiny fraction of the total number of patients, patients who are dying in pain must be left to do so, year after year, against their entreaty to have it ended.

Just how real is the risk? When a new medical discovery is claimed, some time commonly elapses before it becomes tested sufficiently to justify large-scale production of the drug, or training in the techniques involved. This is a warning period when euthanasia in the particular class of case would probably be halted anyway. Thus it is quite probable that when the new discovery becomes available, the euthanasia process would not in fact show any mistakes in this regard.

Kamisar says that in my book I 'did not deign this objection to euthanasia more than a passing reference'. I still do not think it is worth any more than that.

He advances the familiar but hardly convincing arguments that the quantitative need for euthanasia is not large. As one reason for this argument, he suggests that not many patients would wish to benefit from euthanasia, even if it were allowed. I am not impressed by the argument. It may be true, but it is irrelevant. So long as there are *any* persons dying in weakness and grief who are refused their request for a speeding of their end, the argument for legalizing euthanasia remains. Next, he suggests that there is no great need for euthanasia because of the advances made with pain-killing drugs. He has made so many quotations from my book that I cannot complain that he has not made more, but there is one relevant point that he does not mention. In my book, recognizing that medical science does manage to save many dying patients from the extreme of physical pain, I pointed out that it often fails to save them from an artificial, twilight existence, with nausea, giddiness, and extreme restlessness, as well as the long hours of consciousness of a hopeless condition. A dear friend of mine, who died of cancer of the bowel, spent his last months in just this state, under the influence of morphine, which deadened pain, but vomiting incessantly, day in and day out. The question that we have to face is whether the unintelligent brutality of such an existence is to be imposed on one who wishes to end it....

The last part of the essay is devoted to the ancient 'wedge' argument which I have already examined in my book. It is the trump card of the traditionalist, because no proposal for reform, however strong the arguments in its favour, is immune from the wedge objection. In fact, the stronger the argument in favor of a reform, the more likely it is that the traditionalist will take the wedge objection—it is then the only one he has. C.M. Cornford put the argument in its proper place when he said that the wedge objection means this: that you should not act justly today, for fear that you may be asked to act still more justly tomorrow.

We heard a great deal of this type of argument in England in the nineteenth century, when it was used to resist almost every social and economic change. In the present century we have had less of it, but it is still accorded an exaggerated importance in some contexts.

When lecturing on the law of torts in an American university a few years ago, I suggested that just as compulsory liability insurance for automobiles had spread practically throughout the civilized world, so we should in time see the law of tort superseded in this field by a system of state insurance for traffic accidents, administered independently of proof of fault. The suggestion was immediately met by one student with a horrified reference to 'creeping socialism'. That is the standard objection made by many people to any proposal for a new department of state activity. The implication is that you must resist every proposal, however admirable in itself, because otherwise you will never be able to draw the line. On the particular question of socialism, the fear is belied by the experience of a number of countries which have extended state control of the economy without going the whole way to socialistic state regimentation.

Kamisar's particular bogey, the racial laws of Nazi Germany, is an effective one in the democratic countries. Any reference to the Nazis is a powerful weapon to prevent change in the traditional taboo on sterilization as well as euthanasia. The case of sterilization is particularly interesting on this; I dealt with it at length in my book, though Kamisar does not mention its bearing on the argument. When proposals are made for promoting voluntary sterilization on eugenic and other grounds, they are immediately condemned by most people as the thin end of a wedge leading to involuntary sterilization; and then they point to the practices of the Nazis. Yet a more persuasive argument pointing in the other direction can easily be found. Several American states have sterilization laws, which for the most part were originally drafted in very wide terms to cover desexualization as well as sterilization, and authorizing involuntary as well as voluntary operations. This legislation goes back long before the Nazis; the earliest statute was in Indiana in 1907. What has been its practical effect? In several American states it has hardly been used. A few have used it, but in practice they have progressively restricted it until now it is virtually confined to voluntary sterilization. This is so, at least, in North Carolina, as Mrs Woodside's study strikingly shows. In my book I summed up the position as follows:

The American experience is of great interest because it shows how remote from reality in a democratic community is the fear—frequently voiced by Americans themselves—that voluntary sterilization may be the 'thin end of the wedge', leading to a large-scale violation of human rights as happened in Nazi Germany. In fact, the American experience is the precise opposite—starting with compulsory sterilization, administrative practice has come to put the operation on a voluntary footing.

But it is insufficient to answer the 'wedge' objection in general terms; we must consider the particular fears to which it gives rise. Kamisar professes to fear certain other measures that the Euthanasia Societies may bring up if their present measure is conceded to them. Surely these other measures, if any, will be debated on their merits. Does he seriously fear that anyone in the United States or in Great Britain is going to propose the extermination of people of a minority race or religion? Let us put aside such ridiculous fancies and discuss practical politics.

Kamisar is quite right in thinking that a body of opinion would favour the legalization of the involuntary euthanasia of hopelessly defective infants, and some day a proposal of this kind may be put forward. The proposal would have distinct limits, just as the proposal for voluntary euthanasia of incurable sufferers has limits. I do not think that any responsible body of opinion would now propose the euthanasia of insane adults, for the perfectly clear reason that any such practice would greatly increase the sense of insecurity felt by the borderline insane and by the large number of insane persons who have sufficient understanding on this particular matter.

Kamisar expresses distress at a concluding remark in my book in which I advert to the possibility of old people becoming an overwhelming burden on mankind. I share his feeling that there are profoundly disturbing possibilities here; and if I had been merely a propagandist, intent upon securing agreement for a specific measure of law reform, I should have done wisely to have omitted all reference to this subject. Since, however, I am merely an academic writer, trying to bring such intelligence as I have to bear on moral and social issues, I deemed the topic too important and threatening to leave without a word. I think I have made it clear, in the passages cited, that I am not for one moment proposing any euthanasia of the aged in present society; such an idea would shock me as much as it shocks Kamisar and would shock everybody else. Still, the fact that we may one day have to face is that medical science is more successful in preserving the body than in preserving the mind. It is not impossible that, in the foreseeable future, medical men will be able to preserve the mindless body until the age, say, of a thousand, while the mind itself will have lasted only a tenth of that time. What will mankind do then? It is hardly possible to imagine that we shall establish huge hospital-mausolea where the aged are kept in a kind of living death. Even if it is desired to do this, the cost of the undertaking may make it impossible.

This is not an immediately practical problem, and we need not yet face it. The problem of maintaining persons afflicted with senile dementia is well within our economic resources as the matter stands at present. Perhaps some barrier will be found to medical advance which will prevent the problem becoming more acute. Perhaps, as time goes on, and as the alternatives become more clearly realized, men will become more resigned to human control over the mode of termination of life. Or the solution may be that after the individual has reached a certain age, or a certain degree of decay, medical science will hold its hand, and allow him to be carried off by natural causes. But what if these natural causes are themselves painful? Would it not then be kinder to substitute human agency?

In general, it is enough to say that we do not have to know the solutions to these problems. The only doubtful moral question upon which we have to make an immediate decision in relation to involuntary euthanasia is whether we owe a moral duty to terminate the life of an insane person who is suffering from a painful and incurable disease. Such a person is left unprovided for under the legislative proposal formulated in my book. The objection to any system of involuntary euthanasia of the insane is that it may cause a sense of insecurity. It is because I think that the risk of this fear is a serious one that a proposal for the reform of the law must exclude its application to the insane.

The Treatment of Defective Newborns

To Save or Let Die: The Dilemma of Modern Medicine

Richard A. McCormick

A biographical sketch of Richard A. McCormick is found on page 196.

McCormick directly confronts the issue of the moral justifiability of allowing severely defective newborns to die. After insisting on the necessity of formulating substantive guidelines to govern decisions as to which infants should be allowed to die, McCormick argues that we must squarely face quality-of-life judgments. He would allow infants having *no significant potential for human relationships* to die. Although McCormick argues primarily as a moral theologian, within the context of the Judeo-Christian tradition, his overall argument would seem not to be limited to that tradition. Life, he maintains, is a relative good. Life is valuable as a condition of other goods, principally human relationships. Hence, where there is no significant potential for human relationships, where life is "meaningless," there is no moral obligation to preserve life. McCormick insists, however, that the decision to allow an infant to die "must be made in terms of the child's good, this alone." That is, he would exclude utilitarian considerations such as the emotional and financial burden of caring for a severely defective child.

On February 24, the son of Mr. and Mrs. Robert H.T. Houle died following court-ordered emergency surgery at Maine Medical Center. The child was born February 9, horribly deformed. His entire left side was malformed; he had no left eye, was practically without a left ear, had a deformed left hand; some of his vertebrae were not fused. Furthermore, he was afflicted with a tracheal esophageal fistula and could not be fed by mouth. Air leaked into his stomach instead of going to the lungs, and fluid from the stomach pushed up into the lungs. As Dr. André Hellegers recently noted, "It takes little imagination to think there were further internal deformities" (*Obstetrical and Gynecological News*, April 1974).

As the days passed, the condition of the child deteriorated. Pneumonia set in. His reflexes became impaired and because of poor circulation, severe brain damage was suspected. The tracheal esophageal fistula, the immediate threat to his survival, can be corrected with relative ease by surgery. But in view of the associated complications and deformities, the parents refused their consent to surgery on "Baby Boy Houle." Several doctors in the Maine Medical Center felt dif-

ferently and took the case to court. Maine Superior Court Judge David G. Roberts ordered the surgery to be performed. He ruled: "At the moment of live birth there does exist a human being entitled to the fullest protection of the law. The most basic right enjoyed by every human being is the right to life itself."

"MEANINGFUL LIFE"

Instances like this happen frequently. In a recent issue of the *New England Journal of Medicine*, Drs. Raymond S. Duff and A.G.M. Campbell[1] reported on 299 deaths in the special-care nursery of the Yale-New Haven Hospital between 1970 and 1972. Of these, 43 (14%) were associated with discontinuance of treatment for children with multiple anomalies, trisomy, cardiopulmonary crippling, meningomyelocele, and other central nervous system defects. After careful consideration of each of these 43 infants, parents and physicians in a group decision concluded that the prognosis for "meaningful life" was extremely poor or hopeless, and therefore rejected further treatment. The abstract of the Duff-Campbell report states: "The awesome finality

Reprinted with permission of the author and the publisher from *Journal of the American Medical Association*, vol. 229 (July 8, 1974), pp. 172–176.

of these decisions, combined with a potential for error in prognosis, made the choice agonizing for families and health professionals. Nevertheless, the issue has to be faced, for not to decide is an arbitrary and potentially devastating decision of default."

In commenting on this study in the *Washington Post* (October 28, 1973), Dr. Lawrence K. Pickett, chief-of-staff at the Yale-New Haven Hospital, admitted that allowing hopelessly ill patients to die "is accepted medical practice." He continued: "This is nothing new. It's just being talked about now."

It has been talked about, it is safe to say, at least since the publicity associated with the famous "Johns Hopkins Case"[2] some three years ago. In this instance, an infant was born with Down's syndrome and duodenal atresia. The blockage is reparable by relatively easy surgery. However, after consultation with spiritual advisors, the parents refused permission for this corrective surgery, and the child died by starvation in the hospital after 15 days. To feed him by mouth in this condition would have killed him. Nearly everyone who has commented on this case has disagreed with the decision.

It must be obvious that these instances—and they are frequent—raise the most agonizing and delicate moral problems. The problem is best seen in the ambiguity of the term "hopelessly ill." This used to and still may refer to lives that cannot be saved, that are irretrievably in the dying process. It may also refer to lives that can be saved and sustained, but in a wretched, painful, or deformed condition. With regard to infants, the problem is, which infants, if any, should be allowed to die? On what grounds or according to what criteria, as determined by whom? Or again, is there a point at which a life that can be saved is not "meaningful life," as the medical community so often phrases the question?...

Thus far, the ethical discussion of these truly terrifying decisions has been less than fully satisfactory. Perhaps this is to be expected since the problems have only recently come to public attention. In a companion article to the Duff-Campbell report,[1] Dr. Anthony Shaw[3] of the Pediatric Division of the Department of Surgery, University of Virginia Medical Center, Charlottesville, speaks of solutions "based on the circumstances of each case rather than by means of a dogmatic formula approach." Are these really the only options available to us? Shaw's statement makes it appear that the ethical alternatives are narrowed to dogmatism (which imposes a formula that prescinds from circum-

stances) and pure concretism (which denies the possibility of usefulness of any guidelines).

ARE GUIDELINES POSSIBLE?

Such either-or extremism is understandable. It is easy for the medical profession, in its fully justified concern with the terrible concreteness of these problems and with the issue of who makes these decisions, to trend away from any substantive guidelines. As *Time* remarked in reporting these instances: "Few, if any, doctors are willing to establish guidelines for determining which babies should receive lifesaving surgery or treatment and which should not" (*Time*, March 25, 1974). On the other hand, moral theologians, in their fully justified concern to avoid total normlessness and arbitrariness wherein the right is "discovered," or really "created," only in and by brute decision, can easily be insensitive to the moral relevance of the raw experience, of the conflicting tensions and concerns provoked through direct cradleside contact with human events and persons.

But is there no middle course between sheer concretism and dogmatism? I believe there is. Dr. Franz J. Ingelfinger,[4] editor of the *New England Journal of Medicine*, in an editorial on the Duff-Campbell-Shaw articles, concluded, even if somewhat reluctantly: "Society, ethics, institutional attitudes and committees can provide the broad guidelines, but the onus of decision-making ultimately falls on the doctor in whose care the child has been put." Similarly, Frederick Carney of Southern Methodist University, Dallas, and the Kennedy Institute...stated of these cases: "What is obviously needed is the development of substantive standards to inform parents and physicians who must make such decisions" (*Washington Post*, March 20, 1974).

"Broad guidelines," "substantive standards." There is the middle course, and it is the task of a community broader than the medical community. A guideline is not a slide rule that makes the decision. It is far less than that. But it is far more than the concrete decision of the parents and the physician, however seriously and conscientiously this is made. It is more like a light in a room, a light that allows the individual objects to be seen in the fullness of their context. Concretely, if there are certain infants that we agree ought to be saved in spite of illness or deformity, and if there are certain infants that we agree should be allowed to die, then there is a line to be drawn. And if there is a line to be drawn, there ought to be some criteria, even if very general, for doing this. Thus, if nearly every commentator has disagreed with the Hopkins decision, should we not be able to distill from such consensus some general wisdom that will inform and guide future decisions? I think so.

The task is not easy. Indeed, it is so harrowing that the really tempting thing is to run from it. The most sensitive, balanced, and penetrating study of the Hopkins case that I have seen is that of the University of Chicago's James Gustafson.[2] Gustafson disagreed with the decision of the Hopkins physicians to deny surgery to the mongoloid infant. In summarizing his dissent, he notes: "Why would I draw the line on a different side of mongolism than the physician did? While reasons can be given, one must recognize that there are intuitive elements, grounded in beliefs and profound feelings, that enter into particular judgments of this sort." He goes on to criticize the assessment made of the child's intelligence as too simplistic, and he proposes a much broader perspective on the meaning of suffering than seemed to have operated in the Hopkins decision. I am in full agreement with Gustafson's reflections and conclusions. But ultimately, he does not tell us where he would draw the line or why, only where he would *not*, and why.

This is very helpful already, and perhaps it is all that can be done. Dare we take the next step, the combination and analysis of such negative judgments to extract from them the positive criterion or criteria inescapably operative in them? Or more startlingly, dare we *not* if these decisions are already being made? Gustafson is certainly right in saying that we cannot always establish perfectly rational accounts and norms for our decisions. But I believe we must never cease trying, in fear and trembling to be sure. Otherwise, we have exempted these decisions in principle from the one critique and control that protects against abuse. Exemption of this sort is the root of all exploitation whether personal or political. Briefly, if we must face the frightening task of making quality-of-life judgments—and we must—then we must face the difficult task of building criteria for these judgments.

FACING RESPONSIBILITY

What has brought us to this position of awesome responsibility? Very simply, the sophistication of modern medicine. Contemporary resuscitation and life-sustaining devices have brought a remarkable change in the state of the question. Our duties toward the care

and preservation of life have been traditionally stated in terms of the use of ordinary and extraordinary means. For the moment and for purposes of brevity, we may say that, morally speaking, ordinary means are those whose use does not entail grave hardships to the patient. Those that would involve such hardship are extraordinary. Granted the relativity of these terms and the frequent difficulty of their application, still the distinction has had an honored place in medical ethics and medical practice. Indeed, the distinction was recently reiterated by the House of Delegates of the American Medical Association in a policy statement. After disowning intentional killing (mercy killing), the AMA statement continues: "The cessation of the employment of extraordinary means to prolong the life of the body when there is irrefutable evidence that biological death is imminent is the decision of the patient and/or his immediate family. The advice and judgment of the physician should be freely available to the patient and/or his immediate family" (JAMA 227:728, 1974).

This distinction can take us just so far—and thus the change in the state of the question. The contemporary problem is precisely that the question no longer concerns only those for whom "biological death is imminent" in the sense of the AMA statement. Many infants who would have died a decade ago, whose "biological death was imminent," can be saved. Yesterday's failures are today's successes. Contemporary medicine with its team approaches, staged surgical techniques, monitoring capabilities, ventilatory support systems, and other methods, can keep almost anyone alive. This has tended gradually to shift the problem from the means to reverse the dying process to the quality of the life sustained and preserved. The questions, "Is this means too hazardous or difficult to use" and "Does this measure only prolong the patient's dying," while still useful and valid, now often become "Granted that we can easily save the life, what kind of life are we saving?" This is a quality-of-life judgment. And we fear it. And certainly we should. But with increased power goes increased responsibility. Since we have the power, we must face the responsibility.

A RELATIVE GOOD

In the past, the Judeo-Christian tradition has attempted to walk a balanced middle path between medical vitalism (that preserves life at any cost) and medical pessimism (that kills when life seems frustrating, burdensome, "useless"). Both of these extremes root in an identical idolatry of life—an attitude that, at least by inference, views death as an unmitigated, absolute evil, and life as the absolute good. The middle course that has structured Judeo-Christian attitudes is that life is indeed a basic and precious good, but a good to be preserved precisely as the condition of other values. It is these other values and possibilities that found the duty to preserve physical life and also dictate the limits of this duty. In other words, life is a relative good, and the duty to preserve it a limited one. These limits have always been stated in terms of the *means* required to sustain life. But if the implications of this middle position are unpacked a bit, they will allow us, perhaps, to adapt to the type of quality-of-life judgment we are now called on to make without tumbling into vitalism or a utilitarian pessimism.

A beginning can be made with a statement of Pope Pius XII[5] in an allocution to physicians delivered November 24, 1957. After noting that we are normally obliged to use only ordinary means to preserve life, the Pontiff stated: "A more strict obligation would be too burdensome for most men and would render the attainment of the higher, more important good too difficult. Life, death, all temporal activities are in fact subordinated to spiritual ends." Here it would be helpful to ask two questions. First, what are these spiritual ends, this "higher, more important good"? Second, how is its attainment rendered too difficult by insisting on the use of extraordinary means to preserve life?

The first question must be answered in terms of love of God and neighbor. This sums up briefly the meaning, substance and consummation of life from a Judeo-Christian perspective. What is or can easily be missed is that these two loves are not separable. St. John wrote: "If any man says 'I love God' and hates his brother, he is a liar. For he who loves not his brother, whom he sees, how can he love God whom he does not see?" (I John 4:20–21). This means that our love of neighbor is in some very real sense our love of God. The good our love wants to do Him and to which He enables us, can be done only for the neighbor, as Karl Rahner has so forcefully argued. It is in others that God demands to be recognized and loved. If this is true, it means that, in Judeo-Christian perspective, the meaning, substance, and consummation of life is found in human *relationships*, and the qualities of justice, respect, concern, compassion, and support that surround them.

Second, how is the attainment of this "higher, more important (than life) good" rendered "too difficult" by

life-supports that are gravely burdensome? One who must support his life with disproportionate effort focuses the time, attention, energy, and resources of himself and others not precisely on relationships, but on maintaining the condition of relationships. Such concentration easily becomes overconcentration and distorts one's view of and weakens one's pursuit of the very relational goods that define our growth and flourishing. The importance of relationships gets lost in the struggle for survival. The very Judeo-Christian meaning of life is seriously jeopardized when undue and unending effort must go into its maintenance....

THE QUALITY OF LIFE

...Life's potentiality for other values is dependent on two factors, those external to the individual, and the very condition of the individual. The former we can and must change to maximize individual potential. That is what social justice is all about. The latter we sometimes cannot alter. It is neither inhuman nor unchristian to say that there comes a point where an individual's condition itself represents the negation of any truly human—i.e., relational—potential. When that point is reached, is not the best treatment no treatment? I believe that the *implications* of the traditional distinction between ordinary and extraordinary means point in this direction.

In this tradition, life is not a value to be preserved in and for itself. To maintain that would commit us to a form of medical vitalism that makes no human or Judeo-Christian sense. It is a value to be preserved precisely as a condition for other values, and therefore insofar as these other values remain attainable. Since these other values cluster around and are rooted in human relationships, it seems to follow that life is a value to be preserved only insofar as it contains some potentiality for human relationships. When in human judgment this potentiality is totally absent or would be, because of the condition of the individual, totally subordinated to the mere effort for survival, that life can be said to have achieved its potential.

HUMAN RELATIONSHIPS

If these reflections are valid, they point in the direction of a guideline that may help in decisions about sustaining the lives of grossly deformed and deprived infants. That guideline is the potential for human relationships associated with the infant's condition. If that potential is simply nonexistent or would be utterly submerged and undeveloped in the mere struggle to survive, that life has achieved its potential. There are those who will want to continue to say that some terribly deformed infants may be allowed to die *because* no extraordinary means need be used. Fair enough. But they should realize that the term "extraordinary" has been so relativized to the condition of the patient that it is this condition that is decisive. The means are extraordinary because the infant's condition is extraordinary. And if that is so, we must face this fact head-on—and discover the substantive standard that allows us to say this of some infants, but not of others.

Here several caveats are in order. First, this guideline is not a detailed rule that preempts decisions; for relational capacity is not subject to mathematical analysis but to human judgment. However, it is the task of physicians to provide some more concrete categories or presumptive biological symptoms for this human judgment. For instance, nearly all would very likely agree that the anencephalic infant is without relational potential. On the other hand, the same cannot be said of the mongoloid infant. The task ahead is to attach relational potential to presumptive biological symptoms for the gray area between such extremes. In other words, individual decisions will remain the anguishing onus of parents in consultation with physicians.

Second, because this guideline is precisely that, mistakes will be made. Some infants will be judged in all sincerity to be devoid of any meaningful relational potential when that is actually not quite the case. This risk of error should not lead to abandonment of decisions; for that is to walk away from the human scene. Risk of error means only that we must proceed with great humility, caution, and tentativeness. Concretely, it means that if err we must at times, it is better to err on the side of life—and therefore to tilt in that direction.

Third, it must be emphasized that allowing some infants to die does not imply that "some lives are valuable, other not" or that "there is such a thing as a life not worth living." Every human being, regardless of age or condition, is of incalculable worth. The point is not, therefore, whether this or that individual has value. Of course he has, or rather *is* a value. The only point is whether this undoubted value has any potential at all, in continuing physical survival, for attaining a share, even if reduced, in the "higher, more important good." This is not a question about the inherent value of the individual. It is a question about whether this

worldly existence will offer such a valued individual any hope of sharing those values for which physical life is the fundamental condition. Is not the only alternative an attitude that supports mere physical life as long as possible with every means?

Fourth, this whole matter is further complicated by the fact that this decision is being made for someone else. Should not the decision on whether life is to be supported or not be left to the individual? Obviously, wherever possible. But there is nothing inherently objectionable in the fact that parents with physicians must make this decision at some point for infants. Parents must make many crucial decisions for children. The only concern is that the decision not be shaped out of the utilitarian perspectives so deeply sunk into the consciousness of the contemporary world. In a highly technological culture, an individual is always in danger of being valued for his function, what he can do, rather than for who he is.

It remains, then, only to emphasize that these decisions must be made in terms of the child's good, this alone. But that good, as fundamentally a relational good, has many dimensions. Pius XII,[5] in speaking of the duty to preserve life, noted that this duty "derives from well-ordered charity, from submission to the Creator, from social justice, as well as from devotion towards his family." All of these considerations pertain to that "higher, more important good." If that is the case with the duty to preserve life, then the decision not to preserve life must likewise take all of these into account in determining what is for the child's good.

Any discussion of this problem would be incomplete if it did not repeatedly stress that it is the pride of the Judeo-Christian tradition that the weak and defenseless, the powerless and unwanted, those whose grasp on the goods of life is most fragile—that is, those whose potential is real but reduced—are cherished and protected as our neighbor in greatest need. Any application of a general guideline that forgets this is but a racism of the adult world profoundly at odds with the gospel, and eventually corrosive of the humanity of those who ought to be caring and supporting as long as that care and support has human meaning. It has meaning as long as there is hope that the infant will, in relative comfort, be able to experience our caring and love. For when this happens, both we and the child are sharing in that "greater, more important good."

Were not those who disagreed with the Hopkins decision saying, in effect, that for the infant, involved human relationships were still within reach and would not be totally submerged by survival? If that is the case, it is potential for relationships that is at the heart of these agonizing decisions.

REFERENCES

1 Duff S., Campbell A.G.M.: "Moral and ethical dilemmas in the special-care nursery." *N Engl J Med* 289:890–894, 1973.

2 Gustafson J.M.: "Mongolism, parental desires, and the right to life." *Perspect Biol Med* 16:529–559, 1973.

3 Shaw A.: "Dilemmas of 'informed' consent in children." *N Engl J Med* 289:885–890, 1973.

4 Ingelfinger F.: "Bedside ethics for the hopeless case." *N Engl J Med* 289:914, 1973.

5 Pope Pius XII: *Acta Apostolicae Sedis* 49:1031–1032, 1957.

Ethical Issues in Aiding the Death of Young Children

H. Tristram Engelhardt, Jr.

A biographical sketch of H. Tristram Engelhardt, Jr., is found on page 254.

After reviewing the differences between the euthanasia of adults and the euthanasia of children, Engelhardt focuses attention on the status of children. In his view, young children are not persons in a strict sense. Rather, they are persons only in "a social sense," by virtue of their role in a family and society. Since young children "belong" to their parents, it is the parents who are the proper decision makers with regard to the treatment or nontreatment of severely defective newborns. Engelhardt finds it morally acceptable to allow a severely defective newborn to die when (1) it is unlikely that the child can attain a "good quality of life" (i.e., a developed personal life) and/or (2) it seems clear that providing continued care for the child would constitute a "severe burden" for the family. It is Engelhardt's incorporation of a cost factor that principally distinguishes his view from that of McCormick. Engelhardt goes on to develop the concept of "the injury of continued existence," arguing that a child has a right not to have its life prolonged in those cases where life would be painful and futile. Thus, he maintains, allowing a severely defective newborn to die (in some cases) is not only *morally acceptable* but indeed *morally demanded*. In concluding, Engelhardt briefly discusses the justifiability of active euthanasia of severely defective newborns.

Euthanasia in the pediatric age group involves a constellation of issues that are materially different from those of adult euthanasia.[1] The difference lies in the somewhat obvious fact that infants and young children are not able to decide about their own futures and thus are not persons in the same sense that normal adults are. While adults usually decide their own fate, others decide on behalf of young children. Although one can argue that euthanasia is or should be a personal right, the sense of such an argument is obscure with respect to children. Young children do not have any personal rights, at least none that they can exercise on their own

behalf with regard to the manner of their life and death. As a result, euthanasia of young children raises special questions concerning the standing of the rights of children, the status of parental rights, the obligations of adults to prevent the suffering of children, and the possible effects on society of allowing or expediting the death of seriously defective infants.

What I will refer to as the euthanasia of infants and young children might be termed by others infanticide, while some cases might be termed the withholding of extraordinary life-prolonging treatment.[2] One needs a term that will encompass both death that results from active intervention and death that ensues when one simply ceases further therapy.[3] In using such a term, one must recognize that death is often not directly but only obliquely intended. That is, one often intends only to treat no further, not actually to have death follow, even though one knows death will follow.[4]

Finally, one must realize that deaths as the result of withholding treatment constitute a significant proportion of neonatal deaths. For example, as high as 14 percent of children in one hospital have been identified as dying after a decision was made not to treat further, the presumption being that the children would have lived longer had treatment been offered.[5]

Even popular magazines have presented accounts of parental decisions not to pursue treatment.[6] These decisions often involve a choice between expensive treatment with little chance of achieving a full, normal life for the child and "letting nature take its course," with the child dying as a result of its defects. As this suggests, many of these problems are products of medical progress. Such children in the past would have died. The quandaries are in a sense an embarrassment of riches; now that one *can* treat such defective children, *must* one treat them? And, if one need not treat such defective children, may one expedite their death?

I will here briefly examine some of these issues. First, I will review differences that contrast the euthanasia of adults to euthanasia of children. Second, I will review the issue of the rights of parents and the status of children. Third, I will suggest a new notion, the concept of the "injury of continued existence," and draw out some of its implications with respect to a duty to prevent suffering. Finally, I will outline some important questions that remain unanswered even if the foregoing issues can be settled. In all, I hope more to display the issues involved in a difficult question than to advance a particular set of answers to particular dilemmas.

For the purpose of this paper, I will presume that adult euthanasia can be justified by an appeal to freedom. In the face of imminent death, one is usually choosing between a more painful and more protracted dying and a less painful or less protracted dying, in circumstances where either choice makes little difference with regard to the discharge of social duties and responsibilities. In the case of suicide, we might argue that, in general, social duties (for example, the duty to support one's family) restrain one from taking one's own life. But in the face of imminent death and in the

presence of the pain and deterioration of a fatal disease, such duties are usually impossible to discharge and are thus rendered moot. One can, for example, picture an extreme case of an adult with a widely disseminated carcinoma, including metastases to the brain, who because of severe pain and debilitation is no longer capable of discharging any social duties. In these and similar circumstances, euthanasia becomes the issue of the right to control one's own body, even to the point of seeking assistance in suicide. Euthanasia is, as such, the issue of assisted suicide, the universalization of a maxim that all persons should be free, *in extremis*, to decide with regard to the circumstances of their death.

Further, the choice of positive euthanasia could be defended as the more rational choice: the choice of a less painful death and the affirmation of the value of a rational life. In so choosing, one would be acting to set limits to one's life in order not to live when pain and physical and mental deterioration make further rational life impossible. The choice to end one's life can be understood as a noncontradictory willing of a smaller set of states of existence for oneself, a set that would not include a painful death. As such, it would not involve a desire to destroy oneself. That is, adult euthanasia can be construed as an affirmation of the rationality and autonomy of the self.[7]

The remarks above focus on the active or positive euthanasia of adults. But they hold as well concerning what is often called passive or negative euthanasia, the refusal of life-prolonging therapy. In such cases, the patient's refusal of life-prolonging therapy is seen to be a right that derives from personal freedom, or at least from a zone of privacy into which there are no good grounds for social intervention.[8]

Again, none of these considerations apply directly to the euthanasia of young children, because they cannot participate in such decisions. Whatever else pediatric, in particular neonatal, euthanasia involves, it surely involves issues different from those of adult euthanasia. Since infants and small children cannot commit suicide, their right to assisted suicide is difficult to pose. The difference between the euthanasia of young children and that of adults resides in the difference between children and adults. The difference, in fact, raises the troublesome question of whether young children are persons, or at least whether they are persons in the sense in which adults are. Answering that question will resolve in part at least the right of others to decide whether a young child should live or die and whether he should receive life-prolonging treatment.

THE STATUS OF CHILDREN

Adults belong to themselves in the sense that they are rational and free and therefore responsible for their actions. Adults are *sui juris*. Young children, though, are neither self-possessed nor responsible. While adults exist in and for themselves, as self-directive and self-conscious beings, young children, especially newborn infants, exist for their families and those who love them. They are not, nor can they in any sense be, responsible for themselves. If being a person is to be a responsible agent, a bearer of rights and duties, children are not persons in a strict sense. They are, rather, persons in a social sense: others must act on their behalf and bear responsibility for them. They are, as it were, entities defined by their place in social roles (for example, mother-child, family-child) rather than beings that define themselves as persons, that is, in and through themselves. Young children live as persons in and through the care of those who are responsible for them, and those responsible for them exercise the children's rights on their behalf. In this sense children belong to families in ways that most adults do not. They exist in and through their family and society.

Treating young children with respect has, then, a sense different from treating adults with respect. One can respect neither a newborn infant's or very young child's wishes nor its freedom. In fact, a newborn infant or young child is more an entity that is valued highly because it will grow to be a person and because it plays a social role as if it were a person.[9] That is, a small child is treated as if it were a person in social roles such as mother-child and family-child relationships, though strictly speaking the child is in no way capable of claiming or being responsible for the rights imputed to it. All the rights and duties of the child are exercised and "held in trust" by others for a future time and for a person yet to develop.

Medical decisions to treat or not to treat a neonate or small child often turn on the probability and cost of achieving that future status—a developed personal life. The usual practice of letting anencephalic children (who congenitally lack all or most of the brain) die can be understood as a decision based on the absence of the possibility of achieving a personal life. The practice of refusing treatment to at least some children born with meningomyelocele can be justified through a similar, but more utilitarian, calculus. In the case of anencephalic children one might argue that care for them as persons is futile since they will never be persons. In the case of a child with meningomyelocele, one might argue that when the cost of cure would likely be very high and the probable lifestyle open to attainment very truncated, there is not a positive duty to make a large investment of money and suffering. One should note that the cost here must include not only financial costs but also the anxiety and suffering that prolonged and uncertain treatment of the child would cause the parents.

This further raises the issue of the scope of positive duties not only when there is no person present in a strict sense, but when the likelihood of a full human life is also very uncertain. Clinical and parental judgment may and should be guided by the expected lifestyle and the cost (in parental and societal pain and money) of its attainment. The decision about treatment, however, belongs properly to the parents because the child belongs to them in a sense that it does not belong to anyone else, even to itself. The care and raising of the child falls to the parents, and when considerable cost and little prospect of reasonable success are present, the parents may properly decide against life-prolonging treatment.

The physician's role is to present sufficient information in a usable form to the parents to aid them in making a decision. The accent is on the absence of a positive duty to treat in the presence of severe inconvenience (costs) to the parents; treatment that is very costly is not obligatory. What is suggested here is a general notion that there is never a duty to engage in extraordinary treatment and that "extraordinary" can be defined in terms of costs. This argument concerns children (1) whose future quality of life is likely to be seriously compromised and (2) whose present treatment would be very costly. The issue is that of the circumstances under which parents would not be obliged to take on severe burdens on behalf of their children or those circumstances under which society would not be so obliged. The argument should hold as well for those cases where the expected future life would surely be of normal quality, though its attainment would be extremely costly. The fact of little likelihood of success in attaining a normal life for the child makes decisions to do without treatment more plausible because the hope of success is even more remote and therefore the burden borne by parents or society becomes in that sense more extraordinary. But very high costs themselves could be a sufficient criterion, though in actual cases judgments in that regard would be very difficult when a normal life could be expected.[10]

The decisions in these matters correctly lie in the hands of the parents, because it is primarily in terms of the family that children exist and develop—until children become persons strictly, they are persons in virtue of their social roles. As long as parents do not unjustifiably neglect the humans in those roles so that the value and purpose of that role (that is, child) stands to be eroded (thus endangering other children), society need not intervene. In short, parents may decide for or against the treatment of their severely deformed children.

However, society has a right to intervene and protect children for whom parents refuse care (including treatment) when such care does not constitute a severe burden and when it is likely that the child could be brought to a good quality of life. Obviously, "severe burden" and "good quality of life" will be difficult to define and their meanings will vary, just as it is always difficult to say when grains of sand dropped on a table constitute a heap. At most, though, society need only intervene when the grains clearly do not constitute a heap, that is, when it is clear that the burden is light and the chance of a good quality of life for the child is high. A small child's dependence on his parents is so essential that society need intervene only when the absence of intervention would lead to the role "child" being undermined. Society must value mother-child and family-child relationships and should intervene only in cases where (1) neglect is unreasonable and therefore would undermine respect and care for children, or (2) where societal intervention would prevent children from suffering unnecessary pain.[11]

THE INJURY OF CONTINUED EXISTENCE

But there is another viewpoint that must be considered: that of the child or even the person that the child might become. It might be argued that the child has a right not to have its life prolonged. The idea that forcing existence on a child could be wrong is a difficult notion, which, if true, would serve to amplify the foregoing argument. Such an argument would allow the construal of the issue in terms of the perspective of the child, that is, in terms of a duty not to treat in circumstances where treatment would only prolong suffering. In particular, it would at least give a framework for a decision to stop treatment in cases where, though the costs of treatment are not high, the child's existence would be characterized by severe pain and deprivation.

A basis for speaking of continuing existence as an injury to the child is suggested by the proposed legal concept of "wrongful life." A number of suits have been initiated in the United States and in other countries on the grounds that life or existence itself is, under certain circumstances, a tort or injury to the living person.[12] Although thus far all such suits have ultimately failed, some have succeeded in their initial stages. Two examples may be instructive. In each case the ability to receive recompense for the injury (the tort) presupposed the existence of the individual, whose existence was itself the injury. In one case a suit was initiated on behalf of a child against his father alleging that his father's siring him out of wedlock was an injury to the child.[13] In another case a suit on behalf of a child born of an inmate of a state mental hospital impregnated by rape in that institution was brought against the state of New York.[14] The suit was brought on the grounds that being born with such historical antecedents was itself an injury for which recovery was due. Both cases presupposed that nonexistence would have been preferable to the conditions under which the person born was forced to live.

The suits for tort for wrongful life raise the issue not only of when it would be preferable not to have been born but also of when it would be *wrong* to cause a person to be born. This implies that someone should have judged that it would have been preferable for the child never to have had existence, never to have been in the position to judge that the particular circumstances of life were intolerable.[15] Further, it implies that the person's existence under those circumstances should have been prevented and that, not having been prevented, life was not a gift but an injury. The concept of tort for wrongful life raises an issue concerning the responsibility for giving another person existence, namely, the notion that giving life is not always necessarily a good and justifiable action. Instead, in certain circumstances, so it has been argued, one may have a duty *not* to give existence to another person. This concept involves the claim that certain qualities of life have a negative value, making life an injury, not a gift; it involves, in short, a concept of human accountability and responsibility for human life. It contrasts with the notion that life is a gift of God and thus similar to other "acts of God" (that is, events for which no man is accountable). The concept thus signals the fact that humans can now control reproduction and that where rational control is possible humans are accountable. That is, the expansion of human capabilities has resulted in an expansion of human responsibilities such that one must now decide when and under what circumstances persons will come into existence.

The concept of tort for wrongful life is transferable in part to the painfully compromised existence of children who can only have their life prolonged for a short, painful, and marginal existence. The concept suggests that allowing life to be prolonged under such circumstances would itself be an injury of the person whose painful and severely compromised existence would be made to continue. In fact, it suggests that there is a duty not to prolong life if it can be determined to have a substantial negative value for the person involved.[16] Such issues are moot in the case of adults, who can and should decide for themselves. But small children cannot make such a choice. For them it is an issue of justifying prolonging life under circumstances of painful and compromised existence. Or, put differently, such cases indicate the need to develop social canons to allow a decent death for children for whom the only possibility is protracted, painful suffering.

I do not mean to imply that one should develop a new basis for civil damages. In the field of medicine, the need is to recognize an ethical category, a concept of wrongful continuance of existence, not a new legal right. The concept of injury for continuance of existence, the proposed analogue of the concept of tort for wrongful life, presupposes that life can be of a negative value such that the medical maxim *primum non nocere* ("first do no harm") would require not sustaining life.[17]

The idea of responsibility for acts that sustain or prolong life is cardinal to the notion that one should not under certain circumstances further prolong the life of a child. Unlike adults, children cannot decide with regard to euthanasia (positive or negative), and if more than a utilitarian justification is sought, it must be sought in a duty not to inflict life on another person in circumstances where that life would be painful and futile. This position must rest on the facts that (1) medicine now can cause the prolongation of the life of seriously deformed children who in the past would have died young and that (2) it is not clear that life so prolonged is a good for the child. Further, the choice is

made not on the basis of costs to the parents or to society but on the basis of the child's suffering and compromised existence.

The difficulty lies in determining what makes life not worth living for a child. Answers could never be clear. It seems reasonable, however, that the life of children with diseases that involve pain and no hope of survival should not be prolonged. In the case of Tay-Sachs disease (a disease marked by a progressive increase in spasticity and dementia usually leading to death at age three or four), one can hardly imagine that the terminal stages of spastic reaction to stimuli and great difficulty in swallowing are at all pleasant to the child (even insofar as it can only minimally perceive its circumstances). If such a child develops aspiration pneumonia and is treated, it can reasonably be said that to prolong its life is to inflict suffering. Other diseases give fairly clear portraits of lives not worth living: for example, Lesch-Nyhan disease, which is marked by mental retardation and compulsive self-mutilation.

The issue is more difficult in the case of children with diseases for whom the prospects for normal intelligence and a fair lifestyle do exist, but where these chances are remote and their realization expensive. Children born with meningomyelocele present this dilemma. Imagine, for example, a child that falls within Lorber's fifth category (an IQ of sixty or less, sometimes blind, subject to fits, and always incontinent). Such a child has little prospect of anything approaching a normal life, and there is a good chance of its dying even with treatment.[18] But such judgments are statistical. And if one does not treat such children, some will still survive and, as John Freeman indicates, be worse off if not treated.[19] In such cases one is in a dilemma. If one always treats, one must justify extending the life of those who will ultimately die anyway and in the process subjecting them to the morbidity of multiple surgical procedures. How remote does the prospect of a good life have to be in order not to be worth great pain and expense?[20] It is probably best to decide, in the absence of a positive duty to treat, on the basis of the cost and suffering to parents and society. But, as Freeman argues, the prospect of prolonged or even increased suffering raises the issue of active euthanasia.[21]

If the child is not a person strictly, and if death is inevitable and expediting it would diminish the child's pain prior to death, then it would seem to follow that, all else being equal, a decision for active euthanasia would be permissible, even obligatory.[22] The difficulty lies with "all else being equal," for it is doubtful that active euthanasia could be established as a practice without eroding and endangering children generally, since, as John Lorber has pointed out, children cannot speak in their own behalf.[23] Thus, although there is no argument in principle against the active euthanasia of small children, there could be an argument against such practices based on questions of prudence. To put it another way, even though one might have a duty to hasten the death of a particular child, one's duty to protect children in general could override that first duty. The issue of active euthanasia turns in the end on whether it would have social consequences that refraining would not, on whether (1) it is possible to establish procedural safeguards for limited active euthanasia and (2) whether such practices would have a significant adverse effect on the treatment of small children in general. But since these are procedural issues dependent on sociological facts, they are not open to an answer within the confines of this article. In any event, the concept of the injury of continued existence provides a basis for the justification of the passive euthanasia of small children—a practice already widespread and somewhat established in our society—beyond the mere absence of a positive duty to treat.[24]

CONCLUSION

Though the lack of certainty concerning questions such as the prognosis of particular patients and the social consequence of active euthanasia of children prevents a clear answer to all the issues raised by the euthanasia of infants, it would seem that this much can be maintained: (1) Since children are not persons strictly but exist in and through their families, parents are the appropriate ones to decide whether or not to treat a deformed child when *(a)* there is not only little likelihood of full human life but also great likelihood of suffering if the life is prolonged, or *(b)* when the cost of prolonging life is very great. Such decisions must be made in consort with a physician who can accurately give estimates of cost and prognosis and who will be able to help the parents with the consequences of their decision. (2) It is reasonable to speak of a duty not to treat a small child when such treatment will only prolong a painful life or would in any event lead to a painful death. Though this does not by any means answer all the questions, it does point out an important fact—that

medicine's duty is not always to prolong life doggedly but sometimes is quite the contrary.

NOTES

1 I am grateful to Laurence B. McCullough and James P. Morris for their critical discussion of this paper. They may be responsible for its virtues, but not for its shortcomings.

2 The concept of extraordinary treatment as it has been developed in Catholic moral theology is useful: treatment is extraordinary and therefore not obligatory if it involves great costs, pain, or inconvenience, and is a grave burden to oneself or others without a reasonable expectation that such treatment would be successful. See Gerald Kelly, S.J., *Medico-Moral Problems* (St. Louis: The Catholic Hospital Association Press, 1958), pp. 128–141. Difficulties are hidden in terms such as "great costs" and "reasonable expectation," as well as in terms such as "successful." Such ambiguity reflects the fact that precise operational definitions are not available. That is, the precise meaning of "great," "reasonable," and "successful" are inextricably bound to particular circumstances, especially particular societies.

3 I will use the term euthanasia in a broad sense to indicate a deliberately chosen course of action or inaction that is known at the time of decision to be such as will expedite death. This use of euthanasia will encompass not only positive or active euthanasia (acting in order to expedite death) and negative or passive euthanasia (refraining from action in order to expedite death), but acting and refraining in the absence of a direct intention that death occur more quickly (that is, those cases that fall under the concept of double effect). See note 4.

4 But, both active and passive euthanasia can be appreciated in terms of the Catholic moral notion of double effect. When the doctrine of double effect is invoked, one is strictly not intending euthanasia, but rather one intends something else. That concept allows actions or omissions that lead to death (1) because it is licit not to prolong life *in extremis* (allowing death is not an intrinsic evil), (2) if death is not actually willed or actively sought (that is, the evil is not directly willed), (3) if that which is willed is a major good (for example, avoiding useless major expenditure of resources or serious pain),

and (4) if the good is not achieved by means of the evil (for example, one does not will to save resources or diminish pain *by* the death). With regard to euthanasia the doctrine of double effect means that one need not expend major resources in an endeavor that will not bring health but only prolong dying and that one may use drugs that decrease pain but hasten death. See Richard McCormick, *Ambiguity in Moral Choice* (Milwaukee: Marquette University Press, 1973). I exclude the issue of double effect from my discussion because I am interested in those cases in which the good may follow directly from the evil—the death of the child. In part, though, the second section of this paper is concerned with the concept of proportionate good.

5 Raymond S. Duff and A.G.M. Campbell, "Moral and Ethical Dilemmas in the Special-Care Nursery," *The New England Journal of Medicine*, 289 (Oct. 25, 1973), pp. 890–894.

6 Roger Pell, "The Agonizing Decision of Joanne and Roger Pell," *Good Housekeeping* (January 1972), pp. 76–77, 131–135.

7 This somewhat Kantian argument is obviously made in opposition to Kant's position that suicide involves a default of one's duty to oneself "...to preserve his life simply because he is a person and must therefore recognize a duty to himself (and a strict one at that)," as well as a contradictory volition: "that man ought to have the authorization to withdraw himself from all obligation, that is, to be free to act as if no authorization at all were required for this withdrawal, involves a contradiction. To destroy the subject of morality in his own person is tantamount to obliterating from the world..." Immanuel Kant, *The Metaphysical Principles of Virtue: Part II of the Metaphysics of Morals*, trans. James Ellington (Indianapolis: Bobbs-Merrill, 1964), p. 83; Akademie Edition, VI, 422–423.

8 Norman L. Cantor, "A Patient's Decision To Decline Life-Saving Medical Treatment: Bodily Integrity Versus the Preservation of Life," *Rutgers Law Review*, 26 (Winter 1972), p. 239.

9 By "young child" I mean either an infant or child so young as not yet to be able to participate, in any sense, in a decision. A precise operational definition of "young child" would clearly be difficult to develop. It is also not clear how one would bring older children into such decisions. See, for example, Milton Viederman. "Saying 'No' to Hemodialysis:

Exploring Adaptation," and Daniel Burke, "Saying 'No' to Hemodialysis: An Acceptable Decision," both in *The Hastings Center Report*, 4 (September 1974), pp. 8–10, and John E. Schowalter, Julian B. Ferholt, and Nancy M. Mann, "The Adolescent Patient's Decision to Die," *Pediatrics*, 51 (January 1973), pp. 97–103.

10 An appeal to high costs alone is probably hidden in judgments based on statistics: even though there is a chance for a normal life for certain children with apparently severe cases of meningomyelocele, one is not obliged to treat since that chance is small, and the pursuit of that chance is very expensive. Cases of the costs being low but the expected suffering of the child being high will be discussed under the concept of the injury of continued existence. It should be noted that none of the arguments in this paper bear on cases where neither the cost nor the suffering of the child is considerable. Cases in this last category probably include, for example, children born with mongolism complicated only by duodenal atresia.

11 I have in mind here the issue of physicians, hospital administrators, or others being morally compelled to seek an injunction to force treatment of the child in the absence of parental consent. In these circumstances, the physician, who is usually best acquainted with the facts of the case, is the natural advocate of the child.

12 G. Tedeschi, "On Tort Liability for 'Wrongful Life,'" *Israel Law Review*, 1 (1966), p. 513.

13 Zepeda v. Zepeda: 41 Ill. App. 2d 240, 190 N.E. 2d 849 (1963).

14 Williams v. State of New York: 46 Misc. 2d 824, 260 N.Y.S. 2d 953 (Ct.Cl., 1965).

15 Torts: "Illegitimate Child Denied Recovery against Father for 'Wrongful Life,'" *Iowa Law Review*, 49 (1969), p. 1009.

16 It is one thing to have a conceptual definition of the injury of continued existence (for example, causing a person to continue to live under circumstances of severe pain and deprivation when there are no alternatives but death) and another to have an operational definition of that concept (that is, deciding what counts as such severe pain and deprivation). This article has focused on the first, not the second, issue.

17 H. Tristram Engelhardt, Jr., "Euthanasia and Children: The Injury of Continued Existence,"

The Journal of Pediatrics, 83 (July 1973), pp. 170–171.

18 John Lorber, "Results of Treatment of Myelomeningocele,' *Developmental Medicine and Child Neurology*, 13 (1971), p. 286.

19 John M. Freeman, "The Shortsighted Treatment of Myelomeningocele: A Long-Term Case Report," *Pediatrics*, 53 (March 1974), pp. 311–313.

20 John M. Freeman, "To Treat or Not to Treat," *Practical Management of Meningomyelocele,* ed. John Freeman (Baltimore: University Park Press, 1974), p. 21.

21 John Lorber, "Selective Treatment of Myelomeningocele: To Treat or Not to Treat," *Pediatrics*, 53 (March 1974), pp. 307–308.

22 I am presupposing that no intrinsic moral distinctions exist in cases such as these, between acting and refraining, between omitting care in the hope that death will ensue (that is, rather than the child living to be even more defective) and acting to ensure that death will ensue rather than having the child live under painful and seriously compromised circumstances. For a good discussion of the distinction between acting and refraining, see Jonathan Bennett, "Whatever the Consequences," *Analysis*, 26 (January 1966), pp. 83–102; P.J. Fitzgerald, "Acting and Refraining," *Analysis*, 27 (March 1967), pp. 133–139; Daniel Dinello, "On Killing and Letting Die," *Analysis*, 31 (April 1971), pp. 83–86.

23 Lorber, "Selective Treatment of Myelomeningocele," p. 308.

24 Positive duties involve a greater constraint than negative duties. Hence it is often easier to establish a duty not to do something (not to treat further) than a duty to do something (to actively hasten death). Even allowing a new practice to be permitted (for example, active euthanasia) requires a greater attention to consequences than does establishing the absence of a positive duty. For example, at common law there is no basis for action against a person who watches another drown without giving aid; this reflects the difficulty of establishing a positive duty.

Involuntary Euthanasia of Defective Newborns

John A. Robertson

John A. Robertson is professor of law at the School of Law, University of Texas at Austin. He is the author of *The Rights of the Critically Ill* (1983) and has published such articles as "Compensating Injured Research Subjects: The Law," "Medical Ethics in the Courtroom," and "Taking Consent Seriously: IRB Intervention in the Consent Process."

Robertson, in vivid contrast to Engelhardt, denies that the undesirable consequences of treating a severely defective newborn can morally justify the decision to withhold ordinary medical treatment. The consequentialist argument directly under attack by Robertson has two versions. One version is based on the suffering of the severely defective newborn, whereas the other version is based on the suffering of others (principally the family but also health professionals and society as a whole). The first version of the consequentialist argument, identified by Robertson as the "quality-of-life argument," maintains that withholding treatment is morally justified because the severely defective newborn is better off dead.

Although Robertson insists that it is often false that death is a better fate than continued life for the severely defective newborn, his fundamental objection to the quality-of-life argument stems from his reluctance to accept proxy assessments of quality-of-life. The second version of the consequentialist argument holds that withholding treatment is morally justified because of the emotional and financial burden falling on those who would have to provide the continued care for a severely defective child. Robertson's central objection to this version of the consequentialist argument has to do with its utilitarian spirit, but he also argues that it is seldom plausible to think that the suffering of others is so grave as to outweigh the defective newborn's interest in life.

One of the most perplexing dilemmas of modern medicine concerns whether "ordinary"[1] medical care justifiably can be withheld from defective newborns. Infants with malformations of the central nervous system[2] such as anencephaly,[3] hydrocephaly,[4] Down's syndrome,[5] spina bifida,[6] and myelomeningocele[7] often require routine surgical or medical attention[8] merely to stay alive. Until recent developments in surgery and pediatrics, these infants would have died of natural causes. Today with treatment many will survive for long periods, although some will be severely handicapped and limited in their potential for human satisfaction and interaction. Because in the case of some defective newborns, the chances are often slim that they will ever lead normal human lives, it is now common practice for parents to request, and for physicians to agree, not to treat such infants. Without treatment the infant usually dies....

If we reject the argument that defective newborns are not persons, the question remains whether circumstances exist in which the consequences of treatment as compared with nontreatment are so undesirable that the omission of care is justified....

... Many parents and physicians deeply committed to the loving care of the newborn think that treating severely defective infants causes more harm than good, thereby justifying the withholding of ordinary care. In their view the suffering and diminished quality of the child's life do not justify the social and economic costs of treatment. This claim has a growing commonsense appeal, but it assumes that the utility or quality of one's life can be measured and compared with other lives, and that health resources may legitimately be allocated to produce the greatest personal utility. This argument will now be analyzed from the perspective of the defective patient and others affected by his care.

A THE QUALITY OF THE DEFECTIVE INFANT'S LIFE

Comparisons of relative worth among persons, or between persons and other interests, raise moral and methodological issues that make any argument that relies on such comparisons extremely vulnerable. Thus the strongest claim for not treating the defective newborn is that treatment seriously harms the infant's own interests, whatever may be the effects on others. When maintaining his life involves great physical and psychosocial suffering for the patient, a reasonable person might conclude that such a life is not worth living. Presumably the patient, if fully informed and able to communicate, would agree. One then would be morally justified in withholding lifesaving treatment if such action served to advance the best interests of the patient.

Congenital malformations impair development in several ways that lead to the judgment that deformed retarded infants are "a burden to themselves."[9] One is the severe physical pain, much of it resulting from repeated surgery that defective infants will suffer. Defective children also are likely to develop other pathological features, leading to repeated fractures, dislocations, surgery, malfunctions, and other sources of pain. The shunt, for example, inserted to relieve hydrocephalus, a common problem in defective children, often becomes clogged, necessitating frequent surgical interventions.

Pain, however, may be intermittent and manageable with analgesics. Since many infants and adults experience great pain, and many defective infants do not, pain alone, if not totally unmanageable, does not sufficiently show that a life is so worthless that death is preferable. More important are the psychosocial deficits resulting from the child's handicaps. Many defective children never can walk even with prosthesis, never interact with normal children, never appreciate growth, adolescence, or the fulfillment of education and employment, and seldom are even able to care for themselves. In cases of severe retardation, they may be left with a vegetative existence in a crib, incapable of choice or the most minimal response to stimuli. Parents or others may reject them, and much of their time will be spent in hospitals, in surgery, or fighting the many illnesses that beset them. Can it be said that such a life is worth living?

There are two possible responses to the quality-of-life argument. One is to accept its premises but to question the degree of suffering in particular cases, and thus restrict the justification for death to the most extreme cases. The absence of opportunities for schooling, career, and interaction may be the fault of social attitudes and the failings of healthy persons, rather than a necessary result of congenital malformations. Psychosocial suffering occurs because healthy, normal persons reject or refuse to relate to the defective, or hurry them to poorly funded institutions. Most nonambulatory, mentally retarded persons can be trained for satisfying roles. One cannot assume that a nonproductive existence is necessarily unhappy: even social rejection and nonacceptance can be mitigated. Moreover, the psychosocial ills of the handicapped often do not differ in kind from those experienced by many persons. With training and care, growth, development, and a full range of experiences are possible for most people with physical and mental handicaps. Thus, the claim that death is a far better fate than life cannot in most cases be sustained.

This response, however, avoids meeting the quality-of-life argument on its strongest grounds. Even if many defective infants can experience growth, interaction, and most human satisfactions if nurtured, treated, and trained, some infants are so severely retarded or grossly deformed that their response to love and care, in fact their capacity to be conscious, is always minimal. Although mongoloid and nonambulatory spina bifida children may experience an existence we would hesitate to adjudge worse than death, the profoundly retarded, nonambulatory, blind, deaf infant who will spend his few years in the back-ward cribs of a state institution is clearly a different matter.

To repudiate the quality-of-life argument, therefore, requires a defense of treatment in even these extreme cases. Such a defense would question the validity of any surrogate or proxy judgments of the worth or quality of life when the wishes of the person in question cannot be ascertained. The essence of the quality-of-life argument is a proxy's judgment that no reasonable person can prefer the pain, suffering, and loneliness of, for example, life in a crib at an IQ level of 20, to an immediate, painless death.

But in what sense can the proxy validly conclude that a person with different wants, needs, and interests, if able to speak, would agree that such a life were worse than death? At the start one must be skeptical of the proxy's claim to objective disinterestedness. If the proxy is also the parent or physician, as has been the case in pediatric euthanasia, the impact of treatment on the proxy's interests, rather than solely on those of the child, may influence his assessment. But even if the proxy were truly neutral and committed only to caring for the child, the problem of egocentricity and knowing another's mind remains. Compared with the situation and life prospects of a "reasonable man," the child's potential quality of life indeed appears dim. Yet a standard based on healthy, ordinary development may be entirely inappropriate to this situation. One who has never known the pleasures of mental operation, ambulation, and social interaction surely does not suffer from their loss as much as one who has. While one who has known these capacities may prefer death to a life without them, we have no assurance that the handicapped person, with no point of comparison, would agree. Life, and life alone, whatever its limitations, might be of sufficient worth to him.

One should also be hesitant to accept proxy assessments of quality-of-life because the margin of error in such predictions may be very great. For instance, while one expert argues that by a purely clinical assessment he can accurately forecast the minimum degree of future handicap an individual will experience, such forecasting is not infallible, and risks denying care to infants whose disability might otherwise permit a reasonably acceptable quality-of-life. Thus given the problems in ascertaining another's wishes, the proxy's bias to personal or culturally relative interests, and the unreliability of predictive criteria, the quality-of-life argument is open to serious question. Its strongest appeal arises in the case of a grossly deformed, retarded, institutionalized child, or one with incessant unmanageable pain, where continued life is itself torture. But these cases are few, and cast doubt on the utility of any such judgment. Even if the judgment occasionally may be defensible, the potential danger of quality-of-life assessments may be a compelling reason for rejecting this rationale for withholding treatment.

B   THE SUFFERING OF OTHERS

In addition to the infant's own suffering, one who argues that the harm of treatment justifies violation of the defective infant's right to life usually relies on the psychological, social, and economic costs of maintaining his existence to family and society. In their view the minimal benefit of treatment to persons incapable of full social and physical development does not justify the burdens that care of the defective infant imposes on parents, siblings, health professionals, and other patients. Matson, a noted pediatric neurosurgeon, states:

> [I]t is the doctor's and the community's responsibility to provide [custodial] care and to minimize suffering; but, at the same time, it is also their responsibility not to prolong such individual, familial, and community suffering unnecessarily, and not to carry out multiple procedures and prolonged, expensive, acute hospitalization in an infant whose chance for acceptable growth and development is negligible.[10]

Such a frankly utilitarian argument raises problems. It assumes that because of the greatly curtailed orbit of his existence, the costs or suffering of others is greater than the benefit of life to the child. This judgment, however, requires a coherent way of measuring and comparing interpersonal utilities, a logical-practical problem that utilitarianism has never surmounted. But even if such comparisons could reliably show a net loss from treatment, the fact remains that the child must sacrifice his life to benefit others. If the life of one individual, however useless, may be sacrificed for the benefit of any person, however useful, or for the benefit of any number of persons, then we have acknowledged the principle that rational utility may justify any outcome. As many philosophers have demonstrated, utilitarianism can always permit the sacrifice of one life for other interests, given the appropriate arrangement of utilities on the balance sheet. In the absence of principled grounds for such a decision, the social equation involved in mandating direct, involuntary euthanasia becomes a difference of degree, not kind, and we reach the point where protection of life depends solely on social judgments of utility.

These objections may well be determinative. But if we temporarily bracket them and examine the extent to which care of the defective infant subjects others to suffering, the claim that inordinate suffering outweighs the infant's interest in life is rarely plausible. In this regard we must examine the impact of caring for defective infants on the family, health professions, and society-at-large.

The Family

The psychological impact and crisis created by birth of a defective infant is devastating. Not only is the mother denied the normal tension release from the stresses of pregnancy, but both parents feel a crushing blow to their dignity, self-esteem and self-confidence. In a very short time, they feel grief for the loss of the normal expected child, anger at fate, numbness, disgust, waves of helplessness, and disbelief. Most feel personal blame for the defect, or blame their spouse. Adding to the shock is fear that social position and mobility are permanently endangered. The transformation of a "joyously awaited experience into one of catastrophe and profound psychological threat"[11] often will reactivate unresolved maturational conflicts. The chances for social pathology—divorce, somatic complaints, nervous and mental disorders—increase and hard-won adjustment patterns may be permanently damaged.

The initial reactions of guilt, grief, anger, and loss, however, cannot be the true measure of family suffering caused by care of a defective infant, because these costs are present whether or not the parents choose treatment. Rather, the question is to what degree treatment imposes psychic and other costs greater than would occur if the child were not treated. The claim that care is more costly rests largely on the view that parents and family suffer inordinately from nurturing such a child.

Indeed, if the child is treated and accepted at home, difficult and demanding adjustments must be made. Parents must learn how to care for a disabled child, confront financial and psychological uncertainty, meet the needs of other siblings, and work through their own conflicting feelings. Mothering demands are greater than with a normal child, particularly if medical care and hospitalization are frequently required. Counseling or professional support may be nonexistent or difficult to obtain. Younger siblings may react with hostility and guilt, older with shame and anger. Often the normal feedback of child growth that renders the turmoil of childrearing worthwhile develops more slowly or not at all. Family resources can be depleted (especially if medical care is needed), consumption patterns altered, or standards of living modified. Housing may have to be found closer to a hospital, and plans for further children changed. Finally, the anxieties, guilt, and grief present at birth may threaten to recur or become chronic.

Yet, although we must recognize the burdens and frustrations of raising a defective infant, it does not necessarily follow that these costs require nontreatment, or even institutionalization. Individual and group counseling can substantially alleviate anxiety, guilt, and frustration, and enable parents to cope with underlying conflicts triggered by the birth and the adaptations required. Counseling also can reduce psychological pressures on siblings, who can be taught to recognize and accept their own possibly hostile feelings and the difficult position of their parents. They may even be taught to help their parents care for the child.

The impact of increased financial costs also may vary. In families with high income or adequate health insurance, the financial costs are manageable. In others, state assistance may be available. If severe financial problems arise or pathological adjustments are likely, institutionalization, although undesirable for the child, remains an option. Finally, in many cases, the experience of living through a crisis is a deepening and enriching one, accelerating personality maturation, and giving one a new sensitivity to the needs of spouse, siblings, and others. As one parent of a defective child states: "In the last months I have come closer to people and can understand them more. I have met them more deeply. I did not know there were so many people with troubles in the world."[12]

Thus, while social attitudes regard the handicapped child as an unmitigated disaster, in reality the problem may not be insurmountable, and often may not differ from life's other vicissitudes. Suffering there is, but seldom is it so overwhelming or so imminent that the only alternative is death of the child.

Health Professionals

Physicians and nurses also suffer when parents give birth to a defective child, although, of course, not to the degree of the parents. To the obstetrician or general practitioner the defective birth may be a blow to his professional identity. He has the difficult task of informing the parents of the defects, explaining their causes, and dealing with the parents' resulting emotional shock. Often he feels guilty for failing to produce a normal baby. In addition, the parents may project anger or hostility on the physician, questioning his professional competence or seeking the services of other doctors. The physician also may feel that his expertise and training are misused when employed to maintain the life of an infant whose chances for a productive existence are so diminished. By neglecting other patients, he may feel that he is prolonging rather than alleviating suffering.

Nurses, too, suffer role strain from care of the defective newborn. Intensive-care-unit nurses may work with only one or two babies at a time. They face the daily ordeals of care—the progress and relapses—and often must deal with anxious parents who are themselves grieving or ambivalent toward the child. The situation may trigger a nurse's own ambivalence about death and mothering, in a context in which she is actively working to keep alive a child whose life prospects seem minimal.

Thus, the effects of care on physicians and nurses are not trivial, and must be intelligently confronted in medical education or in management of a pediatric unit. Yet to state them is to make clear that they can but weigh lightly in the decision of whether to treat a defective newborn. Compared with the situation of the parents, these burdens seem insignificant, are short term, and most likely do not evoke such profound emotions. In any case, these difficulties are hazards of the profession—caring for the sick and dying will always produce strain. Hence, on these grounds alone it is difficult to argue that a defective person may be denied the right to life.

Society

Care of the defective newborn also imposes societal costs, the utility of which is questioned when the infant's expected quality-of-life is so poor. Medical resources that can be used by infants with a better prognosis, or throughout the health-care system generally, are consumed in providing expensive surgical and intensive-care services to infants who may be severely retarded, never lead active lives, and die in a few months or years. Institutionalization imposes costs on taxpayers and reduces the resources available for those who might better benefit from it, while reducing further the quality of life experienced by the institutionalized defective.

One answer to these concerns is to question the impact of the costs of caring for defective newborns. Precise data showing the costs to taxpayers or the trade-offs with health and other expenditures do not exist. Nor would ceasing to care for the defective necessarily lead to a reallocation within the health budget that would produce net savings in suffering or life; in fact, the released resouces might not be reallocated for health at all. In any case, the trade-offs within the health budget may well be small. With advances in prenatal diagnosis of genetic disorders many deformed infants who would formerly require care will be aborted beforehand. Then, too, it is not clear that the most technical and expensive procedures always constitute the best treatment for certain malformations. When compared with the almost seven percent of the GNP now spent on health, the money in the defense budget, or tax revenues generally, the public resources required to keep defective newborns alive seem marginal, and arguably worth the commitment to life that such expenditures reinforce. Moreover, as the Supreme Court recently recognized,[13] conservation of the taxpayer's purse does not justify serious infringement of fundamental rights. Given legal and ethical norms against sacrificing the lives of nonconsenting others, and the imprecisions in diagnosis and prediction concerning the eventual outcomes of medical care, the social cost argument does not compel nontreatment of defective newborns....

NOTES

1 Few persons would argue that "extraordinary" care must be provided a defective newborn, or indeed, to any person. The difficult question, however, is to distinguish "ordinary" from "extraordinary" care.... In this Article "ordinary" care refers to those medical and surgical procedures that would normally be applied in situations not involving physically or mentally handicapped persons.

2 The need for ordinary treatment will also arise with noncentral nervous system malformations such as malformations of the cardiovascular, respiratory, orogastrointestinal, urogenital, muscular and skeletal systems, as well as deformities of the eye, ear, face, endocrine glands, and skin. *See generally* J. WARKANY, CONGENITAL MALFORMATIONS (1971). Often these defects will accompany central nervous system malformations. The medical-ethical dilemma discussed in this Article has arisen chiefly with regard to central nervous system problems, perhaps because the presence of such defects seriously affects

intelligence, social interaction, and the potential for development and growth, and will be discussed only in the context of the major central nervous system malformations. Parents of physically deformed infants with normal intelligence might face the same choice, but because of the child's capacity for development, pressure to withhold ordinary treatment will be less severe.

3 Anencephaly is partial or total absence of the brain. J. WARKANY, *supra* note 2, at 189–99.

4 Hydrocephaly is characterized by an increase of free fluid in the cranial cavity which results in a marked enlargement of the head. *Id.* at 217. It is a symptom of many diverse disorders, and is associated with hereditary and chromosomal syndromes. *Id.* at 217–18. Warkany describes the symptoms as follows: "Bulging of the forehead, protrusion of the parietal areas and extension of the occipital region are characteristic changes.... The skin of the scalp is thin and stretched and its veins are dilated.... The head cannot be held up, and walking and talking are delayed. The legs are spastic, the tendon reflexes increased and convulsions may occur. Anorexia, vomiting and emaciation complicate severe cases. As a rule, hydrocephalic children are dull and lethargic. Blindness can develop, but hearing and the auditory memory may be good. Physical and mental development depend on several factors, such as rapidity of onset, intracranial pressure, compensatory growth of the head, nature of the basic malformations and progress or arrest of the process. Such variability makes the prognosis and evaluation of therapeutic measures difficult. Pressure on the hypothalamic area can cause obesity or precocious puberty in exceptional cases." *Id.* at 226–27.

5 Down's syndrome or mongolism is a chromosomal disorder producing mental retardation caused by the presence of 47 rather than 46 chromosomes in a patient's cells, and marked by a distinctively shaped head, neck, trunk, and abdomen. *Id.* at 311–12, 324. For summary of clinical and pathological characteristics, *see id.* at 324–31.

6 Spina bifida refers generally to midline defects of the osseous spine. The defect usually appears in the posterior aspects of the vertebral canal, and may be marked by an external saccular protrusion (spina bifida cystica). *Id.* at 272. Spina bifida is often seriously involved with urinary tract deficiency, hydrocephaly, and may involve paralysis of the lower extremities. *Id.* at 286–88. While there are important differences between spina bifida, meningoceles, and myelomeningocele, the terms will be used interchangeably in discussing and evaluating the duty to treat.

7 The saccular enlargements of spina bifida cystica protruding through osseous defects of the vertebral column that contain anomalous meninges and spinal fluid but do not have neural elements affixed to their walls are called meningoceles. If the spinal cord or nerves are included in the formation of the sac, the anomaly is called myelomeningocele. *Id.* at 272. As with spina bifida, myelomeningocele may substantially interfere with locomotion, sphincter and bladder control, and may be accompanied by kyphoscoliosis and hydrocephaly leading to mental retardation. For a description of symptoms and treatment alternatives, *see* Lorber, *Results of Treatment of Myelomeningocele*, 13 DEVELOP. MED. & CHILD NEUROL. 279–303 (1971).

8 The infant might suffer from duodenal atresia and need surgery to connect the stomach to the intestine; or need an appendectomy; or antibiotics to fight pneumonia; or suffer from Respirator Distress Syndrome and need breathing assistance. In some cases the question is whether to begin or continue feeding.

9 Smith & Smith, *Selection for Treatment in Spina Bifida Cystica*, 4 BRIT. MED. J. 189, 195 (1973).

10 Matson, *Surgical Treatment of Myelomeningocele*, 42 PEDIATRICS 225, 226 (1968).

11 Goodman, *Continuing Treatment of Parents with Congenitally Defective Infants*, SOCIAL WORK, Vol. 9, No. I, at 92 (1964).

12 *Quoted in* Johns, *Family Reactions to the Birth of a Child with a Congenital Abnormality*, 26 OBSTET. & GYNECOL. SURVEY 635, 637 (1971).

13 *Memorial Hosp. v. Maricopa County*, 415 U.S. 250 (1974).

ANNOTATED BIBLIOGRAPHY: CHAPTER 8

Beauchamp, Tom L., and Seymour Perlin, eds.: *Ethical Issues in Death and Dying* (Englewood Cliffs, N.J.: Prentice-Hall, 1978). Chapter 1 and Chapter 4 of this book are especially useful. Chapter 1 contains a wide range of readings on "The Definition and Determination of Death." Chapter 4 includes subsections on "The Quinlan Case" and "Natural Death and Living Wills." Also noteworthy is "A Reply to Rachels on Active and Passive Euthanasia" (pp. 246–258), in which Beauchamp suggests that rule-utilitarian considerations may provide a basis for defending the moral significance of the distinction between active and passive euthanasia.

Cranford, Ronald E., and Harmon L. Smith: "Some Critical Distinctions between Brain Death and the Persistent Vegetative State," *Ethics in Science & Medicine* 6 (1979), pp. 199–209. In this article, factual differences between (whole) brain death and the persistent vegetative state are emphasized. The appropriate treatment of patients with each of these neurologic conditions is also discussed.

Downing, A. B., ed.: *Euthanasia and the Right to Death: The Case for Voluntary Euthanasia* (New York: Humanities Press; London: Peter Owen, 1969). This collection of euthanasia articles is written from many perspectives—philosophical, humanitarian, sociological, legal, and medical. Especially noteworthy is an article by Antony Flew, "The Principle of Euthanasia." Flew constructs "a general moral case for the establishment of a legal right" to voluntary (active) euthanasia.

Duff, Raymond S., and A. G. M. Campbell: "Moral and Ethical Dilemmas in the Special-Care Nursery," *New England Journal of Medicine* 289 (Oct. 25, 1973), pp. 890–894. This article, a frequent reference point in ethical discussions of the treatment of defective newborns, provides helpful descriptions of the ethical attitudes and actual practices associated with one hospital's special-care nursery. Duff and Campbell make clear that in actual practice some infants are allowed to die.

Fleishman, Alan R., and Thomas H. Murray: "Ethics Committees for Infants Doe?" *Hastings Center Report* 13 (December 1983), pp. 5–9. The authors recommend the establishment of hospital ethics committees for the purpose of reviewing nontreatment decisions for seriously ill newborns. They provide an overall sketch of how such committees might function.

Gustafson, James M.: "Mongolism, Parental Desires, and the Right to Life," *Perspectives in Biology and Medicine* 16 (Summer 1973), pp. 529–557. Gustafson provides a thorough discussion and ethical analysis of a case in which a Down's syndrome infant, suffering from an intestinal blockage, was allowed to die. Gustafson emphasizes that a Down's syndrome child has some significant potential for a satisfying life and suggests that the infant should have been saved.

Kohl, Marvin, ed.: *Beneficent Euthanasia* (Buffalo, N.Y.: Prometheus Books, 1975). This anthology includes a number of helpful articles on the moral aspects of euthanasia. Also included are articles that provide statements of various religious positions on euthanasia. Other articles address the medical and legal aspects of euthanasia.

Lynn, Joanne, and James F. Childress: "Must Patients Always Be Given Food and Water?" *Hastings Center Report* 13 (October 1983), pp. 17–21. The authors argue that nutrition and hydration may be withheld in cases where their provision would not offer the patient a net benefit.

President's Commission for the Study of Ethical Problems in Medicine and Biomedical and Behavioral Research: *Deciding to Forego Life-Sustaining Treatment* (1983). This document is valuable in its entirety, but two chapters are especially noteworthy. Chapter 5 deals with patients who have permanently lost consciousness but are not "brain-dead," and Chapter 6 deals with seriously ill newborns.

———: *Defining Death* (1981). In this document, the Commission provides an overall account of its deliberations leading to the recommendation that the Uniform Determination of Death Act be adopted in each of the states.

Rachels, James: "Euthanasia." In Tom Regan, ed., *Matters of Life and Death* (New York: Random House, 1980), pp. 28–66. In this long essay, Rachels evaluates (1) arguments for and against the morality of active euthanasia and (2) arguments for and against legalizing it. He concludes that active euthanasia is morally acceptable and that it ought to be legalized.

Sherlock, Richard: "Selective Non-Treatment of Defective Newborns: A Critique," *Ethics in Science & Medicine* 7 (1980), pp. 111–117. Sherlock contends, against those who advocate nontreatment of newborns whose life "is not worth living anyway," that no one has succeeded in specifying reasonable, nonarbitrary criteria for the identification of such lives.

Steinbock, Bonnie, ed.: *Killing and Letting Die* (Englewood Cliffs, N.J.: Prentice-Hall, 1980). This anthology provides a wealth of material on the killing/letting die distinction.

Trammell, Richard L.: "Euthanasia and the Law," *Journal of Social Philosophy* 9 (January 1978), pp. 14–18. Trammell contends that the legalization of voluntary positive (i.e., active) euthanasia would probably not "result in overall positive utility for the class of people eligible to choose." He emphasizes the unwelcome pressures that would be created by legalization.

Veatch, Robert M.: *Death, Dying, and the Biological Revolution: Our Last Quest for Responsibility* (New Haven, Conn.: Yale University Press, 1976). The first two chapters of this book provide an extensive discussion of the definition of death. Veatch himself favors an analysis according to which death is the "irreversible loss of consciousness or the capacity for social interaction." Two other chapters are especially notable in the context of euthanasia discussions. Chapter 3 considers many of the prominent conceptual difficulties. Chapter 5 considers various public policy options.

Weir, Robert F.: *Selective Nontreatment of Handicapped Newborns: Moral Dilemmas in Neonatal Medicine* (New York: Oxford University Press, 1984). Weir surveys and critically analyzes a wide range of views (advanced by various pediatricians, attorneys, and ethicists) on the subject of selective nontreatment. He then presents and defends an overall policy for the guidance of decision making in this area.

Chapter 9

Abortion

INTRODUCTION

With the landmark abortion decision of the United States Supreme Court in *Roe v. Wade* (1973), restrictive abortion laws, except under narrowly defined conditions, have been ruled unconstitutional. Thus abortion is *legally* available. However, the ethical (moral) acceptability of abortion remains a hotly contested issue. This chapter focuses attention on abortion as an ethical issue, that is, on the morality of abortion. In addition, some attention is given to the social policy aspects of abortion.

Abortion: The Ethical Issue

Discussions of the ethical acceptability of abortion often take for granted (1) an awareness of the various kinds of reasons that may be given for having an abortion and (2) a minimal sort of acquaintance with the biological development of a human fetus.

Reasons for Abortion Why would a woman have an abortion? The following catalog, not meant to provide an exhaustive survey, is sufficient to indicate that there is a wide range of potential reasons for abortion. (*a*) In certain extreme cases, if the fetus is allowed to develop normally and come to term, the mother herself will die. (*b*) In other cases it is not the mother's life but her health, physical or mental, that will be severely endangered if the pregnancy is allowed to continue. (*c*) There are also cases in which the pregnancy will probably, or surely, produce a severely deformed child,[1] and (*d*) there are others in which the pregnancy is the result of rape or incest.[2] (*e*) There are instances in which the mother is unmarried and there will be the social stigma of illegitimacy. (*f*) There are other instances in which having a child, or having another child, will be an unbearable financial burden. (*g*) Certainly common, and perhaps most common of all, are those instances in which having a child will interfere with the happiness of the woman, or the joint happiness of the parents, or even the joint happiness of a family unit that already includes children. Here there are almost endless possibilities. The woman may desire a professional career. A couple may be content and happy together and feel their relationship would be damaged by the intrusion of a child. Parents may have older children and not feel up to raising another child, and so forth.

The Biological Development of a Human Fetus During the course of a human pregnancy, in the nine-month period from conception to birth, the product of conception undergoes a continual process of change and development. *Conception* takes place when a male germ cell (the spermatozoon) combines with a female germ cell (the ovum), resulting in a single cell (the single-cell zygote), which embodies the full genetic code, twenty-three pairs of chromosomes. The single-cell zygote soon begins a process of cellular division. The resultant multi-cell zygote, while continuing to grow and beginning to take shape, proceeds to move through the fallopian tube and then to undergo gradual *implantation* at the uterine wall. The unborn entity is formally designated a zygote up until the time that implantation is complete, almost two weeks after conception. Thereafter, until the end of the eighth week, roughly the point at which brain waves can be detected, the unborn entity is formally designated an *embryo*. It is in this embryonic period that organ systems and other human characteristics begin to undergo noticeable development. From the end of the eighth week until birth, the unborn entity is formally designated a *fetus*. (The term "fetus," however, is commonly used as a general term to designate the unborn entity, whatever its stage of development.) Two other points in the development of the fetus are especially noteworthy as relevant to discussions of abortion. Somewhere between the twelfth and the sixteenth week there usually occurs *quickening*, the point at which the mother begins to feel the movements of the fetus. And somewhere between the twentieth and the twenty-eighth week the fetus reaches *viability*, the point at which it is capable of surviving outside the womb. In this chapter's opening selection, André E. Hellegers describes in detail the various stages of fetal development.

With the facts of fetal development in view, it may be helpful to indicate the various medical techniques of abortion. Early (first trimester) abortions were at one time performed by *dilatation and curettage* (D&C) but are now commonly performed by *uterine aspiration*, also called "suction curettage." The D&C features the stretching (dilatation) of the cervix and the scraping (curettage) of the inner walls of the uterus. Uterine aspiration simply involves sucking the fetus out of the uterus by means of a tube connected to a suction pump. Later abortions require *dilatation and evacuation* (D&E), *induction techniques*, or *hysterotomy*. In the D&E, which is the abortion procedure commonly used in the early stages of the second trimester, a forceps is used to dismember the fetus within the uterus; the fetal remains are then withdrawn through the cervix. In one commonly-employed induction technique, a saline solution injected into the amniotic cavity induces labor, thus expelling the fetus. Another induction technique employs prostaglandins (hormonelike substances) to induce labor. Hysterotomy—in essence a miniature cesarean section—is a major surgical procedure and is uncommonly employed in the United States.

A brief discussion of fetal development together with a cursory survey of various reasons for abortion has prepared the way for a formulation of the ethical issue of abortion in its broadest terms. *Up to what point of fetal development, if any, and for what reasons, if any, is abortion ethically acceptable?* Some hold that abortion is *never* ethically acceptable, or at most is acceptable only where abortion is necessary to save the life of the mother. This view is frequently termed the *conservative* view on abortion. Others hold that abortion is *always* ethically acceptable—at any point of fetal development and for any of the standard reasons. This view is frequently termed the *liberal* view on abortion. Still others are anxious to defend more *moderate* views, holding that abortion is ethically acceptable up to a certain point of fetal development *and/or* holding that some reasons provide a sufficient justification for abortion whereas others do not.

The Conservative View and the Liberal View

The *moral status* of the fetus has been a pivotal issue in discussions of the ethical acceptability of abortion. The concept of moral status is commonly explicated in terms of rights. On this construal, to say that a fetus has moral status is to say that the fetus has rights. What kind of rights, if any, does the fetus have? Does it have the same rights as more visible humans, and thus *full moral status*, as conservatives typically contend? Does it have no rights, and thus *no (significant) moral status*, as liberals typically contend? (Or perhaps, as some moderates argue, does the fetus have a subsidiary or *partial moral status*, however this is to be conceptualized?) If the fetus has no rights, the liberal is prone to argue, then it does not have any more right to life than a piece of tissue such as an appendix, and an abortion is no more morally objectionable than an appendectomy. If the fetus has the same rights as any other human being, the conservative is prone to argue, then it has the same right to life as the latter, and an abortion, except perhaps when the mother's life is endangered, is as morally objectionable as any other murder.

Discussions of the moral status of the fetus often refer directly to the biological development of the fetus and pose the question: At what point in the continuous development of the fetus do we have a human life? In the context of such discussions, "human" implies full moral status, "nonhuman" implies no (significant) moral status, and any notion of partial moral status is systematically excluded. To distinguish the human from the non-human, to "draw the line," and to do so in a nonarbitrary way, is the central matter of concern. The *conservative* on abortion typically holds that the line must be drawn at conception. Usually the conservative argues that conception is the only point at which the line can be nonarbitrarily drawn. Against attempts to draw the line at points such as implantation, quickening, viability, or birth, considerations of continuity in the development of the fetus are pressed. The conservative is sometimes said to employ "slippery slope arguments," that is, to argue that a line cannot be securely drawn anywhere along the path of fetal development. It is said that the line will inescapably slide back to the point of conception in order to find objective support. John T. Noonan argues in this fashion, at least in part, as he provides a defense of the conservative view in one of the selections in this chapter.

With regard to "drawing the line," the *liberal* typically contends that the fetus remains nonhuman even in its most advanced stages of development. The liberal, of course, does not mean to deny that a fetus is biologically a human fetus. Rather the claim is that the fetus is not human in any morally significant sense, that is, the fetus has no (significant) moral status. This point is often made in terms of the concept of personhood. Mary Anne Warren, who defends the liberal view on abortion in one of this chapter's selections, argues that the fetus is not a person. She also contends that the fetus bears so little resemblance to a person that it cannot be said to have a significant right to life. It is important to notice that, as Warren analyzes the concept of personhood, even a newborn baby is not a person. This conclusion, as might be expected, prompts Warren to a consideration of the moral justifiability of infanticide, an issue closely related to the problem of abortion.

Although the conservative view on abortion is most commonly predicated upon the straightforward contention that the fetus is a person from conception, there are at least two other lines of argument that have been advanced in its defense. One conservative, advancing what might be labeled "The Presumption Argument," writes:

> In being willing to kill the embryo, we accept responsibility for killing what we must admit *may* be a person. There is some reason to believe it is—namely the *fact* that it is a living, human individual and the inconclusiveness of arguments that try to exclude it from the protected circle of personhood.
>
> *To be willing to kill what for all we know could be a person is to be willing to kill it if it is a person.* And since we cannot absolutely settle if it is a person except by a metaphysical postulate, for all practical purposes we must hold that to be willing to kill the embryo is to be willing to kill a person.[3]

In accordance with this line of argument, although it may not be possible to conclusively show that the fetus is a person from conception, we must presume that it is. Another line of argument that has been advanced by some conservatives emphasizes the potential rather than the actual personhood of the fetus. Even if the fetus is not a person, it is said, there can be no doubt that it is a potential person. Accordingly, by virtue of its potential personhood, the fetus must be accorded a right to life. Mary Anne Warren, in response to this line of argument, argues that the potential personhood of the fetus provides no basis for the claim that it has a significant right to life.

Moderate Views

The conservative and liberal views, as explicated, constitute two extreme poles on the spectrum of ethical views of abortion. Each of the extreme views is marked by a formal simplicity. The conservative proclaims abortion to be immoral, irrespective of the stage of fetal development and irrespective of alleged justifying reasons. The one exception, admitted by some conservatives, is the case in which abortion is necessary to save the life of the mother.[4] The liberal proclaims abortion to be morally acceptable, irrespective of the stage of fetal development.[5] Moreover, there is no need to draw distinctions between those reasons that are sufficient to justify abortion and those that are not. No justification is needed. The moderate, in vivid contrast to both the conservative and the liberal, is unwilling to sweepingly condemn or condone abortion. Some abortions are morally justifiable; some are morally objectionable. In some moderate views, the stage of fetal development is a relevant factor in the assessment of the moral acceptability of abortion. In other moderate views, the alleged justifying reason is a relevant factor in the assessment of the moral acceptability of abortion. In still other moderate views, both the stage of fetal development and the alleged justifying reason are relevant factors in the assessment of the moral acceptability of abortion.

Moderate views have been developed in accordance with the following clearly identifiable strategies:

1   Moderation of the Conservative View   One strategy for generating a moderate view presumes the typical conservative contention that the fetus has full moral status from conception. What is denied, however, is that we must conclude to the moral impermissibility of abortion in *all* cases. In one of this chapter's readings, Jane English attempts to moderate the conservative view in just this way. She argues that certain abortion cases may be assimilated to cases of self-defense. Thus, for English, on the presumption that the fetus from conception has full moral status, some reasons are sufficient to justify abortion whereas others are not.

2 Moderation of the Liberal View A second strategy for generating a moderate view presumes the liberal contention that the fetus has no (significant) moral status even in the latest stages of pregnancy. What is denied, however, is that we must conclude to the moral permissibility of abortion in *all* cases. It might be said, in accordance with this line of thought, that abortion, even though it does not violate the rights of the fetus (which is presumed to have no rights), remains ethically problematic because of the negative social consequences of the practice of abortion. Such an argument seems especially forceful in the later stages of pregnancy, when the fetus increasingly resembles a newborn infant. It is argued that very late abortions have a brutalizing effect on those involved and, in various ways, lead to the breakdown of attitudes associated with respect for human life. Jane English, in an effort to moderate the liberal view, advances an argument of this general type. Even if the fetus is not a person, she holds, it is gradually becoming increasingly personlike. Appealing to a "coherence of attitudes," she argues that abortion in the later stages of pregnancy demands more weighty justifying reasons than it does in the earlier stages.

3 Moderation in "Drawing the Line" A third strategy for generating a moderate view, in fact a whole range of moderate views, is associated with "drawing the line" discussions. Whereas the conservative typically draws the line between human (full moral status) and nonhuman (no moral status) at conception and the liberal typically draws that same line at birth (or sometime thereafter), a moderate view may be generated by drawing the line somewhere between these two extremes. For example, one might draw the line at implantation, at the point where brain activity begins, at quickening, at viability, and so forth. Whereas drawing the line at implantation would tend to generate a rather "conservative" moderate view, drawing the line at viability would tend to generate a rather "liberal" moderate view. Wherever the line is drawn, it is the burden of any such moderate view to show that the point specified is a nonarbitrary one. Once such a point has been specified, however, it might be argued that abortion is ethically acceptable before that point and ethically unacceptable after that point. Or further stipulations may be added in accordance with strategies (1) and (2) above.

4 Moderation in the Assignment of Moral Status A fourth strategy for generating a moderate view is dependent upon assigning the fetus some sort of subsidiary or *partial moral status*, an approach taken by Daniel Callahan in one of this chapter's readings. It would seem that anyone who defends a moderate view based on the concept of partial moral status must first of all face the problem of explicating the nature of such partial moral status. Second, and closely related, there is the problem of showing how the interest of those with partial moral status is to be weighed against the interest of those with full moral status.

Abortion and Social Policy

In the United States, the Supreme Court's decision in *Roe v. Wade* (1973) is at the core of existing social policy on abortion. This case had the effect, for all practical purposes, of legalizing "abortion-on-request." The Court held that it was unconstitutional for a state to have laws prohibiting the abortion of a previable fetus. According to the Court, a woman has a constitutionally guaranteed right to decide to terminate a pregnancy (prior to viability), although a state, for reasons related to maternal health, may restrict the manner and circumstances in which abortions are performed subsequent to the end of the first trimester. The reasoning underlying the Court's holding in *Roe* can be found in the majority opinion reprinted in this chapter.

Since the action of the Court in *Roe* had the practical effect of establishing a woman's legal right to choose whether or not to abort, it was enthusiastically received by "right-to-choose" forces. On the other hand, "right-to-life" forces, committed to the conservative view on the morality of abortion, vehemently denounced the Court for "legalizing murder." In response to *Roe*, right-to-life forces have adopted a number of political strategies. Three of the most significant of these strategies will be discussed here.

For right-to-life forces, the enactment of a constitutional amendment directly overruling *Roe* and banning abortion is the most desirable political outcome. (Less desirable would be the enactment of an amendment allowing Congress and/or each state to decide whether or not to restrict abortion.) The proposed Human Life Amendment, worded so as to declare the personhood of the fetus, is calculated to achieve the legal prohibition of abortion, allowing an exception only when abortion is necessary to save the life of the mother. Right-to-choose forces typically argue that the Human Life Amendment represents an illicit attempt to impose the moral views of one group (conservatives on abortion) on those who have different views. Thus, to some extent, the justifiability of such an amendment is bound up with a much broader question, whether or not it is justifiable to employ the law in an effort to "enforce morality." (Cf. the discussion of the principle of legal moralism in Chapter 1.)

Right-to-life forces have been successful in achieving a more limited political aim, the cutoff of Medicaid funding for abortion. Medicaid is a social program designed to provide public funds to pay for the medical care of impoverished people. At issue in *Harris v. McRae*, decided by the Supreme Court in 1980, was the constitutionality of the so-called Hyde Amendment, legislation that had passed Congress with vigorous right-to-life support. The Hyde Amendment, in the version considered by the Court, restricted federal Medicaid funding to (1) cases in which the mother's life is endangered and (2) cases of rape and incest. The Court, in a five-to-four decision, upheld the constitutionality of the Hyde Amendment. According to the Court, a woman's right to an abortion does not entail *the right to have society fund the abortion.* But if there is no constitutional obstacle to the cutoff of Medicaid funding for abortion, it must still be asked if society's refusal to fund the abortions of poor women is an ethically sound social policy. Considerations of social justice are often pressed by those who argue that it is not.

Right-to-life forces have also made efforts to secure the passage of statutes designed (in various ways) to place obstacles in the path of women seeking an abortion. In *Akron v. Akron Center for Reproductive Health* (1983), the Supreme Court considered the constitutionality of a local ordinance of this sort. The Court's reasoning in this case is reviewed by George J. Annas in this chapter's last selection.

T. A. M.

NOTES

1 The first subsection of Chapter 10 provides an extensive discussion of prenatal diagnosis and selective abortion.

2 The expression "therapeutic abortion" suggests abortion for medical reasons. Accordingly, abortions corresponding to (*a*), (*b*), and (*c*) are usually said to be therapeutic. More problematically, abortions corresponding to (*d*) have often been identified as therapeutic. Perhaps it is presumed that pregnancies resulting from rape or incest are traumatic, thus a threat to mental health. Or perhaps calling such an abortion "therapeutic" is just a way of indicating that it is thought to be justifiable.

3 Germain Grisez, *Abortion: The Myths, the Realities, and the Arguments* (New York: Corpus Books, 1970), p. 306.

4 One especially prominent conservative view is associated with the Roman Catholic Church. In accordance with Catholic moral teaching, the *direct* killing of innocent human life is forbidden. Hence, abortion is forbidden. Even if the mother's life is in danger, perhaps because her heart or kidney function is inadequate, abortion is impermissible. In two special cases, however, procedures resulting in the death of the fetus are allowable. In the case of an ectopic pregnancy, where the developing fetus is lodged in the fallopian tube, the fallopian tube may be removed. In the case of a pregnant woman with a cancerous uterus, the cancerous uterus may be removed. In these cases, the death of the fetus is construed as *indirect* killing, the foreseen but unintended by-product of a surgical procedure designed to protect the life of the mother. As the exchange between James Rachels and Thomas D. Sullivan in Chapter 8 makes clear, the distinction between direct and indirect killing is a controversial one. Sullivan relies on the distinction between intentional and nonintentional terminations of life whereas Rachels contends that the distinction has no moral significance. If, however, the distinction between direct and indirect killing is a defensible one, it might still be suggested that the distinction is not rightly applied in the Roman Catholic view of abortion. For example, some critics contend that abortion may be construed as indirect killing, indeed an allowable form of indirect killing, in at least all cases where it is necessary to save the life of the mother. For one helpful exposition and critical analysis of the Roman Catholic position on abortion, see Daniel Callahan, *Abortion: Law, Choice and Morality* (New York: Macmillan, 1970), chap. 12, pp. 409–447.

5 In considering the liberal contention that abortions are morally acceptable irrespective of the stage of fetal development, we should take note of an ambiguity in the concept of abortion. Does "abortion" refer merely to the termination of a pregnancy in the sense of detaching the fetus from the mother, or does "abortion" entail the death of the fetus as well? Whereas the abortion of a *previable* fetus entails its death, the "abortion" of a *viable* fetus, by means of hysterotomy (a miniature cesarean section), does not entail the death of the fetus and would seem to be tantamount to the birth of a baby. With regard to the "abortion" of a *viable* fetus, liberals can defend the woman's right to detach the fetus from her body without contending that the woman has the right to insist on the death of the child.

The Biology of Fetal Development

Fetal Development

André E. Hellegers

André E. Hellegers (1926–1979), M.D., was professor of obstetrics and gynecology at Georgetown University Hospital. He was also the first director of the Kennedy Institute of Ethics, Georgetown University. As the author of a monthly column that appeared in *Ob. Gyn. News*, he had turned his attention to a wide range of issues in biomedical ethics. One example of his other published work in biomedical ethics is "Abortion: 'Another Form of Birth Control'?"

In this exclusively descriptive selection, Hellegers makes clear the various stages of fetal development.

No [discussion of] abortion would be complete without a chapter on the fetus. He or she (in the absence of knowledge of the sex, we shall use the neutral "it") is, after all, one of the subjects in the debate. Frequently in the discussions on abortion, the physician is asked when life begins. Some seem to imply that there would be no problem of abortion if only a definitive statement could be made about the beginning of human life. This, however, is far from so, for the presence of human life has never precluded our taking it if we felt justified in doing so. [Here] the question (when life begins) is therefore asked not to endorse or prohibit abortion, but rather because the layman is baffled by the fetus, since he cannot see it.

Since society has imagery and definitions of its own, which it has inherited from the past, it may be well in the description which follows to highlight those stages of development to which, for one reason or another, men have attached importance in the past.[1]

I

First, let us ask in what way the ovum, or female egg, and the sperm, or male eggs, differ from the fertilized ovum. The essential difference is that an ovum or a sperm will inevitably die unless they are combined together in the process of fertilization, while the fertilized egg will automatically develop unless untoward events occur. The first definition of life, then, could be the ability to reproduce oneself, and this the fertilized

egg has while the individual ovum and sperm do not.

How is this process of fertilization brought about? At intercourse, about 300,000,000 sperm are deposited in the vagina and will begin their journey upwards through the uterus, or womb, and up into the tube leading from the uterus towards the ovary. If an ovum has been released from the woman's ovary, it in turn will pass from the ovary down the same tube towards the uterus. The survival time of this ovum will be about twenty-four hours. If fertilization has not occurred in that time, both the ovum and the sperm will die. From a variety of mammalian species it has been learned that the sperm, as ejaculated, are not capable of immediately fertilizing an ovum. They must undergo a chemical change called "capacitation," without which they cannot fertilize the ovum.[2] The process is as yet little understood, but it is thought that a substance in the female uterus or tube changes the sperm in such a way that they gain the ability to fertilize. In most species this process occurs in a matter of hours, say six or eight. Although the process has not yet been proven in the human, it is commonly assumed to exist, since it occurs in other mammalian species studied. Following intercourse, there would therefore be a period of several hours in which interference with reproduction would fall under the generally recognized heading of contraception rather than abortion, since no ovum would yet have been fertilized. Several hours after intercourse, then, fertilization may occur. The significance of this event lies in the fact that a totally new genetic package is now produced. The fertilized ovum contains genetic

Reprinted with permission of the author and the publisher from *Theological Studies*, vol. 31, no. 1 (March 1970), pp. 3–9.

information brought from the father through the sperm, and from the mother through the ovum, so that a new combination of genetic information is created. This newly fertilized egg, sometimes called a zygote, has within it the hereditary characteristics of both the father and the mother, one half from each. The characteristics are derived from the genetic thread of life called DNA, contained in each.

This single fertilized cell will then proceed to divide into two cells, then four, then eight, etc., and this it will do at a rate of almost one division per day.[3]

It is well known that in this early stage of development the sphere of cells may split into identical parts to form identical twins. Twinning in the human may occur until the fourteenth day, when conjoined twins can still be produced. Less well known is the fact that it is also in these first few days that twins or triplets may be recombined into one single individual.

Experiments carried out in mice by Mintz showed that it was possible to recombine the early dividing cell stages from black parents and from white parents into a single black-and-white-striped mouse.[4] The significance of this phenomenon would seem to be that up until this stage the new individual mammal is not as yet irreversibly an individual, since it still may be recombined with others into one new, final being.

In the last few years this phenomenon has also been found in man. From the genetic make-up of these human individuals and from the make-up of their red blood cells it is clear that these human so-called chimeras, whose genetic type is XX-XY, are in fact recombinations into one human being of the products of more than one fertilization. The subject has recently been extensively reviewed by Benirschke,[5] and a prototype case can be found in the report of Myhre *et al.*[6] It is not as yet clear up to precisely what stage of development this can occur in the human, but in mice the recombination can still be performed at the 32-cell stage. The diagnostic criteria for such cases are that their genetic karyotype is XX-XY, that they are gonadally disturbed consisting as they do of a genetic mixture of male and female, that they can contain two different populations of red blood cells, and that they may have heterochromia of the eyes. Six human cases meeting these requirements have been reported up to the present time.

The initial stages of cell division of the fertilized egg do not seem to be dependent on any paternal genetic material brought to the fertilized egg by the sperm. It would seem as if genetic material brought to the fertil-

ized egg in the mother's ovum suffices to take the fertilized egg through the earliest stages of cell division.

All these matters are brought forth to point out that, although at fertilization a new genetic package is brought into being within the confines of one cell, this anatomical fact does not necessarily mean that all of the genetic material in it becomes crucially activated at that point, or that final irreversible individuality has been achieved.

Modern genetic studies therefore suggest that, in old standard Catholic language, one could say: "If by means of two fertilizations two souls are infused, and if a single body only contains one soul, then we are beginning to see cases in which one of the two souls must have disappeared without any fertilized egg having died."

It is also important to realize that in these first few days of life it is quite impossible for the women to know that she is pregnant, or for the doctor to diagnose the condition by a pregnancy test.

The fact that the first seven days of the reproductive process take place entirely in the tube, and not in the uterus itself, has several major implications for the subject of abortion. These should be fully understood. If within seven days of intercourse, as for instance following rape, the lining of the uterus is removed by curettage, abortion, in its legal sense, has not taken place. It would be impossible to prove that an abortion had been performed when all pregnancy tests were shown to be negative and the lining of the uterus was shown, under the microscope, to have contained no pregnancy. Indeed the operation of curettage is a common gynecological one, which is frequently carried out in the second half of the menstrual cycle, when a fertilized ovum may well be present in the tube. There has never been a medical tradition to perform the curettage only immediately following menstruation, in order to assure that no fertilized egg could be present in the tube (since ovulation would not as yet have occurred). By the same token, women scheduled to undergo a curettage are not instructed to forego intercourse lest there be present in the tube a fertilized ovum which would be unable to implant into the uterus due to the removal of its lining. Moreover, there is some evidence that modern "contraceptive" techniques such as the intrauterine loop, and even some of the steroid pills, may well exert their effect in pregnancy prevention by acting after fertilization of the ovum has occurred, but before implantation in the uterus.[7] Although the action of these agents is not yet fully understood, there has never been a suggestion that they would be considered abortifacient under the civil law, since no evidence of pregnancy could possibly be obtained.

II

After approximately six or seven days of this cell-division process (all of which occurs in the tube), the next critical stage of development starts. The sphere of cells will now enter the uterus and implant itself into the uterine lining. This process of implantation is highly critical, for it is during these days that one pole of the sphere of cells, the trophoblast (later to become the placenta), burrows its way into the lining of the uterus. The opposite pole of this sphere will become the fetus. The part which becomes the placenta produces hormones. These enter the maternal blood stream and serve a critical function in preventing the mother from menstruating. Since the time interval between ovulation and menstruation is approximately fourteen days, and since the first seven days of the new life have been passed in the tube, it is obvious that the implanting trophoblast only has about seven days to produce enough hormone to stop the mother from menstruating and thus sloughing off the fetal life. These same hormones, circulating in the mother, form the basis for the chemical tests which enable us to diagnose pregnancy. After this second week of pregnancy the zygote rapidly becomes more complex and is now called the embryo. Somewhere between the third and fourth week the differentiation of the embryo will have been sufficient for heart pumping to occur,[8] although the heart will by no means yet have reached its final configuration. At the end of six weeks all of the internal organs of the fetus will be present, but as yet in a rudimentary stage. The blood vessels leading from the heart will have been fully deployed, although they too will continue to grow in size with growth of the fetus. By the end of seven weeks tickling of the mouth and nose of the developing embryo with a hair will cause it to flex its neck, while at the end of eight weeks there will be readable electrical activity coming from the brain.[9] The meaning of the activity cannot be interpreted. By now also the fingers and toes will be fully recognizable. Sometime between the ninth and tenth week local reflexes appear such as swallowing, squinting, and tongue retraction. By the tenth week spontaneous movement is seen, independent of stimulation. By the eleventh week thumb-sucking

has been observed and X rays of the fetus at this time show clear details of the skeleton. After twelve weeks the fetus, now 3½ inches in size, will have completed its brain structure, although growth of course will continue. By this time also it has become possible to pick up the fetal heart by modern electrocardiographic techniques, via the mother.

The twelve-week stage is also important for an entirely different reason. It is after this stage that the performance of an abortion by the relatively simple D&C (scraping of the womb) becomes dangerous. Thereafter abortion must be performed either by abdominal operation or by the more recently developed technique of the injection of a concentrated fluid into the amniotic cavity.*

Sometime between the twelfth and sixteenth week "quickening" will occur. This event, long considered important in law, denotes the fact that fetal movements are first felt by the mother. Quickening, therefore, is a phenomenon of maternal perception rather than a fetal achievement. It is subjective and varies with the degree of experience and obesity of the mother.

Sometime between the sixteenth and twentieth week it will also become possible to hear the fetal heart, not just by the refined EKG, but also by the simple stethoscope.

The twentieth-week stage again has definite importance. Before this date delivery of the product of conception is called an abortion in medical terminology. After this date we no longer speak of abortion but of premature delivery. The fetus at this stage will weigh about one pound. Between the twentieth and twenty-eighth week fetuses born have an approximately 10% chance of survival. At twenty-eight weeks the fetus will weigh slightly over two pounds. In former days the medical profession defined fetuses of less than twenty-eight weeks of age as abortions, but this was impossible to maintain when 10% of such infants might survive. As a consequence, a discrepancy may now exist between possible definitions of viability in legal and in medical circles; at least the ability to ensure survival of fetuses has progressively occurred at earlier stages.

After the twenty-eighth week little change in outward appearance of the fetus occurs, although growth obviously continues, and with this growth the chances of survival also increase.

*Editor's note: Another abortion procedure, the D&E (dilatation and evacuation), is now commonly employed up to the sixteenth week.

These, then, are the major stages of fetal development in the order of their occurrence. Grouped systematically, and therefore rather arbitrarily, by genetic factors, by cardiovascular or nervous system development, and by chances of survival, they can be summarized as in the accompanying Table.

Throughout the analysis of the beginning of life it is important to bear several factors in mind. First, the understanding of the processes described is the understanding of today. The eliciting of fetal responses depends on the methods available today. Second, it is not a function of science to prove, or disprove, where in this process *human* life begins, in the sense that those discussing the abortion issue so frequently use the word "life," i.e., human dignity, human person-hood, or human inviolability. Such entities do not pertain to the science or art of medicine, but are rather a societal judgment. Science cannot prove them; it can only describe the biological development and predict what will occur to it with an accuracy that depends on the stage of development of the particular science. In the ultimate analysis the question is not just to forecast

Some Major Normal Stages in Fetal Development

Time	Cardiovascular system	Nervous system	Other criterion
Some hours	—	—	Intercourse followed by "capacitation"
0 hours	—	—	Fertilization; 1 cell, often called zygote
About 22 hours	—	—	2 cell ⎞ Possible recombination
About 44 hours	—	—	4 cell ⎟ until day?
About 66 hours	—	—	8 cell ⎟ Possible twinning
About 4 days	—	—	16 cell ⎠ until day 14 "Morula" stage
About 6–7 days	—	—	Implantation—often called "blastocyst" stage
2 weeks	—	—	Name changed from zygote to embryo
3–4 weeks	Heart pumping	—	—
6 weeks	—	—	All organs present
7–8 weeks	—	Mouth or nose tickling, neck flexing	—
8 weeks	—	Readable brain electric activity	Name changed from embryo to fetus. Length 3 cm
9–10 weeks	—	Swallowing, squinting, local reflexes	—
10 weeks	—	Spontaneous movement	—
11 weeks	—	—	Thumb sucking
12 weeks	Fetal EKG via mother	—	Brain structure complete Length 10 cm
13 weeks*	—	—	D&C contraindicated hereafter
12–16 weeks*	—	—	"Quickening." Length 18 cm at 16 weeks
16–20 weeks*	Fetal heart heard	—	Length 25 cm at 20 weeks
20 weeks*	—	—	Name changed from abortus to premature infant
20–28 weeks*	—	—	10% survive
28 weeks*	—	—	Fetus said to be "viable" in some definitions
40 weeks*	—	—	Birth

*Calculated from the first day of the last menstrual period.

when life begins, but rather: How should one behave when one does not know whether dignity is or is not present in the fetus?

NOTES

1 I shall stress heavily the new biology on the developmental processes in the first seven days, while the "fetus" is in the tube. This is crucial, I believe, (1) by reason of its own biological interest; (2) because of the action of the pill and intrauterine devices, which may act during these seven days; (3) because this stage precedes the period when a diagnosis of pregnancy can be made, i.e., it is the stage commonly described as "the normal second half of the normal menstrual cycle"; (4) because it is the stage when the "morning-after pill" may act; (5) because it is not presently covered under abortion laws, inasmuch as it precedes the stage when the woman knows she is pregnant (for she has not yet missed a period) and precedes the stage when a diagnosis can be made; (6) because it is a stage upon which the Catholic Hospital Association has not yet reflected, since we frequently do operations after ovulation but before a period is missed, i.e., during these seven days.

2 Cf. C. E. Adams, "The Influence of Maternal Environment on Preimplantation Stages of Pregnancy in the Rabbit," in *Preimplantation Stages of Pregnancy*, ed. G. E. W. Wolstenholme and M. O'Connor (Boston, 1965) p. 345; K. A. Rafferty, "The Beginning of Development," in *Intrauterine Development*, ed. A. C. Barnes (Philadelphia, 1968).

3 Cf. Rafferty, *op. cit.*

4 Cf. B. Mintz, "Experimental Genetic Mosaicism in the Mouse," in *Preimplantation Stages of Pregnancy* (n. 2 above) p. 194.

5 Cf. K. Benirschke, *Current Topics in Pathology*, (1969) 1.

6 Cf. A. Myhre, T. Meyer, J. N. Opitz, R. R. Race, R. Sanger, and T. J. Greenwalt, "Two Populations of Erythrocytes Associated with XX-XY Mosaicism," *Transfusion* 5 (1965) 501.

7 Cf. P. A. Corfman and S. J. Segal, "Biologic Effects of Intrauterine Devices," *American Journal of Obstetrics and Gynecology* 100 (1968) 448; also "Hormonal Steroids in Contraception," *WHO Technical Report Series* 1968 (Geneva, 1968) p. 386.

8 Cf. J. W. C. Johnson, "Cardio-Respiratory Systems," in *Intrauterine Development* (n. 2 above).

9 Cf. D. Goldblatt, "Nervous System and Sensory Organs," in *Intrauterine Development* (n. 2 above).

The Morality of Abortion

An Almost Absolute Value in History

John T. Noonan, Jr.

John T. Noonan, Jr., is professor of law at the University of California, Berkeley. His academic interests extend beyond matters of law to philosophical and theological issues, and his intellectual allegiance in this regard is with the Roman Catholic tradition. Among his books are *Contraception: A History of Its Treatment by the Catholic Theologians and Canonists* (1965), *Persons and Masks of the Law* (1976), and *A Private Choice: Abortion in America in the Seventies* (1979).

Noonan, defending the conservative view on abortion, immediately raises the question of how to determine the *humanity* of a being. In an updated version of the traditional theological view he contends that, if a being is conceived by human parents and thereby has a human genetic code, then that being is a *human being*.

Conception is the point at which the nonhuman becomes the human. Noonan argues that other alleged criteria of humanity are inadequate. He also argues, primarily through an analysis of probabilities, that his own criterion of humanity is objectively based and nonarbitrary. Finally, Noonan contends, once the humanity of the fetus is recognized, we must judge abortion morally wrong, except in those rare cases where the mother's life is in danger.

The most fundamental question involved in the long history of thought on abortion is: How do you determine the humanity of a being? To phrase the question that way is to put in comprehensive humanistic terms what the theologians either dealt with as an explicitly theological question under the heading of "ensoulment" or dealt with implicitly in their treatment of abortion. The Christian position as it originated did not depend on a narrow theological or philosophical concept. It had no relation to theories of infant baptism. It appealed to no special theory of instantaneous ensoulment. It took the world's view on ensoulment as that view changed from Aristotle to Zacchia. There was, indeed, theological influence affecting the theory of ensoulment finally adopted, and, of course, ensoulment itself was a theological concept, so that the position was always explained in theological terms. But the theological notion of ensoulment could easily be translated into humanistic language by substituting "human" for "rational soul"; the problem of knowing when a man is a man is common to theology and humanism.

If one steps outside the specific categories used by the theologians, the answer they gave can be analyzed as a refusal to discriminate among human beings on the basis of their varying potentialities. Once conceived, the being was recognized as man because he had man's potential. The criterion for humanity, thus, was simple and all-embracing: if you are conceived by human parents, you are human.

The strength of this position may be tested by a review of some of the other distinctions offered in the contemporary controversy over legalizing abortion. Perhaps the most popular distinction is in terms of viability. Before an age of so many months, the fetus is not viable, that is, it cannot be removed from the mother's womb and live apart from her. To that extent, the life of the fetus is absolutely dependent on the life of the mother. This dependence is made the basis of denying recognition to its humanity.

There are difficulties with this distinction. One is that the perfection of artificial incubation may make the fetus viable at any time: it may be removed and artificially sustained. Experiments with animals already show that such a procedure is possible. This hypothetical extreme case relates to an actual difficulty: there is considerable elasticity to the idea of viability. Mere length of life is not an exact measure. The viability of the fetus depends on the extent of its anatomical and functional development. The weight and length of the fetus are better guides to the state of its development than age, but weight and length vary. Moreover, different racial groups have different ages at which their fetuses are viable. Some evidence, for example, suggests that Negro fetuses mature more quickly than white fetuses. If viability is the norm, the standard would vary with race and with many individual circumstances.

The most important objection to this approach is that dependence is not ended by viability. The fetus is still absolutely dependent on someone's care in order to continue existence; indeed a child of one or three or even five years of age is absolutely dependent on another's care for existence; uncared for, the older fetus or the younger child will die as surely as the early fetus detached from the mother. The unsubstantial lessening in dependence at viability does not seem to signify any special acquisition of humanity.

A second distinction has been attempted in terms of experience. A being who has had experience, has lived and suffered, who possesses memories, is more human than one who has not. Humanity depends on formation by experience. The fetus is thus "unformed" in the most basic human sense.

This distinction is not serviceable for the embryo which is already experiencing and reacting. The embryo is responsive to touch after eight weeks and at least at that point is experiencing. At an earlier stage the zygote is certainly alive and responding to its environment. The distinction may also be challenged by the rare case where aphasia has erased adult memory: has it erased humanity? More fundamentally, this distinction leaves even the older fetus or the younger child to be treated as an unformed inhuman thing. Finally, it is not clear why experience as such confers humanity. It could be argued that certain central experiences such as loving or learning are necessary to make a man human. But then human beings who have failed to love or to learn might be excluded from the class called man.

A third distinction is made by appeal to the sentiments of adults. If a fetus dies, the grief of the parents is not the grief they would have for a living child. The fetus is an unnamed "it" till birth, and is not perceived as personality until at least the fourth month of existence when movements in the womb manifest a vigorous presence demanding joyful recognition by the parents.

Yet feeling is notoriously an unsure guide to the humanity of others. Many groups of humans have had difficulty in feeling that persons of another tongue, color, religion, sex, are as human as they. Apart from reactions to alien groups, we mourn the loss of a ten-year-old boy more than the loss of his one-day-old brother or his 90-year-old grandfather. The difference felt and the grief expressed vary with the potentialities extinguished, or the experience wiped out; they do not seem to point to any substantial difference in the humanity of baby, boy, or grandfather.

Distinctions are also made in terms of sensation by the parents. The embryo is felt within the womb only after about the fourth month. The embryo is seen only at birth. What can be neither seen nor felt is different from what is tangible. If the fetus cannot be seen or touched at all, it cannot be perceived as man.

Yet experience shows that sight is even more untrustworthy than feeling in determining humanity. By sight, color became an appropriate index for saying who was a man, and the evil of racial discrimination was given foundation. Nor can touch provide the test: a being confined by sickness, "out of touch" with others, does not thereby seem to lose his humanity. To the extent that touch still has appeal as a criterion, it appears to be a survival of the old English idea of "quickening"—a possible mistranslation of the Latin *animatus* used in the canon law. To that extent touch as a criterion seems to be dependent on the Aristotelian notion of ensoulment, and to fail when this notion is discarded.

Finally, a distinction is sought in social visibility. The fetus is not socially perceived as human. It cannot communicate with others. Thus, both subjectively and objectively, it is not a member of society. As moral rules are rules for the behavior of members of society

to each other, they cannot be made for behavior toward what is not yet a member. Excluded from the society of men, the fetus is excluded from the humanity of men.

By force of the argument from the consequences, this distinction is to be rejected. It is more subtle than that founded on an appeal to physical sensation, but it is equally dangerous in its implications. If humanity depends on social recognition, individuals or whole groups may be dehumanized by being denied any status in their society. Such a fate is fictionally portrayed in *1984* and has actually been the lot of many men in many societies. In the Roman empire, for example, condemnation to slavery meant the practical denial of most human rights; in the Chinese Communist world, landlords have been classified as enemies of the people and so treated as nonpersons by the state. Humanity does not depend on social recognition, though often the failure of society to recognize the prisoner, the alien, the heterodox as human has led to the destruction of human beings. Anyone conceived by a man and a woman is human. Recognition of this condition by society follows a real event in the objective order, however imperfect and halting the recognition. Any attempt to limit humanity to exclude some group runs the risk of furnishing authority and precedent for excluding other groups in the name of the consciousness or perception of the controlling group in the society.

A philosopher may reject the appeal to the humanity of the fetus because he views "humanity" as a secular view of the soul and because he doubts the existence of anything real and objective which can be identified as humanity. One answer to such a philosopher is to ask how he reasons about moral questions without supposing that there is a sense in which he and the others of whom he speaks are human. Whatever group is taken as the society which determines who may be killed is thereby taken as human. A second answer is to ask if he does not believe that there is a right and wrong way of deciding moral questions. If there is such a difference, experience may be appealed to: to decide who is human on the basis of the sentiment of a given society has led to consequences which rational men would characterize as monstrous.

The rejection of the attempted distinctions based on viability and visibility, experience and feeling, may be buttressed by the following considerations: Moral judgments often rest on distinctions, but if the distinctions are not to appear arbitrary fiat, they should relate to some real difference in probabilities. There is a kind of continuity in all life, but the earlier stages of the elements of human life possess tiny probabilities of development. Consider for example, the spermatozoa in any normal ejaculate: There are about 200,000,000 in any single ejaculate, of which one has a chance of developing into a zygote. Consider the oocytes which may become ova: there are 100,000 to 1,000,000 oocytes in a female infant, of which a maximum of 390 are ovulated. But once spermatozoon and ovum meet and the conceptus is formed, such studies as have been made show that roughly in only 20 percent of the cases will spontaneous abortion occur. In other words, the chances are about 4 out of 5 that this new being will develop. At this stage in the life of the being there is a sharp shift in probabilities, an immense jump in potentialities. To make a distinction between the rights of spermatozoa and the rights of the fertilized ovum is to respond to an enormous shift in possibilities. For about twenty days after conception the egg may split to form twins or combine with another egg to form a chimera, but the probability of either event happening is very small.

It may be asked, What does a change in biological probabilities have to do with establishing humanity? The argument from probabilities is not aimed at establishing humanity but at establishing an objective discontinuity which may be taken into account in moral discourse. As life itself is a matter of probabilities, as most moral reasoning is an estimate of probabilities, so it seems in accord with the structure of reality and the nature of moral thought to found a moral judgment on the change in probabilities at conception. The appeal to probabilities is the most commonsensical of arguments, to a greater or smaller degree all of us base our actions on probabilities, and in morals, as in law, prudence and negligence are often measured by the account one has taken of the probabilities. If the chance is 200,000,000 to 1 that the movement in the bushes into which you shoot is a man's, I doubt if many persons would hold you careless in shooting; but if the chances are 4 out of 5 that the movement is a human being's, few would acquit you of blame. Would the argument be different if only one out of ten children conceived came to term? Of course this argument would be different. This argument is an appeal to probabilities that actually exist, not to any and all states of affairs which may be imagined.

The probabilities as they do exist do not show the humanity of the embryo in the sense of a demonstration in logic any more than the probabilities of the movement in the bush being a man demonstrate beyond all doubt that the being is a man. The appeal is a "buttressing" consideration, showing the plausibility of the standard adopted. The argument focuses on the decisional factor in any moral judgment and assumes that part of the business of a moralist is drawing lines. One evidence of the nonarbitrary character of the line drawn is the difference of probabilities on either side of it. If a spermatozoon is destroyed, one destroys a being which had a chance of far less than 1 in 200 million of developing into a reasoning being, possessed of the genetic code, a heart and other organs, and capable of pain. If a fetus is destroyed, one destroys a being already possessed of the genetic code, organs, and sensitivity to pain, and one which had an 80 percent chance of developing further into a baby outside the womb who, in time, would reason.

The positive argument for conception as the decisive moment of humanization is that at conception the new being receives the genetic code. It is this genetic information which determines his characteristics, which is the biological carrier of the possibility of human wisdom, which makes him a self-evolving being. A being with a human genetic code is man.

This review of current controversy over the humanity of the fetus emphasizes what a fundamental question the theologians resolved in asserting the inviolability of the fetus. To regard the fetus as possessed of equal rights with other humans was not, however, to decide every case where abortion might be employed. It did decide the case where the argument was that the fetus should be aborted for its own good. To say a being was human was to say it had a destiny to decide for itself which could not be taken from it by another man's decision. But human beings with equal rights often come in conflict with each other, and some decision must be made as to whose claims are to prevail. Cases of conflict involving the fetus are different only in two respects: the total inability of the fetus to speak for itself and the fact that the right of the fetus regularly at stake is the right to life itself.

The approach taken by the theologians to these conflicts was articulated in terms of "direct" and "indirect." Again, to look at what they were doing from outside their categories, they may be said to have been drawing lines or "balancing values." "Direct" and "indirect" are spatial metaphors; "line-drawing" is another. "To weigh" or "to balance" values is a metaphor of a more complicated mathematical sort hinting at the process which goes on in moral judgments. All the metaphors suggest that, in the moral judgments made, comparisons were necessary, that no value completely controlled. The principle of double effect was no doctrine fallen from heaven, but a method of analysis appropriate where two relative values were being compared. In Catholic moral theology, as it developed, life even of the innocent was not taken as an absolute. Judgments on acts affecting life issued from a process of weighing. In the weighing, the fetus was always given a value greater than zero, always a value separate and independent from its parents. This valuation was crucial and fundamental in all Christian thought on the subject and marked it off from any approach which considered that only the parents' interests needed to be considered.

Even with the fetus weighed as human, one interest could be weighed as equal or superior: that of the mother in her own life. The casuists between 1450 and 1895 were willing to weigh this interest as superior. Since 1895, that interest was given decisive weight only in the two special cases of the cancerous uterus and the ectopic pregnancy. In both of these cases the fetus itself had little chance of survival even if the abortion were not performed. As the balance was once struck in favor of the mother whenever her life was endangered, it could be so struck again. The balance reached between 1895 and 1930 attempted prudentially and pastorally to forestall a multitude of exceptions for interests less than life.

The perception of the humanity of the fetus and the weighing of fetal rights against other human rights constituted the work of the moral analysts. But what spirit animated their abstract judgments? For the Christian community it was the injunction of Scripture to love your neighbor as yourself. The fetus as human was a neighbor; his life had parity with one's own. The commandment gave life to what otherwise would have been only rational calculation.

The commandment could be put in humanistic as well as theological terms: Do not injure your fellow man without reason. In these terms, once the humanity of the fetus is perceived, abortion is never right except in self-defense. When life must be taken to save life, reason alone cannot say that a mother must prefer a child's life to her own. With this exception, now of great rarity, abortion violates the rational humanist tenet of the equality of human lives.

For Christians the commandment to love had received a special imprint in that the exemplar proposed of love was the love of the Lord for his disciples. In the light given by this example, self-sacrifice carried to the point of death seemed in the extreme situations not without meaning. In the less extreme cases, preference for one's own interest to the life of another seemed to express cruelty or selfishness irreconcilable with the demands of love.

On the Moral and Legal Status of Abortion

Mary Anne Warren

Mary Anne Warren is a philosopher who teaches at San Francisco State University. Feminist-related issues provide one focal point of her philosophical work. Among her published articles are "Secondary Sexism and Quota Hiring," "Do Potential People Have Moral Rights?" and "Is Androgyny the Answer to Sexual Stereotyping?" She is also the author of *The Nature of Woman: An Encyclopedia and Guide to the Literature* (1980).

Warren, defending the liberal view of abortion, promptly distinguishes two senses of the term "human": (1) One is *human in the genetic sense* when one is a member of the biological species *Homo sapiens*. (2) One is *human in the moral sense* when

Reprinted by permission from vol. 57, no. 1 of *The Monist*, LaSalle, Illinois 61301. "Postscript on Infanticide" reprinted with permission of the author from *The Problem of Abortion*, Second Edition, edited by Joel Feinberg (Belmont, Calif.: Wadsworth, 1984).

one is a full-fledged member of the moral community. Warren attacks the presupposition underlying Noonan's argument against abortion—that the fetus is human in the moral sense. She contends that the moral community, the set of beings with full and equal moral rights, consists of all and only people (persons). (Thus she takes the concept of personhood to be equivalent to the concept of humanity in the moral sense.) After analyzing the concept of person, she concludes that a fetus is so unlike a person as to have no significant right to life. Nor, she argues, does the fetus's *potential* for being a person provide us any basis for ascribing to it any significant right to life. It follows, she contends, that a woman's right to obtain an abortion is absolute. Abortion is morally justified at any stage of fetal development. It also follows, she contends, that no legislation against abortion can be justified on the grounds of protecting the rights of the fetus. In a concluding postscript, Warren briefly assesses the moral justifiability of infanticide.

The question which we must answer in order to produce a satisfactory solution to the problem of the moral status of abortion is this: How are we to define the moral community, the set of beings with full and equal moral rights, such that we can decide whether a human fetus is a member of this community or not? What sort of entity, exactly, has the inalienable rights to life, liberty, and the pursuit of happiness? Jefferson attributed these rights to all *men*, and it may or may not be fair to suggest that he intended to attribute them *only* to men. Perhaps he ought to have attributed them to all human beings. If so, then we arrive, first, at Noonan's problem of defining what makes a being human, and, second, at the equally vital question which Noonan does not consider, namely, What reason is there for identifying the moral community with the set of all human beings, in whatever way we have chosen to define that term?

1 ON THE DEFINITION OF "HUMAN"

One reason why this vital second question is so frequently overlooked in the debate over the moral status of abortion is that the term 'human' has two distinct, but not often distinguished, senses. This fact results in a slide of meaning, which serves to conceal the fallaciousness of the traditional argument that since (1) it is wrong to kill innocent human beings, and (2) fetuses are innocent human beings, then (3) it is wrong to kill fetuses. For if 'human' is used in the same sense in both (1) and (2) then, whichever of the two senses is meant, one of these premises is question-begging. And if it is used in two different senses then of course the conclusion doesn't follow.

Thus, (1) is a self-evident moral truth,[1] and avoids begging the question about abortion, only if 'human being' is used to mean something like 'a full-fledged member of the moral community.' (It may or may not also be meant to refer exclusively to members of the species *Homo sapiens*.) We may call this the *moral* sense of 'human.' It is not to be confused with what we will call the *genetic* sense, i.e., the sense in which *any* member of the species is a human being, and no member of any other species could be. If (1) is acceptable only if the moral sense is intended, (2) is non-question-begging only if what is intended is the genetic sense.

In "Deciding Who is Human," Noonan argues for the classification of fetuses with human beings by pointing to the presence of the full genetic code, and the potential capacity for rational thought.[2] It is clear that what he needs to show, for his version of the traditional argument to be valid, is that fetuses are human in the moral sense, the sense in which it is analytically true that all human beings have full moral rights. But, in the absence of any argument showing that whatever is genetically human is also morally human, and he gives none, nothing more than genetic humanity can be demonstrated by the presence of the human genetic code. And, as we will see, the *potential* capacity for rational thought can at most show that an entity has the potential for *becoming* human in the moral sense.

2 DEFINING THE MORAL COMMUNITY

Can it be established that genetic humanity is sufficient for moral humanity? I think that there are very good reasons for not defining the moral community in this way. I would like to suggest an alternative way of defining the moral community, which I will argue for only to the extent of explaining why it is, or should be, self-evident. The suggestion is simply that the moral community consists of all and only *people*, rather than all and only human beings,[3] and probably the best way of demonstrating its self-evidence is by considering the concept of personhood, to see what sorts of entity are and are not persons, and what the decision that a being is or is not a person implies about its moral rights.

What characteristics entitle an entity to be considered a person? This is obviously not the place to attempt a complete analysis of the concept of personhood, but we do not need such a fully adequate analysis just to determine whether and why a fetus is or isn't a person. All we need is a rough and approximate list of the most basic criteria of personhood, and some idea of which, or how many, of these an entity must satisfy in order to properly be considered a person.

In searching for such criteria, it is useful to look beyond the set of people with whom we are acquainted, and ask how we would decide whether a totally alien being was a person or not. (For we have no right to assume that genetic humanity is necessary for personhood.) Image a space traveler who lands on an unknown planet and encounters a race of beings utterly unlike any he has ever seen or heard of. If he wants to be sure of behaving morally toward these beings, he has to somehow decide whether they are people, and hence have full moral rights, or whether they are the sort of thing which he need not feel guilty about treating as, for example, a source of food.

How should he go about making this decision? If he has some anthropological background, he might look for such things as religion, art, and the manufacturing of tools, weapons, or shelters, since these factors have been used to distinguish our human from our prehuman ancestors, in what seems to be closer to the moral than the genetic sense of 'human.' And no doubt he would be right to consider the presence of such factors as good evidence that the alien beings were people, and morally human. It would, however, be overly anthropocentric of him to take the absence of these things as adequate evidence that they were not, since we can imagine people who have progressed beyond, or evolved without ever developing, these cultural characteristics.

I suggest that the traits which are most central to the concept of personhood, or humanity in the moral sense, are, very roughly, the following:

1 Consciousness (of objects and events external and/or internal to the being), and in particular the capacity to feel pain;

2 Reasoning (the *developed* capacity to solve new and relatively complex problems);

3 Self-motivated activity (activity which is relatively independent of either genetic or direct external control);

4 The capacity to communicate, by whatever means, messages of an indefinite variety of types, that is, not just with an indefinite number of possible contents, but on indefinitely many possible topics;

5 The presence of self-concepts, and self-awareness, either individual or racial, or both.

Admittedly, there are to apt to be a great many problems involved in formulating precise definitions of these criteria, let alone in developing universally valid behavioral criteria for deciding when they apply. But I will assume that both we and our explorer know approximately what (1)–(5) mean, and that he is also able to determine whether or not they apply. How, then, should he use his findings to decide whether or not the alien beings are people? We needn't suppose that an entity must have *all* of these attributes to be properly considered a person; (1) and (2) alone may well be sufficient for personhood, and quite probably (1)–(3) are sufficient. Neither do we need to insist that any one of these criteria is *necessary* for personhood, although once again (1) and (2) look like fairly good candidates for necessary conditions, as does (3), if 'activity' is construed so as to include the activity of reasoning.

All we need to claim, to demonstrate that a fetus is not a person, is that any being which satisfies *none* of (1)–(5) is certainly not a person. I consider this claim to be so obvious that I think anyone who denied it, and claimed that a being which satisfied none of (1)–(5) was a person all the same, would thereby demonstrate that he had no notion at all of what a person is—perhaps because he had confused the concept of a person with that of genetic humanity. If the opponents of abortion were to deny the appropriateness of these five criteria, I do not know what further arguments would convince them. We would probably have to admit that our conceptual schemes were indeed irreconcilably different, and that our dispute could not be settled objectively.

I do not expect this to happen, however, since I think that the concept of a person is one which is very nearly universal (to people), and that it is common to both proabortionists and antiabortionists, even though neither group has fully realized the relevance of this concept to the resolution of their dispute. Furthermore, I think that on reflection even the antiabortionists ought to agree not only that (1)–(5) are central to the concept of personhood, but also that it is a part of this concept that all and only people have full moral rights. The concept of a person is in part a moral concept; once we have admitted that *x* is a person we have recognized, even if we have not agreed to respect, *x's* right to be treated as a member of the moral community. It is true that the claim that *x* is a *human being* is more commonly voiced as part of an appeal to treat *x* decently than is the claim that *x* is a person, but this is either because 'human being' is here used in the sense which implies personhood, or because the genetic and moral sense of 'human' have been confused.

Now if (1)–(5) are indeed the primary criteria of personhood, then it is clear that genetic humanity is neither necessary nor sufficient for establishing that an entity is a person. Some human beings are not people, and there may well be people who are not human beings. A man or woman whose consciousness has been permanently obliterated but who remains alive is a human being which is no longer a person; defective human beings, with no appreciable mental capacity, are not and presumably never will be people; and a fetus is a human being which is not yet a person, and which therefore cannot coherently be said to have full moral rights. Citizens of the next century should be prepared to recognize highly advanced, self-aware robots or computers, should such be developed, and intelligent inhabitants of other worlds, should such be found, as people in the fullest sense, and to respect their moral rights. But to ascribe full moral rights to an entity which is not a person is as absurd as to ascribe moral obligations and responsibilities to such an entity.

3   FETAL DEVELOPMENT AND THE RIGHT TO LIFE

Two problems arise in the application of these suggestions for the definition of the moral community to the determination of the precise moral status of a human fetus. Given that the paradigm example of a person is a normal adult human being, then (1) How like this paradigm, in particular how far advanced since conception, does a human being need to be before it begins to have a right to life by virtue, not of being fully a person as of yet, but of being *like* a person? and (2) To

what extent, if any, does the fact that a fetus has the *potential* for becoming a person endow it with some of the same rights? Each of these questions requires some comment.

In answering the first question, we need not attempt a detailed consideration of the moral rights of organisms which are not developed enough, aware enough, intelligent enough, etc., to be considered people, but which resemble people in some respects. It does seem reasonable to suggest that the more like a person, in the relevant respects, a being is, the stronger is the case for regarding it as having a right to life, and indeed the stronger its right to life is. Thus we ought to take seriously the suggestion that, insofar as "the human individual develops biologically in a continuous fashion...the rights of a human person might develop in the same way."[4] But we must keep in mind that the attributes which are relevant in determining whether or not an entity is enough like a person to be regarded as having some of the same moral rights are no different from those which are relevant to determining whether or not it is fully a person—i.e., are no different from (1)–(5)—and that being genetically human, or having recognizable human facial and other physical features, or detectable brain activity, or the capacity to survive outside the uterus, are simply not among these relevant attributes.

Thus it is clear that even though a seven- or eight-month fetus has features which make it apt to arouse in us almost the same powerful protective instinct as is commonly aroused by a small infant, nevertheless it is not significantly more personlike than is a very small embryo. It is *somewhat* more personlike; it can apparently feel and respond to pain, and it may even have a rudimentary form of consciousness, insofar as its brain is quite active. Nevertheless, it seems safe to say that it is not fully conscious, in the way that an infant of a few months is, and that it cannot reason, or communicate messages of indefinitely many sorts, does not engage in self-motivated activity, and has no self-awareness. Thus, in the *relevant* respects, a fetus, even a fully developed one, is considerably less personlike than is the average mature mammal, indeed the average fish. And I think that a rational person must conclude that if the right to life of a fetus is to be based upon its resemblance to a person, then it cannot be said to have any more right to life than, let us say, a newborn guppy (which also seems to be capable of feeling pain), and that a right of that magnitude could never override a woman's right to obtain an abortion, at any stage of her pregnancy.

There may, of course, be other arguments in favor of placing legal limits upon the stage of pregnancy in which an abortion may be performed. Given the relative safety of the new techniques of artificially inducing labor during the third trimester, the danger to the woman's life or health is no longer such an argument. Neither is the fact that people tend to respond to the thought of abortion in the later stages of pregnancy with emotional repulsion, since mere emotional responses cannot take the place of moral reasoning in determining what ought to be permitted. Nor, finally, is the frequently heard argument that legalizing abortion, especially late in the pregnancy, may erode the level of respect for human life, leading, perhaps, to an increase in unjustified euthanasia and other crimes. For this threat, if it is a threat, can be better met by educating people to the kinds of moral distinctions which we are making here than by limiting access to abortion (which limitation may, in its disregard for the rights of women, be just as damaging to the level of respect for human rights).

Thus, since the fact that even a fully developed fetus is not personlike enough to have any significant right to life on the basis of its personlikeness shows that no legal restrictions upon the stage of pregnancy in which an abortion may be performed can be justified on the grounds that we should protect the rights of the older fetus; and since there is no other apparent justification for such restrictions, we may conclude that they are entirely unjustified. Whether or not it would be *indecent* (whatever that means) for a women in her seventh month to obtain an abortion just to avoid having to postpone a trip to Europe, it would not, in itself, be *immoral*, and therefore it ought to be permitted.

4   POTENTIAL PERSONHOOD AND THE RIGHT TO LIFE

We have seen that a fetus does not resemble a person in any way which can support the claim that it has even some of the same rights. But what about its *potential*, the fact that if nurtured and allowed to develop naturally it will very probably become a person? Doesn't that alone give it at least some right to life? It is hard to deny that the fact that an entity is a potential person is a strong prima facie reason for not destroying it; but we need not conclude from this that a potential person has a right to life, by virtue of that potential. It may be that our feeling that it is better, other things being

equal, not to destroy a potential person is better explained by the fact that potential people are still (felt to be) an invaluable resource, not to be lightly squandered. Surely, if every speck of dust were a potential person, we would be much less apt to conclude that every potential person has a right to become actual.

Still, we do not need to insist that a potential person has no right to life whatever. There may well be something immoral, and not just imprudent, about wantonly destroying potential people, when doing so isn't necessary to protect anyone's rights. But even if a potential person does have some prima facie right to life, such a right could not possibly outweigh the right of a woman to obtain an abortion, since the rights of any actual person invariably outweigh those of any potential person, whenever the two conflict. Since this may not be immediately obvious in the case of a human fetus, let us look at another case.

Suppose that our space explorer falls into the hands of an alien culture, whose scientists decide to create a few hundred thousand or more human beings, by breaking his body into its component cells, and using these to create fully developed human beings, with, of course, his genetic code. We may imagine that each of these newly created men will have all of the original man's abilities, skills, knowledge, and so on, and also have an individual self-concept, in short that each of them will be a bona fide (though hardly unique) person. Imagine that the whole project will take only seconds, and that its chances of success are extremely high, and that our explorer knows all of this, and also knows that these people will be treated fairly. I maintain that in such a situation he would have every right to escape if he could, and thus to deprive all of these potential people of their potential lives; for his right to life outweighs all of theirs together, in spite of the fact that they are all genetically human, all innocent, and all have a very high probability of becoming people very soon, if only he refrains from acting.

Indeed, I think he would have a right to escape even if it were not his life which the alien scientists planned to take, but only a year of his freedom, or, indeed, only a day. Nor would he be obligated to stay if he had gotten captured (thus bringing all these people-potentials into existence) because of his own carelessness, or even if he had done so deliberately, knowing the consequences. Regardless of how he got captured, he is not morally obligated to remain in captivity for *any* period of time for the sake of permitting any number of potential people to come into actuality, so great is the margin by which one actual person's right to liberty outweighs whatever right to life even a hundred thousand potential people have. And it seems reasonable to conclude that the rights of a woman will outweigh by a similar margin whatever right to life a fetus may have by virtue of its potential personhood.

Thus, neither a fetus's resemblance to a person, nor its potential for becoming a person provides any basis whatever for the claim that it has any significant right to life. Consequently, a woman's right to protect her health, happiness, freedom, and even her life,[5] by terminating an unwanted pregnancy, will always override whatever right to life it may be appropriate to ascribe to a fetus, even a fully developed one. And thus, in the absence of any overwhelming social need for every possible child, the laws which restrict the right to obtain an abortion, or limit the period of pregnancy during which an abortion may be performed, are a wholly unjustified violation of a woman's most basic moral and constitutional rights.[6]

POSTSCRIPT ON INFANTICIDE, FEBRUARY 26, 1982

One of the most troubling objections to the argument presented in this article is that it may appear to justify not only abortion but infanticide as well. A newborn infant is not a great deal more personlike than a nine-month fetus, and thus it might seem that if late-term abortion is sometimes justified, then infanticide must also be sometimes justified. Yet most people consider that infanticide is a form of murder, and thus never justified.

While it is important to appreciate the emotional force of this objection, its logical force is far less than it may seem at first glance. There are many reasons why infanticide is much more difficult to justify than abortion, even though if my argument is correct neither constitutes the killing of a person. In this country, and in this period of history, the deliberate killing of viable newborns is virtually never justified. This is in part because neonates are so very *close* to being persons that to kill them requires a very strong moral justification—as does the killing of dolphins, whales, chimpanzees, and other highly personlike creatures. It is certainly wrong to kill such beings just for the sake of convenience, or financial profit, or "sport."

Another reason why infanticide is usually wrong, in our society, is that if the newborn's parents do not want it, or are unable to care for it, there are (in most cases) people who are able and eager to adopt it and to provide a good home for it. Many people wait years for the opportunity to adopt a child, and some are unable to do so even though there is every reason to believe that they would be good parents. The needless destruction of a viable infant inevitably deprives some person or persons of a source of great pleasure and satisfaction, perhaps severely impoverishing their lives. Furthermore, even if an infant is considered to be unadoptable (e.g., because of some extremely severe mental or physical handicap) it is still wrong in most cases to kill it. For most of us value the lives of infants, and would prefer to pay taxes to support orphanages and state institutions for the handicapped rather than to allow unwanted infants to be killed. So long as most people feel this way, and so long as our society can afford to provide care for infants which are unwanted or which have special needs that preclude home care, it is wrong to destroy any infant which has a chance of living a reasonably satisfactory life.

If these arguments show that infanticide is wrong, at least in this society, then why don't they also show that late-term abortion is wrong? After all, third trimester fetuses are also highly personlike, and many people value them and would much prefer that they be preserved; even at some cost to themselves. As a potential source of pleasure to some family, a viable fetus is just as valuable as a viable infant. But there is an obvious and crucial difference between the two cases: once the infant is born, its continued life cannot (except, perhaps, in very exceptional cases) pose any serious threat to the woman's life or health, since she is free to put it up for adoption, or, where this is impossible, to place it in a state-supported institution. While she might prefer that it die, rather than being raised by others, it is not clear that such a preference would constitute a right on her part. True, she may suffer greatly from the knowledge that her child will be thrown into the lottery of the adoption system, and that she will be unable to ensure its well-being, or even to know whether it is healthy, happy, doing well in school, etc.: for the law generally does not permit natural parents to remain in contact with their children, once they are adopted by another family. But there are surely better ways of dealing with these problems than by permitting infanticide in such cases. (It might help, for instance, if the natural parents of adopted children could at least receive some information about their progress, without necessarily being informed of the identity of the adopting family.)

In contrast, a pregnant woman's right to protect her own life and health clearly outweighs other people's desire that the fetus be preserved—just as, when a person's life or limb is threatened by some wild animal, and when the threat cannot be removed without killing the animal, the person's right to self-protection outweighs the desires of those who would prefer that the animal not be harmed. Thus, while the moment of birth may not mark any sharp discontinuity in the degree to which an infant possesses a right to life, it does mark the end of the mother's absolute right to determine its fate. Indeed, if and when a late-term abortion could be safely performed without killing the fetus, she would have no absolute right to insist on its death (e.g., if others wish to adopt it or pay for its care), for the same reason that she does not have a right to insist that a viable infant be killed.

It remains true that according to my argument neither abortion nor the killing of neonates is properly considered a form of murder. Perhaps it is understandable that the law should classify infanticide as murder or homicide, since there is no other existing legal category which adequately or conveniently expresses the force of our society's disapproval of this action. But the moral distinction remains, and it has several important consequences.

In the first place, it implies that when an infant is born into a society which—unlike ours—is so impoverished that it simply cannot care for it adequately without endangering the survival of existing persons, killing it or allowing it to die is not necessarily wrong—provided that there is no *other* society which is willing and able to provide such care. Most human societies, from those at the hunting and gathering stage of economic development to the highly civilized Greeks and Romans, have permitted the practice of infanticide under such unfortunate circumstances, and I would argue that it shows a serious lack of understanding to condemn them as morally backward for this reason alone.

In the second place, the argument implies that when an infant is born with such severe physical anomalies that its life would predictably be a very short and/or very miserable one, even with the most heroic of medical treatment, and where its parents do not choose to bear the often crushing emotional, financial and other burdens attendant upon the artificial prolongation of

such a tragic life, it is not morally wrong to cease or withhold treatment, thus allowing the infant a painless death. It is wrong (and sometimes a form of murder) to practice involuntary euthanasia on persons, since they have the right to decide for themselves whether or not they wish to continue to live. But terminally ill neonates cannot make this decision for themselves, and thus it is incumbent upon responsible persons to make the decision for them, as best they can. The mistaken belief that infanticide is always tantamount to murder is responsible for a great deal of unnecessary suffering, not just on the part of infants which are made to endure needlessly prolonged and painful deaths, but also on the part of parents, nurses, and other involved persons, who must watch infants suffering needlessly, helpless to end that suffering in the most humane way.

I am well aware that these conclusions, however modest and reasonable they may seem to some people, strike other people as morally monstrous, and that some people might even prefer to abandon their previous support for women's right to abortion rather than accept a theory which leads to such conclusions about infanticide. But all that these facts show is that abortion is not an isolated moral issue; to fully understand the moral status of abortion we may have to reconsider other moral issues as well, issues not just about infanticide and euthanasia, but also about the moral rights of women and of nonhuman animals. It is a philosopher's task to criticize mistaken beliefs which stand in the way of moral understanding, even when—perhaps especially when—those beliefs are popular and widespread. The belief that moral strictures against killing should apply equally to *all* genetically human entities, and *only* to genetically human entities, is such an error. The overcoming of this error will undoubtedly require long and often painful struggle; but it must be done.

NOTES

1 Of course, the principle that it is (always) wrong to kill innocent human beings is in need of many other modifications, e.g., that it may be permissible to do so to save a greater number of other innocent human beings, but we may safely ignore these complications here.

2 John Noonan, "Deciding Who is Human," *Natural Law Forum*, 13 (1968), 135.

3 From here on, we will use 'human' to mean genetically human, since the moral sense seems closely connected

to, and perhaps derived from, the assumption that genetic humanity is sufficient for membership in the moral community.

4 Thomas L. Hayes, "A Biological View," *Commonweal*, 85 (March 17, 1967), 677–78; quoted by Daniel Callahan, in *Abortion: Law, Choice and Morality* (London: Macmillan & Co., 1970).

5 That is, insofar as the death rate, for the woman, is higher for childbirth than for early abortion.

6 My thanks to the following people, who were kind enough to read and criticize an earlier version of this paper: Herbert Gold, Gene Glass, Anne Lauterbach, Judith Thomson, Mary Mothersill, and Timothy Binkley.

Abortion Decisions: Personal Morality

Daniel Callahan

A biographical sketch of Daniel Callahan is found on page 244.

Callahan defends one kind of moderate view on the problem of the ethical acceptability of abortion. On the issue of the moral status of the fetus, he steers a middle course. He rejects the "tissue" theory, the view that the fetus has negligible moral status, on the grounds that such a theory is out of tune with both the biological evidence and a respect for the sanctity of human life. On the other hand, he contends that the fetus does not qualify as a person and thus rejects the view that the fetus has full moral status. His contention that the fetus is nevertheless an "important and valuable form of human life" can be understood as implying that the fetus has some kind of *partial* moral status. In Callahan's view, a respect for the sanctity of human life should incline every woman to a strong initial (moral) bias against abortion. Yet, he argues, since a woman has duties to herself, her family, and her society, there may be circumstances in which such duties would override the prima facie duty not to abort.

...To press the problem to a finer point, what ought [women] to think about as they try to work out their own views on abortion?

Only a few suggestions will be made here, taking the form of arguing for an ethic of personal responsibility which tries, in the process of decision-making, to make itself aware of a number of things. The biological evidence should be considered, just as the problem of methodology must be considered; the philosophical assumptions implicit in different uses of the word "human" need to be considered; a philosophical theory of biological analysis is required; the social consequences of different kinds of analyses and different meanings of the word "human" should be thought

through; consistency of meaning and use should be sought to avoid *ad hoc* and arbitrary solutions.

It is my own conviction that the "developmental school" offers the most helpful and illuminating approach to the problem of the beginning of human life, avoiding, on the one hand, a too narrow genetic criterion of human life and, on the other, a too broad and socially dangerous social definition of the "human." Yet the kinds of problems which appear in any attempt to decide upon the beginning of life suggest that no one position can be either proved or disproved from biological evidence alone. It becomes a question of trying to do justice to the evidence while, at the same time, realizing that how the evidence is approached and used will be a function of one's way of looking at reality, one's moral policy, the values and rights one believes need balancing, and the type of questions one thinks need to be asked. At the very least, however, the genetic evidence for the uniqueness of zygotes and embryos (a uniqueness of a different kind than that of the uniqueness of sperm and ova), their potentiality for development into a human person, their early development of human characteristics, their genetic and organic distinctness from the organism of the mother, appear to rule out a treatment even of zygotes, much less the more developed stages of the conceptus, as mere pieces of "tissue," of no human significance or value. The "tissue" theory of the significance of the conceptus can only be made plausible by a systematic disregard of the biological evidence. Moreover, though one may conclude that a conceptus is only potential human life, in the process of continually actualizing its potential through growth and development, a respect for the sanctity of life, with its bias in favor even of undeveloped life, is enough to make the taking of such life a moral problem. There is a choice to be made and it is a moral choice....

It is possible to imagine a huge number of situations where a woman could, in good and sensitive conscience, choose abortion as a moral solution to her personal or social difficulties. But, at the very least, the bounds of morality are overstepped when either through a systematic intellectual negligence or a willful choosing of that moral solution most personally convenient, personal choice is deliberately made easy and problem-free....

...Abortion is *one* way to solve the problem of an unwanted or hazardous pregnancy (physically, psychologically, economically or socially), but it is rarely the only way, at least in affluent societies (I would be considerably less certain about making the same statement about poor societies). Even in the most extreme cases—rape, incest, psychosis, for instance—alternatives will usually be available and different choices, open. It is not necessarily the end of every woman's chance for a happy, meaningful life to bear an illegitimate child. It is not necessarily the automatic destruction of a family to have a seriously defective child born into it. It is not necessarily the ruination of every family living in overcrowded housing to have still another child. It is not inevitable that every immature woman would become even more so if she bore a child or another child. It is not inevitable that a

gravely handicapped child can hope for nothing from life. It is not inevitable that every unwanted child is doomed to misery. It is not written in the essence of things, as a fixed law of human nature, that a woman cannot come to accept, love and be a good mother to a child who was initially unwanted. Nor is it a fixed law that she could not come to cherish a grossly deformed child. Naturally, these are only generalizations. The point is only that human beings are as a rule flexible, capable of doing more than they sometimes think they can, able to surmount serious dangers and challenges, able to grow and mature, able to transform inauspicious beginnings into satisfactory conclusions. Everything in life, even in procreative and family life, is not fixed in advance; the future is never wholly unalterable....

Assuming...that most women would seek a broader ethical horizon than that of their exclusively personal self-interest, what might they think about when faced with an abortion decision? A respect for the sanctity of human life should, I believe, incline them toward a general and strong bias against abortion. Abortion is an act of killing, the violent, direct destruction of potential human life, already in the process of development. That fact should not be disguised, or glossed over by euphemism and circumlocution. It is not the destruction of a human person—for at no stage of its development does the conceptus fulfill the definition of a person, which implies a developed capacity for reasoning, willing, desiring and relating to others—but it is the destruction of an important and valuable form of human life. Its value and its potentiality are not dependent upon the attitude of the woman toward it; it grows by its own biological dynamism and has a genetic and morphological potential distinct from that of the woman. It has its own distinctive and individual future. If contraception and abortion are both seen as forms of birth limitation, they are distinctly different acts; the former precludes the possibility of a conceptus being formed, while the latter stops a conceptus already in existence from developing. The bias implied by the principle of the sanctity of human life is toward the protection of all forms of human life, especially, in ordinary circumstances, the protection of the right to life. That right should be accorded even to doubtful life; its existence should not be wholly dependent upon the personal self-interest of the woman.

Yet she has her own rights as well, and her own set of responsibilities to those around her; that is why she may have to choose abortion. In extreme situations of overpopulation, she may also have a responsibility for the survival of the species or of a people. In many circumstances, then, a decision in favor of abortion—one which overrides the right to life of that potential human being she carries within—can be a responsible moral decision, worthy neither of the condemnation of others nor of self-condemnation. But the bias of the principle of the sanctity of life is against a routine, unthinking employment of abortion; it bends over backwards not to take life and gives the benefit of the doubt to life. It does not seek to diminish the range of responsibility toward life—potential or actual—but to extend it. It does not seek the narrowest definition of life, but the widest and the richest. It is mindful of individual possibility, on the one hand, and of a destructive human tendency, on the other, to exclude from the category of "the human" or deny rights to those beings whose existence is or could prove burdensome to others....

...Moral seriousness presupposes one is concerned with the protection and furthering of life. This means that, out of respect for human life, one bends over backwards not to eliminate human life, not to desensitize oneself to the meaning and value of potential life, not to seek definitions of the "human" which serve one's self-interest only. A desire to respect human life in all of its forms means, therefore, that one voluntarily imposes upon oneself a pressure against the taking of life; that one demands of oneself serious reasons for doing so, even in the case of a very early embryo; that one use not only the mind but also the imagination when a decision is being made; that one seeks not to evade the moral issues but to face them; that one

searches out the alternatives and conscientiously entertains them before turning to abortion. A bias in favor of the sanctity of human life in all of its forms would include a bias against abortion on the part of women; it would be the last rather than the first choice when unwanted pregnancies occurred. It would be an act to be avoided if at all possible.

A bias of this kind, voluntarily imposed by a woman upon herself, would not trap her; for it is also part of a respect for the dignity of life to leave the way open for an abortion when other reasonable choices are not available. For she also has duties toward herself, her family and her society. There can be good reasons for taking the life even of a very late fetus; once that also is seen and seen as a counterpoise in particular cases to the general bias against the taking of potential life, the way is open to choose abortion. The bias of the moral policy implies the need for moral rules which seek to preserve life. But, as a policy which leaves room for choice—rather than entailing a fixed set of rules—it is open to flexible interpretation when the circumstances point to the wisdom of taking exception to the normal ordering of the rules in particular cases. Yet, in that case, one is not genuinely taking exception to the rules. More accurately, one would be deciding that, for the preservation or furtherance of other values or rights—species-right, person-rights—a choice in favor of abortion would be serving the sanctity of life. That there would be, in that case, conflict between rights, with one set of rights set aside (reluctantly) to serve another set, goes without saying. A subversion of the principle occurs when it is made out that there is no conflict and thus nothing to decide.

Abortion and the Concept of a Person

Jane English

Jane English was a philosopher whose life came to a tragic end, at the age of 31, in a 1978 mountain climbing accident on the Matterhorn. She had taught at the University of North Carolina, Chapel Hill and had published such articles as "Justice between Generations" and "Sex Equality in Sports." She was also the editor of *Sex Equality* (1977).

Reprinted from vol. 5, no. 2 (October 1975) of the *Canadian Journal of Philosophy*, by permission of the Canadian Association for Publishing in Philosophy.

English begins by arguing that one of the central issues in the abortion debate, whether a fetus is a person, cannot be decisively resolved. However, she contends, whether we presume that the fetus is or is not a person, we must arrive at a moderate stance on the problem of abortion. In an effort to moderate the *conservative* view, English argues that it is unwarranted to conclude, from the presumption that the fetus is a person, that abortion is always morally impermissible. Reasoning on the basis of a self-defense model, she finds abortion morally permissible in many cases. In an effort to moderate the *liberal* view, English argues that it is unwarranted to conclude, from the presumption that the fetus is not a person, that abortion is always morally permissible. Even if the fetus is not a person, she argues, the similarity between a fetus and a baby is sufficient to make abortion problematic in the later stages of pregnancy.

The abortion debate rages on. Yet the two most popular positions seem to be clearly mistaken. Conservatives maintain that a human life begins at conception and that therefore abortion must be wrong because it is murder. But not all killings of humans are murders. Most notably, self defense may justify even the killing of an innocent person.

Liberals, on the other hand, are just as mistaken in their argument that since a fetus does not become a person until birth, a woman may do whatever she pleases in and to her own body. First, you cannot do as you please with your own body if it affects other people adversely.[1] Second, if a fetus is not a person, that does not imply that you can do to it anything you wish. Animals, for example, are not persons, yet to kill or torture them for no reason at all is wrong.

At the center of the storm has been the issue of just when it is between ovulation and adulthood that a person appears on the scene. Conservatives draw the line at conception, liberals at birth. In this paper I first examine our concept of a person and conclude that no single criterion can capture the concept of a person and no sharp line can be drawn. Next I argue that if a fetus is a person, abortion is still justifiable in many cases; and if a fetus is not a person, killing it is still wrong in many cases. To a large extent, these two solutions are in agreement. I conclude that our concept of a person cannot and need not bear the weight that the abortion controversy has thrust upon it.

I

The several factions in the abortion argument have drawn battle lines around various proposed criteria for determining what is and what is not a person. For example, Mary Anne Warren[2] lists five features (capacities for reasoning, self-awareness, complex communication, etc.) as her criteria for personhood and argues for the permissibility of abortion because a fetus falls outside this concept. Baruch Brody[3] uses brain waves. Michael Tooley[4] picks having-a-concept-of-self as his criterion and concludes that infanticide and abortion are justifiable, while the killing of adult animals is not. On the other side, Paul Ramsey[5] claims a certain gene structure is the defining characteristic. John Noonan[6] prefers conceived-of-humans and presents counterexamples to various other candidate criteria. For instance, he argues against viability as the criterion because the newborn and infirm would then be non-persons, since they cannot live without the aid of others. He rejects any criterion that calls upon the sorts of sentiments a being can evoke in adults on the grounds that this would allow us to exclude other races as non-persons if we could just view them sufficiently unsentimentally.

These approaches are typical: foes of abortion propose sufficient conditions for personhood which fetuses satisfy, while friends of abortion counter with necessary conditions for personhood which fetuses lack. But these both presuppose that the concept of a person can be captured in a strait jacket of necessary and/or sufficient conditions.[7] Rather, "person" is a cluster of features, of which rationality, having a self concept and being conceived of humans are only part.

What is typical of persons? Within our concept of a person we include, first, certain biological factors: descended from humans, having a certain genetic makeup, having a head, hands, arms, eyes, capable of locomotion, breathing, eating, sleeping. There are psychological factors: sentience, perception, having a concept of self and of one's own interests and desires, the ability to use tools, the ability to use language or symbol systems, the ability to joke, to be angry, to doubt. There are rationality factors: the ability to reason and draw conclusions, the ability to generalize and to learn from past experience, the ability to sacrifice present interests for greater gains in the future. There are social factors: the ability to work in groups and respond to peer pressures, the ability to recognize and consider as valuable the interests of others, seeing oneself as one among "other minds," the ability to sympathize, encourage, love, the ability to evoke from others the responses of sympathy, encouragement, love, the ability to work with others for mutual advantage. Then there are legal factors: being subject to the law and protected by it, having the ability to sue and enter contracts, being counted in the census, having a name and citizenship, the ability to own property, inherit, and so forth.

Now the point is not that this list is incomplete, or that you can find counterinstances to each of its points. People typically exhibit rationality, for instance, but someone who was irrational would not thereby fail to qualify as a person. On the other hand, something could exhibit the majority of these features and still fail to be a person, as an advanced robot might. There is no single core of necessary and sufficient features which we can draw upon with the assurance that they constitute what really makes a person; there are only features that are more or less typical.

This is not to say that no necessary or sufficient conditions can be given. Being alive is a necessary condition for being a person, and being a U.S. Senator is sufficient. But rather than falling inside a sufficient condition or outside a necessary one, a fetus lies in the penumbra region where our concept of a person is not so simple. For this reason I think a conclusive answer to the question whether a fetus is a person is unattainable.

Here we might note a family of simple fallacies that proceed by stating a necessary condition for personhood and showing that a fetus has that characteristic. This is a form of the fallacy of affirming the consequent. For example, some have mistakenly reasoned from the premise that a fetus is human (after all, it is a human fetus rather than, say, a canine fetus), to the conclusion that it is *a* human. Adding an equivocation on "being," we get the fallacious argument that since a fetus is something both living and human, it is a human being.

Nonetheless, it does seem clear that a fetus has very few of the above family of characteristics, whereas a newborn baby exhibits a much larger proportion of them—and a two-year-old has even more. Note that one traditional anti-abortion argument has centered on pointing out the many ways in which a fetus resembles a baby. They emphasize its development ("It already has ten fingers...") without mentioning its dissimilarities to adults (it still has gills and a tail). They also try to evoke the sort of sympathy on our part that we only feel toward other persons ("Never to laugh...or feel the sunshine?"). This all seems to be a relevant way to argue, since its purpose is to persuade us that a fetus satisfies so many of the important features on the list that it ought to be treated as a person. Also note that a fetus near the time of birth satisfies many more of these factors than a fetus in the early months of development. This could provide reason for making distinctions among the different stages of pregnancy, as the U.S. Supreme Court has done.[8]

Historically, the time at which a person has been said to come into existence has varied widely. Muslims date personhood from fourteen days after conception. Some medievals followed Aristotle in placing ensoulment at forty days after conception for a male fetus and eighty days for a female fetus.[9] In European common law since the Seventeenth Century, abortion was considered the killing of a person only after quickening, the time when a pregnant woman first feels the fetus move on its own. Nor is this variety of opinions surprising. Biologically, a human being develops gradually. We shouldn't expect there to be any specific time or sharp dividing point when a person appears on the scene.

For these reasons I believe our concept of a person is not sharp or decisive enough to bear the weight of a solution to the abortion controversy. To use it to solve that problem is to clarify *obscurum per obscurius*.

II

Next let us consider what follows if a fetus is a person after all. Judith Jarvis Thomson's landmark article, "A Defense of Abortion,"[10] correctly points out that some additional argumentation is needed at this point in the conservative argument to bridge the gap between the premise that a fetus is an innocent person and the conclusion that killing it is always wrong. To arrive at this conclusion, we would need the additional premise that killing an innocent person is always wrong. But killing an innocent person is sometimes permissible, most notably in self defense. Some examples may help draw out our intuitions or ordinary judgments about self defense.

Suppose a mad scientist, for instance, hypnotized innocent people to jump out of the bushes and attack innocent passers-by with knives. If you are so attacked, we agree you have a right to kill the attacker in self defense, if killing him is the only way to protect your life or to save yourself from serious injury. It does not seem to matter here that the attacker is not malicious but himself an innocent pawn, for your killing of him is not done in a spirit of retribution but only in self defense.

How severe an injury may you inflict in self defense? In part this depends upon the severity of the injury to be avoided: you may not shoot someone merely to avoid having your clothes torn. This might lead one to the mistaken conclusion that the defense may only equal the threatened injury in severity; that to avoid death you may kill, but to avoid a black eye you may only inflict a black eye or the equivalent. Rather, our laws and customs seem to say that you may create an injury somewhat, but not enormously, greater than the injury to be avoided. To fend off an attack whose outcome would be as serious as rape, a severe beating or the loss of a finger, you may shoot; to avoid having your clothes torn, you may blacken an eye.

Aside from this, the injury you may inflict should only be the minimum necessary to deter or incapacitate the attacker. Even if you know he intends to kill you, you are not justified in shooting him if you could equally well save yourself by the simple expedient of running away. Self defense is for the purpose of avoiding harms rather than equalizing harms.

Some cases of pregnancy present a parallel situation. Though the fetus is itself innocent, it may pose a threat to the pregnant woman's well-being, life prospects or health, mental or physical. If the pregnancy presents a slight threat to her interests, it seems self defense cannot justify abortion. But if the threat is on a par with a serious beating or the loss of a finger, she may kill the fetus that poses such a threat, even if it is an innocent person. If a lesser harm to the fetus could have the same defensive effect, killing it would not be justified. It is unfortunate that the only way to free the woman

from the pregnancy entails the death of the fetus (except in very late stages of pregnancy). Thus a self defense model supports Thomson's point that the woman has a right only to be freed from the fetus, not a right to demand its death.[11]

The self defense model is most helpful when we take the pregnant woman's point of view. In the pre-Thomson literature, abortion is often framed as a question for a third party; do you, a doctor, have a right to choose between the life of the woman and that of the fetus? Some have claimed that if you were a passer-by who witnessed a struggle between the innocent hypnotized attacker and his equally innocent victim, you would have no reason to kill either in defense of the other. They have concluded that the self defense model implies that a woman may attempt to abort herself, but that a doctor should not assist her. I think the position of the third party is somewhat more complex. We do feel some inclination to intervene on behalf of the victim rather than the attacker, other things equal. But if both parties are innocent, other factors come into consideration. You would rush to the aid of your husband whether he was attacker or attackee. If a hypnotized famous violinist were attacking a skid row bum, we would try to save the individual who is of more value to society. These considerations would tend to support abortion in some cases.

But suppose you are a frail senior citizen who wishes to avoid being knifed by one of these innocent hypnotics, so you have hired a bodyguard to accompany you. If you are attacked, it is clear we believe that the bodyguard, acting as your agent, has a right to kill the attacker to save you from a serious beating. Your rights of self defense are transferred to your agent. I suggest that we should similarly view the doctor as the pregnant woman's agent in carrying out a defense she is physically incapable of accomplishing herself.

Thanks to modern technology, the cases are rare in which a pregnancy poses as clear a threat to a woman's bodily health as an attacker brandishing a switchblade. How does self defense fare when more subtle, complex and long-range harms are involved?

To consider a somewhat fanciful example, suppose you are a highly trained surgeon when you are kidnapped by the hypnotic attacker. He says he does not intend to harm you but to take you back to the mad scientist who, it turns out, plans to hypnotize you to have a permanent mental block against all your knowledge of medicine. This would automatically destroy your career which would in turn have a serious adverse impact on your family, your personal relationships and your happiness. It seems to me that if the only way you can avoid this outcome is to shoot the innocent attacker, you are justified in so doing. You are defending yourself from a drastic injury to your life prospects. I think it is no exaggeration to claim that unwanted pregnancies (most obviously among teenagers) often have such adverse life-long consequences as the surgeon's loss of livelihood.

Several parallels arise between various views on abortion and the self defense model. Let's suppose further that these hypnotized attackers only operate at night, so that it is well known that they can be avoided completely by the considerable inconvenience of never leaving your house after dark. One view is that since you could stay home at night, therefore if you go out and are selected by one of these hypnotized people, you have no right to defend yourself. This parallels the view that abstinence is the only acceptable way to avoid pregnancy. Others might hold that you ought to take along some defense such as Mace which will deter the hypnotized person without killing him, but that if this defense fails, you are obliged to submit to the resulting injury, no matter how severe it is. This parallels the view that contraception is all right but abortion is always wrong, even in cases of contraceptive failure.

A third view is that you may kill the hypnotized person only if he will actually kill you, but not if he will only injure you. This is like the position that abortion is permissible only if it is required to save a woman's life. Finally we have the view that it is all right to kill the attacker, even if only to avoid a very slight inconvenience to yourself and even if you knowingly walked down the very street where all these incidents have been taking place without taking along any Mace or protective escort. If we assume that a fetus is a person, this is the analogue of the view that abortion is always justifiable, "on demand."

The self defense model allows us to see an important difference that exists between abortion and infanticide, even if a fetus is a person from conception. Many have argued that the only way to justify abortion without justifying infanticide would be to find some characteristic of personhood that is acquired at birth. Michael Tooley, for one, claims infanticide is justifiable because

the really significant characteristics of person are acquired some time after birth. But all such approaches look to characteristics of the developing human and ignore the relation between the fetus and the woman. What if, after birth, the presence of an infant or the need to support it posed a grave threat to the woman's sanity or life prospects? She could escape this threat by the simple expedient of running away. So a solution that does not entail the death of the infant is available. Before birth, such solutions are not available because of the biological dependence of the fetus on the woman. Birth is the crucial point not because of any characteristics the fetus gains, but because after birth the women can defend herself by a means less drastic than killing the infant. Hence self defense can be used to justify abortion without necessarily thereby justifying infanticide.

III

On the other hand, supposing a fetus is not after all a person, would abortion always be morally permissible? Some opponents of abortion seem worried that if a fetus is not a full-fledged person, then we are justified in treating it in any way at all. However, this does not follow. Non-persons do get some consideration in our moral code, though of course they do not have the same rights as persons have (and in general they do not have moral responsibilities), and though their interests may be overridden by the interests of persons. Still, we cannot treat them in any way at all.

Treatment of animals is a case in point. It is wrong to torture dogs for fun or to kill wild birds for no reason at all. It is wrong Period, even though dogs and birds do not have the same rights persons do. However, few people think it is wrong to use dogs as experimental animals, causing them considerable suffering in some cases, provided that the resulting research will probably bring discoveries of great benefit to people. And most of us think it all right to kill birds for food or to protect our crops. People's rights are different from the consideration we give to animals, then, for it is wrong to experiment on people, even if others might later benefit a great deal as a result of their suffering. You might volunteer to be a subject, but this would be supererogatory; you certainly have a right to refuse to be a medical guinea pig.

But how do we decide what you may or may not do to non-persons? This is a difficult problem, one for which I believe no adequate account exists. You do not want to say, for instance, that torturing dogs is all right whenever the sum of its effects on people is good—when it doesn't warp the sensibilities of the torturer so much that he mistreats people. If that were the case, it would be all right to torture dogs if you did it in private, or if the torturer lived on a desert island or died soon afterward, so that his actions had no effect on people. This is an inadequate account, because whatever moral consideration animals get, it has to be indefeasible, too. It will have to be a general proscription of certain actions, not merely a weighing of the impact on people on a case-by-case basis.

Rather, we need to distinguish two levels on which consequences of actions can be taken into account in moral reasoning. The traditional objections to Utilitarianism focus on the fact that it operates solely on the first level, taking all the consequences into account in particular cases only. Thus Utilitarianism is open to "desert island" and "lifeboat" counterexamples because these cases are rigged to make the consequences of actions severely limited.

Rawls' theory could be described as a teleological sort of theory, but with teleology operating on a higher level.[12] In choosing the principles to regulate society from the original position, his hypothetical choosers make their decision on the basis of the total consequences of various systems. Furthermore, they are constrained to choose a general set of rules which people can readily learn and apply. An ethical theory must operate by generating a set of sympathies and attitudes toward others which reinforces the functioning of that set of moral principles. Our prohibition against killing people operates by means of certain moral sentiments including sympathy, compassion and guilt. But if these attitudes are to form a coherent set, they carry us further: we tend to perform supererogatory actions, and we tend to feel similar compassion toward person-like non-persons.

It is crucial that psychological facts play a role here. Our psychological constitution makes it the case that for our ethical theory to work, it must prohibit certain treatment of non-persons which are significantly person-like. If our moral rules allowed people to treat some person-like non-persons in ways we do not want people to be treated, this would undermine the system

of sympathies and attitudes that makes the ethical system work. For this reason, we would choose in the original position to make mistreatment of some sorts of animals wrong in general (not just wrong in the cases with public impact), even though animals are not themselves parties in the original position. Thus it makes sense that it is those animals whose appearance and behavior are most like those of people that get the most consideration in our moral scheme.

It is because of "coherence of attitudes," I think, that the similarity of a fetus to a baby is very significant. A fetus one week before birth is so much like a newborn baby in our psychological space that we cannot allow any cavalier treatment of the former while expecting full sympathy and nurturative support for the latter. Thus, I think that anti-abortion forces are indeed giving their strongest arguments when they point to the similarities between a fetus and a baby, and when they try to evoke our emotional attachment to and sympathy for the fetus. An early horror story from New York about nurses who were expected to alternate between caring for six-week premature infants and disposing of viable 24-week aborted fetuses is just that—a horror story. These beings are so much alike that no one can be asked to draw a distinction and treat them so very differently.

Remember, however, that in the early weeks after conception, a fetus is very much unlike a person. It is hard to develop these feelings for a set of genes which doesn't yet have a head, hands, beating heart, response to touch or the ability to move by itself. Thus it seems to me that the alleged "slippery slope" between conception and birth is not so very slippery. In the early stages of pregnancy, abortion can hardly be compared to murder for psychological reasons, but in the latest stages it is psychologically akin to murder.

Another source of similarity is the bodily continuity between fetus and adult. Bodies play a surprisingly central role in our attitudes toward persons. One has only to think of the philosophical literature on how far physical identity suffices for personal identity or Wittgenstein's remark that the best picture of the human soul is the human body. Even after death, when all agree the body is no longer a person, we still observe elaborate customs of respect for the human body; like people who torture dogs, necrophiliacs are not to be trusted with people.[13] So it is appropriate that we show respect to a fetus as the body continuous with the body of a person. This is a degree of resemblance to persons that animals cannot rival.

Michael Tooley also utilizes a parallel with animals. He claims that it is always permissible to drown new-born kittens and draws conclusions about infanticide.[14] But it is only permissible to drown kittens when their survival would cause some hardship. Perhaps it would be a burden to feed and house six more cats or to find other homes for them. The alternative of letting them starve produces even more suffering than the drowning. Since the kittens get their rights second-hand, so to speak, *via* the need for coherence in our attitudes, their interests are often overridden by the interests of full-fledged persons. But if their survival would be no inconvenience to people at all, then it is wrong to drown them, *contra* Tooley.

Tooley's conclusions about abortion are wrong for the same reason. Even if the fetus is not a person, abortion is not always permissible, because of the resemblance of a fetus to a person. I agree with Thomson that it would be wrong for a woman who is seven months pregnant to have an abortion just to avoid having to postpone a trip to Europe. In the early months of pregnancy when the fetus hardly resembles a baby at all, then, abortion is permissible whenever it is in the interests of the pregnant woman or her family. The reasons would only need to outweigh the pain and inconvenience of the abortion itself. In the middle months, when the fetus comes to resemble a person, abortion would be justifiable only when the continuation of the pregnancy or the birth of the child would cause harms—physical, psychological, economic or social—to the woman. In the late months of pregnancy, even on our current assumption that a fetus is not a person, abortion seems to be wrong except to save a woman from significant injury or death.

The Supreme Court has recognized similar gradations in the alleged slippery slope stretching between conception and birth. To this point, the present paper has been a discussion of the moral status of abortion only, not its legal status. In view of the great physical, financial and sometimes psychological costs of abortion, perhaps the legal arrangement most compatible with the proposed moral solution would be the absence of restrictions, that is, so-called abortion "on demand."

So I conclude, first, that application of our concept of a person will not suffice to settle the abortion issue. After all, the biological development of a human being is gradual. Second, whether a fetus is a person or not, abortion is justifiable early in pregnancy to avoid modest harms and seldom justifiable late in pregnancy except to avoid significant injury or death.[15]

NOTES

1. We also have paternalistic laws which keep us from harming our own bodies even when no one else is affected. Ironically, anti-abortion laws were originally designed to protect pregnant women from a dangerous but tempting procedure.
2. Mary Anne Warren, "On the Moral and Legal Status of Abortion," *Monist* 57 (1973), p. 55.
3. Baruch Brody, "Fetal Humanity and the Theory of Essentialism," in Robert Baker and Frederick Elliston (eds.), *Philosophy and Sex* (Buffalo, N.Y., 1975).
4. Michael Tooley, "Abortion and Infanticide," *Philosophy and Public Affairs* 2 (1971).
5. Paul Ramsey, "The Morality of Abortion," in James Rachels, ed., *Moral Problems* (New York, 1971).
6. John Noonan, "Abortion and the Catholic Church: A Summary History," *Natural Law Forum* 12 (1967), pp. 125–131.
7. Wittgenstein has argued against the possibility of so capturing the concept of a game, *Philosophical Investigations* (New York, 1958), § 66–71.
8. Not because the fetus is partly a person and so has some of the rights of persons, but rather because of the rights of person-like non-persons. This I discuss in part III below.
9. Aristotle himself was concerned, however, with the different question of when the soul takes form. For historical data, see Jimmye Kimmey, "How the Abortion Laws Happened," *Ms.* 1 (April, 1973), pp. 48ff, and John Noonan, *loc. cit.*
10. J. J. Thomson, "A Defense of Abortion," *Philosophy and Public Affairs* 1 (1971).
11. *Ibid.*, p. 52.
12. John Rawls, *A Theory of Justice* (Cambridge, Mass., 1971), § 3–4.
13. On the other hand, if they can be trusted with people, then our moral customs are mistaken. It all depends on the facts of psychology.
14. *Op. cit.*, pp. 40, 60–61.
15. I am deeply indebted to Larry Crocker and Arthur Kuflik for their constructive comments.

Abortion and Social Policy

Majority Opinion in *Roe v. Wade*

Justice Harry Blackmun

Harry Blackmun, associate justice of the United States Supreme Court, is a graduate of Harvard Law School. After some fifteen years in private practice he became legal counsel to the Mayo Clinic (1950–1959). Justice Blackmun also served as United States circuit judge (1959–1970) before his appointment in 1970 to the Supreme Court.

In this case, a pregnant single woman, suing under the fictitious name of Jane Roe, challenged the constitutionality of the existing Texas criminal abortion law. According to the Texas Penal Code, the performance of an abortion, except to save the life of the mother, constituted a crime that was punishable by a prison sentence of two to five years. At the time this case was finally resolved by the Supreme Court, abortion legislation varied widely from state to state. Some states, principally New York, had already legalized abortion on demand. Most other states, however, had legalized various forms of therapeutic abortion but had retained some measure of restrictive abortion legislation.

Justice Blackmun, writing an opinion concurred in by six other justices, argues that a woman's decision to terminate a pregnancy is encompassed by a *right to privacy*—but only up to a certain point in the development of the fetus. As the right to privacy is not an absolute right, it must yield at some point to the state's legitimate interests. Justice Blackmun contends that the state has a legitimate interest in protecting the health of the mother and that this interest becomes compelling at approximately the end of the first trimester in the development of the fetus. He also contends that the state has a legitimate interest in protecting potential life and that this interest becomes compelling at the point of viability.

It is...apparent that at common law, at the time of the adoption of our Constitution, and throughout the major portion of the 19th century, abortion was viewed with less disfavor than under most American statutes currently in effect. Phrasing it another way, a woman enjoyed a substantially broader right to terminate a pregnancy than she does in most States today. At least with respect to the early stage of pregnancy, and very possibly without such a limitation, the opportunity to make this choice was present in this country well into the 19th century. Even later, the law continued for some time to treat less punitively an abortion procured in early pregnancy....

Three reasons have been advanced to explain historically the enactment of criminal abortion laws in the 19th century and to justify their continued existence.

It has been argued occasionally that these laws were the product of a Victorian social concern to discourage illicit sexual conduct. Texas, however, does not advance this justification in the present case, and it appears that no court or commentator has taken the argument seriously....

A second reason is concerned with abortion as a medical procedure. When most criminal abortion laws were first enacted, the procedure was a hazardous one for the woman. This was particularly true prior to the

United States Supreme Court; January 22, 1973. 410 U.S. 113, 93 S.Ct. 705.

development of antisepsis. Antiseptic techniques, of course, were based on discoveries by Lister, Pasteur, and others first announced in 1867, but were not generally accepted and employed until about the turn of the century. Abortion mortality was high. Even after 1900, and perhaps until as late as the development of antibiotics in the 1940's, standard modern techniques such as dilation and curettage were not nearly so safe as they are today. Thus it has been argued that a State's real concern in enacting a criminal abortion law was to protect the pregnant woman, that is, to restrain her from submitting to a procedure that placed her life in serious jeopardy.

Modern medical techniques have altered this situation. Appellants and various *amici* refer to medical data indicating that abortion in early pregnancy, that is, prior to the end of first trimester, although not without its risk, is now relatively safe. Mortality rates for women undergoing early abortions, where the procedure is legal, appear to be as low as or lower than the rates for normal childbirth. Consequently, any interest of the State in protecting the woman from an inherently hazardous procedure, except when it would be equally dangerous for her to forego it, has largely disappeared. Of course, important state interests in the area of health and medical standards do remain. The State has a legitimate interest in seeing to it that abortion, like any other medical procedure, is performed under circumstances that insure maximum safety for the patient. This interest obviously extends at least to the performing physician and his staff, to the facilities involved, to the availability of after-care, and to adequate provision for any complication or emergency that might arise. The prevalence of high mortality rates at illegal "abortion mills" strengthens, rather than weakens, the State's interest in regulating the conditions under which abortions are performed. Moreover, the risk to the woman increases as her pregnancy continues. Thus the State retains a definite interest in protecting the woman's own health and safety when an abortion is performed at a late stage of pregnancy.

The third reason is the State's interest—some phrase it in terms of duty—in protecting prenatal life. Some of the argument for this justification rests on the theory that a new human life is present from the moment of conception. The State's interest and general obligation to protect life then extends, it is argued, to prenatal life. Only when the life of the pregnant mother herself is at stake, balanced against the life she carries within her, should the interest of the embryo or fetus not prevail. Logically, of course, a legitimate state interest in this area need not stand or fall on acceptance of the belief that life begins at conception or at some other point prior to live birth. In assessing the State's interest, recognition may be given to the less rigid claim that as long as at least *potential* life is involved, the State may assert interests beyond the protection of the pregnant woman alone.

Parties challenging state abortion laws have sharply disputed in some courts the contention that a purpose of these laws, when enacted, was to protect prenatal life. Pointing to the absence of legislative history to support the contention, they claim that most state laws were designed solely to protect the woman. Because medical advances have lessened this concern, at least with respect to abortion in early pregnancy, they argue that with respect to such abortions the laws can no longer be justified by any state interest. There is some scholarly support for this view of original purpose. The few state courts called upon to interpret their laws in the late 19th and early 20th centuries did focus on the State's interest in protecting the woman's health rather than in preserving the embryo and fetus....

The Constitution does not explicitly mention any right of privacy. In a line of decisions, however, going back perhaps as far as *Union Pacific R. Co. v. Botsford* (1891), the Court has recognized that a right of personal privacy, or a guarantee of certain areas or zones of privacy, does exist under the constitution. In varying contexts the Court or individual Justices have indeed found at least the roots of that right in the First Amendment,...in the Fourth and Fifth Amendments ...in the penumbras of the Bill of Rights...in the Ninth Amendment...or in the concept of liberty guaranteed by the first section of the Fourteenth Amendment.... These decisions make it clear that only personal rights that can be deemed "fundamental" or "implicit in the concept of ordered liberty,"...are included in this guarantee of personal privacy. They also make it clear that the right has some extension to activities relating to marriage,...procreation,...contraception, ...family relationships,...and child rearing and education,...

This right of privacy, whether it be founded in the Fourteenth Amendment's concept of personal liberty and restrictions upon state action, as we feel it is, or, as the District Court determined, in the Ninth Amendment's reservation of rights to the people, is broad enough to encompass a woman's decision whether or not to terminate her pregnancy....

...[A]ppellants and some *amici* argue that the woman's right is absolute and that she is entitled to terminate her pregnancy at whatever time, in whatever way, and for whatever reason she alone chooses. With this we do not agree. Appellants' arguments that Texas either has no valid interest at all in regulating the abortion decision, or no interest strong enough to support any limitation upon the woman's sole determination, is unpersuasive. The Court's decisions recognizing a right of privacy also acknowledge that some state regulation in areas protected by that right is appropriate. As noted above, a state may properly assert important interests in safe-guarding health, in maintaining medical standards, and in protecting potential life. At some point in pregnancy, these respective interests become sufficiently compelling to sustain regulation of the factors that govern the abortion decision. The privacy right involved, therefore, cannot be said to be absolute....

We therefore conclude that the right of personal privacy includes the abortion decision, but that this right is not unqualified and must be considered against important state interests in regulation.

We note that those federal and state courts that have recently considered abortion law challenges have reached the same conclusion....

Although the results are divided, most of these courts have agreed that the right of privacy, however based, is broad enough to cover the abortion decision; that the right, nonetheless, is not absolute and is subject to some limitations; and that at some point the state interests as to protection of health, medical standards, and prenatal life, become dominant. We agree with this approach....

The appellee and certain *amici* argue that the fetus is a "person" within the language and meaning of the Fourteenth Amendment. In support of this they outline at length and in detail the well-known facts of fetal development. If this suggestion of personhood is established, the appellant's case, of course, collapses, for the fetus' right to life is then guaranteed specifically by the Amendment. The appellant conceded as much on reargument. On the other hand, the appellee conceded on reargument that no case could be cited that holds that a fetus is a person within the meaning of the Fourteenth Amendment....

All this, together with our observation, *supra*, that throughout the major portion of the 19th century prevailing legal abortion practices were far freer than they are today, persuades us that the word "person," as used in the Fourteenth Amendment, does not include the unborn.... Indeed, our decision in *United States v. Vuitch* (1971) inferentially is to the same effect, for we there would not have indulged in statutory interpretation favorable to abortion in specified circumstances if the necessary consequence was the termination of life entitled to Fourteenth Amendment protection.

... As we have intimated above, it is reasonable and appropriate for a State to decide that at some point in time another interest, that of health of the mother or that of potential human life, becomes significantly involved. The woman's privacy is no longer sole and any right of privacy she possesses must be measured accordingly.

Texas urges that, apart from the Fourteenth Amendment, life begins at conception and is present throughout pregnancy, and that, therefore, the State has a compelling interest in protecting that life from and after conception. We need not resolve the difficult question of when life begins. When those trained in the respective disciplines of medicine, philosophy, and theology are unable to arrive at any consensus, the judiciary, at this point in the development of man's knowledge, is not in a position to speculate as to the answer.

It should be sufficient to note briefly the wide divergence of thinking on this most sensitive and difficult question. There has always been strong support for the view that life does not begin until live birth. This was the belief of the Stoics. It appears to be the predominant, though not the unanimous, attitude of the Jewish faith. It may be taken to represent also the position of a large segment of the Protestant community, insofar as that can be ascertained; organized groups that have taken a formal position on the abortion issue have generally regarded abortion as a matter for the conscience of the individual and her family. As we have noted, the common law found greater significance in quickening. Physicians and their scientific colleagues have regarded that event with less interest and have tended to focus either upon conception or upon live birth or upon the interim point at which the fetus becomes "viable," that is, potentially able to live outside the mother's womb, albeit with artificial aid. Viability is usually placed at about seven months (28 weeks) but may occur earlier, even at 24 weeks....

In areas other than criminal abortion the law has been reluctant to endorse any theory that life, as we recognize it, begins before live birth or to accord legal rights to the unborn except in narrowly defined situations and except when the rights are contingent upon live birth....In short, the unborn have never been recognized in the law as persons in the whole sense.

In view of all this, we do not agree that, by adopting one theory of life, Texas may override the rights of the pregnant woman that are at stake. We repeat, however, that the State does have an important and legitimate interest in preserving and protecting the health of the pregnant woman, whether she be a resident of the State or a nonresident who seeks medical consultation and treatment there, and that it has still *another* important and legitimate interest in protecting the potentiality of human life. These interests are separate and distinct. Each grows in substantiality as the woman approaches term and, at a point during pregnancy, each becomes "compelling."

With respect to the State's important and legitimate interest in the health of the mother, the "compelling" point, in the light of present medical knowledge, is at approximately the end of the first trimester. This is so because of the now established medical fact...that until the end of the first trimester mortality in abortion is less than mortality in normal childbirth. It follows that, from and after this point, a State may regulate the abortion procedure to the extent that the regulation reasonably relates to the preservation and protection of maternal health. Examples of permissible state regulation in this area are requirements as to the qualifications of the person who is to perform the abortion; as to the licensure of that person; as to the facility in which the procedure is to be performed, that is, whether it must be a hospital or may be a clinic or some other place of less-than-hospital status; as to the licensing of the facility; and the like.

This means, on the other hand, that, for the period of pregnancy prior to this "compelling" point, the attending physician, in consultation with his patient, is free to determine, without regulation by the State, that in his medical judgment the patient's pregnancy should be terminated. If that decision is reached, the judgment may be effectuated by an abortion free of interference by the State.

With respect to the State's important and legitimate interest in potential life, the "compelling" point is at viability. This is so because the fetus then presumably has the capability of meaningful life outside the mother's womb. State regulation protective of fetal life after viability thus has both logical and biological justifications. If the State is interested in protecting fetal life after viability, it may go so far as to proscribe abortion during that period except when it is necessary to preserve the life or health of the mother....

To summarize and repeat:

1 A state criminal abortion statute of the current Texas type, that excepts from criminality only a *life saving* procedure on behalf of the mother, without regard to pregnancy stage and without recognition of the other interests involved, is violative of the Due Process Clause of the Fourteenth Amendment.

a For the stage prior to approximately the end of the first trimester, the abortion decision and its effectuation must be left to the medical judgment of the pregnant woman's attending physician.

b For the stage subsequent to approximately the end of the first trimester, the State, in promoting its interest in the health of the mother, may, if it chooses, regulate the abortion procedure in ways that are reasonably related to maternal health.

c For the stage subsequent to viability the State, in promoting its interest in the potentiality of human life, may, if it chooses, regulate, and even proscribe, abortion except where it is necessary, in appropriate medical judgment, for the preservation of the life or health of the mother.

2 The State may define the term "physician," as it has been employed [here], to mean only a physician currently licensed by the State, and may proscribe any abortion by a person who is not a physician as so defined.

...The decision leaves the State free to place increasing restrictions on abortion as the period of pregnancy lengthens, so long as those restrictions are tailored to the recognized state interests. The decision vindicates the right of the physician to administer medical treatment according to his professional judgment up to the points where important state interests provide compelling justifications for intervention. Up to those points the abortion decision in all its aspects is inherently, and primarily, a medical decision, and basic responsibility for it must rest with the physician. If an individual practitioner abuses the privilege of exercising proper medical judgment, the usual remedies, judicial and intraprofessional, are available....

Roe v. Wade Reaffirmed

George J. Annas

A biographical sketch of George J. Annas is found on page 114.

Annas interprets the decision of the U.S. Supreme Court in *Akron v. Akron Center for Reproductive Health* (1983) as a strong reaffirmation of the principles enunciated by the Court in *Roe v. Wade* (1973). At issue in *Akron* was a local abortion ordinance that, among other things, incorporated a *hospitalization requirement* (for all abortions after the first trimester) and a very demanding *consent requirement*. Annas traces the reasoning used by the Court in rejecting both of these requirements as unconstitutional. He also briefly considers the point of view expressed by Justice O'Connor in a dissenting opinion.

The Supreme Court's message is clear: if states continue to pass statutes that restrict a woman's access to abortion in ways not permitted by its 1973 *Roe v. Wade* decision, the Court will strike them down. Efforts to persuade the Court to overrule or curtail *Roe* have failed, and the Court's commitment to a pregnant woman's liberty interest in her decision regarding childbirth or abortion can no longer be questioned.

In *Roe v. Wade* (410 U.S. 113) the Court held that the Constitution protected the woman's right to decide, with her physician, to have an abortion. As long as abortion was safer than childbirth (until about the end of the first trimester), the state could not demonstrate any interest in maternal health compelling enough to interfere with the decision. Until the fetus was considered viable, that is, had "the capability of meaningful life outside the mother's womb" (usually about the beginning of the third trimester), the interests of the mother continued to outweigh those of the fetus.

At viability, however, the state's interest in protecting fetal life became compelling enough to permit the state to prohibit abortions, "except when necessary to preserve the life or health of the mother." Sometimes denoted the "trimester system," the actual dividing lines regarding permissible state regulation were two: the time when abortion became more dangerous to the pregnant woman than childbirth, and the time when the fetus became viable.

THE AKRON OPINION

Until the Court's decision in *Akron v. Akron Center for Reproductive Health* (51 LW 4767), decided by a vote of six to three on June 15, 1983, it was possible to argue that the Supreme Court was slowly backing away from its most controversial decision of the past twenty-five years. In 1977, for example, the Court ruled that the Constitution did not require a state's Medicaid program to pay for nontherapeutic abortions if it paid for childbirth.[1] In 1980 the Court held that the Constitution did not require Medicaid funding of *any* abortions, even medically necessary ones, because failure to fund them did not place any state-created obstacle in the path of a poor woman who elected to terminate her pregnancy by abortion.[2]

But these cases were limited to the issue of government funding; those commentators who, like me, interpreted them as signaling a retreat from *Roe v. Wade*, have now been proven incorrect. Indeed, one could probably not write a stronger reaffirmation of the principles of *Roe* than Justice Louis Powell's majority opinion in *Akron*.

At issue was a detailed ordinance of the City of Akron, Ohio, that attempted to place numerous obstacles in the way of a woman who wished to have an abortion. The ordinance's provisions relating to in-hospital abortions and informed consent probably best illustrate the court's overall position.

Reprinted with permission of the author and the publisher from *Hastings Center Review*, vol. 13 (August 1983), pp. 21–22.

THE HOSPITALIZATION REQUIREMENT

The ordinance required that all abortions after the first trimester be performed in a hospital. This would have been acceptable in 1973, when such abortions were considered more dangerous to a woman's health than childbirth. However, in 1983 medical evidence indicates that when the method of dilation and evacuation (D&E) is used, abortions may be safer than childbirth up to a gestational age of sixteen weeks. While continuing to put the line for the state's interest in protecting maternal health "at approximately the end of the first trimester," the Court notes that this interest no longer justifies a blanket hospital rule because: (1) the safety of second-trimester abortions has "increased dramatically" since *Roe*; (2) the American Public Health Association and the American College of Obstetricians and Gynecologists both agree that second-trimester abortions using dilation and evacuation can be safely performed in nonhospital facilities; and (3) the additional cost of an in-hospital abortion, $850–900 *versus* $350–400 for a clinic abortion, places "a significant obstacle in the path of women seeking abortion."[3]

The Court concludes:

By preventing the performance of D&E abortions in an appropriate nonhospital setting, Akron has imposed a heavy, and unnecessary, burden on women's access to a relatively inexpensive, otherwise accessible, and safe abortion procedure...and therefore unreasonably infringes upon a woman's constitutional right to obtain an abortion.

THE CONSENT REQUIREMENT

Another portion of the ordinance, mislabeled "informed consent," required the physician personally to inform the pregnant woman of a number of specific items, including the statement that "the unborn child is a human life from the moment of conception"; a description detailing the "anatomical and physiological characteristics of the particular unborn child...including appearance, mobility, tactile sensitivity, including pain, perception, or response..."; the warning that "abortion is a major surgical procedure, which can result in serious complications...and can result in severe emotional problems"; and the suggestion that "numerous public and private agencies are available to assist her during pregnancy and after the birth of her child if she chooses not to have an abortion...."

Although agreeing that informed consent is an essential part of the abortion decision, the Court concludes that the relevant information can vary based on the patient's "particular circumstances" and that it should remain "primarily the responsibility of the physician to ensure that appropriate information is conveyed to the patient." The information required by the Akron ordinance, the Court concludes, is "designed not to inform the woman's consent but rather to persuade her to withhold it altogether."

Equally decisive, the Court says, is that it intrudes "upon the discretion of the pregnant woman's physician." The state "may require that the physician make certain that the pregnant woman understands the physical and emotional implications of having an abortion," but it places unconstitutional "obstacles in the path of the doctor upon whom the woman is entitled to rely for advice in connection with her decision" when it insists "upon the recitation of a lengthy and inflexible list of information."

The Court also rejects the requirement that the physician always obtain informed consent personally, because it does not believe the state could demonstrate that such a requirement was reasonably designed to further the state's interest in the woman's health: "the critical factor is whether she obtains the necessary information and counseling from a qualified person, not the identity of the person from whom she obtains it."

THE DISSENT

Roe v. Wade was a seven-to-two decision. Justice Sandra O'Connor wrote the dissent in *Akron*, joined by the original two dissenters in *Roe*, Justices White and Rehnquist. Justice O'Connor's primary arguments center on the "completely unworkable" trimester system that requires courts and legislatures "to continuously and conscientiously study contemporary medical and scientific literature" to determine the acceptability of current practice, the safety of abortion at a given period in pregnancy, and the point of viability. She argues that the *Roe* approach turns the court into a "science review board" and violates a primary principle of judicial decision making: the application of neutral principles "sufficiently absolute to give them roots throughout the community and continuity over significant periods of time...."

While this is the framework she outlines, her dissent makes clear that she is not upset with the changing nature of *Roe* (which *is* tied to the state of medical technology) but with its outcome. She would be no happier with a decision that supported the woman's liberty interest in abortion on some more permanent basis; her goal was a decision that permitted the states to heavily regulate or outlaw abortion altogether.

Her central argument is that *Roe*'s trimester framework "is clearly on a collision course with itself" and therefore should be abandoned. She correctly notes that abortion will probably keep getting safer later in pregnancy, and may even become safer than childbirth up to and after fetal viability. As a result, states will be prohibited from enacting unreasonable and burdensome restrictions on abortion up to fetal viability. But the state will still have the ability to proscribe abortion altogether *after* viability, even if abortion is (at some future date) always safer or as safe as continuing the pregnancy to term. At this point the *Roe* trimester test will collapse into a two-period test: pre- and post-viability.

The real issue, therefore, is fetal viability and the effect of improved technology, which may permit younger and younger fetuses to survive to "meaningful lives." Under *Roe* such technological improvements will enhance the state's ability to regulate abortion, and will require women seeking abortions to have them prior to fetal viability (as they must now) and thus earlier and earlier in pregnancy. I have difficulty seeing, however, why such a result is either discontinuous with *Roe* or socially undesirable. Perhaps Justice O'Connor is worried about the day—surely in the distant future—when it may be possible not only to conceive a child in the laboratory, but also to grow the fetus to viability in an "artificial placenta." Then, since

the fetus is "immediately viable" the *Roe* framework will provide no basis for distinguishing between any of the phases of pregnancy, and a new analytical framework will be necessary. In an area in which scientific advances are central concerns it is perfectly appropriate for both courts and legislatures to reconsider their rules in light of these advances.

Reaffirming *Roe v. Wade*, the Supreme Court takes a strong stand on the side of our being a government of law. As Justice Powell put it for the Court: "The doctrine of *stare decisis* [following precedents]...is a doctrine that demands respect in a society governed by the rule of law." *Roe v. Wade* was the law in 1973, has been the law since, and remains the law. Debate will continue as to its wisdom, its moral basis, and its effect. The debate as to its legal status in the Supreme Court, however, is over.

NOTES

1 George J. Annas, "Let Them Eat Cake," *Hastings Center Report*, vol. 7, August 1977, pp. 8–9.
2 George J. Annas, "The Supreme Court and Abortion: The Irrelevance of Medical Judgment," *Hastings Center Report*, vol. 10, October 1980, pp. 23–24.
3 In a companion case the Court approved a state requirement that all fetal remains be examined by a pathologist because of the health rationale and the "comparatively small added cost" put at $19.40. On the other hand, an Akron requirement involving a twenty-four-hour waiting period between consent and the abortion procedure was struck down because of the cost involved in making two separate trips to the clinic. Small costs with health rationales are permitted; burdensome and unnecessary added costs are not.

ANNOTATED BIBLIOGRAPHY: CHAPTER 9

Armstrong, Robert L.: "The Right to Life," *Journal of Social Philosophy* 8 (January 1977), pp 13–19. Armstrong develops an interesting and somewhat distinctive moderate view on the morality of abortion. Although fetuses are not actual persons, he contends, they may be said to have a right to life on the basis of their potential personhood, but *only* if they have what he calls "real or serious" potentiality.

Bok, Sissela: "Ethical Problems of Abortion," *Hastings Center Studies* 2 (January 1974), pp. 33–52. Rejecting efforts to define "humanity," Bok suggests that various reasons for protecting life gain in strength as the fetus develops. Thus, she holds, while early abortions are relatively unproblematic, later abortions raise serious ethical difficulties.

Brody, Baruch: "On the Humanity of the Foetus." In Robert L. Perkins, ed., *Abortion: Pro and Con* (Cambridge, Mass.: Schenkman, 1974), pp. 69–90. Brody critically examines the various proposals for "drawing the line" on the humanity of the fetus, ultimately suggesting that the most defensible view would draw the line at the point where fetal brain activity begins.

Callahan, Daniel: *Abortion: Law, Choice and Morality* (New York: Macmillan, 1970). Callahan provides a wealth of useful data relevant to deciding various medical, social, and legal questions about abortion. Against this background, he discusses the ethical acceptability of abortion and ultimately defends a moderate position.

Engelhardt, H. Tristram, Jr.: "The Ontology of Abortion," *Ethics* 84 (April 1974), pp. 217–234. Engelhardt focuses attention on the issue of "whether or to what extent the fetus is a person." He argues that, strictly speaking, a human person is not present until the later stages of infancy. However, he finds the point of viability significant in that, with viability, an infant can play the social role of "child" and thus be treated "as if it were a person."

Feinberg, Joel: "Abortion." In Tom Regan, ed., *Matters of Life and Death* (New York: Random House, 1980), pp. 183–217. In this long essay, Feinberg analyzes the strengths and weaknesses of alternative views about the moral status of the fetus. He also considers the extent to which abortion is morally justifiable *if* it is granted that the fetus is a person.

————, ed.: *The Problem of Abortion*, 2nd ed. (Belmont, Calif.: Wadsworth, 1984). This excellent anthology features a wide range of articles on the moral justifiability of abortion.

Grisez, Germain: *Abortion: The Myths, The Realities, and the Arguments* (New York: Corpus Books, 1970). Early chapters of this long book provide discussions of a number of factual and historical aspects of abortion. Grisez's conservative view on the morality of abortion appears in Chapter 6, "Ethical Arguments." Chapter 7, also notable, is entitled "Toward a Sound Public Policy."

Humber, James M.: "Abortion: The Avoidable Moral Dilemma," *Journal of Value Inquiry* 9 (Winter 1975), pp. 282–302. Humber, defending the conservative view on the morality of abortion, examines and rejects what he identifies as the major defenses of abortion. He also contends that proabortion arguments are typically so poor that they can only be viewed as "after-the-fact-rationalizations."

Langerak, Edward A.: "Abortion: Listening to the Middle," *Hastings Center Report* 9 (October 1979), pp. 24–28. Langerak suggests a theoretical framework for a moderate view that incorporates two "widely shared beliefs": (1) that there is something about the fetus *itself* that makes abortion morally problematic and (2) that late abortions are significantly more problematic than early abortions.

Noonan, John T., Jr., ed.: *The Morality of Abortion: Legal and Historical Perspectives* (Cambridge, Mass.: Harvard University Press, 1970). This book contains a series of readings representing various theological perspectives on abortion. The conservative view is prominent.

Ross, Steven L.: "Abortion and the Death of the Fetus," *Philosophy and Public Affairs* 11 (Summer 1982), pp. 232–245. Ross draws a distinction between abortion as the termination of pregnancy and abortion as the termination of the life of the fetus. He proceeds to defend abortion in the latter sense, insisting that it is justifiable for a woman to desire not only the termination of pregnancy but also the death of the fetus.

Sumner, L. W.: "Toward a Credible View of Abortion," *Canadian Journal of Philosophy* 4 (September 1974), pp. 163–181. Rejecting both the conservative and liberal views on the morality of abortion, Sumner develops a "more credible, because more moderate, alternative." Following a developmental approach, he holds that the moral status of the fetus increases as the fetus develops.

Thomson, Judith Jarvis: "A Defense of Abortion," *Philosophy and Public Affairs* 1 (Fall 1971), pp. 47–66. In this widely discussed article, Thomson attempts to "moderate the conservative view." For the sake of argument, she grants the premise that the fetus (from conception) is a person. Still, she argues, under certain conditions abortion remains morally permissible.

Tooley, Michael: "Abortion and Infanticide," *Philosophy and Public Affairs* 2 (Fall 1972), pp. 37–65. Tooley, in this landmark defense of the liberal view on the morality of abortion, investigates the question of what properties an organism must possess in order to qualify as having a serious right to life. On his analysis, neither a fetus nor an infant can be said to have a serious right to life, and thus both abortion and infanticide are ethically acceptable.

———: *Abortion and Infanticide* (New York: Oxford, 1983). In this long book, Tooley defends the liberal view on the morality of abortion. He insists that the question of the morality of abortion cannot be satisfactorily resolved "in isolation from the questions of the morality of infanticide and of the killing of nonhuman animals."

Chapter 10

Genetics and Human Reproduction

INTRODUCTION

With the rapid advance of knowledge and techniques in genetics and the biology of human reproduction, a number of complex and troubling ethical issues have arisen. This chapter is designed to address some of the most important of these issues.

Genetic Disease and the Language of Genetics

Tay-Sachs disease is one prominent example of a genetic disease. This disease, which most commonly affects Jewish children of Eastern European heritage, is characterized by progressive neurological degeneration and death in early childhood. Although a child afflicted with Tay-Sachs disease has the disease by virtue of his or her genetic inheritance, the child's parents do not have the disease. (Those afflicted with Tay-Sachs disease do not survive to reproduce.) The parents are "carriers." Tay-Sachs carriers are those persons who have one normal gene and one variant or defective gene (the Tay-Sachs gene) at the same location on paired chromosomes. The Tay-Sachs gene is a *recessive* gene. When it is paired with a normal gene, as is the case with the carrier, the normal gene is dominant. As a result, the carrier does not manifest the disease. However, if a child inherits the Tay-Sachs gene from both parents, then the child will be afflicted with Tay-Sachs disease.

Since Tay-Sachs disease is traceable to a recessive gene, it is said to be a recessive disease. Moreover, it is said to be an *autosomal* recessive disease, where the word "autosomal" simply indicates that the defective genes are located on some pair of chromosomes other than the sex chromosomes. Further, in the language of genetics, Tay-Sachs carriers are said to be in the *heterozygous* state, whereas a child afflicted with Tay-Sachs disease is said to be in the *homozygous* state, with regard to the Tay-Sachs gene. Carriers, having the Tay-Sachs gene paired with a different (normal) gene, are heterozygous with regard to the Tay-Sachs gene. The afflicted child, having two identical Tay-Sachs genes, is homozygous with regard to the Tay-Sachs gene. The carrier is sometimes termed a "heterozygote," the afflicted child a "homozygote."

According to the laws of heredity, when two carriers of a trait associated with an autosomal recessive disease produce offspring, there is one chance in four (25 percent) that their child will be afflicted with the genetic disease in question. There are two chances in four (50 percent) that their child will be, like them, a carrier. Finally, there is one chance in four (25 percent) that their child will be free both of the disease and of the carrier status.

The genetic disease usually called "sickle-cell anemia" is, like Tay-Sachs disease, a well-known autosomal recessive disease. Most commonly affecting blacks, sickle-cell anemia is characterized by acute attacks of abdominal pain and exhibits a range of severity. It is estimated that 10–12 percent of blacks in the United States carry the sickle-cell trait. As is typical of autosomal recessive diseases, if two carriers of the sickle-cell trait produce offspring, there is one chance in four (25 percent) that their child will be afflicted with sickle-cell anemia.

Huntington's chorea provides a leading example of a genetic disease in the category of autosomal *dominant* diseases. Typically, the symptoms of Huntington's chorea emerge only in the prime of life, between the ages of 35 and 50. It is characterized by mental and physical deterioration, leading to death within a period of several years. The defective gene responsible for Huntington's chorea is a dominant one. If a person has the defective gene, that person will eventually fall victim to the disease. Moreover, there is one chance in two (50 percent) that the person carrying the defective gene will pass it on to each of his or her children.

In contrast to *autosomal* genetic diseases, some genetic diseases are linked to mutant genes located on the sex chromosomes. Prominent among the genetic diseases in this latter category are the so-called X-linked diseases. Hemophilia, a well-known disease characterized by uncontrollable bleeding, is a leading example of an X-linked disease. Of the forty-six chromosomes that constitute the normal complement of genetic material in human beings, there are two sex chromosomes. A female has two X chromosomes and a male has one X and one Y chromosome. In human reproduction, if the sperm fertilizing the egg provides an X chromosome, the child will be female. If the sperm fertilizing the egg provides a Y chromosome, the child will be male. (The egg always provides an X chromosome.) Now, hemophilia is a *recessive* X-linked disease. A female, therefore, will have the disease of hemophilia only if she has the mutant gene on both of her X chromosomes. If a female has one normal gene and one mutant gene, however, she will be a carrier. Since a male has only one X chromosome, if he has the mutant gene associated with hemophilia, he will have the disease. On the assumption that a female carrier mates with a male who is free of the disease, there is no risk that their female children will have the disease. Female children will inherit a normal gene from their father and thus themselves be free of the disease, although there is one chance in two (50 percent) that they will inherit their mother's mutant gene and be, like her, a carrier. In contrast, there is one chance in two (50 percent) that male children will have the disease of hemophilia.

Prenatal Diagnosis and Selective Abortion

A number of recently developed techniques are now being utilized to detect chromosomal abnormalities, some genetic diseases, and certain serious anatomical abnormalities in the fetus *in utero*. Among these techniques, amniocentesis has been the most prominent, although ultrasound (a noninvasive technique) has been more commonly employed. In amniocentesis, a needle is inserted through a pregnant woman's abdomen, and a sample of the amniotic fluid surrounding the fetus is withdrawn. Because there are fetal cells in the amniotic fluid, a continually increasing number of genetic diseases in the fetus can be detected through biochemical studies and (more recently) recombinant DNA techniques. Also detectable, via chromosomal analysis, are conditions associated with an abnormal number of chromosomes or an abnormal arrangement of chromosomes. Down's syndrome, for example, is associated with the presence of an extra chromosome, namely, three instead of two number 21 chromosomes. Amniocentesis can also be applied for purposes of sex determination, thus creating the troubling possibility of abortion on the basis of sex selection. In one of this chapter's selections, John C. Fletcher considers the issue of whether amniocentesis should be made available to those who request it for reasons of sex selection. But whatever might be thought of the potential for sexist choices, it is essential to realize that the prenatal determination of sex has been of crucial importance in regard to diseases such as hemophilia, for which no method of prenatal diagnosis has been available, but only male children typically are at risk for the disease.

Amniocentesis has achieved wide acceptance among physicians as a relatively low-risk medical procedure. However, it cannot be performed prior to fourteen to sixteen weeks' gestation, and selective abortion must await the results of diagnostic testing, usually available around the twentieth week. Since second-trimester abortions are in many ways more problematic than first-trimester abortions, a procedure capable of combining the prenatal diagnostic value of amniocentesis with the possibility of first-trimester abortion is much to be desired. *Chorionic villi sampling,* a procedure developed in Europe and first introduced in the United States in 1983, is considered very promising in this regard. Although there are presently unresolved concerns about safety and accuracy, it is possible that chorionic villi sampling will in large part take the place of amniocentesis.

Since prenatal diagnosis is ordinarily undertaken with an eye toward selective abortion, it is clear that the practice of prenatal diagnosis confronts us with one particular aspect of the more general problem of abortion, as discussed in Chapter 9. (There is also a close link with the problem of the treatment of defective newborns, as discussed in Chapter 8.) Is the practice of selective abortion, on grounds of genetic defect, ethically acceptable? Leon R. Kass, in one of this chapter's selections, abstracts from the problem of abortion in general and raises some ethical difficulties for the practice of genetic abortion. Laurence E. Karp, who clarifies some of the technical aspects of prenatal diagnosis, with a focus on amniocentesis, also discusses some of the ethical dimensions of prenatal diagnosis and selective abortion.

Reproductive Risk, Morality, and Coercion

One important ethical issue associated with genetics has to do with the morality of reproduction under circumstances of genetic risk. In one of this chapter's selections, L. M. Purdy argues that it is surely morally wrong to reproduce in those cases where there is high risk of serious genetic disease. If it is justifiable to maintain that we have a moral obligation of the sort that Purdy outlines, we may find ourselves once more faced with the problem of prenatal diagnosis and selective abortion. Clearly, in those cases where prenatal diagnosis is available, abortion offers a means of sidestepping the risk of serious genetic disease.

Purdy considers in detail the case of Huntington's chorea. A special complication of this autosomal dominant disease is that its victims reach a reproductive age well before the time at which symptoms of the disease emerge. In the absence of a presymptomatic test for

Huntington's chorea, a characteristic dilemma has confronted a potential parent who knows that he or she is at 50 percent risk for Huntington's chorea. If the deleterious gene is present, there is a 50 percent chance that it will be inherited by any offspring. In such circumstances, since there is a high risk (25 percent) of serious genetic disease, Purdy argues that reproduction is immoral. But recent developments seem on the verge of easing the dilemma of reproduction that has heretofore confronted a person at risk for Huntington's chorea. Researchers have been developing recombinant DNA techniques that will provide not only a presymptomatic test but also a prenatal diagnostic test for Huntington's chorea. When these tests are available, Purdy would presumably require the employment of one or both as a condition of responsible reproduction for those at risk for Huntington's chorea.

Closely associated with the issue of the morality of reproduction under circumstances of genetic risk is another ethical issue, the justifiability of the use of coercive measures to achieve social control over individual reproductive decisions. It is one thing to say that certain reproductive choices are immoral and quite another to say that coercive measures for the control of reproductive choices are justified. Such coercive controls as compulsory sterilization and mandatory amniocentesis followed by forced abortion are widely rejected as invasive of fundamental rights. Mandatory screening programs for the identification of carriers, while surely less intrusive than other coercive measures, are also widely opposed as unjustifiable. Those who argue in support of coercive measures sometimes introduce claims, difficult to assess, about the dangers of uncontrolled reproduction leading to a deterioration of the human gene pool. Thus proposals for coercive measures often reflect a "negative eugenics" rationale.[1] Such proposals are rejected by those who maintain that there is no clear and present danger of genetic deterioration.[2]

Programs of Genetic Screening

In discussing the ethical acceptability of genetic screening programs, we should distinguish programs for the detection of genetic disease from programs for the identification of the carrier state. There would seem to be little ethical difficulty with screening programs for the detection of genetic disease to the extent that such programs feature voluntary participation and function to detect genetic diseases for which there is some significant medical treatment. However, screening programs become somewhat problematic when they function to detect genetic diseases for which there is no significant medical treatment. Moreover, even presuming that a certain genetic screening program would function to detect genetic diseases for which there is some significant medical treatment, mandatory participation (in the case of adults) raises the familiar issue of paternalistic interference with individual liberty. Screening for phenylketonuria (PKU) provides the most prominent example of a screening program instituted for the detection of genetic disease. Most states have passed legislation making screening for this disease in newborn infants mandatory. Upon detection of PKU, dietary measures can be introduced in order to mitigate the mental retardation associated with the disease.

The most prominent examples of screening programs whose purpose is the identification of the carrier state are Tay-Sachs carrier screening and sickle-cell carrier screening. Tay-Sachs carrier screening has had a less-troubled history than sickle-cell carrier screening. For one thing, the benefits of carrier identification are far less compelling in the absence of a complementary prenatal test. And a prenatal test for Tay-Sachs disease has been available since the time that carrier screening was first initiated, but a prenatal test for sickle-cell anemia was not available in the early years of sickle-cell screening. For another thing, Tay-Sachs carrier screening programs have uniformly been voluntary, but sickle-cell screening programs, while mostly voluntary, have on occasion been made mandatory by state legislation. While mandatory carrier identification programs are not without proponents, most commentators take a dim view of the coercion that they embody. In this chapter, Neil A. Holtzman even warns against subtle forms of coercion in voluntary programs of carrier screening. Moreover, Holtzman is troubled by the potential for stigmatization that attends carrier screening programs. In another selection in this chapter, the President's Commission for the Study of Ethical Problems in Medicine and Biomedical and Behavioral Research attempts to come to grips, in a forward-looking manner, with the possibility of instituting genetic screening programs for *cystic fibrosis*. Cystic fibrosis, like Tay-Sachs disease and sickle-cell anemia, is a well-known autosomal recessive disease.

Reproductive Technologies and the Treatment of Infertility

Human reproduction, as it naturally occurs, is characterized by sexual intercourse, tubal fertilization, implantation in the uterus, and subsequent *in utero* gestation. The expression "reproductive technologies" can be understood as applicable to an array of technical procedures that would replace the various steps in the natural process of reproduction, to a lesser or greater extent.

Artificial insemination is a procedure that replaces sexual intercourse as a means of achieving tubal fertilization. Artificial insemination has long been available, primarily as a means of overcoming infertility on the part of a male, usually a husband. It is sometimes possible that the husband's infertility may be overcome by AIH, artificial insemination with the sperm of the *husband*. More often, the couple must turn to AID, artificial insemination with the sperm of a *donor*. AID has also been employed when it has been established that the husband carries a mutant gene that would place a couple's offspring at genetic risk. Moreover, it has been suggested, most prominently in the work of the well-known geneticist Hermann J. Muller, that AID be voluntarily employed as a way of achieving the aims of positive eugenics.[3] Muller recommended the formation of sperm banks, which would collect and store the sperm of men judged to be "outstanding" in various ways. His idea was that an "enlightened" couple, desiring a child, would then have recourse to one of these banks in order to arrange for the wife's artificial insemination. Another controversial use of AID is its employment by unmarried women. Probably even more controversial is the employment of artificial insemination within the context of a "surrogate motherhood arrangement." In the most typical case, a wife's infertility motivates a couple to seek out a so-called "surrogate mother." The surrogate agrees to be artificially inseminated with the husband's sperm, in order to bear a child for the couple.

In vitro fertilization literally means fertilization "in glass." The sperm of a husband (or a donor) is united, in a laboratory, with the ovum of a wife (or a donor). Whereas artificial insemination is a technically simple procedure, *in vitro* fertilization followed by embryo transfer (to the uterus for implantation) is a system of reproductive technology that features a high degree of technical sophistication. The first documented "test tube baby," Louise Brown, was born in England in July 1978. Her birth was the culmination of years of collaboration between a gynecologist, Patrick Steptoe, and an embryologist, Robert Edwards. This pioneering team developed methods for obtaining mature eggs from a woman's ovaries (via a minor surgical procedure called a laparoscopy), effectively fertilizing eggs in the laboratory, cultivating them to the eight-cell stage, and then transferring a developing embryo to the uterus for implantation.

A number of reproductive centers in the United States now provide *in vitro* procedures for the treatment of infertility. It is expected that success rates, originally quite low, will improve as techniques are further refined. A very important development in this regard is the achievement of the first frozen embryo birth by an Australian team in 1984. Since it is now also possible, with the use of fertility drugs, to harvest a crop of mature eggs (perhaps ten or so) from a woman's ovaries, embryos frozen at the eight-cell stage can be thawed over a period of several months in an effort to achieve a successful implantation. Of course, the freezing of embryos is a technique that seems to suggest a number of ominous possibilities. But the freezing of unfertilized eggs, which at face value seems preferable to the freezing of embryos, has proven to be technically more difficult.

In vitro fertilization followed by embryo transfer is a system of reproductive technology that replaces not only sexual intercourse but also tubal fertilization in the natural process of reproduction. But consider also the future possibility of dispensing with implantation and *in utero* gestation as well. There seems to be no theoretical obstacle to totally artificial gestation, which would take place within the confines of an artificial womb. If *ectogenesis,* the process of artificial gestation, becomes a reality, then the combination of *in vitro* fertilization and ectogenesis would provide us with a system of reproductive technology in which each element in the natural process of reproduction has been effectively replaced. At the present time, however, *in vitro* fertilization (accompanied by embryo transfer) is seen primarily as a means of overcoming female infertility due to obstruction of the fallopian tubes.

In contrast to a woman whose infertility can be traced to fallopian-tube obstruction, consider a woman whose ovaries are either absent or nonfunctional. Since she has no ova, she cannot produce genetic offspring. If her uterus is functional, however, there is no biological obstacle to her bearing a child. Let us suppose that she very much wants to bear a child that is her husband's genetic offspring. Her problem can be addressed by some form of *egg donation;* and there are three major possibilities to consider. (1) *In vitro* fertilization of a donor egg with the husband's sperm, followed by embryo transfer to the wife. (2) Artificial insemination of an egg donor with the husband's sperm, producing *in vivo* (in the living situation) fertilization; nonsurgical removal of the embryo via lavage (a washing out) of the donor's uterus; recovery of the embryo and transfer to the uterus of the wife. (3) Transfer of a donor egg to the wife's fallopian tube, to be followed by sexual intercourse in an effort to achieve tubal fertilization and subsequent implantation. Since both (1) and (2), in contrast to (3), entail embryo transfers that involve a donated egg, the expressions "surrogate embryo transfer" and "prenatal adoption" are sometimes used to describe them. Presently, (1) and (2) are established procedures, but (3) is still in a developmental stage.

In the case just discussed, a woman has a functional uterus but nonfunctional ovaries. Consider now the converse case: a woman has functional ovaries but a nonfunctional uterus. Perhaps she has had a hysterectomy. She is capable of becoming, in a manner of speaking, the *genetic* but not the *gestational* mother of a child. Now, suppose that she and her husband desire a child "of their own." This situation gives rise to the possibility of a surrogate motherhood arrangement somewhat different than the kind predicated upon artificial insemination. In this case, *in vitro* fertilization could be employed to fertilize the wife's egg with the husband's sperm. The embryo could then be transferred to the uterus of a surrogate who would agree to bear the child for the couple.

Probably the most dramatic of the emerging reproductive technologies is cloning, a form of asexual reproduction. Many scientists believe that the techniques necessary for successful human cloning will be available in the not-too-distant future. Accordingly, it is thought that the first cloned man or woman would come about in the following manner. A mature human egg will be obtained from a woman and enucleated in a laboratory—that is, the nucleus of the egg cell will be removed. Meanwhile, a body cell from a donor (who may be anyone including the woman who has provided the egg) will be obtained and enucleated. The resultant nucleus, which contains the donor's heretofore unique genotype, will be inserted into the egg cell. From this point, the renucleated egg will develop in the way that a newly fertilized egg ordinarily develops. Implantation (not necessarily into the uterus of the woman from whom the original egg was obtained) and subsequent *in utero* gestation would then lead to the birth of the first cloned human individual. In contrast to offspring resulting from sexual reproduction, where the resultant genotype is the result of contributions by two parents, the "clone" will have the same genotype as his or her "parent."

Reproductive Technologies: Ethical Concerns

To what extent, if at all, is the employment of the various reproductive technologies ethically acceptable? A host of ethical concerns have been expressed about these technologies, and a brief survey of the most prominent of these concerns should prove helpful.

Most of the ethical opposition to artificial insemination derives from religious views. AID especially has been attacked on the grounds that it illicitly separates procreation from the marriage relationship. Inasmuch as AID introduces a third party (the sperm donor) into a marriage relationship, it has been called a form of adultery. Even AIH, which cannot be accused of separating procreation from the marriage relationship, has not uniformly escaped attack. Some religious ethicists have gone so far as to contend that procreation is morally illicit whenever it is not the product of personal lovemaking. Although these sorts of objections frequently recur in discussions of *in vitro* fertilization, the various forms of egg donation, and cloning, they seem to have little force for those who do not share the basic worldview from which they proceed.

In one of this chapter's selections, Herbert T. Krimmel argues that it is wrong for a person to create a child with the intention of abdicating parental responsibility for it. The argument is meant to apply both to egg donation and sperm donation. Krimmel also objects to an unmarried woman resorting to AID, on the grounds that it is unfair to intentionally deprive a child of a father. But his primary concern is to develop the case against surrogate motherhood. In another selection in this chapter, John A. Robertson contends that surrogate motherhood is an ethically acceptable practice. Since the Krimmel-Robertson exchange serves very effectively to introduce the many strands of argument in the continuing debate over surrogate motherhood, no further discussion of this controversial practice will be provided here.

Some of the ethical opposition to *in vitro* fertilization is based on the perceived "unnaturalness" of the procedure. Closely related is the charge that the procedure depersonalizes or dehumanizes procreation. Other opponents of *in vitro* fertilization argue that we must abstain from any intervention that inflicts unknown risks on developing offspring. Another recurrent argument against *in vitro* fertilization is that its acceptance by society would lead to the acceptance of more and more objectionable developments in reproductive technology. In one of this chapter's selections, Clifford Grobstein considers the force of this "slippery slope" argument.

In addition to arguments advanced in support of a wholesale rejection of *in vitro* fertilization, a number of concerns having a more limited scope can be identified. Some commentators have been quite willing to endorse the employment of *in vitro* fertilization and embryo transfer within the framework of a marital relationship but find any third-party involvement, such as egg donation or surrogate motherhood, objectionable. Other critics object primarily to a frequent concomitant of *in vitro* procedures, the discarding of embryos considered unneeded or unsuitable for implantation. (Those who consider even an early embryo a person are especially vocal on this score.) Although the practice of freezing embryos offers a partial solution to the problem of surplus embryos, some would argue that, in this case, the "solution" creates more problems than it solves.

In terms of ethical acceptability, cloning would seem to be the most problematic of all the reproductive technologies. Whereas the fundamental value of the other reproductive technologies under discussion can be located in the relief of infertility, the connection between cloning and the relief of infertility is a more tenuous one. Related to this consideration is the argument that cloning is the reproductive technology most likely to be misused, to the detriment of society. Of course, the stock charges against reproductive technology—that it is "unnatural" and depersonalizes reproduction—are also raised against cloning. But probably the most important arguments against cloning are those that emphasize difficulties associated with a clone's lack of genetic uniqueness. Hans Jonas, in one of this chapter's selections, declares his opposition to cloning on the basis of an argument of this sort. One other noteworthy argument calls attention to the biological danger that would attend widespread cloning. Widespread cloning would have the effect of limiting the variety of genotypes in the species and thus limit species adaptability in the face of changing circumstances.

T. A. M.

NOTES

1 Roughly, positive eugenics aims at enhancing the genetic heritage of the species, whereas negative eugenics aims at preventing deterioration of the gene pool.
2 This view is defended by Marc Lappé, "Moral Obligations and the Fallacies of 'Genetic Control,'" *Theological Studies* 33 (September 1972), pp. 411–427.
3 See, for example, Hermann J. Muller, "Means and Aims in Human Genetic Betterment," in T. M. Sonneborn, ed., *The Control of Human Heredity and Evolution* (New York: Macmillan, 1965), pp. 100–122.

Prenatal Diagnosis and Selective Abortion

The Prenatal Diagnosis of Genetic Disease

Laurence E. Karp

Laurence E. Karp, M.D., is associate professor of obstetrics and gynecology at the University of Washington School of Medicine. In addition to teaching, he is involved in research on the origins of chromosomal diseases and is the author of many medical and scientific articles. He is also the author of *Genetic Engineering: Threat or Promise?* (1976), from which this selection is excerpted.

Karp provides a discussion of the medical aspects of amniocentesis, which has been the most prominent procedure in prenatal diagnosis. He describes the clinical and laboratory techniques associated with amniocentesis, takes note of potential hazards, and discusses various medical indications for the procedure. Then, from his point of view as a genetic counselor, Karp identifies and briefly discusses a number of controversial (ethical) issues in prenatal diagnosis.

Until the late 1960s, genetic counseling was usually a frustrating experience. Couples at risk could be told the name of the genetic disorder that might appear in their offspring, along with the clinical manifestations of the disease. In most cases, the counselor could also make an accurate estimation of the magnitude of the risk.

Faced with these facts, such couples had only two options. Based on the clinical severity of the disease, the magnitude of the risk, and how badly they wanted to have children, they could either go ahead and hope for a lucky roll of the genetic dice, or they could decide to remain childless. All together, this was an unsatisfactory situation.

But changes were in the making. [In the mid-sixties], efforts to liberalize abortion laws were getting under way, and within a few years, most people had come to agree that abortion should be permitted where there existed a good chance that the child would suffer serious mental or physical impairment. Then, in 1966, two groups of scientists simultaneously reported that it was possible to perform chromosomal analyses of fetal cells removed from the amniotic sac. The next year, both Dr. Carlo Valenti of Brooklyn and Dr. Henry Nadler of Chicago used this new technique to diagnose Down's syndrome (mongolism) in a fetus. The two pregnancies were terminated, and in each case, the diagnosis of Down's syndrome was confirmed by examination of the abortus.

To date, this has been the greatest breakthrough in the field of medical genetics. At last, genetic counseling possesses a practical technique to permit at least some couples at risk to have children free of the fear that the offspring might be gravely malformed or mentally retarded....

Innumerable superstitious practices have long been employed in attempts to ward off birth defects, but until recently, the antenatal diagnosis of such problems has been a concept far beyond available methodology. In 1900, the British obstetrician Ballantyne could speak of attempts to diagnose both fetal heart disease and anencephaly by the character of the heart sounds. This represented a tentative beginning.

Prenatal diagnosis turned the corner in the late 1950s and early 1960s, with the work of Dr. D. C. A. Bevis in Britain, and Dr. A. W. Liley in New Zealand. These physicians performed *amniocentesis* (transabdominal puncture of the amniotic sac) to obtain fluid which they then analyzed for the quantity of degraded blood pigments. These data allowed them to determine the severity of Rh-incompatibility disease of the fetus. A few years later, Valenti and Nadler combined the technique of amniocentesis with recent major advances in laboratory cell culture and chromosomal analysis to make the first prenatal diagnosis of genetic disease.

Today, amniocentesis remains the primary tool in prenatal diagnosis. Other currently utilized techniques are ultrasound scanning and X-ray.

PRENATAL DIAGNOSIS TECHNIQUES: AMNIOCENTESIS

Amniocentesis should not be considered an entity unto itself, but a technique used in prenatal diagnosis, which is itself a branch of genetic counseling. Amniocentesis or other prenatal diagnostic procedures should never be performed without antecedent thorough genetic counseling by someone expert in the field. Most patients are not familiar with the risks and problems of amniocentesis itself. Some patients do not realize that abortion is the only alternative should chromosomal or most biochemical diseases be diagnosed; they believe that intrauterine therapy is possible. Genetic counseling permits the couple at risk to ask questions, consider the alternatives, weigh the risks, and finally come to an informed decision. Only then should investigative procedures be undertaken.

Amniocentesis was long considered dangerous, and was used only sparingly and as a last resort, usually in hydramnios, a condition of obscure causation in which dangerous excesses of amniotic fluid accumulate. But when Liley and Bevis popularized the use of amniocentesis in the assessment of Rh-incompatibility disease, it was realized that the procedure was relatively innocuous. So, the use of amniocentesis was extended to include assessment of fetal maturity, by analysis for creatinine content and for the presence of mature skin cells.

Clinical and Laboratory Techniques of Amniocentesis

For the assessment of both fetal maturity and the severity of Rh-incompatibility disease, amniocentesis is performed during the later weeks of pregnancy. However, to detect genetic disease in the fetus, the tap must be done between fourteen and twenty weeks after the last menstrual period. At this time, there is enough amniotic fluid to permit easy removal of a sample, but it is still early enough to perform an abortion, if disease is discovered.

After appropriate genetic counseling, the patient is instructed to empty her bladder. This is done so that the bladder will not obstruct the path of the needle to the uterus, and also because amniotic fluid at this stage of pregnancy looks exactly like clear, yellow urine. Next, a pelvic examination is performed, to determine the size and position of the uterus, and the optimal site for puncture. During the examination, if an area of unusual softness and prominence is noted in the uterine wall, this region is avoided, since it probably represents the placental implantation site. Many doctors routinely localize the placenta by ultrasound, but the necessity of doing this has not been established.

The patient's lower abdomen is then cleaned with an antiseptic solution, and the skin and the underlying lower abdominal wall are injected with a local anesthetic. After a few minutes, a four-inch-long needle is passed through the anesthetized region and into the uterus; as the amniotic sac is entered, the operator usually feels a distinct lessening of resistance or "give." About twenty cubic centimeters, or two-thirds of a fluid ounce, are drawn into a syringe, and then the needle is removed. The patient sometimes is kept under observation for about an hour after the procedure; if at that time there is no pain, bleeding, or vaginal leakage of fluid, she is sent home to await results.

Amniotic fluid contains small numbers of living body cells. The exact sites of origin of these cells have not yet been determined, but they do arise from the fetus and are probably sloughed off from the skin, the amniotic membrane, the urinary tract, and the respiratory system. When the fluid with its suspended cells is mixed with nutrient-containing tissue-culture fluid, and then maintained in an incubator at 37° C (normal human body temperature), the living cells will attach to the walls of the plastic culture dish and reproduce, forming colonies. Fetal cells grow slowly at first, reaching large numbers in one and one-half to two weeks. Occasionally, the cultures are contaminated by maternal uterine cells, but fortunately, these proliferate me rapidly than fetal cells and then die out in about a week. The cultured fetal cells can be analyzed chromosomally after about two weeks of growth; about four weeks are necessary before enough cells accumulate to permit the performance of tests for biochemical abnormalities.

Although most prenatal diagnoses are made by analysis of the cultured cells, occasionally the fluid itself is utilized.

Problems and Hazards of Amniocentesis

Although it sounds highly distasteful and probably a bit scary to have a long needle thrust deep into one's lower belly, the vast majority of patients have expressed surprise at the lack of discomfort. Most of them have said that it was no more unpleasant than a blood test.

Nor is amniocentesis at fourteen to twenty weeks of pregnancy a particularly dangerous procedure. At first, it was feared that needling the uterus this early in pregnancy might provoke miscarriage. However, it is now apparent that the rate of miscarriage after genetic amniocentesis is no higher than the 1 to 3 percent spontaneous abortion rate at this time of pregnancy.

A more real risk is that of striking the fetus with the needle. This has occurred on several occasions, leaving a small punctate or linear depression in the skin. However, since only the trunk or the extremities have been hit, the scars have been of no importance. Only if the face or an eye were punctured might such an accident assume significance. This has not yet been documented to have occurred in a genetic amniocentesis, and is not likely to happen, since at this point in pregnancy, the fetal body is well flexed, with the face "looking down" at the chest.

Other complications have been reported infrequently. Hemorrhage has resulted from the inadvertent puncture of a large vessel in the uterus or in the abdominal wall, and intrauterine infection has occurred, presumably secondary to bacteria introduced via the needle. In addition, there is concern that Rh-incompatibility disease might be initiated by puncture of a placental vessel, allowing the escape of blood cells from an Rh-positive fetus into the circulation of an Rh-negative mother. So far, however, this has only been reported sporadically.

Lastly, there is as yet no definite proof that the removal of fluid at this stage of pregnancy is totally without effect on the fetus. Although infants born after amniocentesis seem to develop normally during the first couple of years of life, the concern has been expressed that the sudden change in intrauterine pressure caused by the fluid withdrawal might adversely affect the developing brain, perhaps causing the loss of a few points of IQ. Studies are now under way in many centers to evaluate this possibility. I believe that these studies will provide reassuring information....

Patients must always be told that there is no prenatal diagnostic procedure, including amniocentesis, that will screen for *all* birth defects. About 3 percent of newborns suffer from major physical or mental abnormalities, most of which cannot be identified before birth. Therefore, the counseled couple must understand that prenatal diagnosis will not guarantee them a normal baby.

Perhaps the most controversial aspect of prenatal diagnosis is that it leads to the abortion of fetuses doomed to be born malformed and/or mentally retarded. Reams of paper have been filled with thoughtful analyses of the questions as to whether abortion is murder, when the fetus acquires legal rights, and whether women should be forced to continue unwanted pregnancies. The disagreement arises basically from the unresolved issue of when a fetus becomes a human being (whatever that is). The fields of law, religion, and ethics have not been able to provide anything resembling an unequivocal answer: however, many people seem to feel reasonably comfortable using the average time of viability (capacity for independent existence) as the milestone for this fetal achievement. In the face of such widespread, fundamental disagreement, I can only conclude that the issue of abortion ought to remain a matter for individual decision.

A generally unappreciated sidelight to the abortion issue is the fact that prenatal diagnosis undoubtedly saves more fetal lives than it terminates. My own experience and that of other workers in the field is that a large number of pregnant women carrying high genetic-risk pregnancies would resort to abortion if diagnostic techniques were unavailable. This is in contrast to the small number of patients who are discovered to be carrying a seriously defective fetus.

A related question is whether abortion should be performed upon diagnosis of a disease that is treatable postnatally. The critical issues to be considered in this situation are the cost and complexity of the therapy, and to what degree it will permit the patient to lead a normal life. This problem is illustrated by galactosemia, which, untreated, leads to cataracts in the eye, liver damage, mental retardation, and eventually death. However, if milk and milk products are avoided, for example, by the use of soy bean formula in infants, patients with galactosemia can lead quite normal lives. Prenatal diagnosis is possible for galactosemia, and it could be followed either by abortion of the affected fetus or by continuation of the pregnancy and immediate postnatal treatment. Since simple dietary therapy permits galactosemics to live with little or no difficulty related to their disease, most prospective parents decide to continue the pregnancy. On the contrary, the treatment of hemophilia involves frequent, expensive intravenous infusions, and most families choose not to risk this possibility.

Sometimes there is a problem with the so-called unexpected result. A case has been reported involving a forty-two-year-old woman whose fetus was found to have not Down's syndrome, but a 47, XYY, chromosomal arrangement. This is the so-called "supermale karyotype" first discovered among maximum security prisoners and therefore linked to aggressive, antisocial behavior. Later work has revealed that about one of every 800 men has an extra Y chromosome, and that most of them are perfectly normal, law-abiding citizens. The patient's doctors debated whether to tell her simply that her child did not have Down's syndrome, or whether she should be given all the facts. The doctors believed that an XYY karyotype did not constitute a good reason for abortion, and that if the patient were to continue the pregnancy, her relationship with her child might be severely affected in that she might interpret as pathological every normal act of childhood aggression. In the end, it was decided that not to tell the patient everything would constitute unethical withholding of information. I think that this was the proper decision. The patient should be entitled to all information obtained, and it ought to be the continuing responsibility of her physicians to help her understand it and cope with it. Furthermore, the patient, not the doctor, must have the final say as to which condition would justify abortion *for her*. Other sex chromosomal abnormalities, such as 47, XXX, are associated with relatively low rates of mental and physical problems. Most patients would want to continue such pregnancies, but others might not wish to risk any deviation from a normal karyotype. I believe that the choice should remain an individual option, based on receipt and consideration of accurate risk figures.

The question sometimes arises as to whether we should use amniocentesis to help us abort carriers for autosomal or X-linked genetic diseases. While I would support the right of any couple to have any pregnancy terminated, I think that the attempted eradication of asymptomatic carriers is based upon specious reasoning. For one thing, it is estimated that all of us carry three to five mutated, defective genes, capable of causing disease in a child conceived by a "wrong" mate. So, a strong effort to wipe out "bad genes" would lead to its being pretty lonely here on earth. Furthermore, genes known to cause disease in a double (homozygous) dose may actually be advantageous in the single (heterozygous) state. For example, a single dose of the recessive gene for sickle cell anemia confers upon its carrier a relative immunity to malaria. Moreover, as previously mentioned, despite the concern that present practice conditions may lead to an increase in the number of deleterious gene carriers in the population, it has been calculated that any such increase would be small, and most likely, of no practical significance. A request for abortion of a gene carrier is usually either based upon misinformation, or represents a conscious or a subconscious attempt to utilize a "socially acceptable reason" for termination of an unwanted pregnancy.

Sometimes, couples request amniocentesis but state that under no circumstance will they elect to abort the pregnancy. In this situation, some geneticists are reluctant to perform the procedure, since this would imply acceptance of the small but definite risk of amniocentesis without any hope of being able to use the information obtained to influence the management of the pregnancy. This objection is answered by the couples' assertions to the effect that prior knowledge of the presence of a birth defect would give them five months to adjust to the fact before the arrival of the baby. Considering both this attitude and the fact that most taps will provide reassuring information, it becomes difficult to deny amniocentesis to such patients, as long as they recognize and accept the intrinsic risks of the procedure.

Some patients request amniocentesis for sex determination, in order that they may abort a fetus of the undesired sex. Even though these requests are perfectly legal, very few geneticists are now honoring them. The reason usually given for refusal is that the laboratory facilities and manpower are not sufficient to handle the volume of work that would accrue if sex determination on request were to become routine, and that preference must be given to families seeking to avoid having children with genetic diseases. This is certainly true enough, but it would not be true to say that the attitude of the doctors is neutral regarding the idea. In fact, all geneticists with whom I've discussed the issue have expressed a negative opinion, ranging from mild distaste to frank revulsion. Eventually, however, I believe the point will become moot: it seems apparent that before laboratory space and technicians proliferate to the point where another excuse would have to be found, a reliable method of preconceptual sex determination will have been made available. This will constitute an option far safer, and more palatable to both patients and doctors than postconceptual diagnosis and selective abortion.

Much has been made of the implications of the use of prenatal diagnosis in regard to the relationship of the individual to society. For example, it has been suggested that couples at risk for genetic disease in their offspring might be penalized by higher insurance rates if they will not have their pregnancies screened and selectively aborted. That may indeed come to pass, but what of it? Insurance companies routinely increase their rates to meet high risk situations. Persons with hypertension or diabetes pay higher life insurance premiums, but no one suggests that we should stop checking patients' blood pressures and blood sugars. To frame another analogy, it's quite lawful to build your house at a great distance from fire hydrants, but you should expect to pay for the privilege with increased fire insurance costs. And what of the couple who elect to use prenatal diagnosis? Since their children will be at lower risk for birth defects, they might qualify for reduced insurance premiums.

Ethicists have expressed the concern that the government eventually might make diagnostic amniocentesis mandatory, and then order abortion of all fetuses diagnosed as defective. I think this is unlikely. In our society, Jehovah's Witnesses are free to reject Rho-GAM, the medication that prevents Rh-incompatibility disease. Members of various cults may invoke their beliefs to avoid compulsory vaccinations. It seems much more likely that anti-abortionists will succeed in imposing their morality by fiat on pro-abortionists than the other way around. Furthermore, if our government does indeed reach the stage of being able to mandate abortion, then I suspect that will be one of our lesser problems.

Implications of Prenatal Diagnosis for the Human Right to Life

Leon R. Kass

Leon R. Kass, a biologist as well as a medical doctor, is Henry R. Luce Professor in the College, University of Chicago. He has served as executive secretary of the Committee on the Life Sciences and Social Policy, National Academy of Sciences. Among the more prominent of his many articles on issues in biomedical ethics are "Regarding the End of Medicine and the Pursuit of Health," "Making Babies—The New Biology and the 'Old' Morality," and "The New Biology: What Price Relieving Man's Estate?"

Setting aside a discussion of the moral problem of abortion in general, Kass focuses on some of the ethical difficulties associated with the abortion of fetuses known by amniocentesis to be genetically defective. He maintains that the practice of *genetic* abortion, inasmuch as it involves a qualitative assessment of fetuses, represents a threat to the "radical moral equality of all human beings." As a result of the practice of genetic abortion, Kass suggests, we will be inclined to take a more negative view of those who are genetically defective or otherwise "abnormal." Thus we will be inclined to treat them in a second-class manner. Moreover, he contends, to commit ourselves to the practice of genetic abortion is to reflect acceptance of a very dangerous principle, that "defectives should not be born."

It is especially fitting on this occasion to begin by acknowledging how privileged I feel and how pleased I am to be a participant in this symposium. I suspect that I am not alone among the assembled in considering myself fortunate to be here. For I was conceived after antibiotics yet before amniocentesis, late enough to have benefited from medicine's ability to prevent and control fatal infectious diseases, yet early enough to have escaped from medicine's ability to prevent me from living to suffer from my genetic diseases. To be sure, my genetic vices are, as far as I know them, rather modest, taken individually—myopia, asthma and other allergies, bilateral forefoot adduction, bowleggedness, loquaciousness, and pessimism, plus some four to eight as yet undiagnosed recessive lethal genes in the heterozygous condition—but, taken together, and if diagnosable prenatally, I might never have made it.

Just as I am happy to be here, so am I unhappy with what I shall have to say. Little did I realize when I first conceived the topic, "Implications of Prenatal Diagnosis for the Human Right to Life," what a painful and difficult labor it would lead to. More than once while this paper was gestating, I considered obtaining permission to abort it, on the grounds that, by prenatal diagnosis, I knew it to be defective. My lawyer told me that I was legally in the clear, but my conscience reminded me that I had made a commitment to deliver myself of this paper, flawed or not. Next time, I shall practice better contraception.

Any discussion of the ethical issues of genetic counseling and prenatal diagnosis is unavoidably haunted by a ghost called the morality of abortion. This ghost I shall not vex. More precisely, I shall not vex the reader by telling ghost stories. However, I would be neither surprised nor disappointed if my discussion of an admittedly related matter, the ethics of aborting the genetically defective, summons that hovering spirit to the reader's mind. For the morality of abortion is a matter not easily laid to rest, recent efforts to do so notwithstanding. A vote by the legislature of the State

Reprinted by permission of the author and Plenum Publishing Corporation from *Ethical Issues in Human Genetics,* edited by Bruce Hilton et al., 1973.

of New York can indeed legitimatize the disposal of fetuses, but not of the moral questions. But though the questions remain, there is likely to be little new that can be said about them, and certainly not by me.

Yet before leaving the general question of abortion, let me pause to drop some anchors for the discussion that follows. Despite great differences of opinion both as to what to think and how to reason about abortion, nearly everyone agrees that abortion is a moral issue.[1] What does this mean? Formally, it means that a woman seeking or refusing an abortion can expect to be asked to justify her action. And we can expect that she should be able to give reasons for her choice other than "I like it" or "I don't like it." Substantively, it means that, in the absence of good reasons for intervention, there is some presumption in favor of allowing the pregnancy to continue once it has begun. A common way of expressing this presumption is to say that "the fetus has a right to continued life."[2] In this context, disagreement concerning the moral permissibility of abortion concerns what rights (or interests or needs), and whose, override (take precedence over, or outweigh) this fetal "right." Even most of the "opponents" of abortion agree that the mother's right to live takes precedence, and that abortion to save her life is permissible, perhaps obligatory. Some believe that a woman's right to determine the number and spacing of her children takes precedence, while yet others argue that the need to curb population growth is, at least at this time, overriding.

Hopefully, this brief analysis of what it means to say that abortion is a moral issue is sufficient to establish two points. First, that the fetus is a living thing with some moral claim on us not to do it violence, and therefore, second, that justification must be given for destroying it.

Turning now from the general questions of the ethics of abortion, I wish to focus on the special ethical issues raised by the abortion of "defective" fetuses (so-called "abortion for fetal indications"). I shall consider only the cleanest cases, those cases where well-characterized genetic diseases are diagnosed with a high degree of certainty by means of amniocentesis, in order to sidestep the added moral dilemmas posed when the diagnosis is suspected or possible, but unconfirmed. However, many of the questions I shall discuss could also be raised about cases where genetic analysis gives only a statistical prediction about the genotype of the fetus, and also about cases where the defect has an infectious or chemical rather than a genetic cause (e.g., rubella, thalidomide).

My first and possibly most difficult task is to show that there is anything left to discuss once we have agreed not to discuss the morality of abortion in general. There is a sense in which abortion for genetic defect is, after abortion to save the life of the mother, perhaps the most defensible kind of abortion. Certainly, it is a serious and not a frivolous reason for abortion, defended by its proponents in sober and rational speech—unlike justifications based upon the false notion that a fetus is a mere part of a woman's body, to be used and abused at her pleasure. Standing behind genetic abortion are serious and well-intentioned people, with reasonable ends in view: the prevention of genetic diseases, the elimination of suffering in families, the preservation of precious financial and medical resources, the protection of our genetic heritage. No profiteers, no sex-ploiters, no racists. No arguments about the connection of abortion with promiscuity and licentiousness, no perjured testimony about the mental health of the mother, no arguments about the seriousness of the population problem. In short, clear objective data, a worthy cause, decent men and women. If abortion, what better reason for it?

Yet if genetic abortion is but a happily wagging tail on the dog of abortion, it is simultaneously the nose of a camel protruding under a rather different tent. Precisely because the quality of the fetus is central to the decision to abort, the practice of genetic abortion has implications which go beyond those raised by abortion in general. What may be at stake here is the belief in the radical moral equality of all human beings, the belief that all human beings possess equally and independent of merit certain fundamental rights, one among which is, of course, the right to life.

To be sure, the belief that fundamental human rights belong equally to all human beings has been but an ideal, never realized, often ignored, sometimes shamelessly. Yet it has been perhaps the most powerful moral idea at work in the world for at least two centuries. It is this idea and ideal that animates most of the current political and social criticism around the globe. It is ironic that we should acquire the power to detect and eliminate the genetically unequal at a time when we have finally succeeded in removing much of the stigma and disgrace previously attached to victims of congenital illness, in providing them with improved care and support, and in preventing, by means of education, feelings of guilt on the part of their parents. One might even wonder whether the development of amniocentesis and prenatal diagnosis may represent a backlash against these same humanitarian and egalitarian tendencies in the practice of medicine, which, by helping to sustain to the age of reproduction persons with genetic disease has itself contributed to the increasing incidence of genetic disease, and with it, to increased pressures for genetic screening, genetic counseling, and genetic abortion.

No doubt our humanitarian and egalitarian principles and practices have caused us some new difficulties, but if we mean to weaken or turn our backs on them, we should do so consciously and thoughtfully. If, as I believe, the idea and practice of genetic abortion points in that direction, we should make ourselves aware of it....

GENETIC ABORTION AND THE LIVING DEFECTIVE

The practice of abortion of the genetically defective will no doubt affect our view of and our behavior toward those abnormals who escape the net of detection and abortion. A child with Down's syndrome or with hemophilia or with muscular dystrophy born at a time when most of his (potential) fellow sufferers were destroyed prenatally is liable to be looked upon by the community as one unfit to be alive, as a second-class (or even lower) human type. He may be seen as a person who need not have been, and who would not have been, if only someone had gotten to him in time.

The parents of such children are also likely to treat them differently, especially if the mother would have wished but failed to get an amniocentesis because of ignorance, poverty, or distance from the testing station, or if the prenatal diagnosis was in error. In such cases, parents are especially likely to resent the child. They may be disinclined to give it the kind of care they might have before the advent of amniocentesis and genetic abortion, rationalizing that a second-class specimen is not entitled to first-class treatment. If pressed to do so, say by physicians, the parents might refuse, and the courts may become involved. This has already begun to happen.

In Maryland, parents of a child with Down's syndrome refused permission to have the child operated on for an intestinal obstruction present at birth. The physicians and the hospital sought an injunction to require the parents to allow surgery. The judge ruled in favor of the parents, despite what I understand to be the weight of precedent to the contrary, on the grounds that the child was Mongoloid, that is, had the child been "normal," the decision would have gone the other way. Although the decision was not appealed to and hence not affirmed by a higher court, we can see through the prism of this case the possibility that the new powers of human genetics will strip the blindfold from the lady of justice and will make official the dangerous doctrine that some men are more equal than others.

The abnormal child may also feel resentful. A child with Down's syndrome or Tay-Sachs disease will probably never know or care, but what about a child with hemophilia or with Turner's syndrome? In the past decade, with medical knowledge and power over the prenatal child increasing and with parental authority over the postnatal child decreasing, we have seen the appearance of a new type of legal action, suits for wrongful life. Children have brought suit against their parents (and others) seeking to recover damages for physical and social handicaps inextricably tied to their birth (e.g., congenital deformities, congenital syphilis, illegitimacy). In some of the American cases, the courts have recognized the justice of the child's claim (that he was injured due to parental negligence), although they have so far refused to award damages, due to policy considerations. In other countries, e.g., in Germany, judgments with compensation have gone for the plaintiffs. With the spread of amniocentesis and genetic abortion, we can only expect such cases to increase. And here it will be the soft-hearted rather than the hard-hearted judges who will establish the doctrine of second-class human beings, out of compassion for the mutants who escaped the traps set out for them.

It may be argued that I am dealing with a problem which, even if it is real, will affect very few people. It may be suggested that very few will escape the traps once we have set them properly and widely, once people are informed about amniocentesis, once the power to detect prenatally grows to its full capacity, and once our "superstitious" opposition to abortion dies out or is extirpated. But in order even to come close to this vision of success, amniocentesis will have to become part of every pregnancy—either by making it mandatory, like the test for syphilis, or by making it "routine medical practice," like the Pap smear. Leaving aside the other problems with universal amniocentesis, we could expect that the problem for the few who escape is likely to be even worse precisely because they will be few.

The point, however, should be generalized. How will we come to view and act toward the many "abnormals" that will remain among us—the retarded, the crippled, the senile, the deformed, and the true mutants—once we embark on a program to root out genetic abnormality? For it must be remembered that we shall always have abnormals—some who escape detection or whose disease is undetectable *in utero,* others as a result of new mutations, birth injuries, accidents, maltreatment, or disease—who will require our care and protection. The existence of "defectives" cannot be fully prevented, not even by totalitarian breeding and weeding programs. Is it not likely that our principle with respect to these people will change from "We try harder" to "Why accept second best?" The idea of "the unwanted because abnormal child" may become a self-fulfilling prophecy, whose consequences may be worse than those of the abnormality itself.

GENETIC AND OTHER DEFECTIVES

The mention of other abnormals points to a second danger of the practice of genetic abortion. Genetic abortion may come to be seen not so much as the prevention of genetic disease, but as the prevention of birth of defective or abnormal children—and, in a way, understandably so. For in the case of what other diseases does preventive medicine consist in the elimination of the patient-at-risk? Moreover, the very language used to discuss genetic disease leads us to the easy but wrong conclusion that the afflicted fetus or person is rather than has a disease. True, one is partly defined by his genotype, but only partly. A person is more than his disease. And yet we slide easily from the language of possession to the language of identity, from "He has hemophilia" to "He is a hemophiliac," from "She has diabetes" through "She is diabetic" to "She is a diabetic," from "The fetus has Down's syndrome" to "The fetus is a Down's." This way of speaking supports the belief that it is defective persons (or potential persons) that are being eliminated, rather than diseases.

If this is so, then it becomes simply accidental that the defect has a genetic cause. Surely, it is only because

of the high regard for medicine and science, and for the accuracy of genetic diagnosis, that genotypic defectives are likely to be the first to go. But once the principle, "Defectives should not be born," is established, grounds other than cytological and biochemical may very well be sought. Even ignoring racialists and others equally misguided—of course, they cannot be ignored—we should know that there are social scientists, for example, who believe that one can predict with a high degree of accuracy how a child will turn out from a careful, systematic study of the socio-economic and psychodynamic environment into which he is born and in which he grows up. They might press for the prevention of socio-psychological disease, even of "criminality," by means of prenatal environmental diagnosis and abortion. I have heard rumor that a crude, unscientific form of eliminating potential "phenotypic defectives" is already being practiced in some cities, in that submission to abortion is allegedly being made a condition for the receipt of welfare payments. "Defectives should not be born" is a principle without limits. We can ill-afford to have it established.

Up to this point, I have been discussing the possible implications of the practice of genetic abortion for our belief in and adherence to the idea that, at least in fundamental human matters such as life and liberty, all men are to be considered as equals, that for these matters we should ignore as irrelevant the real qualitative differences amongst men, however important these differences may be for other purposes. Those who are concerned about abortion fear that the permissible time of eliminating the unwanted will be moved forward along the time continuum, against newborns, infants, and children. Similarly, I suggest that we should be concerned lest the attack on gross genetic inequality in fetuses be advanced along the continuum of quality and into the later stages of life.

I am not engaged in predicting the future; I am not saying that amniocentesis and genetic abortion will lead down the road to Nazi Germany. Rather, I am suggesting that the principles underlying genetic abortion simultaneously justify many further steps down that road. The point was very well made by Abraham Lincoln:

> If A can prove, however conclusively, that he may, of right, enslave B—Why may not B snatch the same argument and prove equally, that he may enslave A?

You say A is white, and B is black. It is color, then; the lighter having the right to enslave the darker? Take care. By this rule, you are to be slave to the first man you meet with a fairer skin than your own.

You do not mean color exactly? You mean the whites are intellectually the superiors of the blacks, and, therefore have the right to enslave them? Take care again. By this rule, you are to be slave to the first man you meet with an intellect superior to your own.

But, say you, it is a question of interest; and, if you can make it your interest, you have the right to enslave another. Very well. And if he can make it his interest, he has the right to enslave you.[3]

Perhaps I have exaggerated the dangers; perhaps we will not abandon our inexplicable preference for generous humanitarianism over consistency. But we should indeed be cautious and move slowly as we give serious consideration to the question "What price the perfect baby?"[4] . . .

NOTES

1 This strikes me as by far the most important inference to be drawn from the fact that men in different times and cultures have answered the abortion question differently. Seen in this light, the differing and changing answers themselves suggest that it is a question not easily put under, at least not for very long.

2 Other ways include: one should not do violence to living or growing things; life is sacred; respect nature; fetal life has value; refrain from taking innocent life; protect and preserve life. As some have pointed out, the terms chosen are of different weight, and would require reasons of different weight to tip the balance in favor of abortion. My choice of the "rights" terminology is not meant to beg the questions of whether such rights really exist, or of where they come from. However, the notion of a "fetal right to life" presents only a little more difficulty in this regard than does the notion of a "human right to life," since the former does not depend on a claim that the human fetus is already "human." In my sense of terms "right" and "life," we might even say that a dog or fetal dog has a "right to life," and that it would be cruel and immoral for a man to go around performing abortions even on dogs for no good reason.

3 Lincoln, A. (1854). In *The Collected Works of Abraham Lincoln*, R. P. Basler, editor. New Brunswick, New Jersey, Rutgers University Press, Vol. II, p. 222.

4 For a discussion of the possible biological rather than moral price of attempts to prevent the birth of defective children see Motulsky, A. G., G. R. Fraser, and J. Felsenstein (1971). In Symposium on Intrauterine Diagnosis, D. Bergsma, editor. *Birth Defects: Original Article Series*, Vol. 7, No. 5. Also see Neel, J. (1972). In *Early Diagnosis of Human Genetic Defects: Scientific and Ethical Considerations*, M. Harris, editor. Washington, D.C., U.S. Government Printing Office, pp. 366–380.

Ethics and Amniocentesis for Fetal Sex Identification
John C. Fletcher

John C. Fletcher, an Episcopal priest, is presently assistant for bioethics in the Warren G. Magnuson Clinical Center of the National Institutes of Health. Fletcher has served as associate editor of the *Encyclopedia of Bioethics* (1978) and is the author of several books, including *Coping with Genetic Disorders* (1982). Among his many articles are "Attitudes Toward Defective Newborns" and "Moral Problems in Genetic Counseling."

Reprinted by permission of the *New England Journal of Medicine*, vol. 301 (September 6, 1979), pp. 550–553.

Fletcher explains why he no longer supports a policy according to which physicians discourage those requesting amniocentesis for the purpose of sex selection. His previous endorsement of this policy was based primarily on the conviction that sex choice is a trivial, morally unjustifiable reason for abortion. While maintaining his moral opposition to abortion for sex selection, Fletcher has nevertheless concluded that there is an overriding consideration to take into account—a woman's right to decide whether she will abort or not. In his present view, blocking access to information about the fetus is inconsistent with a recognition of the right of a woman to decide about abortion.

Two types of parents request fetal sex identification by amniocentesis: the first group risk transmitting a sex-linked hereditary disorder and the second want to select the gender of their next child. Physicians generally encourage the first type of parent but discourage the second.

Prenatal diagnosis for sex choice is controversial because of ethical objections to the use of abortion for such a reason and because of the question of whether amniocentesis, a scarce medical resource, can prudently be used for this purpose.[1] The issue is complex and involves many competing ethical claims.

I have re-evaluated my position on this issue as a result of participation in a Hastings Center study group[2] and consultation with staff of the Prenatal Diagnostic Center of the Johns Hopkins Hospital on their policy on amniocentesis for sex choice.

My earlier position was based on four main points. In the first place, I argued that parents with this request ought to be discouraged because sex is not a disease. I saw prenatal diagnosis as a tool that ethically could be used to diagnose hereditary diseases or congenital defects in the fetus. Secondly, I stressed that abortion for sex choice could contribute to social inequality between the sexes because of a preference for male offspring. Thirdly, I criticized sex choice as a "frivolous" reason for abortion that could not be successfully defended in the company of serious moral persons. My fourth point was that amniocentesis was a scarce resource in the light of the total number of pregnancies at risk. Requests for fetal sex identification could swamp an already overloaded system or delay laboratory work in cases of serious genetic diseases.

A legal and a public-relations consideration buttressed these reasons and secured my position. Physicians cannot legally be forced to provide procedures that are not "lifesaving." Furthermore, if parents were accommodated with this request, antiabortion forces might raise a public outcry that would discourage parents genuinely at risk from seeking prenatal testing. I supported the prevailing policy of discouragement and defended the practice in some laboratories of refusing to do karyotyping when fetal sex alone was the presenting indication.

RE-EVALUATION

My re-evaluation assumes that the basis for the policy of discouragement is the belief of most physicians who perform prenatal diagnosis that abortion for sex choice is morally unjustifiable. Those who reason as I did also use the scarce-resource argument[3] and are wary of the use of prenatal diagnosis for "social engineering" to plan the sex of children. In practice, however, discouragement based on opposition to abortion for sex choice is weightier than the other two reasons. Most of us have an uneasy conscience about the number of abortions performed in the United States and about the lack of moral seriousness with which abortion is sometimes requested and carried out. We have preferred to use prenatal diagnosis in the context of saving fetal lives. I personally believe that sex choice is not a compelling reason for abortion. The first moral response of most who think about the issue is close to queasiness. Yet, the issue does not turn on the validity of opposition to abortion for sex choice. The issue turns on the validity of the legal rules on abortion defined by the Supreme Court,[4] which do not require that a woman state reasons in a public or medical forum for early to mid-trimester abortion. No one is presumed to be a public judge of her reasons except herself. Family, friends, counselors or physicians may challenge her reasons if she chooses to confide in them. But the rule is that no public test of reasons is required.

Is this the best rule to apply in abortion? Yes, if one holds, as I do, that the woman's right to decide is the overriding consideration in the abortion issue. The rationale for the legal rule omitting a test of reasons is that a woman has the right to control her reproduction and the risks involved in a pregnancy. To employ public or medical tests of reasons provides opportunities to obstruct and defeat society's obligation to grant women the freedom to determine their own reproductive futures. To prevent obstruction of self-determination, it is better to have no public tests of reasons.

The Supreme Court took the position that the state has no interest in refusing an adult woman the right of self-determination in reproduction through the second trimester of pregnancy. Although a Supreme Court decision is not itself an ethical consideration, the legal guideline on abortion points beyond itself to the principles of justice and respect for persons. Justice in the modern state requires that women be freed from restrictions on their freedom and opportunity to compete for the social and economic rewards of citizenship. Respect for persons requires that a woman's autonomy and personal responsibility be the standards that govern the final resolution of conflicts about reproduction and abortion.

The Supreme Court justices probably did not imagine in 1973 that their decision on abortion was related to the right of parents to choose the sex of children through amniocentesis. However, even if the justices were then aware of the potential use of amniocentesis for this purpose, it did not figure in their reasoning. The position that they took made abortion on request a legal practice and the conscience of the individual woman the sole arbiter of the reasons. Abortion for sex choice is legal, and if we are to act in accordance with the principles that should now inform decision making on abortion, all forms of tests should be removed.

Given the ethical and legal posture discussed above, one must be willing to accept the fact that some abortions will be performed for trivial reasons. The existence of some trivial reasons should not deter us from the larger goal of protecting the right of women to make such decisions in the first place. That is what is at stake in the issue under discussion. My major argument is that it is inconsistent to support an abortion law that protects the absolute right of women to decide and, at the same time, to block access to information about

the fetus because one thinks that an abortion may be foolishly sought on the basis of the information.

AN EXAMPLE

Another way to measure the degree of ethical inconsistency in the policy of discouragement is to reflect on an example. An obstetrician-gynecologist is asked by a 30-year-old woman in the second month of gestation to perform an abortion. The physician does not inquire about her reasons. As it turns out, she desired the abortion so that she could make a trip to Europe. The same physician is a cooperating member of a prenatal diagnostic center in a university hospital with a policy of discouraging access for prenatal sex identification and a prohibition against laboratory cultures for this purpose. The mother of three children of one gender requests fetal sex identification in the fourth pregnancy. The physician must either refer her to another center at some distance or do the amniotic tap in the office and send the sample to a commercial laboratory where no questions are asked.

If the sometimes trivial reason for abortion must be accepted to protect the rights of many women, how could it be acceptable for the same physician to participate in a system that discriminates because of reasons for abortion? To hold to this inconsistency is morally self-defeating and leads to hypocrisy. Furthermore, amniocentesis and laboratory work should be done under the very best of conditions, if done at all. The physician should not be forced to defend an inconsistent policy and practice less than optimum medicine and science.

INFORMED CONSENT

When physicians counsel parents who want to know the sex of the fetus, they should carefully inform them about several areas of risk.

Amniocentesis carries a small but nonetheless real risk of death to the fetus and injury to the mother. The risk of fetal death from amniocentesis has been shown to be less than 1 per cent in controlled studies in the United States and Canada.[5,6] A British study that suggested a 1.5 percent fetal loss[7] has been challenged on the ground that selection of controls was biased. Until this controversy is resolved, the previous risk figures and the fact that risk factors are still being studied should be communicated to the parents.

A very small number of technical errors are still made in laboratories. A recent review of 3000 consecutive amniocenteses showed the karyotyping-error rate to be 0.07 percent, or 7 in 10,000.[8]

Mid-trimester abortion is a major procedure, and depression has been reported in both parents after genetically indicated abortions.[9]

Finally, an unknown risk of insult to other members of the family and to the wider society is involved in a decision to abort for sex choice. The physician can, if he or she chooses, state an opposing view in moral terms. What the physician should not do is withhold amniocentesis if informed parents desire to proceed. To do so would be to test the parents' reasons for abortion. The parents may or may not decide on abortion on the basis of the information gained. In any event, that decision remains theirs to make, legally and morally.

PUBLIC AND PRIVATE OPPOSITION

Individuals and groups who want to test the reasoning of those who may seek abortions are free to do so within the limits of the law. Religious groups opposed to abortion can attempt to convince anyone in society that abortion is morally wrong. Any group is free to work toward amending the Constitution so that public tests of reasons on abortion are required. Parents are free to instruct children about human sexuality in a manner that reduces the likelihood that abortion will ever be needed in their families. Spouses and companions are free to challenge the reasoning used in any instance of contemplation of abortion. Social critics and moralists are free to write and speak against the current rules on abortion and the ethical perspective behind the rules. What none of these persons is free to do is to construct a public or medical test of a woman's reasons.

COMPETING ETHICAL CLAIMS

Wherever possible, competing ethical claims should be acknowledged in practice. There are three major ethical claims on the other side of the issue: scarcity of amniocentesis, risks and costs of the procedure and social engineering without full appreciation of the consequences.

When there is a genuine scarcity of amniocentesis in any center, its use for sex choice should be given the lowest priority. Parents who request amniocentesis for sex choice should bear all expenses, since society is not confronted with a disease in the fetus that should be prevented in the interest of the family in society. Because of risks to the mother and fetus, the procedure should only be performed when there is adequate counseling and access to high-quality laboratory work.

Forecasting the long-range consequences of sex preselection is a complex task[10] that deserves more encouragement and support. An earlier study based on data from the 1970 National Fertility Survey showed that the major consequence of sex determination would be planning the order of children (male first, female second) rather than increasing the number of boys.[11] Coombs's excellent study of the preferences for sex of children among American couples showed that wives are much more likely to prefer a son than a daughter and more likely to prefer either one than to have a positive underlying desire for an equal number of boys and girls.[12] The exceptions to this finding were wives of Hispanic heritage, who preferred girls. These findings suggest that if a safe, inexpensive preconception method of sex selection were available, firstborns would increasingly be male. Would these firstborn boys receive such a disproportionate share of the emotional and economic resources of their parents that secondborn girls would be seriously disadvantaged? More work needs to be done connecting forecasts of technologic advances in sex control with psychologic research in gender roles and birth order. The immediate ethical question is whether a more permissive policy on amniocentesis for sex choice will precipitate a social experiment in sex selection before there is sufficient study of the consequences. The parents who now need amniocentesis for sex choice are presumably motivated to have one child of the opposite gender from their living children. If this is true, these parents and their needs are not accurate predictors of the long-range consequences of sex determination in a planned birth order. Those consequences should be researched in the framework of sex-control methods that are more easily diffused and involve fewer risks than abortion.

CONCLUSIONS

In my revised view, it is not ethically required that physicians withhold amniocentesis from fully informed parents who may use the results in deciding to abort for sex choice. Even though the physician may personally disapprove of the request, it is fairer to the parents to grant it within the limits of availability of amniocentesis. Physicians who agree with the social-ethical perspective that informs the legal rules on abortion will finally want to keep faith with the moral intent of the law. Policymakers in this field should now reconsider their obligation to be responsive and consistent in their beliefs. I include myself in the company of those who need to be changed.

REFERENCES

1 Fletcher, J. C.: Prenatal diagnosis: ethical issues, *Encyclopedia of Bioethics.* New York, Macmillan, 1978, pp. 1336–1346.

2 Powledge, T. M., Fletcher, J.: Guidelines for the ethical, social and legal issues in prenatal diagnosis: a report from the Genetics Research Group of the Hastings Center, Institute of Society, Ethics and the Life Sciences. *N Engl J Med* 300:168–172, 1979.

3 Milunsky, A.: *Know Your Genes.* Boston, Houghton Mifflin Company, 1977.

4 Roe v. Wade. 410 US 113, 35 L.Ed.2d, 147.93 S.Ct. 705 (1973); Doe v. Bolton, 410 US 179, 35 L.Ed.2d, 201.93 S.Ct. 739 (1973).

5 The NICHD National Registry for Amniocentesis Study Group: Mid-trimester amniocentesis for prenatal diagnosis: safety and accuracy. *JAMA* 236: 1471–1476, 1976.

6 Simpson, N. E., Dallaire L., Miller J. R., et al.: Prenatal diagnosis of genetic disease in Canada: report of a collaborative study. *Can Med Assoc J* 115:739–748, 1976.

7 An assessment of the hazards of amniocentesis: report to the Medical Research Council by their Working Party on Amniocentesis. *Br J Obstet Gynaecol* 85:Suppl 2:1–41, 1978.

8 Golbus, M. S., Loughman, W. D., Epstein, C. J., et al.: Prenatal genetic diagnosis in 3000 amniocenteses. *N Engl J Med* 300:157–163, 1979.

9 Blumberg, B. D., Golbus, M. S., Hanson, K. H.: The psychological sequelae of abortion performed for a genetic indication. *Am J Obstet Gynecol* 122:799–808, 1975.

10 Largey, G.: Reproductive technologies: sex selection, *Encyclopedia of Bioethics.* New York, Macmillan, 1978, pp. 1439–1444.

11 Westoff, C. F., Rindfuss, R. R.: Sex preselection in the United States: some implications. *Science* 184:633–636, 1974.

12 Coombs, L. C.: Preferences for sex of children among U.S. couples. *Fam Plann Perspect* 9: 259–265, 1977.

Negative and Positive Rights: A Commentary on Fletcher

James F. Childress

James F. Childress is Commonwealth Professor of Religious Studies and also professor of medical education at the University of Virginia. Childress was formerly Joseph P. Kennedy, Sr., Professor of Christian Ethics, Kennedy Institute, Center for Bioethics, Georgetown University. In addition to numerous articles in biomedical ethics, he is the author of *Priorities in Biomedical Ethics* (1981) and *Who Should Decide?* (1982) and the coauthor of *Principles of Biomedical Ethics* (1979).

Childress is not unsympathetic to Fletcher's conclusion that amniocentesis should be provided to women who request it for reasons of sex selection, but he does argue that Fletcher has failed to provide an adequate argument in support of this

Reprinted with permission of the author and the publisher from *Hastings Center Report*, vol. 10 (February 1980), p. 19.

conclusion. Childress charges Fletcher with overlooking the distinction between a *negative* right and a *positive* right. According to Childress, *Roe v. Wade* (1973) establishes only a woman's negative right to an abortion, her right to be free of interference in procuring an abortion. Thus one can consistently affirm the Court's decision while denying that a woman has a right to the assistance of others in securing an abortion for reasons of sex selection.

A strong case can be made for Fletcher's conclusion, but it cannot be made simply or primarily by an appeal to consistency, ethical or otherwise. It requires a substantive moral principle such as fairness. Fletcher supposes that the appeal to consistency is sufficient only because he overlooks some important distinctions (especially the distinction between negative and positive rights) that negate the charge of inconsistency.

Fletcher describes his "major argument":

> it is inconsistent to support an abortion law that protects the absolute right of women to decide and, at the same time, to block access to information about the fetus because one thinks that an abortion may be foolishly sought on the basis of the information.

Fletcher's reading of the Supreme Court decisions is curiously one-sided. I can clarify this point by distinguishing negative from positive rights. A negative right is a justified claim to noninterference. If X has a negative right, Y has a duty not to interfere with X's exercise of that right. A positive right is a justified claim to someone's assistance.

Fletcher considers only the 1973 Supreme Court decisions on abortion—decisions that recognize only a negative right to an abortion. The woman, in consultation with her physician, has a right, based on privacy, to decide whether to have an abortion. The state has a duty not to prohibit it (at least until the last trimester). Subsequent Supreme Court decisions indicated that husbands and parents (in the case of mature minors) may not veto the woman's decision to have an abortion. But the Court has consistently refused to recognize a positive right to abortion, i.e., a justified claim that the state or others such as hospitals and physicians either fund or perform abortions.

Even the negative right is not absolute, for the state may prohibit abortion during the third trimester except where the woman's life or health is threatened. It is not inconsistent to affirm a negative right to an abortion and simultaneously to deny a positive right to an abortion. Thus, Fletcher cannot charge that it is inconsistent to affirm the Supreme Court's decisions in 1973 and to refuse to provide amniocentesis or to perform abortions for sex choice.

Fletcher claims that the issue of amniocentesis and abortion for sex choice "turns on the validity of the legal rules on abortion defined by the Supreme Court, which *do not require* that a woman state reasons in a public or medical forum for early to mid-trimester abortion." This claim is ambiguous. First, "validity" presumably refers not to legal or constitutional validity, but rather to moral justifiability. And for moral justification Fletcher appeals to the principles of justice and respect for persons. Even if we accept his claim (and I do) that these principles establish the negative right to an abortion, his claim that they also establish a positive right is nowhere supported, other than by the appeal to consistency. Second, while Fletcher is right that current legal rules do not *require* public reasons for abortion, he fails to see that they *permit* an inquiry into those reasons for purposes of the distribution of public funds and the physician's determination of his or her own role. No party—the state, the husband, the parents, or the physician—may interfere with the woman's decision to have an abortion, whatever her reasons; indeed, she is not required to state her reasons to prevent others from interfering with her decision. But the state is not legally bound to fund the abortion, and the physician is not legally bound to perform it, except possibly where certain reasons prevail (such as the protection of the mother's health and life). Thus, in the physician-patient relationship, the physician is *permitted* to inquire into the woman's reasons and to refuse to carry out the procedure if he or she chooses. The physician is probably legally and morally bound to *inform* the woman of amniocentesis, but not to provide it. As Fletcher recognizes, physicians "cannot legally be forced to provide procedures that are not 'lifesaving.'" In short, Fletcher is mistaken when he claims that no one is "free...to construct a public or medical test of a woman's reasons." Physicians have this freedom regarding their own actions within the physician-patient relationship. Contrary to Fletcher, the Supreme Court did not make "the conscience of the individual woman the sole arbiter of the reasons." Even if his claim holds for *noninterference,* it does not hold for *assistance.* The physician's conscience is also involved, and he or she is not legally or morally bound to violate conscience by providing amniocentesis (in contrast to providing information about amniocentesis) or by performing the abortion.

It is easier, of course, when appeals to consistency can do the work of substantive moral argument. But the appeal to consistency will not yield Fletcher's conclusion: that amniocentesis should be provided (where conditions permit) to women who request it for sex determination. That conclusion, however, may be established by other arguments. Unfortunately, Fletcher only hints at those arguments, which include the principle of *fairness,* a substantive principle, irreducible to the formal principle of consistency.

Reproductive Risk: Morality and Screening Programs

Genetic Diseases: Can Having Children Be Immoral?

L. M. Purdy

L. M. Purdy is assistant professor of philosophy at Wells College (Aurora, N.Y.). She has also taught at Cornell University, where she was postdoctoral associate in the Program on Science, Technology, and Society. Specializing in ethics and political philosophy, she has published articles such as "On Hiring Apparently Less Qualified Women" and "The Morality of Euthanasia."

Purdy argues that it is morally wrong to reproduce under some circumstances of genetic risk, most clearly in cases where there is high risk of serious genetic disease. Much of her analysis focuses on Huntington's chorea, which she considers a clear case of high-risk, serious genetic disease. To support her basic thesis, Purdy advances and defends the following set of claims: (1) We have an obligation to try to provide every child with a "normal opportunity for health"; (2) In acting on this obligation, we do not do wrong in preventing the existence of possible children; (3) Where there is high risk of serious genetic disease, this obligation overrides the generally recognized right to reproduce. Proceeding on the assumption that victims of Huntington's chorea lead worse than average lives, Purdy maintains that it is morally wrong for those at risk of passing on this disease to reproduce.

I INTRODUCTION

Suppose you know that there is a fifty percent chance you have Huntington's chorea, even though you are still free of symptoms, and that if you do have it, each of your children has a fifty percent chance of having it also.

Should you now have children?

There is always some possibility that a pregnancy will result in a diseased or handicapped child. But certain persons run a higher than average risk of producing such a child. Genetic counselors are increasingly able to calculate the probability that certain problems will occur; this means that more people can find out

Reprinted with permission of the author from *Genetics* Now: *Ethical Issues in Genetic Research,* edited by John J. Buckley, Jr. (Washington, D.C.: University Press of America, 1978).

whether they are in danger of creating unhealthy off-spring *before* the birth of a child.

Since this kind of knowledge is available, we ought to use it wisely. I want in this paper to defend the thesis that it is wrong to reproduce when we know there is a high risk of transmitting a serious disease or defect. My argument for this claim is in three parts. The first is that we should try to provide every child with a normal opportunity for health; the second is that in the course of doing this it is not wrong to prevent possible children from existing. The third is that this duty may require us to refrain from childbearing.[1]

One methodological point must be made. I am investigating a problem in biomedical ethics: this is a philosophical enterprise. But the conclusion has practical importance since individuals do face the choice I examine. This raises a question: what relation ought the outcome of this inquiry bear to social policy?[2] It may be held that a person's reproductive life should not be interfered with. Perhaps this is a reasonable position, but it does not follow from it that it is never wrong for an individual to have children or that we should not try to determine when this is the case. All that does follow is that we may not coerce persons with regard to childbearing. Evaluation of this last claim is a separate issue which cannot be handled here.

I want to deal with this issue concretely. The reason for this is that, otherwise, discussion is apt to be vague and inconclusive. An additional reason is that it will serve to make us appreciate the magnitude of the difficulties faced by diseased or handicapped individuals. Thus it will be helpful to consider a specific disease. For this purpose I have chosen Huntington's chorea.[3]

II HUNTINGTON'S CHOREA: COURSE AND RISK

Let us now look at Huntington's chorea. First we will consider the course of the disease, then its inheritance pattern.

The symptoms of Huntington's chorea usually begin between the ages of thirty and fifty, but young children can also be affected. It happens this way:

> Onset is insidious. Personality changes (obstinancy, moodiness, lack of initiative) frequently antedate or accompany the involuntary choreic movements. These usually appear first in the face, neck, and arms, and are jerky, irregular, and stretching in character. Contractions of the facial muscles result in grimaces; those of the respiratory muscles, lips, and tongue lead to hesitating, explosive speech. Irregular movements of the trunk are present; the gait is shuffling and dancing. Tendon reflexes are increased....Some patients display a fatuous euphoria; others are spiteful, irascible, destructive, and violent. Paranoid reactions are common. Poverty of thought and impairment of attention, memory, and judgment occur. As the disease progresses, walking becomes impossible, swallowing difficult, and dementia profound. Suicide is not uncommon.[4]

The illness lasts about fifteen years, terminating in death.

Who gets Huntington's chorea? It is an autosomal dominant disease; this means it is caused by a single mutant gene located on a non-sex chromosome. It is passed from one generation to the next via affected individuals. When one has the disease, whether one has symptoms and thus knows one has it or not, there is a fifty percent chance that each child will have it also. If one has escaped it then there is no risk to one's children.[5]

How serious is this risk? For geneticists, a ten percent risk is high.[6] But not every high risk is unacceptable: this depends on what is at stake.

There are two separate evaluations in any judgment about a given risk. The first measures the gravity of the worst possible result; the second perceives a given risk as great or small. As for the first, in medicine as elsewhere, people may regard the same result quite differently:

> ...The subjective attitude to the disease or lesion itself may be quite at variance with what informed medical opinion may regard as a realistic appraisal. Relatively minor limb defects with cosmetic overtones are examples here. On the other hand, some patients regard with equanimity genetic lesions which are of major medical importance.[7]

For devastating diseases like Huntington's chorea, this part of the judgment should be unproblematic: no one could want a loved one to suffer so.

There may be considerable disagreement, however, about whether a given probability is big or little. Individuals vary a good deal in their attitude toward this aspect of risk.[8] This suggests that it would be difficult to define the "right" attitude to a particular risk in many circumstances. Nevertheless, there are good grounds for arguing in favor of a conservative approach here. For it is reasonable to take special precautions to avoid very bad consequences, even if the risk is small. But the possible consequences here *are* very bad: a child who may inherit Huntington's chorea is a child with a much larger than average chance of being subjected to severe and prolonged suffering. Even if the child does not have the disease, it may anticipate and fear it, and anticipating an evil, as we all know, may be worse than experiencing it. In addition, if a parent loses the gamble, his child will suffer the consequences. But it is one thing to take a high risk for oneself; to submit someone else to it without his consent is another.

I think that these points indicate that the morality of procreation in situations like this demands further study. I propose to do this by looking first at the position of the possible child, then at that of the potential parent.[9]

III REPRODUCTION: THE POSSIBLE CHILD'S POSITION

The first task in treating the problem from the child's point of view is to find a way of referring to possible future offspring without seeming to confer some sort of morally significant existence upon them. I will call children who might be born in the future but who are not now conceived "possible" children, offspring, individuals, or persons. I stipulate that this term implies nothing about their moral standing.

The second task is to decide what claims about children or possible children are relevant to the morality of childbearing in the circumstances being considered. There are, I think, two such claims. One is that we ought to provide every child with at least a normal opportunity for a good life. The other is that we do not harm possible children if we prevent them from existing. Let us consider both these matters in turn.

A Opportunity for a Good Life

Accepting the claim that we ought to try to provide for every child a normal opportunity for a good life involves two basic problems: justification and practical application.

Justification of the claim could be derived fairly straightforwardly from either utilitarian or contractarian theories of justice, I think, although a proper dis-

cussion would be too lengthy to include here. Of prime importance in any such discussion would be the judgment that to neglect this duty would be to create unnecessary unhappiness or unfair disadvantage for some persons.

The attempt to apply the claim that we should try to provide a normal opportunity for a good life leads to a couple of difficulties. One is knowing what it requires of us. Another is defining "normal opportunity." Let us tackle the latter problem first.

Conceptions of "normal opportunity" vary among societies and also within them: *de rigueur* in some circles are private music lessons and trips to Europe, while in others providing eight years of schooling is a major sacrifice. But there is no need to consider this complication since we are here concerned only with health as a prerequisite for normal opportunity. Thus we can retreat to the more limited claim that every parent should try to ensure normal heath for his child. It might be thought that even this moderate claim is unsatisfactory since in some places debilitating conditions are the norm. One could circumvent this objection by saying that parents ought to try to provide for their children health normal for that culture, even though it may be inadequate if measured by some outside standard. This conservative position would still justify efforts to avoid the birth of children at risk for Huntington's chorea and other serious genetic diseases.

But then what does this stand require of us: is sacrifice entailed by the duty to try to provide normal health for our children? The most plausible answer seems to be that as the danger of serious disability increases, the greater the sacrifice demanded of the potential parent. This means it would be more justifiable to recommend that an individual refrain from childbearing if he risks passing on spina bifida than if he risks passing on webbed feet. Working out all the details of such a schema would clearly be a difficult matter; I do not think it would be impossible to set up workable guidelines, though.

Assuming a rough theoretical framework of this sort, the next question we must ask is whether Huntington's chorea substantially impairs an individual's opportunity for a good life.

People appear to have different opinions about the plight of such persons. Optimists argue that a child born into a family afflicted with Huntington's chorea has a reasonable chance of living a satisfactory life. After all, there is a fifty percent chance it will escape the disease even if a parent has already manifested it, and a still greater chance if this is not so. Even if it does have the illness, it will probably enjoy thirty years of healthy life before symptoms appear; and, perhaps, it may not find the disease destructive. Optimists can list diseased or handicapped persons who have lived fruitful lives. They can also find individuals who seem genuinely glad to be alive. One is Rick Donohue, a sufferer from the Joseph family disease: "You know, if my mom hadn't had me, I wouldn't be here for the life I have had. So there is a good possibility I will have children."[10] Optimists therefore conclude that it would be a shame if these persons had not lived.

Pessimists concede these truths, but they take a less sanguine view of them. They think a fifty percent risk of serious disease like Huntington's chorea appallingly high. They suspect that a child born into an afflicted family is liable to spend its youth in dreadful anticipation and fear of the disease. They expect that the disease, if it appears, will be perceived as a tragic and painful end to a blighted life. They point out that Rick Donohue is still young and has not yet experienced the full horror of his sickness.

Empirical research is clearly needed to resolve this dispute: we need much more information about the psychology and life history of sufferers and potential sufferers. Until we have it we cannot know whether the optimist or the pessimist has a better case; definitive judgment must therefore be suspended. In the meantime, however, common sense suggests that the pessimist has the edge.

If some diseased persons do turn out to have a worse than average life there appears to be a case against further childbearing in afflicted families. To support this claim two more judgments are necessary, however. The first is that it is not wrong to refrain from childbearing. The second is that asking individuals to so refrain is less of a sacrifice than might be thought.[11] I will examine each of these judgments.

B   The Morality of Preventing the Birth of Possible Persons

Before going on to look at reasons why it would not be wrong to prevent the birth of possible persons, let me try to clarify the picture a bit. To understand the claim it must be kept in mind that we are considering a prospective situation here, not a retrospective one: we are trying to rank the desirability of various alternative future states of affairs. One possible future state is this:

a world where nobody is at risk for Huntington's chorea except as a result of random mutation. This state has been achieved by sons and daughters of persons afflicted with Huntington's chorea ceasing to reproduce. This means that an indeterminate number of children who might have been born were not born. These possible children can be divided into two categories: those who would have been miserable and those who would have lived good lives. To prevent the existence of members of the first category it was necessary to prevent the existence of all. Whether or not this is a good state of affairs depends on the morality of the means and the end. The end, preventing the existence of miserable beings, is surely good; I will argue that preventing the birth of possible persons is not intrinsically wrong. Hence this state of affairs is a morally good one.

Why then is it not in itself wrong to prevent the birth of possible persons? It is not wrong because there seems to be no reason to believe that possible individuals are either deprived or injured if they do not exist. They are not deprived because to be deprived in a morally significant sense one must be able to have experiences. But possible persons do not exist. Since they do not exist, they cannot have experiences. Another way to make this point is to say that each of us might not have been born, although most of us are glad we were. But this does not mean that it makes sense to say that we would have been deprived of something had we not been born. For if we had not been born, we would not exist, and there would be nobody to be deprived of anything. To assert the contrary is to imagine that we are looking at a world in which we do not exist. But this is not the way it would be: there would be nobody to look.

The contention that it is wrong to prevent possible persons from existing because they have a right to exist appears to be equally baseless. The most fundamental objection to this view is that there is no reason to ascribe rights to entities which do not exist. It is one thing to say that as-yet-nonexistent persons will have certain rights if and when they exist: this claim is plausible if made with an eye toward preserving social and environmental goods.[12] But what justification could there be for the claim that nonexistent beings have a right to exist?

Even if one conceded that there was a presumption in favor of letting some nonexistent beings exist, stronger claims could surely override it.[13] For one thing, it would be unfair not to recognize the prior claim of already existing children who are not being properly cared for. One might also argue that it is simply wrong to prevent persons who might have existed from doing so. But this implies that contraception and population control are also wrong.

It is therefore reasonable to maintain that because possible persons have no right to exist, they are not injured if not created. Even if they had that right, it could rather easily be overridden by counterclaims. Hence, since possible persons are neither deprived nor injured if not conceived, it is not wrong to prevent their existence.

C   Conclusion of Part III

At the beginning of Part III I said that two claims are relevant to the morality of childbearing in the circumstances being considered. The first is that we ought to provide every child with at least a normal opportunity for a good life. The second is that we do not deprive or injure possible persons if we prevent their existence.

I suggested that the first claim could be derived from currently accepted theories of justice: a healthy body is generally necessary for happiness and it is also a prerequisite for a fair chance at a good life in our competitive world. Thus it is right to try to ensure that each child is healthy.

I argued, with regard to the second claim, that we do not deprive or injure possible persons if we fail to create them. They cannot be deprived of anything because they do not exist and hence cannot have experiences. They cannot be injured because only an entity with a right to exist could be injured if prevented from existing; but there are no good grounds for believing that they are such entities.

From the conjunction of these two claims I conclude that it is right to try to ensure that a child is healthy even if by doing so we preclude the existence of certain possible persons. Thus it is right for individuals to prevent the birth of children at risk for Huntington's chorea by avoiding parenthood. The next question is whether it is seriously wrong *not* to avoid parenthood.

IV   REPRODUCTION: THE POTENTIAL PARENT'S SITUATION

I have so far argued that if choreics live substantially worse lives than average, then it is right for afflicted families to cease reproduction. But this conflicts with the generally recognized freedom to procreate and so it does not automatically follow that family members ought not to have children. How can we decide whether the duty to try to provide normal health for one's child should take precedence over the right to reproduce?

This is essentially the same question I asked earlier: how much must one sacrifice to try to ensure that one's offspring is healthy? In answer to this I suggested that the greater the danger of serious disability, the more justifiable considerable sacrifice is.

Now asking someone who wants a child to refrain from procreation seems to be asking for a large sacrifice. It may, in fact, appear to be too large to demand of anyone. Yet I think it can be shown that it is not as great as it initially seems.

Why do people want children? There are probably many reasons, but I suspect that the following include some of the most common. One set of reasons has to do with the gratification to be derived from a happy family life—love, companionship, watching a child grow, helping mold it into a good person, sharing its pains and triumphs. Another set of reasons centers about the parents as individuals—validation of their place within a genetically continuous family line, the conception of children as a source of immortality, being surrounded by replicas of themselves.

Are there alternative ways of satisfying these desires? Adoption or technological means provide ways to satisfy most of the desires pertaining to family life without passing on specific genetic defects. Artificial insemination by donor is already available; implantation of donor ova is likely within a few years. Still another option will exist if cloning becomes a reality. In the meantime, we might permit women to conceive and bear babies for those who do not want to do so themselves.[14] But the desire to extend the genetic line, the desire for immortality, and the desire for children that physically resemble one cannot be met by these methods.

Many individuals probably feel these latter desires strongly. This creates a genuine conflict for persons at risk for transmitting serious genetic diseases like Huntington's chorea. The situation seems especially unfair because, unlike normal people, through no fault of their own, doing something they badly want to do may greatly harm others.

But if my common sense assumption that they are in grave danger of harming others is true, then it is imperative to scrutinize their options carefully. On the one hand, they can have children: they satisfy their desires but risk eventual crippling illness and death for their offspring. On the other, they can remain childless or seek nonstandard ways of creating a family: they have some unfulfilled desires, but they avoid risking harm to their children.

I think it is clear which of these two alternatives is best. For the desires which must remain unsatisfied if they forgo normal procreation are less than admirable. To see the genetic line continued entails a sinister legacy of illness and death; the desire for immortality cannot really be satisfied by reproduction anyway; and the desire for children that physically resemble one is narcissistic and its fulfillment cannot be guaranteed even by normal reproduction. Hence the only defence of these desires is that people do in fact feel them.

Now, I am inclined to accept William James' dictum regarding desires: "Take any demand, however slight, which any creature, however weak, may make. Ought it not, for its own sole sake be satisfied? If not, prove why not."[15] Thus I judge a world where more desires are satisfied to be better than one in which fewer are. But not all desires should be regarded as legitimate, since, as James suggests, there may be good reasons why these ought to be disregarded. The fact that their fulfillment will seriously harm others is surely such a reason. And I believe that the circumstances I have described are a clear example of the sort of case where a desire must be judged illegitimate, at least until it can be shown that sufferers from serious genetic diseases like Huntington's chorea do not live considerably worse than average lives. Therefore, I think it is wrong for individuals in this predicament to reproduce.

V   CONCLUSION

Let me recapitulate. At the beginning of this paper I asked whether it is wrong for those who risk transmitting severe genetic disease like Huntington's chorea to have "blood" children. Some despair of reaching an answer to this question.[16] But I think such pessimism is not wholly warranted, and that if generally accepted would lead to much unnecessary harm. It is true that in many cases it is difficult to know what ought to be done. But this does not mean that we should throw up our hands and espouse a completely laissez-faire approach: philosophers can help by probing the central issues and trying to find guidelines for action.

Naturally there is no way to derive an answer to this kind of problem by deductive argument from self-evident premises, for it must depend on a complicated interplay of facts and moral judgments. My preliminary exploration of Huntington's chorea is of this nature. In the course of the discussion I suggested that, if it is true that sufferers live substantially worse lives than do normal persons, those who might transmit it should not have children. This conclusion is supported by the judgments that we ought to try to provide for every child a normal opportunity for a good life, that possible individuals are not harmed if not conceived, and that it is sometimes less justifiable for persons to exercise their right to procreate than one might think.

I want to stress, in conclusion, that my argument is incomplete. To investigate fully even a single disease, like Huntington's chorea, empirical research on the lives of members of afflicted families is necessary. Then, after developing further the themes touched upon here, evaluation of the probable consequences of different policies on society and on future generations is needed. Until the results of a complete study are available, my argument could serve best as a reason for persons at risk for transmitting Huntington's chorea and similar diseases to put off having children. Perhaps this paper will stimulate such inquiry.

NOTES

1   There are a series of cases ranging from low risk of mild disease or handicap to high risk of serious disease or handicap. It would be difficult to decide where the duty to refrain from procreation becomes compelling. My point here is that there are some clear cases.

I'd like to thank Lawrence Davis and Sidney Siskin for their helpful comments on an earlier version of this paper.

2   This issue is one which must be faced most urgently by genetic counselors. The proper role of the genetic counselor with regard to such decisions has been the subject of much debate. The dominant view seems to be that espoused by Lytt Gardner who maintains that it is unethical for a counselor to make ethical judgments about what his clients ought to do. ("Counseling in Genetics," *Early Diagnosis of Human Genetic Defects: Scientific & Ethical Considerations,* ed. Maureen Harris, [H.E.W. Publication No. (NIH) 72–25; Fogarty Center Proceedings No. 6]; p. 192.) Typically this view is unsupported by an argument. For other views see

Bentley Glass "Human Heredity and Ethical Problems" *Perspectives in Biology & Medicine,* Vol. 15 (winter '72) 237–53, esp. 242–52; Marc Lappé, "The Genetic Counselor Responsible to Whom?" *Hastings Center Report,* Vol. 1, No. 2 (Sept. '71) 6–8; E. C. Fraser, "Genetic Counseling" *Am. J. of Human Genetics* 26: 636–659, 1974.

3 I have chosen Huntington's chorea because it seems to me to be one of the clearest cases of high risk serious genetic disease known to the public, despite the fact that it does not usually manifest itself until the prime of life. The latter entails two further facts. First an individual of reproductive age may not know whether he has the disease; he therefore does not know the risk of passing on the disease. Secondly, an affected person may have a substantial number of years of healthy life before it shows itself. I do not think that this factor materially changes my case, however. Even if an individual does not in fact risk passing the disease to his children, *he cannot know that this is true.* And even thirty years of healthy life may well be seriously shadowed by anticipation and fear of the disease. Thus the fact that the disease develops late does not diminish its horror. If it could be shown that these factors could be adequately circumvented, my claim that there is a *class* of genetic disease of such severity that it would be wrong to risk passing them on would not be undermined.

It might also be thought that Huntington's chorea is insufficiently common to merit such attention. But, depending on reproductive patterns, the disease could become a good deal more widespread. Consider the fact that in 1916 nine hundred and sixty-two cases could be traced from six seventeenth-century arrivals in America. (Gordon Rattray Taylor, *The Biological Time Bomb,* [New York, 1968], p. 176.) But more importantly, even if the disease did not spread, it would still be seriously wrong, I think, to inflict it unnecessarily on *any* members of new generations. Finally, it should be kept in mind that I am using Huntington's chorea as an example of the sort of disease we should try to eradicate. Thus the arguments presented here would be relevant to a wide range of genetic diseases.

4 *The Merck Manual* (Rahway, N.J.: Merck, 1972), p. 1346.

5 Hymie Gordon, "Genetic Counseling," *JAMA,* Vol. 217 No. 9 (August 30, 1971), 1217.

6 Charles Smith, Susan Holloway, and Alan E. H.

Emery, "Individuals at Risk in Families—Genetic Disease," *J. of Medical Genetics,* 8 (1971), 453. See also Townes in *Genetic Counseling,* ed. Daniel Bergsma, *Birth Defects Original Article Series,* Vol. VI, No. 1 (May 1970).

7 J. H. Pearn, "Patients' Subjective Interpretation of Risks Offered in Genetic Counseling," *Journal of Medical Genetics,* 10 (1973), 131.

8 Pearn, p. 132.

9 There are many important and interesting points that might be raised with respect to future generations and present society. There is no space to deal with them here, although I strongly suspect that conclusions regarding them would support my judgment that it is wrong for those who risk transmitting certain diseases to reproduce—for some discussion of future generations, see Gerald Leach, *The Biocrats,* (Middlesex, England: Penguin Books, 1972), p. 150; M. P. Golding, "Obligations to Future Generations," *Monist* 56 (Jan. 1972) 84–99; Gordon Rattray Taylor, *The Biological Time Bomb* (New York, 1968), esp. p. 176. For some discussions of society, see Daniel Callahan, "The Meaning and Significance of Genetic Disease: Philosophical Perspectives," *Ethical Issues in Human Genetics,* ed. Bruce Hilton et al. (New York, 1973), p. 87ff.; John Fletcher, "The Brink: The Parent-Child Bond in the Genetic Revolution," *Theological Studies* 33 (Sept. '72) 457–485; Glass (supra 2ª); Marc Lappé, "Human Genetics," Annals of the *New York Academy of Sciences,* Vol. 26 (May 18, 1973) 152–59; Marc Lappé, "Moral Obligations and the Fallacies of 'Genetic Control,'" *Theological Studies* Vol. 33, No. 3 (Sept '72), 411–427; Martin P. Golding, "Ethical Issues in Biological Engineering," *UCLA Law Review* Vol. 15: 267 (1968) 443–479; L. C. Dunn, *Heredity and Evolution in Human Populations* (Cambridge, Mass., 1959), p. 145; Robert S. Morison in *Ethical Issues in Human Genetics,* ed. Bruce Hilton et. al. (New York, 1973), p. 208.

10 *The New York Times,* September 30, 1975, p. 1., col. 6. The Joseph family disease is similar to Huntington's chorea except that symptoms start appearing in the twenties. Rick Donohue is in his early twenties.

11 There may be a price for the individuals who refrain from having children. We will be looking at the situation from their point of view shortly.

12 This is in fact the basis for certain parental duties. An example is the maternal duty to obtain proper nutrition before and during pregnancy, for this is

necessary if the child is to have normal health when it is born.

13 One might argue that as many persons as possible should exist so that they may enjoy life.

14 Some thinkers have qualms about the use of some or all of these methods. They have so far failed to show why they are immoral, although, naturally, much careful study will be required before they could be unqualifiedly recommended. See, for example, Richard Hull, "Genetic Engineering:

Comment on Headings," *The Humanist,* Vol. 32 (Sept./Oct. 1972), 13.

15 *Essays in Pragmatism,* ed. A. Castell (New York, 1948), p. 73.

16 For example, see Leach, p. 138. One of the ways the dilemma described by Leach could be lessened would be if society emphasized those aspects of family life not dependent on "blood" relationships and downplayed those that are.

Genetic Screening: For Better or for Worse?

Neil A. Holtzman

Neil A. Holtzman, M.D., is professor of pediatrics at the Johns Hopkins University School of Medicine. In addition to numerous original investigations in the area of biomedical research, Holtzman has also conducted original investigations in the area of epidemiological and health services research. Some of his published work, such as this selection, explicitly reflects a concern with the social and ethical aspects of genetic screening.

After pointing out the importance of identifying carriers before they reproduce, Holtzman warns against adopting screening programs that are "subtly" coercive or have a high potential for the stigmatization of carriers. He discusses the anxiety and fear of stigmatization that arose among some of the identified carriers in one effort (in high schools) to increase voluntary participation in Tay-Sachs screening. Holtzman argues that, in order to ensure that the risks of genetic screening do not outweigh its benefits, increased emphasis must be placed on education about human genetics.

Cystic fibrosis, sickle cell anemia, Tay-Sachs disease, and thalassemia are autosomal-recessive diseases that occur more frequently than once in 4,000 live births in subgroups of the American population. Tay-Sachs disease can be diagnosed by mid-trimester amniocentesis, a safe procedure.[1] Early intrauterine detection of sickle cell anemia and thalassemia by placental aspiration has been reported[2,3]; the safety and accuracy of the techniques require confirmation. In the future, diagnosis of the 16-week fetus with cystic fibrosis will also be possible.

Prenatal diagnosis could drastically reduce the incidence of these disorders, but there are two prerequisites. First, couples in whom both mates are carriers must be identified before they have any children. There is as great a chance of first births being affected as any other, and they constitute over 40 percent of all births in the United States,[4] with the proportion rising. Carrier identification is already possible for all of the conditions mentioned except cystic fibrosis. Second, couples at risk must terminate the pregnancy of affected fetuses. Although few couples would have a child with Tay-

Reprinted with permission of the publisher from *Pediatrics,* vol. 59 (January 1977), pp. 131–133. Copyright © American Academy of Pediatrics, 1977.

Sachs disease if they could avoid it, those at risk for having offspring with cystic fibrosis or sickle cell anemia, in which mental retardation and early death are not the usual outcome, might not make the same choice.[5]

In order to satisfy the two prerequisites screening could be made compulsory and those identified as carriers compelled to avoid the birth of affected children. Although such extreme and opprobrious measures seem unlikely today, coercive pressures could be subtly exerted and carriers could be sufficiently stigmatized so that they become undesirable mates. Thus, model screening programs should be carefully scrutinized for evidence of coercion and stigmatization before they are widely adopted.

Participation has been a problem in Tay-Sachs screening. Programs directed at young married couples often attract only a small proportion of the target population....Clow and Scriver describe an attempt to increase participation by screening in high schools.[6] Fortunately, they provide information that enables the reader to assess some of the effects, both beneficial and harmful.

Although the most intensive effort involved the addition of material on human genetics to the high schools' biology curriculum, coercion and peer pressure cannot be excluded. The chief medical officer of the school system was recruited to recommend testing "in an official letter to all Jewish students...and a school assembly was held to discuss the benefits of testing...."[7] Whether it was education, coercion, peer pressure, a captive audience, or something else, acceptance of screening improved markedly. Whereas the earlier program, directed at newlyweds, attracted only 10.8 percent of the target population,[7] the authors report that 75 percent of the eligible students were screened. Thus, a far greater proportion of the at-risk population now knows whether or not they are carriers. What effect will this new knowledge have?

Let us first consider the effect on non-carriers. Ten percent of them had an improved self-image after testing. A similar percentage said they would not mate with carriers. These attitudes are not consonant with the facts: those who do not carry the Tay-Sachs gene posses, on the average, genes for three or four other "bad" diseases; there is no reason for self-image to improve. Nor is there any risk of having a child with Tay-Sachs disease in matings between a non-carrier and a carrier.

Let us turn to the carriers. All of them indicated they would want to know the results of screening in their intended spouses. Twelve percent, however, said they would "reconsider" if he or she was also a carrier. This group apparently does not understand or accept prenatal diagnosis and abortion as a means of avoiding the birth of affected infants. How many other carriers lack understanding or acceptance is unknown. Until follow-up information on the actions of carriers later in life is available the encouragement of high school screening "as the preferred program" may be premature.

Screening for carriers at a time in life when choice of mate is not imminent and when self-confidence ebbs and flows may cause additional problems. Fear of stigmatization may be the reason why one third of carriers, compared to 15 percent of non-carriers, did not inform their friends of the result. One half of the carriers were worried or depressed immediately after learning their status; several months later 17.7 percent said they were still worried. Nine percent of students identified as carriers had a diminished self-image. Although anxiety also occurs in married individuals identified as carriers, fear of stigmatization is less.[8] The significance of depression or anxiety will only be determined by comparing the subsequent experience of carriers and non-carriers identified by screening. Because of the psychological and social hazards one group of physicians advised their community against Tay-Sachs screening at any age.[9]

Before concluding that risks outweigh benefits, efforts to increase participation in screening that do not endanger the individual's freedom of choice or well-being must be considered. More education about human genetics is fundamental. Greater appreciation of the laws of inheritance might result from teaching about genetic traits of humans rather than those of peas or fruit flies. Clow and Scriver have made a notable contribution by developing in-service training for high school teachers. Further evaluation of changes in students' understanding as a result of the curriculum modification is needed.

Physicians can also educate. Indeed, people in communities involved in Tay-Sachs screening expected them to do so. Yet as the actual source of information about screening, physicians were outranked by synagogues, newspapers, radio, television, and friends.[7,10] One obstacle may be infrequent contact between physicians and young adults. Another may be physicians' preoccupation with the treatment of overt illness. But medical care administered after disease becomes manifest is a less effective way of reducing untimely death and disability than earlier intervention. As a greater number of interventions that do not depend on the presence of overt illness become available, physicians may be expected to take responsibility for them. In the case of genetic screening, the doctor-patient relationship provides a confidential channel for communication of advice and results; coercion and stigmatization might be less of a problem.

Finally, the community must be among those who decide whether screening should be undertaken. It must be presented with the objectives of screening as well as the potential pitfalls. Community input and involvement could serve to reduce the harmful effects. As no group can speak for all of its constituents, each individual should receive information about the benefits and risks before being screened and have the opportunity to refuse screening.

In the immediate future the determination of how inappropriate psychological and social attitudes that result from screening can be minimized is more important than the extension of programs whose effects are still uncertain. With the knowledge that accrues, genetic screening for better, not for worse, will result.

REFERENCES

1 NICHD National Registry for Amniocentesis Study Group: Mid-trimester amniocentesis for prenatal diagnosis. *JAMA* 236:1471, 1976.

2 Kan, Y. W., Golbus, M. S., Trecartin, R.: Prenatal diagnosis of sickle cell anemia. *N Engl J Med* 294:1039, 1976.

3 Alter, B. P., Friedman, S., Hobbins, J. C., *et al.:* Prenatal diagnosis of sickle cell anemia and alpha-G-Philadephia. *N Engl J Med* 294:1040, 1976.

4 National Center for Health Statistics: Advance Report, Final Natality Statistics, 1974. Vital Stat Rep, 1976.

5 Stomatoyannopoulos, G.: Problems of screening and counseling in the hemoglobinopathies. In Motulsky, A. G., Lenz, W. (eds): *Birth Defects.* Amsterdam, Excerpta Medica, 1974, pp. 268–276.

6 Clow, C.L., Scriver, C.R.: Knowledge and attitudes about genetic screening among high school students: The Tay-Sachs experience, *Pediatrics* 59:86, 1977.

7 Beck, E., Blaichman S., Scriver, C. R., Clow, C. L.: Advocacy and compliance in genetic screening, behavior of physicians and clients in a voluntary program of testing for the Tay-Sachs gene. *N Engl J Med* 291:1166, 1974.

8 Childs, B., Gordis, L., Kaback, M. M., Kazazian, H. H.: Tay-Sachs screening: Social and psychological impact. *Am J Hum Genet,* to be published.

9 Kuhr, M. D.: Doubtful benefits of Tay-Sachs screening. *N Engl J Med* 295:113, 1976.

10 Childs, B., Gordis, L., Kaback, M. M., Kazazian, H. H.: Tay-Sachs screening: Motives for participating and knowledge of genetics and probability. *Am J Hum Genet,* to be published.

Cystic Fibrosis Screening: A Case Study

President's Commission for the Study of Ethical Problems in Medicine and Biomedical and Behavioral Research

A descriptive account of the President's Commission is found on page 103.

Anticipating the emergence of reliable methods for both the prenatal detection of cystic fibrosis and the detection of the carrier state, the Commission attempts to identify the advantages and disadvantages of various approaches to cystic fibrosis screening. The Commission distinguishes, in broad terms, between a prospective approach and a retrospective approach. Screening, on a prospective approach, would extend either to the general population or some identified segment of it,

Reprinted from President's Commission for the Study of Ethical Problems in Medicine and Biomedical and Behavioral Research, *Screening and Counseling for Genetic Conditions* (1983), chapter 3, pp. 87–88, 93–100.

perhaps married couples and those planning marriage. Screening, on a retrospective approach, would be limited to families in which cystic fibrosis had already emerged. Within the category of a prospective approach, the Commission further distinguishes between a community-based approach and a physician-based approach. The Commission also briefly considers the likely benefits and harms of screening newborn children for cystic fibrosis.

... By the end of the 1980s the means are likely to be at hand for a new program of mass genetic screening of vast proportions. The disease in question—cystic fibrosis—is the most prevalent known autosomal recessive cause of serious illness and early death among Americans.

Despite intensive research, no definitive way to detect cystic fibrosis (CF) carriers or affected fetuses has been developed as yet. However, methods suitable for large-scale screening are predicted; once available, they are likely to generate great interest. Consequently, [our focus here is] on potential CF screening and counseling programs....

DESCRIPTION OF THE DISEASE

Cystic fibrosis is the most common lethal genetic disease among young people in the United States, affecting about 20,000–30,000 people. Approximately one out of every 1800 infants is born with CF; by comparison, only about one out of every 14,000 babies in the United States is born with PKU, for which newborn screening is routine. The incidence of CF in American blacks is about one-tenth the incidence in Caucasians, and the disease is almost never seen in Orientals or African blacks.

Advances in managing symptoms have increased the life span of people with cystic fibrosis in the 50 years since it was first identified as a distinct disease. Despite this progress, most CF victims today do not survive past their teenage years. Although the improvements in treatment have been palliative and both the causative biochemical defect and the cure for CF remain a mystery, research holds promise for significant advances in treatment and care.

CF is characterized by pulmonary and digestive malfunction and by abnormally high concentrations of electrolytes in a person's sweat. The pancreatic insufficiency, the pulmonary problems, and most of the other clinical manifestations of the disease are largely secondary to CF's main characteristic—a dys-

function of the exocrine (secreting) glands that leads to abnormal amounts of mucus that can obstruct organ passages. Within the first few months of life CF can be diagnosed through a "sweat test" that detects high electrolyte concentrations. In fact, the old wives' tale that a baby whose brow tastes salty when kissed will not live long probably arose from observations of infants who had CF.

CF is inherited in an autosomal recessive pattern. About one in 20 whites and one in 60 blacks in the United States is heterozygous for the CF gene; these carriers do not manifest any identifiable symptoms of the disease. [With random mating, about one white couple in every 400 and one black couple in every 3600 would be a carrier-carrier pairing, and each child they had would face one-in-four odds of having CF.] By comparison, about one Ashkenazi Jew in 30 is a carrier for Tay-Sachs disease and about one black in 12 carries the gene for sickle-cell anemia, the next most common lethal genetic disease in the United States. Due to the proportion of the U.S. population that is Caucasian, the frequency of CF carriers in the entire population is five times that of sickle-cell carriers.

CF affects a vastly larger population than the other genetic diseases for which mass screening programs have been undertaken: essentially the entire U.S. population (at least those with some Caucasian lineage) is "at risk." No "high-risk" subgroup, except individuals with a family history of CF, has been identified. The development of screening tests for CF could, therefore, trigger the largest demand for genetic screening and counseling ever experienced in this country....

PLANNING PROGRAMS FOR CARRIER AND PRENATAL TESTING

If a carrier and/or prenatal test proves acceptable in pilot studies, planners will need to identify who to screen and in what setting. Both the likely benefits and harms to potential screenees and the relative costs and benefits to society will need to be evaluated. Outside a research setting, screening programs ought to be introduced only if they seem likely to offer a net benefit to those being screened. The benefits of carrier and prenatal tests differ and will be influenced by the order in which the tests become available. Clearly, families who have a child with CF view the tests differently from those who do not.

Assessing Potential Benefit and Harm

Prenatal diagnosis for CF is likely to be developed either in conjunction with the discovery of a carrier test or in advance of it, depending upon the method that first proves successful (for example, biochemical or recombinant DNA). The availability of a prenatal test would eliminate some of the difficulties that arise when only carrier testing is available; in the latter case, test results may be used to select mates or to decide whether to forego childbearing but not to determine the outcome of a particular pregnancy. The contrasting experiences of screening for sickle-cell anemia (before the recent development of a means of prenatal diagnosis) and Tay-Sachs disease are illustrative. Some potential sickle-cell screenees found that the availability of carrier screening without prenatal diagnosis was more harmful than helpful since they did not wish to make decisions based on carrier status alone. With Tay-Sachs disease, the simultaneous availability of a carrier test and prenatal diagnosis (and selective abortion) led some carrier couples to try to have children rather than forego reproduction entirely.

Although the experiences with sickle-cell and Tay-Sachs screening are instructive, neither is perfectly analogous to CF testing.[1] Like sickle-cell anemia, CF can be variable and is susceptible to some palliative treatment; although not as rapidly lethal as Tay-Sachs, CF is usually a very burdensome condition. Moreover, there are sociocultural as well as individual differences in the assessment of the benefits of prenatal diagnosis based on the importance people attach to health and to medicine generally and on their attitudes toward abortion.

In this way, the potential for CF screening is a precursor of the many difficult issues of risk and benefit that will increasingly arise in various types of genetic testing. The expanding capability to detect conditions and even predilections toward diseases prenatally— including, perhaps, some that occur later in life— underscores the importance of individuals freely choosing whether to participate in screening.

Deciding Who and When to Screen

Careful consideration will need to be given to the relative advantages and disadvantages of the two possible approaches to CF screening: prospective and retrospective testing. A prospective program would extend to the general population or some segment of it (for example, couples considering childbearing). It would require extensive educational efforts to provide information about CF to people who are unacquainted with the disease. A retrospective program would be limited to families that include someone with CF. These candidates would already have some familiarity with the condition.

There are several ways that prospective screening could be organized. It could be provided in a community-based or mass screening program in which community resources are used to inform people about the disease and the test and in which screening is made widely available. Some experts have questioned this approach for diseases with a low incidence, however, arguing that the anxiety and stigmatization that can result from such a mass screening effort can outweigh the benefits when the likelihood that an individual screenee will produce an affected child is small. This question will need to be addressed in the planning of a CF program, especially in deciding whether to screen populations with a very low incidence of the disease. CF is very rare in American blacks, for example. Just as individuals without eastern Jewish heritage are not screened for Tay-Sachs disease and Caucasians are not screened for sickle-cell anemia, CF screening of American blacks is probably inappropriate. In the past, screening for PKU was discontinued in predominantly black cities (such as Washington, D.C.) because PKU is so rare in blacks that the costs of screening were seen to outweigh the benefits.

In defining the target population a decision will also have to be made about whether to offer screening to people who are unmarried or not of reproductive age. The U.S. experience with sickle-cell screening of schoolchildren—about whom confidentiality was often difficult to maintain—sounds a warning about screening a population in which the benefits are so remote that they are likely to be outweighed by the harm, including the risk of breach of confidence. The young children screened for sickle-cell could do nothing with the information, and serious problems of stigmatization and confusion over the meaning of carrier status injured those screened and gave the whole effort a bad name.

Alternatively, it is at least theoretically possible to obtain nearly as complete an identification of at-risk cases through screening solely married couples and people planning marriage as through general screening. Initially, most Tay-Sachs screening involved only married couples because the programs' organizers (which typically included rabbis and other leaders in the Jewish community) did not want to risk having carrier status influence marital choices (and saw no need for such an influence, since amniocentesis was available for carrier-carrier couples). This policy reflected an understandable sensitivity to the risk that the label "carrier" might stigmatize a person in the eyes of others (including prospective mates and their families) as well as lead to a loss of self-esteem. Since children would not need the information to make reproductive decisions, there was no reason to risk the stigma.[2]

Although concerns over the possible harm of stigmatization are important, they must be weighed against the value of early screening. Many people may wish to know their carrier status prior to marriage (though not all of them may have thorough premarital medical examinations) and some do not wait until marriage to conceive children. This raises the question of whether people would generally regard it as desirable for decisions about dating, marriage, and reproduction to be made (at least in part) on genetic grounds. The outcome of the balancing process in the case of CF screening will depend upon facts about the test and the auspices and procedures for implementing it. The benefits of administrative efficiency in screening easily accessible populations (such as schoolchildren) will need to be weighed against all the harms, including nonphysical risks to individuals and society.

The alternative to a community-based program would be physician-based screening. If both prenatal and carrier tests were available, obstetricians could provide screening. All pregnant women could be offered the heterozygote test, partners of carriers could be screened, and "carrier couples" could be offered prenatal diagnosis. One drawback of this approach is that some couples or individuals, particularly those who would not want prenatal diagnosis, may wish to know whether they are carriers before marrying or conceiving a child. An obstetrics-based screening program would be inadequate in these cases. Screening offered as part of more generalized medical care (internists, gynecologists, and family practitioners) might be more responsive to

this demand, but would still exclude a large number of potential screenees who do not receive regular medical care. Physician-based screening would require improved understanding of genetic diseases among physicians who are not specialists in genetics.

If retrospective instead of prospective screening were used (for example, if a prenatal test were developed before a cost-effective means of carrier screening), the physician-based rather than the community-based approach would have to be employed. In terms of reducing the incidence of CF, the impact of retrospective screening would be much less than large-scale prospective screening.

> Under a scheme of prospective diagnosis the case reduction is 100% (i.e. no cases with the disease are born), as opposed to the less effective reduction which can be achieved with retrospective diagnosis (i.e. following birth of an affected child). Considering only the economic aspects, the saving to society by not having to bear the high costs of supporting patients with cystic fibrosis for the relatively large number of years which they can now survive will probably be substantially greater than the continuing costs of the programs for premarital screening, for intrauterine diagnosis and for selective abortion once the use of automated devices is introduced.[3]

As the Commission has noted throughout this Report, however, the fundamental value of genetic screening and counseling lies in its potential for providing individuals with information they consider beneficial for autonomous decision-making. Therefore, although societal impact and cost-effectiveness are relevant considerations, the benefits and harms that could accrue to individual screenees deserve special consideration if retrospective CF screening is being contemplated.

Distributing Benefits

The potential demand for CF screening is so large that even if a rather sizable portion of it does not materialize an enormous demand for genetic counselors and other health care personnel and services could still be engendered. Since CF tests should not be offered unless support services are adequate, program objectives must either provide for the expansion of needed resources, especially trained personnel, or limit screening initially in a manner that would distribute it equitably.

An important objective, therefore, for those with responsibility for genetic screening programs will be to guarantee that needed resources, or the means of generating them in an orderly fashion, are available as screening is offered....

A rough approximation of the number of tests an obstetrics-based system would involve can be calculated as follows: screening 3.3 million pregnant women (the approximate number of live births each year) would yield about 165,000 carriers (assuming a carrier frequency of 5 percent); if the partner of each carrier is then screened, about 8250 couples who are carriers would be identified. Theoretically, therefore, the capability to perform more than 3.4 million carrier tests and 8250 prenatal tests annually would be needed even under the narrowest form of prospective screening (that it, obstetrics-based). Of course, not all women obtain medical care early enough in pregnancy for prenatal diagnosis, and some pregnant women or their partners may choose not to undergo the carrier or prenatal test, so that demand will not be fully realized. Still, trying to meet even part of that demand would put a considerable strain on the health care system.

Alternatively, a mass screening program to detect carriers that was targeted, for example, at Caucasians of reproductive age could create a demand for many millions of tests in a short period of time. Large numbers of trained counselors and other public health personnel would be required, in addition to widespread public education and community involvement.

Involving and Educating the Public

The generalized nature of the population at risk for cystic fibrosis in the United States has implications for the types of public education programs and local involvement in screening that will be suitable for this disease. A mass screening program will not be able to rely on any preexisting subgroups in the population affected who have special interest in the tests, as has been done with other genetic diseases. Planners would need to turn to a larger and more diverse range of organizations and individuals, both locally and nationally, to achieve public participation. They will have to be very resourceful in identifying how members of the public can become informed about the availability and objectives of the screening and participate in planning local programs....

PLANNING A NEWBORN SCREENING PROGRAM

Assessing Benefits and Harms

The value of the most widely used neonatal genetic test—for PKU—is that early diagnosis and treatment averts serious disease complications. For cystic fibrosis, however, it is not clear that a diagnosis in the neonatal period would usually affect outcome or even alter therapy. CF is not always recognized at the first sign of symptoms but some delay in arriving at a correct diagnosis has not been thought to affect the outcome of treatment adversely.

Families with a child who has CF should already be aware of the possibility of a subsequent CF birth, and therefore newborn screening would primarily benefit those who are not aware they are carriers. The possible benefits of mass newborn CF screening (if an effective method is developed) are that it could eliminate some of the costs, frustration, parental anxiety, and harm of incorrect diagnoses and therapies. Physicians are now studying the possibility that the prognosis for CF patients improves if treatment is begun before the onset of clinical signs. In addition, prospective newborn screening would provide the parents of a CF child with an earlier warning that they are CF carriers and, therefore, that any other children they conceive have a 25 percent chance of having cystic fibrosis. On the other hand, presymptomatic identification of CF may generate needless psychosocial problems within families since infants who would otherwise still be regarded as "normal" would instead be seen as sick and at risk for developing CF symptoms at any moment....

NOTES

1 One reason for the greater acceptance of Tay-Sachs screening is the seriousness of the disorder itself; after a few months of normal development, affected infants begin to undergo a tragic degeneration, followed by death at a very young age. In contrast, the clinical effects of sickle-cell anemia vary considerably; patients can reach adulthood with symptoms ranging from quite mild to very severe.

2 This strict policy in the early Tay-Sachs programs has been relaxed in light of demands for the test

from unmarried individuals, particularly those with a Tay-Sachs victim in the family.

3 Arno G. Motulsky, George R. Fraser, and Joseph Felsenstein, "Public Health and Long-Term Genetic

Implications of Intrauterine Diagnosis and Selective Abortion," 7 *Birth Defects: Original Article Series* (No. 5, 1971) at 24.

Surrogate Motherhood

Surrogate Mothers: Not So Novel After All

John A. Robertson

A biographical sketch of John A. Robertson is found on page 440.

Robertson focuses attention on the most typical kind of surrogate mother arrangement, whereby a woman (the surrogate) contracts with a married couple to be artificially inseminated with the husband's sperm, in order to bear a child for the couple. He analyzes the potential benefits and harms of surrogate motherhood and maintains that the practice is ethically acceptable. Because surrogate motherhood deliberately separates *biological* from *social* parentage, Robertson recognizes the risk of psychosocial harm to the offspring as a serious concern. But problems on this score, he contends, are no more serious than those associated with well-established practices such as ordinary adoption and AID. Against the view that it is wrong for a surrogate to use the reproductive process for selfish ends, Robertson contends that "the mere presence of selfish motives does not render reproduction immoral, as long as it is carried out in a way that respects the child's interests." With regard to public policy, he argues that the state may justifiably regulate but not block surrogate motherhood arrangements.

All reproduction is collaborative, for no man or woman reproduces alone. Yet the provision of sperm, egg, or uterus through artificial insemination, embryo transfer, and surrogate mothering makes reproduction collaborative in another way. A third person provides a genetic or gestational factor not present in ordinary paired reproduction. As these practices grow, we must confront the ethical issues raised and their implications for public policy.

Collaborative reproduction allows some persons who otherwise might remain childless to produce healthy children. However, its deliberate separation of genetic, gestational, and social parentage is troublesome. The offspring and participants may be harmed, and there is a risk of confusing family lineage and personal identity.

In addition, the techniques intentionally manipulate a natural process that many persons want free of technical intervention. Yet many well-accepted practices, including adoption, artificial insemination by donor (AID), and blended families (families where children of different marriages are raised together) intentionally separate biologic and social parenting, and have become an accepted thread in the social fabric. Should all collaborative techniques be similarly treated? When, if ever, are they ethical? Should the law prohibit, encourage, or regulate them, or should the practice be left to private actors? Surrogate motherhood—the controversial practice by which a woman agrees to bear a child conceived by artificial insemination and to relinquish it at birth to others for rearing—illustrates the

Reprinted with permission of the author and the publisher from *Hastings Center Report*, vol. 13 (October 1983), pp. 28–34.

legal and ethical issues arising in collaborative reproduction generally.

HOW SURROGATE MOTHERING WORKS

For a fee of $5,000–10,000 a broker (usually a lawyer) will put an infertile couple (or less often, a single man) in contact with women whom he has recruited and screened who are willing to serve as surrogates. If the parties strike a deal, they will sign a contract in which the surrogate agrees to be artificially inseminated (usually by a physician) with the husband's sperm, to bear the child, and then at or soon after birth to relinquish all parental rights and transfer physical custody of the child to the couple for adoption by the wife. Typically the contract has provisions dealing with prenatal screening, abortion, and other aspects of the surrogate's conduct during pregnancy, as well as her consent to relinquish the child at birth. The husband and wife agree to pay medical expenses related to the pregnancy, to take custody of the child, and to place approximately $10,000 in escrow to be paid to the surrogate when the child is transferred. The lawyer will also prepare papers establishing the husband's paternity, terminating the surrogate's rights, and legalizing the adoption.

AN ALTERNATIVE TO AGENCY ADOPTIONS

Infertile couples who are seeking surrogates hire attorneys and sign contracts with women recruited through newspaper ads. The practice at present probably involves at most a few hundred persons. But repeated attention on *Sixty Minutes* and the *Phil Donahue Show* and in the popular press is likely to engender more demand, for thousands of infertile couples might find surrogate mothers the answer to their reproductive needs. What began as an enterprise involving a few lawyers and doctors in Michigan, Kentucky, and California is now a national phenomenon. There are surrogate mother centers in Maryland, Arizona, and several other states, and even a surrogate mother newsletter.

Surrogate mother arrangements occur within a tradition of family law that gives the gestational mother (and her spouse, if any) rearing rights and obligations. (However, the presumption that the husband is the father can be challenged, and a husband's obligations to his wife's child by AID will usually require his consent.)[1] Although no state has legislation directly on the subject of surrogate motherhood, independently arranged adoptions are lawful in most states. It is no crime to agree to bear a child for another, and then relinquish it for adoption. However, paying the mother a fee for adoption beyond medical expenses is a crime in some states, and in others will prevent the adoption from being approved.[2] Whether termination and transfer of parenting rights will be legally recognized depends on the state. Some states, like Hawaii and Florida, ask few questions and approve independent adoptions very quickly. Others, like Michigan and Kentucky, won't allow surrogate mothers to terminate and assign rearing rights to another if a fee has been paid, or even allow a paternity determination in favor of the sperm donor. The enforceability of surrogate contracts has also not been tested, and it is safe to assume that some jurisdictions will not enforce them. Legislation clarifying many of these questions has been proposed in several states, but has not yet been enacted.

Even this brief discussion highlights an important fact about surrogate motherhood and other collaborative reproductive techniques. They operate as an alternative to the nonmarket, agency system of allocating children for adoption, which has contributed to long queues for distributing healthy white babies. This form of independent adoption is controlled by the parties, planned before conception, involves a genetic link with one parent, and enables both the father and mother of the adopted child to be selected in advance.

Understood in these terms, the term "surrogate mother," which means substitute mother, is a misnomer. The natural mother, who contributes egg and uterus, is not so much a substitute mother as a substitute spouse who carries a child for a man whose wife is infertile. Indeed, it is the adoptive mother who is the surrogate mother for the child, since she parents a child borne by another. What, if anything, is wrong with this arrangement? Let us look more closely at its benefits and harms before discussing public policy.

ALL THE PARTIES CAN BENEFIT

Reproduction through surrogate mothering is a deviation from our cultural norms of reproduction, and to many persons it seems immoral or wrong. But surrogate mothering may be a good for the parties involved.

Surrogate contracts meet the desire of a husband and wife to rear a healthy child, and more particularly, a child with one partner's genes. The need could arise because the wife has an autosomal dominant or sex-linked genetic disorder, such as hemophilia. More likely, she is infertile and the couple feels a strong need to have children. For many infertile couples the inability to conceive is a major personal problem causing marital conflict and filling both partners with anguish and self-doubt. It may also involve multiple medical work-ups and possibly even surgery. If the husband and wife have sought to adopt a child, they may have been told either that they do not qualify or to join the queue of couples waiting several years for agency adoptions (the wait has grown longer due to birth control, abortion, and the greater willingness of unwed mothers to keep their children[3]). For couples exhausted and frustrated by these efforts, the surrogate arrangement seems a godsend. While the intense desire to have a child often appears selfish, we must not lose sight of the deep-seated psychosocial and biological roots of the desire to generate children.[4]

The arrangement may also benefit the surrogate. Usually women undergo pregnancy and childbirth because they want to rear children. But some women want to have the experience of bearing and birthing a child without the obligation to rear. Philip Parker, a Michigan psychiatrist who has interviewed over 275 surrogate applicants, finds that the decision to be a surrogate springs from several motives.[5] Most women willing to be surrogates have already had children, and many are married. They choose the surrogate role primarily because the fee provides a better economic opportunity than alternative occupations, but also because they enjoy being pregnant and the respect and attention that it draws. The surrogate experience may also be a way to master, through reliving, guilt they feel from past pregnancies that ended in abortion or adoption. Some surrogates may also feel pleased, as organ donors do, that they have given the "gift of life" to another couple.[6]

The child born of a surrogate arrangement also benefits. Indeed, but for the surrogate contract, this child would not have been born at all. Unlike the ordinary agency or independent adoption, where a child is already conceived or brought to term, the conception of this child occurs solely as a result of the surrogate agreement. Thus even if the child does suffer identity problems, as adopted children often do because they are not able to know their mothers, this child has benefited, or at least has not been wronged, for without the surrogate arrangement, she would not have been born at all.[7]

BUT PROBLEMS EXIST TOO

Surrogate mothering is also troublesome. Many people think that it is wrong for a woman to conceive and bear a child that she does not intend to raise, particularly if she receives a fee for her services. There are potential costs to the surrogate and her family, the adoptive couple, the child, and even society at large from satisfying the generative needs of infertile couples in this way.

The couple must be willing to spend about $20,000–25,000, depending on lawyers' fees and the supply of and demand for surrogate mothers. (While this price tag makes the surrogate contract a consumption item for the middle classes, it is not unjust to poor couples, for it does not leave them worse off than they were.) The couple must also be prepared to experience, along with the adjustment and demands of becoming parents, the stress and anxiety of participating in a novel social relationship that many still consider immoral or deviant. What do they tell their friends or family? What do they tell the child? Will the child have contact with the mother? What is the couple's relationship with the surrogate and her family during the pregnancy and after? Without established patterns for handling these questions, the parties may experience confusion, frustration, and embarrassment.

A major source of uncertainty and stress is likely to be the surrogate herself. In most cases she will be a stranger, and may never even meet the couple. The lack of a preexisting relation between the couple and surrogate and the possibility that they live far apart enhance the possibility of mistrust. Is the surrogate taking care of herself? Is she having sex with others during her fertile period? Will she contact the child afterwards? What if she demands more money to relinquish the child? To allay these anxieties, the couple could try to establish a relationship of trust with the surrogate, yet such a relationship creates reciprocal rights and duties and might create demands for an undesired relationship after the birth. Even good lawyering that specifies every contingency in the contract is unlikely to allay uncertainty and anxiety about the surrogate's trustworthiness.

The surrogate may also find the experience less satisfying than she envisioned. Conceiving the child may require insemination efforts over several months at inconvenient locations. The pregnancy and birth may entail more pain, unpleasant side effects, and disruption than she expected. The couple may be more intrusive or more aloof than she wishes. As the pregnancy advances and the birth nears, the surrogate may find it increasingly difficult to remain detached by thinking of the child as "theirs" rather than "hers." Relinquishing the baby after birth may be considerably more disheartening and disappointing than she anticipated. Even if informed of this possibility in advance, she may be distressed for several weeks with feelings of loss, depression, and sleep disturbance.[8] She may feel angry at the couple for cutting off all contact with her once the baby is delivered, and guilty at giving up her child. Finally, she will have to face the loss of all contact with "her" child. As the reality of her situation dawns, she may regret not having bargained harder for access to "her baby."

As with the couple, the surrogate's experience will vary with the expectations, needs, and personalities of the parties, the course of the pregnancy, and an advance understanding of the problems that can arise. The surrogate should have a lawyer to protect her interests. Often, however, the couple's lawyer will end up advising the surrogate. Although he has recruited the surrogate, he is paid by and represents the couple. By disclosing his conflicting interest, he satisfies legal ethics, but he may not serve the interests of the surrogate as well as independent counsel.

HARMS TO THE CHILD

Unlike embryo transfer, gene therapy, and other manipulative techniques (some of which are collaborative), surrogate arrangements do not pose the risk of physical harm to the offspring. But there is the risk of psychosocial harm. Surrogate mothering, like adoption and artificial insemination by donor (AID), deliberately separates genetic and gestational from social parentage. The mother who begets, bears, and births does not parent. This separation can pose a problem for the child who discovers it. Like adopted and AID children, the child may be strongly motivated to learn the absent parent's identity and to establish a relationship, in this case with the mother and her family. Inability to make that connection, especially inability to learn who the mother is, may affect the child's self-esteem, create feelings of rootlessness, and

leave the child thinking that he had been rejected due to some personal fault.[9] While this is a serious concern, the situation is tolerated when it arises with AID and adoptive children. Intentional conception for adoption—the essence of surrogate mothering—poses no different issue.

The child can also be harmed if the adoptive husband and wife are not fit parents. After all, a willingness to spend substantial money to fulfill a desire to rear children is no guarantee of good parenting. But then neither is reproduction by paired mates who wish intensely to have a child. The nonbiologic parent may resent or reject the child, but the same possibility exists with adoption, AID, or ordinary reproduction.

There is also the fear, articulated by such commentators as Leon Kass and Paul Ramsey,[10] that collaborative reproduction confuses the lineage of children and destroys the meaning of family as we know it. In surrogate mothering, as with ovum or womb donors, the genetic and gestational mother does not rear the child, though the biologic father does. What implications does this hold for the family and the child's lineage?

The separation of the child from the genetic or biologic parent in surrogate mothering is hardly unique. It arises with adoption, but surrogate arrangements are more closely akin to AID or blended families, where at least one parent has a blood-tie to the child and the child will know at least one genetic parent. He may, as adopted children often do, have intense desires to learn his biologic mother's identity and seek contact with her and her family. Failure to connect with biologic roots may cause suffering. But the fact that adoption through surrogate mother contracts is planned before conception does not increase the chance of identity confusion, lowered self-esteem, or the blurring of lineage that occurs with adoption or AID.

The greatest chance of confusing family lines arises if the child and couple establish relations with the surrogate and the surrogate's family. If that unlikely event occurs, questions about the child's relations with the surrogate's spouse, parents, and other children can arise. But these issues are not unique. Indeed, they are increasingly common with the growth of blended families. Surrogate mothering in a few instances may lead to a new variation on blended families, but its threat to the family is trivial compared to the rapid changes in family structure now occurring for social, economic, and demographic reasons.

In many cases surrogate motherhood and other forms of collaborative reproduction may shore up, rather than undermine, the traditional family by enabling couples who would otherwise be childless to have children. The practice of employing others to assist in child rearing—including wet-nurses, neonatal ICU nurses, day-care workers, and babysitters—is widely accepted. We also tolerate assistance in the form of sperm sales and donation of egg and gestation (adoption). Surrogate mothering is another method of assisting people to undertake child rearing, and thus serves the purposes of the marital union. It is hard to see how its planned nature obstructs that contribution.

USING BIRTH FOR SELFISH ENDS

A basic fear about the new reproductive technologies is that they manipulate a natural physiologic process involved in the creation of human life. When one considers the potential power that resides in our ability to manipulate the genes of embryos, the charges of playing God or arrogantly tampering with nature and the resulting dark Huxleyian vision of genetically engineered babies decanted from bottles are not surprising. While *Brave New World* is the standard text for this fear, the 1982 film *Bladerunner* also evokes it. Trycorp., a genetic engineering corporation, manufactures "replicants," who resemble human beings in most respects, including their ability to remember their childhoods, but who are programmed to die in four years. In portraying the replicants' struggle for long life and full human status, the film raises a host of ethical issues relevant to gene manipulation, from the meaning of personhood to the duties we have in "fabricating" people to make them as whole and healthy as possible.

Such fears, however, are not a sufficient reason to stop splicing genes or relieving infertility through external fertilization.[11] In any event they have no application to surrogate mothering, which does not alter genes or even manipulate the embryo. The only technological aid is a syringe to inseminate and a thermometer to determine when ovulation occurs. Although embryo manipulation would occur if the surrogate received the fertilized egg of another woman, the qualms about surrogate mothering stem less from its potential for technical manipulation, and more from its attitude toward the body and mother-child relations. Mothers bear and give up children for adoption rather frequently when the conception is unplanned. But here

the mother conceives the child for that purpose, deliberately using her body for a fee to serve the needs of others. It is the cold willingness to use her body as a baby-making machine and deny the mother-child gestational bond that bothers. (Ironically, the natural bond may turn out to be deeper and stronger than the surrogate imagined.)

Since the transfer of rearing duties from the natural gestational mother to others is widely accepted, the unwillingness of the surrogate mother to rear her child cannot in itself be wrong. As long as she transfers rearing responsibility to capable parents, she is not acting irresponsibly. Still, some persons assert that it is wrong to use the reproductive process for ends other than the good of the child.[12] But the mere presence of selfish motives does not render reproduction immoral, as long as it is carried out in a way that respects the child's interests. Otherwise most pregnancies and births would be immoral, for people have children to serve individual ends as well as the good of the child. In terms of instrumentalism, surrogate mothering cannot be distinguished from most other reproductive situations, whether AID, adoption, or simply planning a child to experience the pleasures of parenthood.

In this vein the problems that can arise when a defective child is born are cited as proof of the immorality of surrogate mothering. The fear is that neither the contracting couple nor the surrogate will want the defective child. In one recent case (*New York Times*, January 28, 1983, p. 18) a dispute arose when none of the parties wanted to take a child born with microcephaly, a condition related to mental retardation. The contracting man claimed on the basis of blood typing that the baby was not his, and thus he was not obligated under the contract to take it, or to pay the surrogate's fee. It turned out that [the] surrogate had borne her husband's child, for she had unwittingly become pregnant by him before being artificially inseminated by the contracting man. The surrogate and her husband eventually assumed responsibility for the child.

An excessively instrumental and callous approach to reproduction when a less than perfect baby is born is not unique to surrogate mothering. Similar reactions can occur whenever married couples have a defective child, as the Baby Doe controversy, which involved the passive euthanasia of a child with Down syndrome, indicates. All surrogate mothering is not wrong because in some instances a handicapped child will be rejected. Nor is it clear that this reaction is more likely in surrogate mothering than in conventional births for it reflects common attitudes toward handicapped newborns as much as alienation in the surrogate arrangement.

As with most situations, "how" something is done is more important than the mere fact of doing it. The morality of surrogate mothering thus depends on how the duties and responsibilities of the role are carried out, rather than on the mere fact that a couple produces a child with the aid of a collaborator. Depending on the circumstances, a surrogate mother can be praised as a benefactor to a suffering couple (the money is hardly adequate compensation) or condemned as a callous user of offspring to further her selfish ends. The view that one takes of her actions will also influence the role one wants the law to play.

WHAT SHOULD THE STATE'S ROLE BE?

What stance should public policy and the law take toward surrogate mothering? As with all collaborative reproduction, a range of choices exists, from prohibition and regulation to active encouragement.

However, there may be constitutional limits to the state's power to restrict collaborative reproduction. The right not to procreate, through contraception and abortion, is now firmly established.[13] A likely implication of these cases, supported by rulings in other cases, is that married persons (and possibly single persons) have a right to bear, beget, birth, and parent children by natural coital means using such technological aids (microsurgery and in vitro fertilization, for example) as are medically available. It should follow that married persons also have a right to engage in noncoital, collaborative reproduction, at least where natural reproduction is not possible. The right of a couple to raise a child should not depend on their luck in the natural lottery, if they can obtain the missing factor of reproduction from others.[14]

If a married couple's right to procreative autonomy includes the right to contract with consenting collaborators, then the state will have a heavy burden of justification for infringing that right. The risks to surrogate, couple, and child do not seem sufficiently compelling to meet this burden, for they are no different from the harms of adoption and AID. Nor will it suffice to point to a communal feeling that such uses of the body are—aside from the consequences—immoral. Moral distaste alone does not justify interference with a fundamental right.

Although surrogate mothering is not now criminal, this discussion is not purely hypothetical. The ban in Michigan and several other states on paying fees for adoption beyond medical expenses has the same effect as an outright prohibition, for few surrogates will volunteer for altruistic reasons alone. A ban on fees is not necessary to protect the surrogate mother from coercion or exploitation, or to protect the child from abuse, the two objectives behind passage of those laws. Unlike the pregnant unmarried woman who "sells" her child, the surrogate has made a considered, knowing choice, often with the assistance of counsel, before becoming pregnant. She may of course choose to be a surrogate for financial reasons, but offering money to do unpleasant tasks is not in itself coercive.

Nor does the child's welfare support a ban on fees, for the risk is no greater than in natural paired reproduction that the parents will be unfit or abuse the child. The specter of slavery, which some opposed to surrogate mothering have raised, is unwarranted. It is quibbling to question whether the couple is "buying" a child or the mother's personal services. Quite clearly, the couple is buying the right to rear a child by paying the mother to beget and bear one for that very purpose. But the purchasers do not buy the right to treat the child or surrogate as a commodity or property. Child abuse and neglect laws still apply, with criminal and civil sanctions available for mistreatment.

The main concern with fees rests on moral and aesthetic grounds. An affront to moral sensibility arises over paying money for a traditionally noncommercial, intimate function. Even though blood and sperm are sold, and miners, professional athletes, and petrochemical workers sell some of their health and vitality, some persons think it wrong for women to bear children for money, in much the same way that paying money for sex or body organs is considered wrong. Every society excludes some exchanges from the marketplace on moral grounds. But the state's power to block exchanges that interfere with the exercise of a fundamental right is limited. Since blocking this exchange stops infertile couples from reproducing and rearing the husband's child, a harm greater than moral distaste is necessary to justify it.

Although the state cannot block collaborative reproductive exchanges on moral grounds, it need not subsidize or encourage surrogate contracts. One could argue that allowing the parties to a surrogate contract to use the courts to terminate parental rights, certify paternity, and legalize adoption is a subsidy and therefore not required of the state. Similarly, a state's refusal to enforce surrogate contracts as a matter of public policy could be taken as a refusal to subsidize rather than as interference with the right to reproduce. But given the state's monopoly of those functions and the impact its denial will have on the ability of infertile couples to find reproductive collaborators, it is more plausible to view the refusal to certify and effectuate surrogate contracts as an infringement of the right to procreate. Denying an adoption because it was agreed upon in advance for a fee interferes with the couple's procreative autonomy as much as any criminal penalty for paying a fee to or contracting with a collaborator. (The crucial distinction between interfering with and not encouraging the exercise of a right has been overlooked by the Michigan and Kentucky courts that have held constitutional the refusal to allow adoptions or paternity determinations where a fee has been paid to the surrogate mother. This error makes these cases highly questionable precedents.[15])

A conclusion that surrogate contracts must be *enforced*, however, does not require that they be specifically carried out in all instances. As long as damage remedies remain, there is no constitutional right to specific performance. For example, a court need not enjoin the surrogate who changes her mind about abortion or relinquishing the child once it is born. A surrogate who wants to breach the contract by abortion should pay damages, but not be ordered to continue the pregnancy, because of the difficulty in enforcing or monitoring the order. (Whether damages are a practical alternative in such cases will depend on the surrogate's economic situation, or whether bonding or insurance to assure her contractual obligation is possible.) On the other hand, a court could reasonably order the surrogate after birth to relinquish the child. Whether such an order should issue will depend on whether the surrogate's interest in keeping the child is deemed greater than the couple's interest in rearing (assuming that both are fit parents). A commitment to freedom of contract and the rights of parties to arrange collaborative reproduction would favor the adoptive couple, while sympathy for the gestational bond between mother and child would favor the mother. If the mother prevailed, the couple should still have other remedies, including visitation rights for the father, restitution of the surrogate's fee and other expenses, and perhaps money damages as well.

The constitutional status of a married couple's procreative choice shields collaborative arrangements from interference on moral grounds alone, but not from all regulation. While the parties may assign the rearing rights according to contract, the state need not leave the entire transaction to the vagaries of the private sector. Regulation to minimize harm and assure knowing choices would be permissible, as long as the regulation is reasonably related to promoting these goals.

For example, the state could set minimum standards for surrogate brokers, set age and health qualifications for surrogates, and structure the transaction to assure voluntary, knowing choices. The state could also define and allocate responsibilities among the parties to protect the best interests of the offspring—for example, refusing to protect the surrogate's anonymity, requiring that the contracting couple assume responsibility for a defective child, or even transferring custody to another if threats to the child's welfare justify such a move....

ACKNOWLEDGMENTS

The author gratefully acknowledges the comments of Rebecca Dresser, Mark Frankel, Inga Markovits, Phillip Parker, Bruce Russel, John Sampson, and Ted Schneyer on earlier drafts.

REFERENCES

1 People v. Sorenson, 68 Cal. 2d 280, 437 P.2d 495; Walter Wadlington, "Artificial Insemination: The Dangers of a Poorly Kept Secret, *Northwestern Law Review* 64 (1970), 777.

2 See, for example, Michigan Statutes Annotated, 27.3178 (555.54)(555.69) (1980).

3 William Landes and Eleanor Posner, "The Economics of the Baby Shortage," *Journal of Legal Studies* 7 (1978), 323.

4 See Erik Erikson, *The Life Cycle Completed* (New York: Norton, 1980), pp. 122–124.

5 Phillip Parker, "Surrogate Mother's Motivations: Initial Findings," *American Journal of Psychiatry* 140:1 (January 1983), 117–118; Phillip Parker, "The Psychology of Surrogate Motherhood: A Preliminary Report of a Longitudinal Pilot Study" (unpublished). See also Dava Sobel, "Surrogate Mothers: Why Women Volunteer," *New York Times*, June 25, 1981, p. 18.

6 Mark Frankel, "Surrogate Motherhood: An Ethical Perspective," pp. 1–2. (Paper presented at Wayne

State Symposium on Surrogate Motherhood, Nov. 20, 1982.)

7 See John Robertson, "In Vitro Conception and Harm to the Unborn," *Hastings Center Report* 8 (October 1978), 13–14; Michael Bayles, "Harm to the Unconceived," *Philosophy and Public Affairs* 5 (1976), 295.

8 A small, uncontrolled study found these effects to last some four to six weeks. Statement of Nancy Reame, R. N. at Wayne State University, Symposium on Surrogate Motherhood, Nov. 20, 1982.

9 Betty Jane Lifton, *Twice Born: Memoirs of an Adopted Daughter* (New York: Penguin, 1977); L. Dusky, "Brave New Babies," *Newsweek,* Dec. 6, 1982, p. 30.

10 Leon Kass, "Making Babies—the New Biology and the Old Morality," *The Public Interest* 26 (1972), 18; "Making Babies Revisited," *The Public Interest* 54 (1979), 32; Paul Ramsey, *Fabricated Man: The Ethics of Genetic Control* (New Haven: Yale University Press, 1970).

11 The President's Commission for the Study of Ethical Problems in Medicine and Biomedical and Behavioral Research, *Splicing Life: The Social and Ethical Issues of Genetic Engineering with Human Beings* (Washington, D.C., 1982), pp. 53–60.

12 Herbert Krimmel, Testimony before California Assembly Committee on Judiciary, Surrogate Parenting Contracts (November 14, 1982), pp. 89–96.

13 Griswold v. Connecticut, 381 U.S. 479 (1964); Eisenstadt v. Baird, 405 U.S. 438 (1972); Roe v. Wade, 410 U.S. 113 (1973); Planned Parenthood v. Danforth, 428 U.S. 52 (1976); Bellotti v. Baird, 443 U.S. 622 (1979); Carey v. Population Services International, 431 U.S. 678 (1977).

14 Although this article does not address the right of single persons to contract with others for reproductive purposes, it should be noted that the right of married persons to engage in collaborative reproduction does not entail a similar right for unmarried persons. For a more detailed exposition of the arguments for the reproductive rights of married and single persons, see John Robertson, "Procreative Liberty and the Control of Conception, Pregnancy and Childbirth," *Virginia Law Review* 69 (April 1983), 405, 418–420.

15 See Doe v. Kelley, 106 Mich. App. 164, 307 N.W. 2d 438 (1981). Syrkowski v. Appleyard, 9 Family Law Rptr. 2348 (April 5, 1983); In re Baby Girl, 9 Family Law Rptr. 2348 (March 8, 1983).

The Case Against Surrogate Parenting

Herbert T. Krimmel

Herbert T. Krimmel is professor of law at Southwestern University School of Law, Los Angeles. His areas of specialization include jurisprudence and bioethics, and he is the coauthor of "Abortion: an Inspection into the Nature of Human Life and Potential Consequences of Legalizing its Destruction."

In Krimmel's view, it is fundamentally wrong to separate the decision to create a child from the decision to parent it. He does not object to the surrogate mother's role as host for a developing child, but he maintains that it is unethical for her to create a child (via the provision of an ovum) with the intention of abdicating all parental responsibilities. (For analogous reasons, he considers the donation of sperm in AID to be unethical.) "The procreator should desire the child for its own sake, and not as a means to attaining some other end." If surrogate motherhood arrangements are accepted by society, he maintains, there is a great danger that we will come to view children as commodities. He also argues that acceptance of

Reprinted with permission of the author and the publisher from *Hastings Center Report*, vol. 13 (October 1983), pp. 35–39.

surrogate motherhood arrangements would have other negative social consequences, most notably an increased stress upon the family structure. But his
opposition to the legalization of surrogate motherhood arrangements is based
first and foremost on his conviction that it is morally wrong for a person "to create
a child, not because she desired it, but because it could be useful to her."

Is it ethical for someone to create a human life with the intention of giving it up? This seems to be the primary question for both surrogate mother arrangements and artificial insemination by donor (AID), since in both situations a person who is providing germinal material does so only upon the assurance that someone else will assume full responsibility for the child he or she helps to create.

THE ETHICAL ISSUE

In analyzing the ethics of surrogate mother arrangements, it is helpful to begin by examining the roles the surrogate mother performs. First, she acts as a procreator in providing an ovum to be fertilized. Second, after her ovum has been fertilized by the sperm of the man who wishes to parent the child, she acts as host to the fetus, providing nurture and protection while the newly conceived individual develops.

I see no insurmountable moral objections to the functions the mother performs in this second role as host. Her actions are analogous to those of a foster mother or of a wet-nurse who cares for a child when the natural mother cannot or does not do so. Using a surrogate mother as a host for the fetus when the biological mother cannot bear the child is no more morally objectionable than employing others to help educate, train, or otherwise care for a child. Except in extremes, where the parent relinquishes or delegates responsibilities for a child for trivial reasons, the practice would not seem to raise a serious moral issue.

I would argue, however, that the first role that the surrogate mother performs—providing germinal material to be fertilized—does pose a major ethical problem. The surrogate mother provides her ovum, and enters into a surrogate mother arrangement, with the clear understanding that she is to avoid responsibility for the life she creates. Surrogate mother arrangements are designed to separate in the mind of the surrogate mother the decision to create a child from the decision to have and raise that child. The cause of this dissocia-

tion is some other benefit she will receive, most often money.[1] In other words, her desire to create a child is born of some motive other than the desire to be a parent. This separation of the decision to create a child from the decision to parent it is ethically suspect. The child is conceived not because he is wanted by his biological mother, but because he can be useful to someone else. He is conceived in order to be given away.

At their deepest level, surrogate mother arrangements involve a change in motive for creating children: from a desire to have them for their own sake, to a desire to have them because they can provide some other benefit. The surrogate mother creates a child with the intention to abdicate parental responsibilities. Can we view this as ethical? My answer is no. I will explain why by analyzing various situations in which surrogate mother arrangements might be used.

WHY MOTIVE MATTERS

Let's begin with the single parent. A single woman might use AID, or a single man might use a surrogate mother arrangement, if she or he wanted a child but did not want to be burdened with a spouse.[2] Either practice would intentionally deprive the child of a mother or a father. This, I assert, is fundamentally unfair to the child.

Those who disagree might point to divorce or to the death of a parent as situations in which a child is deprived of one parent and must rely solely or primarily upon the other. The comparison, however, is inapt. After divorce or the death of a parent, a child may find herself with a single parent due to circumstances that were unfortunate, unintended, and undesired. But when surrogate mother arrangements are used by a single parent, depriving the child of a second parent is one of the intended and desired effects. It is one thing to ask how to make the best of a bad situation when it is thrust upon a person. It is different altogether to ask whether one may intentionally set out to achieve the same result. The morality of identical results (for example, killings) will oftentimes differ depending upon whether the situation is invited by, or involuntarily thrust upon, the actor. Legal distinctions following and based upon this ethical distinction are abundant. The law of self-defense provides a notable example.[3]

Since a woman can get pregnant if she wishes whether or not she is married, and since there is little that society can do to prevent women from creating children even if their intention is to deprive the children of a father, why should we be so concerned about single men using surrogate mother arrangements if they too want a child but not a spouse? To say that women can intentionally plan to be unwed mothers is not to condone the practice. Besides, society will hold the father liable in a paternity action if he can be found and identified, which indicates some social concern that people should not be able to abdicate the responsibilities that they incur in generating children. Otherwise, why do we condemn the proverbial sailor with a pregnant girlfriend in every port?

In many surrogate mother arrangements, of course, the surrogate mother will not be transferring custody of the child to a single man, but to a couple: the child's biological father and a stepmother, his wife. What are the ethics of surrogate mother arrangements when the child is taken into a two-parent family? Again, surrogate mother arrangements and AID pose similar ethical questions: The surrogate mother transfers her parental responsibilities to the wife of the biological father, while with AID the sperm donor relinquishes his interest in the child to the husband of the biological mother. In both cases the child is created with the intention of transferring the responsibility for its care to a new set of parents. The surrogate mother situation is more dramatic than AID since the transfer occurs after the child is born, while in the case of AID the transfer takes place at the time of the insemination. Nevertheless, the ethical point is the same: creating children for the purpose of transferring them. For a surrogate mother the question remains: Is it ethical to create a child for the purpose of transferring it to the wife of the biological father?

At first blush this looks to be little different from the typical adoption, for what is an adoption other than a transfer of responsibility from one set of parents to another? The analogy is misleading, however, for two reasons. First, it is difficult to imagine anyone conceiving children for the purpose of putting them up for adoption. And, if such a bizarre event were to occur, I doubt that we would look upon it with moral approval. Most adoptions arise either because an undesired conception is brought to term, or because the parents wanted to have the child, but find that they are unable to provide for it because of some unfortunate circumstances that develop after conception.

Second, even if surrogate mother arrangements were to be classified as a type of adoption, not all offerings of children for adoption are necessarily moral. For example, would it be moral for parents to offer their three-year-old for adoption because they are bored with the child? Would it be moral for a couple to offer for adoption their newborn female baby because they wanted a boy?

Therefore, even though surrogate mother arrangements may in some superficial ways be likened to adoption, one must still ask whether it is ethical to separate the decision to create children from the desire to have them. I would answer no. The procreator should desire the child for its own sake, and not as a means to attaining some other end. Even though one of the ends may be stated altruistically as an attempt to bring happiness to an infertile couple, the child is still being used by the surrogate. She creates it not because she desires it, but because she desires something from it.

To sanction the use and treatment of human beings as means to the achievement of other goals instead of as ends in themselves is to accept an ethic with a tragic past, and to establish a precedent with a dangerous future. Already the press has reported the decision of one couple to conceive a child for the purpose of using it as a bone marrow donor for its sibling (*Los Angeles Times*, April 17, 1979, p. I-2). And the bioethics literature contains articles seriously considering whether we should clone human beings to serve as an inventory of spare parts for organ transplants[4] and articles that foresee the use of comatose human beings as self-replenishing blood banks and manufacturing plants for human hormones.[5] How far our society is willing to proceed down this road is uncertain, but it is clear that the first step to all these practices is the acceptance of the same principle that the Nazis attempted to use to justify their medical experiments at the Nuremberg War Crimes Trials: that human beings may be used as means to the achievement of other goals, and need not be treated as ends in themselves.[6]

But why, it might be asked, is it so terrible if the surrogate mother does not desire the child for its own sake, when under the proposed surrogate mother arrangements there will be a couple eagerly desiring to have the child and to be its parents? That this argument may not be entirely accurate will be illustrated in the following section, but the basic reply is that creating a child without desiring it fundamentally changes the way we look at children—instead of viewing them as unique individual personalities to be desired in their own right, we may come to view them as commodities or items of manufacture to be desired because of their utility. A recent newspaper account describes the business of an agency that matches surrogate mothers with barren couples as follows:

> Its first product is due for delivery today. Twelve others are on the way and an additional 20 have been ordered. The "company" is Surrogate Mothering Ltd. and the "product" is babies.[7]

The dangers of this view are best illustrated by examining what might go wrong in a surrogate mother arrangement, and most important, by viewing how the various parties to the contract may react to the disappointment.

WHAT MIGHT GO WRONG

Ninety-nine percent of the surrogate mother arrangements may work out just fine: the child will be born normal, and the adopting parents (that is, the biological father and his wife) will want it. But, what happens when, unforeseeably, the child is born deformed? Since many defects cannot be discovered prenatally by amniocentesis or other means, the situation is bound to arise.[8] Similarly, consider what would happen if the biological father were to die before the birth of the child. Or if the "child" turns out to be twins or triplets. Each of these instances poses an inevitable situation where the adopting parents may be unhappy with the prospect of getting the child or children. Although legislation can mandate that the adopting parents take the child or children in whatever condition they come or whatever the situation, provided the surrogate mother has abided by all the contractual provisions of the surrogate mother arrangement, the important point for our discussion is the attitude that the surrogate mother or the adopting parent might have. Consider the example of the deformed child.

When I participated in the Surrogate Parent Foundation's inaugural symposium in November 1981, I was struck by the attitude of both the surrogate mothers and the adopting parents to these problems. The adopting parents worried, "Do we have to take such a child?" and the surrogate mothers said in response, "Well, we don't want to be stuck with it." Clearly, both groups were anxious not [to] be responsible for the "undesirable child" born of the surrogate mother arrangement. What does this portend?

It is human nature that when one pays money, one expects value. Things that one pays for have a way of being seen as commodities. Unavoidable in surrogate mother arrangements are questions such as: "Did I get a good one?" We see similar behavior with respect to the adoption of children: comparatively speaking, there is no shortage of black, Mexican-American, mentally retarded, or older children seeking homes; the shortage is in attractive, intelligent-looking Caucasian babies.[9] Similarly, surrogate mother arrangements involve more than just the desire to have a child. The desire is for a certain type of child.

But, it may be objected, don't all parents voice these same concerns in the normal course of having children? Not exactly. No one doubts or minimizes the pain and disappointment parents feel when they learn that their child is born with some genetic or congenital birth defect. But this is different from the surrogate mother situation, where neither the surrogate mother nor the adopting parents may feel responsible, and both sides may feel that they have a legitimate excuse not to assume responsibility for the child. The surrogate mother might blame the biological father for having "defective sperm," as the adopting parents might blame the surrogate mother for a "defective ovum" or for improper care of the fetus during pregnancy. The adopting parents desire a normal child, not *this* child in any condition, and the surrogate mother doesn't want it in any event. So both sides will feel threatened by the birth of an "undesirable child." Like bruised fruit in the produce bin of a supermarket, this child is likely to become an object of avoidance.

Certainly, in the natural course of having children a mother may doubt whether she wants a child if the father has died before its birth; parents may shy away from a defective infant, or be distressed at the thought of multiple births. Nevertheless, I believe they are more likely to accept these contingencies as a matter of fate. I do not think this is the case with surrogate mother arrangements. After all, in the surrogate mother arrangement the adopting parents can blame someone outside the marital relationship. The surrogate mother has been hosting this child all along, and she is delivering it. It certainly *looks* far more like a commodity than the child that arrives in the natural course within the family unit.

A DANGEROUS AGENDA

Another social problem, which arises out of the first, is the fear that surrogate mother arrangements will fall prey to eugenic concerns.[10] Surrogate mother contracts typically have clauses requiring genetic tests of the fetus and stating that the surrogate mother must have an abortion (or keep the child herself) if the child does not pass these tests.[11]

In the last decade we have witnessed a renaissance of interest in eugenics. This, coupled with advances in biomedical technology, has created a host of abuses and new moral problems. For example, genetic counseling clinics now face a dilemma: amniocentesis, the same procedure that identifies whether a fetus suffers from certain genetic defects, also discloses the sex of a fetus. Genetic counseling clinics have reported that even when the fetus is normal, a disproportionate number of mothers abort female children.[12] Aborting normal fetuses simply because the prospective parents desire children of a certain sex is one result of viewing children as commodities. The recent scandal at the Repository for Germinal Choice, the so-called "Nobel Sperm Bank," provides another chilling example. Their first "customer" was, unbeknownst to the staff, a woman who "had lost custody of two other children because they were abused in an effort to 'make them smart.'"[13] Of course, these and similar evils may occur whether or not surrogate mother arrangements are allowed by law. But to the extent that they promote the view of children as commodities, these arrangements contribute to these problems. There is nothing wrong with striving for betterment, as long as it does not result in intolerance to that which is not perfect. But I fear that the latter attitude will become prevalent.

Sanctioning surrogate mother arrangements can also exert pressures upon the family structure. First, as was noted earlier, there is nothing technically to prevent the use of surrogate mother arrangements by single males desiring to become parents. Indeed, single females can already do this with AID or even without it. But even if legislation were to limit the use of the surrogate mother arrangement to infertile couples, other pressures would occur: namely the intrusion of a third adult into the marital community.[14] I do not think that

society is ready to accept either single parenting or quasi-adulterous arrangements as normal.

Another stress on the family structure arises within the family of the surrogate mother. When the child is surrendered to the adopting parents it is removed not only from the surrogate mother, but also from her family. They too have interests to be considered. Do not the siblings of that child have an interest in the fact that their little baby brother has been "given" away?[15] One woman, the mother of a medical student who had often donated sperm for artificial insemination, expressed her feelings to me eloquently. She asked, "I wonder how many grandchildren I have that I have never seen and never been able to hold or cuddle."

Intrafamily tensions can also be expected to result in the family of the adopting parents due to the asymmetry of relationship the adopting parents will have toward the child. The adopting mother has no biological relationship to the child, whereas the adopting father is also the child's biological father. Won't this unequal biological claim on the child be used as a wedge in child-rearing arguments? Can't we imagine the father saying, "Well, he is my son, not yours"? What if the couple eventually gets divorced? Should custody in a subsequent divorce between the adopting mother and the biological father be treated simply as a normal child custody dispute? Or should the biological relationship between father and child weigh more heavily? These questions do not arise in typical adoption situations since both parents are equally unrelated biologically to the child. Indeed, in adoption there is symmetry. The surrogate mother situation is more analogous to second marriages, where the children of one party by a prior marriage are adopted by the new spouse. Since asymmetry in second marriage situations causes problems, we can anticipate similar difficulties arising from surrogate mother arrangements.

There is also the worry that the offspring of a surrogate mother arrangement will be deprived of important information about his or her heritage. This also happens with adopted children or children conceived by AID,[16] who lack information about their biological parents, which could be important to them medically. Another less popularly recognized problem is the danger of half-sibling marriages,[17] where the child of the surrogate mother unwittingly falls in love with a half sister or brother. The only way to avoid these problems is to dispense with the confidentiality of parental records; however, the natural parents may not always want their identity disclosed.

The legalization of surrogate mother arrangements may also put undue pressure upon poor women to use their bodies in this way to support themselves and their families. Analogous problems have arisen in the past with the use of paid blood donors.[18] And occasionally the press reports someone desperate enough to offer to sell an eye or some other organ.[19] I believe that certain things should be viewed as too important to be sold as commodities, and I hope that we have advanced from the time when parents raised children for profitable labor, or found themselves forced to sell their children.

While many of the social dilemmas I have outlined here have their analogies in other present-day occurrences such as divorced families or in adoption, every addition is hurtful. Legalizing surrogate mother arrangements will increase the frequency of these problems, and put more stress on our society's shared moral values.[20]

[CONCLUSION]

An infertile couple might prefer to raise a child with a biological relationship to the husband, rather than to raise an adopted child who has no biological relationship to either the husband or the wife. But does the marginal increase in joy that they might therefore experience outweigh the potential pain that they, or the child conceived in such arrangements, or others might suffer? Does their preference outweigh the social costs and problems that the legalization of surrogate mothering might well engender? I honestly do not know. I don't even know on what hypothetical scale such interests could be weighed and balanced. But even if we could weigh such interests, and even if personal preference outweighed the costs, I still would not be able to say that we could justify achieving those ends by these means; that ethically it would be permissible for a person to create a child, not because she desired it, but because it could be useful to her....

REFERENCES

1 See Philip J. Parker, "Motivation of Surrogate Mothers: Initial Findings," *American Journal of Psychiatry* 140:1 (January 1983), 117–18; see also Doe V. Kelley, Circuit Court of Wayne County Michigan (1980) reported in 1980 Rep. on Human Reproduction and Law II-A-1.

2 See, e.g., C. M. v. C. C., 152 N.J. Supp. 160, 377 A.2d 821 (1977); "Why She Went to 'Nobel Sperm Bank' for Child," *Los Angeles Herald Examiner*, Aug. 6, 1982, p. A9; "Womb for Rent," *Los Angeles Herald Examiner*, Sept. 21, 1981, p. A3.

3 See also Richard McCormick, "Reproductive Technologies: Ethical Issues" in *Encyclopedia of Bioethics*, edited by Walter Reich, Vol. 4 (New York: The Free Press, 1978) pp. 1454, 1459; Robert Snowden and G. D. Mitchell, *The Artificial Family* (London: George Allen & Unwin, 1981), p. 71.

4 See, e.g., Alexander Peters, "The Brave New World: Can the Law Bring Order Within Traditional Concepts of Due Process?" *Suffolk Law Review* 4 (1970), 894, 901–02; Roderic Gorney, "The New Biology and the Future of Man," *UCLA Law Review* 15 (1968), 273, 302; J. G. Castel, "Legal Implications of Biomedical Science and Technology in the Twenty-First Century," *Canadian Bar Review* 51 (1973), 119, 127.

5 See Harry Nelson, "Maintaining Dead to Serve as Blood Makers Proposed: Logical, Sociologist Says," *Los Angeles Times,* February 26, 1974, p. II-1; Hans Jonas, "Against the Stream: Comments on the Definition and Redefinition of Death," in *Philosophical Essays: From Ancient Creed to Technological Man* (Chicago: University of Chicago Press, 1974), pp. 132–40.

6 See Leo Alexander, "Medical Science under Dictatorship," *New England Journal of Medicine* 241:2 (1949), 39; United States v. Brandt, Trial of the Major War Criminals, International Military Tribunal: Nuremberg, 14 November 1945–1 October 1946.

7 Bob Dvorchak, "Surrogate Mothers: Pregnant Idea Now a Pregnant Business," *Los Angeles Herald Examiner,* December 27, 1983, p. A1.

8 "Surrogate's Baby Born with Deformities Rejected by All," *Los Angeles Times,* January 22, 1983, p. I-17; "Man Who Hired Surrogate Did Not Father Ailing Baby," *Los Angeles Herald Examiner,* February 3, 1983, p. A6.

9 See, e.g., Adoption in America, Hearing before the Subcommittee on Aging, Family and Human Services of the Senate Committee on Labor and Human Resources, 97th Congress. lst Session (1981), p. 3 (comments of Senator Jeremiah Denton) and pp. 16–17 (statement of Warren Master, Acting Commissioner of Administration for Children, Youth and Families, HHS).

10 Cf. "Discussion: Moral, Social and Ethical Issues," in *Laws and Ethics of A.I.D. and Embryo Transfer*

(1973) (comments of Himmelweit); reprinted in Michael Shapiro and Roy Spece, *Bioethics and Law* (St. Paul: West Publishing Company, 1981), p. 548.

11 See, e.g., Lane (Newsday), "Womb for Rent," *Tucson Citizen* (Weekender), June 7, 1980, p. 3; Susan Lewis, "Baby Bartering? Surrogate Mothers Pose Issues for Lawyers, Courts," *The Los Angeles Daily Journal,* April 20, 1981; see also Elaine Markoutsas, "Women Who Have Babies for Other Women," *Good Housekeeping* 96 (April 1981), 104.

12 See Morton A. Stenchever, "An Abuse of Prenatal Diagnosis," *Journal of the American Medical Association* 221 (1972), 408; Charles Westoff and Ronald R. Rindfus, "Sex Preselection in the United States: Some Implications," *Science* 184 (1974), 633, 636; see also Phyllis Battelle, "Is It a Boy or a Girl"? *Los Angeles Herald Examiner,* Oct. 8, 1981, p. A17.

13 "2 Children Taken from Sperm Bank Mother," *Los Angeles Times,* July 14, 1982; p. I-3; "The Sperm Bank Scandal," *Newsweek* 24 (July 26, 1982).

14 See Helmut Thielicke, *The Ethics of Sex*, John W. Doberstein, trans. (New York: Harper & Row, 1964).

15 According to one newspaper account, when a surrogate mother informed her nine-year-old daughter that the new baby would be given away, the daughter replied, "Oh, good. If it's a girl we can keep it and give Jeffrey [her two-year-old half brother] away." "Womb for Rent," *Los Angeles Herald Examiner,* Sept. 21, 1981, p. A3.

16 See, e.g., Lorraine Dusky, "Brave New Babies"? *Newsweek* 30 (December 6, 1982). Also testimony of Suzanne Rubin before the California Assembly Committee on Judiciary, Surrogate Parenting Contracts, Assembly Publication No. 962, pp. 72–75 (November 19, 1982).

17 This has posed an increasing problem for children conceived through AID. See, e.g., Martin Curie-Cohen, et al., "Current Practice of Artificial Insemination by Donor in the United States," *New England Journal of Medicine* 300 (1979), 585–89.

18 See, e.g., Richard M. Titmuss, *The Gift Relationship: From Human Blood to Social Policy* (New York: Random House, 1971).

19 See, e.g., "Man Desperate for Funds: Eye for Sale at $35,000," *Los Angeles Times,* February 1, 1975, p. II-1; "100 Answer Man's Ad for New Kidney," *Los Angeles Times,* September 12, 1974, p. I-4.

20 See generally Guido Calabresi, "Reflections on Medical Experimentation in Humans," *Daedalus* 98 (1969), 387–93; also see Michael Shapiro and Roy Spece, "On Being 'Unprincipled on Principle': The Limits of Decision Making 'On the Merits,'" in *Bioethics and Law,* pp. 67–71.

Reproductive Technologies

Coming to Terms with Test-Tube Babies

Clifford Grobstein

Clifford Grobstein is professor of biological science and public policy at the University of California, San Diego. He is well known among biologists for his research in developmental biology. He is also the author of *The Strategy of Life* (1965), *A Double Image of the Double Helix* (1979), and *From Chance to Purpose: An Appraisal of External Human Fertilization* (1981).

Grobstein's point of departure is his perception of a "new wave of concern" about the employment of external (*in vitro*) fertilization. Anxiety has arisen because IVF procedures have provided an "open window" on early human development; and,

Reprinted with permission of the publisher from *New Scientist*, October 7, 1982.

closely related, there is a heightened sense that we are being led down a "slippery slope" to the acceptance of more and more unsavory applications of *in vitro* techniques. Grobstein traces the heightened sense of the slippery slope largely to the availability of surplus embryos and to the possibility of freezing them. (At the time this selection was written, the idea of freezing embryos was under consideration; the practice is now well established.) Grobstein contends that we must not allow our fear of the slippery slope to lead us to a wholesale rejection of *in vitro* procedures. The proper response, he argues, is to establish policies that set appropriate boundaries.

The first baby that was conceived by external (*in vitro*) fertilisation was born in England in 1978. The event created much excitement and some controversy. First reactions died down as additional technology-assisted babies were born, not only in England but in Australia and the U.S. More than three years later, however, controversy in England is stirring anew—as though people are suddenly seeing the matter in a new light. This "double-take," sometimes exploited by comedians to get a laugh, in this instance has serious significance.

Earlier misgivings in the U.S. were effectively summarised in the hearings and deliberations of the Ethics Advisory Board, charged in 1978 by Joseph Califano, then Secretary of the Department of Health, Education and Welfare, to evaluate external human fertilisation. Central in the board's consideration were questions of the safety and efficacy of the procedure—designed to relieve female infertility due to blockage or loss of the fallopian tubes. Safety referred largely to possible harmful effects on the offspring, efficacy largely to the percentage of attempts that would yield viable offspring. Three years later, with about a score of babies born, all but one appear to have been normal at birth and the several clinics with greatest experience are projecting a one in five chance of success for each attempt. The trend of the growing clinical experience is, therefore, toward safety and success rates close to those for the natural internal process.

While external fertilisation cannot yet be regarded as an established medical procedure, its trials so far suggest that it will prove reasonably safe and efficacious. The new wave of concern, in fact, centres on broader issues—the "open window" on early human development afforded by the procedure and conceivable procedures that can be visualised as ranging along a "slippery slope" toward applications that are unpalatable to many people. The "open window," of course, is the accessibility external fertilisation provides for observation or manipulation of early human developmental stages, previously rarely obtainable and never before able to be maintained alive while undergoing development. The Cambridge physiologist Robert Edwards and obstetrician Patrick Steptoe and their colleagues, whose arduous and dedicated efforts brought the procedure to realisation, have recently reported on the growth of externally cultured human embryos from fertilisation to the blastocyst ("ball of cells") stage, at which time the embryos normally would be implanting in the wall of the uterus. The objective of these observations is to improve further the safety and efficacy of the procedure. However, such entirely reasonable efforts are further widening the open window and heightening concern in some quarters about the presumed slippery slope. This much more consequential matter undoubtedly is providing the major impetus to calls for a second look, and even a moratorium, on continued research to improve and expand the use of the procedure. The concern stems from the fact that manipulations of fertilisation and early stages in development, comparable with those now accessible in humans, are being practised increasingly widely on other mammalian species, both in the laboratory and in commercial animal production. Two objectives of these practices are to gain greater knowledge of hereditary and developmental processes on one hand and to apply this knowledge to achieve economic benefits on the other. The concern is that the very same manipulations, if applied to human eggs or embryos, raise unprecedented moral issues and, in some minds, the possibility of unanticipated or frankly undesirable social impacts.

The possibility of entering upon a slippery slope has come more sharply into focus largely because of two technical innovations in external fertilisation, one already in effect and the other under consideration. The first is the use of hormonal stimulation to increase the number of mature eggs that can be obtained from a given donor. In humans, of course only a single egg usually matures in each menstrual cycle. Having several eggs mature clearly might increase the success rate for a given procedure for recovering eggs. Edwards and Steptoe in early efforts, however, had poorer success when they obtained multiple eggs by hormonal stimulation than they had with single eggs obtained from a natural cycle. Their first births, in fact, were from eggs obtained in natural cycles. Subsequently, however, other groups using slightly different methods, notably Carl Wood at the Monash University in Australia, have had greater success with multiple eggs hormonally induced from a single donor and are achieving overall improved success rates. The reinsertion of more than one egg has given rise to a few twin pregnancies, and, because up to six mature eggs can be produced hormonally, donors may be stimulated to produce more than the optimal number of eggs for a given cycle.

There are several options for the further fate of such surplus eggs. They might be killed and discarded. They might be used, as the Edwards and Steptoe group has done, to gain more knowledge about these early human stages, in turn perhaps contributing to the safety and efficacy of the procedure. Or they might be frozen and stored for other, later use. Each of the options is controversial, for each raises the knotty issue of the legal and social status of the early human embryo. If one holds, as legislation pending in the U.S. Congress does, that a person exists from conception, then any option other than immediate return to a receptive uterus (and possibly even that) is excluded. If, however, one holds that the early embryo is something other than a person, then the options are admissible, but with a degree of restriction depending upon how close to a person the early embryo is defined to be.

VALUABLE BY-PRODUCTS

Setting aside this question of status for the moment, what do the options offer technically? The first obviously offers nothing other than avoiding the necessity to face the other two. Surplus embryos would be treated as unwanted by-products of the procedure and would be dispatched without further consideration or concern. The second option would assign special value to the early embryos as a source of additional knowledge, not for the benefit of the embryos themselves but possibly to benefit other embryos and humanity in general. The third option is the most complex because

it puts the embryos in temporary stasis for purposes that have not been specified. What might some of these purposes be?

The most immediate purpose and the closest to the original rationale of the basic procedure of external fertilisation would be to provide embryos for insertion into the uterus of the donor in later menstrual cycles. One of the concerns about the hormonal induction of multiple eggs is that the hormonal stimulation may not only affect the ovary but might also disturb the cycle of the uterus. Having obtained the embryos it might be advantageous not to return them immediately to the uterus but to wait for a subsequent cycle uncomplicated by the administration of hormones. At the very least, this would allow successive attempts at reinsertion after only a single extraction of eggs. Obtaining the egg is the most uncomfortable step for the patient, involving a small incision through the abdominal wall under light anaesthesia. Moreover, the reinsertion step also has, at the moment, the lowest success rate. If multiple eggs were obtained by a single extraction from the ovary and if all that were not immediately reinserted were frozen, the thawed embryos could later be inserted in successive cycles until success were achieved. This might enhance the success rate while adding as little as possible to the patient's discomfort.

The pertinent question, of course, is the possible harm done to the embryo by freezing and thawing. Here it is important to note that the freezing and thawing of embryos stems from extensive studies over several decades in what is called cryobiology. It is now possible, as the result of research on the processes of freezing and thawing of living tissues in various media and at different temperatures, to freeze and thaw many microbial, plant and animal cells with minimal damage. In the frozen state metabolism is suspended and even genetic change is slowed down to insignificant levels. Mammalian embryos, including those of mice and cattle, have been kept in frozen storage and shown to continue normal development with high frequency on thawing. Scientifically valuable strains of mice are now being stored in frozen embryo banks to eliminate the effort and cost of constant breeding.

The application of the procedure to human embryos would not, therefore, be a shot in the dark. On the other hand, its application to humans is not the same as its application to mice or cattle. Ninety per cent success rates, for example, may be acceptable for laboratory and domestic animals. In humans it is the 10 per cent failure rate that is of concern—particularly if these are partial failures, not detectable until after birth of even later in life. Clearly these are matters for most careful consideration before frozen-thawed human embryos are reinserted for continued development.

If the safety issue were favourably resolved, we can envisage further technical possibilities. Eggs surplus for the original donor might also be inserted into the receptive uterus of a non-donor. Such embryo transfers are commonly done with high rates of success in laboratory animals and cattle. They are done most effectively with frozen-thawed embryos because these can be held until the uterus of the recipient is in the most receptive stage of the cycle. We can imagine two circumstances in which this might be attempted in humans. The first is based upon the original rationale for external human fertilisation, that is, to relieve infertility. The recipient would be a woman whose ovaries do not produce mature and normal eggs but whose uterus is normal. The insertion of an embryo into her uterus would be comparable with an early adoption. She would have the full experience of pregnancy but with an offspring to which she had made no genetic contribution. If, incidentally, she were to receive a surplus egg fertilised by her husband's sperm the offspring would have genetic kinship at least with the father, a situation exactly the converse of artificial insemination by donor to cope with male infertility.

The slippery slope would begin to steepen if the same technical procedure were to be applied to a non-donor who was not sterile but who acted as a surrogate ("foster mother") for the donor. This might still be a measure to overcome sterility if the donor were without a uterus due to an earlier hysterectomy. It might, however, also be done because the donor might expect a pregnancy to be dangerous to her health or merely inconvenient. In the last instance the original motivation to relieve sterility would have been diluted to the vanishing point, replaced by considerations of maternal preference and convenience.

Having reached this point, further options might be seen that would still employ the same basic techniques. For example, there is a trend in the U.S. for women to postpone pregnancy to avoid interrupting their careers. In addition, the incidence of Down's syndrome in offspring rises sharply as maternal age moves into the last decade of fecundity, between 35 and 45. Suppose a young woman were to have eggs removed from her ovaries to be fertilised externally by sperm from her husband (or other male), and the resulting embryos were to be frozen. These embryos could then be inserted into her uterus at convenient times that fit her career needs, and possibly reduce the risk of developmental defect. Incidentally, with a secure supply in the frozen-embryo bank, a couple could submit to sterilisation procedures without losing the capacity to have a family. This comes close to the ultimate in family planning.

This is but one chain of options along an imaginable and not wildly speculative slippery slope. It is the kind of thing that arouses uneasiness and causes many people to say, "Now wait! What are we rushing into? Let's take another look." A prudent position, but what comes next? Do we attempt to prohibit a procedure that is on the way to being safe and efficacious, and able to bring satisfaction to many people? Could or should such a procedure be effectively prohibited? Would it not simply become covert, more expensive and perhaps less well managed? Should we attempt instead to cut off all further advance by limiting research on reproduction, endocrinology and genetics? If this were seriously to be considered could such a draconian measure be enforced worldwide? Can we, should we, cut off the progress of human knowledge?

Better, it would seem, to examine more carefully the kinds of slippery slopes that can reasonably be anticipated to appear on the rising peak of external human fertilisation. All slopes, after all, do not end in precipices and not all are slippery. We live most of our lives on slopes of one kind or another, sometimes using them to advantage, sometimes by exercise of will moving up them instead of down, sometimes enjoying the very slipperiness of slopes or the challenge to overcome them. We do not invariably forgo something that is basically beneficial because it may be abused or may lead toward something malignant. Rather we move to establish sound guidelines and policies that set appropriate boundaries, limits to rates of progression, or otherwise reassure against over-enthusiasm or irresponsibility.

For example, another identifiable slope is arising in the possible combination of external human fertilisation with molecular genetics. Some human genes have been chemically characterised, can be reproduced in bacteria and can be manipulated to yield their normal product. Human insulin has been produced in this way. Moreover, normal genetic material has been inserted into cultured human cells to correct genetic defect in those cells. This is but one step—though possibly a long one—from gene therapy to correct defects in precursor human red cells that give rise to sickle-cell anaemia and B-thalassaemia. Gene transfers also have been made into mouse embryos, leading to genetic modification not only of the resulting adult but of offspring in the next generation. The embryonic stages used in the mouse experiments are precisely the ones in the open window provided by external human fertilisation. The slope thus points toward a distant capability to influence human evolution in limited ways.

We cannot avoid considering the implications of such slopes, even though they may not have to be faced with full responsibility for a generation or two. We cannot avoid this consideration because anxiety over the possibilities produces the reaction mentioned earlier; stop moving ahead until we know where we are going. A reasonable response is to start thinking ahead even as we move ahead, so as to proceed under agreed consensus as to purposes and precautions. The agreed consensus, if it is to be achieved and effective, must be formulated on a broad social base. It must have the character of a future-sensitive tradition that will soundly guide our growing powers to intervene in human reproduction, heredity and development.

IMPROVING THE SPECIES

This is not a task that will be completed in any definable period while all progress is stopped. It is a task to begin now and to intensify as wider options evolve. It might be started by attempting to formulate principles that allow near-term progress but emphasise awareness on the part of all involved that existing concerns and long-term consequences must be carefully considered. For example, many would be reassured to know that the intent of any intervention in human reproduction would be to benefit individuals and not to "improve" the species as a whole. Though these two are linked, in contemporary thinking the first is generally understood and accepted, the second is burdened by suspicion and fraught with uncertainties as to how "improvement" will be defined—and by whom.

It would also be reassuring to know that defects that *limit* self-realisation and self-satisfaction are the legitimate target; that conservation and fuller fruition of humanity as we know it is the goal, not the "engineering" of new forms of human life. It should be specified most compellingly that no intervention will be countenanced that reduces or limits human potential, regardless of assumed benefits to particular societies, groups or ideologies. On the other hand, interventions to gratify individual desires (for example, to provide offspring of a particular sex) will not be practised without full evaluation of collective consequences (such as distorted sex ratios).

Can such policies be formulated, elevated to the status of social guidelines and implemented? An affirmative answer can be given only if the procedures for establishing such guidelines are soundly formulated. Formulation would have to be by a deliberative body of appropriate integrity, stature and authority. The deliberations must be sufficiently accessible to incorporate all relevant opinion, and yet secluded enough to be free of excessive immediate pressures. The principles must be formulated cogently and emotively, yet simply, so that they can easily gain currency in broad communities. They should not be entangled in statutory legalities but should become matters of individual conscience, of professional ethics and of common law.

This is but a sketch to indicate the nature of the task ahead. The inventiveness of human mind has vastly extended the powers of the human hand; now we are challenged to display equivalent innovativeness in defining human purpose. It is a time for prudence but it is also a time for vision. We must not freeze into immobility but we must step carefully as we move upward to new uncharted ground. At this new level our future will be brought in greater degree into the orbit of our deliberate choice. This will, indeed, take our measure as we move into a new millenium.

Ethical Aspects of Surrogate Embryo Transfer

LeRoy Walters

A biographical sketch of LeRoy Walters is found on page 148.

The first human births resulting from surrogate embryo transfer (SET), following both *in vitro* and *in vivo* fertilization, occurred in late 1983 and early 1984, respectively. As these achievements were unfolding, Walters wrote this essay, in which he proposes a framework for ethical assessment. Mindful of the great value of anti-infertility techniques for those who suffer from involuntary infertility, he endorses the use of such a technique "provided that its benefits are not outweighed by safety considerations and social consequences." In accordance with this underlying framework of evaluation, Walters then provides an initial analysis of the safety considerations and social consequences relevant to the employment of SET.

The article by Hodgen published in this issue of *The Journal* [JAMA, Oct. 28, 1983, 2167–2171] suggests that some infertile women who cannot produce fertilizable ova may one day be able to bear children. Such women may have ovaries that are functionally deficient in a critical respect, or they may lack ovaries entirely. For these women, bearing a child that is genetically "their own" is a physical impossibility.

Any new technique that helps to reduce involuntary infertility is to be welcomed, provided that its benefits are not outweighed by safety considerations and social consequences. The present moment, when surrogate embryo transfer (SET) is being tested in primates and initially attempted in humans[1-3] seems the appropriate time to inventory the ethical issues that the clinical use of this new technique may raise.

Safety considerations in SET and accompanying techniques concern three biologic individuals—the oocyte or embryo donor, the embryo itself, and the embryo recipient. The risk factors vary somewhat, depending on whether SET is employed in conjunction with in vitro or in vivo fertilization. With SET after in vitro fertilization, the physical risks of the procedures to embryo and recipient are for the most part comparable with the risks of in vitro fertilization and embryo transfer without donation. Surrogate embryo transfer after in vivo fertilization may involve less risk to the early embryo than in vitro fertilization and embryo transfer, with or without donation, because the in vivo technique substantially reduces the time during which the early embryo is exposed to an artificial, extrauterine environment. Conversely, with SET after in vivo fertilization, the embryo recipient may be at slightly greater risk of acquiring an infection from the donor via the transfer procedure.

The physical risk differential is most striking in the case of the donor. An oocyte donor must undergo inhalation or conduction anesthesia during the oocyte recovery process. Therefore, it seems unlikely that most women would volunteer to undergo oocyte recovery merely for donation purposes, except under extraordinary circumstances. Much more likely is the scenario in which an oocyte has already been harvested for the woman's own in vitro fertilization and is not needed, thereby becoming available for donation. In contrast, with SET after in vivo fertilization, the physical risks to the donor—in this case, an *embryo* donor—are greatly reduced, but some hazards remain. Most important are the potential risks of uterine lavage—and, in the future, of possible superovulation—to the embryo donor. In veterinary medicine similar nonsurgical techniques have been employed successfully to recover bovine and equine embryos without apparent ill effect, although the nonhuman donors are either anesthesized or sedated.[4,5] Hodgen does note that an ectopic pregnancy occurred in one of the female monkey donors and suggests that the tubal pregnancy may have been an unintended result of retrograde uterine lavage. Hodgen's recommendation that human embryo donors be carefully monitored for possible ectopic pregnancy seems eminently reasonable. A further possibility is that a normal uterine pregnancy may ensue if the lavage procedure fails to retrieve all embryos from the donor's uterus. The embryo donor would then confront a decision about the continuation of an unexpected pregnancy.

The social consequences of a new biomedical technique cannot be predicted in great detail or with total accuracy. However, at least three general arenas of potential social impact for SET can be identified: (1) the family unit, (2) the medical care provision system, and (3) the commercial sphere. Surrogate embryo transfer necessarily involves the introduction of a third party into the relationship between a man and a woman, who will usually be husband and wife. If the woman cannot produce fertilizable ova and if the couple wishes to bear and/or raise children, the members of the couple have no alternative but to select some kind of adoptive procedure. Their three primary options are the adoption of an already born child who is not genetically related to them, the employment of a surrogate mother who would perhaps be inseminated with the husband's sperm, or SET. Of these alternatives, SET most closely approximates the usual process of human reproduction. Both members of the couple are directly involved in the pregnancy, the man through providing semen and the woman through carrying the pregnancy to term and giving birth to the child. In addition, with SET the couple, particularly the woman, has greater control over the physiological environment of the developing fetus and embryo than in either postnatal adoption or surrogate-motherhood arrangements. The embryo recipient herself can determine what work schedule to follow, how much to rest, what foods and drugs to ingest, and whether to smoke cigarettes or drink alcoholic beverages.

Because the embryo or oocyte donor's involvement in SET is temporally limited, preimplantation adoption through SET will quite probably involve fewer psychological and legal complications than surrogate motherhood and subsequent adoption.[6,7] However, as

in the case of surrogate motherhood, the adopting parents know little about the overall health status of the adopted embryo and child to be—far less than parents adopting a newborn infant know. If, after SET, an adopted embryo is delivered as a handicapped newborn, the adopting parents may tend to blame the donor for the infant's defects or even to reject the child. The recent controversy surrounding a handicapped child born to a surrogate mother in Michigan indicates that these possibilities are not merely theoretical (*The New York Times,* Jan. 23, 1983, p. 19).

Even if the neonate born after SET is normal, the adopting family and the health professionals involved will face several generic questions of disclosure and confidentiality that are similar to those raised by artificial insemination by donor and more traditional modes of adoption. For example, will the identity of the donor female be disclosed to the recipient couple, or vice versa? And will the resulting child be told that he or she was adopted before implantation? If so, will the child perhaps be interested in learning more about his or her biologic roots?

In short, preimplantation adoption through SET should be less disruptive to the family unit than surrogate-motherhood arrangements. The impact of SET on the adopting family will probably be comparable with that of artificial insemination by donor or postnatal adoption; it may in fact be less because SET allows both members of the adopting couple to be biologically involved in either the initiation or sustenance of the pregnancy.

The possible impact of SET on the medical care provision system is more difficult to anticipate. A major concern is that SET may join in vitro fertilization as a high-technology anti-infertility technique available only to those able to afford a major expense. Private health insurers have been notably cautious in reimbursing the costs of in vitro fertilization, and state and federal medical assistance programs have made infertility treatment a low or nonexistent priority. According to a recent study published by the National Center for Health Statistics, there are 4.3 million currently married women in the United States aged 15 to 44 years who experience impaired fecundity. Of these, 47.3%, or more than 2 million women, want to bear a first child (840,000), a second child (641,000), or an additional child (556,000) but are prevented by infertility problems from doing so.[8] This situation requires both a national recognition of the devastating impact that involuntary infertility can have on the lives of the couples involved and a public policy on infertility treatment that is more in accord with that recognition.

A final potential social impact of SET is commercial and should be considered merely speculative. If semen donors are paid for their "donations," it is at least conceivable that oocyte or embryo donors, who undergo greater risk, will request equal treatment. Therefore, a group of professional donors could develop among women to parallel the already existing group of professional semen donors among men. Moreover, commercial oocyte or embryo banks (analogous to existing commercial sperm banks) could employ cryopreservation techniques like those recently reported from Australia (*Washington Post,* May 3, 1983, p. A14) to store donated oocytes or embryos until appropriate recipients are found.

The introduction of a commercial dimension into the transfer of human blood, germ cells, or organs between people has occasioned vigorous debate.[9-11] Strenuous opposition would be likely to greet any proposal to establish a commercial human-embryo bank on the ground that the sale of human embryos for adoption is more like the (prohibited) sale of infants for adoption than the (permitted) selling of human semen or blood. At the very least, society may want to require that all prospective germ-cell or embryo donors receive careful screening, including karyotyping and pedigree analysis.

In summary, SET may provide a means for overcoming the involuntary infertility of a new group of patients. The safety of the technique for oocyte or embryo donors should be closely monitored, and its potential social impact on the family unit, the medical care provision system, and the commercial sphere should—even at this early stage of human application—be carefully assessed.

NOTES

1 Buster, J. E., Bustillo, M., Thornycroft, I., et al.: Non-surgical transfer of an in-vivo fertilised donated ovum to an infertility patient. *Lancet* 1983; 1: 816–817.

2 Trounson, A., Leeton, J., Besanko, M., et al.: Pregnancy established in an infertile patient after transfer of a donated embryo fertilised in vitro. *Br Med J* 1983; 286:835–838.

3 Steptoe, P., Edwards, R. G., Trounson, A., et al.: Pregnancy in an infertile patient after transfer of an embryo fertilised in vitro. *Br Med J* 1983; 286: 1351–1352.

4 Rowe, R. F., Del Campo, M. R., Critser, M. S., et al.: Embryo transfer in cattle: Nonsurgical collection techniques. *Am J Vet Res* 1980; 41:106–108.

5 Imel, K. J., Squires, E. L., Elsden, R. P., et al.: Collection and transfer of equine embryos. *J Am Vet Med Assoc* 1981; 179:987–991.

6 Ethical issues in surrogate motherhood. *ACOG Newsletter* 1983; 27:3, 11–12.

7 Parker, P. J.: Motivation of surrogate mothers: Initial findings. *Am J Psychiatry* 1983; 140:117–118.

8 Mosher, W. D., Pratt, W. F.: Reproductive impairments among married couples: United States, *Vital and Health Statistics,* series 23, data from the national survey of family growth; No. 11. National Center for Health Statistics, December 1982, pp. 13, 32.

9 Titmuss, R.: *The Gift Relationship: From Human Blood to Social Policy.* New York, Pantheon Books Inc., 1971.

10 Arrow, K. J.: Gifts and exchanges. *Philosophy Public Affairs* 1972; 1:343–362.

11 Curie-Cohen, M., Luttrell, L., Shapiro, S.: Current practice of artificial insemination by donor in the United States. *N Engl J Med* 1979; 300:585–590.

Questions About Cloning

Hans Jonas

A biographical sketch of Hans Jonas is found on page 185.

From the various reasons that can be given for the desirability of cloning, Jonas singles out the replication of excellence as the most worthy of serious consideration. But cloning, in his view, is morally objectionable even in the name of such a worthy objective. Whereas some opponents of cloning appeal to a "right to a unique genotype," the basis of Jonas's opposition to cloning is his assertion of a "right to ignorance." His principal concern is that the possibility of a person's "authentic growth" would be undermined by the knowledge that he or she is a clone.

The questions we have to ask [about cloning] have nothing to do with the conjectural extents of a practice which—if it comes to it at all—may never reach numerical values that are genetically significant for the population. The most important questions in its hypothetical use on man are those that apply to the single no less than to the multiplied case and must be answered before even the first is allowed to occur. They must, therefore, first of all be asked.

We ask three questions: *What* is brought about by cloning? *Why* is it supposedly to be brought about, i.e., what reasons are there for wishing it? *Ought* it to be brought about, i.e., is its very idea to be accepted or rejected?

A The Physical Outcome of Cloning   What is brought about by cloning? A genetic double of the donor, with the same degree of resemblance of phenotype as is known from identical twins. Clone and donor are indeed identical twins with a time lag: the non-contemporaneity will become a relevant facet in our later appraisal. With identical twins one can speak of mutual mirror images; the clone is unilaterally the copy of a preexisting individual. The time lag is indeterminate: since tissue cultures can be kept alive and growing indefinitely, the clone may be derived from a long dead donor (a new sense of individual immortality). By the same token, many clones may be derived, and may continue to be derived, from the same self-replenishing source, with a mediated twinhood among themselves, in principle not different from that with

the original donor, but allowing for any relation of time lag, overlap, or simultaneity whatsoever. With the genetic potential presumably identical among the replicated genotypes, one pheno-actualization of that potential at least, and possibly more, is already on record before any clone begins his.

B Reasons for Cloning   The last statement provides the main answer to the questions of *why* cloning should be done at all: a known individual life performance sufficiently outstanding in some desired respect to prompt the wish for more of its kind, and rare enough in its (presumed) genetic basis not to expect the desired frequency of it from the chances of ordinary or even selective interbreeding. Indeed, it is the "unique" in some sense which by cloning is to be saved from its uniqueness and secured in its repetition. This has obvious advantages in animal husbandry: the prize milch cow is much more certain to be reproduced by direct asexual replication than by the fortuitous detour of even the most careful mating, and moreover—because not requiring her own motherhood—with the option of incomparably greater numbers (any cow can be made the host bearer of another prize cow); and so for the exquisite race horse, and so on. Thus the perpetuation and multiplication of excellence (peak performance) would be a major reason for cloning. The multiplication of specimens would then also furnish the broadened numerical basis for renewed cross breeding, with the prospect of topping even the previous peak that has become a take-off plateau; and so forth, with appropriate switching between the two methods in an upward curve. In this way, cloning—in itself fixating evolutionary results—would become part of a progressive evolutionary drive. Another goal may be the utility value of uniformity as such; and also the well-balanced mean rather than the more vulnerable, onesided excellence may be made the selective criterion. All this concerns the utility-ruled sphere of animal husbandry, where the interests of the species itself are not consulted. Additional considerations (but ruling out none of the above) enter in the human sphere. I can do no better than reproduce here the "laundry list of possible applications [that] keeps growing, in anticipation of the perfected technology," which Dr. Leon Kass has compiled.

(1) Replication of individuals of great genius or great beauty to improve the species or to make life more pleasant. (2) Replication of the healthy to bypass the risk of genetic disease contained in the lottery of sexual recombination. (3) Provision of large sets of genetically identical humans for scientific studies on the relative importance of nature and nurture for various aspects of human performance. (4) Provision of a child to an infertile couple. (5) Provision of a child with a genotype of one's own choosing—of someone famous, of a departed loved one, of one's spouse or oneself. (6) Control of the sex of future children; the sex of a cloned offspring is the same as that of the adult from whom the donor nucleus was taken. (7) Production of sets of identical persons to perform special occupations in peace and war (not excluding espionage). (8) Production of embryonic replicas of each person, to be frozen away until needed as a source of organs for transplantation to their genetically identical twin. (9) To beat the Russians and the Chinese, to prevent a cloning gap.[1]

The list is less facetious than it sounds; no wish is perverse enough (as, e.g., that for self-replication), or cynically utilitarian enough (as Number 7), or scientifically fanatic enough (as Number 3), that it might not, on the offer of its feasibility, find bidders and defenders among the children of Adam and Eve. On the whole, however, we may assume that the argument for excellence to be perpetuated and multiplied (i.e., Number 1 of the list) will hold sway in the human context and would, if the method ever graduated from the laboratory, confine its practice to the extraordinary. It is

certainly the most exalted of the proposed aims and for that reason not only more seductive than any other, but also more apt to force philosophical comment to its radical declaration. We shall accordingly concentrate on this aspect.

C Replication of Excellence Examined The argument of excellence, though naive, is not frivolous in that it enlists our reverence for greatness and pays tribute to it by wishing that more Mozarts, Einsteins, and Schweitzers might adorn the human race.[2] It is naive in taking it for granted that more than one of each would really be to the good of mankind, let alone of the Mozarts and Einsteins of this world—generally in holding that, if a thing is good, more of it would be better.[3] It is also an unblushing consumer argument, not asking whether the genius, granted that he is a blessing to us, is not a curse to himself, often the unhappiest of men, and whether we have the right to condemn anyone deliberately to this terrible price of our enrichment. If, on the other hand, we let the candidate model himself decide about the worthwhileness of a *da capo* in his case, we may get a selection of the vain.[4] Also, of course, what really would happen with these would-be geniuses of the second and third try, once the star hour favoring the first—the unique constellation of subject and occasion—has passed, nobody can even remotely divine. (Let's find out, opposing counsel will say, at least the odds for superior performance are better than with all knowable alternatives to begin with.) Nor can we foresee how the presence of these precertified ones in their midst will affect their fellow men, including upcoming, *de novo* geniuses among them; even the bygone archetype, once revered, might come to be resented for his greedy intrusion by proxy into the open business of the present.

But all this is speculative and largely extraneous to the one *ethical* issue we wish to raise, namely, what to *be* a clone would mean for the subject concerned; and here the case of the distinguished donor merely serves to bring into sharper light what would apply to all cases, i.e., to the cloning proposition as such. Here, also, we get not caught in conjectural questions of quality, of dosing, of relative merits of selection, of benefits and costs to the rest of us—questions which only experience can settle, but can hope for the transempirical certainty which matters of essence sometimes grant: the single, unspecified case X will be as valid as any number of any specification can be.

Existential Critique

A Contemporaneity of Identical Twins The focal question of essence is that of unprejudiced selfhood, and it can be attacked from the situation of a twinhood that lacks contemporaneity. The situation of identical twins (or triplets, etc.) has its own problems, for which, as a rule, no human agency is responsible. This changes, of course, if it is induced by chemical or other prenatal means which are likely or even intended to cause an incipient embryo to split into multiple equivalents of itself. (This seems to happen now with a statistical frequency as a—still unintended—byproduct of certain fertility drugs and may soon be in our choice to cause deliberately.) Whatever objections of an existential nature can be raised against causing the situation knowingly—and condoning the risk is only a weaker form of doing so—one essential feature shared with the accidents of nature sets its results apart from those of cloning: the "multiplets" who have to face the reiteration of their genotype in one another are strictly contemporaneous, none has a head start, and none has to relive a previously completed life. It is irrelevant to what extent the genotype actually dominates individual history, and how far "identity" here goes in determining the final effect. What matters is that the sexually produced genotype is a novum in itself, unknown to all to begin with and still to reveal itself to owners and fellow men alike. Ignorance is here the precondition of freedom: the new throw of the dice has to discover itself in the guideless efforts of living its life for the first and only time, i.e., to *become* itself in meeting a world as unprepared for the newcomer as this is for himself. None of the siblings, though continually confronted with his likeness, suffers from the precedence of a firstcomer who has already demonstrated the potentials of his being (at least one set of them) and thereby preempted their authenticity for him. It may well be, as has been suggested, that he is still injured in a more transcendental (and on principle unverifiable) right, namely, that to the possession of a unique genotype shared with none. If there is such a right, then its denial would be a wrong already in the case of wilfully induced one-egg sibling sets, their genetic firstness and simultaneity notwithstanding, and *a fortiori* in the case of cloning.[5]

B Uniqueness of Genotype and Uniqueness of Being Much as I am in sympathy with the underlying idea, I will not make it my argument. For if there is a right to uniqueness, it is to uniqueness of being, of which uniqueness of genotype may or may not be a necessary condition: we just don't know. (I myself don't believe it is; in fact, the cloned double of another will on that very count be quite unique in his own, probably miserable, way!) Nor is uniqueness of genotype itself a verifiable fact—though normally of the highest statistical probability—and only its absence is known in the exceptional cases under discussion: but what bearing this absence as such (apart from its being known or believed) has on the objective chances of unique selfhood is hardly determinable. I suspect, the real object of the "right" in question is not genotypes at all. An objective, enabling ground of individual uniqueness is in truth a metaphysical, not a physical, postulate (its name was once "the soul") and as such is not only beyond finding out, but also transcendent to the whole question of rights, which it literally antecedes. But it is a different matter altogether that the existing subject, whatever his objective foundations, has an existential right to certain subjective terms of his being—and these are in question in our present probing. It was deliberate that we spoke of the *situation* of identical twins, not of the objective force of identical genotypes; and so we propose to treat of the *situation* of the human clone—an immanent matter of his experience and that of those around him: this makes for an existential, not a metaphysical, discourse, and one that can entirely waive the moot question of the extent of biological determinism.

C Non-contemporaneity and the Right to Ignorance Contrary to the equality of twins, the replication of a genotype creates inherently unequal conditions for the phenotypes concerned—and an inequality deadly for the clone. Here it is where our argument substitutes a manifest right to ignorance for any hidden right (which we need neither deny nor affirm) to a unique genotype.[6] The invocation of a right to ignorance is, I believe, new to ethical theory, which has consistently deplored lack of knowledge as a deficiency in the human condition and an obstacle on the path of virtue—surely as something to be remedied to the best of our possibility. Self-knowledge above all had from Delphic days been exalted as the mark of a higher life, of which there can be only too little, never too much. Yet knowledge of the future, especially one's own, has always been tacitly excepted and the attempt to gain it by whatever means (astrology is one) disparaged—as futile superstition by the enlightened, but as sin by theologians; and in the latter case with reasons that are also philosophically sound (and, interestingly, not committed on the question of determinism per se). But from thus disputing a right or permission to know, there is still a step to asserting a right not to know; and this step we must take in the face of an entirely novel, still hypothetical, contingency which indeed constitutes the first occasion ever for activating a right which had lain dormant and hidden for lack of a call for it.

The simple and unprecedented fact is that the clone knows (or believes to know) altogether too much about himself and is known (or is believed to be known) altogether too well to others. Both facts are paralyzing for the spontaneity of becoming himself, the second also for the genuineness of others' consorting with him. It is the known donor archetype that will dictate all expectations, predictions, hopes and fears, goal settings, comparisons, standards of success and failure, of fulfillment and disappointment, for all "in the know"—clone and witnesses alike; and this putative knowledge must stifle in the pre-charted subject all immediacy of the groping quest and eventual finding "himself" with which a toiling life surprises itself for good and for ill. It is all a matter much more of supposed than real knowledge, of opinion than truth. Note that it does not matter one jot whether the genotype is really, by its own force, a person's fate: it is *made* his fate by the very assumptions in cloning him, which by their imposition on all concerned become a force themselves. It does not matter whether replication of genotype really entails repetition of life performance: the donor has been chosen with some such idea, and that idea is tyrannical in effect. It does not matter what the real relation of "nature and nurture," of genetic premise and contingent environment is in forming a person and his possibilities: their interplay has been falsified by both the subject and the environment having been "primed."[7] The trial of life has been cheated of its enticing (also frightening) openness; the past has been made to preempt the future as the spurious knowledge of it in the most intimate sphere, that of the question "who am I?" which must be a secret to the seeker after an answer and can find its answer only with the secret there as condition of the search—indeed as a condition of *becoming* what may *then be* the answer. The spurious manifestness at the beginning destroys that condition of all authentic growth. No matter whether the "knowledge" is true or false (there are reasons for saying that

in essence it is false per se), it is pernicious to the task of selfhood: existentially significant is what the cloned individual *thinks*—is compelled to think—of himself, not what he "is" in the substance-sense of being. In brief, he is antecedently robbed of the *freedom* which only under the protection of ignorance can thrive; and to rob a human-to-be of that freedom deliberately is an inexpiable crime that must not be committed even once.

One may object that the clone need not know; but this will not wash, for the secret will out. As long as it is kept from him, it means the existence of others privy to it, who know "all about him"—an intolerable situation in itself and an unsafe one to boot; not to mention the existence of archives, data banks, etc., with their chronic proneness to "leaks." But apart from being thus the object of an illicit knowledge, equally degrading in the success and the failure of keeping it from him, the clone is bound to find out for himself. For the whole point of cloning him was the distinction of his "donor," established by outstanding feats and certified by fame: so that the day must come when the (presumably not stupid) copy makes the connection between himself and the publicly enshrined original. The choice between being told early or discovering later is one between two unacceptable alternatives. The only remedy against the certainty of the second would be random cloning from the anonymous and insignificant: but then, why cloning at all?

D Knowledge, Ignorance, and Freedom We have dwelt on this, still wholly hypothetical, contingency of human cloning so extensively because its theoretical possibility has begun to fascinate biologists, which is in itself alarming; because it may be impending, and we should for once be forewarned; and because its discussion, profiting from the purity of an extreme case without analogy in the previous experience of mankind, breaks new ground in moral theory with a bearing, beyond the special case, on the whole issue of genetic engineering. Even with no agreement on the particular ethics of our deliberation, the simple principle of not experimenting on the unborn (making them means of our gaining knowledge) should interdict already the first try, even bar the "experiments" paving the way to it, for they would have to be performed on human "material" and thus already fall within the forbidden field. Those dazzled by the vision of a glorious specimen emerging from the try should also think of the inevitable failures—abnormal embryos to be discarded, or malformed beings to be guilty for—even if they lack the imagination to foresee the glorious specimen itself (perhaps most of all) become their accuser for abuse of power. But the major gain from our example for ethical theory I see in its demonstrating a *right to ignorance,* which rules the situation in even the technically flawless cases, where no mishap of any sort gives cause for more extraneous complaints. That there can be (and mostly is) too little knowledge has always been realized; that there can be too much of it stands suddenly before us in a blinding light. Obviously, two different kinds of ignorance and knowledge must be at issue. When discussing the responsibilities of technological power we have heretofore pleaded for the modesty of an ignorance conceded: tribute to a failing of ours, the doers; now we plead for the right, and its protection, to an ignorance needed: tribute to the possible freedom of others subject to our deed. In the one case, we may not know enough for doing something which only full knowledge could justify; in the other, we may know too much for doing anything with the guessing spontaneity of true deed. The ethical command here entering the enlarged stage of our powers is: never to violate the right to that ignorance which is a condition for the possibility of authentic action; or: *to respect the right of each human life to find its own way and be a surprise to itself.* How this plea for ignorance about one's presumptive being tallies with the old command of "Know thyself" is a question whose none-too-difficult answer would make it plain that the self-*discovery* enjoined in that command is precisely the process of generating one's self at once with coming to know it in the tests of life which the "knowledge" here repudiated would obstruct.

NOTES

1 Leon R. Kass, "New Beginnings in Life," in *The New Genetics and the Future of Man,* ed. Michael P. Hamilton (Grand Rapids, Mich.: Eerdman's Publishing Company, 1972), pp. 14–63, at 44f. A revised version was published in the Winter 1972 issue of *The Public Interest* under the title "Making Babies—The New Biology and the 'Old' Morality," pp. 18–56 (the "laundry list" on page 41f).

2 Nobody ever mentions Nietzsche in this connection, or Kafka, few even Beethoven or Michelangelo—a revealing symptom of the tacit eudaemonism of the whole dream: one wants his genius happy or at least serene; but most of all, edifying in his "contribution."

3 The vision of a limitless supply from each master die, to cater to this general idea and any private request (the eventuality of commercial tissue banks and an open market for their wares is by no means unthinkable)—the vision thus of many such "identical" issues, of every age from childhood to decrepitude, simultaneously walking the earth and meeting their "own" past or future in the flesh, has an outright ghostly quality about it.

4 See Kass, *op. cit.:* "Indeed, should we not assert as a principle that any so-called great man who *did* consent to be cloned should on that basis be disqualified, as possessing too high an opinion of himself and of his genes? Can we stand an increase in arrogance?"

5 The point has been raised tentatively by Leon Kass, who asks (*loc. cit.*) "Does it make sense to say that each person has a natural right not to be deliberately denied a unique genotype?" and finds parenthetically that, if this right exists, "then the deliberate production of identical human twins...must also be declared morally wrong." The main context of his question, however, is cloning. "Is one inherently injured by having been made the copy of another human being, independent of *which* human being?...Central to this matter is the idea of the dignity and worth of each human being," familiar to us from the Judaeo-Christian tradition with its "notion of the special yet equal relationship of each person to the Creator" and beautifully illustrated by the Midrash: "For a man stamps many coins in one mold and they are all alike; but the King who is king over all kings ...stamped every man in the mold of the first man, yet no one of them resembles his fellow." Kass' own conclusion is: "To answer the question posed above: We may *not* be entitled, in principle, to a unique genotype, but we *are* entitled not to have deliberately weakened the necessary supports for a worthy life. Genetic distinctiveness would seem to me to be one such support" ("New Beginnings in Life," pp. 46–47; the Judaeo-Christian reference and the Midrashic passage were omitted from the *Public Interest* version). With this cautious verdict one may well agree. My discussion in B seeks to make clear *why* a unique genotype, whether we are entitled to it or not, is not the real point at issue.

6 Kass, though not relinquishing genetic distinctiveness, takes in substance the same step when attending next to the "related problem" that the cloned individual "is saddled with a genotype that has already lived": there he touches on all the aspects—surprise,

knowledge, ignorance, and freedom—I am now going to treat as the central issue.

7 Kass: "For example, if a couple decided to clone a

Rubinstein, is there any doubt that early in life young Arthur would be deposited at the piano and 'encouraged' to play?"

ANNOTATED BIBLIOGRAPHY: CHAPTER 10

Bayles, Michael D.: *Reproductive Ethics* (Englewood Cliffs, N.J.: Prentice-Hall, 1984). Chapter 1 of this book includes sections on AID, surrogate motherhood, and *in vitro* fertilization. Chapter 2 includes sections on sex preselection, carrier screening, and prenatal diagnosis.

Chadwick, Ruth F.: "Cloning," *Philosophy* 57 (April 1982), pp. 201–210. Chadwick contends, on utilitarian grounds, that cloning could be morally justified in some circumstances.

Fletcher, John: "Moral and Ethical Problems of Prenatal Diagnosis," *Clinical Genetics* 8 (October 1975), pp. 251–257. Prominent among the ethical problems identified by Fletcher is the problem of selective abortion. He recommends a "holistic approach to ethical problems," paying attention to both principles and consequences.

Fletcher, Joseph: *The Ethics of Genetic Control: Ending Reproductive Roulette* (Garden City, N.Y.: Doubleday Anchor, 1974). In this short and very readable book, Fletcher applies his scheme of "situation ethics" to a wide range of ethical issues associated with genetics and human reproduction. Much of his discussion centers on the various reproductive technologies.

Goodman, Madeleine J., and Lenn E. Goodman: "The Overselling of Genetic Anxiety," *Hastings Center Report* 12 (October 1982), pp. 20–27. The authors contend that mass screening programs for the identification of Tay-Sachs carriers should be abandoned. Concerned to make clear the negative effects of such programs, they emphasize the problem of stigmatization and the promotion of anxiety in the Jewish community.

Hilton, Bruce, et al., eds.: *Ethical Issues in Human Genetics: Genetic Counseling and the Use of Genetic Knowledge* (New York: Plenum, 1973). This extensive work, a record of the proceedings of a 1971 symposium, provides a wealth of material on the ethical aspects of genetic counseling, genetic screening, and related areas.

Holmes, Helen B., et al., eds.: *The Custom-Made Child? Women-Centered Perspectives* (Clifton, N.J.: Humana, 1981). The material in this volume derives from a 1979 conference. There are subsections on prenatal diagnosis, sex preselection, and "manipulative reproductive technologies."

Humber, James M., and Robert F. Almeder, eds.: *Biomedical Ethics Reviews 1983* (Clifton, N.J.: Humana, 1983). Section II of this book (pp. 45–90) contains two long articles on surrogate motherhood. In "Surrogate Gestation: Law and Morality," Theodore M. Benditt concludes that "there is not much of a legal case or moral case" against surrogate gestation. In an exploratory essay, "Surrogate Motherhood: The Ethical Implications," Lisa H. Newton identifies and discusses five areas of moral concern.

Jones, Hardy: "Genetic Endowment and Obligations to Future Generations," *Social Theory and Practice* 4 (1976), pp. 29–46. Jones is concerned with the problem of providing a rationale for the obligation to provide good genetic endowments for future persons. He rejects as conceptually confused any attempt to found this obligation on a "right to a good genetic endowment." He then proceeds to sketch a suggested rationale.

Kass, Leon R.: "New Beginnings in Life." In Michael Hamilton, ed., *The New Genetics and the Future of Man* (Grand Rapids, Mich.: Eerdmans, 1972), pp. 15–63. Kass raises a number of ethical objections to both *in vitro* fertilization and cloning. His principal objections to such reproductive technologies are that (1) the experiments necessary for their development cannot be done in an ethically acceptable way, (2) they are prone to misuse, (3) their acceptance will lead to the acceptance of other undesirable developments, and (4) their employment amounts to "voluntary dehumanization," through the depersonalization of procreation. In addition, against cloning he emphasizes problems of identity and individuality. A largely parallel article by Kass is called "Making Babies: The New Biology and the 'Old' Morality," *The Public Interest* 26 (Winter 1972), pp. 18–56.

————: "'Making Babies' Revisited," *The Public Interest* 54 (Winter 1979), pp. 32–60. In arguing that the federal government should not fund research on *in vitro* fertilization and embryo transfer, Kass introduces a wide range of ethical considerations.

Lappé, Marc: "Moral Obligations and the Fallacies of 'Genetic Control,'" *Theological Studies* 33 (September 1972), pp. 411–427. Lappé reviews the state of our genetic knowledge and argues that there is no evidence of "a clear and present danger of genetic deterioration" in the human species. Accordingly, he insists that society would be unjustified in coercively intervening in reproductive decisions.

Lappé, Marc, et al.: "Ethical and Social Issues in Screening for Genetic Disease," *New England Journal of Medicine* 286 (May 25, 1972), pp. 1129–1132. In this report from a research group (associated with The Hastings Center), a set of principles for guiding the operation of screening programs is proposed.

McCormick, Richard A.: "Reproductive Technologies: Ethical Issues," *Encyclopedia of Bioethics* (1978), vol. 4, pp. 1454–1464. McCormick reviews the ethical issues associated with artificial insemination, *in vitro* fertilization, and cloning. In an extensive discussion of artificial insemination, he makes clear the views of various religious ethicists.

Powledge, Tabitha M.: "Genetic Screening," *Encyclopedia of Bioethics* (1978), vol. 2, pp. 566–573. Powledge reviews the history of genetic screening programs and attempts to clarify some of the ethical issues raised by such programs.

President's Commission for the Study of Ethical Problems in Medicine and Biomedical and Behavioral Research: *Screening and Counseling for Genetic Conditions* (1983). In this report, the Commission provides a helpful review of "the evolution and status of genetic services," then considers "ethical and legal implications." Explicit conclusions and recommendations are also announced.

Ramsey, Paul: *Fabricated Man: The Ethics of Genetic Control* (New Haven, Conn.: Yale University Press, 1970). In Chapter 1 of this short book, Ramsey provides a general discussion of the ethical and religious dimensions of genetic control. In Chapter 2, he considers cloning, raising some ethical objections. In Chapter 3, he raises objections to embracing the "prospect of man's limitless self-modification."

Tiefel, Hans O.: "Human *In Vitro* Fertilization: A Conservative View," *Journal of the American Medical Association* 247 (June 18, 1982), pp. 3235–3242. Tiefel contends that "the decisive objection to clinical uses of [*in vitro* fertilization] lies in the possible and even likely risk of greater than normal harm to offspring." He also argues that nonclinical (purely experimental) uses of *in vitro* fertilization are morally unjustifiable, because such uses fail to accord due respect to human embryos.

Tormey, Judith Farr: "Ethical Considerations of Prenatal Genetic Diagnosis," *Clinical Obstetrics and Gynecology* 19 (December 1976), pp. 957–963. Tormey attempts to clarify some of the unique difficulties associated with the moral justifiability of prenatal genetic diagnosis. She also addresses the closely related issue of the justifiability of therapeutic (genetic) abortion.

Walters, LeRoy: "Human In Vitro Fertilization: A Review of the Ethical Literature," *Hastings Center Report* 9 (August 1979), pp. 23–43. This very helpful review article identifies a host of ethical issues raised by *in vitro* fertilization and related research technology. It also provides an extensive survey of relevant ethical views.

Walters, William A. W., and Peter Singer, eds.: *Test-Tube Babies: A Guide to Moral Questions, Present Techniques and Future Possibilities* (New York: Oxford, 1982). This volume provides a very useful collection of articles on the ethical aspects of *in vitro* fertilization.

Chapter 11

Social Justice and Health-Care Policy

INTRODUCTION

In 1982 the United States spent 10.3 percent of its gross national product on health care. The money invested in health care was not the result of some overall, well-designed health-care policy, but the cumulative effect of decisions made by individuals, employers, hospitals, insurance companies, and local, state, and federal governments. Items paid for were as commonplace as aspirins and appendectomies and as technologically advanced as kidney and lung transplants. At the same time, not all the medical needs of people were met because of factors as diverse as a shortage of organ donors, the dearth of physicians in certain areas, an inadequate supply of highly specialized professionals, and inadequate funding for medical and basic research. The escalating cost of health care and the promise of continuing expensive technological advances in medicine, on the one hand, and the inequitable distribution of medical resources, on the other, give a special sense of urgency to the questions currently being asked in our society regarding the funding and provision of health care. This chapter addresses a few of these questions and explores some of the central moral issues involved.

Macroallocation Decisions

In our society, policy decisions about the allocation of health-care resources are made every day by Congress, state legislatures, health organizations, private foundations, health insurance companies, and federal, state, and local agencies. Federal money, for example, supports much of today's medical research, partly finances medical schools, and provides government-financed insurance to people over 65 (Medicare) and to those below a certain income level (Medicaid). The allocation decisions made by these kinds of groups about health-care expenditures and the distribution of health-care resources are usually called "macroallocation decisions." They are contrasted with "microallocation decisions," those made by particular hospital staffs and individual physicians about the allocation of available health-care resources.

Macroallocation Decisions—Efficiency and Equity   Two of the most important questions raised concerning macroallocation decisions are the following: (1) How much of our total economic resources should go for health care? (2) How should this total be divided among specific areas, such as biomedical research, preventive measures, "crisis care," and the production of new equipment used in treatment and diagnosis? In respect to (1), further questions must be asked about the importance of health care in relation to other goods. For example, current biomedical technology is making it possible to save and prolong lives that could not have been saved before. Is the value of prolonging these lives so great that we should adopt public policies that encourage prolongation no matter what it costs? Should other social goods, such as education, for example, receive less funding in order to prolong individual lives as long as possible? Answers here require decisions about what values society ought to encourage and about the kind of life most worth living. In respect to (2), questions must be answered regarding both the correct method for making macroallocation decisions and the values that should guide those decisions.

The initial readings in this chapter deal with these last two questions. Roger W. Evans briefly explains two methods that could be used for macroallocation decisions—cost-effectiveness analysis (CEA) and cost-benefit analysis (CBA). A CBA requires the assignment of monetary values to both costs and benefits; a CEA does not. A CEA measures benefits in nonmonetary terms such as morbidity, mortality, and quality-adjusted life years. Samuel Gorovitz, who sees a commitment to either of these methods as a commitment to the value of efficiency, analyzes the concept of efficiency to show that any use of this notion presupposes other value assumptions about desirable outcomes. Gorovitz also briefly analyzes the concept of equity (justice or fairness) and explores some of the ethical problems raised when macroallocations that maximize efficiency violate the requirements of equity or vice-versa.

Justice and Health Care

Many of the readings in this chapter, including the readings on macroallocation, assume that society has a moral obligation to make it possible for people to meet at least some of their medical needs and that it is part of the legitimate function of government to ensure some measure of access to medical care for all who need it. Does society have a moral obligation to ensure that everyone in society has access to at least some level of health care? If yes, what is the extent of the obligation? For example, should society ensure that everyone who needs and wants even the most sophisticated and specialized hospital care should have access to it? To every possible life-extending therapy? To only rudimentary care? And just what is the appropriate role of government in regard to funding and providing health care? Answering these kinds of questions requires first an understanding of various conceptions of justice and second, an understanding of the difference between the *public funding* and *public delivery* of health care.

Justice, Liberty, Equality, and the Legitimate Role of Government   Three conceptions of justice are dominant in contemporary social-political theory: libertarian, socialist, and liberal (or liberal-humanitarian). Two moral ideals, liberty and equality, are of key importance. A *libertarian* conception of justice holds liberty to be the ultimate moral ideal; a *socialist* conception of justice takes social equality to be the ultimate moral ideal; and a *liberal* conception of justice tries to combine both equality and liberty into one ultimate moral ideal.

The Libertarian Conception of Justice   On a libertarian view, individuals have certain moral rights to life, liberty, and property, which any just society must recognize and respect. These are conceived as negative rights, or rights of noninterference: If *A* has a right to *X*, no one should prevent *A* from pursuing *X* or deprive *A* of *X*, since *A* is entitled to it. (The distinction between negative and positive rights is discussed in Chapter 1.) According to a libertarian, the sole function of government is to protect the individual's life, liberty, and property against force and fraud. Everything else in society is a matter of individual responsibility, decision, and action. Providing for the welfare of those who cannot or will not provide for themselves is not a morally justifiable function of government. To make such provisions, the government would have to take from some against their will in order to give to others. This is perceived as an unjustifiable limitation on individual liberty. Individuals own their own bodies and, therefore, the labor they exert. It follows, for the libertarian, that individuals have the right to whatever income or wealth their labor can earn in a free marketplace, and no one has the right to take part of that income to provide health care for others. Robert M. Sade, in this chapter, advances a libertarian argument when he attacks the very conception of a right to medical care. On his view, rights of noninterference are the only moral rights whereas a "right to health care" would be a right to the labor of physicians and other medical professionals. No one, Sade argues, has a right to another's labor unless the latter has entered into a voluntary agreement. In rejecting the right to medical care, Sade also rejects any correlative social obligation.

The Socialist Conception of Justice   A direct challenge to libertarians comes from those who defend a socialist conception of justice. Although socialist views differ in many respects, one common element is a commitment to social equality and to government or collective measures furthering that equality. Since social equality is the ultimate ideal, limitations on individual liberty that are necessary to promote equality are seen as justified. Socialists attack the libertarian views on the primacy of liberty in at least two ways. First, they offer defenses of their ideal of social equality. These take various forms and will not concern us here. Second, they point out the meaninglessness of libertarian rights to those who lack adequate food, health care, and so forth. For those who lack the money to buy food and health care needed to sustain life, the libertarian right to life is an empty sham. The rights of liberty, such as the right to freely exchange goods, are a joke to those who cannot exercise such rights because of economic considerations. Where libertarians stress freedom from government interference, socialists stress the government's obligation to promote the welfare of its citizens by ensuring that their most important needs are met. Where libertarians stress *negative rights*, socialists stress *positive rights*. Where libertarians criticize socialism for the limitations it imposes on liberty, socialists criticize libertarianism for allowing gross inequalities among those who are "equally human."

The Liberal Conception of Justice   The liberal rejects the libertarian conception of justice since it fails to include what liberals perceive as a fundamental moral concern. Any purported conception of justice that fails to incorporate the requirement that those who have more than enough must help those in need is morally unacceptable. Like the socialist, the liberal recognizes the extent to which economic coercion in an industrial society actually limits the exercise of negative rights by those lacking economic power. Unlike the socialist, the liberal sees some of the negative rights of the libertarian as extremely important, but advocates institutions that will function to ensure certain basic liberties (e.g., freedom of speech) and yet provide for the basic needs of the disadvantaged members of society. Liberals are not opposed to all social and economic inequalities, but they disagree concerning both the morally acceptable extent of those inequalities and their correct justification. A utilitarian committed to a liberal position, for example, might hold that inequalities are justified to the extent that allowing them maximizes the total amount of good in society. A different approach is taken by an important contemporary philosopher, John Rawls, who maintains that the only justified inequalities in the distribution of primary social goods (e.g., income, opportunities) are those that will benefit everyone in society, especially the least advantaged.[1] The concern here is not with the total amount of good in a society but with the good of the least advantaged. As Gorovitz asserts in this chapter, those who suffer from debilitating diseases are, in one sense, the least advantaged among us. Social institutions that support an inegalitarian system of medical care that does not meet even the most basic needs of all the medically needy would seem to be ruled out by a Rawlsian position, even if they could be justified on utilitarian grounds.

The United States system of health care can be seen as exemplifying, however inadequately, a liberal-humanitarian conception of justice. Theoretically, we have a system in which everyone is supposed to have access to at least some minimum level of health care. Many individuals pay for their own health care, primarily through various insurance schemes including employer-employee funded plans. Medicare, Medicaid and other government programs provide funding for others. A libertarian would criticize the existing system for granting a legal right to medical care to the neediest people in our society. A socialist, on the other hand, would criticize the inequalities in the system, which result from many factors, including the unequal distribution of physicians and the lack of funding for those who can neither afford to pay for their own care nor qualify for existing government programs. Even the liberal-humanitarian would criticize as unjust a system that does not make it possible for all in society to have their basic health-care needs met.

Government Role in Health-Care Delivery: Public Funding versus Public Provision of Health Care   What part should the government in a just society play in the *delivery* of health-care services? It will be useful in answering this question to first compare the health-care delivery systems in the United States and England.[2]

The United States   The United States system is primarily a system of *private medical care*. Most general hospitals are owned by nonprofit corporations, which are sponsored by both sectarian groups and private citizens. Mental hospitals are run primarily by individual states. Some hospitals, especially those giving long-term care, are operated by some grouping of federal, state, and local governments. Most physicians are in private practice. This is true of general practitioners as well as specialists, including those affiliated with hospitals. Physicians own or rent their equipment and their offices, singly or in groups. Dentists are in the same situation. Most physicians and dentists are paid on a fee-for-service basis—so much per office visit, so much per test, and so forth. Pharmacists are usually retail store owners or employees.

Private funds pay for 62 percent of the cost of direct services. This money comes directly from individuals or from both profit-making and non-profit-making insurance companies. Most of the costs of privately funded hospital care are paid for by voluntary health insurance; the rest is paid by individuals directly. Thirty-eight percent of the cost of direct services is paid out of *public funds*—by different levels of government.

Over 70 percent of the population has some form of voluntary health insurance. In many cases this is paid largely or partly by employers' contributions. People over 65 and those below a certain income level have government-financed insurance—Medicare or Medicaid. In addition, special groups such as veterans or those suffering from specific diseases, such as cancer or tuberculosis, are directly cared for in hospitals operated by the government. Veterans' hospitals, for example, are operated by the federal government; other hospitals are supported by federal, local, and state funds. Several years ago when some members of

Congress argued for some forms of compulsory health insurance, they were advocating neither the public funding of insurance coverage nor a system of *public medical care*. On their proposals, part of the funding for this insurance would have come from employee-employer contributions. The government would have paid for insurance coverage for those who were not covered by employee-employer contributions as well as for coverage for catastrophic illnesses for everyone.

England   The English system is primarily a system of *public medical care*. In England, the entire hospital system is owned and operated by the central government. The system provides all goods and services. A very small part of the cost of this system is paid for by payroll deductions. Most of it is paid from general tax funds. In order to have access to this hospital system, individuals need only to sign up with a general practitioner, as 95 percent of the people have done.

General practitioners own or rent their offices, singly or in groups, but they are not paid on a fee-for-service system. They are paid on a *per patient* basis. The charge per patient is decided by negotiations between the government and representatives of the general practitioners. General practitioners are *not* affiliated with hospitals. Dentists, unlike general practitioners, are paid on a fee-for-service basis; here too, however, the fee is decided by negotiation with the government. Specialists are salaried employees of hospital medical staffs. Patients cannot contact them directly. They must be referred by general practitioners. Pharmacists are paid according to a schedule negotiated with the government, and prescription drugs are available for a small fee.

There is a small private sector in medicine. People who wish to do so can use this private sector. In addition, it is possible to carry a limited type of supplementary health insurance. This is carried by a small number of people.

Public or Private Medical Care?   These two examples illustrate the difference between the *public financing of private medical care* (e.g., Medicare in the United States), and the *public offering of medical care* (e.g., the socialized system in England). Those who argue that society has an obligation to make it possible for everyone to meet their health-care needs are not necessarily arguing for a socialized system of medicine. They may simply be arguing for the public financing or partial financing of medical care. One question that cannot be ignored, however, is whether a socialized system of medical care is morally preferable to a private one. On Sade's libertarian position the answer is a definite "no," since both the public funding and the public provision of health care are incompatible with the libertarian conception of justice. In this chapter, Elizabeth Telfer rejects the libertarian position and evaluates three other possible approaches regarding the government's role in the provision of health care: the liberal-humanitarian, the liberal-socialist, and the pure socialist. On her account, the liberal-socialist position is exemplified by the system currently existing in England, whereas a pure-socialist system would prohibit *all* private provision of medical care. Telfer does not attempt to provide any theoretical justification for her claim that the state should ensure that it is possible for everyone needing it to secure medical care. Rather, assuming that the state does have this function, Telfer examines some of the advantages and disadvantages of different government roles in the provision of health care. Her discussion explores both the empirical and the ethical issues involved in debates about the government's role in health-care delivery.

Policy Decisions and Individual Responsibility for Health

If public funds are used to pay for medical care, should individuals whose life-styles are not conducive to good health shoulder a higher share of the tax burden for medical care? More and more evidence supports the contention that one of the most important factors in maintaining good health is individual life-style. Heavy smoking, for example, is linked with cancer; heavy drinking with cirrhosis of the liver; obesity and inadequate exercise with cardiovascular and other diseases. In view of this, should smokers, alcohol consumers, and others indulging in high-risk behavior pay additional taxes on products such as alcohol in order to provide additional money for medical resources?

Answering this question involves complex empirical, conceptual, and ethical considerations. Relevant *empirical* questions include, for example: Do the extra medical costs necessitated by some high-risk behavior, such as heavy smoking, place a greater financial burden on society than the financial costs to society (e.g., to the social security system) of supporting octogenarians and septuagenarians whose lives may have been prolonged by healthy habits? Relevant *conceptual* issues include determining the appropriate criteria for distinguishing voluntary from involuntary high-risk behavior. Relevant *moral* issues include determining what constitutes fairness in the distribution of society's burdens and benefits. Dan E. Beauchamp, in this chapter, attacks the view that those who indulge in "voluntary" high-risk behavior should pay a greater share of the costs of funding medical care. Beauchamp contends that in holding individuals responsible for costs resulting from this kind of "voluntary" behavior, we act unjustly by ignoring the whole social context that encourages and fosters it. In Beauchamp's view, the responsibility at issue is collective and not individual. In this chapter, Robert M. Veatch examines some of the central empirical, conceptual, and moral issues raised by our growing realization of the link between individual life-styles and the need for medical care. His article includes an evaluation of Beauchamp's position.

Microallocation Decisions

Physicians and hospital staffs must often make decisions about scarce medical resources, such as artificial and natural organs. When there are too many medically qualified candidates for some medical procedure, the choice among candidates must be made on the basis of some nonmedical criteria. The central ethical question raised concerning the microallocation of scarce health-care resources is the following: When there are too many medically needy candidates for a scarce lifesaving medical resource, what criteria should be used to choose among the candidates? When the scarce resource is a part of human body tissue (e.g., a kidney, heart, or lung), another important question arises: What policies for increasing the supply are morally permitted or, perhaps, even morally required?

The procedure that focused both popular and philosophical attention on the ethical problems raised by microallocation decisions was the method of kidney dialysis. In the 1960s and early 1970s, the scarcity of artificial kidney machines, which "wash the blood" of patients who have to be connected to them at regular intervals, forced hospitals to limit access to the procedure to a very small percentage of those needing treatment. With dialysis, the patients could not only stay alive, but even live normal lives within limits. Without dialysis, they died. Selection committees, composed of doctors and community leaders, set up their own moral criteria for choosing among competing applicants. In 1972 Congress made a macroallocation decision to fund kidney dialysis for almost everyone who needed it.[3] This decision has, for the most part, eliminated the need for microallocation decisions about kidney dialysis. But several articles written by ethicists prior to the congressional ruling reveal the moral difficulties involved in the microallocation of any scarce lifesaving resource.

Both utilitarian and Kantian considerations are represented in the literature dealing with the morally correct criteria for the microallocation of scarce lifesaving medical resources. (Utilitarian and Kantian views are discussed in Chapter 1.) In this chapter, the criteria advocated by Nicholas P. Rescher are partially based on utilitarian considerations. Rescher argues for the adoption of a complex set of criteria of selection; these include such social value considerations as potential future social contributions. Rescher's approach is not completely utilitarian, however, since he maintains that equity requires the consideration of past services even in the event that these considerations cannot be justified on utilitarian grounds. The Kantian approach is exemplified in this chapter by James F. Childress and Margaret Holmgren. Childress argues for the use of a random selection procedure when the pool of medically qualified candidates exceeds the available resources. Other Kantians take a more extreme approach, maintaining that the principle of respect for persons requires that when everyone cannot be saved, no one should be. In a more recent article, Holmgren attempts to develop another Kantian position, which, contra Childress and the more extreme view noted above, allows the use of selection criteria when the pool of medically qualified candidates exceeds the available resources.

In respect to the policy issue noted earlier concerning the acquisition of human body tissue for transplantation, two major positions have been advanced. The first position advocates an *encouraged voluntarism* approach. This approach is the dominant one exemplified in current policies in the United States. In the 1960s, for example, supporters of encouraged voluntarism advocated laws that would legally enable individuals to donate organs by using "living wills" or donor cards. In 1968 the Uniform Anatomical Gift Act authorized individuals to donate their bodies, or certain organs and tissues, for transplantation or scientific research. Even where no such authorization is given, however, families of the deceased may be approached and asked to consent to the donation. Advocates of the policy of encouraged voluntarism perceive it as the policy that (1) is most compatible with respect for individual freedom and individual rights and (2) fosters the socially desirable virtues of altruism and benevolence. The second position taken on the policy issue advocates a "presumed consent" approach. Defenders of this policy argue that physicians should have state or federal authority to simply take needed tissues and organs from human bodies except when the deceased carries a card specifically prohibiting such transfers or when the family of the deceased objects. Many advocates of presumed consent, including Arthur L. Caplan in this chapter, advance utilitarian arguments, holding that presuming consent, barring evidence to the contrary, would alleviate many of the present scarcities and thus save numerous lives. Giving credence to Caplan's position is the fact that thirteen countries that follow a policy of presumed consent have come closer to meeting the demand for many organs than countries, like the United States, which primarily adopt an encouraged voluntarism approach.[4] Caplan also advances arguments against the encouraged voluntarism approach by challenging the "voluntary" nature of the consent given by bereaved families if they are cajoled, pressured, shamed, or coerced into consenting.

Although the articles on organ donation in this chapter focus primarily on correct social policy, questions can also be raised about whether *individuals* have a *moral duty* to save others' lives. This issue is especially pressing where live donors are needed (e.g., for bone marrow transplants). There may be excellent reasons, including the potentiality for abuse, for not establishing a legal duty to be a donor. Alan Meisel and Loren H. Roth bring out some of these reasons in their discussion of a recent lawsuit filed by a man against his cousin when the latter refused to donate his bone marrow. But the moral question remains: Do duties of beneficence (such as those discussed in Chapter 1) include the duty to provide another person with one's live tissue (e.g., a kidney or bone marrow) to save the latter's life?

NOTES

1 John Rawls, *A Theory of Justice* (Cambridge, Mass.: Harvard, 1970). Philosophers disagree about the correct conclusions to be drawn from Rawls's theory in regard to the distribution of medical care. See, for example, Ronald M. Green, "Health Care and Justice in Contract Theory Perspective," in Robert M. Veatch and Roy Branson, eds., *Ethics and Health Policy* (Cambridge, Mass.: Ballinger, 1976), pp. 111–126; and Norman Daniels, "Health Care Needs and Distributive Justice" in *Philosophy and Public Affairs* 10 (Spring 1981), pp. 146–179.

2 The comparisons below are based on material in Odin W. Anderson, *Health Care: Can There Be Equity?* (New York: Wiley, 1972), pp. 6–8.

3 Individuals and their dependents are entitled to Medicare, which includes a right to dialysis and kidney transplants if (1) they have paid into Social Security for twenty-four quarters or (2) they began paying into Social Security and then became disabled. This covers about 96 percent of the U.S. population eligible for dialysis and transplant (about 60,000 Americans) and costs about $2 billion annually. Individuals not covered by Medicare include many Indians who often work on reservations for each other and are not covered by Social Security. Whether they are eligible for dialysis payment depends on the policies of the Indian Health Service.

4 Countries with a presumed consent approach include Finland, Greece, Italy, Norway, Spain, and Sweden. Despite their greater success in the acquisition of other organs, these countries still have sizable waiting lists for kidney transplants, perhaps because the presumed consent laws do little or nothing to encourage hospital nurses and physicians to aid in identifying potential donors.

Macroallocation Decisions: Efficiency and Equity

Health Care Technology and the Inevitability of Resource Allocation

Roger W. Evans

Roger W. Evans, a sociologist, is clinical assistant professor in the Department of Health Services at the University of Washington in Seattle. He is also a research scientist at the Health and Population Study Center, Battelle Human Affairs Research Centers in Seattle. Evans has published numerous papers dealing with health-care issues. These include "Social and Economic Costs of Heart Transplantation," "Issues in Liver Transplantation," and "Heart Transplants and Priorities."

Evans distinguishes between the allocation and the rationing of health care, using "allocation" as synonymous with "macroallocation" and "rationing" as synonymous with "microallocation." His purpose (in this brief excerpt from a much longer two-part article) is to identify the methods that should be used to assess alternatives when resource allocations must be made. Distinguishing between cost-benefit analysis and cost-effectiveness analysis, Evans describes various types of allocation decisions and argues that in all but one case the method of choice should be cost-effectiveness analysis.

Reprinted with permission of the author and the publisher from *Journal of the American Medical Association*, vol. 249 (April 22/29, 1983), pp. 2208–2210.

ALLOCATION AND RATIONING OF
HEALTH CARE RESOURCES

Of all the resource-shortage crises this nation is expected to confront in the future, the problem of resource distribution is likely to be most acute and problematic in medicine.[2,3,9] Persons will be recognized as in need of, and then denied, benefits that the medical care provision system is capable of providing. Instead of an unidentified mass of persons being denied access to a needed resource, persons whose names have become known to the public will be declared ineligible for a treatment or service they are known to require.[10] Perhaps this scenario is inhumane, but it is undoubtedly a true representation of reality....[T]echnology now permits to be saved the lives of persons who less than a decade ago would have surely died. Moreover, technology has made it exceedingly difficult to specify at precisely what point life ceases. This has prompted Crane[1] to conclude that both medicine and law are moving toward a "social interpretation" of life.

It should come as no surprise that the resources available to meet the demand for health care are limited.[11-16] Weinstein and Stason,[13] for example, have pointed out that decisions are already being made—physicians allocate their time, hospitals ration beds, fiscal intermediaries devise reimbursement policies—all of which suggest that priorities are being set. This is not to deny the recency of problems associated with resource constraints. Even a few decades ago, before the proliferation of medical technology and the pervasiveness of insurance, constraints on health care resources were largely unheard of. In the past, the distribution of health care resources has been accomplished by implicitly limiting their availability or, when available, restricting people's access to them.[17] Thus, the concepts of availability and accessibility are critical to the problem of resource distribution.[18,19] *Rationing* is the term often used to describe the process of differentially distributing resources. *Rationing* has become a value-laden term—one that implies that persons are likely to be treated unequally.[20] *Allocation* is another term often used to describe the unequal distribution of resources. While *Webster's New World Dictionary* defines *rationing* as "a fixed portion; share; allowance," *allocation* is to "set apart for a specific purpose, to distribute according to a plan."

As suggested by the definitions of rationing and allocation, there is merit in distinguishing between the allocation and the rationing of health care resources. Others have used the terms *macroallocation* and *microallocation* to make a similar distinction.[20,21] Regardless of the terms used, it should be recognized that allocation and rationing differ with regard to temporality and level. First, allocation decisions are likely to precede rationing decisions. Second, allocation is a concept that does not apply well at the level of the individual patient but rather is more appropriately applied at the aggregate or health care program level.

In a period when resources available for health care have become increasingly constrained, attention is directed toward making the provision of health care more efficient. For example, although much attention has recently focused on the enormous cost of the End-Stage Renal Disease Program, the question being addressed is not whether patients should have their Medicare benefits cut off but rather how treatment can be provided at less cost. (The total cost of the kidney program in fiscal year 1982 is expected to be $1.8 billion. Stated in other terms, patients with end-stage renal disease (ESRD), representing <0.25% of all Medicare part B beneficiaries, now account for >9% of total Medicare part B expenditures.[22]) Thus, the debate over which type of therapy (primarily home or in-center dialysis) is least costly is again being hotly debated.[23-33] At the same time, there is renewed interest in methods by which donor organ availability can be increased.[34-37] Recent hearings once again have indicated that home dialysis is probably less costly than in-center dialysis but that kidney transplantation is a greater bargain since the cost is not only lower in the long run, but the quality of life of renal transplant recipients is generally thought to be better than that of patients receiving dialysis.[38-41] Since there seems to be room for improving the provision of ESRD services, there is only minimal consideration being given to reduction or discontinuation of benefits that patients with renal disease currently receive. Thus, resources will continue to be allocated to the End-Stage Renal Disease Program, but, in the future, greater attention will focus on the *intraprogram* allocation of resources. It will be expected that the agency responsible for administering the program, the Health Care Financing Administration (HCFA), will write regulations that will maximize the use of those resources made available to the program; that is, the HCFA will be expected to promote the least costly treatment modalities by providing incentives for their adoption.[24]

Should the resources available for health care become

increasingly constrained, the Department of Health and Human Services will be put in a position wherein *interprogram* allocation decisions will become necessary. These allocation decisions would concern how to distribute resources across health and, perhaps, social and other publicly financed programs. For example, a question might be raised as to whether the resources currently used to treat kidney disease might better be allocated to prevention activities or to a maternal and child health care program in which the derived benefits are likely to surpass those currently received by patients with ESRD.[5] In the future, competition for the available resources is likely to be great. The high cost of some new technologies might well make their widespread use prohibitive. Should this prove to be the case, it will then be necessary to consider the rationing of resources within health care programs....

Now that the federal government is at least willing to entertain the possibility of differentially allocating resources to health care programs, it inevitably will also have to entertain the need to ration health care resources once interprogram allocation has occurred and the efficient use of available resources is maximized. Should resources be constrained further and no greater efficiency attained, it would become necessary to ration the available resources to certain persons based on some uniform set of guidelines.

The foregoing raises two important questions that have yet to be addressed—(1) On what basis will resource allocation decisions be made? (2) How are criteria for rationing likely to be developed? [The balance of this paper will focus on the first question.]

ESTABLISHING CRITERIA FOR EXPLICIT RESOURCE ALLOCATION

In the medical literature, one increasingly finds medical procedures, practices, and technology subjected to what is commonly referred to as "cost-effectiveness and cost-benefit analysis."[4,12–16,42–46] Although the two are related, they are different approaches to the assessment of health practices and technology. Nevertheless, both cost-effectiveness analysis (CEA) and cost-benefit analysis (CBA) are presented as tools that can be used by the policymaker to make resource allocation decisions.

A CBA or a benefit-cost analysis requires that both costs and benefits be assigned monetary values.[47] Various methods have been proposed to measure the resource value of health care benefits. These include,

for example, expected productivity loss based on discounted future earnings at the age of death or disability.[7,48,49] The benefit-cost framework thus converts decreased deaths and disability into increases in productivity and treats them as the indirect benefits of a health intervention. Thus, indirect benefits are then combined with any direct savings in health resource consumption (the direct benefits) to yield a net value.

A CEA, unlike a CBA, does not require that both costs and benefits be assessed in monetary terms. Instead, the aim of a CEA is to measure benefits in nonmonetary terms using mortality, morbidity, or quality-adjusted life years. To this extent, a CEA preserves a sense of intangible health care benefits, whereas a CBA typically notes these but fails to assess them.[47] A CEA is particularly useful for comparing alternative approaches with the treatment of a given medical condition. For example, in-center hemodialysis, home hemodialysis, continuous ambulatory peritoneal dialysis, and kidney transplantation all represent alternative approaches to the treatment of ESRD. A CEA allows one to compare these treatments to determine which provides the greatest benefits at the least cost.[49] Similarly, heart transplantation might be compared with its alternative—traditional medical and surgical management—as approaches to the treatment of end-stage cardiac disease (ESCD).[6] Finally, percutaneous transluminal coronary angioplasty might be compared with coronary artery bypass surgery as alternative approaches to the treatment of atherosclerosis.[50,51] In all these instances, the goal of a CEA is the same—to determine which treatment approach to a given condition yields the greatest benefits at the least cost.

Both CEA and CBA can be applied on a larger scale than described herein. This application is critical to both intraprogram and interprogram allocation decisions. A CEA can be used to compare the benefits derived from various health care programs to determine which program (not specific treatment approach) yields the greatest benefit at the least cost, provided the benefits of each program being compared are expressed in the same terms (M. C. Weinstein, PhD, written communication, April 14, 1982). For example, kidney dialysis can be compared with heart transplantation to see which has the greatest benefits, with benefits expressed in terms of mortality, morbidity, or quality-adjusted life years. Weinstein describes this process as follows:

The comparison of cost-effectiveness ratios serves as a basis for allocating resources if the objective is to maximize health benefits. Thus, if kidney dialysis has a cost-effectiveness ratio (relative to the next best alternative for ESRD) of $60,000 per quality-adjusted life year, and cardiac transplant has a cost-effectiveness ratio (relative to the next best alternative for ESCD) of $50,000 per quality-adjusted life year, then resources should be allocated to the latter ahead of the former.

In this case, the proposed interprogram analysis strictly applies to health care programs. Another pertinent example might be to compare the cost of a potential maternal and child health program with the End-Stage Renal Disease Program or a potential ESCD program.

If the goal of the interprogram analysis is to compare the expenditure of health care resources with other socially desirable uses of resources, such as a public assistance program, a cost-benefit analysis is appropriate. Within the CBA framework, all expenditures and benefits are converted to monetary terms, which permits direct comparisons to be made among various diverse programs. The results of such an analysis may indicate that resources should be reallocated from social and other publicly financed programs to support health programs and vice versa. The problem with the CBA framework, however, is the requirement that human lives and quality of life be valued in dollars.[8,13]

Ultimately, the major objective of an interprogram analysis that involves only health programs or health and other publicly financed programs is to ensure that those programs that produce the greatest benefit will be those that receive the greatest support from the federal government. In this regard, it is apparent that, given limited resources and a need to allocate them in the most effective manner possible, a CEA or a CBA allows programs to be ranked according to their effectiveness or benefits derived or both. Weinstein and Stason[13] have summarized how this is done in the case of CEA as follows:

> Alternative programs or services are then ranked from the lowest value of the cost-effectiveness ratio to the highest, and selected from the top until available resources are exhausted. The point on the priority list at which the available resources are exhausted, or at which society is no longer willing to pay the price for the benefits achieved, becomes society's cut-off level of permissible cost per unit effectiveness. Application of this procedure ensures that the maximum health benefit is realized, subject to whatever resource constraint is in effect.

Thus, it is now possible to see that the allocation of health care resources and resources available to other programs as well can be subjected to a formalized set of procedures. By requiring that all assumptions are clearly stated, it is possible to perform the necessary quantitative analyses required to make the appropriate allocation decisions. In those areas where the data are least secure, it is possible to undertake sensitivity analyses to explore further the impact of decisions under differing assumptions.

Table 1 summarizes which type of analysis can be applied to various allocation decisions. If possible to achieve, a CEA should be the method of choice. In only one instance is it likely that a CEA would be inappropriate. This is in the case wherein an interprogram analysis is required to compare health program expenditures and benefits with non-health-related program expenditures and benefits. In this case, it

Table 1 Applying Cost-effectiveness and Cost-Benefit Analysis to Program Allocation Decisions

Type of decision required	Cost-effectiveness analysis (CEA)	Cost-Benefit analysis (CBA)	Method of choice
Intraprogram allocation decision	Yes	Yes	CEA
Interprogram health allocation decision	Yes	Yes	CEA
Interprogram health v. other publicly financed program allocation decision	No	Yes	CBA

would be necessary to express in monetary terms the benefits derived from the program. If an intraprogram allocation decision is required, a CEA should always be the method of choice, while, in principle, both a CBA and CEA could be applied to making an interprogram *health* allocation decision....

REFERENCES

1 Crane, D., *The Sanctity of Social Life: Physicians' Treatment of Critically Ill Patients*. New York, Russell Sage Foundation, 1975.

2 Becker, E. L., Finite resources and medical triage. *Am J Med* 1979;66:549–550.

3 Martin, S. W., Donaldson, M. C., London, C. D., et al., Inputs into coronary care during 30 years: A cost-effectiveness study. *Ann Intern Med* 1974; 81:289–293.

4 Banta, H. D., Behney, C. J., Williams, J. S., *Toward Rational Technology in Medicine*. New York, Springer Publishing Co., Inc., 1981.

5 Hiatt, H. H., Protecting the medical commons: Who is responsible? *N Engl J Med* 1975;293:235–241.

6 Evans, R. W., Economic and social costs of heart transplantation. *Heart Transplantation* 1982; 1:243–251.

7 Cooper, B. S., Rice, D. P., The economic cost of illness revisited. *Soc Secur Bull* 1976;39:21–36.

8 Mushkin, S. J., Dunlop, D. W. (eds.), *Health: What Is it Worth?: Measures of Health Benefits*. New York, Pergamon Press Ltd., 1979.

9 Rescher, N., The allocation of exotic medical lifesaving therapy. *Ethics* 1969;79:173–186.

10 Schelling, T. C., The life you save may be your own, in Chase, S. B., Jr. (ed.): *Problems in Public Expenditure Analysis*. Washington, D.C., The Brookings Institution, 1968, pp. 127–176.

11 Fuchs, V. R., *Who Shall Live?: Health, Economics, and Social Choice*. New York, Basic Books, Inc., 1974.

12 Weinstein, M. C., Stason, W. B., *Hypertension: A Policy Perspective*. Cambridge, Mass., Harvard University Press, 1976.

13 Weinstein, M. C., Stason, W. B., Foundations of cost-effectiveness analysis for health and medical practices. *N Engl J Med* 1977;296:716–721.

14 Weinstein, M. C., Fineberg, H. V., Elstein, A. S., et al., *Clinical Decision Analysis*. Philadelphia, W.B. Saunders Co., 1980.

15 Stason, W. B., Weinstein, M. C., Allocation of resources to manage hypertension. *N Engl J Med* 1977;296:732–739.

16 Weinstein, M. C.: Estrogen use in postmenopausal women—costs, risks and benefits. *N Engl J Med* 1980; 303:308–316.

17 Mechanic, D., The growth of medical technology and bureaucracy: Implications for medical care. *Milbank Mem Fund Q* 1977;55:61–78.

18 Mechanic, D., *Medical Sociology*, ed. 2. New York, Free Press, 1978.

19 Aday, L. A., Anderson, R., *Development of Indices of Access to Medical Care*. Ann Arbor, Mich., Health Administration Press, 1975.

20 Childress, J. F., Rationing of medical treatment, in Reich, W. T. (ed.): *Encyclopedia of Biomedical Ethics*. New York, Oxford University Press, 1979, pp. 1414–1419.

21 Blumstein, J. F., *Constitutional and Legal Constraints on the Rationing of Medical Resources*. Prepared for the President's Commission for the Study of Ethical Problems in Medicine and Biomedical and Behavioral Research, Nashville, Tenn., October 1981.

22 David, C. K., Hearings of the U.S. House of Representatives' Committee on Governmental Operations, Subcommittee on Intergovernmental Relations and Human Resources. *Contemp Dial* 1982;3(April):23–30.

23 Kusserow, R. P., Hearings of the U.S. House of Representatives' Committee on Governmental Operations, Subcommittee on Intergovernmental Relations and Human Resources. *Contemp Dial* 1982;59:12–18.

24 Iglehart, J. K., Health policy report: Funding the End-Stage Renal Disease Program. *N Engl J Med* 1982;306:492–496.

25 Relman, A. S., The new medical-industrial complex. *N Engl J Med* 1980;303:963–970.

26 Rettig, R. A., The politics of health cost containment: End-stage renal disease. *Bull NY Acad Med* 1980;56:115–138.

27 Rettig, R. A., *Implementing the End-Stage Renal Disease Program of Medicare*, Rand publication 2505-HCFA/HEW. Santa Monica, Calif., Rand Corporation, 1980.

28 Kolata, G. B., NMC thrives selling dialysis. *Science* 1980;208:380–382.

29 Kolata, G. B., Dialysis after nearly a decade. *Science* 1980;208:473–476.

30 Lowrie, E. G., Hampers, C. L., The success of Medicare's End-Stage Renal Disease Program: The case for profits and the private marketplace. *N Engl J Med* 1981;305:434–438.

31 Lowrie, E. G., Hampers, C. L., Proprietary dialysis and the End-Stage Renal Disease Program. *Dial Transplant* 1982;11:191–204.

32 Hampers, C. L., Hager, E. B., The delivery of dialysis services on a nationwide basis—can we afford the nonprofit system? *Dial Transplant* 1979;8:417–423, 442.

33 Blagg, C. R., Cui bono?: A response to Drs. Hampers and Hager. *Dial Transplant* 1979;8:501–502, 513.

34 Bart, K. J., Macon, E. J., Humphries, A. L., A response to the shortage of cadaveric kidneys for transplantation. *Transplant Proc* 1979;11:455–457.

35 Bart, K. J., Macon, E. J., Humphries, A. L., Jr., et al., Increasing the supply of cadaveric kidneys for transplantation. *Transplantation* 1981;31:383–387.

36 Bart, K. J., Macon, E. J., Whittier, F. C., et al., Cadaveric kidneys for transplantation. *Transplantation* 1981;31:379–382.

37 Steinbrook, R. L., Kidneys for transplantation. *J Health Polit Policy Law* 1981;6:504–573.

38 Simmons, R. G., Schilling, K. J., Social and psychological rehabilitation of the diabetic transplant patient. *Kidney Int Suppl* 1974;6:S152–S158.

39 Simmons, R. G., Klein, S. D., Simmons, R. L., *The Gift of Life: The Social and Psychological Impact of Organ Transplantation*. New York, John Wiley & Sons, Inc., 1977.

40 Poznanski, E. O., Miller, E., Salguero, C., et al., Quality of life for long-term survivors of end-stage renal disease. *JAMA* 1978;239:2343–2347.

41 Guttmann, R. D., Renal transplantation: II. *N Engl J Med* 1979;301:1038–1048.

42 Office of Technology Assessment, *The Implications of Cost-Effectiveness: Analysis of Medical Technology*. Government Printing Office, 1980.

43 Bunker, J. P., Mosteller, C. F., Barnes, B. A.: *Costs, Risks and Benefits of Surgery*. New York, Oxford University Press, 1977.

44 Fuchs, V. R., What is CBA/CEA and why are they doing this to us? *N Engl J Med* 1980;303:937–938.

45 Lashof, J. C., Behney, C., Banta, D., et al., The role of cost-benefit and cost-effectiveness analyses in controlling health care costs, in McNeil, B. J., Cravalho, E. G. (eds.), *Critical Issues in Medical Technology*. Boston, Auburn House, 1982, pp. 185–189.

46 Warner, K. E., Luce, B. R., *Cost-Benefit and Cost-Effectiveness Analysis in Health Care: Principles, Practice, and Potential*. Ann Arbor, Mich., Health Administration Press, 1982.

47 Fineberg, H. V., Pearlman, L. A., *The Implications of Cost-Effectiveness Analysis of Medical Technology: Case Study #11: Benefit-and-Cost Analysis of Medical Interventions: The Case of Cimetidine and Peptic Ulcer Disease*, stock OTA-BP-H-9(11). Office of Technology Assessment, 1981.

48 Klarman, H. E., Application of cost-benefit analysis to the health services and the special case of technologic innovation. *Int J Health Serv* 1974;4:325–352.

49 Evans, R. W., Garrison, L. P., Manninen, D., The National Kidney Dialysis and Kidney Transplantation Study: Study description, statement of objectives, and project significance. *Contemp Dial* 1982;3(June):55–58.

50 Gruntzig, A. R., Senning, A., Siegenthaler, W. E., Nonoperative dilation of coronary-artery stenosis: Percutaneous transluminal coronary angioplasty. *N Engl J Med* 1979;301:61–68.

51 Levy, R. I., Jesse, M. S., Mock, M. B., Position on percutaneous transluminal coronary angioplasty (PTCA). *Circulation* 1979;59:613.

Equity, Efficiency, and the Distribution of Health Care

Samuel Gorovitz

Samuel Gorovitz is professor of philosophy at the University of Maryland. He has served as senior scholar at the National Center for Health Services Research and has acted as consultant to the National Institutes of Health and the National

Reprinted with permission of the author and the publisher from *Philosophic Exchange* 2 (Summer 1979), pp. 3–12.

Center for Health Care Technology. Gorovitz is the author of *Doctors' Dilemmas: Moral Conflicts and Medical Care* (1982) and coeditor of *Moral Problems in Medicine* (2nd ed., 1983).

Gorovitz analyzes the concepts of efficiency and equity. He discusses the kinds of problems that can arise for health-care policy making when the goals of efficiency and equity conflict. Gorovitz then briefly presents the numerous functions served by the government in the provision of health care and the various principles that might be used in making health-care allocation decisions. Although he does not distinguish between microallocation and macroallocation decisions, Gorovitz's discussion of possible principles provides examples of both.

We spend a stunning amount on health care. That amount is soaring, and there seems no end in sight. Yet a significant portion of the American public suffers from poor health, and a different, but overlapping segment of the American public receives poor health care, or none. The vast sums that are spent on high technology medicine not only benefit just a small number of patients, but do so in ways that raise new and troubling moral dilemmas. Nearly everyone agrees that our total system of health care delivery—including the distribution of costs and benefits—is not in excellent health, in spite of our large investment in it. There is a fair amount of agreement about the symptoms, a scant amount about the diagnosis, and next to none about the treatment. Complicating our attempts to set the matter right is the fact that we want our expenditures to be used efficiently, and we believe in, or at least say we believe in, equity as a value to be reflected in the functioning of all our social arrangements. But we are not very clear about what efficiency and equity are. And we have barely begun to consider the relationship between these two notions in the specific context of our concerns about containing the costs of health care.

I will look first, and separately, at the notions of efficiency and of equity, then at the relationship between them, and finally, briefly, at a few of the issues that arise as we apply these notions to the context of health care....

When we speak of efficiency, we tend to do so in a way that reflects the usage of that notion in physics. There, efficiency is a calculable ratio—the ratio of work input to work output—which approaches the value one as a limiting and unachievable ideal. Every machine has an efficiency, every efficiency is a number, and any two efficiencies can therefore be compared. But when we leave the realm of physics, we leave its precision behind. Our talk of efficiency in other contexts

suffers from the tempting but false assumption that it is still a precise notion, quite serviceable for making quantitative decisions. And it doesn't help to dress the old notion of efficiency up in the fancy new clothes of cost-benefit or cost-effectiveness language.

Consider this illustration. Two automobile engines are mounted on a bench. Engine A, which can propel a two-ton car for twenty five miles on a gallon of gasoline, hums smoothly on the bench. Engine B, in contrast, can propel a two-ton car only for fifteen miles on one gallon of the same gasoline at the same speed. It sits on the bench, clattering and sputtering, whistling and clanging. Which is the more efficient engine? So long as it is propelling cars that is at issue, of course Engine A is more efficient. But if I tell you that I am a movie producer at work on the sound track of a film about antique automobiles, and that what I am after is the most automotive engine clatter I can get per gallon, then it is obviously Engine B that is more efficient.

The point should be clear enough. Implicit in any use of the notion of efficiency is an assumption about what the desired outcome is. In classical physics, it is well defined. In ordinary discourse about cars, it is contextually implied. In the example of the two engines, it was hidden at first, and perhaps surprising when revealed.

When we talk about efficiency in health care, what exactly are the values and the output products in terms of which—and only in terms of which—we can make sense of claims about efficiency? We have not answered this question in any adequate way. But until we can reach some clarity about what the output objectives of medical care are to be, we cannot usefully make more than impressionistic judgments about efficiency.

Lest it be thought that the answer is clear enough, except to the fussing of the philosopher, let me illustrate:

1 If an investment by a hospital in one of those infamous CAT scanners saves 30 additional lives a year, is it an efficient investment as compared with endowing a community diagnostic program that could improve the health of hundreds of people?

2 Is a multi-million dollar public immunization program an efficient investment of health care dollars if it protects most of the population at risk against an epidemic of unknown likelihood?

These questions are not clear yet hard to answer. Rather, the questions themselves are unclear. They utilize a notion of efficiency which is not well defined or well understood.

Regarding the first example: we often spend a great deal to save the life of an identified person. We are less likely to invest in the statistical saving of lives—to incur expenses that will save the lives of persons unspecified. Sometimes, however, we invest heavily to that end—for instance, in the establishment of a shock-trauma unit or in a hospital's acquisition of a hyperbaric chamber. Yet we do not make all the investments that would surely save lives, in part because we are not sure how important to us it is to save all the lives it is medically possible to save. But unless we know how much a life is worth to us, how can we judge the efficiency of an investment that saves the life? Further, it is impossible to compare such an investment with one that provides non-vital medical care without understanding what value we place on good health. It is not obvious, anyway, that we clearly favor saving a few lives over substantially improving the well-being of a large number of people.

Regarding the second example: the problem is not just one of empirical uncertainty about the epidemic and its severity. It is partly an uncertainty about how important it is to relieve anxiety and about what the prevention of symptoms is worth.

These questions, of course, are not for philosophy to answer alone. They are problems of social decision, the answers to which must be fashioned by all those whose risk and whose resources are involved. Further, the question of what to take as the appropriate objective in terms of which to evaluate efficiency is itself a question of value on which considerations of equity can have bearing.

It is time, then, to turn to equity—what common usage and the dictionary both take as equivalent to justice, fairness, doing the right thing. There are various competing views of what constitutes equity. One prominent view is that equity is or requires equality. What might that mean in the context of the distribution of health care? There are at least these choices:

(1) *Equality in the dollar expenditure on each individual.* This interpretation makes little sense. Some lucky people just don't need health care; they thrive until they die, and there isn't anything to spend their health care dollars on. Perhaps we could approximate to equal expenditure by adopting a plan invented, I think, by Dan Callahan, whereby each person is allowed some fixed amount—say $100,000—over his lifetime, with a refund of any unused portion to go to his estate.

(2) *Equality in the state of health of each individual.* The problem here is that this sort of equality is impossible no matter what we spend or how. Some people enjoy robust health, some are sickly or worse all their lives, and we have only limited leverage on the natural distribution of physiological characteristics.

(3) *Equality in the maximum to which each individual is benefited.* This would mean that each person has equal access to medical care up to some limit, to be drawn on as needed, with no pretense of equalizing actual expenditures. We may find this becoming a position to be taken seriously, though the question of what sorts of limits should be set is just beginning to rear its vexsome head.

(4) *Equality in the treatment of like cases.* Under this interpretation, a national health service, for example, could have a program in renal dialysis, treating as needed all medically qualified cases. At the same time, it could refuse to treat cases of hemophilia at all—arguing that such an exclusion was necessary on grounds of economy, and going on to claim that the health care was wholly equitable, thoroughly equal, in the sense that each person had equal claim on such treatments as were made available. Both the patient with kidney failure and the hemophyliac would have equal access to dialysis as needed according to this plan.

So if we interpret equity as equality in some sense or other, we immediately face problems of interpretation. Each interpretation, moreover, is problematic. It is not clear, nor unchallenged, that any sort of egalitarian interpretation of equity is tenable. First, there is the problem of scarcity. There will always be medical treatments or supplies in short supply—at least the ones that have just been developed. How are we to achieve equality here, except by a lottery that provides not equal treatment, but an equal *chance* of getting treatment? Second, there is the problem of entitlement. Consider the research scientist who has devoted his life to the search for a vaccine that is effective against a disease that has slaughtered his ancestors for generations. Now he has the vaccine, but initially in short supply. Are we to deny his claim on a dose for himself or his child because that would violate our commitment to equal access? Many would argue that he has an entitlement that sets him apart from the rest; that to deny it would itself be to abandon our commitment to equity.

So equity, like efficiency—although for different reasons—is an elusive notion. We rely on them both in the rhetoric that surrounds the defense of policy, and we rely on our intuitions about them in the setting and advocacy of policy. But when it comes to a specific case of defending a policy under careful scrutiny, these notions slip away from precise clarification. What, then, is to be said for them?

One way to interpret the notion of efficiency—a way that seems to correspond well with the way we actually use it—is as a measure of the extent to which an action produces good—where good is itself defined as the satisfaction of human needs and desires. That action, program or policy then is the most efficient which, at a given level of expenditure, is the one among all available alternatives that maximizes good. Comparative judgments are then possible to the degree to which we have a clear conception of what is good, and also a clear account of what consequences will flow from the various acts we contemplate.

This is classical utilitarianism, and moral philosophy for the last century, like economics and Anglo-American legislative policy over the same century, has been dominated by the influence of utilitarian theory. The objections to it are numerous and powerful, but its appeal is nonetheless unsurpassed as an account of what we ought to do, individually and collectively, and why. This appeal rests ultimately in the simple fact that we do care about the satisfaction of human wants and needs—about the production of good—and we therefore want our efforts and our resources to produce as much of it as possible. This want translates into our concern with efficiency.

Equity is a more obviously moral notion. It means justice, fairness in our dealings with one another. But how are we to understand what is just? Here, again, there is a historical tradition of thought to guide us. From the ancient Pythagorean rules of conduct and the ten commandments, through the austere moral strictures of Immanuel Kant, to an extensive body of antiutilitarian moral theory, we have nurtured and sustained a sense that some kinds of actions are right and other kinds are wrong, regardless of the consequences they lead to or the ends they serve, simply because of the kinds of acts they are. Thus we condemn the framing of an innocent man, no matter how great the social benefits of the conviction might be, just as we condemn torture, slavery, and other moral abominations without regard to the role they may play in the larger pursuit of noble ends. Or, at least, all of us do except the most intransigent of the hard-core utilitarians. And we do so not because such actions strike us as inefficient in the production of good, but because they violate our sense of justice.

Providing an account of that sense of justice is no small task. But it does seem that Mill's view that justice is derivative from considerations of utility, of efficiency in the production of good results, is in decline. Recent moral philosophy has shown reluctance to consider justice as a derivative concept. Rather, it has come to be largely viewed as a dimension of morality that is separate from and independent of utility, and which can therefore be in conflict with it.

Efficiency as a value thus reflects our concern with the maximum production of good, and equity as a value reflects our concern with doing what is just or fair, regardless of its efficiency. In an ideal world, these values would never be in conflict, but in fact the conflict is notorious. We may want both equity and efficiency, but at least sometimes one may be purchased only at the cost of the other.

To see the conflict between equity and efficiency etched sharply, consider a hypothetical example. Real cases, if they are interesting, involve complexity of the sort that can obscure a simple point; I use an artificial example, just as the physicist does when he speaks of the frictionless plane. Imagine that we are all on a desert island, struggling to survive. Most of us cluster into a village, but a few set out for remote parts of the island where the fishing is perhaps better. There is little rain, so drinking water is a constant problem; there is just marginally enough to keep us alive. Suddenly, a rescue mission flies overhead. Using remote sensing technology, they assess our situation. They depart, then return with a large crate which they parachute to the island. We open the crate and find a tank truck filled with pure water and a message that the water is for all the people on the island. How shall we distribute the water?

There are 100 people on the island; 1000 gallons in the tank. Specify whatever distribution you think is equitable. You can favor ten gallons per person, or more for those who work more, or most for those in positions of authority—it doesn't matter which distribution you favor as most equitable. For you now discover that the tank truck has a steam engine. In order to move it around at all you have to use water. And the conflict between efficiency and equity—however you construe equity—becomes plain. Assuming that each gallon of water is as valuable to each person as any other gallon—that is, there is no diminishing marginal utility of water in the range of quantities at issue—then the most efficient thing to do is not use the engine at all. Let water go to those who come for it—to the able-bodied who live nearby. The weak, the ill, the aged, the distant will get none, but since there is linearity in the good produced by incremental allocations of water, their deprivation is of no consequence, for we produce more good this way than by spending some of the water on operating the delivery truck. It would be hard to argue that justice is served, however, especially given that the water was sent to all the people on the island.

So equity costs something. In some situations the most efficient action and the most equitable action are not the same. Some balance must then be struck between the two competing values. For one who places justice above all, considerations of efficiency may legitimately come into play, but only after justice is fully served. This position would be exemplified by the egalitarian who insisted on an equal distribution of water to all island inhabitants, even if most of the water were used by delivering it. But he could still be seriously concerned with mapping the best route, in order to conserve water, and thus to distribute it most efficiently within the constraints of equity. He would be the mirror image of the complete utilitarian who advocated making the decision solely on the grounds of efficiency and therefore leaving the truck in place. For many people, myself among them, some middle ground is best—some approximation to complete equity, tempered by an unwillingness to let efficiency fall too low.

I have not shown, of course, that equity and efficiency are always in conflict—only that they are competing values in some situations. It is a separate question whether the kinds of situations that arise in regard to the distribution of health care are of the sort in which equity and efficiency are in conflict. But the answer is apparent; one example should suffice to show that the conflict is present.

Assume that considerations of equity—of justice or fairness in the treatment of persons—require that each individual be free to choose the geographical location in which he or she will seek work. Assume further that considerations of equity require that in an affluent industrialized nation like ours a minimally decent level of health care should be available to all citizens, including those in poor, rural communities. Finally, assume that our concern with containing the costs of health care places limits on the amount of financial incentive we can provide to induce physicians to practice in otherwise undesirable locations. Then the conflict is evident: we can resolve the problem only by some sacrifice in the freedom of the physician, the health care of the poor, or the pocketbook of the public. And any such sacrifice will be to some extent a concession with respect either to equity or efficiency.

Having argued that equity and efficiency, however we interpret them, are different and competing values, I want to turn next to some further questions of health care distribution and cost containment.

Since health is not the only thing we care about—nor should it be—we want to have substantial resources available for other expenditures. It may, therefore, seem obvious that we ought to decide how much to spend on health care, and also how it should be spent. It would be a mistake, however, to think that any such determination takes place in any systematic or comprehensive way. Rather, what we spend on health care is the total of the expenditures in diverse sectors ranging from the individual buying a bottle of useless cold pills or a much needed bandage to the government building a useless new 21 million dollar Navy hospital in New Orleans or purchasing essential medical care for a large class of people in need. There simply is no coherent, organized or regulated arrangement regarding how much is spent, what it is spent on, or how care is distributed. Nor is there much effective coordination among the various sectors of health care activity. Therefore there is no overall determination of a total level of expenditure—indeed, we know only approximately what the total expenditure is. And there is no systematic control over the ways in which the funds are spent. Any approach to health care distribution or cost containment must therefore be piecemeal, addressing individual aspects of the health care landscape one locale at a time.

If we are speaking of a single individual or family, it is relatively easy to say how to keep costs down: live prudently, carry a good medical insurance program, and be an alert, informed, active and critical consumer of health care services. Then, most probably, the costs of health care will be reasonably well contained. But that by itself will not relieve the rising costs associated with high technology medicine nor will it keep insurance costs from rising beyond the reach of increasingly many people. For the problem is not fundamentally one of individual choice and action; it is one of a cumulative financial effect that can only be addressed, however piecemeal, by collective response—that is, as a matter of public policy.

Governmental expenditure on health care is approximately 75 billion dollars a year, and the government role is exceedingly diverse. The government functions:

1 *As direct provider of care.* Example: the Veterans Administration's system of nearly 200 hospitals, for which the 1978 fiscal year budget appropriation for medical care is over 4.7 billion dollars.

2 *As provider of medical insurance.* Example: the Medicare and Medicaid programs, through which the government is the largest provider of medical insurance in the country.

3 *As the operator of support systems for health care research and delivery.* Example: the National Center for Disease Control in Atlanta.

4 *As a medical educator.* Example: the Uniformed Services University of the Health Sciences.

5 *As a supporter of medical education.* Example: capitation grants to medical, nursing, and allied health professional schools.

6 *As a sponsor and operator of medical research programs.* Example: the National Institutes of Health.

7 *As a regulator of persons, substances, and institutions.* Example: rulings by the Food and Drug Administration. And finally,

8 *As an indirect influence on health care.* Example: OSHA regulations, automobile safety standards, EPA rulings, and the like.

Each of these functions is itself diverse, and each thus provides a complex context of expenditure wherein questions of efficiency and of equity can be raised. Further, the government's regulatory and legislative powers will play a crucial role in any collective response to the problems associated with cost containment. So the government is the central figure in the story.

Any consideration of containing costs must deal with problems of distribution and supply, among others. Basically, there are just two possibilities for containing costs: one can limit or reduce service, or one can limit or reduce the cost for the average instance of service. One way to reduce or limit service is to distribute it only to a limited portion of those cases where a need is present.

The reduction of service is also possible, however, through the redefinition of need. We can increase or diminish the claims for health care services by broadening or narrowing the definitions of illness, without thereby affecting anyone medically. If our clinics are too crowded, we can thin the crowds by a decision that although people with dandruff, obesity, bizarre noses, and lackadaisical libido may have problems, they are not necessarily sick, and do not qualify to make claims on the health care facilities. The closer we move toward publicly funded health care or health care insurance, the more critical it will become to clarify what is to count as illness for purposes of claiming entitlement to health care resources.

Now consider the notion of limiting costs by leaving some needs unmet. Recall specifically those inevitably cited patients with kidney failure. In the early days of renal dialysis, we had a classic problem of allocating limited vital resources. There were not enough machines to go around. That problem is now essentially past, but a similar situation exists with respect to live organ transplants. Many more patients are medically qualified to receive transplanted kidneys than can be accommodated given the present rate of supply. How shall we respond to this situation?

Various principles of distribution come to mind. Consider:

1 *To each according to his means.* This is a free market policy. Kidneys go to those who can afford them, with the price determined by market phenomena.

2 *To each according to his social utility.* This is roughly the approach adopted in the original dialysis selection in Seattle, where an assessment was made of the social utility of the applicants. It is the utilitarian approach, the one that seeks to maximize efficiency.

3 *To each according to his entitlement or status.* A policy like this might favor veterans, landowners, members of the party in power, or other groups or individuals making special claims.

4 *To each according to his luck.* This is the policy of the strict egalitarian: count every medically qualified individual as an equal, and draw lots to determine who will get the kidneys.

5 *To each according to his need.* To implement this policy, of course, requires an increase in the supply of the resource the scarcity of which presents the problem in the first place.

The choice among these distributional policies will be difficult because our values do not all point to a single choice. In particular, we are sympathetic both to considerations of social utility and to the desirability of meeting everyone's need where we have the ability to meet anyone's. So there is a pressure to increase service to meet demand, thereby to eliminate some of the conflict we feel, and that yields pressure to increase the supply of transplantable kidneys while keeping a lid on the costs. Is there any possibility of doing that?

ABC news reported in the autumn of 1978 that recent legislation in France makes a person's organs available at death for transplantation unless the individual has exercised a prior option of objection. Should we adopt a similar policy? The government could go a step beyond France, requiring organ donation without option of prior objection. Or it could go two steps beyond, drafting people into a national organ bank battalion. These people might be selected if they are in good health, late in life and of low social utility. They would then be required to donate one kidney, with the rest of their organs to be taken at death. The French policy is moderate in the context of what is possible. Still, it is seen as overly coercive by many critics. Milder measures include a proposal made recently by an officer of the American Kidney Foundation, who suggested that each individual agree or decline at the time of registration with the Social Security Administration. But Sidney Wolfe, of the Health Research Group, responded that any such association with a government agency that provides vital support services could be implicitly coercive. Still milder measures are available, however. The government could decide to support the present system of total voluntarism with a campaign aimed at persuading large numbers of people to become donors. Or the government could leave the matter wholly to the workings of the private sector.

For an illuminating comparison, consider briefly a different problem. We provide military manpower in various ways at various times depending not only on our national security needs but also on our moral priorities. The draft, favored in wartime, is the most efficient way to provide the manpower, especially combined with selective deferment. The government conscripts soldiers, paying what it decides to pay—

thereby containing payroll costs, and exempting those whose greater social utility lies elsewhere—thereby maximizing social efficiency. The principle is: *from each according to his usefulness.* But this policy is criticized on grounds of equity. It sends the poor and underprivileged off to battle, favoring further the already favored, while the benefit of national defense—that is, the security of the nation—is equally enjoyed by all. Moved by conscience to provide military manpower more equitably, we change to a lottery. Now the principle is: *from each according to his luck in an equal risk lottery.* But this policy has critics, for it obliterates the freedom of the unlucky draftee, as well as reducing efficiency by drafting some who would be more usefully placed elsewhere. So out of respect for personal liberty, we move to a volunteer service. *From each according to his choice.* Freedom is honored, but the costs soar because the incentive to join is not great for most people in a reasonably sound economy. And now we hear lamentation from the Pentagon: we have liberty, but the price is getting beyond our reach, and the efficiency is low. So once again we may move to another system, striking a different balance among the competing values of efficiency, equality and liberty.

A parallel situation exists in regard to kidney supply and distribution. The various plans clearly exhibit different degrees of respect for different values. A plausible utilitarian case can be made for the very coercive plans to increase supply, and as we move through the shadings of coercion from a draft or universal requirement, to coercion of varying degrees, to persuasion, education, and voluntarism, the level of efficiency seems to drop. At the same time, the level of equity in the treatment of persons seems to rise, especially if we take equity to require respect for personal autonomy and the bodily integrity of individual persons. But now a curious bind seems to emerge. For if the most equitable policy for distribution requires meeting the needs of all patients who require transplants, that policy also seems to require, as a practical matter, a highly efficient policy for obtaining transplantable kidneys. Yet the policies that seem most efficient in this regard seem least equitable from the point of view of potential donors. Thus we see equity not only in opposition to efficiency, but to equity itself.

We need to sustain a systematic inquiry into the considerations of equity and efficiency in health care, and as part of that process we need a more sophisticated understanding of how to assess the value of the outcomes that health care provides. This is particularly important as our concern with cost containment heightens, for although the crisis in health care costs is not primarily a government spending crisis, only the government is in any position to get real leverage on the currents of supply and distribution of health care goods and services. And when we look to government to solve large scale social problems, we should remember that we are looking to a ponderous and unpredictable force, mighty in itself, yet subject to the shifting drifts of political sentiment. We are well advised to understand what we are asking it to do.

My own view is that we have a tendency to weigh efficiency too heavily in its conflict with equity, in part—but only in part—because of the difficulty of measuring the value of considerations of equity. Perhaps the basic mistake is to assume that the kind of assessment needed can be *measurement* at all, as opposed to the informed and sensitive judgment that lies at the heart of leadership and statesmanship.

One final example: imagine a large family next door. They treat all their children well except the youngest. That one is neglected, disdained—an outcast. We would, I think, judge that family harshly, accepting as a mark of its degree of decency the way it treats the one whom it treats least well. John Rawls, in *A Theory of Justice*, argues that equity requires us to use a similar criterion in judging social institutions. The keystone of his theory is respect for liberty conjoined with concern for the least advantaged among us. Those who suffer from debilitating illness or handicap are, in an important sense, the least advantaged among us, and we

neglect them at our own moral risk. There is no way to assign a dollar value to such considerations, and they may in tragic circumstances even be defeasible on grounds of excessive cost. Nonetheless they have a force that should not be underestimated. It may be useful to keep Rawls' criterion in mind as a *prima facie* constraint on our pursuit of efficiency. That constraint would prevent us from assessing health care policies in a purely utilitarian way or in a way that excludes the interests of any segment of the population. It would not by itself determine what policies we should set, but by narrowing the range of choices it would play some role in the process. That larger process of setting public policies for health care that are equitable and affordable will be more complex even than the systems of supply and distribution, and it would be futile to expect any stable resolution of policy to be achieved. Rather, there must be a process of assessment and reassessment in the public and political forums—an on-going exchange of which the perspectives of philosophy are an essential part.

ACKNOWLEDGMENT

I am grateful to Norman Weissman, Ruth Macklin, and Norman Daniels for criticisms of an earlier draft of this essay. They are, of course, wholly innocent in respect to its remaining faults. I am also grateful to the Hastings Center, under whose auspices this work was done with the support of a grant from the National Center for Health Services Research, for permission to provide this essay to the Philosophic Exchange.

Justice and Health Care

Medical Care as a Right: A Refutation

Robert M. Sade

Robert M. Sade, whose speciality is thoracic surgery, is associate professor of thoracic surgery at the Medical University of South Carolina, Charleston. His published articles include "Concept of Rights: Philosophy and Application to Health Care" and "Scarce Medical Resources."

In rejecting the claim that health care is a right, Sade advances his own position on rights. He maintains that the primary right, from which three corollary rights

Reprinted by permission of the *New England Journal of Medicine*, vol. 285, pp. 1288–1292; 1971.

follow, is the right to one's own life. Appealing to these rights, conceived as natural rights of noninterference, Sade advances arguments to support his claim that it would be immoral to enact laws making health care a legal right.

The current debate on health care in the United States is of the first order of importance to the health professions, and of no less importance to the political future of the nation, for precedents are now being set that will be applied to the rest of American society in the future. In the enormous volume of verbiage that has poured forth, certain fundamental issues have been so often misrepresented that they have now become commonly accepted fallacies. This paper will be concerned with the most important of these misconceptions, that health care is a right, as well as a brief consideration of some of its corollary fallacies.

RIGHTS—MORALITY AND POLITICS

The concept of rights has its roots in the moral nature of man and its practical expression in the political system that he creates. Both morality and politics must be discussed before the relation between political rights and health care can be appreciated.

A "right" defines a freedom of action. For instance, a right to a material object is the uncoerced choice of the use to which that object will be put; a right to a specific action, such as free speech, is the freedom to engage in that activity without forceful repression. The moral foundation of the rights of man begins with the fact that he is a living creature: he has the right to his own life. All other rights are corollaries of this primary one; without the right to life, there can be no others, and the concept of rights itself becomes meaningless.

The freedom to live, however, does not automatically ensure life. For man, a specific course of action is required to sustain his life, a course of action that must be guided by reason and reality and has as its goal the creation or acquisition of material values, such as food and clothing, and intellectual values, such as self-esteem and integrity. His moral system is the means by which he is able to select the values that will support his life and achieve his happiness.

Man must maintain a rather delicate homeostasis in a highly demanding and threatening environment, but has at his disposal a unique and efficient mechanism for dealing with it: his mind. His mind is able to perceive, to identify percepts, to integrate them into concepts, and to use those concepts in choosing actions suitable to the maintenance of his life. The rational function of mind is volitional, however; a man must *choose* to think, to be aware, to evaluate, to make conscious decisions. The extent to which he is able to achieve his goals will be directly proportional to his commitment to reason in seeking them.

The right to life implies three corollaries: the right to select the values that one deems necessary to sustain one's own life; the right to exercise one's own judgment of the best course of action to achieve the chosen values; and the right to dispose of those values, once gained, in any way one chooses, without coercion by other men. The denial of any one of these corollaries severely compromises or destroys the right to life itself. A man who is not allowed to choose his own goals, is prevented from setting his own course in achieving those goals and is not free to dispose of the values he has earned is no less than a slave to those who usurp those rights. The right to private property, therefore, is essential and indispensable to maintaining free men in a free society.

Thus, it is the nature of man as a living, thinking being that determines his rights—his "natural rights." The concept of natural rights was slow in dawning on human civilization. The first political expression of that concept had its beginnings in 17th and 18th century England through such exponents as John Locke and Edmund Burke, but came to its brilliant debut as a form of government after the American Revolution. Under the leadership of such men as Thomas Paine and Thomas Jefferson, the concept of man as a being sovereign unto himself, rather than a subdivision of the sovereignty of a king, emperor or state, was incorporated into the formal structure of government for the first time. Protection of the lives and property of individual citizens was the salient characteristic of the Constitution of 1787. Ayn Rand has pointed out that the principle of protection of the individual against the coercive force of government made the United States the first moral society in history.[1]

In a free society, man exercises his right to sustain his own life by producing economic values in the form of goods and services that he is, or should be, free to exchange with other men who are similarly free to trade with him or not. The economic values produced, however, are not given as gifts by nature, but exist only by virtue of the thought and effort of individual men. Goods and services are thus owned as a consequence of the right to sustain life by one's own physical and mental effort.

If the chain of natural rights is interrupted, and the right to a loaf of bread, for example, is proclaimed as primary (avoiding the necessity of earning it), every man owns a loaf of bread, regardless of who produced it. Since ownership is the power of disposal,[2] every man may take his loaf from the baker and dispose of it as he wishes with or without the baker's permission. Another element has thus been introduced into the relation between men: the use of force. It is crucial to observe who has initiated the use of force: it is the man who demands unearned bread as a right, not the man who produced it. At the level of an unstructured society it is clear who is moral and who immoral. The man who acted rationally by producing food to support his own life is moral. The man who expropriated the bread by force is immoral.

To protect this basic right to provide for the support of one's own life, men band together for their mutual protection and form governments. This is the only proper function of government: to provide for the defense of individuals against those who would take their lives or property by force. The state is the repository for retaliatory force in a just society wherein the only actions prohibited to individuals are those of physical harm or the threat of physical harm to other men. The closest that man has ever come to achieving this ideal of government was in this country after its War of Independence.

When a government ignores the progression of natural rights arising from the right to life, and agrees with a man, a group of men, or even a majority of its citizens, that every man has a right to a loaf of bread, it must protect that right by the passage of laws ensuring that everyone gets his loaf—in the process depriving the baker of the freedom to dispose of his own product. If the baker disobeys the law, asserting the priority of his right to support himself by his own rational disposition of the fruits of his mental and physical labor, he will be taken to court by force or threat of force where he will have more property forcibly taken from him (by fine) or have his liberty taken away (by incarceration). Now the initiator of violence is the government itself. The degree to which a government exercises its monopoly on the retaliatory use of force by asserting a claim to the lives and property of its citizens is the degree to which it has eroded its own legitimacy. It is a frequently overlooked fact that behind every law is a policeman's gun or soldier's bayonet. When that gun and bayonet are used to initiate violence, to take property or to restrict liberty by force, there are no longer any rights, for the lives of the citizens belong to the state. In a just society with a moral government, it is clear that the only "right" to the bread belongs to the baker, and that a claim by any other man to that right is unjustified and can be enforced only by violence or the threat of violence.

RIGHTS—POLITICS AND MEDICINE

The concept of medical care as the patient's right is immoral because it denies the most fundamental of all rights, that of a man to his own life and the freedom of action to support it. Medical care is neither a right nor a privilege: it is a service that is provided by doctors and others to people who wish to purchase it. It is the provision of this service that a doctor depends upon for his livelihood, and is his means of supporting his own life. If the right to health care belongs to the patient, he starts out owning the services of a doctor without the necessity of either earning them or receiving them as a gift from the only man who has the right to give them: the doctor himself. In the narrative above substitute "doctor" for "baker" and "medical service" for "bread." American medicine is now at the point in the story where the state has proclaimed the nonexistent "right" to medical care as a fact of public policy, and has begun to pass the laws to enforce it. The doctor finds himself less and less his own master and more and more controlled by forces outside of his own judgment....

Any doctor who is forced by law to join a group or a hospital he does not choose, or is prevented by law from prescribing a drug he thinks is best for his patient, or is compelled by law to make any decision he would not otherwise have made, is being forced to act against his own mind, which means forced to act against his own life. He is also being forced to violate his most fundamental professional commitment, that of using his own best judgment at all times for the greatest benefit of his patient. It is remarkable that this principle has never been identified by a public voice in the medical profession, and that the vast majority of doctors in this country are being led down the path to civil servitude, never knowing that their feelings of uneasy foreboding have a profoundly moral origin, and never recognizing that the main issues at stake are not those being formulated in Washington, but are their own honor, integrity and freedom, and their own survival as sovereign human beings.

SOME COROLLARIES

The basic fallacy that health care is a right has led to several corrollary fallacies, among them the following:

That health is primarily a community or social rather than an individual concern.[3] A simple calculation from American mortality statistics[4] quickly corrects that false concept: 67 per cent of deaths in 1967 were due to diseases known to be caused or exacerbated by alcohol, tobacco smoking or overeating, or were due to accidents. Each of those factors is either largely or wholly correctable by individual action. Although no statistics are available, it is likely that morbidity, with the exception of common respiratory infections, has a relation like that of mortality to personal habits and excesses.

That state medicine has worked better in other countries than free enterprise has worked here. There is no evidence to support that contention, other than anecdotal testimonials and the spurious citation of infant mortality and longevity the other hand, a good deal of evidence to the contrary.[5,6]

That the provision of medical care somehow lies outside the laws of supply and demand, and that government-controlled health care will be free care. In fact, no service or commodity lies outside the economic laws. Regarding health care, market demand, individual want, and medical need are entirely different things, and have a very complex relation with the cost and the total supply of available care, as recently discussed and clarified by Jeffers et al.[7] They point out that "'health is purchaseable', meaning that somebody has to pay for it, individually or collectively, at the expense of foregoing the current or future consumption of other things." The question is whether the decision of how to allocate the consumer's dollar should belong to the consumer or to the state. It has already been shown that the choice of how a doctor's services should be rendered belongs only to the doctor: in the same way the choice of whether to buy a doctor's service rather than some other commodity or service belongs to the consumer as a logical consequence of the right to his own life.

That opposition to national health legislation is tantamount to opposition to progress in health care. Progress is made by the free interaction of free minds developing new ideas in an atmosphere conducive to experimentation and trial. If group practice really is better than solo, we will find out because the success of groups will result in more groups (which has, in fact, been happening); if prepaid comprehensive care really is the best form of practice, it will succeed and the health industry will swell with new Kaiser-Permanente plans. But let one of these or any other form of practice become the law, and the system is in a straight jacket that will stifle progress. Progress requires freedom of action, and that is precisely what national health legislation aims at restricting.

That doctors should help design the legislation for a national health system, since they must live with and within whatever legislation is enacted. To accept this concept is to concede to the opposition its philosophic premises, and thus to lose the battle. The means by which nonproducers and hangers-on throughout history have been able to expropriate material and intellectual values from the producers has been identified only relatively recently: the sanction of the victim.[8] Historically, few people have lost their freedom and their rights without some degree of complicity in the plunder. If the American medical profession accepts the concept of health care as the right of the patient, it will have earned the Kennedy-Griffiths bill by default. The alternative for any health professional is to withhold his sanction and make clear who is being victimized. Any physician can say to those who would shackle his judgment and control his profession: I do not recognize your right to my life and my mind, which belong to me and me alone; I will not participate in any legislated solution to any health problem.

In the face of the raw power that lies behind government programs, nonparticipation is the only way in which personal values can be maintained. And it is only with the attainment of the highest of those values—integrity, honesty and self-esteem—that the physician can achieve his most important professional value, the absolute priority of the welfare of his patients.

The preceding discussion should not be interpreted as proposing that there are no problems in the delivery of medical care. Problems such as high cost, few doctors, low quantity of available care in economically depressed areas may be real, but it is naïve to believe that governmental solutions through coercive legislation can be anything but shortsighted and formulated on the basis of political expediency. The only long-range plan that can hope to provide for the day after tomorrow is a "non-system"—that is, a system that proscribes the imposition by force (legislation) of any one group's conception of the best forms of medical care. We must identify our problems and seek to solve them by experimentation and trial in an atmosphere of freedom from compulsion. Our sanction of anything less will mean the loss of our personal values, the death of our profession, and a heavy blow to political liberty.

NOTES

1 Rand, A., Man's rights, Capitalism: The unknown ideal. New York, New American Library, Inc., 1967, pp. 320–329.

2 Von Mises, L., Socialism: An Economic and Sociological Analysis. New Haven: Yale University Press, 1951, pp. 37–55.

3 Millis, J. S., Wisdom? Health? Can society guarantee them? N Engl J Med 283:260–261, 1970.

4 Department of Health, Education, and Welfare, Public Health Service: Vital Statistics of the United States 1967, Vol II, Mortality. Part A. Washington, D.C., Government Printing Office, 1969, pp. 1–7.

5 Financing Medical Care: An appraisal of foreign programs. Edited by H. Shoeck. Caldwell, Idaho, Caxton Printers, Inc., 1962.

6 Lynch, M. J., Raphael, S. S., Medicine and the State. Springfield, Illinois, Charles C. Thomas, 1963.

7 Jeffers, J. R., Bognanno, M. F., Bartlett, J. C., On the demand versus need for medical services and the concept of "shortage." Am J Publ Health 61:46–63, 1971.

8 Rand, A., Atlas Shrugged. New York, Random House, 1957, p. 1066.

Justice, Welfare, and Health Care

Elizabeth Telfer

Elizabeth Telfer teaches in the Department of Moral Philosophy at the University of Glasgow (Scotland). She is the coauthor of *Respect for Persons* (1970) and *Caring and Curing: A Philosophy of Medicine and Social Work* (1980) and the author of *Happiness* (1980).

Telfer discusses the pros and cons of four possible systems of health-care distribution: (1) laissez faire, (2) liberal-humanitarian, (3) liberal-socialist, and (4) pure socialist. She analyzes each system both for its content and for the views of its antagonists and protagonists. Her purpose is to bring out some of the principles at issue in any discussion of socialized medicine.

In this paper I shall be examining some of the broad principles which are relevant to discussions as to the proper way to provide health care in the community. Such discussions have taken a very pointed turn in recent years, for example, in regard to the 'pay beds' issue.* The state of that practical issue is changing all the time, so I shall not attempt to relate what I say at all closely to the present state of play. Rather I hope to elucidate some of the background of ideas against which the protagonists in that debate pursue their argument.

In my discussion I shall assume the principle that

*Editor's note: At issue in the "pay beds" controversy is whether National Health Service hospitals should have a certain number of beds or wards set aside for "private," i.e., paying, patients. The controversy stems partly from the fact that, for "public" patients, hospital admittance is based on medical priority. Public patients who do not need immediate care may wait much longer for treatment than private patients who need such treatment.

Reprinted with permission of the publisher from *Journal of Medical Ethics*, vol. 2 (September 1976), pp. 107–111.

the state is responsible for the health of the citizens, in the sense that it is bound, insofar as the community's resources permit, to see that it is possible for everyone who needs it to secure medical care. The detailed analysis of this principle, whether in terms of needs, rights or justice, is a matter of controversy, but in broad outline the principle is entailed by any political philosophy which ascribes to a government the positive function of furthering the welfare of its citizens; and such a political philosophy is readily accepted by all but extremists at the present time. Assuming this principle, then, I shall examine the various ways in which a government might try to implement its obligation to see that everyone gets the opportunity of health care. There are of course many possibilities here, but I think four broad types can be distinguished, which I shall call respectively *laissez-faire*, liberal humanitarian, liberal socialist, and pure socialist. I shall briefly describe each system, and then discuss the pros and cons of each.

FOUR POSSIBLE SYSTEMS OF HEALTH CARE

The *laissez-faire* system leaves medical care entirely to private enterprise. Those who can afford it pay for their medical treatment on a business footing, either directly or through insurance schemes. The needy are looked after, if at all, by private charities. The government interferes only to the extent that it interferes in other commercial enterprises: that is to say, it enforces contracts, hears suits for damage and tries to prevent fraud—perhaps in this case by insisting on qualifications of some kind for medical practitioners. The liberal humanitarian system is a modification of this. Those who can afford it pay for themselves, as before. But the needy are looked after not by private charity but by the state, using funds obtained by taxing the less needy. The liberal socialist scheme is what we have in Britain today. Everyone, or everyone who is able, has to contribute to a state scheme which provides for his medical care. But he may if he wishes pay also for private medicine. There can of course be systems between the liberal humanitarian and the liberal socialist, whereby everyone may belong to the state system but anyone may instead if he wishes opt out both of benefiting from it and also from all or part of his share of paying for it. Lastly there is pure socialism, which is what some now advocate: the complete abolition by law of non-state medicine.

I shall take it that the *laissez-faire* system is agreed to be inadequate; indeed, under such a system the state would in my view be abrogating its responsibilities towards the needy. It is true that the needy might be very well provided for if there were a strong enough tradition of charity of this kind. But it seems too haphazard a basis for such an important service. In any case, it might be said that the opportunity for health care is owed to everyone as a basic human right; if this is so, receiving it should not have to depend on people's goodwill, however forthcoming that goodwill is. Of course replacing a *laissez-faire* system with one of the others might mean a loss of that worthwhile thing, exercise of the motive of charity. But there are some things which are so important that getting them done properly is more important than getting them done inadequately from the right motive. In any case, scope would remain on any scheme for the exercise of charity. We have today, for example, charities which support medical research, and which may feel justified in pursuing projects with a high risk of failure which those bodies using taxpayers' extorted money feel unjustified in supporting.

I turn then to a consideration of the more plausible schemes. My strategy will be to mention first some of the advantages people have advanced in favour of liberal humanitarianism, and the criticisms made of it from a socialist point of view. Then I shall turn to the advantages and disadvantages of socialism, considering the liberal and pure versions together for the time being. Finally I shall touch on the vexed and topical question of liberal *versus* pure socialism.

THE LIBERAL HUMANITARIAN SCHEME OF HEALTH CARE

The first advantage attributed to the liberal humanitarian scheme is that it meets everyone's needs with minimum coercion: people are constrained only to the extent of paying taxes for the needy and not made to contribute to their own good, a practice which smacks of unwarranted interference. Secondly, it is said that resources are more usefully distributed: state aid can be concentrated on those who really need special help, and those who are paying for their own services will have an incentive not to squander them, as they do not have under a state scheme.

The third and fourth advantages of the liberal humanitarian scheme are what may be called moral, rather than merely medical. The third is the advantage of preserved incentive. People are encouraged to work harder if they can get what they need only by working, and discouraged if extra work brings no extra reward. Having an incentive to work hard is a double advantage: it benefits the community by increasing prosperity and it cultivates industriousness in the individual's character. The fourth advantage is similarly one of development of character: to have to decide for oneself how to manage such an important department of one's life develops a sense of responsibility and powers of decision.

In criticising this system, the socialist can first point to the problem posed for the liberal humanitarian by those who are perfectly well able to provide for themselves, by means of private insurance, but neglect to do so. If they fall ill even the liberal humanitarian will have to admit that the state must look after them; it is unfair that they should receive this benefit without paying for it, but one cannot leave a man to die because he has been improvident. The socialist can say that for him there is no problem, because everyone has to pay his way.

The second socialist criticism is a denial that the medical needs of the average man can in fact be met by a non-coercive liberal scheme, on the ground that the average man, not just the needy man, could not afford to pay for modern medicine individually, even if he had in his control all that part of his money which at present the state takes from him for general medical care. This assertion, if true, would be a knock-down argument against liberal humanitarianism. I shall not discuss it in detail, as it depends on economic rather than philosophical arguments. One point in its favour is that the distinction on which the liberal humanitarian scheme really rests, between being and not being too poor to buy necessities, does not apply to medical care even roughly, because one person's basic necessities in medical care may be vastly more expensive than another person's luxuries. There may therefore be those who, although quite well off, will not be able to afford, or even necessarily afford the premiums to cover, what is medically necessary for them. At best, then, a scheme which really meets people's needs will require state subsidies not merely for the poorest but also for the illest; and this is already a departure from the basic liberal humanitarian scheme. Apart from this, the question whether a private system would be cheap enough for the consumer depends on such things as the way in

which, and scale on which, it is organized; the level of doctor's fees in such a system; and so on. I shall say a little on the latter question shortly.

The third criticism is that to have some people recipients of state aid when the majority are paying for themselves creates an unfortunately sharp division between haves and have-nots, the independent and the dependent, which is more blurred when all are in a state scheme. However strongly one might insist on the human right to medical care, those who are given it without paying, when others pay, will feel they are recipients of charity; and this feeling is damaging to self esteem, and embittering to those who cannot help their dependent position.

The fourth socialist criticism of liberal humanitarianism is the most important and the most baffling, since it combines many different strands. It can be expressed by saying that the scheme makes medical care a commercial matter, and this is unsuitable. But why might it be thought to be unsuitable? Medicine is not like love, which logically cannot be bought. People say here that it is wrong to 'traffick in,' or to 'exploit,' people's need. This description might, however, apply equally well to those who sell food, or any needed commodity, and no one suggests that they are immoral; a butcher or baker meets a need and in doing so meets his own needs too. There is, all the same, a difference in the medical case, which means that what may be called market safeguards do not protect the patient as well as they do the ordinary consumer. In general, the consumer is not actually suffering, as distinct from needy, and also he understands something of what he is buying; so he can 'shop around' and look for cheap goods and services. But a patient will not want to wait and will not know how to judge, so he can very easily be exploited. Nor would an agreed 'professional fee' system improve his position; on the contrary, if such fees were fixed at an over-high rate (as is perhaps the case with lawyers now) he would have no chance of finding the most favourable price for medical care.

The liberal humanitarian can agree with all these views, but points out that they do not constitute a special difficulty for his scheme as opposed to a socialist one. Given the urgency with which medical care is needed, doctors can on a socialist scheme also blackmail the consumers (here society at large) to pay them too much, so that again everyone suffers. The patient, he will go on, is best safeguarded by a private system, which will at least leave some room for 'shopping around'; apart from that he is protected by the compassion and goodwill of the majority of the profession.

Here, however, the socialist tends to retort that the market system implicit in the liberal humanitarian scheme is deficient precisely in that it leaves no room for compassion or goodwill. Those partaking in a market economy (he goes on) are in business to make a profit, and as large a one as possible, just as the consumer is trying to pay as little as possible: that is what the market is all about. Greed, then, rather than compassion, is the motive of the doctor in a liberal humanitarian scheme.

This socialist doctrine is, however, a muddle. It is true that what we may call a pure market transaction can be defined as one in which each party seeks to do as well as possible. But this is an artificial abstraction from actual practice, where what goes on might be a product of all kinds of forces; doctor and patient will both be governed by many non-market considerations in arriving at a fee. It is also true as a matter of fact that the doctor in commercial medicine must make enough to live on if he is to remain in business; so the bottom end of his scale is fixed. But there is no practical necessity for him to be a pure marketeer, trying to make the largest possible profit, and therefore no reason why his main motive should not be compassion just as much as if he had private means and worked for nothing. Nor does compassion for a person's sufferings entail refusal to take any money from him, any more than sympathy for a stranded motorist entails refusal to accept payment for a gallon of petrol. Of course a doctor in a *laissez-faire* system has a problem if his patients are too poor to pay enough even to support him. But in a liberal humanitarian system such patients are subsidized by the state.

I think then that the claim that medicine should not be a commercial matter cannot be sustained in its crude form. But there is nevertheless a difficulty about commercial medicine which arises less obviously in a socialist system: considerations of cost, rather than of need, will obtrude too much into the doctor's medical thinking. Of course the National Health Service doctor also is constantly being urged to economize. But if he thinks a certain expensive drug or treatment is needed for a patient, not merely useful or beneficial, he can go ahead. With a private patient, however, he will have to think all the time, 'Can this patient afford it?' and this must be very inhibiting to the process of making a balanced decision on treatment.

THE SOCIALIST SYSTEM OF HEALTH CARE

The strengths of the socialist position will already have emerged to some extent through their criticisms of the liberal humanitarian: a socialist scheme can offer very large resources to any individual who needs expensive treatment, in a way which avoids both the stigma suffered by the involuntary non-contributor and the unfair advantages enjoyed by the negligent one. It is also said that a socialist scheme avoids the self-interested motivation of a commercial scheme. But as we have seen there is no need for doctors participating in a commercial scheme to do so out of self interest. Moreover, there is no reason why doctors, and patients, should not be self-interested in a state scheme: patients wanting more than their share of attention, doctors wanting more and more money. No doubt the philosophy behind the socialist scheme is 'from each according to his capacity, to each according to his need'—a kind of fraternal spirit. But there is nothing in the system to ensure that participants in fact see it this way. No doubt they can see their National Insurance contributions and taxes as benefiting the community rather than themselves; but then the liberal humanitarian can see his taxes in that way too.

It is also maintained in favour of a socialist system that it ensures equal treatment for equal needs. This unqualified claim is probably rather optimistic. On a socialist scheme influence, aggressiveness and articulateness will to some extent win more attention and care than is fair, just as money may do on a commercial scheme. But to claim an advantage over liberal humanitarianism on grounds of equality the socialist has only to show that his scheme has more equal results than the liberal alternative; and this he can probably do. The question does arise, however, what importance is to be attached to achieving equality if everyone's basic needs are met; it might be maintained that above the level of basic needs the demands of equality are rather controversial. The real issue, then, is whether a socialist system meets people's needs more satisfactorily than its rivals. We have seen that where a large expenditure for one person is concerned this may be the case. But many would maintain that a socialist system is necessarily too wasteful of resources to be able to give a satisfactory routine service to all, on the grounds that the removal of any need to pay at the time encourages over-extravagant use. How far this common charge is borne out in practice is a question for the sociologist rather than for the philosopher. But it should be noted that 'unnecessary' calls upon the doctor's time are often due to ignorance rather than to selfishness: an educated person does not think of calling in a doctor for a cold or flu or bleeding nose, not because he is too public-spirited, but because he himself knows what to do. It should therefore be possible for the socialist to lessen abuses without needing the deterrent of payment, by educating the public rather more than doctors at present seem to be willing to do.

I suggest then that the socialist might be able to escape the charge that his system is necessarily inefficient. But there are two other charges that are perhaps even more serious: that a socialist scheme is an unwarranted infringement of liberty, and that it undermines individual responsibility. The first charge is not so easy to maintain as some of those who make it seem to think. Obviously the scheme is a curtailment of liberty; but it would presumably be justified nevertheless if it promoted a great common good that could be achieved in no other way. The issue of liberty, then, is partly the issue of whether the alternative liberal humanitarian system is economically viable. But even if it were, we must still ask whether the unhappiness of those who are stigmatized under it is a price worth paying for retaining greater freedom. And to this there is no easy answer.

The second criticism is that socialized medicine undermines individual responsibility for health. On a socialist system, it may be said, the state takes over that responsibility for health care which under a private system the individual possesses: the need to plan how his health care (and that of his family) is to be paid for, and to decide his priorities accordingly. Why is this said to be a bad thing? Many reasons are advanced. One is that the individual will come to think that all aspects of health care are now looked after by Them, and so cease to 'take responsibility' for those things which on any system only he can provide: a sensible diet, adequate sleep and so on. Whether this happens in fact is an empirical question; it seems to me likely that those people who do take this kind of responsibility for themselves are too individualistic to be affected one way or the other.

A second reason for criticising the removal of responsibility is that it trivializes the individual's concern for his life: the more the important areas of life are taken over by the government, the more people see their main business in life as the contriving of amuse-ments. Instead of thinking about health and education, they think about clothes and holidays. Now this is perhaps a tendentious description of the situation: if one were to say that state control of the utilities of life gives people more chance to cultivate their talents and develop their personal relationships, to think about things worthwhile in themselves rather than merely useful, the argument against state control would be less clear. But perhaps most people's capacity to achieve the aristocratic ideal of leisure, as opposed to mere amusements, is limited; if so, it might in general be true that too much socialism leads people to give trivial things undue importance in life.

The third and most important argument advanced against this kind of removal of responsibility is the claim that it saps character. On a liberal humanitarian scheme people have to make decisions and live with the results of them, whereas on a socialist scheme decisions are taken out of their hands. The argument is that a person who does not have to make decisions cannot express his individuality, because it is in making one's own choices, different from anyone else's, that individuality is both shown and fostered; and moreover he loses his autonomy, the capacity for self-determination which makes him a person in the full sense.

The socialist can reply that these considerations apply unqualifiedly only when every area of life is governed by the state; the nationalization of some aspects of life—such as education, housing, health—leaves plenty of scope for individual choice and decision. He might admit that there is even so a measure of deterioration in character, but think it amply compensated for by the increased benefits; or he might take the line that there is no need to assume that people's characters suffer at all. But even if he is right in this latter claim about what actually happens, the liberal can object on moral grounds: even supposing that character remains intact in a socialist world, is it appropriate to treat adults as though they were like children, capable of deciding only unimportant matters? This is where the liberty and responsibility arguments coincide; liberty, it might be said, is liberty in the exercise of responsibility. Treating people properly involves respecting their liberty, or treating them as responsible creatures. But, as I said earlier, even the claims of liberty may have to bow to those of utility, or of humanity to those who would suffer under a libertarian scheme.

THE LIBERAL SOCIALIST VERSUS THE PURE SOCIALIST SYSTEMS OF HEALTH CARE

I come now to the final section of my discussion: the issue of pure *versus* liberal socialism. At present our own system is a liberal version, which allows those who wish and are able to do so to buy extra services on a private basis. Many people now advocate that this should be forbidden by law, and pure socialized medicine imposed. The issue is very complex. In Great Britain the question is whether people should be allowed to supplement the services they can get under the National Health Service. But there is also the possibility of a system whereby people can opt out of the National Health Service altogether. I cannot go into the pros and cons of this latter system. Again, even in Great Britain there are two separate questions: whether private medicine in state hospitals should be forbidden, and whether private medicine should be forbidden altogether. I shall not be able to distinguish between these two positions with the exactness which they really require. A further complexity is that the degree of extra service which is available for private purchase varies very much. I shall assume that it consists only of earlier appointments and more leisurely consultations with general practitioners and specialists, freer choice of specialist, prompter hospital treatment for non-emergencies and more privacy in hospital. Private treatment is not necessarily better in any respect other than these, and the degree to which it is better even in these will vary from place to place.

The usual argument concerns the right to private treatment. But I would suggest that for some people on some occasions private treatment may be not merely a right but a duty. Whatever the arguments against it, they can surely on occasion be morally outweighed, for those who can manage to afford private treatment, by obligations to others: the obligation to be restored to full health quickly and not be a drag on family or colleagues; the obligation to arrange a hospital stay at the least difficult time for family or colleagues; the obligation to continue working in hospital and to secure the privacy which makes this possible. The fact that not everyone can afford private medicine does not absolve those who can from this kind of duty. It would sometimes be true to say, contrary to the normal view, that a person who insisted on public medicine when he could afford private was being selfish and unpublic spirited.

Of course the usual defence of private medicine is in terms not of duties but of rights. People have a right, it is said, to spend their money on what they like: some, it is often added, spend their spare money on bingo or drinking, why should I not spend mine on health insurance? This is basically an appeal to liberty. The mention of those who spend their money on smoking or drinking is an attempt to add considerations of equality. It is salutary to be reminded that there are now a great many ordinary people who could afford private treatment if they gave it high priority. But there are still some who could not, and while this is so, a man cannot claim the right to buy private treatment merely on grounds of equality. What he has to say instead is, Why is it thought that people should be free to spend far more than the poorest can spend on every other kind of goods, but not on medical care?

One reply might be that people should not be free to spend unequally in any sphere: in other words, wealth should be redistributed equally. I have already refused to enter into discussion of this general question and suggested that what is uncontroversial and of paramount importance is the meeting of needs. But this is precisely why some people who are by no means egalitarians in general are against private medicine. The public system, they maintain, does not at present meet people's basic needs, especially their need of reasonably prompt treatment. The so-called 'extras' which private medicine provides are on this view not mere luxuries but basic necessities, open to the rich but too expensive for the poor. Assertions that we are free to buy everything other than medical care are thus beside the point, insofar as there is no other basic necessity beyond the reach of the poorest.

If this account is true, there are some medical necessities which can at present be got only by paying extra. But it does not follow that everyone's basic needs will more nearly be met if no one is allowed to pay extra. It is said that private patients use up a disproportionate amount of scarce resources; if they were done away with, queues would shorten and beds would multiply. But the extra services they receive are surely small in comparison with the extra money they pay; in other words, they are subsidizing the other patients. Without their money, resources would therefore be scarcer and queues longer, especially as some doctors would leave the profession, or the country, if there were no private patients. I suggest then that private medicine is one of those inequalities which are justified in that everyone, including the worst off, benefits from them.

The sensitive individual may still feel reluctant to avail himself of private medicine, even if he is convinced that the National Health Service can do with his money. I think this is to do with a sense of the fraternity of suffering: a wish not to cut oneself off from fellow-sufferers by having an easier time, even if one's easier time is of use to them. Such a feeling is certainly likeable, just as is a person's reluctance to eat his Christmas dinner when he thinks of those who are starving. But if I am right about the value of the private patient's contributions he should ignore his feelings on this matter.

In this long paper I have reached few conclusions.

As always in real-life issues, the philosophical aspect is too intertwined with the empirical, and the empirical too elusive in any case, to permit any dogmatism. What I have hoped to do is simply to bring out some of the principles at issue in any discussion of the rights and wrongs of socialized medicine.[1]

NOTE

1 This paper owes much to the following: Acton, H. B. (1971), *The Morals of Markets* (London, Longman Group), especially chapters III and IV, and Barry, Brian (1965), *Political Argument* (London, Routledge and Kegan Paul), chapter VII.

Policy Decisions and Individual Responsibility for Health

Public Health as Social Justice

Dan E. Beauchamp

Dan E. Beauchamp teaches in the Department of Health Administration, School of Public Health and in the Department of Community Medicine and Hospital Administration, both at the University of North Carolina at Chapel Hill. His numerous articles on public health policy include "Alcoholism as Blaming the Alcoholic," "Public Health: Alien Ethic in a Strange Land?" and "Exploring New Ethics for Public Health: Developing a Fair Alcohol Policy."

Beauchamp rejects the attempt to hold individuals and not the social group as a whole responsible for the illnesses resulting from "voluntary" behavior. Aware of the need for effective preventive measures in health care, Beauchamp criticizes the resistance found in society against public funding of such measures. He argues that this resistance is rooted in a mistaken conception of justice—market justice—which emphasizes individual responsibility and ignores the social preconditions that strongly influence behavior. Beauchamp advocates the adoption of a different conception of justice—social justice—which will emphasize society's and not the individual's responsibility for illness. Only under this kind of system, Beauchamp argues, can there be any real assurance of full and equal protection of all human life. He concludes his article by attacking the notion of freedom involved in attempts to limit the kinds of programs needed to maximize the health and safety of all members of society.

Anthony Downs[1] has observed that our most intractable public problems have two significant characteristics. First, they occur to a relative minority of our population (even though that minority may number millions of people). Second, they result in significant part from arrangements that are providing substantial benefits or advantages to a majority or to a powerful minority of citizens. Thus solving or minimizing these problems requires painful losses, the restructuring of society and the acceptance of new burdens by the most powerful and the most numerous on behalf of the least powerful or the least numerous. As Downs notes, this bleak reality has resulted in recent years in cycles of public attention to such problems as poverty, racial discrimination, poor housing, unemployment or the abandonment of the aged; however, this attention and interest rapidly wane when it becomes clear that solving these problems requires painful costs that the dominant interests in society are unwilling to pay. Our public ethics do not seem to fit our public problems.

It is not sufficiently appreciated that these same bleak realities plague attempts to protect the public's health. Automobile-related injury and death; tobacco, alcohol and other drug damage; the perils of the workplace; environmental pollution; the inequitable and ineffective distribution of medical care services; the hazards of biomedicine—all of these threats inflict death and disability on a minority of our society at any given time. Further, minimizing or even significantly reducing the death and disability from these perils entails that the majority or powerful minorities accept new burdens or relinquish existing privileges that they presently enjoy. Typically, these new burdens or restrictions involve more stringent controls over these and other hazards of the world.

This somber reality suggests that our fundamental attention in public health policy and prevention should not be directed toward a search for new technology, but rather toward breaking existing ethical and political barriers to minimizing death and disability. This is not to say that technology will never again help avoid painful social and political adjustments.[2] Nonetheless, only the technological Pollyannas will ignore the mounting evidence that the critical barriers to protecting the public against death and disability are not the barriers to technological progress—indeed the evidence is that it is often technology itself that is our own worst enemy. The critical barrier to dramatic reductions in death and disability is a social ethic that unfairly protects the most numerous or the most powerful from the burdens of prevention.

This is the issue of justice. In the broadest sense, justice means that each person in society ought to receive his due and that the burdens and benefits of society should be fairly and equitably distributed.[3] But what criteria should be followed in allocating burdens and benefits: Merit, equality or need?[4] What end or goal in life should receive our highest priority: Life, liberty or the pursuit of happiness? The answer to these questions can be found in our prevailing theories or models of justice. These models of justice, roughly speaking, form the foundation of our politics and public policy in general, and our health policy (including our prevention policy) specifically. Here I am speaking of politics not as partisan politics but rather the more ancient and venerable meaning of the political as the search for the common good and the just society.

These models of justice furnish a symbolic framework or blueprint with which to think about and react to the problems of the public, providing the basic rules to classify and categorize problems of society as to whether they necessitate public and collective protection, or whether individual responsibility should prevail. These models function as a sort of map or guide to the common world of members of society, making visible some conditions in society as public issues and concerns, and hiding, obscuring or concealing other conditions that might otherwise emerge as public issues or problems were a different map or model of justice in hand.

In the case of health, these models of justice form the basis for thinking about and reacting to the problems of disability and premature death in society. Thus, if public health policy requires that the majority or a powerful minority accept their fair share of the burdens of protecting a relative minority threatened with death or disability, we need to ask if our prevailing model of justice contemplates and legitimates such sacrifices.

MARKET-JUSTICE

The dominant model of justice in the American experience has been market-justice.[5] Under the norms of market-justice people are entitled only to those valued ends such as status, income, happiness, etc., that they have acquired by fair rules of entitlement, e.g., by their own individual efforts, actions or abilities. Market-justice emphasizes individual responsibility, minimal collective action and freedom from collective obligations except to respect other persons' fundamental rights.

While we have as a society compromised pure market-justice in many ways to protect the public's health, we are far from recognizing the principle that death and disability are collective problems and that all persons are entitled to health protection. Society does not recognize a general obligation to protect the individual against disease and injury. While society does prohibit individuals from causing direct harm to others, and has in many instances regulated clear public health hazards, the norm of market-justice is still dominant and the primary duty to avert disease and injury still rests with the individual. The individual is ultimately alone in his or her struggle against death.

Barriers to Protection

This individual isolation creates a powerful barrier to the goal of protecting all human life by magnifying the power of death, granting to death an almost supernatural reality.[6] Death has throughout history presented a basic problem to humankind,[7] but even in an advanced society with enormous biomedical technology, the individualism of market-justice tends to retain and exaggerate pessimistic and fatalistic attitudes toward death and injury. This fatalism leads to a sense of powerlessness, to the acceptance of risk as an essential element of life, to resignation in the face of calamity, and to a weakening of collective impulses to confront the problems of premature death and disability.

Perhaps the most direct way in which market-justice undermines our resolve to preserve and protect human life lies in the primary freedom this ethic extends to all individuals and groups to act with minimal obligations to protect the common good.[8] Despite the fact that this rule of self-interest predictably fails to protect adequately the safety of our workplaces, our modes of transportation, the physical environment, the commodities we consume, or the equitable and effective distribution of medical care, these failures have resulted so far in only half-hearted attempts at regulation and control. This response is explained in large part by the powerful sway market-justice holds over our imagination, granting fundamental freedom to all individuals to be left alone—even if the "individuals" in question

are giant producer groups with enormous capacities to create great public harm through sheer inadvertence. Efforts for truly effective controls over these perils must constantly struggle against a prevailing ethical paradigm that defines as threats to fundamental freedoms attempts to assure that all groups—even powerful producer groups—accept their fair share of the burdens of prevention.

Market-justice is also the source of another major barrier to public health measures to minimize death and disability—the category of voluntary behavior. Market-justice forces a basic distinction between the harm caused by a factory polluting the atmosphere and the harm caused by the cigarette or alcohol industries, because in the latter case those that are harmed are perceived as engaged in "voluntary" behavior.[9] It is the radical individualism inherent in the market model that encourages attention to the individual's behavior and inattention to the social preconditions of that behavior. In the case of smoking, these preconditions include a powerful cigarette industry and accompanying social and cultural forces encouraging the practice of smoking. These social forces include norms sanctioning smoking as well as all forms of media, advertising, literature, movies, folklore, etc. Since the smoker is free in some ultimate sense to not smoke, the norms of market-justice force the conclusion that the individual voluntarily "chooses" to smoke; and we are prevented from taking strong collective action against the powerful structures encouraging this so-called voluntary behavior.

Yet another way in which the market ethic obstructs the possibilities for minimizing death and disability, and alibis the need for structural change, is through explanations for death and disability that "blame the victim."[10] Victim-blaming misdefines structural and collective problems of the entire society as individual problems, seeing these problems as caused by the behavioral failures or deficiencies of the victims. These behavioral explanations for public problems tend to protect the larger society and powerful interests from the burdens of collective action, and instead encourage attempts to change the "faulty" behavior of victims.

Market-justice is perhaps the major cause for our over-investment and over-confidence in curative medical services. It is not obvious that the rise of medical science and the physician, taken alone, should become fundamental obstacles to collective action to prevent death and injury. But the prejudice found in market-justice against collective action perverts these scientific advances into an unrealistic hope for "technological shortcuts"[11] to painful social change. Moreover, the great emphasis placed on individual achievement in market-justice has further diverted attention and interest away from primary prevention and collective action by dramatizing the role of the solitary physician-scientist, picturing him as our primary weapon and first line of defense against the threat of death and injury.

The prestige of medical care encouraged by market-justice prevents large-scale research to determine whether, in fact, our medical care technology actually brings about the result desired—a significant reduction in the damage and losses suffered from disease and injury. The model conceals questions about our pervasive use of drugs, our intense specialization, and our seemingly boundless commitment to biomedical technology. Instead, the market model of justice encourages us to see problems as due primarily to the failure of individual doctors and the quality of their care, rather than to recognize the possibility of failure from the structure of medical care itself.[12] Consequently, we seek to remedy problems by trying to change individual doctors through appeals to their ethical sensibilities, or by reshaping their education, or by creating new financial incentives.

Government Health Policy

The vast expansion of government in health policy over the past decades might seem to signal the demise of the market ethic for health. But it is important to remember that the preponderance of our public policy for health continues to define health care as a consumption good to be allocated primarily by private decisions and markets, and only interferes with this market with public policy to subsidize, supplement or extend the market system when private decisions result in sufficient imperfections or inequities to be of public concern. Medicare and Medicaid are examples. Other examples include subsidizing or stimulating the private sector through public support for research, education of professionals, limited areawide planning, and the construction of facilities. Even national health insurance is largely a public financing mechanism to subsidize private markets in the hope that curative health services will be more equitably distributed. None of these policies is likely to bring dramatic reductions in rates of death and disability.

Our current efforts to reform the so-called health system are little more than the use of public authority to perpetuate essentially private mechanisms for allocating curative health services. These reforms are paraded as evidence that the system is capable of functioning equitably. But, as Barthes[13] points out (in a different context), reform measures may merely serve to "inoculate" the larger society against the suspicion that it is the model itself (in our case, market-justice) that is at fault. In fact, the constant reform efforts designed to "save the system" may better be viewed as an attempt to expand the hegemony of the key actors in the present system—especially the medical care complex. As McKnight says, the medical care complex may need the hot air of reform if its ballooning empire is to continue to inflate.[14]

Public Health Measures

I have saved for last an important class of health policies—public health measures to protect the environment, the workplace, or the commodities we purchase and consume. Are these not signs that the American society is willing to accept collective action in the face of clear public health hazards?

I do not wish to minimize the importance of these advances to protect the public in many domains. But these separate reforms, taken alone, should be cautiously received. This is because each reform effort is perceived as an isolated exception to the norm of market-justice; the norm itself still stands. Consequently, the predictable career of such measures is to see enthusiasm for enforcement peak and wane. These public health measures are clear signs of hope. But as long as these actions are seen as merely minor exceptions to the rule of individual responsibility, the goals of public health will remain beyond our reach. What is required is for the public to see that protecting the public's health takes us beyond the norms of market-justice categorically, and necessitates a completely new health ethic.

I return to my original point: Market-justice is the primary roadblock to dramatic reductions in preventable injury and death. More than this, market-justice is a pervasive ideology protecting the most powerful or the most numerous from the burdens of collective action. If this be true, the central goal of public health should be ethical in nature: The challenging of market-justice as fatally deficient in protecting the health of the public. Further, public health should advocate a "counter-ethic" for protecting the public's health, one articulated in a different tradition of justice and one designed to give the highest priority to minimizing death and disability and to the protection of all human life against the hazards of this world.

SOCIAL JUSTICE

The fundamental critique of market-justice found in the Western liberal tradition is social justice. Under social justice all persons are entitled equally to key ends such as health protection or minimum standards of income. Further, unless collective burdens are accepted, powerful forces of environment, heredity or social structure will preclude a fair distribution of these ends.[15-PV] While many forces influenced the development of public health, the historic dream of public health that preventable death and disability ought to be minimized is a dream of social justice.[18] Yet these egalitarian and social justice implications of the public health vision are either still not widely recognized or are conveniently ignored.

Seeing the public health vision as ultimately rooted in an egalitarian tradition that conflicts directly with the norms of market-justice is often glossed over and obscured by referring to public health as a general strategy to control the "environment." For example, Canada's "New Perspectives on the Health of Canadians"[19] correctly notes that major reductions in death and disability cannot be expected from curative health services. Future progress will have to result from alterations in the "environment" and "lifestyle." But if we substitute the words "market-justice" for environment or lifestyle, "New Perspectives" becomes a very radical document indeed.

Ideally, then, the public health ethic[20] is not simply an alternative to the market ethic for health—it is a fundamental critique of that ethic as it unjustly protects powerful interests from the burdens of prevention and as that ethic serves to legitimate a mindless and extravagant faith in the efficacy of medical care. In other words, the public health ethic is a *counter-ethic* to market-justice and the ethics of individualism as these are applied to the health problems of the public.

This view of public health is admittedly not widely accepted. Indeed, in recent times the mission of public health has been viewed by many as limited to that minority of health problems that cannot be solved by the market provision of medical care services and that necessitate organized community action.[21] It is interesting to speculate why many in the public health profession have come to accept this narrow view of public health—a view that is obviously influenced and shaped by the market model as it attempts to limit the burdens placed on powerful groups.[22]

Nonetheless, the broader view of public health set out here is logically and ethically justified if one accepts the vision of public health as being the protection of all human life. The central task of public health, then, is to complete its unfinished revolution: The elaboration of a health ethic adequate to protect and preserve all human life. This new ethic has several key implications which are referred to here as "principles"[23]: (1) Controlling the hazards of this world, (2) to prevent death and disability, (3) through organized collective action, (4) shared equally by all except where unequal burdens result in increased protection of everyone's health and especially potential victims of death and disability.

These ethical principles are not new to public health. To the contrary, making the ethical foundations of public health visible only serves to highlight the social justice influences at work behind pre-existing principles.

Controlling the Hazards

A key principle of the public health ethic is the focus on the identification and control of the hazards of this world rather than a focus on the behavioral defects of those individuals damaged by these hazards. Against this principle it is often argued that today the causes of death and disability are multiple and frequently behavioral in origin.[24] Further, since it is usually only a minority of the public that fails to protect itself against most known hazards, additional controls over these perilous sources would not seem to be effective or just. We should look instead for the behavioral origins of most public health problems,[25] asking why some people expose themselves to known hazards or perils, or act in an unsafe or careless manner.

Public health should—at least ideally—be suspicious of behavioral paradigms for viewing public health problems since they tend to "blame the victim" and unfairly protect majorities and powerful interests from the burdens of prevention.[26] It is clear that behavioral models of public health problems are rooted in the tradition of market-justice, where the emphasis is upon individual ability and capacity, and individual success and failure.

Public health, ideally, should not be concerned with explaining the successes and failures of differing individuals (dispositional explanations)[27] in controlling the hazards of this world. Rather these failures should be seen as signs of still weak and ineffective controls or limits over those conditions, commodities, services, products or practices that are either hazardous for the health and safety of members of the public, or that are vital to protect the public's health.

Prevention

Like the other principles of public health, prevention is a logical consequence of the ethical goal of minimizing the numbers of persons suffering death and disability. The only known way to minimize these adverse events is to prevent the occurrence of damaging exchanges or exposures in the first place, or to seek to minimize damage when exposures cannot be controlled.

Prevention, then, is that set of priority rules for restructuring existing market rules in order to maximally protect the public. These rules seek to create policies and obligations to replace the norm of market-justice, where the latter permits specific conditions, commodities, services, products, activities or practices to pose a direct threat or hazard to the health and safety of members of the public, or where the market norm fails to allocate effectively and equitably those services (such as medical care) that are necessary to attend to disease at hand.

Thus, the familiar public health options:[28]

1 Creating rules to minimize exposure of the public to hazards (kinetic, chemical, ionizing, biological, etc.) so as to reduce the rates of hazardous exchanges.

2 Creating rules to strengthen the public against damage in the event damaging exchanges occur anyway, where such techniques (fluoridation, seat-belts, immunization) are feasible.

3 Creating rules to organize treatment resources in the community so as to minimize damage that does occur since we can rarely prevent all damage.

Collective Action

Another principle of the public health ethic is that the control of hazards cannot be achieved through voluntary mechanisms but must be undertaken by governmental or non-governmental agencies through planned, organized and collective action that is obligatory or non-voluntary in nature. This is for two reasons.

The first is because market or voluntary action is typically inadequate for providing what are called public goods.[29] Public goods are those public policies (national defense, police and fire protection, or the protection of all persons against preventable death and disability) that are universal in their impacts and effects, affecting everyone equally. These kinds of goods cannot easily be withheld from individuals in the community who choose not to support these services (this is typically called the "free rider" problem). Also, individual holdouts might plausibly reason that their small contribution might not prevent the public good from being offered.

The second reason why self-regarding individuals might refuse to voluntarily pay the costs of such public goods as public health policies is because these policies frequently require burdens that self-interest or self-protection might see as too stringent. For example, the minimization of rates of alcoholism in a community clearly seems to require norms or controls over the substance of alcohol that limit the use of this substance to levels that are far below what would be safe for individual drinkers.[30]

With these temptations for individual noncompliance, justice demands assurance that all persons share equally the costs of collective action through obligatory and sanctioned social and public policy.

Fair-Sharing of the Burdens

A final principle of the public health ethic is that all persons are equally responsible for sharing the burdens—as well as the benefits—of protection against death and disability, except where unequal burdens result in greater protection for every person and especially potential victims of death and disability.[31] In practice this means that policies to control the hazards of a given substance, service or commodity fall unequally (but still fairly) on those involved in the production, provision or consumption of the service, commodity or substance. The clear implication of this principle is that the automotive industry, the tobacco industry, the coal industry and the medical care industry—to mention only a few key groups—have an unequal responsibility to bear the costs of reducing death and disability since their actions have far greater impact than those of individual citizens....

CONCLUSION

I have attempted to show the broad implications of a public health commitment to protect and preserve human life, setting out tentatively the logical consequences of that commitment in the form of some general principles....

Nothing written here should be construed as a per se attack on the market system. I have, rather, surfaced the moral and ethical norms of that system and argued that, whatever other benefits might accrue from those norms, they are woefully inadequate to assure full and equal protection of all human life....

Finally, it is a peculiarity of the word freedom that its meaning has become so distorted and stretched as to lend itself as a defense against nearly every attempt to extend equal health protection to all persons. This is the ultimate irony. The idea of liberty should mean, above all else, the liberation of society from the injustice of preventable disability and early death. Instead, the concept of freedom has become a defense and protection of powerful vested interests, and the central issue is viewed as a choice between freedom on the one hand, and health and safety on the other. I am confident that ultimately the public will come to see that extending life and health to all persons will require some diminution of personal choices, but that such restrictions are not only fair and do not constitute abridgement of fundamental liberties, they are a basic sign and imprint of a just society and a guarantee of that most basic of all freedom—protection against man's most ancient foe.

NOTES

1 Downs, A., "The Issue-Attention Cycle and the Political Economy of Improving Our Environment," revised version of the Royer Lectures presented at the University of California at Berkeley, April 13–14, 1970.

2 Etzioni, A. and Remp, R., "Technological 'Shortcuts' to Social Change," *Science* 175:31–38 (1972).

3 Jonsen, A. R. and Hellegers, A. E., "Conceptual Foundations for an Ethics of Medical Care," in: Tancredi, L. R. (ed.) *Ethics of Health Care* (Washington, D.C.: National Academy of Sciences, 1974).

4 Outka, E., "Social Justice and Equal Access to Health Care," *The Journal of Religious Ethics* 2:11–32 (1974).

5 Some might object strenuously to the marriage of the two terms "market" and "justice." One theory of the market holds that it is a blind hand that rewards without regard to merit or individual effort. For this point of view, see: Friedman, M., *Capitalism and Freedom* (Chicago: University of Chicago Press, 1962); and Hayek, F., *The Constitution of Liberty* (Chicago: University of Chicago Press, 1960). But Irving Kristol, in his "When Virtue Loses All Her Loveliness," [*The Public Interest* 21:3–15 (1970)], argues that this is a minority view; most accept the marriage of the market ideal and the merits of individual effort and performance. I agree with this point of view—which is to say I see the dominant model of justice in America as a merger of the notions of meritarian and market norms.

6 Marcuse, H., "The Ideology of Death," in: Feifel, H., *The Meaning of Death* (New York: McGraw-Hill, 1959).

7 Illich, I., "The Political Uses of Natural Death," *Hastings Center Studies* 2:3–20 (1974).

8 For excellent discussions of the notion of market "externalities," see: Hardin, G., *Exploring New Ethics for Survival* (Baltimore, Md.: Penguin Books, 1972); Mishan, E., *The Costs of Economic Growth* (New York: Praeger, 1967); and Kapp, W., *Social Costs of Business Enterprise*, 2d ed. (New York: Asia Publishing House, 1964).

9 Brotman, R. and Suffet, F., "The Concept of Prevention and Its Limitations," *The Annals of the American Academy of Political and Social Science* 417:53–65 (1975).

10 Ryan, W., *Blaming the Victim* (New York: Vintage Books, 1971). See Barry, P., "Individual Versus Community Orientation in the Prevention of Injuries," *Preventive Medicine* 4:45–56 (1975), for an excellent discussion of "victim-blaming" in the field of injury-control. Also, see Beauchamp, D., "Alcoholism As Blaming the Alcoholic," *The International Journal of Addictions* 11 (1) (1976); and "The Alcohol Alibi: Blaming Alcoholics," *Society* 12:12–17 (1975), for discussion of the process of victim-blaming in the area of alcoholism policy.

11 Etzioni and Remp, *op. cit.*

12 Freidson, E., *Professional Dominance* (Chicago: Aldine, 1971).

13 Barthes, R., *Mythologies* (New York: Hill and Wang, 1972).

14 McKnight, J., "The Medicalization of Politics," *Christian Century* 92:785–787 (1975).

15 Tawney, R., *Equality* (London: G. Allen and Unwin, 1964).

16 Hobhouse, L. T., *Liberalism* (New York: Oxford University Press, 1964).

17 Rawls, J., *A Theory of Justice* (Cambridge: Harvard University Press, 1971).

18 I am aware that I am passing too quickly over a very complex subject: The formative influences for public health. I am simply asserting that the dream of eliminating or minimizing preventable death and disability involves a radical commitment to the protection and preservation of human life and that this vision ultimately belongs to the tradition of social justice. Further, one can clearly find social justice influences in the classics of the public health literature. For example, see: Smith, S., *The City That Was* (Metuchen, N.J.: Scarecrow Reprint Corporation, 1973); and Winslow, C.- E. A., *The Life of Hermann Biggs, Physician and Statesman of the Public Health* (Philadelphia: Lea and Febiger, 1929).

There are several reasons why public health has seldom been treated as standing in the tradition of social justice. Public health usually entails public or collective goods (such as clean air and water supplies) where the question of distributive shares seems not important. However, for collective goods and in the case of death and disability, the key distributive questions are the *numbers* or *rates* of persons who suffer these fates, that no group or individual be unfairly or arbitrarily excluded from protection, and that the *burdens* of collective policies be fairly distributed. Writers in the tradition of social justice (such as Rawls) do not pay sufficient attention to the social justice implications of public or collective goods. This helps explain in part why many in the public health movement seldom saw themselves as involved in a drive for social justice—their work was defined as protection for the entire community (and often the entire community, rather than a minority, seem threatened in the age of acute infectious epidemics or in the drive for sanitary reform). Further, while there was opposition to even these reforms, the question of distributing the burdens of collective action did not arise so acutely as it does in the present period.

19 Government of Canada. *A New Perspective on the Health of Canadians* (Ottawa, Ontario, Canada: Ministry of National Health and Welfare, 1974).

20 By the "public health ethic" I mean several things: The assignment of the highest priority to the preservation of human life, the assurance that this protection is extended maximally (consistent with maintaining basic political liberties: See Rawls, *op. cit.*,....), that no person or group should be arbitrarily excluded, and finally that all persons ought accept these burdens of preserving life as just.

21 Two examples of this point: A standard text in health administration, John Hanlon's *Public Health Administration and Practice* (St. Louis, Missouri: C. V. Mosby, 1974), does reference very broad definitions of public health but quickly settles down to discussing public health in terms of those various programs designed to deal with market failures or inadequacies. Nowhere does Hanlon seem to view the concept of public health as an ethical concept standing as a fundamental critique of the existing measures to protect human life. Second, a recent proposed policy statement on prevention for adoption by the American Public Health Association (*The Nation's Health*, October 1975), does give a very high priority to prevention but contains within it a major concession to the norm of market-justice—the category of voluntary or self-imposed risks and the treatment of this category as distinctively different from other public health hazards.

22 Beauchamp, D., "Public Health: Alien Ethic in a Strange Land?" *American Journal of Public Health* 65:1338–1339 (December 1975).

23 I hasten to add that I am not arguing that there are exactly four principles of the public health ethic. Actually, the four offered here can be easily collapsed to two—controls over the hazards of this world and the fair sharing of the burdens of these controls. However, the reason for expanding these two key principles is to draw out the character of the public health ethic as a counter-ethic or counter-paradigm to the market model, and to demonstrate that the public health ethic focuses on different aspects of the world, asserts different priorities and imposes different obligations than the market ethic.

24 Brotman and Suffet, *op. cit.*

25 Sade, R., "Medical Care As A Right: A Refutation," *The New England Journal of Medicine* 285:1288–1292 (1971).

26 Ryan, *op. cit.* See also: Terris, M., "A Social Policy for Health," *American Journal of Public Health* 58:5–12 (1968).

27 See Brown, R., *Explanation in Social Science* (Chicago: Aldine, 1963) for an excellent discussion of the limitations of dispositional explanations in social science. Also, see Beauchamp, D., "Alcoholism as Blaming the Alcoholic," *op. cit.*, for a further discussion of the pitfalls of dispositional explanations in the specific area of alcohol policy.

28 For excellent discussions of the strategies of public health, see: Haddon, W., Jr., "Energy Damage and the Ten Countermeasure Strategies," *The Journal of Trauma* 13:321–331 (1973); Haddon, W., Jr.,

"The Changing Approach to the Epidemiology, Prevention, and Amelioration of Trauma," *American Journal of Public Health* 58:1431–1438 (1968); and Terris, M., "Breaking the Barriers to Prevention," paper presented to the Annual Health Conference, New York Academy of Medicine, April 26, 1974.

29 Olson, M., *The Logic of Collective Action* (Cambridge: Harvard University Press, 1965).

30 Beauchamp, D., "Federal Alcohol Policy: Captive to an Industry and a Myth," *Christian Century* 92:788–791 (1975).

31 This principle is similar to Rawls' "difference principle." See Rawls, *op. cit.*

Voluntary Risks to Health: The Ethical Issues

Robert M. Veatch

A biographical sketch of Robert M. Veatch is found on page 56.

Veatch explores some of the empirical, conceptual, and ethical issues raised by the correlation between life-styles and health. He first addresses a question whose answer embodies both empirical and conceptual considerations: "Are health risks voluntary?" In response, Veatch presents four conceptual approaches, or models: (1) the voluntary model, (2) the medical model, (3) the psychological model, and (4) the social structural model. Citing the limitations of each of these models, Veatch argues for the adoption of a multicausal model. He then distinguishes between responsibility and culpability and explores some of the pro and con arguments regarding the just treatment of individuals who squander their opportunity for good health. Veatch defends the view that if individuals have equal opportunities to be healthy, it is just to treat those who waste their opportunities by engaging in voluntary high-risk behavior differently from those who do not. Policies adopted in keeping with such differential treatment might include taxes on cigarettes or special insurance plans for those on an unhealthy diet.

In an earlier era, one's health was thought to be determined by the gods or by fate. The individual had little responsibility for personal health. In terms of the personal responsibility for health and disease, the modern medical model has required little change in this view. One of the primary elements of the medical model was the belief that people were exempt from responsibility for their condition.[1] If one had good health in old age,

from the vantage point of the belief system of the medical model, one would say he had been blessed with good health. Disease was the result of mysterious, uncontrollable microorganisms or the random process of genetic fate.

A few years ago we developed a case study[2] involving a purely hypothetical proposal that smokers should be required to pay for the costs of their extra health care

Reprinted with permission of the author and the publisher from *Journal of the American Medical Association*, vol. 243 (January 4, 1980), pp. 50–55.

required over and above that of nonsmokers. The scheme involved taxing tobacco at a rate calculated to add to the nation's budget an amount equal to the marginal health cost of smoking.

Recently a number of proposals have been put forth that imply that individuals are in some sense personally responsible for the state of their health. The town of Alexandria, Va., refuses to hire smokers as fire fighters, in part because smokers increase the cost of health and disability insurance (*The New York Times*, Dec. 18, 1977, p. 28). Oral Roberts University insists that students meet weight requirements to attend school. Claiming that the school was concerned about the whole person, the school dean said that the school was just as concerned about the students' physical growth as their intellectual and spiritual growth (*The New York Times*, Oct. 9, 1977, p. 77). Behaviors as highly diverse as smoking, skiing, playing professional football, compulsive eating, omitting exercise, exposing oneself excessively to the sun, skipping needed immunizations, automobile racing, and mountain climbing all can be viewed as having a substantial voluntary component. Health care needed as a result of any voluntary behavior might generate very different claims on a health care system from care conceptualized as growing out of some other causal nexus. Keith Reemtsma, M.D., chairman of the Department of Surgery at Columbia University's College of Physicians and Surgeons, has called for "a more rational approach to improving national health," involving "a reward/ punishment system based on individual choices." Persons who smoked cigarettes, drank whiskey, drove cars, and owned guns would be taxed for the medical consequences of their choices (*The New York Times*, Oct. 14, 1976, p. 37). That individuals should be personally responsible for their health is a new theme, implying a new model for health care and perhaps for funding of health care.[3-6]

Some data correlating life-style to health status are being generated. They seem to support the conceptual shift toward a model that sees the individual as more personally responsible for his health status. The data of Belloc and Breslow[7-9] make those of us who lead the slovenly life-style very uncomfortable. As Morison[3] has pointed out, John Wesley and his puritan brothers of the covenant may not have been far from wrong after all. Belloc and Breslow identify seven empirical correlates of good health: eating moderately, eating regularly, eating breakfast, no cigarette smoking, moderate or no use of alcohol, at least moderate exercise, and seven to eight hours of sleep nightly. They all seem to be well within human control, far less mysterious than the viruses and genes that exceed the comprehension of the average citizen. The authors found that the average physical health of persons aged 70 years who reported all of the preceding good health practices was about the same as persons aged 35 to 44 years who reported fewer than three.

We have just begun to realize the policy implications and the ethical impact of the conceptual shift that begins viewing health[7] status as, in part, a result of voluntary risk taking in personal behavior and life-style choices. If individuals are responsible to some degree for their health and their need for health resources, why should they not also be responsible for the costs involved? If national health insurance is on the horizon, it will be even more questionable that individuals should have such health care paid for out of the same money pool generated by society to pay for other kinds of health care. Even with existing insurance plans, is it equitable that all persons contributing to the insurance money pool pay the extra costs of those who voluntarily run the risk of increasing their need for medical services?

The most obvious policy proposals—banning from the health care system risky behaviors and persons who have medical needs resulting from such risks—turns out to be the least plausible.[10,11] For one thing, it is going to be extremely difficult to establish precisely the cause of the lung tumor at the time the patient is standing at the hospital door. Those who have carcinoma of the lung possibly from smoking or from unknown causes should not be excluded.

Even if the voluntary component of the cause could be determined, it is unlikely that our society could or would choose to implement a policy of barring the doors. While we have demonstrated a capacity to risk statistical lives or to risk the lives of citizens with certain socioeconomic characteristics, it is unlikely that we would be prepared to follow an overall policy of refusing medical service to those who voluntarily brought on their own conditions. We fought a similar battle over social security and concluded that—in part for reasons of the stress placed on family members and on society as a whole—individuals would not be permitted to take the risk of staying outside the social security system.

A number of policy options are more plausible. Additional health fees on health-risk behavior calculated to reimburse the health care system would redistribute the burden of the cost of such care to those who have chosen to engage in it. Separating health insurance pools for persons who engage in health-risk behavior and requiring them to pay out of pocket the marginal cost of their health care is another alternative. In some cases the economic cost is not the critical factor, it may be scarce personnel or equipment. Some behaviors might have to be banned to free the best neurosurgeons or orthopedic specialists for those who need their services for reasons other than for injuries suffered from the motorcycle accident or skiing tumble. Of course, all of these policy options require not only judgments about whether these behaviors are truly voluntary, but also ethical judgments about the rights and responsibilities of the individual and the other, more social components of the society.

There are several ethical principles that could lead us to be concerned about these apparently voluntary behaviors and even lead us to justify decisions to change our social policy about paying for or providing health care needed as a result of such behavior. The most obvious, the most traditional, medical ethical basis for concern is that the welfare of the individual is at stake. The Hippocratic tradition is committed to having the physician do what he thinks will benefit the patient. If one were developing an insurance policy or a mode of approaching the individual patient for private practice, paternalistic concern about the medical welfare of the patient might lead to a conclusion that, for the good of the patient, this behavior ought to be prevented or deferred. The paternalistic Hippocratic ethic, however, is suspect in circles outside the medical profession and is even coming under attack from within the physician community itself.[12] The Hippocratic ethic leaves no room for the principle of self-determination—a principle at the core of liberal Western thought. The freedom of choice to smoke, ski, and even race automobiles may well justify avoiding more coercive policies regarding these behaviors—assuming that it is the individual's own welfare that is at stake. The hyperindividualistic ethics of Hippocratism also leaves no room for concern for the welfare of others or the distribution of burdens within the society. A totally different rationale for concern is being put forward, however. Some, such as Tom Beauchamp,[13] have argued that we have a right to be concerned about such behaviors because of their social costs. He leaves unanswered the question of why it would be considered fair or just to regulate these voluntary behaviors when and only when their total social costs exceed the total social benefits of the behavior. This is a question we must explore.

Clearly, the argument is a complex one requiring many empirical, conceptual, and ethical judgments. Those judgments will have to be made regardless of whether we decide to continue the present policy or adopt one of the proposed alternatives. At this point, we need a thorough statement of the kinds of questions that must be addressed and the types of judgments that must be made.

ARE HEALTH RISKS VOLUNTARY?

The first question, addressed to those advocating policy shifts based on the notion that persons are in some sense responsible for their own health, melds the conceptual and empirical issues. Are health risks voluntary? Several models are competing for the conceptual attention of those working in the field.

The Voluntary Model

The model that considers the individual as personally responsible for his health has a great deal going for it. The empirical correlations of life-style choices with health status are impressive. The view of humans as personally responsible for their destiny is attractive to those of us within modern Western society. Its appeal extends beyond the view of the human as subject to the forces of fate and even the medical model, which as late as the 1950s saw disease as an attack on the individual coming from outside the person and outside his control.

The Medical Model

Of course, that it is attractive cannot justify opting for the voluntarist model if it flies in the face of the empirical reality. The theory of external and uncontrollable causation is central to the medical model.[14] It is still probably the case that organic causal chains almost totally outside human control account now and then for a disease. But the medical model has been under such an onslaught of reality testing in the last decade that it can hardly provide a credible alternative to the voluntarist model. Even for those conditions that undeniably have an organic causal component, the luxury of human innocence is no longer a plausible defense against human accountability. The more we learn about disease and health and their causal chains, the more we have the possibility of intervening to change those chains of causation. Since the days of the movement for public health, sanitation, and control of contagion, there has been a rational basis for human responsibility. Even for those conditions that do not yet lend themselves to such direct voluntary control, the chronic diseases and even genetic diseases, there exists the possibility of purposeful, rational decisions that have an indirect impact on the risk. Choices can be made to minimize our exposure to potential carcinogens and risk factors for cardiovascular disease. Parents now have a variety of potential choices to minimize genetic disease risk and even eliminate it in certain cases. We may not be far from the day when we can say that all health problems can be viewed as someone's fault—if not our own fault for poor sanitary practices and life-style choices, then the fault of our parents for avoiding carrier status diagnosis, amniocentesis, and selective abortion; the fault of industries that pollute our environment; or the fault of the National Institutes of Health for failing to make the scientific breakthroughs to understand the causal chain so that we could intervene. Although there remains a streak of plausibility in the medical model as an account of disease and health, it is fading rapidly and may soon remain only as a fossil-like trace in our model of health.

The Psychological Model

While the medical model seems to offer at best a limited counter to the policy options rooted in the voluntarist model, other theories of determinism may be more plausible. Any policy to control health care services that are viewed as necessitated by voluntary choices to risk one's health is based on the judgment that the behavior is indeed voluntary. The primary argument countering policies to tax or control smoking to be fair in distributing the burdens for treating smokers' health problems is that the smoker is not really responsible for his medical problems. The argument is not normally based on organic or genetic theories of determinism, but on more psychological theories. The smoker's personality and even the initial pattern of smoking are developed at such an early point in life that they could be viewed as beyond voluntary control. If the smoker's behavior is the result of toilet training rather than rational decision making, then to blame the smoker for the toilet training seems odd.

Many of the other presumably voluntary risks to health might also be seen as psychologically determined and therefore not truly voluntary. Compulsive eating, the sedentary life-style, and the choice of a high-stress life pattern may all be psychologically determined.

Football playing is a medically risky behavior. For the professional, the choice seems to be made consciously and voluntarily. But the choice to participate in high school and even grade school competitive leagues may not really be the voluntary choice of the student. Then, if reward systems are generated from these early choices, certainly college level football could be the result. The continuum from partially nonvoluntary choices of the youngster to the career choice of professional athlete may have a heavy psychological overlay after all.

If so-called voluntary health risks are really psychologically determined, then the ethical and policy implications collapse. But it must seriously be questioned whether the model of psychological determinism is a much more plausible monocausal explanation of these behaviors than the medical model. Choosing to be a professional football player, or even to continue smoking, simply cannot be viewed as determined and beyond personal choice because of demonstrated irresistible psychological forces. The fact that so many people have stopped smoking or drinking or even playing professional sports reveals that such choices are fundamentally different from monocausally determined behaviors. Although state of mind may be a component in all disease, it seems that an attempt to will away pneumonia or a carcinoma of the pancreas is much less likely to be decisively influential than using the will to control the behaviors that are now being grouped as voluntary.

The Social Structural Model

Perhaps the most plausible competition to the voluntarist model comes not from a theory of organic or even psychological determinism, but from a social structural model. The correlations of disease, mortality, and even so-called voluntary health-risk behavior with socioeconomic class are impressive. Recent data from Great Britain and from the Medicaid system in the United States[15] reveal that these correlations persist even with elaborate schemes that attempt to make health care more equitably available to all social classes. In Great Britain, for instance, it has recently been revealed that differences in death rates by social class continue, with inequalities essentially undiminished, since the advent of the National Health Service. Continuing to press the voluntarist model of personal responsibility for health risk in the face of a social structural model of the patterns of health and disease could be nothing more than blaming the victim,[16-19] avoiding the reality of the true causes of disease, and escaping proper social responsibility for changing the underlying social inequalities of the society and its modes of production.

This is a powerful counter to the voluntarist thesis. Even if it is shown that health and disease are governed by behaviors and risk factors subject to human control, it does not follow that the individual should bear the sole or even primary responsibility for bringing about the changes necessary to produce better health. If it is the case that for virtually every disease, those who are the poorest, those who are in the lowest socioeconomic classes, are at the greatest risk,[20-22] then there is a piously evasive quality to proposals that insist on individuals changing their life-styles to improve their positions and their health potential. The smoker may not be forced into his behavior so much by toilet training as by the social forces of the workplace or the society. The professional football player may be forced into that role by the work alternatives available to him, especially if he is a victim of racial, economic, and educational inequities.

If one had to make a forced choice between the voluntarist model and the social structural model, the choice would be difficult. The knowledge that some socially deprived persons have pulled themselves up by their bootstraps is cited as evidence for the voluntarist model, but the overwhelming power of the social system to hold most individuals in their social place cannot be ignored.

A Multicausal Model and Its Implications

The only reasonable alternative is to adopt a multicausal model; one that has a place for organic, psychological, and social theories of causation, as well as voluntarist elements, in an account of the cause of a disease or health pattern. One of the great conceptual issues confronting persons working in this area will be whether it is logically or psychologically possible to maintain simultaneously voluntarist and deterministic theories. In other areas of competing causal theories, such as theories of crime, drug addiction, and occupational achievement, we have not been very successful in maintaining the two types of explanation simultaneously. I am not convinced that it is impossible. A theory of criminal behavior that simultaneously lets the individual view criminal behavior as voluntary while the society views it as socially or psychologically determined has provocative and attractive implications. In the end it may be no more illogical or implausible than a reductionistic, monocausal theory.

The problem parallels one of the classic problems of philosophy and theology: How is it that there can be freedom of the will while at the same time the world is orderly and predictable? In more theological language, how can humans be free to choose good and evil while at the same time affirming that they are dependent on divine grace and that there is a transcendent order to the world? The tension is apparent in the Biblical authors, the Pelagian controversy of the fourth century, Arminius's struggle with the Calvinists, and contemporary secular arguments over free will. The conclusion that freedom of choice is a pseudo-problem, that it is compatible with predictability in the social order, may be the most plausible of the alternative, seemingly paradoxical answers.

The same conclusions may be reached regarding voluntary health risks. It would be a serious problem if a voluntarist theory led to abandoning any sense of social structural responsibility for health patterns. On the other hand, it seems clear that there are disease and health differentials even within socioeconomic classes and that some element of voluntary choice of life-style remains that leads to illness, even for the elite of the capitalist society and even for the members of the classless society. The voluntarist model seems at least to apply to differentials in behavior within socioeconomic classes or within groups similarly situated. Admitting the possibility of a theory of causation that includes a voluntary element may so distract the society from attention to the social and economic components in the causal nexus that the move would become counterproductive. On the other hand, important values are affirmed in the view that the human is in some sense responsible for his own medical destiny, that he is not merely the receptacle for external forces. These values are important in countering the trend toward the professionalization of medical decisions and the reduction of the individual to a passive object to be manipulated. They are so important that some risk may well be necessary. This is one of the core problems in any discussion of the ethics of the voluntary health-risk perspective. One of the most difficult research questions posed by the voluntary health-risk theme is teasing out the implications of the theme for a theory of the causation of health patterns.

RESPONSIBILITY AND CULPABILITY

Even in cases where we conclude that the voluntarist model may be relevant—where voluntary choices are at least a minor component of the pattern of health—it is still unclear what to make of the voluntarist conclusion. If we say that a person is responsible for his health, it still does not follow that the person is culpable for the harm that comes from voluntary choices. It may be that society still would want to bear the burden of providing health care needed to patch up a person who has voluntarily taken a health risk.

To take an extreme example, a member of a community may choose to become a professional fire fighter. Certainly this is a health-risking choice. Presumably it could be a relatively voluntary one. Still it does not follow that the person is culpable for the harms done to his health. Responsible, yes, but culpable, no.

To decide in favor of any policy incorporating the so-called presumption that health risks are voluntary, it will be necessary to decide not only that the risk is voluntary, but also that it is not worthy of public subsidy. Fire fighting, an occupation undertaken in the public interest, probably would be worthy of subsidy. It seems that very few such activities, however, are so evaluated. Professional automobile racing, for instance, hardly seems socially ennobling, even if it does provide entertainment and diversion. A more plausible course would be requiring auto racers to purchase a license for a fee equal to their predicted extra health costs.

But what about the health risks of casual automobile driving for business or personal reasons? There are currently marginal health costs that are not built into the insurance system, e.g., risks from automobile exhaust pollution, from stress, and from the discouraging of exercise. It seems as though, in principle, there would be nothing wrong with recovering the economic part of those costs, if it could be done. A health tax on gasoline, for instance, might be sensible as a progressive way of funding a national health service. The evidence for the direct causal links and the exact costs will be hard, probably impossible, to discover. That difficulty, however, may not be decisive, provided there is general agreement that there are some costs, that the behavior is not socially ennobling, and that the funds are obtained more or less equitably in any case. It would certainly be no worse than some other luxury tax.

THE ARGUMENTS FROM JUSTICE

The core of the argument over policies deriving from the voluntary health-risks thesis is the argument over what is fair or just. Regardless of whether individuals have a general right to health care, or whether justice in general requires the social provision of health services, it seems as though what justice requires for a risk voluntarily assumed is quite different from what it might require in the more usual medical need.

Two responses have been offered to the problem of justice in providing health care for medical needs resulting from voluntarily assumed risks. One by Dan Beauchamp[19,23] and others resolves the problem by attacking the category of voluntary risk. He implies that so-called voluntary behaviors are, in reality, the result of social and cultural forces. Since voluntary behavior is a null set, the special implications of meritorious or blameworthy behavior for a theory of justice are of no importance. Beauchamp begins forcefully with a somewhat egalitarian theory of social justice, which leads to a moral right to health for all citizens. There is no need to amend that theory to account for fairness of the claims of citizens who bring on their need for health care through their voluntary choices, because there are no voluntary choices.

It seems reasonable to concede to Dan Beauchamp that the medical model has been overly individualistic, that socioeconomic and cultural forces play a much greater role in the causal nexus of health problems than is normally assumed. Indeed, they probably play the dominant role. But the total elimination of voluntarism from our understanding of human behavior is quite implausible. Injuries to the socioeconomic elite while mountain climbing or waterskiing are not reasonably seen as primarily the result of social structural determinism. If there remains a residuum of the voluntary theory, then one of justice for health care will have to take that into account.

A second approach is that of Tom Beauchamp,[13] who goes further than Dan Beauchamp. He attacks the principle of justice itself. Dan Beauchamp seems to hold that justice or fairness requires us to distribute resources according to need. Since needs are not the result of voluntary choices, a subsidiary consideration of whether the need results from foolish, voluntary behavior is unnecessary. Tom Beauchamp, on the other hand, rejects the idea that needs per se have a claim on us as a society. He seems to accept the idea that at least occasionally behaviors may be voluntary. He questions whether need alone provides a plausible basis for deciding what is fair in cases where the individual has voluntarily risked his health and is subsequently in need of medical services. He offers a utilitarian alternative, claiming that the crucial dimension is the total social costs of the behaviors. He argues:

> Hazardous personal behaviors should be restricted if, and only if: (1) the behavior creates risks of harm to persons other than those who engage in such activities, and (2) a cost-benefit analysis reveals that the social investment in controlling such behaviors would produce a net increase in social utility, rather than a net decrease.

The implication is that any social advantage to the society that can come from controlling these behaviors would justify intervention, regardless of how the benefits and burdens of the policy are distributed.

A totally independent, nonpaternalistic argument is based much more in the principle of justice. This approach examines not only the impact of disease, but also questions of fairness. It is asked, is it fair that society as a whole should bear the burden of providing medical care needed only because of voluntarily taken risks to one's health? From this point of view, even if the net benefit of letting the behavior continue exceeded the benefits of prohibiting it, the behavior justifiably might be prohibited, or at least controlled, on nonpaternalistic grounds. Consider the case, for instance, where the benefits accrue overwhelmingly to persons who do engage in the behavior and the costs to those who do not. If the need for medical care is the result of the voluntary choice to engage in the behavior, then those arguing from the standpoint of equity or fairness might conclude that the behavior should still be controlled even though it produces a net benefit in aggregate.

Both Beauchamps downplay a secondary dimension of the argument over the principle of justice. Even those who accept the egalitarian formula ought to concede that all an individual is entitled to is an equal opportunity for a chance to be as healthy, insofar as possible, as other people.[24] Since those who are volun-

tarily risking their health (assuming for the moment that the behavior really is voluntary) do have an opportunity to be healthy, it is not the egalitarian dimensions of the principle of justice that are relevant to the voluntary health-risks question. It is the question of what is just treatment of those who have had opportunity and have not taken advantage of it. The question is one of what to do with persons who have not made use of their chance. Even the most egalitarian theories of justice—of which I consider myself to be a proponent—must at times deal with the secondary question of what to do in cases where individuals voluntarily have chosen to use their opportunities unequally. Unless there is no such thing as voluntary health-risk behavior, as Dan Beauchamp implies, this must remain a problem for the more egalitarian theories of justice.

In principle I see nothing wrong with the conclusion, which even an egalitarian would hold, that those who have not used fairly their opportunities receive inequalities of outcome. I emphasize that this is an argument in principle. It would not apply to persons who are truly not equal in their opportunity because of their social or psychological conditions. It would not apply to those who are forced into their health-risky behavior because of social oppression or stress in the mode of production.

From this application of a subsidiary component of the principle of justice, I reach the conclusion that it is fair, that it is just, if persons in need of health services resulting from true, voluntary risks are treated differently from those in need of the same services for other reasons. In fact, it would be unfair if the two groups were treated equally.

For most cases this would justify only the funding of the needed health care separately in cases where the need results from voluntary behavior. In extreme circumstances, however, where the resources needed are scarce and cannot be supplemented with more funds (e.g., when it is the skill that is scarce), then actual prohibition of the behavior may be the only plausible option, if one is arguing from this kind of principle of justice.

This essentially egalitarian principle, which says that like cases should be treated alike, leaves us with one final problem under the rubric of justice. If all voluntary risks ought to be treated alike, what do we make of the fact that only certain of the behaviors are monitorable? Is it unfair to place a health tax on smoking, automobile racing, skiing at organized resorts with ski lifts, and other organized activities that one can monitor, while letting slip by failing to exercise, mountain climbing, skiing on the hill on one's farm, and other behaviors that cannot be monitored? In a sense it may be. The problem is perhaps like the unfairness of being able to treat the respiratory problems of pneumonia, but not those of trisomy E syndrome or other incurable diseases. There may be some essential unfairness in life. This may appear in the inequities of policy proposals to control or tax monitorable behavior, but not behavior that cannot be monitored. Actually some ingenuity may generate ways to tax what seems untaxable— taxing gasoline for the health risks of automobiles, taxing mountain climbing equipment (assuming it is not an ennobling activity), or creating special insurance pools for persons who eat a bad diet. The devices probably would be crude and not necessarily in exact proportion to the risks involved. Some people engaged in equally risky behaviors probably would not be treated equally. That may be a necessary implication of the crudeness of any public policy mechanism. Whether the inequities of not being able to treat equally people taking comparable risks constitute such a serious problem that it would be better to abandon entirely the principle of equality of opportunity for health is the policy question that will have to be resolved.

COST-SAVING HEALTH-RISK BEHAVIORS

Another argument is mounted against the application of the principle of equity to voluntarily health-risking behaviors. What ought to be done with behaviors that are health risky, but that end up either not costing society or actually saving society's scarce resources? This question will separate clearly those who argue for intervention on paternalistic grounds from those who argue on utilitarian grounds or on the basis of the principle of justice. What ought to be done about a behavior that would risk a person's health, but risk it in such a way that he would die rapidly and cheaply at about retirement age? If the concern is from the unfair burden that these behaviors generate on the rest of society, and, if the society is required to bear the costs and to use scarce resources, then a health-risk behavior that did not involve such social costs would surely be exempt from any social policy oriented to controlling such unfair behavior. In fact, if social utility were the only concern, then this particular type of risky behavior

ought to be encouraged. Since our social policy is one that ought to incorporate many ethical concerns, it seems unlikely that we would want to encourage these behaviors even if such encouragement were cost-effective. This, indeed, shows the weakness of approaches that focus only on aggregate costs and benefits.

REVULSION AGAINST THE RATIONAL, CALCULATING LIFE

There is one final, last-ditch argument against adoption of a health policy that incorporates an equitable handling of voluntary health risks. Some would argue that, although the behavior might be voluntary and supplying health care to meet the resulting needs unfair to the rest of the society, the alternative would be even worse. Such a policy might require the conversion of many decisions in life from spontaneous expressions based on long tradition and life-style patterns to cold, rational, calculating decisions based on health and economic elements.

It is not clear to me that that would be the result. Placing a health fee on a package of cigarettes or on a ski-lift ticket may not make those decisions any more rational calculations than they are now. The current warning on tobacco has not had much of an impact. Even if rational decision making were the outcome, however, I am not sure that it would be wrong to elevate such health-risking decisions to a level of consciousness in which one had to think about what one was doing. At least it seems that as a side effect of a policy that would permit health resources to be paid for and used more equitably, this would not be an overwhelming or decisive counterargument.

CONCLUSION

The health policy decisions that must be made in an era in which a multicausal theory is the only plausible one are going to be much harder than the ones made in the simpler era of the medical model—but then, those were harder than some of the ones that had to be made in the era where health was in the hands of the gods. Several serious questions remain to be answered. These are both empirical and normative. They may constitute a research agenda for pursuing the question of ethics and health policy for an era when some risks to health may be seen, at least by some people, as voluntary.

REFERENCES

1 Parsons, T., *The Social System*. New York, The Free Press, 1951, p. 437.
2 Steinfels, P., Veatch, R. M., Who should pay for smokers' medical care? *Hastings Cent. Rep.* 4:8–10, 1974.
3 Morison, R. S., Rights and responsibilities: Redressing the uneasy balance. *Hastings Cent. Rep.* 4:1–4, 1974.
4 Vayda, E., Keeping people well: A new approach to medicine. *Hum. Nature* 1:64–71, 1978.
5 Somers, A. R., Hayden, M. C., Rights and responsibilities in prevention. *Health Educ.* 9:37–39, 1978.
6 Kass, L., Regarding the end of medicine and the pursuit of health. *Public Interest* 40:11–42, 1975.
7 Belloc, N. B., Breslow, L., Relationship of physical status health and health practices. *Prev. Med.* 1:409–421, 1972.
8 Belloc, N. B., Relationship of health practices and mortality. *Prev. Med.* 2:68–81, 1973.
9 Breslow, L., Prospects for improving health through reducing risk factors. *Prev. Med.* 7:449–458, 1978.
10 Wikler, D., Coercive measures in health promotion: Can they be justified? *Health Educ. Monogr.* 6:223–241, 1978.
11 Wikler, D., Persuasion and coercion for health: Ethical issues in government efforts to change lifestyles. *Milbank Mem. Fund Q.* 56:303–338, 1978.
12 Veatch, R. M., The Hippocratic ethic: Consequentialism, individualism and paternalism, in Smith, D. H., Bernstein, L. M. (eds.), *No Rush to Judg-ment: Essays on Medical Ethics*. Bloomington, Ind., The Poynter Center, Indiana University, 1978, pp. 238–264.
13 Beauchamp, T., The regulation of hazards and hazardous behaviors. *Health Educ. Monogr.* 6:242–257, 1978.
14 Veatch, R. M., The medical model: Its nature and problems. *Hastings Cent. Rep.* 1:59–76, 1973.
15 Morris, J. N., Social inequalities undiminished. *Lancet* 1:87–90, 1979.
16 Ryan, W., *Blaming the Victim*. New York, Vintage Books, 1971.
17 Crawford, R., Sickness as sin. *Health Policy Advisory Center Bull.* 80:10–16, 1978.
18 Crawford, R., You are dangerous to your health. *Social Policy* 8:11–20, 1978.
19 Beauchamp, D. E., Public health as social justice. *Inquiry* 13:3–14, 1976.
20 Syme, L., Berkman, I., Social class, susceptibility and sickness. *Am. J. Epidemiol.* 104:1–8, 1976.
21 Conover, P. W., Social class and chronic illness. *Int. J. Health Serv.* 3:357–368, 1973.
22 *Health of the Disadvantaged: Chart Book*, publication (HRA) 77-628. Hyattsville, Md., U.S. Dept. of Health, Education, and Welfare, Public Health Service, Health Resources Administration, 1977.
23 Beauchamp, D. E., Alcoholism as blaming the alcoholic. *Int. J. Addict.* 11:41–52, 1976.
24 Veatch, R. M., What is a "just" health care delivery? in Branson, R., Veatch, R. M. (eds.), *Ethics and Health Policy*. Cambridge, Mass., Ballinger Publishing Co., 1976, pp. 127–153.

Microallocation Decisions

The Allocation of Exotic Medical Lifesaving Therapy

Nicholas P. Rescher

Nicholas P. Rescher is professor of philosophy at the University of Pittsburgh. Among his many books are *The Logic of Commands* (1966), *Distributive Justice: A Constructive Critique of the Utilitarian Theory of Distribution* (1966), *Welfare: The Social Issues in Philosophical Perspective* (1972), *Unselfishness: The Role of the Vicarious Affects in Moral Philosophy* (1975), and *Dialectics: A Controversy*

Reprinted with permission of the author and the publisher from *Ethics*, vol. 79, no. 3 (April 1969), pp. 173–86. Copyright © 1969 by The University of Chicago.

Oriented Approach to the Theory of Knowledge (1977). Rescher's published articles include "Ethical Issues Regarding the Delivery of Health-Care Services."

Rescher focuses on *microallocation* decisions regarding scarce medical lifesaving therapies. He attempts to set forth the criteria that should govern the selection process when the decisions made determine who will be given and who will be denied the opportunity to survive. Rescher advocates a two-tiered, cluster-of-criteria system. He suggests one set of criteria that should be used to determine who will be placed in the pool of applicants from which some will be chosen to receive treatment. The main criterion here seems to be the "prospect of success factor." Rescher then proposes a second set of criteria that should be used to select individuals from the first pool. In presenting this second set of criteria, Rescher appeals to both utility and justice. He concludes by arguing that if there are no really significant disparities within the pool of candidates selected by this two-step process, a random selection process should be used in making the final decisions.

I THE PROBLEM

Technological progress has in recent years transformed the limits of the possible in medical therapy. However, the elevated state of sophistication of modern medical technology has brought the economists' classic problem of scarcity in its wake as an unfortunate side product. The enormously sophisticated and complex equipment and the highly trained teams of experts requisite for its utilization are scarce resources in relation to potential demand. The administrators of the great medical institutions that preside over these scarce resources thus come to be faced increasingly with the awesome choice: *Whose life to save?*

A (somewhat hypothetical) paradigm example of this problem may be sketched within the following set of definitive assumptions: We suppose that persons in some particular medically morbid condition are "mortally afflicted": It is virtually certain that they will die within a short time period (say ninety days). We assume that some very complex course of treatment (e.g., a heart transplant) represents a substantial probability of life prolongation for persons in this mortally afflicted condition. We assume that the facilities available in terms of human resources, mechanical instrumentalities, and requisite materials (e.g., hearts in the case of a heart transplant) make it possible to give a certain treatment—this "exotic (medical) lifesaving therapy," or ELT for short—to a certain, relatively small number of people. And finally we assume that a substantially greater pool of people in the mortally afflicted condition is at hand. The problem then may be formulated as follows: How is one to select within the pool of afflicted patients the ones to be given the ELT treatment in question: how to select those "whose lives are to be saved"? Faced with many candidates for an ELT process that can be made available to only a few, doctors and medical administrators confront the decision of who is to be given a chance at survival and who is, in effect, to be condemned to die.

As has already been implied, the "heroic" variety of spare-part surgery can pretty well be assimilated to this paradigm. One can foresee the time when heart transplantation, for example, will have become pretty much a routine medical procedure, albeit on a very limited basis, since a cardiac surgeon with the technical competence to transplant hearts can operate at best a rather small number of times each week and the elaborate facilities for such operations will most probably exist on a modest scale. Moreover, in "spare-part" surgery there is always the problem of availability of the "spare parts" themselves. A report in one British newspaper gives the following picture: "Of the 150,000 who die of heart disease each year [in the U.K.], Mr. Donald Longmore, research surgeon at the National Heart Hospital [in London] estimates that 22,000 might be eligible for heart surgery. Another 30,000 would need heart and lung transplants. But there are probably only between 7,000 and 14,000 potential donors a year."[1] Envisaging this situation in which at the very most something like one in four heart-malfunction victims can be saved, we clearly confront a problem in ELT allocation.

A perhaps even more drastic case in point is afforded by long-term haemodialysis, an ongoing process by which a complex device—an "artificial kidney machine"—is used periodically in cases of chronic renal failure to substitute for a non-functional kidney in "cleaning" potential poisons from the blood. Only a few major institutions have chronic haemodialysis units, whose complex operation is an extremely expensive proposition. For the present and the foreseeable future the situation is that "the number of places available for chronic haemodialysis is hopelessly inadequate."[2]

The traditional medical ethos has insulated the physician against facing the very existence of this problem. When swearing the Hippocratic Oath, he commits himself to work for the benefit of the sick in "whatsoever house I enter."[3] In taking this stance, the physician substantially renounces the explicit choice of saving certain lives rather than others. Of course, doctors have always in fact had to face such choices on the battlefield or in times of disaster, but there the issue had to be resolved hurriedly, under pressure, and in circumstances in which the very nature of the case effectively precluded calm deliberation by the decision maker as well as criticism by others. In sharp contrast, however, cases of the type we have postulated in the present discussion arise predictably, and represent choices to be made deliberately and "in cold blood."

It is, to begin with, appropriate to remark that this problem is not fundamentally a medical problem. For when there are sufficiently many afflicted candidates for ELT then—so we may assume—there will also be more than enough for whom the purely medical grounds for ELT allocation are decisively strong in any individual case, and just about equally strong throughout the group. But in this circumstance a selection of some afflicted patients over and against others cannot *ex hypothesi* be made on the basis of purely medical considerations.

The selection problem, as we have said, is in substantial measure not a medical one. It is a problem *for* medical men, which must somehow be solved by them, but that does not make it a medical issue—any more than the problem of hospital building is a medical issue. As a problem it belongs to the category of philosophical problems—specifically a problem of moral philosophy or ethics. Structurally, it bears a substantial kinship with those issues in this field that revolve about the notorious whom-to-save-on-the-lifeboat and whom-to-throw-to-the-wolves-pursuing-the-sled questions. But whereas questions of this just-indicated sort are artificial, hypothetical, and far-fetched, the ELT issue poses a *genuine* policy question for the responsible administrators in medical institutions, indeed a question

that threatens to become commonplace in the foreseeable future.

Now what the medical administrator needs to have, and what the philosopher is presumably *ex officio* in a position to help in providing, is a body of *rational guidelines* for making choices in these literally life-or-death situations. This is an issue in which many interested parties have a substantial stake, including the responsible decision maker who wants to satisfy his conscience that he is acting in a reasonable way. Moreover, the family and associates of the man who is turned away—to say nothing of the man himself—have the right to an acceptable explanation. And indeed even the general public wants to know that what is being done is fitting and proper. All of these interested parties are entitled to insist that a reasonable code of operating principles provides a defensible rationale for making the life-and-death choices involved in ELT.

II THE TWO TYPES OF CRITERIA

Two distinguishable types of criteria are bound up in the issue of making ELT choices. We shall call these *Criteria of Inclusion* and *Criteria of Comparison*, respectively. The distinction at issue here requires some explanation. We can think of the selection as being made by a two-stage process: (1) the selection from among all possible candidates (by a suitable screening process) of a group to be taken under serious consideration as candidates for therapy, and then (2) the actual singling out, within this group, of the particular individuals to whom therapy is to be given. Thus the first process narrows down the range of comparative choice by eliminating *en bloc* whole categories of potential candidates. The second process calls for a more refined, case-by-case comparison of those candidates that remain. By means of the first set of criteria one forms a selection group; by means of the second set, an actual selection is made within this group.

Thus what we shall call a "selection system" for the choice of patients to receive therapy of the ELT type will consist of criteria of these two kinds. Such a system will be acceptable only when the reasonableness of its component criteria can be established.

III ESSENTIAL FEATURES OF AN ACCEPTABLE ELT SELECTION SYSTEM

To qualify as reasonable, an ELT selection must meet two important "regulative" requirements: it must be *simple* enough to be readily intelligible, and it must be *plausible*, that is, patently reasonable in a way that can be apprehended easily and without involving ramified subtleties. Those medical administrators responsible for ELT choices must follow a modus operandi that virtually all the people involved can readily understand to be acceptable (at a reasonable level of generality, at any rate). Appearances are critically important here. It is not enough that the choice be made in a *justifiable* way; it must be possible for people—*plain* people—to "see" (i.e., understand without elaborate teaching or indoctrination) that *it is justified*, insofar as any mode of procedure can be justified in cases of this sort.

One "constitutive" requirement is obviously an essential feature of a reasonable selection system: all of its component criteria—those of inclusion and those of comparison alike—must be reasonable in the sense of being *rationally defensible*. The ramifications of this requirement call for detailed consideration. But one of its aspects should be noted without further ado: it must be *fair*—it must treat relevantly like cases alike, leaving no room for "influence" or favoritism, etc.

IV   THE BASIC SCREENING STAGE: CRITERIA OF INCLUSION (AND EXCLUSION)

Three sorts of considerations are prominent among the plausible criteria of inclusion/exclusion at the basic screening stage: the constituency factor, the progress-of-science factor, and the prospect-of-success factor.

A   The Constituency Factor

It is a "fact of life" that ELT can be available only in the institutional setting of a hospital or medical institute or the like. Such institutions generally have normal clientele boundaries. A veterans' hospital will not concern itself primarily with treating nonveterans, a children's hospital cannot be expected to accommodate the "senior citizen," an army hospital can regard college professors as outside its sphere. Sometimes the boundaries are geographic—a state hospital may admit only residents of a certain state. (There are, of course, indefensible constituency principles—say race or religion, party membership, or ability to pay; and there are cases of borderline legitimacy, e.g., sex.[4]) A medical institution is justified in considering for ELT only persons within its own constituency, provided this constituency is constituted upon a defensible basis. Thus the haemodialysis selection committee in Seattle "agreed to con-

sider only those applicants who were residents of the state of Washington.... They justified this stand on the grounds that since the basic research...had been done at...a state-supported institution—the people whose taxes had paid for the research should be its first beneficiaries."[5]

While thus insisting that constituency considerations represent a valid and legitimate factor in ELT selection, I do feel there is much to be said for minimizing their role in life-or-death cases. Indeed a refusal to recognize them at all is a significant part of medical tradition, going back to the very oath of Hippocrates. They represent a departure from the ideal arising with the institutionalization of medicine, moving it away from its original status as an art practiced by an individual practitioner.

B   The Progress-of-Science Factor

The needs of medical research can provide a second valid principle of inclusion. The research interests of the medical staff in relation to the specific nature of the cases at issue is a significant consideration. It may be important for the progress of medical science—and thus of potential benefit to many persons in the future—to determine how effective the ELT at issue is with diabetics or persons over sixty or with a negative RH factor. Considerations of this sort represent another type of legitimate factor in ELT selection.

A very definitely *borderline* case under this head would revolve around the question of a patient's willingness to pay, not in monetary terms, but in offering himself as an experimental subject, say by contracting to return at designated times for a series of tests substantially unrelated to his own health, but yielding data of importance to medical knowledge in general.

C   The Prospect-of-Success Factor

It may be that while the ELT at issue is not without *some* effectiveness in general, it has been established to be highly effective only with patients in certain specific categories (e.g., females under forty of a specific blood type). This difference in effectiveness—in the absolute or in the probability of success—is (we assume) so marked as to constitute virtually a difference in kind rather than in degree. In this case, it would be perfectly legitimate to adopt the general rule of making the ELT at issue available only or primarily to persons in this substantial-promise-of-success category. (It is on grounds of this sort that young children and persons over fifty are generally ruled out as candidates for haemodialysis.)

We have maintained that the three factors of constituency, progress of science, and prospect of success
represent legitimate criteria of inclusion for ELT selection. But it remains to examine the considerations
which legitimate them. The legitimating factors are in
the final analysis practical or pragmatic in nature.
From the practical angle, it is advantageous—indeed
to some extent necessary—that the arrangements governing medical institutions should embody certain constituency principles. It makes good pragmatic and

utilitarian sense that progress-of-science considerations
should be operative here. And, finally, the practical
aspect is reinforced by a whole host of other considerations—
including moral ones—in supporting the prospect-of-
success criterion. The workings of each of these factors
are of course conditioned by the ever-present element
of limited availability. They are operative only in this
context, that is, prospect of success is a legitimate
consideration at all only because we are dealing with a
situation of scarcity.

V   THE FINAL SELECTION STAGE:
CRITERIA OF SELECTION

Five sorts of elements must, as we see it, figure primarily
among the plausible criteria of selection that are to be
brought to bear in further screening the group constituted after application of the criteria of inclusion: the
relative-likelihood-of-success factor, the life-expectancy
factor, the family role factor, the potential-contributions
factor, and the services-rendered factor. The first two
represent the *biomedical* aspect, the second three the
social aspect.

A   The Relative-Likelihood-of-Success Factor

It is clear that the relative likelihood of success is a
legitimate and appropriate factor in making a selection
within the group of qualified patients that are to receive
ELT. This is obviously one of the considerations that
must count very significantly in a reasonable selection
procedure.

The present criterion is of course closely related to
item C of the preceding section. There we were concerned with prospect-of-success considerations categorically and *en bloc*. Here at present they come into
play in a particularized case-by-case comparison among
individuals. If the therapy at issue is not a once-and-
for-all proposition and requires ongoing treatment,

cognate considerations must be brought in. Thus, for
example, in the case of a chronic ELT procedure such
as haemodialysis it would clearly make sense to give
priority to patients with a potentially reversible condition (who would thus need treatment for only a fraction
of their remaining lives).

B   The Life-Expectancy Factor

Even if the ELT is "successful" in the patient's case he
may, considering his age and/or other aspects of his
general medical condition, look forward to only a very
short probable future life. This is obviously another
factor that must be taken into account.

C   The Family Role Factor

A person's life is a thing of importance not only to
himself but to others—friends, associates, neighbors,
colleagues, etc. But his (or her) relationship to his
immediate family is a thing of unique intimacy and
significance. The nature of his relationship to his wife,
children, and parents, and the issue of their financial
and psychological dependence upon him, are obviously
matters that deserve to be given weight in the ELT
selection process. Other things being anything like
equal, the mother of minor children must take priority
over the middle-aged bachelor.

D   The Potential Future-Contributions Factor
(Prospective Service)

In "choosing to save" one life rather than another, "the
society," through the mediation of the particular medical institution in question—which should certainly
look upon itself as a trustee for the social interest—is
clearly warranted in considering the likely pattern of
future *services to be rendered* by the patient (adequate
recovery assumed), considering his age, talent, training,
and past record of performance. In its allocations of
ELT, society "invests" a scarce resource in one person
as against another and is thus entitled to look to the
probable prospective "return" on its investment.

It may well be that a thoroughly egalitarian society
is reluctant to put someone's social contribution into
the scale in situations of the sort at issue. One popular
article states that "the most difficult standard would be
the candidate's value to society," and goes on to quote
someone who said: "You can't just pick a brilliant
painter over a laborer. The average citizen would be
quickly eliminated."[6] But what if it were not a brilliant
painter but a brilliant surgeon or medical researcher
that was at issue? One wonders if the author of the

obiter dictum that one "can't just pick" would still feel equally sure of his ground. In any case, the fact that the standard is difficult to apply is certainly no reason for not attempting to apply it. The problem of ELT selection is inevitably burdened with difficult standards.

Some might feel that in assessing a patient's value to society one should ask not only who if permitted to continue living can make the greatest contribution to society in some creative or constructive way, but also who by dying would leave behind the greatest burden on society in assuming the discharge of their residual responsibilities.[7] Certainly the philosophical utilitarian would give equal weight to both these considerations. Just here is where I would part ways with orthodox utilitarianism. For—though this is not the place to do so—I should be prepared to argue that a civilized society has an obligation to promote the furtherance of positive achievements in cultural and related areas even if this means the assumption of certain added burdens.[8]

E   The Past Services-Rendered Factor (Retrospective Service)

A person's services to another person or group have always been taken to constitute a valid basis for a claim upon this person or group—of course a moral and not necessarily a legal claim. Society's obligation for the recognition and reward of services rendered—an obligation whose discharge is also very possibly conducive to self-interest in the long run—is thus another factor to be taken into account. This should be viewed as a morally necessary correlative of the previously considered factor of *prospective* service. It would be morally indefensible of society in effect to say: "Never mind about services you rendered yesterday—it is only the services to be rendered tomorrow that will count with us today." We live in very future-oriented times, constantly preoccupied in a distinctly utilitarian way with future satisfactions. And this disinclines us to give much recognition to past services. But parity considerations of the sort just adduced indicate that such recognition should be given *on grounds of equity*. No doubt a justification for giving weight to services rendered can also be attempted along utilitarian lines. ("The reward of past services rendered spurs people on to greater future efforts and is thus socially advantageous in the long-run future.") In saying that past services should be counted "on grounds of equity"—rather than "on grounds of utility"—I take the view that even

if shown to be fallacious, I should still be prepared to maintain the propriety of taking services rendered into account. The position does not rest on a utilitarian basis and so would not collapse with the removal of such a basis.[9]

As we have said, these five factors fall into three groups: the biomedical factors A and B, the familial factor C, and the social factors D and E. With items A and B the need for a detailed analysis of the medical considerations comes to the fore. The age of the patient, his medical history, his physical and psychological condition, his specific disease, etc., will all need to be taken into exact account. These biomedical factors represent technical issues: they call for the physicians' expert judgment and the medical statisticians' hard data. And they are ethically uncontroversial factors—their legitimacy and appropriateness are evident from the very nature of the case.

Greater problems arise with the familial and social factors. They involve intangibles that are difficult to judge. How is one to develop subcriteria for weighing the relative social contributions of (say) an architect or a librarian or a mother of young children? And they involve highly problematic issues. (For example, should good moral character be rated a plus and bad a minus in judging services rendered?) And there is something strikingly unpleasant in grappling with issues of this sort for people brought up in times greatly inclined towards maxims of the type "Judge not!" and "Live and let live!" All the same, in the situation that concerns us here such distasteful problems must be faced, since a

failure to choose to save some is tantamount to sentencing all. Unpleasant choices are intrinsic to the problem of ELT selection; they are of the very essence of the matter.[10]

But is reference to all these factors indeed inevitable? The justification for taking account of the medical factors is pretty obvious. But why should the social aspect of services rendered and to be rendered be taken into account at all? The answer is that they must be taken into account not from the *medical* but from the *ethical* point of view. Despite disagreement on many fundamental issues, moral philosophers of the present day are pretty well in consensus that the justification of human actions is to be sought largely and primarily—if not exclusively—in the principles of utility and of justice.[11] But utility requires reference of services to be rendered and justice calls for a recognition of services that have been rendered. Moral considerations would thus demand recognition of these two factors. (This, of course, still leaves open the question of whether the point of view provides a valid basis of action: Why base one's actions upon moral principles?—or, to put it bluntly—Why be moral? The present paper is, however, hardly the place to grapple with so fundamental an issue, which has been canvassed in the literature of philosophical ethics since Plato.)

VI MORE THAN MEDICAL ISSUES ARE INVOLVED

An active controversy has of late sprung up in medical circles over the question of whether non-physician laymen should be given a role in ELT selection (in the specific context of chronic haemodialysis). One physician writes: "I think that the assessment of the candidates should be made by a senior doctor on the [dialysis] unit, but I am sure that it would be helpful to him—both in sharing responsibility and in avoiding personal pressure—if a small unnamed group of people [presumably including laymen] officially made the final decision. I visualize the doctor bringing the data to the group, explaining the points in relation to each case, and obtaining their approval of his order of priority.[12]

Essentially this procedure of a selection committee of laymen has for some years been in use in one of the most publicized chronic dialysis units, that of the Swedish Hospital of Seattle, Washington.[13] Many physicians are apparently reluctant to see the choice of allocation of medical therapy pass out of strictly medical hands. Thus in a recent symposium on the "Selection of Patients for Haemodialysis,"[14] Dr. Ralph Shakman writes: "Who is to implement the selection? In my opinion it must ultimately be the responsibility of the consultants in charge of the renal units...I can see no reason for delegating this responsibility to lay persons. Surely the latter would be better employed if they could be persuaded to devote their time and energy to raise more and more money for us to spend on our patients."[15] Other contributors to this symposium strike much the same note. Dr. F. M. Parsons writes: "In an attempt to overcome...difficulties in selection some have advocated introducing certain specified lay people into the discussions. Is it wise? I doubt whether a committee of this type can adjudicate as satisfactorily as two medical colleagues, particularly as successful therapy involves close cooperation between doctor

and patient."[16] And Dr. M. A. Wilson writes in the same symposium: "The suggestion has been made that lay panels should select individuals for dialysis from among a group who are medically suitable. Though this would relieve the doctor-in-charge of a heavy load of responsibility, it would place the burden on those who have no personal knowledge and have to base their judgments on medical or social reports. I do not believe this would result in better decisions for the group or improve the doctor-patient relationship in individual cases."[17]

But no amount of flag waving about the doctor's facing up to his responsibility—or prostrations before the idol of the doctor-patient relationship and reluctance to admit laymen into the sacred precincts of the conference chambers of medical consultations—can obscure the essential fact that ELT selection is not a wholly medical problem. When there are more than enough places in an ELT program to accommodate all who need it, then it will clearly be a medical question to decide who does have the need and which among these would successfully respond. But when an admitted gross insufficiency of places exists, when there are ten or fifty or one hundred highly eligible candidates for each place in the program, then it is unrealistic to take the view that purely medical criteria can furnish a sufficient basis for selection. The question of ELT selection becomes serious as a phenomenon of scale—because, as more candidates present themselves, strictly medical factors are increasingly less adequate as a selection criterion precisely because by numerical category-crowding there will be more and more cases whose "status is much the same" so far as purely medical considerations go.

The ELT selection problem clearly poses issues that transcend the medical sphere because—in the nature of the case—many residual issues remain to be dealt with once *all* of the medical questions have been faced. Because of this there is good reason why laymen as well as physicians should be involved in the selection process. Once the medical considerations have been brought to bear, fundamental social issues remain to be resolved. The instrumentalities of ELT have been created through the social investment of scarce resources, and the interests of the society deserve to play a role in their utilization. As representatives of their social interests, lay opinions should function to complement and supplement medical views once the proper arena of medical considerations is left behind.[18] Those physicians who have urged the presence of lay members on selection panels can, from this point of view, be recognized as having seen the issue in proper perspective.

One physician has argued against lay representation on selection panels for haemodialysis as follows: "If the doctor advises dialysis and the lay panel refuses, the patient will regard this as a death sentence passed by an anonymous court from which he has no right of appeal."[19] But this drawback is not specific to the use of a lay panel. Rather, it is a feature inherent in every selection procedure, regardless of whether the selection is done by the head doctor of the unit, by a panel of physicians, etc. No matter who does the selecting among patients recommended for dialysis, the feelings of the patient who has been rejected (and knows it) can be expected to be much the same, provided that he recognizes the actual nature of the choice (and is not deceived by the possibly convenient but ultimately poisonous fiction that because the selection was made by physicians it was made entirely on medical grounds).

In summary, then, the question of ELT selection would appear to be one that is in its very nature heavily laden with issues of medical research, practice, and administration. But it will not be a question that can be resolved on solely medical grounds. Strictly social issues of justice and utility will invariably arise in this area— questions going outside the medical area in whose resolution medical laymen can and should play a substantial role.

VII THE INHERENT IMPERFECTION (NON-OPTIMALITY) OF ANY SELECTION SYSTEM

Our discussion to this point of the design of a selection system for ELT has left a gap that is a very fundamental and serious omission. We have argued that five factors must be taken into substantial and explicit account:

A *Relative likelihood of success.*—Is the chance of the treatment's being "successful" to be rated as high, good, average, etc.?[20]

B *Expectancy of future life.*—Assuming the "success" of the treatment, how much longer does the patient stand a good chance (75 per cent or better) of living—considering his age and general condition?

C *Family role.*—To what extent does the patient have responsibilities to others in his immediate family?

D *Social contributions rendered.*—Are the patient's past services to his society outstanding, substantial, average, etc.?

E *Social contributions to be rendered.*—Considering his age, talents, training, and past record of performance, is there a substantial probability that the patient will—*adequate recovery being assumed*—render in the future services to his society that can be characterized as outstanding, substantial, average, etc.?

This list is clearly insufficient for the construction of a reasonable selection system, since that would require not only *that these factors be taken into account* (somehow or other), but—going beyond this—would specify *a specific set of procedures for taking account of them*. The specific procedures that would constitute such a system would have to take account of the interrelationship of these factors (e.g., B and E), and to set out exact guidelines as to the relevant weight that is to be given to each of them. This is something our discussion has not as yet considered.

In fact, I should want to maintain that there is no such thing here as a single rationally superior selection system. The position of affairs seems to me to be something like this: (1) It is necessary (for reasons already canvassed) to *have* a system, and to have a system that is rationally defensible, and (2) to be rationally defensible, this system must take the factors A–E into substantial and explicit account. But (3) the exact manner in which a rationally defensible system takes account of these factors cannot be fixed in any one specific way on the basis of general considerations. Any of the variety of ways that give A–E "their due" will be acceptable and viable. One cannot hope to find within this range of workable systems some one that is *optimal* in relation to the alternatives. There is no one system that does "the (uniquely) best"—only a variety of systems that do "as well as one can expect to do" in cases of this sort.

The situation is structurally very much akin to that of rules of partition of an estate among the relations of a decedent. It is important *that there be* such rules. And it is reasonable that spouse, children, parents, siblings, etc., be taken account of in these rules. But the question of the exact method of division—say that when the decedent has neither living spouse nor living children then his estate is to be divided, dividing 60 per cent between parents, 40 per cent between siblings versus dividing 90 per cent between parents, 10 per cent between siblings—cannot be settled on the basis of any general abstract considerations of reasonableness. Within broad limits, a *variety* of resolutions are all perfectly acceptable—so that no one procedure can justifiably be regarded as "the (uniquely) best" because it is superior to all others.[21]

VIII   A POSSIBLE BASIS FOR A REASONABLE SELECTION SYSTEM

Having said that there is no such thing as the *optimal* selection system for ELT, I want now to sketch out the broad features of what I would regard as *one acceptable* system.

The basis for the system would be a point rating. The scoring here at issue would give roughly equal weight to the medical considerations (A and B) in comparison with the extramedical considerations (C = family role, D = services rendered, and E = services to be rendered), also giving roughly equal weight to the three items involved here (C, D, and E). The result of such a scoring procedure would provide the essential *starting point* of our ELT selection mechanism. I deliberately say "starting point" because it seems to me that one should not follow the results of this scoring in an *automatic* way. I would propose that the actual selection should only be guided but not actually be dictated by this scoring procedure, along lines now to be explained.

IX   THE DESIRABILITY OF INTRODUCING AN ELEMENT OF CHANCE

The detailed procedure I would propose—not of course as optimal (for reasons we have seen), but as eminently acceptable—would combine the scoring procedure just discussed with an element of chance. The resulting selection system would function as follows:

1 First the criteria of inclusion of Section IV above would be applied to constitute a *first phase selection group*—which we shall suppose) is substantially larger than the number n of persons who can actually be accommodated with ELT.

2 Next the criteria of selection of Section V are brought to bear via a scoring procedure of the type described in Section VIII. On this basis a *second phase selection group* is constituted which is only *somewhat* larger—say by a third or a half—than the critical number n at issue.

3 If this second phase selection group is relatively homogeneous as regards rating by the scoring procedure—that is, if there are no really major disparities within this group (as would be likely if the initial group was

significantly larger than n)—then the final selection is made by *random* selection of n persons from within this group.

This introduction of the element of chance—in what could be dramatized as a "lottery of life and death"—must be justified. The fact is that such a procedure would bring with it three substantial advantages.

First as we have argued above (in Section VII), any acceptable selection system is inherently non-optimal. The introduction of the element of chance prevents the results that life-and-death choices are made by the automatic application of an admittedly imperfect selection method.

Second, a recourse to chance would doubtless make matters easier for the rejected patient and those who have a specific interest in him. It would surely be quite hard for them to accept his exclusion by relatively mechanical application of objective criteria in whose implementation subjective judgment is involved. But the circumstances of life have conditioned us to accept the workings of chance and to tolerate the element of luck (good or bad): human life is an inherently contingent process. Nobody, after all, has an absolute right to ELT—but most of us would feel that we have "every bit as much right" to it as anyone else in significantly similar circumstances. The introduction of the element of chance assures a like handling of like cases over the widest possible area that seems reasonable in the circumstances.

Third (and perhaps least), such a recourse to random selection does much to relieve the administrators of the selection system of the awesome burden of ultimate and absolute responsibility.

These three considerations would seem to build up a substantial case for introducing the element of chance into the mechanism of the system for ELT selection in a way limited and circumscribed by other weightier considerations, along some such lines as those set forth above.[22]

It should be recognized that this injection of *man-made* chance supplements the element of *natural* chance that is present inevitably and in any case (apart from the role of chance in singling out certain persons as victims for the affliction at issue). As F. M. Parsons has observed: "any vacancies [in an ELT program—specifically haemodialysis] will be filled immediately by the first suitable patients, even though their claims for therapy may subsequently prove less than those of other patients refused later."[23] Life is a chancy business and even the most rational of human arrangements can cover this over to a very limited extent at best.[24]

NOTES

1 Christine Doyle, "Spare-Part Heart Surgeons Worried by Their Success," *Observer*, May 12, 1968.

2 J. D. N. Nabarro, "Selection of Patients for Haemodialysis," *British Medical Journal* (March 11, 1967), p. 623. Although several thousand patients die in the U.K. each year from renal failure—there are about thirty new cases per million of population—only 10 per cent of these can for the foreseeable future be accommodated with chronic haemodialysis. Kidney transplantation—itself a very tricky procedure—cannot make a more than minor contribution here. As this article goes to press, I learn that patients can be maintained in home dialysis at an operating cost about half that of maintaining them in a hospital dialysis unit (roughly an $8,000 minimum). In the United States, around 7,000 patients with terminal uremia who could benefit from haemodialysis evolve yearly. As of mid-1968, some 1,000 of these can be accommodated in existing hospital units. By June 1967, a world-wide total of some 120 patients were in treatment by home dialysis. (Data from a forthcoming paper, "Home Dialysis," by C. M. Conty and H. V. Murdaugh. See also R. A. Baillod *et al.*, "Overnight Haemodialysis in the Home," *Proceedings of the European Dialysis and Transplant Association*, VI [1965], 99 ff.).

3 For the Hippocratic Oath see *Hippocrates: Works* (Loeb ed.; London, 1959), I, p. 298.

4 Another example of borderline legitimacy is posed by an endowment "with strings attached," e.g., "In accepting this legacy the hospital agrees to admit and provide all needed treatment for any direct descendant of myself, its founder."

5 Shana Alexander, "They Decide Who Lives, Who Dies," *Life*, LIII (November 9, 1962), 102–25 (see p. 107).

6 Lawrence Lader, "Who Has the Right To Live?" *Good Housekeeping* (January 1968), p. 144.

7 This approach could thus be continued to embrace the previous factor, that of family role, the preceding item (C).

8 Moreover a doctrinaire utilitarian would presumably be willing to withdraw a continuing mode of ELT such as haemodialysis from a patient to make room for a more promising candidate who came to view at a later stage and who could not otherwise be accommodated. I should be unwilling to adopt this course, partly on grounds of utility (with a view to the demoralization of insecurity), partly on the non-utilitarian ground that a "moral commitment" has been made and must be honored.

9 Of course the difficult question remains of the relative weight that should be given to prospective and retrospective service in cases where these factors conflict. There is a good reason to treat them on a par.

10 This in the symposium on "Selection of Patients for Haemodialysis," *British Medical Journal* (March 11, 1967), pp. 622–24. F. M. Parsons writes: "But other forms of selecting patients [distinct from first come, first served] are suspect in my view if they imply evaluation of man by man. What criteria could be used? Who could justify a claim that the life of a mayor would be more valuable than that of the humblest citizen of his borough? Whatever we may think as individuals none of us is indispensable." But having just set out this hard-line view he immediately backs away from it: "On the other hand, to assume that there was little to choose between Alexander Fleming and Adolf Hitler... would be nonsense, and we should be naive if we were to pretend that we could not be influenced by their achievements and characters if we had to choose between the two of them. Whether we like it or not we cannot escape the fact that this kind of selection for long-term haemodialysis will be required until very large sums of money become available for equipment and services [so that *everyone* who needs treatment can be accommodated]."

11 The relative fundamentality of these principles is, however, a substantially disputed issue.

12 J. D. N. Nabarro, *op. cit.*, p. 622.

13 See Shana Alexander, *op. cit.*

14 *British Medical Journal* (March 11, 1967), pp. 622–24.

15 *Ibid.*, p. 624. Another contributor writes in he same symposium, "The selection of the few [to receive haemodialysis] is proving very difficult—a true 'Doctor's Dilemma'—for almost everybody would agree that this must be a medical decision, preferably reached by consultation among colleagues" (Dr. F. M. Parsons, *ibid.*, p. 623).

16 "Selection of Patients for Haemodialysis," *op. cit.* (n. 10 above), p. 623.

17 Dr. Wilson's article concludes with the perplexing suggestion—wildly beside the point given the structure of the situation at issue—that "the final decision will be made by the patient." But this contention is only marginally more ludicrous than Parsons' contention that in selecting patients for haemodialysis "gainful employment in a well chosen occupation is necessary to achieve the best results" since "only the minority wish to live on charity" (*ibid.*).

18 To say this is of course not to deny that such questions of applied medical ethics will invariably involve a host of medical considerations—it is only to insist that extramedical considerations will also invariably be at issue.

19 M. A. Wilson, "Selection of Patients for Haemodialysis," *op. cit.*, p. 624.

20 In the case of an ongoing treatment involving complex procedure and dietary and other mode-of-life restrictions—and chronic haemodialysis definitely falls into this category—the patient's psychological makeup, his willpower to "stick with it" in the face of substantial discouragements—will obviously also be a substantial factor here. The man who gives up, takes not his life alone, but (figuratively speaking) also that of the person he replaced in the treatment schedule.

21 To say that acceptable solutions can range over broad limits is *not* to say that there are no limits at all. It is an obviously intriguing and fundamental problem to raise the question of the factors that set these limits. This complex issue cannot be dealt with adequately here. Suffice it to say that considerations regarding precedent and people's expectations, factors of social utility, and matters of fairness and sense of justice all come into play.

22 One writer has mooted the suggestion that: "Perhaps the right thing to do, difficult as it may be to accept, is to select [for haemodialysis] from among the medically and psychologically qualified patients on a strictly random basis" (S. Gorovitz, "Ethics and the Allocation of Medical Resources," *Medical Research Engineering*, V [1966], p. 7). Outright random selection would, however, seem indefensible because of its refusal to give weight to considerations which, under the circumstances, *deserve* to be given weight. The proposed procedure of superimposing a certain degree of randomness upon the rational-choice criteria would seem to combine the advantages of the two without importing the worst defects of either.

23 "Selection of Patients for Haemodialysis," *op. cit.*, p. 623. The question of whether a patient for chronic treatment should ever be terminated from the program (say if he contracts cancer) poses a variety of difficult ethical problems with which we need not at present concern ourselves. But it does seem plausible to take the (somewhat anti-utilitarian) view that a patient should not be terminated simply because a "better qualified" patient comes along later on. It would seem that a quasi-contractual relationship has been created through established expectations and reciprocal understandings, and that the situation is in this regard akin to that of the man who, having undertaken to sell his house to one buyer, cannot afterward unilaterally undo this arrangement to sell it to a higher bidder who "needs it worse" (thus maximizing the over-all utility).

24 I acknowledge with thanks the help of Miss Hazel Johnson, Reference Librarian at the University of Pittsburgh Library, in connection with the works cited.

Who Shall Live When Not All Can Live?

James F. Childress

A biographical sketch of James F. Childress is found on page 511.

Childress, like Rescher, focuses on the microallocation of scarce lifesaving medical resources. Advocating a two-stage selection process, he suggests that medical criteria be used to establish a pool of "medically-acceptable" candidates. He

Reprinted with permission of the publisher from *Soundings*, vol. 53 (Winter 1970), pp. 339–355.

criticizes and rejects, however, any attempt to use utilitarian reasoning to establish criteria for the second stage of the selection process. Rather, he argues, selection should be made by some sort of random selection procedure ("first come, first served" or a lottery). For Childress, random selection procedures are in keeping with some of our important values—individual dignity, trust, and fairness.

Who shall live when not all can live? Although this question has been urgently forced upon us by the dramatic use of artificial internal organs and organ transplantations, it is hardly new. George Bernard Shaw dealt with it in *The Doctor's Dilemma*:

Sir Patrick: Well, Mr. Savior of Lives: which is it to be? that honest decent man Blenkinsop, or that rotten blackguard of an artist, eh?

Ridgeon: It's not an easy case to judge, is it? Blenkinsop's an honest decent man; but is he any use? Dubedat's a rotten blackguard; but he's a genuine source of pretty and pleasant and good things.

Sir Patrick: What will he be a source of for that poor innocent wife of his, when she finds him out?

Ridgeon: That's true. Her life will be a hell.

Sir Patrick: And tell me this. Suppose you had this choice put before you: either to go through life and find all the pictures bad but all the men and women good, or go through life and find all the pictures good and all the men and women rotten. Which would you choose?[1]

A significant example of the distribution of scarce medical resources is seen in the use of penicillin shortly after its discovery. Military officers had to determine which soldiers would be treated—those with venereal disease or those wounded in combat.[2] In many respects such decisions have become routine in medical circles. Day after day physicians and others make judgments and decisions "about allocations of medical care to various segments of our population, to various types of hospitalized patients, and to specific individuals,"[3] for example, whether mental illness or cancer will receive the higher proportion of available funds. Nevertheless, the dramatic forms of "Scarce Life-Saving Medical Resources" (hereafter abbreviated as SLMR) such as hemodialysis and kidney and heart transplants have compelled us to examine the moral questions that have been concealed in many routine decisions. I shall not attempt [here] to show how a resolution of SLMR cases can help us in the more routine ones that do not involve a conflict of life with life. Rather I shall develop an argument for a particular method of determining who shall live when not all can live. No conclusions are implied about criteria and procedures for determining who shall receive medical resources that are not directly related to the preservation of life (e.g., corneal transplants) or about standards for allocating money and time for studying and treating certain diseases.

Just as current SLMR decisions are not totally discontinuous with other medical decisions, so we must ask whether some other cases might, at least by analogy, help us develop the needed criteria and procedures. Some have looked at the principles at work in our responses to abortion, euthanasia, and artificial insemination.[4] Usually they have concluded that these cases do not cast light on the selection of patients for artificial and transplanted organs. The reason is evident: in abortion, euthanasia, and artificial insemination, there is no conflict of life with life for limited but indispensable resources (with the possible exception of therapeutic abortion). In current SLMR decisions, such a conflict is inescapable, and it makes them morally perplexing and fascinating. If analogous cases are to be found, I think that we shall locate them in moral conflict situations.

ANALOGOUS CONFLICT SITUATIONS

An especially interesting and pertinent one is *U.S. v. Holmes.*[5] In 1841 an American ship, the *William Brown*, which was near Newfoundland on a trip from Liverpool to Philadelphia, struck an iceberg. The crew and half the passengers were able to escape in the two available vessels. One of these, a longboat, carrying too many passengers and leaking seriously, began to founder in the turbulent sea after about twenty-four hours. In a desperate attempt to keep it from sinking, the crew threw overboard fourteen men. Two sisters of one of the men either jumped overboard to join their brother in death or instructed the crew to throw them over. The criteria for determining who should live were "not to part man and wife, and not to throw over any woman." Several hours later the others were rescued. Returning to Philadelphia, most of the crew disappeared, but one, Holmes, who had acted upon orders from the mate, was indicted, tried, and convicted on the charge of "unlawful homicide."

We are interested in this case from a moral rather than a legal standpoint, and there are several possible responses to and judgments about it. The judge contended that lots should have been cast, for in such conflict situations, there is no other procedure "so consonant both to humanity and to justice." Counsel for Holmes, on the other hand, maintained that the "sailors adopted the only principle of selection which was possible in an emergency like theirs—a principle more humane than lots."

Another version of selection might extend and systematize the maxims of the sailors in the direction of "utility"; those are saved who will contribute to the greatest good for the greatest number. Yet another possible option is defended by Edmond Cahn in *The Moral Decision.* He argues that in this case we encounter the "morals of the last days." By this phrase he indicates that an apocalyptic crisis renders totally irrelevant the normal differences between individuals. He continues,

> In a strait of this extremity, all men are reduced—or raised, as one may choose to denominate it—to members of the genus, mere congeners and nothing else. Truly and literally, all were "in the same boat," and thus none could be saved separately from the others. I am driven to conclude that otherwise—that is, if none sacrifice themselves of free will to spare the others—they must all wait and die together. For where all have become congeners, pure and simple, no one can save himself by killing another.[6]

Cahn's answer to the question "who shall live when not all can live" is "none" unless the voluntary sacrifice by some persons permits it.

Few would deny the importance of Cahn's approach, although many, including this writer, would suggest that it is relevant mainly as an affirmation of an elevated and, indeed, heroic or saintly morality that one hopes would find expression in the voluntary actions of many persons trapped in "borderline" situations involving a conflict of life with life. It is a maximal demand that some moral principles impose on the individual in the

recognition that self-preservation is not a good that is to be defended at all costs. The absence of this saintly or heroic morality should not mean, however, that everyone perishes. Without making survival an absolute value and without justifying all means to achieve it, we can maintain that simply letting everyone die is irresponsible. This charge can be supported from several different standpoints, including society at large as well as the individuals involved. Among a group of self-interested individuals, none of whom volunteers to relinquish his life, there may be better and worse ways of determining who shall survive. One task of social ethics, whether religious or philosophical, is to propose relatively just institutional arrangements within which self-interested and biased men can live. The question then becomes: which set of arrangements—which criteria and procedures of selection—is most satisfactory in view of the human condition (man's limited altruism and inclination to seek his own good) and the conflicting values that are to be realized?

There are several significant differences between the *Holmes* and SLMR cases, a major one being that the former involves *direct* killing of another person, while the latter involve only *permitting* a person to die when it is not possible to save all. Furthermore, in extreme situations such as *Holmes*, the restraints of civilization have been stripped away, and something approximating a state of nature prevails, in which life is "solitary, poor, nasty, brutish and short." The state of nature does not mean that moral standards are irrelevant and that might should prevail, but it does suggest that much of the matrix that normally supports morality has been removed. Also, the necessary but unfortunate decisions about who shall live and die are made by men who are existentially and personally involved in the outcome. Their survival too is at stake. Even though the institutional role of sailors seems to require greater sacrificial actions, there is obviously no assurance that they will adequately assess the number of sailors required to man the vessel or that they will impartially and objectively weigh the common good at stake. As the judge insisted in his defense of casting lots in the *Holmes* case: "In no other than this [casting lots] or some like way are those having equal rights put upon an equal footing, and in no other way is it possible to guard against partiality and oppression, violence, and conflict." This difference should not be exaggerated, since self-interest, professional pride, and the like obviously affect the outcome of many medical decisions. Nor do the remaining differences cancel *Holmes's* instructiveness.

CRITERIA OF SELECTION FOR SLMR

Which set of arrangements should be adopted for SLMR? Two questions are involved: Which standards and criteria should be used? and, Who should make the decision? The first question is basic, since the debate about implementation, e.g., whether by a lay committee or physician, makes little progress until the criteria are determined.

We need two sets of criteria, which will be applied at two different stages in the selection of recipients of SLMR. First, medical criteria should be used to exclude those who are not "medically acceptable." Second, from this group of "medically acceptable" applicants, the final selection can be made. Occasionally in current American medical practice, the first stage is omitted, but such an omission is unwarranted. Ethical and social responsibility would seem to require distributing these SLMR only to those who have some reasonable prospect of responding to the treatment. Furthermore, in transplants such medical tests as tissue and blood typing are necessary, although they are hardly fully developed.

"Medical acceptability" is not as easily determined as many nonphysicians assume, since there is considerable debate in medical circles about the relevant factors (e.g., age and complicating diseases). Although ethicists can contribute little or nothing to this debate, two proposals may be in order. First, "medical acceptability" should be used only to determine the group from which the final selection will be made, and the attempt to establish fine degrees of prospective response to treatment should be avoided. Medical criteria, then, would exclude some applicants but would not serve as a basis of comparison between those who pass the first stage. For example, if two applicants for dialysis were medically acceptable, the physicians would *not* choose the one with the *better* medical prospects. Final selection would be made on other grounds. Second, psychological and environmental factors should be kept to an absolute minimum and should be considered only when they are without doubt critically related to medical acceptability (e.g., the inability to cope with the requirements of dialysis, which might lead to suicide).[7]

The most significant moral questions emerge when we turn to the final selection. Once the pool of medically acceptable applicants has been defined and still the number is larger than the resources, what other criteria should be used? How should the final selection be made? First, I shall examine some of the difficulties that stem from efforts to make the final selection in terms of social value; these difficulties raise serious doubts about the feasibility and justifiability of the utilitarian approach. Then I shall consider the possible justification for random selection or chance.

Occasionally criteria of social worth focus on past contributions, but most often they are primarily future-oriented. The patient's potential and probable contribution to the society is stressed, although this obviously cannot be abstracted from his present web of relationships (e.g., dependents) and occupational activities (e.g., nuclear physicist). Indeed, the magnitude of his contribution to society (as an abstraction) is measured in terms of these social roles, relations, and functions. Enough has already been said to suggest the tremendous range of factors that affect social value or worth. (I am excluding from consideration the question of the ability to pay, because most of the people involved have to secure funds from other sources, public or private, anyway. Legislation in 1972 provided payment for most persons who need kidney dialysis or transplantation.) Here we encounter the first major difficulty of this approach: How do we determine the relevant criteria of social value?

The difficulties of quantifying various social needs are only too obvious. How does one quantify and compare the needs of the spirit (e.g., education, art, religion), political life, economic activity, technological development? Joseph Fletcher suggests that "some day we may learn how to 'quantify' or 'mathematicate' or 'computerize' the value problem in selection, in the same careful and thorough way that diagnosis has been."[8] I am not convinced that we can ever quantify values, or that we should attempt to do so. But even if the various social and human needs, in principle, could be quantified, how do we determine how much weight we will give to each one? Which will have priority in case of conflict? Or even more basically, in the light of which values and principles do we recognize social "needs"?

One possible way of determining the values that should be emphasized in selection has been proposed by Leo Shatin.[9] He insists that our medical decisions about allocating resources are already based on an unconscious scale of values (usually dominated by material worth). Since there is really no way of escaping this, we should be self-conscious and critical about it. How should we proceed? He recommends that we discover the values that most people in our society hold and then use them as criteria for distributing SLMR. These values can be discovered by attitude or opinion surveys. Presumably if 51 percent in this testing period put a greater premium on military needs than technological development, military men would have a greater claim on our SLMR than experimental researchers. But valuations of what is significant change, and the student revolutionary who was denied SLMR in 1970 might be celebrated in 1990 as the greatest American hero since George Washington.

Shatin presumably is seeking criteria that could be applied nationally, but at the present, regional and local as well as individual prejudices tincture the criteria of social value that are used in selection. Nowhere is this more evident than in the deliberations and decisions of the anonymous selection committee of the Seattle Artificial Kidney Center, where such factors as church membership and Scout leadership have been deemed significant for determining who shall live.[10] As two critics conclude after examining these criteria and procedures, they rule out "creative nonconformists, who rub the bourgeoisie the wrong way but who historically have contributed so much to the making of America. The Pacific Northwest is no place for a Henry David Thoreau with bad kidneys."[11]

Closely connected to this first problem of determining social value is a second one. Not only is it difficult if not impossible to reach agreement on social value, but it is also rarely easy to predict what our needs will be in a few years and what the consequences of present actions will be. Furthermore it is difficult to predict which persons will fulfill their potential function in society. Admissions committees in colleges and universities experience the frustrations of predicting realization of potential. For these reasons, as someone has indicated, God might be a utilitarian, but we cannot be. We simply lack the capacity to predict very accurately the consequences which we then must evaluate. Our incapacity is never more evident than when we think in societal terms.

Other difficulties make us even less confident that such an approach to SLMR is advisable. Many critics raise the specter of abuse, but this should not be overemphasized. The fundamental difficulty appears on another level: the utilitarian approach would in effect reduce the person to his social role, relations, and functions. Ultimately it dulls and perhaps even eliminates the sense of the person's transcendence, his dignity as a person that cannot be reduced to his past or future contribution to society. It is not at all clear that we are willing to live with these implications of utilitarian selection. Wilhelm Kolff, who invented the artificial kidney, has asked: "Do we really subscribe to the principle that social standing should determine selection? Do we allow patients to be treated with dialysis only when they are married, go to church, have children, have a job, a good income and give to the Community Chest?"[12]

The German theologian Helmut Thielicke contends that any search for "objective criteria" for selection is already a capitulation to the utilitarian point of view which violates man's dignity.[13] The solution is not to let all die, but to recognize that SLMR cases are "borderline situations" which inevitably involve guilt. The agent, however, can have courage and freedom (which, for Thielicke, come from justification by faith) and can

> go ahead anyway and seek for criteria for deciding the question of life or death in the matter of the artificial kidney. Since these criteria are...questionable, necessarily alien to the meaning of human existence, the decision to which they lead can be little more than that arrived at by casting lots.[14]

The resulting criteria, he suggests, will probably be very similar to those already employed in American medical practice.

He is most concerned to preserve a certain *attitude* or *disposition* in SLMR—the sense of guilt that arises when man's dignity is violated. With this sense of guilt, the agent remains "sound and healthy where it really counts."[15] Thielicke uses man's dignity only as a judgmental, critical, and negative standard. It only tells us how all selection criteria and procedures (and even the refusal to act) implicate us in the ambiguity of the human condition and its metaphysical guilt. This approach is consistent with his view of the task of theological ethics: "to teach us how to understand and endure—not 'solve'—the borderline situation."[16] But ethics, I would contend, can help us discern the factors and norms in whose light relative, discriminate judgments can be made. Even if all actions in SLMR should involve guilt, some may preserve human dignity to a greater extent than others. Thielicke recognizes that a decision based on any criteria is "little more than that arrived at by casting lots." But perhaps selection by chance would come the closest to embodying the moral and nonmoral values that we are trying to maintain (including a sense of man's dignity).

THE VALUES OF RANDOM SELECTION

My proposal is that we use some form of randomness or chance (either natural, such as "first come, first served," or artificial, such as a lottery) to determine who shall be saved. Many reject randomness as a surrender to nonrationality when responsible and rational judgments can and must be made. Edmond Cahn criticizes "Holmes' judge" who recommended the casting of lots because, as Cahn puts it, "the crisis involves stakes too high for gambling and responsibilities too deep for destiny."[17] Similarly, other critics see randomness as a surrender to "non-human" forces which necessarily vitiates human values. Sometimes these values are identified with the process of decision-making (e.g., it is important to have persons rather than impersonal forces determining who shall live). Sometimes they are identified with the outcome of the process (e.g., the features such as creativity and fullness of being that make human life what it is are to be considered and respected in the decision). Regarding the former, it must be admitted that the use of chance seems cold and impersonal. But presumably the defenders of utilitarian criteria in SLMR want to make their application as objective and impersonal as possible so that subjective bias does not determine who shall live.

Such criticisms, however, ignore the moral and nonmoral values that might be supported by selection by randomness or chance. A more important criticism is that the procedure that I develop draws the relevant moral context too narrowly. That context, so the argument might run, includes the society and its future and not merely the individual with his illness and claim upon SLMR. But my contention is that the values and principles at work in the narrower context may well take precedence over those operative in the broader context, both because of their weight and significance and because of the weaknesses of selection in terms of social worth. As Paul Freund rightly insists, "The more nearly total is the estimate to be made of an individual, and the more nearly the consequence determines life and death, the more unfit the judgment

becomes for human reckoning....Randomness as a moral principle deserves serious study."[18] Serious study would, I think, point toward its implementation in certain conflict situations, primarily because it preserves a significant degree of *personal dignity* by providing *equality* of opportunity. Thus it cannot be dismissed as a "nonrational" and "nonhuman" procedure without an inquiry into the reasons, including human values, which might justify it. Paul Ramsey stresses this point about the *Holmes* case:

> Instead of fixing our attention upon "gambling" as the solution—with all the frivolous and often corrupt associations the word raises in our minds—we should think rather of *equality* of opportunity as the ethical substance of the relations of those individuals to one another that might have been guarded and expressed by casting lots.[19]

The individual's personal and transcendent dignity, which on the utilitarian approach would be submerged in his social role and function, can be protected and witnessed to by a recognition of his equal right to be saved. Such a right is best preserved by procedures which establish equality of opportunity. Thus selection by chance more closely approximates the requirements established by human dignity than does utilitarian calculation. It is not infallibly just, but it is preferable to the alternatives of letting all die or saving only those who have the greatest social responsibilities and potential contribution.

This argument can be extended by examining values other than individual dignity and equality of opportunity. Another basic value in the medical sphere is the relationship of trust between physician and patient. Which selection criteria are most in accord with this relationship of trust? Which will maintain, extend, and deepen it? My contention is that selection by randomness or chance is preferable from this standpoint too.

Trust, which is inextricably bound to respect for human dignity, is an attitude of expectation about another. It is not simply the expectation that another will perform a particular act, but more specifically that another will act toward him in certain ways—which will respect him as a person. As Charles Fried writes:

> Although trust has to do with reliance on a disposition of another person, it is reliance on a disposition of a special sort: the disposition to act morally, to deal fairly with others, to live up to one's undertak-

ings, and so on. Thus to trust another is first of all to expect him to accept the principle of morality in his dealings with you, to respect your status as a person, your personality.[20]

This trust cannot be preserved in life-and-death situations when a person expects decisions about him to be made in terms of his social worth, for such decisions violate his status as a person. An applicant rejected on grounds of inadequacy in social value or virtue would have reason for feeling that his "trust" had been betrayed. Indeed, the sense that one is being viewed not as an end in himself but as a means in medical progress or the achievement of a greater social good is incompatible with attitudes and relationships of trust. We recognize this in the billboard which was erected after the first heart transplants: "Drive Carefully. Christiaan Barnard Is Watching You." The relationship of trust between the physician and patient is not only an instrumental value in the sense of being an important factor in the patient's treatment. It is also to be endorsed because of its intrinsic worth as a relationship.

Thus the related values of individual dignity and trust are best maintained in selection by chance. But other factors also buttress the argument for this approach. Which criteria and procedures would men agree upon? We have to suppose a hypothetical situation in which several men are going to determine for themselves and their families the criteria and procedures by which they would want to be admitted to and excluded from SLMR if the need arose.[21] We need to assume two restrictions and then ask which set of criteria and procedures would be chosen as the most rational and, indeed, the fairest. The restrictions are these: (1) The men are *self-interested.* They are interested in their own welfare (and that of members of their families), and this, of course, includes survival. Basically, they are not motivated by altruism. (2) Furthermore, they are *ignorant* of their own talents, abilities, potential, and probable contribution to the social good. They do not know how they would fare in a competitive situation, e.g., the competition for SLMR in terms of social contribution. Under these conditions which institution would be chosen—letting all die, utilitarian selection, or the use of chance? Which would seem the most rational? the fairest? By which set of criteria would they want to be included in or excluded from the list of those who will be saved? The rational choice in this setting (assuming self-interest and igno-

rance of one's competitive success) would be random selection or chance since this alone provides equality of opportunity. A possible response is that one would prefer to take a "risk" and therefore choose the utilitarian approach. But I think not, especially since I added that the participants in this hypothetical situation are choosing for their children as well as for themselves; random selection or chance could be more easily justified to the children. It would make more sense for men who are self-interested but uncertain about their relative contribution to society to elect a set of criteria that would build in equality of opportunity. They would consider selection by chance as relatively just and fair.[22]

An important psychological point supplements earlier arguments for using chance or random selection. The psychological stress and strain among those who are rejected would be greater if the rejection is based on insufficient social worth than if it is based on chance. Obviously stress and strain cannot be eliminated in these borderline situations, but they would almost certainly be increased by the opprobrium of being judged relatively "unfit" by society's agents using society's values. Nicholas Rescher makes this point very effectively:

> a recourse to chance would doubtless make matters easier for the rejected patients and those who have a specific interest in him. It would surely be quite hard for them to accept his exclusion by relatively mechanical application of objective criteria in whose implementation subjective judgment is involved. But the circumstances of life have conditioned us to accept the workings of chance and to tolerate the element of luck (good or bad): human life is an inherently contingent process. Nobody, after all, has an absolute right to ELT [Exotic Lifesaving Therapy]—but most of us would feel that we have "every bit as much right" to it as anyone else in significantly similar circumstances.[23]

Although it is seldom recognized as such, selection by chance is already in operation in practically every dialysis unit. I am not aware of any unit that removes some of its patients from kidney machines in order to make room for later applicants who are better qualified in terms of social worth. Furthermore, very few people would recommend it. Indeed, few would even consider removing a person from a kidney machine on the grounds that a person better qualified *medically* had just applied. In a discussion of the treatment of chronic renal failure by dialysis at the University of Virginia Hospital Renal Unit from November 15, 1965 to November 15, 1966, Dr. Harry Abram writes: "Thirteen patients sought treatment but were not considered because the program had reached its limit of nine patients."[24] Thus, in practice and theory, natural chance is accepted, at least within certain limits.

My proposal is that we extend this principle (first come, first served) to determine who among the medically acceptable patients shall live or that we utilize artificial chance such as a lottery or randomness. "First come, first served" would be more feasible than a lottery since the applicants make their claims over a period of time rather than as a group at one time. This procedure would be in accord with at least one principle in our present practices and with our sense of individual dignity, trust, and fairness. Its significance in relation to these values can be underlined by asking how the decision can be justified to the rejected applicant. Of course, one easy way of avoiding this task is to maintain the traditional cloak of secrecy, which works to a great extent because patients are often not aware that they are being considered for SLMR in addition to the usual treatment. But whether public justification is instituted or not is not the significant question; it is rather what reasons for rejection would be most acceptable to the unsuccessful applicant. My contention is that rejection can be accepted more readily if equality of opportunity, fairness, and trust are preserved, and that they are best preserved by selection by randomness or chance.

This proposal has yet another advantage since it would eliminate the need for a committee to examine applicants in terms of their social value. This onerous responsibility can be avoided.

Finally, there is a possible indirect consequence of widespread use of random selection which is interesting to ponder, although I do *not* adduce it as a good reason for adopting random selection. It can be argued, as Professor Mason Willrich of the University of Virginia Law School has suggested, that SLMR cases would practically disappear if these scarce resources were distributed randomly rather than on social worth grounds. Scarcity would no longer be a problem because the holders of economic and political power would make certain that they would not be excluded by a random selection procedure; hence they would help to redirect public priorities or establish private funding so that life-saving medical treatment would be widely and perhaps universally available.

In the framework that I have delineated, are the decrees of chance to be taken without exception? If we recognize exceptions, would we not open Pandora's box again just after we had succeeded in getting it closed? The direction of my argument has been against any exceptions, and I would defend this as the proper way to go. But let me indicate one possible way of admitting exceptions, while at the same time circumscribing them so narrowly that they would be very rare indeed.

An obvious advantage of the utilitarian approach is that occasionally circumstances arise that make it necessary to say that one man is practically indispensable for a society in view of a particular set of problems it faces (e.g., the president when the nation is waging a war for survival). Certainly the argument to this point has stressed that the burden of proof would fall on those who think that the social danger in this instance is so great that they simply cannot abide by the outcome of a lottery or a first come, first served policy. Also, the reason must be negative rather than positive; that is, we depart from chance in this instance not because we want to take advantage of this person's potential contribution to the improvement of our society, but because his immediate loss would possibly (even probably) be disastrous (again, the president in a grave national emergency). Finally, social value (in the negative sense) should be used as a standard of exception in dialysis, for example, only if it would provide a reason strong enough to warrant removing another person from a kidney machine if all machines were taken. Assuming this strong reluctance to remove anyone once the commitment has been made to him, we would be willing to put this patient ahead of another applicant for a vacant machine only if we would be willing (in circumstances in which all machines are being used) to vacate a machine by removing someone from it. These restrictions would make an exception almost impossible.

While I do not recommend this procedure of recognizing exceptions, I think that one can defend it while accepting my general thesis about selection by randomness or chance. If it is used, a lay committee (perhaps advisory, perhaps even stronger) would be called upon to deal with the alleged exceptions, since the doctors or others would in effect be appealing the outcome of chance (either natural or artificial). This lay committee would determine whether this patient was so indispensable at this time and place that he had to be saved even by sacrificing the values preserved by random selection. It would make it quite clear that exception is warranted, if at all, only as the "lesser of two evils." Such a defense would be recognized only rarely, if ever, primarily because chance and randomness preserve so many important moral and nonmoral values in SLMR cases.[25]

NOTES

1 George Bernard Shaw, *The Doctor's Dilemma* (New York, 1941), pp. 132–33.

2 Henry K. Beecher, "Scarce Resources and Medical Advancement," *Daedalus* (Spring 1969), 279–80.

3 Leo Shatin, "Medical Care and the Social Worth of a Man," *American Journal of Orthopsychiatry*, 36 (1967), 97.

4 Harry S. Abram and Walter Wadlington, "Selection of Patients for Artificial and Transplanted Organs," *Annals of Internal Medicine*, 69 (September 1968), 615–20.

5 *United States v. Holmes*, 26 Fed. Cas. 360 (C.C.E.D. Pa. 1842). All references are to the text of the trial as reprinted in Philip E. Davis, ed., *Moral Duty and Legal Responsibility: A Philosophical-Legal Casebook* (New York, 1966), pp. 102–18.

6 *The Moral Decision* (Bloomington, Ind., 1955), p. 71.

7 For a discussion of the higher suicide rate among dialysis patients than among the general population and an interpretation of some of the factors at work, see H. S. Abram, G. L. Moore, and F. B. Westervelt, "Suicidal Behavior in Chronic Dialysis Patients," *American Journal of Psychiatry*, 127 (1971): 1119–1204. This study shows that even "if one does not include death through not following the regimen the incidence of suicide is still more than 100 times the normal population."

8 Joseph Fletcher, "Donor Nephrectomies and Moral Responsibility," *Journal of the American Medical Women's Association*, 23 (December 1968), 1090.

9 Leo Shatin, pp. 96–101.

10 For a discussion of the Seattle selection committee, see Shana Alexander, "They Decide Who Lives, Who Dies," *Life*, 53 (November 9, 1962), 102. For an examination of general selection practices in dialysis see "Scarce Medical Resources," *Columbia Law Review* 69:620 (1969) and Abram and Wadlington.

11 David Sanders and Jesse Dukeminier, Jr., "Medical Advance and Legal Lag: Hemodialysis and Kidney

Transplantation," *UCLA Law Review* 15:367 (1968), 378.

12 "Letters and Comments," *Annals of Internal Medicine*, 61 (August 1964), 360. Dr. G. E. Schreiner contends that "if you really believe in the right of society to make decisions on medical availability on these criteria you should be logical and say that when a man stops going to church or is divorced or loses his job, he ought to be removed from the programme and somebody else who fulfills these criteria substituted. Obviously no one faces up to this logical consequence" (G. E. W. Wolstenholme and Maeve O'Connor, eds., *Ethics in Medical Progress: With Special Reference to Transplantation*, A Ciba Foundation Symposium [Boston, 1966], p. 127).

13 Helmut Thielicke, "The Doctor as Judge of Who Shall Live and Who Shall Die," *Who Shall Live?* ed. by Kenneth Vaux (Philadelphia, 1970), p. 172.

14 Ibid., pp. 173–74.

15 Ibid., p. 173.

16 Thielicke, *Theological Ethics*, Vol. I, *Foundations* (Philadelphia, 1966), p. 602.

17 Cahn, op. cit., p. 71.

18 Paul Freund, "Introduction," *Daedalus* (Spring 1969), xiii.

19 Paul Ramsey, *Nine Modern Moralists* (Englewood Cliffs, N.J., 1962), p. 245.

20 Charles Fried, "Privacy," in *Law, Reason, and Justice*, ed. by Graham Hughes (New York, 1969), p. 52.

21 My argument is greatly dependent on John Rawls's version of justice as fairness, which is a reinterpretation of social contract theory. Rawls, however, would probably not apply his ideas to "borderline situations." See "Distributive Justice: Some Addenda," *Natural Law Forum*, 13 (1968), 53. For Rawls's general theory, see "Justice as Fairness," *Philosophy, Politics and Society* (Second Series), ed. by Peter Laslett and W. G. Runciman (Oxford, 1962), pp. 132–57 and *A Theory of Justice* (Cambridge, Mass., 1971).

22 Occasionally someone contends that random selection may reward vice. Leo Shatin (op. cit., p. 100) insists that random selection "would reward socially disvalued qualities by giving their bearers the same special medical care opportunities as those received by the bearers of socially valued qualities. Personally I do not favor such a method." Obviously society must engender certain qualities in its members, but

not all of its institutions must be devoted to that purpose. Furthermore, there are strong reasons, I have contended, for exempting SLMR from that sort of function.

23 Nicholas Rescher, "The Allocation of Exotic Medical Lifesaving Therapy," *Ethics*, 79 (April 1969), 184. He defends random selection's use only after utilitarian and other judgments have been made. If there are no "major disparities" in terms of utility, etc., in the second stage of selection, then final selection could be made randomly. He fails to give attention to the moral values that random selection might preserve.

24 Harry S. Abram, M.D., "The Psychiatrist, the Treatment of Chronic Renal Failure, and the Prolongation of Life: II" *American Journal of Psychiatry* 126:157–67 (1969), 158.

25 I read a draft of this paper in a seminar on "Social Implications of Advances in Biomedical Science and Technology: Artificial and Transplanted Internal Organs," sponsored by the Center for the Study of Science, Technology, and Public Policy of the University of Virginia, Spring 1970. I am indebted to the participants in that seminar, and especially to its leaders, Mason Willrich, Professor of Law, and Dr. Harry Abram, Associate Professor of Psychiatry, for criticisms which helped me to sharpen these ideas. Good discussions of the legal questions raised by selection (e.g., equal protection of the law and due process) which I have not considered can be found in "Scarce Medical Resources," *Columbia Law Review*, 69:620 (1969); "Patient Selection for Artificial and Transplanted Organs," *Harvard Law Review*, 82:1322 (1969); and Sanders and Dukeminier, op. cit.

The Microallocation of Scarce Medical Lifesaving Resources

Margaret Holmgren

Margaret Holmgren is assistant professor of philosophy at Iowa State University of Science and Technology. Holmgren's areas of specialization are ethics, social and political philosophy, and philosophy of law. She serves on The Governor's Advisory Committee on Organ Transplants in Iowa. Her publications include "Punishment as Restitution: The Rights of the Community."

In her discussion of microallocation decisions, Holmgren adopts a Kantian approach in criticizing some of the first-stage and second-stage criteria proposed by Rescher. She also rejects the random selection procedure advocated by Childress and others partly because it may generate results that violate strong moral intuitions. She criticizes some of the arguments that have been offered in defense of such procedures and conclusions by attempting to develop an alternative position. Holmgren's Kantian analysis yields a set of principles for microallocation decisions in life or death situations from which some of Rescher's criteria follow.

One of the most urgent questions in medical ethics today arises in situations in which we have enough resources to save some of those who might be saved by a particular medical treatment, but not enough to save everyone who could be saved. Here we are forced to decide who will be given the opportunity to live and who will die. These situations have arisen in the past, perhaps most dramatically in connection with hemodialysis. We face them now in connection with organ transplants. And, we can expect to face them regularly in the future as scientists develop the artificial heart, perfect techniques for organ transplantations, and invent other costly medical procedures for saving lives. Thus it is important that we find a morally defensible procedure for determining which patients ought to be saved under these circumstances.

As we might expect, philosophers and others have had very different ideas about how this type of choice ought to be made. Utilitarians and moral pluralists have suggested a comparative approach, in which patients in the applicant pool are evaluated and selected on the basis of a set of criteria such as social worth, family role, life-expectancy, etc. Kantians, or those who advocate an ethics of respect for persons,[1] have responded that such a procedure fails to recognize the equal right of each individual to live. Only a random selection can adequately reflect the equal moral status of persons. In the essay that follows, I argue that Kantians have legitimate worries about several of the criteria proposed in the context of the comparative approach, but that they have not given adequate arguments in support of random selection. I go on to suggest an alternative Kantian analysis of this issue which yields a set of principles for determining who will live and who will die.

I

Let us first consider the comparative selection system often advocated by utilitarians and moral pluralists. A system of this sort has been formulated by Nicholas Rescher.[2] His concern is to provide a rationally defensible selection procedure which incorporates utilitarian considerations but which is also fair, in that "it must treat relevant cases alike, leaving no room for 'influence' or favoritism, etc."[3] Because Rescher's proposal incorporates almost all of the major criteria that have been considered relevant in the allocation of medical lifesaving procedures (MLP's), it may be regarded as a paradigm example of the comparative approach.

Rescher divides the selection process into two phases: first, selecting a group of suitable applicants, and second, choosing the patients to receive MLP's from within this group. For the first phase, he proposes the criteria of constituency, progress of science, and prospect of success. The first two criteria, at least as he has articulated them, do not constitute legitimate bases for

deciding who will live and who will die from the perspective of an ethics of respect for persons. There are two aspects of the criteria referred to as "constituency." First, Rescher claims that a hospital's "normal clientele boundaries" may constitute grounds for narrowing the applicant pool. For example, an army hospital need not consider an applicant who is a college professor and a children's hospital need not accept a senior citizen. Although such a criterion leaves no room for favoritism, it fails to constitute a just basis for denying individuals access to an MLP, assuming that they have nowhere else to turn for the medical treatment they need. There may be a utilitarian justification for employing this criterion: *ceteris paribus*, welfare will be maximized if the hospital staff can be spared the inconveniences of treating those who are outside its normal clientele boundaries. However, to deny individuals the opportunity to live on these grounds is a paradigm case of using them as mere means to our own ends. Each person who needs an MLP has a very significant interest at stake in becoming a member of the applicant pool. If we are to accord these individuals the respect they are due as persons, we cannot require them to sacrifice this major interest in order to avoid minor inconveniences for others.

The second aspect of "constituency" is initially more plausible. Rescher suggests that the well-known hemodialysis selection committee in Seattle was justified in excluding non-residents of the state of Washington on the grounds that the hemodialysis units were financed from state revenues. Because Washington residents paid for the units, they should be given priority for their use.

This argument raises some complex questions about legitimate forms of taxation, and it warrants more attention than I can give it here. Briefly, however, I think it fails for the following reason. Residents of a state are free at any time to combine resources and produce MLP's, if they wish to make their futures more secure in this way. If some of them choose to do so, they are then entitled to work out their own system of allocation. It is not a legitimate function of government, however, to *force* citizens to produce MLP's simply as a kind of insurance policy against fatal diseases they may contract in the future. Such an action would be paternalistic, and it would constitute an undue infringement of individual autonomy. The government is justified in requiring persons to provide revenues for MLP's only if they have a moral obligation to produce them—an obligation that would presumably stem from an obligation to help others in need. In this case, though, the taxpayers have no prior entitlement to the units produced, and I see no reason why a resident of Washington should have priority over anyone else as a recipient of this aid. Further, even if the argument were successful, it would show only that tax-paying residents of the state have priority (priority would not extend to a resident on welfare who did not help pay for the MLP), and it would imply that those in higher tax brackets should have priority over those in lower tax brackets. Thus I believe that Rescher's constituency criterion is properly rejected by the Kantian ethicist, although I will argue below that there is a closely related criterion of selection that is morally defensible.

The factor of progress of science, as Rescher conceives it, is also problematic in that its use may evidence a basic lack of respect for individuals. He cites the "research interests of the medical staff" as a significant consideration if they pertain to the MLP in question. Again, a utilitarian defense of this criterion could be constructed, since any gain we make in scientific knowledge can be expected to contribute to the general welfare. However, the benefits for others stemming from much of this type of research will not be comparable to the fundamental interest at stake on the part of the person in need of the MLP. To require her to give up her chance to live in order to secure these lesser benefits for others seems to be another clear instance of using her as a mere means to promote our own ends. I will argue that progress of science can be a relevant consideration when it is subsumed under another principle of selection: that *ceteris paribus*, we must save more lives rather than fewer.

Rescher's third criterion for this phase of the selection, that an individual must have a reasonable prospect of success to be considered for lifesaving therapy, seems to be valid and could be supported by anyone who would like to see someone saved by an MLP rather than no one.

Rescher proposed five criteria for the final phase of the selection procedure. The first two, relative likelihood of success and life-expectancy, he characterizes as biomedical factors. Again, a determination on the basis of these factors rules out favoritism, but it is not clear that it would satisfy the more substantive demands of justice of an ethics of respect for persons. Further argument is required to show that the use of these criteria adequately reflects the equal moral status of persons and the equal right of each individual to live. If all persons have an equal right to life, on what grounds can we give a 20-year-old priority over a 70-year-old? On an intuitive basis, it does seem as if life-expectancy and relative prospect of success are morally significant when the differences between patients are great. However, in order to provide a sound justification for using these criteria to determine who will live and who will die, an adequate answer will have to be given to the question we have raised here from the Kantian perspective.

Finally, Rescher proposes three "social factors": family role, potential future contribution, and past services rendered. Once again, an advocate of an ethics of respect for persons will reject the first two of these criteria, in spite of the obvious utilitarian justification for them, on the grounds that employing them will entail using persons as mere means to our own ends under many circumstances. If we employ these criteria, applicants will often be required to sacrifice their fundamental interest in the opportunity to live so that others can benefit in less important ways. For example, if we select a member of a symphony orchestra over a garbage collector, we would be requiring the garbage collector to sacrifice his or her chance to live so that others will be able to hear higher quality music.

Rescher's final criterion, past services rendered, is not a utilitarian consideration. There are two arguments that might be given to support it. The first (and the one Rescher has in mind) is that society has an obligation to reward individuals for their past contributions, and in order to pay this debt, we ought to give them priority in receiving MLP's. However, even if society does owe citizens rewards for contributions they have chosen to make (and I find this claim questionable), we cannot legitimately discharge this debt by denying other citizens the chance to live. To do so would be to allocate an unjustifiably large share of the burden of paying the debt to a handful of unfortunate individuals—those who will die without our help. Further, if we really believe that society owes these individuals a reward for their contributions, we should provide the reward when the services are rendered instead of waiting until the recipient contracts a fatal disease.

A more interesting argument in support of this criterion is that persons who have gone out of their way to make contributions to society, or who have demonstrated themselves to be of exceptional moral worth, deserve to be saved before the others because they are better persons. Those who make this claim reject the fundamental claim on which an ethics of respect for persons is based: that all persons have an equal moral status and ought to be treated as equals. Clearly, we cannot resolve here the fundamental question of whether a meritarian or an egalitarian ethics is correct. I will simply point out two difficult tasks that face those who wish to allocate MLP's on the basis of desert. First, they will have to identify the characteristic (or well-ordered set of characteristics) in virtue of which persons deserve to live, and second, they will have to provide us with a reasonably reliable method for ascertaining the extent to which each applicant possesses this characteristic. Neither of these tasks is easy, given the present limitations of human knowledge; hence, making this type of determination is often referred to as "playing God."

To summarize, then, the Kantian ethicist would reject (and for good reasons) the criteria of constituency, progress of science, family role, social worth and past services rendered, at least as Rescher has articulated them. (S)he would also have serious concerns about the criteria of life-expectancy and relative prospect of success—concerns that must be met before we can establish the moral legitimacy of using these criteria in selecting patients for MLP's.

II

In view of the injustices that inhere in the comparative approach, advocates of an ethics of respect for persons have turned to random selection.[4] Ramsey and Childress (among others) have argued that patients ought to be selected at random from among those who would have a reasonably good chance of recovery if given access to an MLP.[5] Ramsey believes that exceptions to random selection are defensible only in extraordinary situations such as wars, plagues, and natural disasters. Childress admits even fewer exceptions than Ramsey, arguing that they are legitimate only if an individual is "practically indispensable" for a society in a particular situation, such that we would be willing to withdraw an MLP from someone who is already using it in order to save her.

A selection system of this sort can be called into question, however, because it may generate results that violate strong moral intuitions. Our intuitions tell us that it would be wrong to save a hopeless heroin addict, a mass murderer, or a senile 95-year-old instead of a responsible 30-year-old who is leading a rewarding life. This problem with the unconstrained lottery indicates the need for further analysis of the issue from a Kantian perspective. The inference from the premise that all individuals are of equal worth to the conclusion that we must institute a random selection system requires mediation in any case, and it is not clear that we are driven to this conclusion if we reject the criteria proposed by Rescher.

Let us take a closer look at two arguments that might support the type of selection system Ramsey and Childress advocate. The first is suggested by Ramsey. He points out that in reference to a narrowly focused goal of the sort that emerges in disasters, we can determine that one person is worth more than another. However, in the absence of such a goal we have no grounds for saying that A is worth more than B. Therefore, we have no grounds for giving A priority over B, and we must resort to random selection.

This argument is not convincing. As Ronald Dworkin has pointed out, it is important to distinguish between treating persons as equals and treating persons equally.[6] We are required to treat persons as equals (in the context of an egalitarian ethics), but we need not treat everyone in exactly the same way in order to fulfill this requirement. For example, we may offer assistance to a quadriplegic but not to Superman, not because the quadriplegic is of greater intrinsic worth than Superman, but because (s)he has a greater interest at stake in receiving our aid. Thus there may be reasons for giving patient A priority over patient B that are not based on the claim that A is worth more than B.

A second argument may be constructed as follows. Each person is of equal worth, and therefore has an equal right to life. If each of us has an equal right to life, it follows that each of us has the right to an equal opportunity to live, or to be saved by an MLP. Because of the extreme importance of the opportunity to live, this right can only be overridden in cases of disaster. This analysis is in conflict with our ordinary understanding of rights, though, in that other rights, including the right to life itself, can be overridden in circumstances far less dramatic than disasters. For example, the right to life may be overridden if we must shoot a sniper to prevent him from killing someone else. Further, we do not always reason from the claim that all persons are of equal worth to the claim that all persons have the right to an equal opportunity to receive X. We need not institute a lottery to guarantee everyone an equal opportunity to receive a Harvard education because we are all of equal moral worth. Other types of moral considerations may disrupt such an inference. Neither of these arguments, then, provides conclusive support for unconstrained random selection.

III

At this point, I would like to suggest an alternative approach to the allocation of scarce lifesaving resources. This approach is based on an egalitarian conception of justice that can be described as Kantian in that it demands that we never treat persons as mere means, but always also as ends in themselves. I propose to unpack the Kantian injunction, roughly, as requiring that the most fundamental interests in life be secured for each individual, compatible with like benefits for all, and that no individual be required to sacrifice a fundamental interest so that another person or group of persons can benefit in a less important way.

From this basic moral position, we might derive the following three lexically ordered principles to govern the allocation of scarce lifesaving resources, assuming that A and B are persons in the same pool of applicants who wish to receive scarce resource S:

1 If B bears a significant amount of responsibility for the scarcity of resources available for saving lives and A does not, then A has priority over B in receiving S.

2 If A clearly has a greater interest at stake than B in receiving S, then A has priority over B.

3 If we can predict with a reasonable degree of certainty that we can save a greater number of lives if we save A rather than B, then A has priority over B in receiving S.

These principles are to be applied in order, and random selection procedures are to be instituted, if necessary, to choose among candidates who are not excluded on the basis of them. For example, suppose that we have 100 applicants for 10 MLP's, and 90 receive priority over the other 10 by application of the first principle. We then apply the second principle, and 30 applicants receive priority over the remaining 60. Application of the third principle finally gives 15 of these 30 priority. At this point, we must apply a random selection procedure to determine which 10 of these 15 will be saved. Or, suppose that after the application of the

third principle, we have narrowed the field to 8 applicants. We must then backtrack and choose by random selection 2 more candidates from among the 30 remaining after the application of the second principle to receive the two additional MLP's. Finally, since we have no moral obligation to help those who do not need our help, I will assume that these principles serve to allocate MLP's only among those who cannot provide the necessary resources to save themselves.

Some comments are in order on each of these principles of selection. The responsibility principle can be derived from the principle of justice cited above because it can be shown to provide a fundamental interest for each person compatible with like benefits for all. It secures for each of us the *opportunity* to put ourselves in the best possible position to secure an MLP, should we need one in order to survive. If this principle is adopted, we can maximize our chances of receiving an MLP by making good decisions, and we will not be disadvantaged in this regard by other persons' wrong choices—a factor over which we have no control. It is important to stress that the responsibility principle does not give priority to A over B because B has made a bad choice and is therefore less fit to live than A. This principle is consistent with the claim that A or B are of equal worth as persons. We give priority to A here only because in doing so we secure an important interest for everyone.

The responsibility principle would assign priority to A over B in cases such as the following:

1 B attacks A, and A is forced to defend himself. As a result of the fight, both A and B need an MLP in order to survive.

2 A has done everything she could throughout her life to take care of her health. B, although she was aware of the potential consequences, has chosen to adopt a very degenerate life style. Doctors tell us that B would be fine today if she had taken reasonable steps to protect her health, but now both A and B need a heart-lung-transplant in order to survive.

3 B has chosen to commit a series of rapes, and as a result, the taxpayers have had to spend a great deal of money tracking him down, giving him a trial, and supporting him in prison. This money could have gone instead towards financing artificial hearts. Now A, who has never wasted public money, and B both need an artificial heart in order to survive.

In each of these cases, B bears a significant degree of responsibility for generating or aggravating a scarcity of lifesaving resources. It is important to specify that *B's* responsibility for aggravating the scarcity must be significant. We would not give *A* priority over *B*, for example, if *B* had only wasted $5 of the taxpayers' money, which could have gone instead towards an MLP. All of us make mistakes from time to time, and we have an interest in being able to recover and go on with our lives after we make them. As the impact of our mistakes on others becomes more trivial, or as it becomes more difficult for us to avoid making the mistake in question, the interest we have in recovering begins to outweigh the interest we have in protecting ourselves from other persons' wrong choices.

Finally, it is interesting to note that the responsibility criterion may generate results that coincide to some extent with Rescher's constituency criterion. *B*, a wealthy citizen of a country that levies very few taxes and does not finance MLP's, may have a moral obligation to provide assistance for persons who need these operations, regardless of where they live. If she is aware that she has this responsibility but chooses not to meet it, she is aggravating the scarcity through her wrong choice. *A*, a conscientious taxpayer of a country that does finance MLP's, would then receive priority over *B* if they both need an MLP and neither can afford to pay for it. (Perhaps *B* has lost her money in a revolution.)

The second principle of selection, which gives *A* priority over *B* if *A* has a more important interest at stake in receiving an MLP than *B*, follows directly from our conception of justice. This principle requires us to consider three factors: prospect of successful recovery, life-expectancy, and quality of life. *Ceteris paribus*, if *B* has a 10% chance of recovery if given access to an MLP and *A* has a 90% chance, *A* has a greater interest at stake in receiving the MLP; if *A* can expect to live 50 more years if (s)he receives an MLP and *B* can expect to live only 2 years longer, *A* has the greater interest at stake; and if *A* looks forward to a wonderful life if (s)he gains access to an MLP and *B's* life would be severely restricted and miserable, *A* has the greater interest at stake.

If we could quantify the quality of life precisely, we could use the following formula to calculate the importance of the interest each patient has in receiving an MLP: probability of recovery × projected number of years left to live × average quality of life per year. Thus all three factors must be considered together. Unfortunately, it is often very difficult to determine how much an individual values life under any given set of

circumstances. One person may place a high value on an existence that appears to the rest of us to be very low quality. Nevertheless, we are not completely in the dark when it comes to making determinations of this sort. There will be many cases in which we can say beyond a reasonable doubt that *A* has a more significant interest at stake in receiving an MLP than *B*. In these cases it is important that we give priority to *A*.

This principle accounts for a case that Marc Basson constructs to provide support for the social worth criterion. He points out that we would prefer to save Mr. Jones, a 27-year-old married nuclear physicist who is a father of three and serves on the school board, rather than Mr. Smith, a senile 92-year-old paraplegic who is terminally ill with another disease and has no friends or relatives.[7] The Kantian principle I have proposed here gives priority to Jones, but *not* on the basis of social worth. Again, this principle is fully compatible with the claim that Jones and Smith have an equal status as persons. Jones receives priority not because he is worth more than Smith, but because he has a more fundamental interest at stake than Smith in continuing to live.

The third principle can also be derived from our conception of justice. If we view our lives from a pre-illness perspective, this principle secures an important interest for each of us. It increases the probability that any one of us will be saved if we happen to need an MLP in the future.[8]

Several implications follow from the requirement that *ceteris paribus*, we must save more lives rather than fewer. First, Rescher's progress of science criterion becomes a relevant consideration under some circumstances. If we can claim with some assurance that giving an MLP to *A* rather than *B* will yield medical knowledge that can be used to save additional lives, and that lives will be lost if we do not obtain the knowledge at this time and in this way, then *A* ought to receive priority over *B*.

Second, there will be some cases, although not many, in which considerations of social worth become relevant under this principle. Suppose that if we save *A*, she, in turn, will be able to save other individuals. *B*, on the other hand, would not be able to save anyone if he were saved. Further, if *A* does not save these other persons, they cannot be saved in any other way. In this case, we ought to give *A* priority over *B*. This line of reasoning provides a theoretical framework for the "disaster exceptions" to random selection suggested by Ramsey and Childress.

Third, this principle dictates that if *A* needs an MLP immediately in order to survive and *B* can survive on his own for six months, and if we can expect an additional MLP to become available within the six-month period, then *A* ought to receive priority over *B* for the MLP that is available now.

Fourth, if it costs less to save *A* than to save *B*, and if we could generate enough funds to save other lives by saving *A* rather than *B*, then we ought to do so.

Finally, if we live in a society in which there is a just distribution of resources, we may be required to save more lives by giving priority to those who can pay for part of their own treatment. If *A* and *B* can each pay for half of their treatment, thereby generating enough funds to save a third person *C*, our principle requires that we save *A* and *B* before we save *D* and *E*, who are completely destitute. In our society, however, resources are not justly distributed, and therefore this policy is not defensible. We could easily save *C*, *D* and *E* by making a small cut in defense spending or by closing an unjust tax loophole.

Clearly, more work needs to be done to develop the principles of selection that have been proposed here. These principles make the problem of allocating MLP's far more complex than it is in the context of the Kantian position adopted by Ramsey and Childress. Nevertheless, the analysis given here may come closer to capturing our moral convictions in specific cases than an unconstrained random selection. Unfortunately, one additional complication must now be introduced. We must recognize that the lexical ordering of the three principles will not hold under all circumstances, although I believe it will hold in a large majority of cases. Our basic conception of justice demands that the most fundamental interests in life be secured for each individual compatible with like interests for all. If we are on the verge of World War III and a top diplomat requires an MLP in order to survive and return to negotiations,[9] the interests secured for each of us by the first two principles will pale into insignificance in comparison with the interests secured by the third. Likewise, if we have an applicant pool of 10 senile 95-year-olds and one happy but somewhat irre-

sponsible 25-year-old, the interest secured by the second principle is more fundamental than the interest secured by the first. Thus there must be some flexibility in the order in which we apply the three principles of selection, and the lexical ordering suggested here should be viewed only as a general guideline.

NOTES

1 I will use these terms interchangeably, to refer to those theorists who take seriously Kant's second formulation of the categorical imperative: that we ought never treat persons as mere means, but always also as ends in themselves.

2 Nicholas Rescher, "The Allocation of Exotic Medical Lifesaving Therapy," *Ethics* 70 (April 1969): 173–80.

3 *Ibid.*, p. 174.

4 Rescher also advocates random selection, but of a much more restricted sort. He believes that we ought to select at random only among those who receive roughly similar evaluations on the basis of the criteria of selection he has proposed.

5 See Paul Ramsey, *The Patient as Person* (New Haven: Yale University Press, 1975), pp. 239–76; and James Childress, "Who Shall Live When Not All Can Live?" in *Ethics and Health Policy*, edited by Robert M. Veatch and Roy Brown (Cambridge, MA: Ballinger Publishing Co., 1975): 199–211.

6 Dworkin draws this distinction in a number of places. For one discussion of it, see *Taking Rights Seriously* (Cambridge, MA: Harvard University Press, 1977), p. 227.

7 Marc D. Basson, "Choosing Among Candidates for Scarce Medical Resources," *Journal of Medicine and Philosophy*, 4 (September 1979): 273.

8 John F. Kilner advocates this principle in his article "A Moral Allocation of Scarce Lifesaving Medical Resources," *The Journal of Religious Ethics* 9, 2 (Fall 1981): 245–85. He also points out that this principle would probably be accepted by all from a pre-illness perspective.

9 Again, Basson proposes this case to support a social worth criterion. See Basson, p. 316.

Must a Man Be His Cousin's Keeper?

Alan Meisel and Loren H. Roth

Alan Meisel is assistant professor of law and psychiatry, University of Pittsburgh School of Law and Western Psychiatric Institute and Clinic. Loren H. Roth is associate professor of psychiatry, University of Pittsburgh School of Medicine, and director, Law and Psychiatry Program, Western Psychiatric Institute and Clinic. Meisel and Roth have coauthored several articles including "What We Do and Do Not Know About Informed Consent" and "Patient Access to Records: Tonic or Toxin?" Roth's articles also include "The Right to Refuse Treatment" and "A Commitment Law for Patients, Doctors, and Lawyers." Meisel's work includes a two-part published article on informed consent, "The Exceptions to Informed Consent. Part I: The Exceptions" and "Part II: Proxy Decision-Making."

Meisel and Roth discuss a recent legal case in which Robert McFall sought an injunction to compel his cousin, David Shimp, to provide the bone marrow for a transplant that physicians considered necessary to save McFall's life. Some of the moral issues underlying the arguments they discuss can be expressed in the following questions: Do individuals have a "duty to donate" live body tissue when a life hangs in the balance? Would it ever be morally correct to compel the donation of live body tissue?

Although the average citizen may not have committed to memory Cardozo's dictum, "Every human being of adult years and sound mind has a right to determine what shall be done with his body," it still seems unthinkable that an American court could entertain a lawsuit seeking to compel one person to donate a portion of his body to another. Yet recent events in Pittsburgh raised just that question. Robert McFall, a thirty-nine-year-old, unmarried asbestos worker, suffering from a usually fatal aplastic anemia, filed a suit in Judge Flaherty's court seeking an injunction to compel David Shimp, his unwilling cousin, to undergo a bone marrow transplant that doctors claimed was necessary to save McFall's life....

Before McFall's suit, there had never been a case in this country (or possibly anywhere in the world) seeking to extract bodily tissue from an objecting donor. There had been a scattering of transplant cases, including some bone marrow transplantation, where the potential donor was either mentally incompetent and unable either to consent or object, or a child who was willing to make the donation but because of legal minority required judicial sanction to do so. In one such case, a

kidney was sought from a mentally retarded man because another relative had refused to donate his. There is no mention in that case of compelling a donation from that relative, a forty-three-year-old farmer with nine children who refused on the grounds that his first duty was to his family. In another case, one involving bone marrow transplantation, a thirteen-year-old mentally retarded boy (and the only compatible donor) was selected to be the donor following a court hearing. The parents of the children (the donor and recipient were siblings) refused to consider the possibility of a third normal sibling, an only daughter, becoming the donor.

Yet here it was—the unthinkable being sought and brought to court. Some would say that McFall never had any real chance because the law is so well settled. As Judge Flaherty stated in his opinion denying the transplant request, "Our society, contrary to many others, has as its first principle, the respect for the individual, and that society and government exist to protect the individual from being invaded and hurt by another." Yet the vitality of our legal system lies in its continual potential for change, and knowing this,

Reprinted with permission of the authors and the publisher from *Hastings Center Report*, vol. 8 (October 1978), pp. 5–6.

McFall's lawyer was ineluctably tempted to break new ground, as indeed it was arguably his professional responsibility to do.

A DUTY TO 'RESCUE'?

Probably realizing the futility of a head-on assault on the legal inviolability of the individual, McFall's attorney took a quite inventive tack, perhaps the only one realistically available to him. Before an individual can become a candidate for donating bone marrow, two tests of tissue compatibility must be performed. Shimp voluntarily underwent the first test but refused to undergo the second. The lawsuit was brought to compel him to submit to the second test, and should the results indicate compatibility, eventually to the transplant. The results of the first test showed that there was an excellent chance that Shimp would be a suitable donor and that no other family member would be appropriate. McFall contended that Shimp first led him to believe that he would help, but later reneged, causing "a delay of critical proportions." As a result of this delay, McFall claimed that Shimp was responsible for McFall's current danger.

Behind this somewhat strained argument is the Anglo-American common law tradition that has consistently refused to impose a general duty on citizens to come to the aid of others *unless* one has created the peril. I am perfectly free, legally speaking, to ignore a drowning child's cries for help even though I am an Olympic swimmer. However, if I voluntarily go to that child's aid, I become legally obliged not to increase the danger in which he has been placed. Thus, if I assure other bystanders that there is no need for them to help because I am an excellent swimmer, when in fact I am mediocre, and this assurance causes them to refrain from rescue attempts and my weak efforts fail to save the child, I have breached a legal duty to him.

This may be, as Judge Flaherty remarked, a *morally* revolting rule of law, but as the legal scholar William Prosser explains: "The difficulties of setting any standards of unselfish service to fellow men, and of making a workable rule to cover possible situations where fifty people might fail to rescue one, has limited any tendency to depart from the rule...." According to McFall's argument, Shimp had no duty to come to his aid at the outset, but having done so and having arguably worsened his lot by having done so—presumably because valuable time was lost in seeking another donor—Shimp was now under a duty to "rescue" McFall.

In the end, the court rejected McFall's plea to compel Shimp to donate the marrow. McFall claimed not to be surprised at the outcome, probably having been prepared for it by his lawyer. McFall died of intracranial bleeding two weeks later. While his tendency to bleed might eventually have been corrected by a successful transplant, it was unclear whether a successful transplant or other concurrent medical treatments could have reversed McFall's condition in time to have been effective. At the time of his death, McFall's doctors were considering giving him an experimental drug, antithymocyte globulin, but according to the newspapers they had not yet completed the steps necessary to clear the substance for use as an experimental treatment. Prior to his death, McFall evidenced no public malice, only compassion for Shimp. Shimp did not attend the funeral, but he granted a television interview to explain his position.

THE PROSPECT OF COMPELLED DONATIONS

Now that the unthinkable has not only been thought, but adjudicated, will the same or a similar case arise again? Will the result be the same? Or can we look forward to the prospect of compelled donations of body parts?

McFall's attorney did not try to establish a duty to donate; however, that approach may be the only one available in future cases. Certain arguments can be made in favor of such a direct effort. First, although somewhere between 100 and 150 punctures of a pelvic bone must be made to extract the necessary amount of bone marrow, the procedure is painlessly performed under general anesthesia. The major risk is the anesthesia, which carries a one in ten thousand risk of death. More important, the bone marrow regenerates itself. Thus the fears that are raised in discussion of involuntary organ donation may be misplaced in the case of bone marrow. "[T]he spectre of the swastika and the Inquisition" raised in Judge Flaherty's opinion may just not be a very good analogy when it comes to forced transfusions of marrow. Not only are the risks minimal to the donor, but the potential benefits to the recipient are momentous.[1] Aplastic anemia is almost certainly fatal if untreated—there is only a 25 percent chance of surviving one year, but with a transfusion of compatible marrow there is a 50 to 60 percent chance of survival.

The procedure is not, however, without some risk to the recipient. There is a possibility of rejection even with compatible bone marrow and immunosuppressive drugs must be administered both prior to and following the transplant. These drugs leave the transplant recipient susceptible to infection. Prior radiation therapy is also necessary to suppress the possibility of rejection, and there is a small chance that the recipient may develop a cancer.

If it were not enough that the risks to the donor are small and the potential benefits to the recipient great, there is yet another consideration to be thrown into the balance: Shimp, the unwilling cousin, did not state, prior to the court's ruling his reasons for refusing to go through with the second compatibility test.... Only a week after Judge Flaherty's decision did Shimp reveal his reasons for refusal. Shimp said he refused because the anesthesia might result in a heart attack, and that the procedure might aggravate already present aches and pains, thus interfering with his ability to work. Because he worked with chemicals, Shimp also worried that his bone marrow might not regenerate. Recently divorced and remarried, Shimp has a teenage daughter to support. There was no evidence that Shimp was "irrational." "It was my decision alone. I talked to my wife about it. But ultimately I decided. My cousin could still pull through without my bone marrow.... If he was my child and if my health was right, I would consider doing it" (*Pittsburgh Press*, August 2, 1978, p. 1).

If there were ever a case to be made for ordering a compelled donation of live body tissue, this would be one of the easier ones to decide in favor of ordering the procedure—second only, perhaps, to the donation of blood. Yet the court refused to do so, and in our view its decision was unquestionably proper. Despite the high potential benefits to the recipient, the relatively low risks (objectively speaking) to the donor, and the distinguishability of this case from other kinds of transplants, irreparable harm would be done to the values of individual autonomy, privacy, and bodily and psychic integrity from compelling a transplant of any kind. We need not even conjure up the spectre of robbing organs from the elderly to aid the young, from the mentally deficient to aid the mentally efficient, or from oppressed minorities to aid the power elite. Assuming the best of faith from our doctors and judicial authorities, we still cannot tolerate an involuntary invasion of the body of one individual—adult, competent, and objecting—to aid another.

No matter how idiosyncratic Shimp's reasons for refusal, his mere wish not to donate marrow should not be overridden. In fact, we must be willing to respect his decision even if he could articulate no reasons whatsoever for refusing. Who are we to judge the import of his reasons? It is he who would have had to bear the risks of donation, even if they were relatively slight, and it is he who now bears the costs of refusing—public notoriety, guilt, family discord. These are inherently personal choices. Who is to say that the death of a cousin is inherently more serious than the breakup of one's marriage or the chance of one's own death or incapacitation from general anesthesia? Shimp decided that, placed in this obviously difficult situation, the costs of donation were greater than the costs of refusing to be a donor. His choice must be honored.

NOTE

1 The arguments by McFall's doctors, however, may be open to some question on the basis of the recent medical literature. Matched siblings and not more distant family members are the persons routinely employed as donors. (E. D. Thomas et al., "Current Status of Bone Marrow Transplantation for Aplastic Anemia and Acute Leukemia," *Blood* 49:671–81, 1977). While the use of Shimp as a donor (if he were compatible) would have been medically proper and McFall's best chance for survival, the circumstances of this case suggest it was a choice of last resort for McFall as much as one of providing a well established treatment for him.

Organ Transplants: The Cost of Success

Arthur L. Caplan

Arthur L. Caplan is associate for the humanities at The Hastings Center. His published writings include "The Artificial Heart," "Ethical Engineers Need Not Apply: The State of Applied Ethics Today," and "When Liberty Meets Authority: Ethical Aspects of the Laetrile Controversy."

Caplan argues that given the inadequate supply of organs for transplantation, new governmental policies need to be established. He notes that a policy adopted in the 1960s—"encouraged voluntarism"—has failed to supply the organs needed for transplants. Caplan advances arguments for the moral superiority of a different policy—the policy of "presumed consent"—and rejects the claim that encouraged voluntarism policies are morally superior to presumed consent policies. Defenders of encouraged voluntarism see it as preserving free choice, protecting individual rights, and fostering socially desirable virtues. Caplan questions the voluntariness of the "informed" consent given by family members, asked to donate the organs of someone who has just died. He argues, that in the case of cadavers, a public policy of presumed consent is more just and humane to both medical personnel and family members. He concludes by arguing for a national registry of consenting organ donors and public policies that will ensure that the strictest standards regarding informed consent be followed in the case of live organ donation.

Just thirty years after the first kidney transplant between identical twins was undertaken in 1954, organ transplantation has come of age. Today many transplant surgeons have attained success rates of over 80 percent survival for at least five years among those who have received kidneys from live related donors. The survival rate for recipients of cadaver kidneys five years after surgery is 60 percent. More than 95 percent of cornea transplant recipients have their sight restored. Aided by new immunosuppressive drugs such as Cyclosporin, better tissue-matching capabilities, and improved surgical techniques, medicine has also made great strides in the past ten years in transplanting bone marrow, hearts, livers, lungs, pancreases, and spleens. In the course of one recent week at the University of Minnesota transplant center, says Chief Surgeon John Najarian, "We transplanted eight kidneys, two hearts, two pancreases, and one liver."

But technological progress has also created a wide range of moral problems. Whereas thirty years ago the primary moral question raised by organ transplantation was whether to subject patients to experimental, last-resort procedures, today the ethical questions concern the inadequate supply of organs and their inequitable distribution, the high cost of transplantation, and the lack of adequate governmental regulation and control over the technique. The policies developed in the early stages of organ transplantation—a system of what might be best termed "encouraged voluntarism" for donations, and government subsidization of the costs of kidney transplantation—were geared toward a small-scale effort involving only the kidney and a few, carefully screened patients. A system designed for a technology in its infancy, it was, in retrospect, limited in its vision. Today new policies are needed to confront the challenge posed by a technology on the verge of widespread success in an era of increasingly scarce resources.

THE EMERGENCE OF "ENCOURAGED VOLUNTARISM"

Since the 1950s American courts have emphasized voluntarism and informed consent as the key moral

Reprinted with permission of the author and the publisher from *Hastings Center Report*, vol. 13 (December 1983), pp. 23–29, 32.

guidelines that ought to govern the procurement of organs. State and federal courts ruled that rational adults could volunteer to donate their organs to their relatives. The courts also permitted minors to donate organs with the consent of their parents and with judicial approval.

In the 1960s advances in medical technology allowed doctors to artificially maintain vital biological functions in dead patients. Respirators and heart-lung machines permitted many organs to be salvaged for transplantation. These technological advances were partially responsible for the shift in the legal definition of death toward the so-called "brain death" standard, which was advanced largely in response to the urgings of the transplantation community. Brain-death statutes permitted organs to be harvested from those who had suffered an irreversible loss of brain function if there was no objection by the next of kin.

By the end of the 1960s it had become clear that simply making voluntary organ donation legal was not sufficient to assure the supply of organs needed by recipients. A variety of policy options were advanced. One option, favored by writers such as Paul Ramsey, Alfred and Blair Sadler, Jay Katz, and Renée Fox and Judith Swazey, was to move from a system of pure voluntarism to one of "encouraged" voluntarism by legally enabling individuals to donate organs through the use of "living wills" or donor cards.[1]

Critics of encouraged voluntarism pointed out that the high costs of promoting such a policy through public and professional education were unnecessary, given the willingness of Americans, as revealed in various public opinion polls, to have their organs utilized upon their deaths. They also worried that a dependence upon encouraged voluntarism would eventually produce a commercial market in organs. Both the living and the next-of-kin of dead people would have an interest in selling organs for transplantation.

As an alternative, scholars such as Jesse Dukeminier and David Sanders argued for a different policy—that of presumed consent—whereby physicians, acting with state or federal authority, would simply take needed tissues and organs from cadavers unless an individual carried a card prohibiting such tissue transfers or unless the deceased person's next-of-kin objected.[2] This system treated bodily organs as property and based its legal justification upon the constitutional authority of the state to mandate that bodies be treated in certain specified ways upon death.

Critics of presumed consent, such as Paul Ramsey and Leon Kass, argued that such a policy was too coercive and could result in the abuse of the rights of religious minorities, who were opposed to any form of autopsy or "mutilation" of dead bodies.[3]

In the end, public policy tipped toward encouraged voluntarism. The Uniform Anatomical Gift Act of 1968 recognized the legal status of donor cards and living wills, as well as the right of next-of-kin to make donations for relatives who had never indicated an unwillingness to serve as an organ donor. The moral argument that carried the day was that voluntarism encouraged socially desirable virtues, such as altruism and benevolence, without running the risk of abusing individual rights. Moreover, proponents noted, such a policy did not require as strong a governmental role as did a policy of presumed consent. Therefore it merited a trial, since it seemed to preserve free choice while posing less of a risk to the rights of religious minorities. . . .

Throughout the 1970s a number of court cases reaffirmed the centrality of voluntarism in adjudicating the ethical quandaries raised by organ transplantation. In the *Shimp* case, for example, a Pennsylvania court refused to order a life-saving bone marrow donation between cousins even though the transplant was relatively safe and entailed no major risks to the donor.[4]

THE GROWING GAP BETWEEN SUPPLY AND DEMAND

The effort to capitalize on encouraged voluntarism as the driving moral force behind organ transplantation may have been a noble experiment in 1968, but fifteen years later it is clear that this effort has failed. Continued progress in organ transplantation has widened the gap between the demand for organs and the number actually available for use. The gap has grown so wide that medical hucksters now offer to "solve" the problem by importing organs from paid donors overseas.

In the New York City area approximately 450 people are waiting for corneal transplants to restore their failing sight. Some of them have been on waiting lists for six months or more. Nationwide, more than 4,000 blind people are waiting for corneas.

The New York City area waiting list for kidney transplants numbers well over 600 individuals, including some who have been waiting over six years. Nationwide, somewhere between 6,000 to 10,000 people are on waiting lists. Dialysis is an alternative treatment, to be sure, but it is considerably more expensive. It costs approximately $35,000 per year to treat an individual with dialysis, whereas the cost of maintaining someone on a kidney transplant is $5,000 to $8,000 per year postsurgery. Moreover, the quality of life enjoyed by transplant recipients is usually much better than that afforded those who receive dialysis treatments.

In the New York area, with a population base of over 12 million, only 100 kidneys per year are salvaged from cadaver donors. Of the 120 area hospitals that could supply cadaver donors, less than 40 percent have provided one kidney during the past five years.[5] Statistics from other regions are similar. During the past year in the Pittsburgh area, which has an extensive and aggressive procurement network, only thirty hospitals out of 135 provided kidneys from cadavers for use in transplantation. Organs for less well-established transplant procedures are even scarcer. In the past year alone the parents of Jamie Fiske, Brandon Hall, and others have conducted campaigns through the national media in order to obtain livers for their children. John Najarian commented recently: "Had Mr. Fiske not made a special plea, the chance of finding a suitable liver [for his daughter Jamie] would have been very remote."

Lungs for transplant are just as rare. The waiting list at Montefiore Medical Center in the Bronx, where the vast majority of lung transplants have been undertaken, numbers over fifty individuals at any given time. Some persons have waited for a suitable lung for over ten months and many have died without any attempt at transplant. Last year Montefiore was able to do only seven lung transplants even though the hospital has the staff and equipment to perform many more.[6]

Bone marrow transplantation between nonrelated donors is another evolving area of transplant research where supply simply does not approximate demand. Edgar Frenkel, a Long Island physician, recently offered a $25,000 reward from privately generated funds in order to locate a suitable matched marrow donor. He also mounted his own (successful) procurement campaign, in the press, complete with press releases and taped appeals.

While not all experts accept the figure, the Center for Disease Control in Atlanta estimates that approximately 20,000 people die each year from causes such as brain injuries, tumors, or strokes, which would permit them to serve as organ donors. Yet, in 1982 no more than 2,500 cadavers were utilized as organ donors.

The time has come for seriously reexamining the alternative option of a policy based upon presumed consent. A centralized system for the mandatory salvaging of organs, with protections for those who wish to dissent, could help to increase the supply, reduce the cost, and alleviate the emotional problems that encouraged voluntarism has produced.

THE CHARADE OF CONSENT

A public policy that insists upon informed consent by the families of those recently deceased has been considered the only means by which personal autonomy can be protected against the powerful demands of both the medical profession and those desperately in need of a transplant. But there are many reasons for doubting whether informed consent does or can protect personal autonomy.

Consider the psychologically wrenching circumstances under which family members must be approached about the possibility of organ donation. Almost always the potential organ donor has died suddenly and unexpectedly. Relatives or friends are in a state of shock, grief, and confusion.

In such situations it is difficult to see how families can have a real opportunity to make an informed or voluntary choice. Basic factors ordinarily held to be absolutely necessary for any choice to be informed and free—time and a suitable decision-making environment—are often absent in a busy hospital corridor or emergency room. The capacity of bereaved family members to comprehend information under such circumstances is highly questionable.

Moreover, it is very difficult to know when encouragement to donate becomes pressure or coercion to do so. Those involved in organ procurement are well aware of the strategies that are most likely to produce a donation—identifying a specific recipient for a particular donation whenever possible; painting an overly optimistic picture of the chances of benefiting others; downplaying the possibility that the organs that are obtained will not be suitable for transplant; and talking in a general way about the overall success rates for organ transplantation rather than about the particular rate of success in the program or hospital where the organ will be utilized. Given these kinds of biases, do individuals really choose to have a loved one serve as an organ donor, or are they pressured, cajoled, shamed, or even coerced into consenting?

It is also difficult to understand how recruiters, faced with the urgent demand to produce a suitable supply of organs for desperately ill people, can present full and complete information to bereaved family members. Those working for organ procurement agencies are under severe pressures from both their own organizations and the transplant hospitals to locate and obtain organs.

Another difficulty with informed consent arises from the varying attitudes of hospital personnel. In many hospitals medical personnel never ask permission from bereaved family members to harvest organs. Some do not ask out of ignorance; others are understandably reluctant to broach the subject with people who are emotionally devastated. Comments like "I feel like a vulture" and "the requests make me feel too ghoulish" are typical of the burdens voluntarism places on those who must confront families under the most trying circumstances imaginable for obtaining informed consent. However, in other hospitals medical personnel are well trained and quite willing to make a request. Some hospitals have a policy of asking every family member; some do so only on a selective basis.

Fairness alone demands a more equitable distribution of the burdens of decision making among the relatives of potential donors. The reliance on a public policy of encouraged voluntarism produces a situation where geography and chance play the key roles in determining which families are asked and which are not.

THE ADVANTAGES OF PRESUMED CONSENT

Not only has voluntarism failed to meet the existing demand for organs; it has also produced decisions that are highly suspect because they are made in an emotional climate of sudden death, grief, and vulnerability. Given the obvious burdens that voluntarism places on both medical personnel and family members, a public policy of presumed consent with respect to cadaver donation would be far more just and humane to both.

Families should be asked not whether they will consent to the donation of organs but whether they have any objections. As James Muyskens has rightly observed,

> When we find ourselves in... "boundary situations"— when our lives have become unraveled—we need ritual, routine, and automatic procedures. These

procedures ought to be those that reflect our collective judgment expressed in more normal times.[7]

Every opinion poll taken over the years shows a majority of citizens willing to serve as organ donors upon their death. If it is possible to fully and adequately protect the interests of those who do not wish to so serve, then it makes no sense to force a small minority of families to confront the question of donation under conditions that make rational deliberation not only difficult but also painful.

If all hospitals were required by law to utilize all suitable cadaver organs for donation unless an individual had (a) placed his or her name on a central computer registry indicating an objection to transplantation; (b) carried a card indicating that he or she did not wish to be a donor; or unless (c) family members had raised an objection to donation, we would create a public policy far more likely to bridge the current gap between supply and demand, while assuring the autonomy and free choice of every citizen. Even if we adopt the most conservative position and do not take organs in the rare situations where there is no indication of the individual's wishes and no family members can be located, there would still be a sufficient supply.

Under such a system the burden of decision with respect to cadaver donation would be equitably allocated. Anyone suffering the tragic and unexpected loss of a loved one would know that organ donation was routine. Medical personnel would be asked to perform the far more psychologically manageable task of inquiring whether the potential donor or family had any objection to ordinary practice. Governmental and regulatory authorities would be responsible for assuring that all hospitals complied with the society's frequently expressed desire to utilize organs to save lives and restore vital biological functions whenever possible. Moreover, such a system might reduce major costs that are involved in maintaining a system based upon encouraged voluntarism. First, massive advertising and public education campaigns must be constantly maintained to remind individuals about the need for organ donation. Though it is difficult to obtain exact figures, the Red Cross, the National Kidney Foundation, and the numerous eye banks located throughout the United States estimate their advertising and promotional costs to be in the millions of dollars.

A voluntary system must also educate emergency room staff to be on the watch for potential organ donors. This "in-service" professional education is very expensive since trained personnel must visit hospitals on a regular and continuous basis if the training is to be effective. The frequent turnover of emergency room staff in most hospitals further adds to the cost of continuing professional education. The New York Regional Transplant program estimates that the cost of education for procuring one kidney is $3,500.

NEW POLICIES TO PROTECT LIVING DONORS

A policy of presumed consent would improve the system by which organs are procured from cadavers; but what about living donors? One of the central problems of organ donation by living donors is the need for access to medical records in order to locate suitable donors. This is especially so for transplantation involving renewable tissues such as bone marrow where it may be necessary to search through biological information on literally millions of candidates in order to establish a suitable match. Much of the information about tissue types now contained in medical records and data banks was gathered for purposes other than organ donation—for routine blood donation, for example. When a patient requires a transplant, searches of existing data banks are often conducted surreptitiously—and unethically.

It is difficult to protect the identity of those whose names are stored in hospital computers. Staff leaks are not uncommon, and the media pressure can be intense to release the name of a person who may be able to make a life-saving tissue donation. For example, William Head, a victim of a fatal form of leukemia, recently attempted to pressure an anonymous California woman to make a donation of bone marrow to him, first through the courts and then later through the media.[8] He learned of the woman's existence as a possible donor as a result of an inadvertent disclosure during a telephone conversation with a hospital technician at the University of Iowa. The mother had been tissue-typed as a potential donor for her child who later died of leukemia.

The Head case illustrates the need for creating a national registry of consenting organ donors. A serious effort must be made to obtain appropriate consent from those whose names are already listed on existing tissue registries. This could be done by phoning or writing to all of them and deleting the names of those who do not wish to be listed as potential organ donors.

But when new people are entered into the data banks, a policy of presumed consent should govern. That is, when information concerning a person's blood type, HLA type, or other biological markers is collected, that person should be told that this information will automatically be stored for purposes of possible organ donation at a future date. Those who do not wish to participate in organ donation should be given the opportunity to withhold their consent to information storage for such purposes and their names should not be included in any tissue registries.

While the costs of compiling and maintaining such tissue registries may be high, it makes sense to institute a policy of automatically storing biological information unless an objection is raised. Such a policy would significantly increase the number of candidates available as potential donors while helping to alleviate further conflicts between those in need of transplants from living donors and the privacy and confidentiality interests of possible donors.

Many of the transplant procedures now being attempted fall into the category of experimentation. Living donors, like any other human subjects involved in experimental procedures, should be able to make free, voluntary, informed choices about whether they wish to participate. Free choice requires adequate time and a suitable environment for making decisions. Voluntariness means that no coercion or duress should be brought to bear. And subjects can only be said to be informed when they comprehend all relevant and reasonable facts about the procedure that is being proposed. Thus it seems inappropriate to allow potential donors to be approached by courts or harangued by the media concerning their willingness to serve as organ donors for someone who needs a transplant.

Some organ transplants, such as those involving kidneys, have been so successful that it seems odd to view them as experimental. Nevertheless, from the live donor's point of view, removing an organ for transplantation does not meet the ordinary definition of what constitutes therapy in medicine. There is no direct benefit for the donor other than, perhaps, some emotional or psychological rewards. The intent of transplantation is never to benefit the donor medically; it is always to benefit an identified or potential recipient.

In light of the nontherapeutic status of live organ donation it seems reasonable to adhere to the strictest standards available in deciding what values should govern informed consent even in proven forms of transplantation. The current procedures and protections inherent in existing informed consent doctrines seem to satisfy this requirement, but public policy must be modified to insure that they are always strictly followed.

In the heated and stressful environment that surrounds a request for transplantation from a living donor, there is a tendency to forget that time is needed for someone to make a voluntary choice. Cooling-off periods, access to privacy, and time to consult with friends, relatives, or experts all appear to be necessary conditions for informed choice.

Voluntariness is also difficult to achieve. Potential donors can be and have been—as in the Head case—subject to tremendous pressures, especially when the needs of a particular person have been widely publicized. Direct personal appeals can be tremendously coercive. Given the kinds of pressures a needy person can bring upon a donor it seems reasonable to institute policies that discourage or minimize direct contacts between organ recipients and potential donors, to the extent that this is possible.

It is equally important to respect the potential donor's right to say no. Once a person has been given all pertinent information and a reasonable opportunity to decide, those attempting to obtain informed consent—be they family, clergy, medical personnel, or the recipient—must be willing to accept the decision, whatever it may be. Once a donor has said no to a reasonable request, continued approaches constitute coercion. Courts, health professionals, and legislators must understand that a commitment to voluntarism as the policy governing donations from living donors requires that individuals be given the chance to say no as well as yes....

THE NEW ERA OF TRANSPLANTATION

Progress in transplanting has highlighted the inadequacy of existing public policy. There is too great a gap between supply and demand, too little protection for families and prospective donors, and too much potential for economic abuse to continue to rely on a system built around encouraged voluntarism and laissez-faire in the procurement and allocation of scarce organs.

A policy of presumed consent both for cadaver donations and for determining the eligibility of living donors with respect to data banks and registries could help to alleviate the shortage of organs that permits so many to die without an opportunity for treatment. Presumed consent would also routinize the procurement of organs in a way that best protects the interests of all parties involved in organ transplantation—donors, families of donors, recipients, and medical personnel....

REFERENCES

1 A. M. Sadler, et al., "Transplantation: A Case for Consent," *New England Journal of Medicine* 280 (1969), 862–67.

2 J. Dukeminier and D. Sanders, "Organ Transplantation: A Proposal for Routine Salvaging of Cadaver Organs," *New England Journal of Medicine* 279 (1968), 413–19.

3 P. Ramsey, *The Patient as Person* (New Haven: Yale University Press, 1970).

4 A. Meisel and L. Roth, "Must a Man Be His Cousin's Keeper?" *Hastings Center Report* 8 (October 1978), pp. 5–6.

5 1981 Annual Report of the New York Regional Transplant Program, Inc.

6 F. J. Veith, "Lung Transplantation, 1983," *Transplantation* 34:4 (1983), 271–78.

7 J. Muyskens, "An Alternative Policy for Obtaining Cadaver Organs for Transplantation," *Philosophy and Public Affairs* 8:1 (1978), 96.

8 A. Caplan; C. Lidz, A. Meisel, L. Roth; and D. Zimmerman, "Mrs. X and the Bone Marrow Transplant," *Hastings Center Report* 13 (June 1983), pp. 17–19.

ANNOTATED BIBLIOGRAPHY: CHAPTER 11

Blackstone, William R.: "On Health Care as a Legal Right: An Exploration of Legal and Moral Grounds," *Georgia Law Review* 10 (1976), pp. 391–418. Blackstone examines a number of legal and moral positions that can be used to argue for or against some kind of right to health care. He argues in favor of a public, socialized, or nationalized health system.

Childress, James F.: "Priorities in the Allocation of Health Care Resources," *Soundings* 62 (Fall 1979), pp. 258–269. Childress focuses on macroallocation decisions that require making choices between (1) health care and other social goods and (2) prevention and crisis or rescue medicine.

Daniels, Norman: "Health-Care Needs and Distributive Justice," *Philosophy and Public Affairs* 10 (1981), pp. 146–179. Daniels defends the following claim: If an acceptable theory of justice includes a principle providing for fair equality of opportunity, then health-care institutions should be among those governed by the principle of fair equality of opportunity. His article includes an account of basic needs in general and health-care needs in particular. He identifies basic needs, including health-care needs, with those important to maintaining normal species functioning and sees such normal functioning as an important determinant of the range of opportunity open to an individual.

Ehrenreich, Barbara, and John Ehrenreich: "Health Care and Social Control," *Social Policy* 5 (May/June 1974), pp. 26–40. In this radical critique of the American health-care system, the Ehrenreichs provide a historical and critical analysis of the ways in which our medical system functions as an instrument of social control.

Fein, Rashi: "On Achieving Access and Equity in Health Care," *Milbank Memorial Fund Quarterly/Health and Society* 50 (October 1972), pp. 157–190. Fein provides a historical and critical analysis of some of the economic criteria used to set a value on human life and to allocate medical resources.

Fried, Charles: "Equality and Rights in Medical Care," *Hastings Center Report* 6 (February 1976), pp. 29–34. Fried argues that a right to health care does not imply a right to equal access. He does, however, argue that it is profoundly wrong not to afford a decent standard of care to all our citizens.

Fuchs, Victor R.: *Who Shall Live?: Health, Economics, and Social Choice* (New York: Basic Books, 1974). Fuchs surveys some important aspects of the American health system, such as physicians and hospitals, the system of drug manufacture and distribution, and payment and insurance plans. He relates all this to what the data reveal about our health needs. Fuchs concludes that heredity, life-style, and environment have more impact on individual health than the money spent on medical care.

Guttmann, Amy: "For and Against Equal Access to Health Care," *Milbank Memorial Fund Quarterly/Health and Society* 59 (Fall 1981), pp. 542–560. Guttmann rejects the free-market approach of Sade and the decent minimum approach of Fried. Drawing on the values of self-respect, equal relief from pain, and equality of opportunity, she argues for equal access to health care as a moral ideal.

Illich, Ivan: *Medical Nemesis* (New York: Pantheon, 1976). Illich's book is an extended criticism of our "misguided overreliance" on health-care professionals. He attacks the "medical establishment," which he sees as a threat to health and as responsible for numerous iatrogenic ills. According to Illich, health care in our society can be improved only if individuals take the responsibility for their own health away from the professionals. He criticizes national health-care schemes whose purpose is to increase the provision of treatment. Such programs, he maintains, will further diminish the individual's responsibility for his or her own health.

Leichter, Howard M.: "Public Policy and the British Experience," *Hastings Center Report* 11 (October 1981), pp. 32–39. Leichter presents some of the assumptions implicit in the new perspective on health care, which emphasizes the relation between life-style and disease. However, the major portion of this article describes the British confrontation between the theoretical assumptions of this perspective and the practical realities of politics and economics.

Rexed, Bror, and Daniel Juda: "Planning for Scarcity in Sweden: An Interview with Bror Rexed," *Hastings Center Report* 7 (June 1977), pp. 5–7. Bror Rexed is the director general of the Swedish National Board of Health. In this interview, Rexed discusses the social impact of the Arab oil embargo of 1973. The interview is especially interesting in relation to this chapter because it shows the kind of public policy decisions regarding the provision of medical care that can only be made and implemented in a society in which the whole medical system is under government control.

Sparer, Edward V.: "The Legal Right to Health Care: Public Policy and Equal Access," *Hastings Center Report* 6 (October 1976), pp. 39-47. Sparer is concerned with the "legal" right to medical care. He examines the legal rights we do have in regard to medical care and various public policy decisions regarding the right to medical care (e.g., decisions regarding Medicare and Medicaid). He concludes with a list of recommendations whose purpose is to promote the achievement of a broad public right to good medical care.

Steiner, Hillel: "The Just Provision of Health Care: A Reply to Elizabeth Telfer," *Journal of Medical Ethics* 2 (1976), pp. 185–189. Steiner examines the four positions offered by Elizabeth Telfer in the article reprinted in this chapter. He criticizes Telfer and argues for a fifth position, which incorporates the important elements of Telfer's two extreme positions—the laissez faire and *pure* socialist approaches to health-care delivery. A brief reply by Telfer follows Steiner's article.

Stern, Lawrence: "Opportunity and Health Care: Criticisms and Suggestions," *The Journal of Medicine and Philosophy* 8 (1983), pp. 339–361. Stern criticizes Norman Daniels's proposal that health care should be distributed on the basis of fair equality of opportunity. He then advances his own position on health care and justice and argues for a health-voucher system that will provide roughly equal access to health care for all classes.

Veatch, Robert M., and Roy Branson, eds.: *Ethics and Health Policy* (Cambridge, Mass.: Ballinger, 1976). Included in this collection of articles are several dealing with justice and health-care delivery. Those interested in John Rawls's theory of distributive justice will be especially interested in the article by Ronald M. Green, "Health Care and Justice in Contract Theory Perspective."

Wikler, Daniel I.: "Persuasion and Coercion for Health," *Milbank Memorial Fund Quarterly/ Health and Society* 56 (Summer 1978), pp. 303–335. Wikler examines two of the central arguments invoked in discussions of the government's role in promoting health-preserving personal behavior: the argument from paternalism and the fair distribution of burdens argument.

Appendix: Case Studies

This appendix contains a set of case studies for analysis and discussion. Most of the cases are essentially records of actual situations. Others, however, are only loosely based on actual happenings, and a few have been constructed simply for their perceived pedagogical value. Most of the cases are developed only up to a crucial "decision point," but some are supplemented by information about what happened after a decision was actually made. In assessing a decision that was actually made in a given case, it is important to focus on the information available to the decision maker prior to the decision and not be overly influenced by the element of hindsight. Case studies of the type presented here may pose another problem. Individuals involved in analyzing such cases often feel that it would be desirable to have more factual details, especially clinical ones. This recurrent desire reflects the well-based axiom that good decision making must be based on "good facts." However, a perceived lack of factual detail should not be allowed to paralyze analysis and discussion. If the proper decision in a certain case is thought to be dependent on information not provided in the case description, and if it is reasonable to believe that the desired information would or could be available to those confronted with the decision, a discussion of the case can include an examination of the precise way in which the desired information is relevant to the decision.

Two final points are worth noting. First, the last paragraph of each case study identifies some questions raised by the case. These questions are not the only ones worthy of consideration, but they can be used to facilitate analysis and discussion. Second, the title of each case study is followed by a number or numbers within brackets. These numbers refer to the various chapters in this book. Thus the chapter or chapters most directly relevant to each case are identified.

Case 1

A Patient's Role in Determining Therapy [2]

Andrew W. is a 56-year-old male who has contracted colon cancer. He is an intelligent man who has considerable research skills. The cancer is in its early stages, and Andrew W. could benefit from the proper chemotherapy. Andrew W. has read that the National Institutes of Health has developed a test to determine the sensitivity of cancer cells to the combinations of chemotherapy. This test (while still somewhat experimental) has proven effective to the point that NIH is offering it as a service to physicians around the country. Andrew W. talks to his physician, Dr. M., about sending a sample of his cancer cells to NIH to determine the most effective form of chemotherapy. Dr. M. is upset by the suggestion and says that treatment determination is the prerogative of the physician and that he knows what is effective for the treatment of colon cancer. He tells Andrew W. that, if he wants the NIH test, he will have to find another oncologist. Andrew W. goes to another physician, undergoes the test, and has the chemotherapy indicated by the test. Three years later Andrew W. is still disease free.

(1) Was Andrew W. within his rights in asking for or even demanding the test? (2) Did Dr. M. act professionally toward Andrew W.? Did Dr. M. act in the best interests of his patient?

Case 2

A Physician's Abandonment of a Patient [2]

Todd Z. is a 75-year-old male who has been diagnosed as having lung cancer with brain metastases. His physician of thirty years, Dr. S., is seriously concerned that, if told of his diagnosis, Todd Z. will go into a deep depression and spend the remainder of his life in that state. Dr. S. keeps the information from Todd Z. and orders Todd Z.'s wife and three sons not to tell Todd Z. of the diagnosis. He tells them that he wants to keep Todd Z. in the hospital for a couple of weeks for brain radiation and promises to make up some excuse for the treatment. After the treatment is concluded, the family can take him home to die. Dr. S. promises that he will visit Todd Z. at his home every week and care for him until he dies because he has been very fond of Todd Z. and lives nearby. Todd Z. becomes increasingly persistent with his questions about his physical condition. By the third week the family breaks down and tells him about the diagnosis. Todd Z. does go into the predictable depression, but it is not as severe as Dr. S. had feared. Dr. S. is angered by the fact that the family had disobeyed his orders. He releases Todd Z. from the hospital and does not keep his promise to visit him at home. He never visits Todd Z. during the six-month period from Todd Z.'s departure from the hospital to the day of his death. During that six-month period Dr. S. is very uncooperative. When the family contacts him to discuss the medication program, he is very curt with them, and when they ask him about a particular condition that is developing, he asserts that they will have to bring Todd Z. to the office or to the hospital. He even refuses to talk with Todd Z. on the telephone.

(1) Did Dr. S. break his fiduciary relationship with the patient and abandon him? (2) Is it appropriate for a physician to set conditions such as deception for full involvement in caring for a patient?

Case 3

Withholding Information About Risks [2]

Marcia W. is a 40-year-old female with multiple myeloma, who upon diagnosis shows great interest in having all the information that is necessary to make a decision about further treatment. Dr. C. tells her that the response rates to chemotherapy with this disease are very good and that recent research has shown that 50 percent of patients can hope for long-term survival rates, which are tantamount to cure. The other 50 percent of patients die within a year or two. What Dr. C. neglects to tell her is that preliminary studies are showing that in twenty years, 10 percent of the 50 percent who survive contract a form of leukemia that is highly resistant to treatment. When her treatment is discussed in a staff meeting, Dr. C. says that he did not want to tell Marcia W. about the 10 percent because he was afraid that it might unduly alarm her and cause her not to take treatment, thereby spoiling her chances for long-term survival. Moreover, he states *(a)* that the research is not conclusive enough to suit him and *(b)* that 10 percent is such a low figure that he is not morally required to communicate the risk. After all, he suggests, one cannot inform a patient of *every* risk.

(1) Did Marcia W. have a right to the information about the possible risk of leukemia? (2) Is this 10 percent chance of contracting leukemia significant for her decision making? (3) Will this information harm her by making it impossible for her to make an autonomous decision? (4) Is the low 10 percent figure counter-balanced by the seriousness of the consequences?

Case 4

Voluntary Sterilization and a Young Unmarried Man [2]

Gregory X., who is 25 years old, unmarried, and childless, wants a vasectomy. (Vasectomy is a sterilization procedure that is considered irreversible, although research is being done to make it reversible.) He comes to Dr. H., a urologist in a clinic in a large city hospital because he cannot afford the surgery elsewhere. He tells Dr. H. that he has decided, after several years of thought, never to be a parent. The vasectomy will now ensure that and make it unnecessary for any woman he loves to run the various risks associated with the available means of contraception. Dr. H. has doubts about performing the surgery on a young, unmarried man. He asks Gregory X. to consider the feelings of a possible future wife who will not have any say about the sterilization decision. Gregory X. insists on the surgery.

(1) Should Dr. H. accede to Gregory X.'s request despite his reservations, since Gregory X. cannot afford the vasectomy otherwise? (2) Is there anything morally problematic about Gregory X.'s request?

Case 5

The Nurse and Informed Consent [2, 3]

Michael G., who is dying of leukemia, is in a hospital where he is receiving chemotherapy. A registered nurse involved in his care, Mary L., learns that he has never received information about alternative natural therapies. She gives Michael G. the information and discusses the advantages and disadvantages of the various alternatives. After extensive reflection and consultation with his family, Michael G. decides to leave the hospital and to make arrangements to try one of the alternative therapies. He informs the attending oncologist of his decision. When the oncologist learns about the source of Michael G.'s information, he charges Mary L. with unprofessional conduct and asks that her nursing license be revoked. Mary L. argues that the patient has the right to know about the alternatives and that a failure to inform him vitiates his "informed consent" to the chemotherapy.

(1) Was Mary L. acting in a morally correct way when she gave Michael G. the information? (2) Should the physician in charge have the final word about the information a patient should receive? (3) If Michael G. did not know about the alternative therapies, was his assent to the chemotherapy *informed* consent?

Case 6

A Nurse's Obligations and a Patient's Living Will [2, 3]

George G., who is 70 years old and has no family, has a history of coronary disease and myocardial infarctions. He is also suffering from a large and advanced carcinoma of the stomach. George G. tells a nurse, Robin C., that he has given his physician, Dr. E., a copy of a living will, which requests that no heroic measures be taken to prolong his life. After a further myocardial collapse occurs, Robin C. learns that Dr. E.'s orders had called for maximum therapeutic efforts in the event of such a collapse, including resuscitation, if necessary. The patient is resuscitated, and his life continues. George G. expresses a desire to die, but his condition has deteriorated to such an extent that his competence to make decisions on his behalf is questionable. If the existence of his living will were known, his present expressions of a desire not to be subjected to further therapy would be given more credence. There is no explicit hospital policy regarding living wills; such matters are left to the physician's discretion.

(1) Does Robin C. have an obligation to inform other hospital personnel about George G.'s living will? (2) Does Robin C. have an obligation to defend George G.'s interests even if this means challenging Dr. E.'s course of treatment? (3) Has Dr. E. violated George G.'s rights?

Case 7

Who Communicates with the Patient? [2, 3]

Thomas P. is a 56-year-old male with head and neck cancer. After radical surgery, which left him quite disfigured, he was apparently disease free. However, the disease reoccurred two years later, and the tumor grew in such a way that it eventually closed off his trachea. He agreed to a tracheotomy to allow him to breathe, but due to complications in surgery he became respirator dependent. His daughter, and only relative, Wanda G., asked the physician in charge, Dr. Z., to extubate Thomas P., that is, remove him from the respirator. Dr. Z. agreed that it might be appropriate to extubate Thomas P. but stated that Thomas P. should be consulted during his conscious periods. Wanda G. agreed that this was the proper procedure and told Dr. Z. to ask her father as quickly as possible. Dr. Z. protested, saying that he had no intention of asking the father. Since the extubation was the daughter's idea, the physician asserted, she should discuss the matter with her father. Wanda G., already grieving because of her father's long illness and impending death, said that she could not discuss the matter with her father. She subsequently asked the nurse taking care of her father to discuss the extubation with him. The nurse refused, saying that it was not her job.

(1) Who has the primary responsibility to discuss this decision with the patient? (2) If the person who has primary responsibility refuses to act on that responsibility, how should the patient's best interests be protected?

Case 8

A Randomized Clinical Trial and a Physician's Responsibility to a Patient [2, 4]

One of the ways of testing the effectiveness of a therapy is to set up a randomized clinical trial (RCT). This involves the random assignment of patients to different therapies, including the one being tested. The reason for the randomization is to eliminate the possibility that variables other than the therapies will affect the results. One of the problems that arises when alternative therapies are being tested in this way is that at a certain point one of the therapies appears to be superior, but if the experiment is stopped and all the patients given the apparently superior therapy, the results may not be considered sufficiently validated. Dr. L. has agreed to include his patients in a RCT designed to test a new drug whose purpose is to treat and cure a disease that is about 70 percent fatal. One of the participants in the trial, Bruce W., has been a patient of Dr. L.'s for eleven years. There are a total of thirty participants in the RCT. Twelve are given placebos. The other eighteen are given the new drug. None of the patients are told which treatment they are receiving, although all know that they are taking part in a randomized clinical trial. After eight of the twelve patients on placebos and five of those receiving the new drug die, Dr. L. is asked by Bruce W. whether he is one of the placebo recipients and whether there is any good reason to think that the new drug is effective. Dr. L. knows that Bruce W. is a placebo recipient and that the data so far support the view that the experimental drug may be effective and prevent death. Dr. L. and the other physicians involved in the trial are unwilling to end the experiment because of their concern about the validity of the study if it is terminated too soon.

(1) Should the experiment be ended and the remaining patients put on the new therapy immediately? (2) Should Dr. L. lie to Bruce W., if necessary, in order to continue the experiment? (3) Does Dr. L. have an obligation to his patient, Bruce W., which should take precedence over his concern with establishing the validity of the results of the RCT?

Case 9

Placebos, Fertility Control, and Human Experimentation [2, 4]

Dr. W., who works part-time as a volunteer in a public health clinic but also has a private practice, wishes to test a new male birth control pill. He solicits volunteers from among his health clinic patients. Each of the patients chosen must be sexually active, in relatively good health, and desirous of controlling his fertility. Dr. W. does not tell the volunteers that half of them will be receiving placebos that have nothing to do with fertility control. He does inform them, however, that the drug is experimental and that there is no guarantee that they will not father children while participating in the experiment. George K. agrees to participate. He and his wife, Melissa K., have two children. Both parents are employed in low-paying jobs, and neither has finished high school. Melissa K. has been advised that she should not get pregnant again for at least a couple of years because of complications with both her pregnancies and a recent miscarriage. She has also been advised not to take birth control pills for reasons related to her physical health. Neither George K. nor Melissa K. wants to be sterilized because they hope to have more children in the future. Dr. W.'s male birth control pill seems to promise them what they need at this time.

(1) Has Dr. W. given George K. sufficient information so that his consent is an informed one? (2) Is there anything morally questionable about Dr. W.'s use of public health clinic patients as volunteers rather than his private patients? (3) Should the research design screen out those who might be (substantially) harmed by a pregnancy?

Case 10

Human Experimentation Without Informed Consent [4]

Henrietta F. is a 51-year-old woman with a grown daughter, Nancy, who was born in 1952. While pregnant with Nancy, Henrietta F. received prenatal care at the University of Chicago's Lying-In Hospital. As part of that "care" Henrietta F.'s obstetrician gave her pills, which he told her were vitamins. Actually these were DES (diethylstilbestrol) pills, a form of medication believed to be effective in preventing miscarriage. Without her consent, Henrietta F. was participating in a controlled experiment. The study being conducted required giving DES to two groups of women: those with a history of miscarriages, and a control group—those without such a history. Henrietta F. belonged in the second group.

In 1971 there was sufficient evidence to establish a link between DES and vaginal cancer and cervical cell abnormalities in the daughters of women given the drug. One-hundred-twenty daughters of the roughly one million women given DES had been shown to have cancer. Sons had not been shown to develop cancer, but as a group they had a higher than average proportion of sterility and genital abnormalities.

In 1975 Henrietta F. was finally informed that she had taken DES during her pregnancy in 1951. She immediately advised Nancy to undergo a medical examination. Nancy was diagnosed as having a condition that is a precursor of cancer—adenosis. Henrietta F. expressed outrage at the treatment she had been accorded by her physician and the hospital. She claimed that her rights had been violated when she was used in an experiment without her consent. She claimed, furthermore, that the physician had no right to give her anything that had nothing to do with her and her prospective child's well-being.

(1) Did Henrietta F.'s physician act immorally? (2) In 1951 no one knew about DES's harmful effects. Is this fact relevant in evaluating the ethical acceptability of the experiment, which involved using human beings as research subjects without their consent? (3) Suppose Henrietta F. had been told about the DES and had consented to the participation in the trial. Would the experimentation have been morally acceptable despite its harmful consequences?

Case 11

Voluntary Consent and Research in Prisons [4]

Michael H. is serving a two-to-five year prison term for armed robbery. He has a sixth-grade education and has difficulty reading and writing. Michael H. suffers from arthritis. Dr. J., who works for a pharmaceutical company, has received permission from the prison authorities to test a new drug intended to alleviate the pain accompanying arthritis. He plans to solicit volunteers who suffer from arthritis and divide them into two groups. One group will receive the drug; the other will receive a placebo. Dr. J. believes that the drug does carry some risks including possible liver damage but that the risk is slight. Michael H. is among the volunteers. Along with the other experimental subjects, Michael H. is informed about both the possibility that he will receive the placebo and the possibility of liver damage. He states that he wants to volunteer because he believes that the Parole Review Board, which will discuss his case in another six months, will be pleased by his participation. When asked whether he understands that he may receive a placebo and not the drug itself and that if he gets the drug he does run a risk of possible liver damage, Michael H. says, "Yes." When asked whether his consent is voluntary, he asserts that it is.

   (1) Is Michael H.'s consent voluntary? Is it informed? (2) Is Dr. J. doing anything that is morally unacceptable?

Case 12

The Dentist and Patient Autonomy [2, 5]

A 36-year-old man, Patrick M., contacts the office of an endodontist. (Endodontics is a specialized field of dentistry.) Patrick M. wants to arrange for a procedure commonly called a "root canal" to be performed on each of his teeth. A root canal is a common (somewhat involved) procedure used as an alternative to extracting a diseased tooth. It consists of removing the damaged or diseased blood vessels and nerves contained within the tooth. The tooth is thus "devital" but functions normally. If this procedure is not done on a diseased tooth or if the tooth is not extracted, infection will very likely develop in the necrotic tissue and spread into the jaw bone and surrounding tissues.

   The endodontist is startled by the idea of performing a root canal on all of Patrick M.'s teeth. Further discussion makes Patrick M.'s motivation clear. He a fervent survivalist, dedicated to planning for every contingency in the expectation that some conflagration is about to destroy society. Patrick M. is attempting to ensure—by having all of his teeth desensitized—that he will never suffer a toothache. Although the endodontist cannot escape a sense of amusement over what he considers a bizarre situation, Patrick M. seems fully prepared both to undergo a difficult set of procedures and to pay what will be a huge overall bill. Still, the endodontist feels that it would be unethical to remove healthy tissue. He feels that he is being asked to perform a procedure that is not indicated by the existing conditions and may never be indicated, judging by the excellent overall health of the teeth.

   (1) Is there any significant difference between dentist-patient relationship and the physician-patient relationship? (2) Should the endodontist accede to Patrick M.'s desires?

Case 13

Privacy and Monitoring Systems in a Mental Institution [3, 6]

The new superintendent of the Meller Valley Mental Institute, Dr. R., has decided to install television monitoring devices in all the patients' rooms as well as in the hallways and visiting rooms of the Institute. His primary purposes are to make it easier to locate personnel when they are needed in a hurry and to help the staff, which is short-handed, keep an eye on the doings of patients, a small number of whom are prone to violence.

Patients know about the surveillance, but visitors are not informed. Some of the members of Dr. R.'s staff object, arguing that the system is a gross violation of the privacy of both patients and visitors.

(1) Is Dr. R. morally justified in establishing the monitoring system? (2) Are patients' and visitors' rights being violated?

Case 14

Autonomy and Mental Illness [5, 6]

Humphrey W., a 40-year-old businessman, is committed to a mental hospital at the instigation of his wife and without his consent after repeated manic episodes in public and a suicide attempt. During some of his manic episodes he has thrown money around on street corners, harangued passers-by, raged aganst his fellow employees, and boasted of nonexistent business deals to his boss. After commitment, Humphrey W. refuses tranquilizing medication, which psychiatrists consider necessary to control his "manic flights" and strengthen his own control over his behavior.

(1) Would it be morally correct for the psychiatrists to give him the tranquilizers (e.g., by means of a syringe) against his expressed dissent? (2) Was it morally correct to commit him to the institution without his consent?

Case 15

A Schizophrenic Son's Refusal of Therapy [5, 6]

William T., who is 22 years old, has a troubled history. He has been diagnosed as suffering from chronic undifferentiated schizophrenia. He has been expelled from several schools due to his severely disruptive conduct and a continuing serious deterioration in his school performance. William T. has been a multiple drug abuser, he has threatened various members of his family, and his behavior has sometimes been catatonic. He has persistently refused to take any medication and has rejected all other forms of treatment. Now William T. is in a state hospital after being charged with attempted armed robbery, assault, and battery. He continues to reject all treatment. William T.'s father, Joseph T., who has been appointed his temporary guardian, wants to consent to the administration of medication to William T. The father thinks that William T. may pose a danger to others if he is discharged without treatment and thereby poses a threat of harm both to himself and others. Joseph T. maintains that he is acting in the best interests of his son, who is incompetent to decide what is best for himself.

(1) Should parents in such cases be allowed to make treatment decisions that go against the expressed wishes of their children? (2) Is William T.'s autonomy sufficiently diminished so that his father's actions on his behalf are an example of weak rather than strong paternalism? (3) Is forcing medication on patients inconsistent with respecting them as persons?

Case 16

Sterilization and the Mentally Retarded [6]

The parents of a 19-year-old, Mindy G., with Down's syndrome and an I.Q. in the upper-30s range, ask a gynecologist to sterilize her by means of a tubal ligation. (In a tubal ligation, a woman's fallopian tubes are tied, making conception impossible.) The parents argue that sterilization would be in Mindy's interest, since if she becomes pregnant she will neither understand her condition nor be able to care for the baby on her own. Furthermore, they are concerned about what will happen to Mindy after they die. They would like to see her settled in a group home for retarded adults and working in a sheltered workshop. They argue that continuous and dependable contraception is a prerequisite for these kinds of changes in her life.

(1) Putting aside any legal complications, would it be *morally* correct for the physician to sterilize Mindy? (2) Is it plausible to see sterilization in this case as a "least restrictive" alternative?

Case 17

Refusal of Life-Sustaining Treatment by a Minor [2, 7]

Charlie R. is an 11-year-old boy who suffers from lymphoma with a prognosis of six months to live. The oncologist has indicated that the condition is terminal and that aggressive chemotherapy can be done, but its results would be at best a three-month to six-month extension of his life. Charlie is also compromised by a neurological disease that he has had for several years. The neurological disease will eventually make it impossible for him to walk, talk, use his hands effectively, or control his excretory functions. Already his speech is slurred, and he cannot hold a pencil. Even without the lymphoma, the prognosis for him because of the neurological disease is death by age 18 at the latest. Charlie has been raised in a strong religious environment, and his belief in God has been an important comforting factor in the course of his disease. He has accepted his disease and his impending death after having the facts fully explained to him. He has said that he is ready to "go to God," and he does not want the chemotherapy. His father has consulted with his local parish priest who says that the Catholic Church requires that in such cases chemotherapy be used because it is seen as therapeutic and not as merely prolonging the dying process. As a result of this consultation the father decides to override Charlie's decision and agrees to the chemotherapy.

(1) Did the priest represent the Catholic Church's position accurately? (2) Should minors of Charlie's age be permitted to participate in decisions of this magnitude? (3) Whose decision, the father's or the child's, should be decisive?

Case 18

Brain Metastases, Memory Continuity, and Autonomy [2, 7]

Thomas P. is a 64-year-old male who has cancer, with a primary site in the lung and metastases to the brain and bone. It has been determined that nothing genuinely therapeutic can be done for the lung disease. He has already had the maximum amount of radiation for the brain metastases. Now he faces a decision as to whether he should have radiation to the bones to reduce the possibility of fractures. The radiation proposed had already been used once in the course of the disease, and it had made the patient very ill for about six weeks. There is every reason to believe that the same morbidity will occur this time. Thomas P. must now decide if he wants to undergo a similar treatment, with its accompanying side effects, for the bone metastases. He is cared for at home by his wife, and he has five children who have genuine loving concern for him.

Thomas P.'s situation is complicated by the fact that, due to the brain metastases, his memory does not always serve him well. He remembers the side effects of the previous radiation, and he seems to be well acquainted with the disease process. However, he does not always remember what his physician tells him and then is forced to make decisions based upon incomplete or unrecalled information. Furthermore, he cannot always remember what he has consented to and what he has not consented to. His locutions sometimes take the form of "Did I agree to that?" He sometimes seems to be persuaded by whomever he is discussing the matter with at the time. This ambivalence, together with the lapses in memory continuity, raises questions about his competence in making decisions.

(1) Is Thomas P. sufficiently autonomous to make decisions about his care? (2) How seriously should his health-care professionals consult with him about his mode of treatment? To what extent should the family be involved?

Case 19

Depression and Autonomy [2, 7]

John Q. is a 56-year-old male with a wife and two grown children. He has just suffered his third heart attack in five years, and his cardiologist, Dr. Y., has told him that he must have bypass surgery if he is going to live. Dr. Y. has also told him that because of the already existent damage to the heart muscles he will be a semi-invalid for the rest of his life even with the surgery. John Q. had been an active businessman until his first attack, and he has resentfully had to cut back on his activity since that attack. Now the possibility of extensive surgery and living as a semi-invalid is too much for him to bear. He goes into a depressed state and refuses the surgery saying that he is "tired of being sick" and that life holds no meaning for him any longer. He is adamant about not having the surgery. The family asks for a psychiatric consultation, and Dr. Y. supports the idea because he believes that the psychiatrist might be able to talk John Q. into the surgery. The psychiatrist says the depression obviously indicates that John Q. is incapable of making a rational judgment and that the family and Dr. Y. should make the decision and ignore the patient's wishes.

(1) Does depression after hearing "bad news" automatically indicate that a patient is incompetent to make decisions regarding treatment? (2) Is it the consulting psychiatrist's role to try to talk the patient into doing what the attending physician wants to do? (3) How can the family serve the best interests of the patient in this situation?

Case 20

Suicide and Pain Control [2, 7]

Beverly S., a 67-year-old female, is suffering the terminal stages of breast cancer with metastases to the bone. The bone pain has become a major problem in the management of her disease. She is cared for at home by her husband, a daughter, and a nurse from a home health service. She has been troubled so much by the pain that she talks frequently of suicide. She has even made three suicide attempts. After the third attempt, which was almost successful, a health-care counselor was called. In the ensuing discussions, it is determined that Beverly S.'s physician is probably not paying sufficient attention to her pain medication needs. When it is suggested that she might want to change to another physician in the area who is well known for her ability to control pain in cancer patients, Beverly S. replies that she does not want to offend her current physician. Eventually, she agrees to contact the other physician who begins to care for her immediately. She dies, relatively pain free, about six weeks later.

(1) Was intervention in Beverly S.'s suicide attempts appropriate? (2) Should health-care counselors encourage patients to explore alternatives with other physicians, or will such encouragement tend to undermine the trust patients have in their physicians? Are patient trust and loyalty to the physician important elements in fostering the patient's well-being?

Case 21

Physician Disagreement Regarding a Patient's Wishes [2, 7]

John H., a 59-year-old male, has been diagnosed as having cancer, the primary site of which is the pancreas. His condition is rapidly deteriorating. John H. has requested that he not be resuscitated if he should go into cardiac arrest. He has also stated that he wishes no further treatment. Dr. W., who is John H.'s personal physician, and Dr. R., the oncologist in the case, agree that he should not be resuscitated, and "Do not resuscitate" is written on his chart. However, when John H. begins to experience severe internal bleeding, he asks his physicians if they can do something. Dr. W. does not want to take measures to stop the bleeding, in keeping with John H.'s request for no further treatment. Dr. R. sees the request "to do something" as taking precedence over the earlier request for no additional treatment. If they do not act quickly to stop the internal bleeding, John H. will die as a result of blood loss.

(1) When the personal physician and the attending specialist disagree, who should decide the course of treatment? (2) When a patient who is in a great deal of pain, weak, and close to death makes a request that seems at odds with a decision he made when he may have been more fully autonomous, which request should guide those caring for him?

Case 22

NG Tube, Battery, and a Nursing Dilemma [2, 3, 7]

Paul F. is a 68-year-old male who is suffering from pancreatic cancer with liver metastases. He is in the final stages of the disease and has been admitted to the hospital for pain control. Paul F. is started on a morphine drip, which is continually increased until pain control is achieved. Upon admission he was coherent and clear-minded when he asserted that he wanted nothing to prolong his dying. He specifically refused antibiotics, tube feeding, and the use of a respirator. As the morphine drip is increased, he becomes confused, but his family adamantly stands by his wishes. The physician, Dr. D., on the other hand, decides that antibiotic therapy is necessary and orders the nurse to begin the therapy. Paul F. develops severe diarrhea, which makes his care very difficult. Dr. D. orders the nurse to insert an NG tube for the administration of Lomotil to control the diarrhea, and he also orders the nurse, Amanda F., to begin feeding the patient through the NG tube. Amanda F. protests. She asserts that she was willing to give the antibiotics to the patient because they did not intrude too much on the patient's well-being, but the NG tube will. She, therefore, refuses to insert the NG tube. Paul F. fights the tube, and the family supports the patient. The family calls Dr. D. protesting the plan, but he refuses to change his orders. After debating the issue at a staff meeting, Amanda F. is told to insert the tube to keep Dr. D. happy. The patient dies nine days later.

(1) In what kind of dilemma does Amanda F. find herself? Has the staff given her appropriate support? (2) Is the staff failing to act in the best interests of the patient by giving priority to the desires of the physician? (3) Does the confusion of the patient reduce the physician's responsibility to honor the patient's wishes? (4) Is there any way that the NG tube can be seen as palliative? To what extent was battery committed against this patient?

Case 23

Honoring the Living Will [2, 7, 8]

Ester K., a 65-year-old woman with a long history of diabetes, has been diagnosed as having pancreatic cancer. At the time of diagnosis, she refused all aggressive therapies and later wrote a "living will," in which she stated clearly that she did not want any "extraordinary means" used to prolong her life. She specified the "extraordinary means" as chemotherapy, respirators, or resuscitation efforts. Three months after diagnosis, Ester K. was admitted to the hospital in a confused state with discoloration on her foot and some evidence of necrotic tissue on the top of her foot. Observation over the next couple of days revealed that the necrosis had spread, and the surgeon, Dr. P., diagnosed gangrene. Dr. P. wanted to remove the foot before the gangrene spread. Ester K. was still somewhat confused but nonetheless agreed to the surgery. The family was very upset with Dr. P. for suggesting the surgery and for considering her competent to give consent. The family thinks that in the spirit of the "living will" she would not want the surgery, which would fall into the class of "extraordinary means." Furthermore, the family thinks that Ester K. is too confused to give reflective consent, and this may be borne out by the fact that the patient whispered to the nurse that she consented only because she was afraid Dr. P. would no longer take care of her and might order her out of the hospital.

(1) How specific should the "living will" be in order for it to be binding? (2) Is there a danger of assuming that a consent is valid merely because it coincides with what the physician wishes to do? (3) What weight should be given to the family's judgment in this case?

Case 24

Discriminating Among Life-Sustaining Therapies [2, 7, 8]

Shirley W. is a 26-year-old female, unmarried with no dependents. She has reached the end stage of leukemia, has accepted her impending death, and wishes to have no heroic measures used to preserve her life, but she wishes to be kept comfortable. Her physician, Dr. Q., wants to honor her request but is concerned with her rapidly falling platelet count. The lower the platelet count, the greater the chance of hemorrhage. The physician does not know whether to interpret possible platelet transfusions as "heroic measures." On the one hand, a hemorrhage would cause Shirley W. to die soon, and a transfusion would extend the dying process. On the other hand, if the hemorrhage occurred in the mouth, the death would be very uncomfortable because the patient would choke. If the latter were allowed to happen, Dr. Q.'s promise to keep the patient comfortable would be broken.

Not knowing quite how to proceed, Dr. Q. consults with the staff and as a result offers the patient the following mode of treatment. If a hemorrhage were to occur in the mouth, the patient would be given platelets as a comfort-producing measure. Thus the platelets would be seen as serving a palliative function in keeping with the patient's desire to be kept comfortable and would not be seen as a heroic measure whose primary function is to prolong life. However, if the hemorrhage were to occur in some other part of the body, the priorities would be reversed, the platelets would be seen as heroic measures, and they would not be given. Shirley W. agreed to this approach and died two days later as the result of a cerebral hemorrhage.

(1) How should one determine "heroic measures" in general? (2) What clinical factors should be utilized in discriminating among life-sustaining therapies? (3) To what extent should the patient be involved in making judgments that discriminate among life-sustaining therapies?

Case 25

Refusing Life-Sustaining Treatment [7, 8]

Rita M., a 78-year-old female, has suffered from chronic obstructive pulmonary disease for about twenty years. She comes to the hospital in crisis about once a year and spends some time on a respirator. Currently, she is a resident of a nursing home where there is decent care for residents but little in the way of diversionary activity. Rita M. says that she is bored there most of the time. She seems decently attached to her son, but he cannot visit her frequently because he lives some distance from the nursing home. Another crisis occurs, and she is admitted to the hospital. This crisis, however, is worse than usual, and Rita M. is told that she will have to remain on a respirator for the rest of her life. The attending physician, Dr. E., informs her that a tracheotomy can make the respirator dependency more comfortable and that she can then return to the nursing home to live out the rest of her life. After several days, Rita M. informs Dr. E. that she does not want to have the tracheotomy and that she wants to be removed from the respirator and allowed to die. Dr. E., who is concerned about this decision, develops the following options in consultation with the house staff who accompany him on rounds: (1) the patient could have the tracheotomy and return to the nursing home; (2) the patient could be removed from the respirator, and nature would then take its course; (3) the patient could be removed from the respirator and receive morphine injections to alleviate pain when it occurred; or (4) the patient could receive a morphine injection prior to removal from the respirator and subsequent injections as needed. Dr. E. presented these options to Rita M. who chose the fourth one. She was subsequently given the injection and extubated. She died twenty hours later.

(1) Is this a case of suicide? Is this a case of euthanasia? (2) Was Rita M.'s refusal of treatment based on her assessment of what constitutes an acceptable quality of life?

Case 26

Is Nutrition Expendable? [7, 8]

Mildred D., a 78-year-old woman, suffers from diabetes, which has been controlled largely by diet. She has a history of heart disease and has suffered two heart attacks. She has now had a stroke, which has rendered her semicomatose and paralyzed. She must be fed through an NG tube, and the sustenance that she receives in this way is the only thing that keeps her going. Mildred D. has previously indicated to her family that in such a circumstance she would not want to be resuscitated. Her condition is slowly deteriorating, but it looks as though the dying process will be a long one. It seems that she will never return from the twilight zone in which she now resides. Angiography indicates that a substantial portion of the brain has been destroyed by the stroke. Her three children want to stop the tube feedings, but the physician objects that it is unethical to "starve" a patient so that she will die sooner.

(1) Is nutrition "extraordinary means" in this case? (2) Does the family have the right to make such a decision for the patient? (3) Should the refusal of resuscitation be considered an indicator that the patient would also refuse nutrition?

Case 27

Neonatal Care and the Problem of Uncertainty [8]

Bobbie C. is now six months old. He was born prematurely with a birth weight of 800 grams and had multiple problems from the beginning. Bobbie developed Hyaline Membrane disease due to his undeveloped lungs and the need for a respirator. He also developed rickets. A CAT scan revealed some calcium deposits in the brain that might or might not compromise his mental functions. Within the first month, Bobbie developed thrombocytopenia (low platelet count), for which he was given transfusions. He now suffers from a depression of his immunological system, the cause of which may be AIDS contracted through the blood transfusions. He shows little interest in eating, and all attempts to bottle feed him have failed after a couple of days. His health-care costs are being supported by Medicaid, and they are estimated to be in the neighborhood of $550,000 for his six months of hospitalization. Now the health-care staff and the attending physician are considering the possibility of a bone marrow transplant to deal with the thrombocytopenia and the immunosuppression. The chances of success in an infant this small are minimal, and the procedure is largely experimental in infants having this condition. If the transplant is successful, it will only alleviate one of his many problems.

(1) In view of the many uncertainties in this case, what is the proper treatment decision? (2) Should society be expected to shoulder such an expense for an infant who is so physiologically and, perhaps, mentally compromised? (3) Do the parents have a right to reject further aggressive therapies?

Case 28

A Brain-Dead Mother Gives Birth [8, 9]

Rosa J. suffered a fatal seizure while she was twenty-three weeks pregnant. Fetuses have a chance to survive at twenty-five to twenty-six weeks. After the seizure, Rosa J. was hooked to life-support systems but was declared brain-dead the next day. She was kept on life-support systems for nine weeks, however, until she gave birth to a healthy baby girl by cesarean section. During this time the physicians used steroids to help the lungs of the fetus to mature and monitored fetal growth with ultrasound examinations. Rosa J. was fed intravenously and given antibiotics for infections when necessary. After the birth, the woman's life-support systems were disconnected. The baby was given an excellent chance to survive, although she weighed only three pounds. From the time of the seizure, all decisions about Rosa J. and the fetus she was carrying were made by physicians in consultation with Rosa J.'s family.

(1) Should Rosa J. have been kept on life-support systems for nine weeks after being declared brain-dead simply in order to give the child she was carrying a better chance to survive? (2) Was Rosa J. being used merely as a means to others' ends? (3) Is someone who is brain-dead a "person" and, therefore, on a Kantian account an individual who cannot be used merely as a means to others' ends?

Case 29

Amniocentesis and Sex Selection [9, 10]

A 32-year-old woman, Lisa B., comes to the prenatal diagnostic center of a major hospital. She is intent on arranging for amniocentesis in order to determine the sex of the fetus she is carrying. A genetic counselor explains to her that the Center has an established policy against making amniocentesis available for purposes of sex selection. The genetic counselor, in defending the policy, tells her that there is a collective sense at the Center that abortion purely on grounds of sex selection is both morally and socially problematic. There is also the conviction that amniocentesis (to some extent a scarce resource) should be reserved for concerns more compelling than sex selection.

Lisa B. proceeds to explain her situation. She and her husband already have three children, all of whom are girls. They want very much to have a male child but, for economic reasons, are determined to have no more than one more child. Indeed, if they had a boy among their three children, they would not even consider having a fourth. They feel so strongly about this fourth child being a boy that if they cannot gain assurance that it is a male they will elect abortion. Lisa B. insists that it is unfair for the Center to deny her access to amniocentesis.

(1) Should the Center consider this case an exceptional one and make amniocentesis available? (2) Would the Center be well advised to develop a different policy regarding the availability of amniocentesis for purposes of sex selection?

Case 30

Sickle-Cell Disease and a Question of Paternity [10]

Harry B. is a one-year-old black male who has been admitted to the hospital in extreme distress and pain. Hematology has discovered that Harry is suffering from sickle-cell crisis. Harry is the first child born in this marriage. Sickle-cell disease is genetic in origin and is passed on in an autosomal recessive pattern of inheritance. This means that for the child to be born with the disease, both parents must either have the disease or be carriers (with a recessive trait). The offspring cannot inherit the disease from one carrier parent, although the child of such a parent might be a carrier. The hospital initiates treatment for Harry, a treatment he will have to undergo every time he goes into crisis. At the physicians' suggestion, the parents undergo a screening blood test to determine their carrier status. The results from the laboratory indicate that the mother is a carrier of the sickle-cell trait but that her husband is not. This means it is virtually certain the husband cannot be Harry's father, although Harry was born after the couple had been married about two years.

(1) Was it necessary for the hospital to run the screening tests on the parents? Did the screening tests assist in the treatment of the child? (2) Should the results of the tests be communicated to the parents, thereby jeopardizing their young marriage?

Case 31

Children at Risk for Huntington's Chorea [10]

Marcia C. is a thirty-eight-year-old female who has just been diagnosed with Huntington's chorea, an autosomal dominant genetic disease whose symptoms first emerge (ordinarily) sometime between the ages of 30 and 50. Because her father was a victim of Huntington's chorea, Marcia C. had known since she was a teenager that she was at 50 percent risk for the disease. But now her worst fears have been confirmed. Like her father before her, she can expect an extended period of progressive physical and mental deterioration leading inevitably to death in ten to fifteen years. Although Marcia C. is deeply distressed, and experiences bouts of depression, her mental capacities appear to be essentially uncompromised at the present time.

One of Marcia C.'s principal concerns is the well-being of her children, a girl 10 years old and a boy 8 years old. If Marcia C. had not inherited the disease from her father, her own children would not have been at risk, but now it is clear that each of her children is at 50 percent risk for the disease. A genetic counselor has told Marcia C. and her husband that it is very likely that a reliable presymptomatic test for Huntington's chorea will soon be available. Thus it would be possible to determine if Marcia C.'s children have inherited the disease. Neither Marcia C. nor her husband regret the fact that they had decided to have children, but Marcia C. feels that she has a special obligation to decide with her husband (before her mental powers become too badly compromised) what is best for her children. Should the children be tested when the presymptomatic test becomes available? If so, should they be informed of the results? Or perhaps the testing should be postponed, thus allowing the children to decide for themselves when they are grown whether or not to have the testing done. When the genetic counselor is asked what should be done, the counselor responds that it is for Marcia C. and her husband to decide.

(1) What course of action is in the best interests of Marcia C.'s children? (2) Should the genetic counselor have adopted a more "directive" approach in this case?

Case 32

A Feminist Sperm Bank [10]

The Oakland (California) Feminist Women's Health Center is a sperm bank that was founded in order to make AID (artificial insemination by donor) available in a manner that is consistent with feminist ideals. Although genetic and medical screening is provided, the keynote of the Center's operation is the fact that no *social* screening of applicants is done. Lesbians and unmarried women are expressly invited, along with more traditional candidates for AID, to make use of the Center's services. In addition, neither standards of economics nor standards of intelligence are employed to exclude applicants, and racial matching is not done.

(1) Is the operational philosophy of this sperm bank morally sound? (2) Should a sperm bank be held accountable to society for a social screening of its applicants for AID? If so, what factors would be sufficient to disqualify an applicant?

Case 33

Patient Responsibility [2, 11]

Brian B., a 57-year-old male, has been a patient of Dr. L.'s for thirty years. Every time he has come to Dr. L. for assistance, Dr. L. has inquired about his smoking habits and has repeatedly advised him to curtail his smoking. Despite repeated warnings, Brian B. has continued his heavy smoking, even after developing signs of emphysema in his early fifties. Now at age 57, Brian B. has developed lung cancer. He is very angry because the cancer was not detected earlier so that effective treatment could have been given, and he blames Dr. L. Now he has become very passive in the treatment decisions for the cancer. He first tells Dr. L. to decide whether to initiate treatment. When the physician refuses to make the decision,

Brian B. tells his wife and two children to make the decision. The family does not know what to do as Brian B. sinks more and more into a depressed state.

(1) What is Brian B.'s responsibility for contracting the cancer? (2) What is Brian B.'s responsibility for his depressed state? (3) Can Brian B. morally surrender his role in the decision-making process leading to treatment?

Case 34

Justice, the Elderly, and Health Care [3, 11]

Miranda B., who is 81 years old, has lived in the Greenmount Nursing Home for nearly ten years. The costs of her care are paid by state and federal funds. Miranda B. moved into the home after she had surgery for an eye disease. She is partly deaf and partly blind and has severe arthritis, but she is capable of some self-care. Miranda B. can feed and dress herself and requires only a little assistance getting in and out of a bathtub. Miranda B. considers Greenmount her home, sees the staff and other patients as family, and maintains that she would be unwilling to move to another institution.

In order to save on the costs of medical care, the state in which Miranda B. lives is considering a policy that would not allow patients who need primarily custodial care to reside in nursing homes such as Greenmount, which are designed and staffed to provide expensive medical care. If the policy is adopted, Miranda B. is one of the patients who will be required to move into another, less expensive facility adequate to her medical and custodial needs. Studies have shown that when people Miranda B.'s age are uprooted against their will and forced to adjust to new institutions, they seldom live long.

(1) Would a public policy that necessitated moving Miranda B. against her will be morally acceptable? (2) Is a cost-benefit analysis appropriate in determining these kinds of policies? A cost-effectiveness analysis? If a cost-benefit analysis is appropriate, what factors should be taken into account in terms of costs and benefits?

Case 35

The Severely Mentally Retarded and Funding Home Care [6, 11]

Leona S. is a severely brain-damaged 3-year-old. She is confined to a hospital where her care, paid for by Medicaid, costs approximately $15,000 a month. Her parents would prefer to care for her at home, but home care would be about $3,000 a month. Medicaid will not pay for home care, and the parents cannot afford that cost.

(1) What kind of public policy should be adopted regarding the funding of care for the severely mentally retarded? (2) Should costs be the primary concern when determinations are made about the care of the severely mentally retarded? What other considerations are relevant?

Case 36

Justice, Mental Retardation, and Public Policy [6, 11]

State representative Amanda S. has introduced a state bill that calls for the establishment of community-based homes for the care and education of the mentally retarded. The bill would provide one home for every fifteen persons presently institutionalized in five state institutions for the mentally retarded. The present annual cost of maintaining the five institutions is 90 million dollars. Providing the new kind of care for the present institutionalized population of 8,000 is expected to cost about $112 million annually.

Amanda S. argues that the mentally retarded who are presently in the five state institutions live in antiquated buildings lacking basic human necessities and amenities. Many of them are unclothed, spending their days huddled in dark, drab rooms, supervised by an overworked staff, many of whom have no professional training. She contends that justice requires that the mentally retarded be taken out of such subhuman surroundings and given at least a minimal chance for a "normal" life.

A physician, Dr. M., testifying before the House of Representatives, argues that the money required to make the change could be used more efficiently to provide health care for three groups: normal or more nearly normal children, pregnant women, and individuals potentially engaged in productive labor. He argues that a great deal of mental retardation can be eliminated through prenatal diagnosis, which would cost about $400 per case for Down's syndrome, compared to the suggested $14,000 needed for each mentally retarded individual annually in the proposed facilities and $11,250 in the present facilities. Even if some of those presently institutionalized might be gainfully employed if they were in the proposed high-quality community homes, the savings from spending the funds on detection rather than on more expensive forms of institutionalized care are enormous.

(1) Should the proposed bill be enacted into law? (2) Do the mentally retarded have a "right" to lead a life as "normal" as possible given their limitations?

Case 37

Justice, Kidney Dialysis and a Mentally Retarded Boy [6, 7, 8, 11]

Joey C. is a 13-year-old retarded boy living in a state-supported home for the mentally retarded. He has no relatives. Joey is suffering from uremic poisoning. Ordinarily someone in Joey's condition would be treated by dialysis three times a week. If Joey does not receive dialysis treatments, he will die. Joey is examined by four kidney experts, all of whom decide against dialysis. They give two reasons for their decision. (1) Joey will not understand the need for the therapy; he will consider the needles and the frequent confinements to the machine as torture, and, as a result, he will be unmanageable. (2) The state institution cannot provide Joey with the necessary hygienic and dietary care required for dialysis. The physicians conclude that the alternative to adopt for Joey is a slow, easy death.

Several employees of the institution protest and argue that Joey should not simply be allowed to die but should be given dialysis treatments. They offer the following reasons: (1) Retardation should not be a criterion for dialysis. (2) Any form of therapy can be perceived as a form of torture by a patient, depending on how the health professionals in charge handle the patient. (3) Other retarded children on dialysis have often been model patients. In fact, retarded young adults are sometimes perceived as overly compliant, meticulously following orders about their care.

(1) When a child has no parents or close relatives and is not competent to understand what is at issue in a life or death decision, who should make the decision for the child? Physicians? The courts? A guardian appointed by the courts? (2) Is severe mental retardation a morally relevant criterion when decisions are made about the use of expensive medical resources?

Case 38

Determining the Quality of Life [7, 8, 11]

George K. is a 25-year-old male who is unmarried and has no dependents. Medicaid supports him in his health-care needs, which are considerable since he suffers from muscular dystrophy. George K. is totally paralyzed and therefore confined to bed. In addition to being quadriplegic, he cannot speak, and he is respirator dependent through a tracheotomy. Ordinarily he resides in a nursing home, but periodically he must be brought to the intensive care unit of a local hospital for crisis care related to the respirator dependency. He has a girl friend who visits him occasionally as well as a mother who visits him regularly. George K. communicates through smiles and raising and lowering his eyebrows. He seems to enjoy watching television and is a great fan of the Dallas Cowboys and the Detroit Tigers.

(1) What assessment should be made of George K.'s quality of life? (2) Should discussions be initiated with George K. about withholding treatment in the case of future crises? (3) Can society afford to support, for long periods of time, individuals who constitute such a drain on health-care resources?

Case 39

Justice and Abortion Funding [9, 11]

Sara G. is a 35-year-old mother of four children whose husband deserted her about a month after she became pregnant with her fifth child. The age of her four children ranges from 1 year old to 6 years old. She knows nothing about her husband's whereabouts and is currently being supported by welfare payments including Aid to Dependent Children (ADC). Sara G. is less than three months pregnant and wants an abortion. Her reasons are as follows. (1) She does not have the skills to get a job that will even come close to the welfare payments she receives. If she has to pay for child care from whatever meager wages she could earn, the money left could not support her family at even the subsistence level. So, at least until the children are older, she will be dependent on welfare and ADC. The sums she receives are barely adequate to take care of her present family. Adding another member would mean even further deprivation for her present family. (2) Her welfare caseworker has agreed that when the four children are a bit older, Sara G. will go into a job-training program that will enable her to get a job paying enough to get the family off public assistance and to give her children a better start in life. Sara G. has undergone a battery of psychological tests to help determine what kind of work she should be capable of doing with the right education and training. The social worker and psychological counselor are both confident that Sara G. can do the work necessary to make a good living for herself and her family. Having another child would only postpone the time when Sara G. will be self-supporting, and in the meantime her family would be living at a very inadequate level.

Because Sara G. is on welfare, she must get an authorization from the social work agency for any medical procedure that is not necessitated by an emergency. In cases involving abortion, the final decision is made by a social worker.

(1) Should the social worker authorize the abortion? (2) What moral justification could be advanced to support an authorization? A refusal to authorize the abortion? (3) What social policy should be adopted to deal with such cases?

Case 40

Justice, Financial Incentives, and Organ Donations [11]

According to a report issued by the American Society of Transplant Surgeons, around 30,000 of the 55,000 patients who currently undergo dialysis because of end-stage renal disease could dispense with the machines and live a relatively normal life with a kidney transplant. However, the supply of cadaver kidneys is severely limited. To meet the need, a member of the U.S. Congress introduces a bill that would provide a tax incentive for "gifts of life." Any individual who donates an organ such as a heart, liver, or kidney, would gain the following financial benefits: (1) a $30,000 deduction on his or her last taxable year and (2) a $30,000 exclusion from estate taxes. In order to qualify for these benefits, the individual's organ would have to be in a condition suitable for transplantation and removed from the cadaver for the purposes of transplantation. If the source of the organ is a dependent, the same tax incentives would be granted to the parents. Since renal dialysis costs the United States government almost $2 billion a year, the projected savings are enormous. In addition, those patients who received a transplant could lead a more satisfactory life because they would no longer need dialysis three times a week.

(1) Will the financial incentive affect families' decisions to donate organs in the case of both children and adults who have not expressed any desire to make such a donation? If yes, is this a good reason not to enact the bill into law? (2) Is there something morally questionable about offering significant cash benefits for consent to organ donation? Since poorer individuals with no estate to leave and much lower tax bills would not have the same opportunities to gain financially from organ donation, is the proposed bill unjust?